Essentials of
Clinical Psychopharmacology

Essentials of
Clinical Psychopharmacology

Edited by
Alan F. Schatzberg, M.D.
Charles B. Nemeroff, M.D., Ph.D.

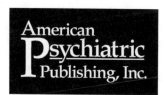

Washington, DC
London, England

Copyright © 2001 American Psychiatric Publishing, Inc.
ALL RIGHTS RESERVED
Manufactured in the United States of America on acid-free paper
03   02   01   4   3   2
American Psychiatric Publishing, Inc.
1400 K Street, N.W.
Washington, DC   20005
www.appi.org

Library of Congress Cataloging-in-Publication Data
Essentials of clinical psychopharmacology   :   based on the American Psychiatric Press textbook of psychopharmacology, second edition   /   edited by Alan F. Schatzberg, Charles B. Nemeroff.—1st ed.
       p.   cm.
     Includes bibliographical references and index.
     ISBN 1-58562-017-3 (alk. paper)
     1. Mental illness—Chemotherapy.   2. Psychotropic drugs. 3. Psychopharmacology.
   I. Schatzberg, Alan F. II. Nemeroff, Charles B. III. American Psychiatric Press.
   IV. American Psychiatric Press textbook of psychopharmacology.
     [DNLM: 1. Mental Disorders—drug therapy. 2. Psychopharmacology. 3. Psychotropic
   Drugs. WM 402 E78 2001}
   RC483.E86   2001
   616.89′18—dc21
                                                                    00-055834

British Library Cataloguing in Publication Data
A CIP record is available from the British Library.

To my wife, Nancy, and my daughters,
Melissa and Lindsey,
who have provided me with
great happiness and support over the years.
A.F.S.

To Gayle Applegate and my two daughters,
Gigi and Mandy,
who taught me to enjoy life again.
C.B.N.

Contents

SECTION I

Classes of Psychiatric Treatments

Dennis S. Charney, M.D., and Herbert Y. Meltzer, M.D., Section Editors

Antidepressants and Anxiolytics

Antipsychotics

SECTION II

Psychopharmacological Treatment

Donald F. Klein, M.D., Section Editor

Contributors

W. Stewart Agras, M.D.
Professor of Psychiatry, Department of
Psychiatry and Behavioral Sciences,
Stanford University School of Medicine,
Stanford, California

James C. Ballenger, M.D.
Professor and Chair, Department of
Psychiatry and Behavioral Sciences; and
Director, Institute of Psychiatry, Medical
University of South Carolina, Charleston

Joseph M. Bebchuk, M.D., F.R.C.P.C.
Assistant Professor of Psychiatry, Wayne
State University School of Medicine,
Detroit, Michigan

Joseph K. Belanoff, M.D.
Acting Assistant Professor of Psychiatry and
Behavioral Sciences, Department of
Psychiatry and Behavioral Sciences,
Stanford University School of Medicine,
Stanford, California

Robert M. Berman, M.D.
Assistant Professor of Psychiatry, Yale
University School of Medicine, New Haven,
Connecticut

Charles L. Bowden, M.D.
Nancy U. Karren Professor and Chairman,
Department of Psychiatry; and Professor,
Department of Pharmacology, The
University of Texas Health Science Center
at San Antonio

Joel Bregman, M.D.
Associate Clinical Professor of Psychiatry,
University of Connecticut; and Assistant
Professor of Child Psychiatry, Yale
University, New Haven, Connecticut

Adam B. Burrows, M.D.
Assistant Professor of Medicine, Boston
University School of Medicine; and Medical
Director, Elder Service Plan, Upham's
Corner Health Center, Boston,
Massachusetts

Katie A. Busch, M.D.
Assistant Professor of Psychiatry,
Rush-Presbyterian-St. Luke's Medical
Center, Chicago, Illinois

Dennis S. Charney, M.D.
Professor of Psychiatry, Yale University
School of Medicine, New Haven,
Connecticut

Jonathan O. Cole, M.D.
Professor of Psychiatry, Harvard Medical
School, Boston, Massachusetts; and Senior
Staff Consultant, McLean Hospital,
Affective Disorders Program, Belmont,
Massachusetts

James W. Cornish, M.D.
Assistant Professor of Psychiatry and
Director of Pharmacotherapy, Treatment
Research Center, University of
Pennsylvania and Department of Veterans
Affairs Medical Center, Philadelphia,
Pennsylvania

Kenneth L. Davis, M.D.
Professor and Chairman, Department of
Psychiatry, Mt. Sinai School of Medicine,
New York City

Karon Dawkins, M.D.
Assistant Professor, Department of
Psychiatry, University of North Carolina,
Chapel Hill

William C. Dement, M.D., Ph.D.
Lowell W. and Josephine Q. Berry
Professor, Department of Psychiatry and
Behavioral Sciences, Stanford University
School of Medicine, Stanford, California;
and Director, Stanford Sleep Disorders
Center, Palo Alto, California

C. Lindsay DeVane, Pharm.D.
Professor of Psychiatry and Behavioral
Sciences and Professor of Pharmaceutical
Sciences, Medical University of South
Carolina, Charleston

Marie deVegvar, M.D.
Fellow, Department of Psychiatry, Mt. Sinai
School of Medicine, New York City

Mina K. Dulcan, M.D.
Margaret C. Osterman Professor of Child
Psychiatry, Children's Memorial Hospital,
Northwestern University Medical School,
Chicago, Illinois

Dwight L. Evans, M.D.
Professor and Chairman, Department of
Psychiatry, University of Pennsylvania
School of Medicine, Philadelphia

S. Hossein Fatemi, M.D., Ph.D.
Associate Professor, Departments of
Psychiatry, Cell Biology, and
Neuroanatomy, Division of Neuroscience
Research, University of Minnesota Medical
School, Minneapolis

Jan Fawcett, M.D.
Professor and Chairman, Department of
Psychiatry, Rush-Presbyterian-St. Luke's
Medical Center; and Grainger Director,
Rush Institute for Mental Well-Being,
Chicago, Illinois

Gary S. Figiel, M.D.
Director, The Mood Disorders Center,
Eastside Heritage Center, Atlanta, Georgia

Ira D. Glick, M.D.
Professor of Psychiatry and Behavioral
Sciences, Department of Psychiatry and
Behavioral Sciences, Stanford University
School of Medicine, Stanford, California

Robert N. Golden, M.D.
Professor and Chair, Department of
Psychiatry, University of North Carolina,
Chapel Hill

Jack M. Gorman, M.D.
Professor of Psychiatry, Department of
Psychiatry, Columbia University; and
Deputy Director, New York State
Psychiatric Institute, New York City

Robert E. Hales, M.D., M.B.A.
Professor and Vice Chair, Department of
Psychiatry, University of California, Davis,
School of Medicine; and Medical Director,
Sacramento County Mental Health Services

Paul E. Keck Jr., M.D.
Associate Professor of Psychiatry and
Pharmacology, and Vice Chairman for
Research, Department of Psychiatry,
University of Cincinnati College of
Medicine, Cincinnati, Ohio

Justine M. Kent, M.D.
Fellow, Affective and Anxiety Disorders
Research Program, New York State
Psychiatric Institute; and Department of
Psychiatry, Columbia University, New York
City

Donald F. Klein, M.D.
Director, Psychiatric Research, Office of
Mental Health, New York State Psychiatric
Institute, New York City

K. Ranga Rama Krishnan, M.D.
Professor of Psychiatry; Head, Division of
Biological Psychiatry; and Director,
Affective Disorders Program, Duke
University Medical Center, Durham, North
Carolina

Robert H. Lenox, M.D.
Professor of Psychiatry, Pharmacology and Neuroscience; and Director of Molecular Neuropsychopharmacology Program, University of Florida College of Medicine and Brain Institute, Gainesville

Husseini K. Manji, M.D., F.R.C.P.C.
Director, Molecular Pathophysiology Program, and Schizophrenia and Mood Disorders Clinical Research Division, Departments of Psychiatry and Behavioral Neurosciences, and Pharmacology, Wayne State University School of Medicine, Detroit, Michigan

Stephen R. Marder, M.D.
Professor and Vice Chair, Department of Psychiatry and Biobehavioral Sciences, UCLA School of Medicine; and Chief, Psychiatry Department, West Los Angeles Veterans Affairs Medical Center, Los Angeles, California

Deborah B. Marin, M.D.
Assistant Professor, Department of Psychiatry, Mt. Sinai School of Medicine, New York City

W. Vaughn McCall, M.D.
Associate Professor, Bowman-Gray School of Medicine, Winston-Salem, North Carolina

William M. McDonald, M.D.
Assistant Professor, Department of Psychiatry, Emory University School of Medicine, Atlanta, Georgia

Susan L. McElroy, M.D.
Associate Professor of Psychiatry, and Director, Biological Psychiatry Program, Department of Psychiatry, University of Cincinnati College of Medicine, Cincinnati, Ohio

Laura F. McNicholas, M.D., Ph.D.
Assistant Professor of Psychiatry, University of Pennsylvania; and Director, Department of Veterans Affairs Center of Excellence in Substance Abuse Treatment, Philadelphia, Pennsylvania

Herbert Y. Meltzer, M.D.
Professor of Psychiatry and Pharmacology and Director of Psychopharmacology Division, Department of Psychiatry, Vanderbilt University School of Medicine, Nashville, Tennessee

Emmanuel Mignot, M.D., Ph.D.
Associate Professor of Psychiatry and Behavioral Sciences, Stanford University School of Medicine, Stanford, California; and Director, Center for Narcolepsy, Stanford Sleep Research Center, Palo Alto, California

Helen L. Miller, M.D.
Department of Psychiatry, Veterans Administration Connecticut Healthcare System, West Haven Campus, West Haven, Connecticut

Michael G. Moran, M.D.
Associate Professor, University of Colorado; and National Jewish Medical and Research Center, Denver, Colorado

Charles B. Nemeroff, M.D., Ph.D.
Reunette W. Harris Professor and Chairman, Department of Psychiatry and Behavioral Sciences, Emory University School of Medicine, Atlanta, Georgia

Linda Nicholas, M.D.
Assistant Professor, Department of Psychiatry, University of North Carolina, Chapel Hill

Philip T. Ninan, M.D.
Associate Professor, Department of
Psychiatry and Behavioral Sciences; and
Director, Mood and Anxiety Disorders
Program, Emory University School of
Medicine, Atlanta, Georgia

Seiji Nishino, M.D., Ph.D.
Senior Research Scientist of Psychiatry and
Behavioral Sciences, Stanford University
School of Medicine, Stanford, California;
and Associate Director, Center for
Narcolepsy, Stanford Sleep Research
Center, Palo Alto, California

Charles P. O'Brien, M.D., Ph.D.
Professor and Vice Chairman, Department
of Psychiatry, University of Pennsylvania;
ACOS, Behavioral Health Services,
Department of Veterans Affairs Medical
Center, Philadelphia, Pennsylvania

Michael J. Owens, Ph.D.
Associate Professor, Department of
Psychiatry and Behavioral Sciences,
Laboratory of Neuropsychopharmacology,
Emory University School of Medicine,
Atlanta, Georgia

Elaine R. Peskind, M.D.
Associate Professor, Department of
Psychiatry and Behavioral Sciences,
University of Washington School of
Medicine, and Veterans Affairs Puget Sound
Health Care System, Seattle, Washington

William Z. Potter, M.D., Ph.D.
Lilly Research Fellow, Lilly Research
Laboratories, Eli Lilly and Company,
Indianapolis, Indiana

Murray A. Raskind, M.D.
Professor and Vice Chair, Department of
Psychiatry and Behavioral Sciences,
University of Washington School of
Medicine, and Veterans Affairs Puget Sound
Health Care System, Seattle, Washington

Martin Reite, M.D.
Professor of Psychiatry, University of
Colorado Health Sciences Center, Denver

S. Craig Risch, M.D.
Professor of Psychiatry and Behavioral
Sciences, Department of Psychiatry and
Behavioral Sciences, Clinical
Neuropharmacology Program, Medical
University of South Carolina, Charleston

Jerrold F. Rosenbaum, M.D.
Director of Outpatient Psychiatry, and
Chief, Clinical Psychopharmacology Unit,
Massachusetts General Hospital, Boston

Matthew V. Rudorfer, M.D.
Assistant Chief, Adult and Geriatric
Treatment and Preventive Interventions
Research Branch, National Institute of
Mental Health, Rockville, Maryland

Carl Salzman, M.D.
Professor of Psychiatry, Harvard Medical
School; and Director of Education and
Director of Psychopharmacology,
Massachusetts Mental Health Center,
Boston

Andrew Satlin, M.D.
Associate Director, Nervous System Clinical
Research, Novartis Pharmaceuticals
Corporation, East Hanover, New Jersey

Alan F. Schatzberg, M.D.
Kenneth T. Norris, Jr., Professor in
Psychiatry and Behavioral Sciences; and
Chairman, Department of Psychiatry and
Behavioral Sciences, Stanford University
School of Medicine, Stanford, California

Larry J. Siever, M.D.
Professor of Psychiatry and Director,
Out-Patient Psychiatry Division, Mt. Sinai
School of Medicine, Bronx VA Medical
Center, New York City

Jonathan M. Silver, M.D.
Chief, Ambulatory Services, Department of Psychiatry, Lenox Hill Hospital; and Clinical Professor of Psychiatry, New York University School of Medicine, New York City

George M. Simpson, M.D.
Professor of Psychiatry, Director of Research Psychiatry, and Interim Chair, Department of Psychiatry, University of Southern California School of Medicine, Los Angeles

Joseph K. Stanilla, M.D.
Department of Psychiatry, MCP-Hahnemann School of Medicine at Eastern Pennsylvania Psychiatric Institute, and Allegheny University–Norristown State Hospital, Clinical Research Unit at Norristown State Hospital, Norristown, Pennsylvania

Alan Stoudemire, M.D.
Department of Psychiatry, Emory University School of Medicine, Atlanta, Georgia

Zachary N. Stowe, M.D.
Department of Psychiatry and Behavioral Sciences, Department of Gynecology and Obstetrics, Emory University School of Medicine, Atlanta, Georgia

James R. Strader Jr., B.S.
Department of Psychiatry and Behavioral Sciences, Emory University School of Medicine, Atlanta, Georgia

C. Barr Taylor, M.D.
Professor of Psychiatry, Department of Psychiatry and Behavioral Sciences, Stanford University School of Medicine, Stanford, California

Gary D. Tollefson, M.D., Ph.D.
Vice President, Lilly Research Laboratories, Eli Lilly and Company, Indianapolis, Indiana

Robert L. Trestman, Ph.D., M.D.
Associate Professor, Department of Psychiatry, Mt. Sinai School of Medicine, New York City

Michael J. Tueth, M.D.
Associate Professor of Psychiatry, University of Florida College of Medicine, Gainesville

Elizabeth B. Weller, M.D.
Professor of Psychiatry, University of Pennsylvania, Philadelphia

Ronald Weller, M.D.
Professor of Psychiatry, University of Pennsylvania, Philadelphia

Ann Marie Woo-Ming, M.D.
Fellow, Department of Psychiatry, Mt. Sinai School of Medicine, New York City

Kimberly A. Yonkers, M.D.
Assistant Professor, Departments of Psychiatry and Obstetrics and Gynecology, University of Texas Southwestern Medical Center, Dallas

Stuart C. Yudofsky, M.D.
D.C. and Irene Ellwood Professor and Chairman, Department of Psychiatry and Behavioral Sciences, Baylor College of Medicine; and Chief, Psychiatry Service, The Methodist Hospital, Houston, Texas

Charles Zorumpski, M.D.
Professor and Chairman, Department of Psychiatry, Washington University School of Medicine, St. Louis, Missouri

Introduction

Psychopharmacology has developed as a medical discipline over approximately the past four decades. The discoveries of the earlier effective antidepressants, antipsychotics, and mood stabilizers were frequently based on serendipitous observations. The repeated demonstration of efficacy of these agents then served as an impetus for considerable research into the neurobiological bases of their therapeutic effects and of emotion and cognition themselves, as well as the biological basis of the major psychiatric disorders. Moreover, the emergence of an entire new multidisciplinary field, neuropsychopharmacology, which has led to newer specific agents to alter maladaptive central nervous system processes or activity, was another by-product of these early endeavors. The remarkable proliferation of information in this area—coupled with the absence of any comparable, currently available text—led us to edit the first edition of *The American Psychiatric Press Textbook of Psychopharmacology*. The response to that edition was overwhelmingly positive. However, since psychopharmacology remains a burgeoning field, in the second edition we expanded considerably on the first edition, covering a number of areas in much greater detail, adding several new chapters, and updating all of the previous material.

For some potential readers, the textbook appeared to provide more material than they felt they needed at a particular point in time. Thus, we decided to develop an abridged essentials version—Essentials of Clinical Psychopharmacology—that focuses on the key aspects of clinical psychopharmacology. We have organized this book around two major sections of the textbook.

The first section, "Classes of Psychiatric Treatments," presents information by classes of drugs. For each drug within a class, data are reviewed on preclinical and clinical pharmacology, pharmacokinetics, indications, dosages, and the like. This section is pharmacopoeia-like. We include data on currently available drugs in the United States and medications that will almost certainly become available in the near future. New chapters or subsections on electroconvulsive therapy, new antipsychotics, new antidepressants (e.g., dual reuptake inhibitors), and nonbenzodiazepine anxiolytics were added to the second edition of the textbook and are included in the essentials.

The second section, "Psychopharmacological Treatment," reviews state-of-the-art therapeutic approaches to patients with major psychiatric disorders as well as to those in specific age groups or circumstances: childhood disorders, emergency psychiatry, pregnancy and postpartum, medically ill patients, and so forth. This section provides the reader with specific information about drug selection and their prescription.

Because of the gap between publishing the second edition of the textbook and the first edition of the essentials, we have updated material and references in the chapters.

This book would not have been possible without the superb work of the chapter authors, who edited and updated their chapters. In addition, we wish to thank Claire Reinburg of American Psychiatric Publishing, Inc., and her staff for their editorial efforts. In particular, we appreciate the major efforts of Stacy Jobb, Book Acquisitions Manager; Pam Harley, Managing Editor; Anne Barnes, Graphics and Prepress Manager; and our project editor, Greg Kuny. Finally, we extend our thanks to Gertrud Cory at Stanford University and Anne Griswell at Emory University for their invaluable assistance.

Alan F. Schatzberg, M.D.
Charles B. Nemeroff, M.D., Ph.D.

SECTION I

Classes of Psychiatric Treatments

Dennis S. Charney, M.D., and
Herbert Y. Meltzer, M.D., Section Editors

Antidepressants and Anxiolytics

ONE

Tricyclics and Tetracyclics

William Z. Potter, M.D., Ph.D.,
Husseini K. Manji, M.D., F.R.C.P.C., and
Matthew V. Rudorfer, M.D.

From the 1960s until the late 1980s, tricyclic antidepressants (TCAs) represented the major pharmacological treatment for depression. They still provide the surest antidepressant response for moderately to severely nondelusionally depressed patients, especially those who may be candidates for hospitalization (Potter et al. 1991). Furthermore, the original tricyclics all included in their biochemical spectrum of effects at least a moderate degree of serotonin reuptake inhibition, a fact that led to the development of the selective serotonin reuptake inhibitors (SSRIs). Thus, the clinical pharmacology of the tricyclics forms the basis of our current understanding of how to best use antidepressants.

In this chapter, we selectively review what has been learned about tricyclics and the subsequently introduced tetracyclics over the past three decades. We focus on their comparative pharmacology and on those findings most relevant to deciding when to treat a patient's condition with any of these compounds.

The synthesis of iminodibenzyl, the "tricyclic" core of imipramine, dates to 1889 (Baldessarini 1985). As Baldessarini noted, it was only after 1948, when Hafliger and Schindler synthesized a series of more than 40 derivatives of iminodibenzyl to be screened as possible antihistamines, sedatives, analgesics, and antiparkinsonian drugs, that the pharmacological properties were investigated. Out of this effort emerged imipramine, distinguished from the phenothiazines only by replacement of the sulfur with an ethylene linkage. Interestingly, the best-known phenothiazine, chlorpromazine, was not synthesized until 1952 (Laborit et al. 1952). Following their screening in animals, a few iminodibenzyl derivatives, including imipramine, were selected on the basis of their sedative or hypnotic properties for therapeutic trials as agents to calm agitated and/or psychotic patients.

In the meantime, a wide variety of clinical effects of chlorpromazine were described, including an ameliorative effect on psychosis. Thus,

The authors thank Melanie Wadman for her editorial assistance in preparing this chapter revision.

with a view toward imipramine as a phenothiazine analogue, Kuhn (1958) assessed its ability to quiet agitated psychotic patients but found it ineffective. On the other hand, he noticed that imipramine seemed to produce remarkable improvement in a subset of patients who were identified as depressed. Kuhn followed up on this chance observation with subsequent administration of imipramine to patients with various depressive syndromes. He suggested that imipramine was most useful in "endogenous" depressions, an impression not that different from what is held today (see Chapter 18 of this volume).

STRUCTURE-ACTIVITY RELATIONS

As shown in Figure 1–1, nine antidepressants are marketed in the United States as tricyclics, and one (maprotiline) is a tetracyclic. (Clomipramine is approved only for obsessive-compulsive disorder.) In most instances, the nature of the side chain rather than the cyclic structure is most easily related to function.

To clarify this point, the first two compounds in Figure 1–1, imipramine and desipramine, are distinguished only by a methyl group on the propylamine side chain. As we discuss later in detail, this simple alteration from a tertiary amine (3°; e.g., imipramine) to a secondary amine (2°; e.g., desipramine) side chain has widespread effects. This is the case in terms of both monoamine uptake inhibition—3° amines are more potent as inhibitors of serotonin, and 2° amines are more potent as inhibitors of norepinephrine uptake—and interaction with α_1-adrenergic, histaminergic, and muscarinic receptors—3° amines are more than an order of magnitude more potent.

Consideration of the next two compounds in Figure 1–1, amitriptyline and nortriptyline, makes these concepts about the structure-activity relation even clearer. Given the same propylamine side chains, the profile of pharmacological effects is qualitatively the same for the

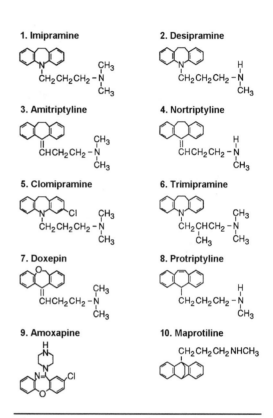

Figure 1–1. Drugs marketed in the United States as tricyclics (1–9) and tetracyclic (10).

respective 3° and 2° amine forms, amitriptyline and nortriptyline, as for imipramine and desipramine. However, absolute potencies in terms of monoamine reuptake and receptor inhibitions are affected by modification of the tricyclic structure. For instance, amitriptyline is more potent than imipramine in terms of cholinergic, α_1-adrenergic, and histaminergic receptor blockade, as well as serotonin uptake inhibition.

The fifth compound, clomipramine, differs from imipramine only in the addition of a chloride atom, which confers an increase in potency as an inhibitor of serotonin reuptake as well as an inhibitor of histaminergic receptors (Hall and Ogren 1981). Clomipramine's demethylated 2° amine metabolite, however, is a potent norepinephrine uptake inhibitor, formed extensively in humans (see section "Pharmacokinetics" later in this chapter).

Trimipramine, the sixth compound, is also closely related to imipramine with the addition of a methyl group to the second carbon of the propylamine side chain. Available data show that in its parent form trimipramine is somewhat less potent than imipramine as a norepinephrine uptake inhibitor (Randrup and Braestrup 1977) but more potent as an antihistamine (Psychoyos 1981).

Doxepin, the seventh compound, is structurally most closely related to amitriptyline. Serotonin uptake inhibition is decreased in comparison to that produced by amitriptyline, and norepinephrine uptake inhibition is somewhat increased (Pinder et al. 1977). In other words, doxepin's biochemical profile functionally most closely resembles that of imipramine, consistent with the retention of the 3° amine side chain.

The eighth compound in Figure 1–1, protriptyline, is closely related to nortriptyline, from which it is distinguished by desaturation of two saturated central ring carbons. This change further enhances this 2° amine's potency as a norepinephrine uptake inhibitor. It also greatly reduces the metabolism, such that protriptyline has a three- to fourfold longer half-life than nortriptyline (Moody et al. 1977; Ziegler et al. 1978).

The last tricyclic in the figure, amoxapine, deviates the most because it is derived more directly from an active neuroleptic, loxapine, which has a very different middle ring. Although amoxapine has two benzene rings (one with a chlorine as for clomipramine), the central ring and side chain have little similarity to the other tricyclic structures. Nonetheless, amoxapine does show potent norepinephrine uptake inhibition (Richelson and Pfenning 1984). Consistent with its close relationship to loxapine, amoxapine and its metabolite, 7-hydroxy-amoxapine, also produce dopamine receptor blockade (Coupet et al. 1979).

The last compound shown in Figure 1–1, maprotiline, is called a tetracyclic. Maprotiline has an ethylene-type bridge between the two central carbons of a six-member middle ring

that produces a more rigid core structure but a compound similar in biochemical properties to desipramine, nortriptyline, and protriptyline, given the presence of the identical 2° amine side chain (Wells and Gelenberg 1981).

PHARMACOLOGICAL PROFILE

Primary Biochemical Effects

The "classic" TCAs are imipramine, amitriptyline, and their close structural analogues. Observations of their ability to block the reuptake of the neurotransmitters serotonin and norepinephrine into their respective nerve terminals formed the basis of the monoamine hypothesis of depression (Bunney and Davis 1965; Prange 1965; Schildkraut 1965). These biochemical activities are still considered the pharmacological essence of their therapeutic effect. Amitriptyline and imipramine are metabolized to the 2° amine antidepressants nortriptyline and desipramine (Figure 1–1).

Of these four compounds, desipramine is the most biochemically selective with respect to both neurotransmitter uptake inhibition and relative lack of interaction with other systems. In actual clinical use, nortriptyline is almost as specific, since it is effective at low plasma concentrations (see below); also, the tetracyclic maprotiline is relatively specific for norepinephrine uptake inhibition (Turner and Ehsanullah 1977). Compared with other tricyclic compounds, desipramine and maprotiline block the reuptake of norepinephrine at concentrations unlikely to affect the uptake of serotonin. Moreover, desipramine has little affinity for muscarinic-cholinergic, histaminergic, and α-adrenergic receptors (Table 1–1), although its potency in these cases is still considerably higher than that seen with the SSRIs, bupropion, venlafaxine, and nefazodone.

The availability of TCAs that showed relative specificity and/or potency with regard to inhibition of norepinephrine or serotonin uptake, together with the clinical impression that

Table 1–1.   **In vitro acute biochemical activity of tricyclic antidepressants**[a]

	Reuptake inhibition			Receptor affinity				
	NE	**5-HT**	**DA**	**α_1**	**α_2**	**H_1**	**MUSC**	**D_2**
Imipramine	+	+	0	++	0	+	++	0
Desipramine	+++	0	0	+	0	0	+	0
Amitriptyline	±	++	0	+++	±	++++	++++	0
Nortriptyline	++	±	0	+	0	+	++	0
Clomipramine	+	+++	0	++	0	+	++	0
Trimipramine	+	0	0	++	±	+++	++	+
Doxepin	++	+	0	++	0	+++	++	0
Protriptyline	++	0	0	+	0	+	++	0
Amoxapine	++	0	0	++	±	±	0	++
Maprotiline	++	0	0	+	0	++	+	0

Note. NE = norepinephrine; 5-HT = serotonin; DA = dopamine; α_1 = α_1-adrenergic receptor; α_2 = α_2-adrenergic receptor; H_1 = histamine-1 receptor; MUSC = muscarinic cholinergic receptor; D_2 = dopamine-2 receptor. + to ++++ = active to strongly active; ± = weakly active; 0 = lacking.
[a]Relative potencies from earlier reviews (i.e., Potter 1984; Potter et al. 1991; Richelson and Nelson 1984; Richelson and Pfenning 1984).

different compounds were effective in different patients, led to the theory that there were noradrenergic and serotonergic forms of depression (Beckmann and Goodwin 1975; Maas et al. 1972). Convincing evidence to support this hypothesis has not been forthcoming. Treatment responses to desipramine (the most selective norepinephrine reuptake inhibitor) compared with those of an early SSRI, zimeldine, and later with those of fluoxetine and other SSRIs have not been consistently different (Potter 1984). Thus, specific pharmacology has not translated into specific antidepressant effects. The rationale for selecting a tricyclic on the basis of its specific biochemical pharmacology is weakened further by findings that even drugs with *acute* biochemical specificity have common effects on multiple biochemical systems with *chronic* administration in humans (Aberg-Wistedt et al. 1982; Golden et al. 1988; Potter et al. 1985).

This brings us to a consideration of the diverse biochemical effects associated with the use of tricyclic compounds. These medications are considered pharmacologically "dirty drugs." That is, in addition to exertion of their pre-

sumed desired mode of action (i.e., inhibition of monoamine neurotransmitter uptake), they interact with a host of receptors in the brain and periphery (Table 1–1), with consequent unwanted actions. The relationships of these diverse biochemical actions to side effects and toxicity are discussed in the next section.

PHARMACOKINETICS

From a clinical point of view, the most important advances from studying the pharmacology of TCAs have emerged from studies of their pharmacokinetics (Amsterdam et al. 1981; Rudorfer and Potter 1987). TCAs are well absorbed following oral administration, although peak plasma levels occur over the relatively wide range of 2–6 hours. Most TCAs have a half-life of approximately 24 hours, which allows for once-a-day dosing (Table 1–2).

Less than 5% of a dose is excreted unchanged; metabolism occurs primarily in the liver through the mixed-function oxidases. The tricyclics undergo demethylation, aromatic hydroxylation, and glucuronide conjugation of

Table 1–2. **Elimination half-lives of tricyclic antidepressants**

	Half-life (hours)	
	Mean	Range
Imipramine	12	7–22
	28	18–34
Desipramine	18	10–31
Amitriptyline	24	20–30
	36	31–46
Nortriptyline	28	22–39
	33	18–58
Clomipramine	24	20–39
Trimipramine	24	16–38
Doxepin	16	8–24
	17	10–47
Protriptyline	74	54–92
Amoxapine	10	8–18
Maprotiline	43	27–58

Source. Adapted from Rudorfer and Potter 1987 with values from one or more studies using more sensitive high-performance liquid chromatography and/or gas chromatography/mass spectrometry assays, with added information on trimipramine and amoxapine from Abernethy et al. 1984 and Calvo et al. 1985, respectively.

the hydroxy metabolite (Figure 1–2). The demethylated metabolites of 3° amines are pharmacologically active, as are the hydroxy metabolites of both 3° and 2° amines (Bertilsson et al. 1979; Potter et al. 1979). The glucuronide metabolites are inactive, both because they have no identified effects on biological systems in the concentrations achieved and because they do not cross the blood-brain barrier (reviewed in detail in Potter et al. 1980).

The metabolism rates of TCAs are determined by individual genetics and vary 30- to 40-fold; 7%–9% of a Caucasian population may be classified as "slow hydroxylators" (Brosen et al. 1985; Evans et al. 1980). Great progress has been made recently in understanding the exact source of slow hydroxylation. Individuals can be so classified on the basis of the urinary ratio of debrisoquin to 4-hydroxydebrisoquin in an

8-hour collection following an oral 10-mg dose of debrisoquin (an antihypertensive). A high ratio means that a person is a "slow hydroxylator."

Cytochrome P450-2D6 (CYP2D6), a specific isozyme of the P450 microsomal enzymes, has been explicitly shown to be responsible for the 2-hydroxylation of imipramine and desipramine, and mutations of the *CYP2D6* gene are responsible for slow metabolism through these pathways (Brosen et al. 1991; Daly et al. 1996). The P450 isozymes involved in TCA demethylation reactions may include CYP1A2, CYP2C19, and CYP3A4 (Madsen et al. 1997; Shen 1997). Of interest, most SSRIs are potent inhibitors of one or another P450 isozymes (Nemeroff et al. 1996). For instance, fluoxetine and norfluoxetine inhibit the CYP2D6 isozyme at therapeutic doses such that parent TCA concentrations can be more than doubled during concurrent use (Brosen and Skjelbo 1991). Paroxetine is also a potent inhibitor of CYP2D6, fluvoxamine is an inhibitor of CYP3A4, and chronic treatment with sertraline (150 mg/day) clearly inhibits CYP2D6 (Kurtz et al. 1997; Shen 1997) (see also section "Drug-Drug Interactions" later in this chapter).

Some of the demethylated metabolites of TCAs that show differential pharmacodynamics as discussed here actually exceed concentrations of the parent compound. For example, the 3° amine and potent serotonin uptake inhibitor clomipramine is metabolized to desmethylclomipramine concentrations that exceed those of the parent compound at steady state (Traskman et al. 1979). Because desmethylclomipramine (as would be expected for a 2° amine) is a potent norepinephrine uptake inhibitor, the in vitro selectivity of clomipramine as a serotonin uptake inhibitor is lost on administration to patients.

Other metabolic pathways may also be relevant to clinical effects (Rudorfer and Potter 1997). Results of both animal and clinical studies suggested that hydroxy-TCA metabolites, which are rarely assayed, may be more cardiotoxic than their parent precursors

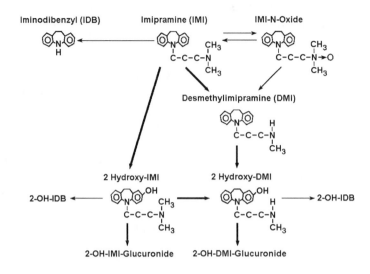

Figure 1–2. Known metabolic pathways for the major tricyclic antidepressant (TCA) imipramine in humans. Similar pathways apply to other TCAs.

(Jandhyala et al. 1977; Young et al. 1984); however, more evidence shows that no such generalization is possible (Pollock et al. 1992a).

Although TCA pharmacokinetics also may be influenced by age, changes in pharmacodynamic responses as a function of aging are more important. Elderly patients are more sensitive to at least the anticholinergic and α_1-antagonistic effects of tricyclics, as reflected in drug-induced delirium (Sunderland et al. 1987) and orthostatic hypotension (Glassman et al. 1979, 1987), respectively. Increased concentrations must, of course, be considered, because secondary decreases in P450 activity and hepatic blood flow are more likely to occur in elderly patients from either concomitant medical illness or medication. Thus, in earlier more naturalistic studies, elevated concentrations of TCAs were sometimes reported as a function of age (Linnoila et al. 1981; Nies et al. 1977; Ziegler and Biggs 1977). However, in more controlled prospective studies, concentrations of parent TCAs or rates of hydroxylation activity do not differ between otherwise healthy old and young subjects (Asberg et al. 1971; Cutler et al. 1981; Pollock et al. 1992b; Young et al. 1984).

With regard to active metabolites, however, the known decline of renal clearance with age predictably reduces the urinary excretion of unconjugated hydroxy metabolites, resulting in substantially increased steady-state concentrations in elderly patients (Kitanaka et al. 1982; Pollock and Perel 1989; Young et al. 1984). These concentrations, especially in the case of nortriptyline, are elevated to a toxic or countertherapeutic range of hydroxynortriptyline (Young et al. 1988). At the other end of the spectrum, in many studies of prepubescent children, TCA clearance is higher than that in adults (Geller 1991; Rapoport and Potter 1981).

Despite the great variability in metabolism of tricyclic drugs and a consequent need to individualize treatment, definitive therapeutic concentrations are not well established. Most critical analyses agree that therapeutic levels have been defined for only nortriptyline, imipramine, and desipramine (American Psychiatric Association Task Force 1985; Perry et al. 1987; Rudorfer and Potter 1987). Nonetheless, attempts have been made to provide estimates of reasonable therapeutic ranges for all marketed TCAs (Orsulak 1989). Lack of response, toxicity, minimizing adverse effects by using the minimal effective dose, and suspected pharmacokinetic interactions (e.g., with neuroleptics or SSRIs) are indications for measurement of plasma drug levels. Even without such measurements, daily doses of tricyclic drugs other than nortriptyline or protriptyline can be increased to 300–350 mg if side effects allow. Dose increases of nortriptyline require monitoring, because plasma levels greater than 150 ng/mL are as ineffective as those yielding a subtherapeutic (<50 ng/mL) level.

TCAs also have a narrow therapeutic index with considerable risk of significant toxicity when blood concentrations are two to six times therapeutic levels; thus, a 1-week supply may be fatal if taken all at once (Gram 1990; Rudorfer and Robins 1982). In general, concentrations greater than 1,000 ng/mL are associated with prolongation of the QRS interval, an effect that may be seen even at 500 ng/mL (Preskorn and Irwin 1982; Rudorfer and Young 1980; Spiker et al. 1975). This relatively narrow therapeutic index is of special concern for depressed patients with suicide potential who may intentionally take an overdose. Central nervous system toxicity in terms of coma, shock, respiratory depression, delirium, seizures, and hyperpyrexia may well contribute as much to fatalities as the quinidine-like effects on cardiac conduction of the TCAs.

MECHANISM OF ACTION

Our discussion of pharmacology so far has been primarily in terms of clomipramine and the four most closely related TCAs marketed in the United States. Because all of these drugs reduce indices of norepinephrine and serotonin synthesis and/or metabolism in humans, all other TCAs are assumed to do the same.

Several major flaws in the original hypothesis about the mechanism of action of TCAs as simply enhancing intrasynaptic norepinephrine and/or serotonin are briefly outlined here. First, compounds with antidepressant activity such as bupropion, nefazodone, and mirtazapine are weak inhibitors of monoamine uptake at best (Ferris et al. 1981; Zis and Goodwin 1979). Second, several potent reuptake inhibitors, most notably cocaine and amphetamine, are not effective antidepressants. Finally, the most compelling objection—and the one raised most frequently—is the large temporal discrepancy between the rapid drug-induced biochemical effects on monoamine uptake, which occur within hours, and the antidepressant response, which generally occurs after at least 7–14 days.

This has led to extensive research and the formulation of the "receptor sensitivity hypothesis of antidepressant drug action," which postulates that alterations in the sensitivity of various receptors after chronic drug administration are directly related to the mechanism of antidepressant drug action (Charney et al. 1991; Heninger and Charney 1987; Sugrue 1983; Sulser 1984). Most recently, alterations of receptor systems have been studied in the context of antidepressant effects on specific messenger RNAs (mRNAs), thereby extending theories of action to long-term molecular changes at the level of the cell nucleus (Duman et al. 1997).

Chronic administration of chemically diverse and unrelated antidepressants can decrease the density of β-adrenoceptors and/or the responsiveness of the β-adrenoceptor-coupled adenylate cyclase system. In contrast, other drugs that share common pharmacological properties with the TCAs, such as various anticholinergic and antihistaminergic agents, do not. Finally, other neurotransmitter receptors including muscarinic-cholinergic, histaminergic, and dopaminergic receptors are not consistently altered during chronic administration of antidepressants to animals (Hauger and Paul 1983).

The time course of the antidepressant-induced decrease in β-adrenoceptors in animals is in keeping with the delayed therapeutic effects of these drugs in humans. Interestingly, both electroconvulsive therapy (ECT) and rapid eye movement (REM) sleep deprivation (which are both clinically effective antidepressants) decrease cerebral β-adrenoceptors in animals somewhat faster than the chemical antidepressants do (Mogilnicka et al. 1980; Sulser et al. 1978), a finding that may be related to their relatively rapid antidepressant effects in patients.

In addition to reducing the number of central β-adrenoceptors, TCAs (as well as SSRIs and monoamine oxidase inhibitors [MAOIs]) appear to alter the number and/or function of serotonin receptors in various forebrain regions (Charney et al. 1991; Heninger and Charney 1987). In particular, evidence indicates that there is increased throughput at the serotonin-1A (5-HT_{1A}) receptor in the hippocampus in the absence of consistent alterations in the density of the receptors themselves, suggesting an enhancement of the coupling to second-messenger-generating systems.

Serotonin receptors have multiple subtypes, among them the broadly inclusive 5-HT_2 class as well as the 5-HT_{1A} class. Chronic administration of antidepressants to rats decreases the number of 5-HT_2 receptors in the brain, and with some drugs, this reduction is quite dramatic (Peroutka and Snyder 1980). Indeed, many antidepressants are far more potent in reducing 5-HT_2 receptors than β-adrenoceptors (with the possible exception of desipramine, which is more effective in reducing β-adrenoceptors). However, because the most effective treatment, electroconvulsive shock (ECS), increases the density of rat cortical 5-HT_2 receptors, direct antidepressant properties clearly cannot be ascribed to a reduction in 5-HT_2 receptor numbers.

Evidence also suggests that a functional linkage exists between the noradrenergic and serotonergic neurotransmitter systems, although how this relates to receptor regulation remains to be defined. For instance, destruction of the noradrenergic system (with 6-hydroxydopamine) markedly reduces the ability of several antidepressants (including ECS) to enhance serotonin-mediated behaviors in rats (Green

and Deakin 1980). Monoamine neurotransmitter system interactions may provide a basis for unifying several major hypotheses of depression and the mechanism of action of antidepressants (Hsiao et al. 1987; Potter et al. 1985).

The potential clinical relevance of these studies designed to explore the mechanisms of action of TCAs in comparison with those of other antidepressants lies in their highlighting two phenomena. First, whatever the balance of acute biochemical effects, all TCAs produce qualitatively similar chronic changes and hence would not be expected to show major differences in degree or type of antidepressant efficacy. Second, biochemical changes occur over a period of 1–2 weeks and may take even longer to stabilize with extended escalation of dose—a phenomenon that argues against any therapeutic advantage of one compound over another in speed of response.

The preceding notwithstanding, the possibility remains that norepinephrine (and serotonin) uptake inhibition may not be necessary or a sufficient condition to initiate and sustain the chain of biochemical events leading to therapeutic response. Complementary in vitro and/or in vivo preclinical studies provide evidence for effects of tricyclics and other antidepressants distal to the receptor whereby coupling of β-adrenoceptors to guanine nucleotide binding proteins (G proteins) (Lesch and Manji 1992; Manji and Potter 1995), coupling of the G protein to the enzyme adenylate cyclase (Chen and Rasenick 1995; Rasenick et al. 1996), and the activity of membrane phospholipases (Manji et al. 1991; Nakamura 1994; Pandey et al. 1991) and protein kinase C (Li and Hrdina 1997; Morishita and Watanabe 1997; Nalepa and Vetulani 1996) are altered. More recently, novel targets of antidepressant drug action have been explored (discussed in Owens 1996), including glucocorticoid receptors (Barden 1996) and neurotrophic factors (Duman et al. 1997; Smith et al. 1995). In addition, one of the most exciting areas of research pertaining to the mechanisms of action of agents used in the treatment of mood disorders has been the study of these agents at the genomic level (Duman et al. 1997; Hyman and Nestler 1996; Manji and Lenox 1994; Manji et al. 1995). It is noteworthy that the chronic administration of TCAs has been demonstrated to modulate glucocorticoid receptor gene expression (Barden 1996), G protein gene expression (Lesch and Manji 1992), and cyclic adenosine monophosphate (cAMP) response element binding (CREB) protein/cAMP response element directed gene transcription both in vitro and ex vivo (Nibuya et al. 1996; Schwaninger et al. 1995).

In terms of core biochemical effects, TCAs are best distinguished from SSRIs by their universal ability to potently inhibit norepinephrine uptake and to more variably inhibit serotonin uptake. Thus, TCAs are more "broad spectrum" in their effects on neurotransmitter systems than are SSRIs and likely have a different spectrum of clinical effects.

In keeping with this suggestion, a series of Danish studies concluded that SSRIs may not be as effective in treatment of severely depressed inpatients as a TCA (Bech 1988; Danish University Antidepressant Group 1990). Indeed, there is a paucity of studies of SSRIs in inpatients; even in outpatients, it is often difficult to distinguish effects of SSRIs from those of placebo. Several clinical predictors help to identify the most appropriate patients to receive TCAs, and some of these are highlighted below.

INDICATIONS

Major Depression and Melancholia

Patients with major depressive disorder, with melancholic features, require pharmacotherapy or ECT (Potter et al. 1991). Earlier studies suggested that major depressive disorder, with melancholic features, responded better to TCAs than did other forms of DSM-IV depression (American Psychiatric Association 1994; Paykel

1972; Raskin and Crook 1976), although more recent data do not support such selectivity of response (Paykel 1989). Still, allowing for the limitations of the research base, a good premorbid personality (i.e., absence of significant personality pathology), psychomotor retardation, and moderate severity with melancholia predict good response to tricyclic drug therapy (Joyce and Paykel 1989). Severity has long been identified as a predictor of response to TCAs (Stewart et al. 1989), whereas good premorbid personality is consistent with observations that primary depression (i.e., depression not preceded by other psychiatric diagnoses or medical illness) responds best to drugs (Coryell and Turner 1985; Fairchild et al. 1986).

Overall, TCAs produce an antidepressant response rate of 80% in nonpsychotic patients who have major depressive disorder, with melancholic features; have an illness duration of less than 1 year; and are maintained at plasma levels in selected ranges for 4–6 weeks. Estimates of lower response rates in these patients most likely result from inadequate dosage over too short a time. The critical importance of adjusting for wide interindividual differences in the pharmacokinetics of the TCAs has already been described.

Atypical Depression

Atypical forms of depression were not formally considered before DSM-IV. The term *atypical* previously referred simply to the absence of melancholic features. However, according to DSM-IV, major depressive disorder, with atypical features, is characterized by a combination of mood reactivity (i.e., inability to experience a positive response to favorable events), overeating, oversleeping, and chronic oversensitivity to rejection (Liebowitz et al. 1988). Patients with atypical depression have a lower response rate to TCAs than to MAOIs (Paykel et al. 1982; Quitkin et al. 1991; Ravaris et al. 1980).

Delusional (With Psychotic Features) Depression

Patients who have symptoms that meet the criteria for major depression and have delusions (DSM-IV major depressive disorder, severe with psychotic features) show a very poor response rate to monotherapy with traditional TCAs (Glassman et al. 1977; Perry et al. 1982). Successful pharmacotherapy for such delusional or psychotic depressions requires a combination of a neuroleptic and a TCA (Spiker et al. 1985). Because amoxapine, the tricyclic metabolite of loxapine, has dopamine-blocking as well as monoamine-uptake-inhibitory properties, it may be effective alone in treating delusional depression (Anton et al. 1985; Coupet et al. 1979). However, the opportunity to adjust the neuroleptic and antidepressant components independently is lost. A potentially important detail regarding combination therapy concerns the ability of some neuroleptic drugs to block the metabolism of TCAs, which necessitates special attention to doses and possibly to blood-level monitoring (Gram et al. 1974). Alternatively, the response rates to ECT among patients with delusional depression are excellent (86% in the aggregate from a dozen studies; Kroessler 1985).

Obsessive-Compulsive Disorder

Only one TCA, clomipramine, has been shown to produce significant therapeutic benefit in patients with obsessive-compulsive disorder, despite attempts to treat this disorder with other members of the drug class (Ananth et al. 1981; Insel et al. 1985; Leonard et al. 1989; Thoren et al. 1980). This effect is believed to be a function of the potent serotonin-reuptake-inhibiting properties of clomipramine because most SSRIs tested to date also produce benefit in obsessive-compulsive disorder. The specified upper dose limit of clomipramine in United States product labeling is 250 mg because the incidence of seizures is increased at higher doses. Unfortunately, studies reporting seizures did not include data on blood levels, and it is almost certain that those patients who are rapid metabolizers of clomipramine will require higher doses. These higher doses (up to 450 mg/day) may well be safe in such rapid metabolizers (Collins 1973).

Enuresis

Nocturnal enuresis in children can clearly benefit from TCAs. Imipramine is the one member of the class that has received United States product labeling for this indication. Recommended doses are low (i.e., 25–50 mg at bedtime in children younger than 12 years and up to 75 mg in those age 12 years or older). Controlled trials with plasma blood-level monitoring provide strong evidence of an antienuretic effect of imipramine (Rapoport et al. 1980). Earlier studies support the use of amitriptyline and nortriptyline for the treatment of nocturnal enuresis in children (Forsythe and Merrett 1969; Lake 1968). Suggested amitriptyline doses are 10–20 mg at bedtime for children ages 6–10 years and 25–50 mg at bedtime for children age 11 years or older.

Panic Disorder

Although we have referred to tricyclic *antidepressants* in this chapter, at least some members of this class clearly are effective treatments for panic disorder. Such use has played a considerable role in the treatment of panic disorder (including that with agoraphobia); controlled studies support the use of both the 3° amine imipramine and the 2° amine nortriptyline (Jobson et al. 1978; Munjack et al. 1988; Uhde and Nemiah 1989; Zitrin et al. 1980). Doses are the same as used in the treatment of depression.

One special consideration in the treatment of panic disorder with TCAs is that, particularly with the 2° amines, too rapid escalation of dose may increase anxiety and even precipitate a panic attack. Therefore, treatment should begin with low doses (e.g., 10–20 mg) and then build up to typical therapeutic doses (100–250 mg) over weeks rather than days.

Attention-Deficit/Hyperactivity Disorder

Spencer and colleagues (1996) reviewed 29 studies of pharmacotherapy for attention-deficit/hyperactivity disorder (ADHD) in children and adolescents (*N* = 1,016) that had been done as of 1995. Most reported modest to robust response rates, at least over a few-week to few-month period.

Earlier controlled studies of imipramine and desipramine reported relatively modest degrees of response (Donnelly et al. 1986; Rapoport et al. 1974). Subsequent studies relied on longer durations of treatment (at least 3–4 weeks) and higher doses (>4 mg/kg in preadolescent children). With this approach, more than two-thirds of children with ADHD treated with desipramine were very much or much improved (Biederman et al. 1989). A recent comparison of desipramine (200 mg/day or as tolerated) and placebo in adults with ADHD produced very similar results (Wilens et al. 1996).

In light of the short half-life and abuse potential of methylphenidate and dextroamphetamine, TCAs, especially the 2° amine desipramine, are argued to be of use for both children and adults with ADHD (Spencer et al. 1996).

Other Indications

A surprisingly diverse number of uses for TCAs is recorded not only in the clinical literature but also in a current authoritative American reference such as the *United States Pharmacopeia Dispensing Information* (USPDI 1997) and an international pharmacopoeia, *Therapeutic Drugs* (Dollery 1991, 1992). In Table 1–3, off-label uses of the TCAs are listed in alphabetical order.

Use in Pregnancy

All medications are best avoided during pregnancy and breast-feeding, but when antidepressant treatment is required at such times, tricyclics have been used safely. Physiological changes during pregnancy lead to a gradual decline in steady-state plasma tricyclic concentrations, requiring upward titration in dosage by mid-pregnancy (Altshuler and Hendrick 1996). Following delivery, TCAs have been used with care in nursing mothers, whose breast milk contains negligible amounts of these drugs (Rudorfer and Potter 1997; Wisner et al. 1997).

Table 1–3. Uses of one or more tricyclic antidepressants (TCAs) not included in product labeling

Use	Specified TCA(s)[a]
Anxiety/panic	Clomipramine, desipramine, doxepin, imipramine
Bulimia	Amitriptyline, desipramine, imipramine
Cataplexy/narcolepsy	Clomipramine, desipramine, imipramine, protriptyline
Enuresis	Amitriptyline, clomipramine, nortriptyline
Migraine (prophylaxis)	Amitriptyline
Nausea with chemotherapy	Nortriptyline
Neuralgia (chronic pain)	Amitriptyline, desipramine, doxepin, imipramine, nortriptyline
Peptic ulcer	Amitriptyline, doxepin, imipramine
Urticaria/pruritus	Doxepin, nortriptyline

[a]At least one mention in USPDI (1997) or *Therapeutic Drugs* (Dollery 1991, 1992).

SIDE EFFECTS AND TOXICOLOGY

As indicated in Table 1–4, there are distinctions among TCAs in the expected frequency and severity of adverse effects. Thus, as predicted from the greater receptor affinities of 3° amine tricyclics (Table 1–1), they produce more pronounced anticholinergic, antihistaminic (H_1 and H_2), sedative, and hypotensive actions than their 2° amine counterparts (Rudorfer et al. 1994).

Cardiovascular Effects

TCAs commonly produce a benign rise in heart rate, often on the order of 15–20 beats per minute. It occurs most consistently after use of 2° amine tricyclics, such as desipramine, for which

Table 1–4. Possible clinical side effects of blocking various receptors

Property	Possible clinical consequences
Blockade of muscarinic receptors	Blurred vision Dry mouth Sinus tachycardia Constipation Urinary retention Cognitive dysfunction
Blockade of α_1-adrenergic receptors	Potentiation of the antihypertensive effect of prazosin and terazosin Postural hypotension, dizziness, drowsiness Reflex tachycardia
Blockade of α_2-adrenergic receptors	Blockade of the antihypertensive effects of clonidine and α-methyldopa
Blockade of dopamine D_2 receptors	Extrapyramidal movement disorders
Blockade of histamine (H_1) receptors	Sedation Weight gain

norepinephrine reuptake blockade clearly plays a role (Ross et al. 1983). α_1-Adrenergic antagonism is more marked after administration of 3° amine TCAs and is the most likely basis for orthostatic hypotension, which can lead to falls and injury in older individuals (Ray 1992). Some experts prefer nortriptyline among the TCAs to minimize orthostatic hypotension in elderly patients because it has relatively less potency at α_1 receptors and achieves therapeutic effects at low blood levels.

The most potentially dangerous TCA cardiac effect (i.e., of a quinidine-like membrane stabilization resulting in slowed impulse conduction) was discussed in the earlier section, "Pharmacokinetics." Although such slowed impulse conduction produces only an innocuous prolongation of electrocardiogram (ECG) parameters during routine TCA dosing in physically healthy individuals (Laird et al. 1993; Rudorfer and Young 1980)—and can suppress preexisting premature atrial or ventricular contractions—it may precipitate frank bundle branch or complete heart block in cardiac patients (Glassman et al. 1987), with consequent morbidity or mortality. This property may relate to cases of sudden death, such as those reported in several children taking desipramine (Riddle et al. 1993). However, despite comprehensive 24-hour monitoring, no evidence of desipramine-associated cardiac abnormalities was found in a subsequent intensive study of 71 pediatric patients, and cardiac parameters failed to correlate with desipramine dose or plasma level (Biederman et al. 1993).

Widening of the QRS complex on the ECG, which has been correlated with red blood cell concentrations of tricyclic desmethyl metabolites (Amitai et al. 1993), has become a standard index of serious TCA poisoning, especially in overdose situations (Jarvis 1991). Recent data have raised concern that the risk of sudden death during TCA treatment among patients with ventricular arrhythmias or ischemic heart disease may be greater than previously appreciated (Glassman et al. 1993).

Anticholinergic Effects

Especially with 3° amine TCAs, antimuscarinic actions of TCAs are universal, presenting minor annoyances to most young healthy patients but posing major hazards to physically compromised individuals. Even the commonly experienced side effect of dry mouth has been associated with serious dental pathology. Reduced tear flow and impaired visual accommodation, with resultant blurred vision, may impair daily function and pose a hazard to contact lens wearers (reviewed by Nierenberg and Cole 1991). Constipation may be a minor discomfort that responds to increased fluids and bulk laxatives, or it could progress to life-threatening paralytic ileus in medically vulnerable patients. A similar spectrum exists for urinary retention, a major risk of TCA use in older men with prostatic hypertrophy. Narrow-angle glaucoma may constitute a contraindication to the use of medications with any anticholinergic effects.

3° Amine TCAs are particularly prone to produce cognitive toxicity, ranging from confusion and memory impairment to frank delirium in elderly patients who have increased sensitivity to anticholinergics (Sunderland et al. 1987). Although some cases of TCA-related sexual dysfunction have been ascribed to anticholinergic effects, such a correlation was not observed in a recent survey (Balon et al. 1993). Indeed, sexual dysfunction has emerged as a more prominent adverse effect associated with the use of SSRIs. Thus, the potent serotonin-uptake-inhibiting property of clomipramine, rather than its strong anticholinergic effects, may explain the high incidence of sexual dysfunction caused by this TCA (Aizenberg et al. 1991).

Anticholinergic side effects are maximal at subtherapeutic plasma concentrations of 3° amine forms (Preskorn and Fast 1991), rendering dosage adjustment inefficient in combating them. Although counteracting cholinergic agents, such as bethanechol, are sometimes used (Rosen et al. 1993), and symptomatic relief can be obtained with the use of artificial saliva or tears, most clinically significant problems re-

quire change of medication. Thus, the 3° amine TCAs should be avoided in standard antidepressant doses, or used judiciously (Rahman et al. 1991), in geriatric patients.

Sedation

The sedative action of the tricyclics, reflecting antihistaminic and α-blocking as well as anticholinergic activity—particularly the 3° amines (Table 1–2)—is one of the few side effects that can be used therapeutically in drug selection. Thus, the 3° amine TCAs are commonly used in a once-daily nighttime dose to address symptomatic sleep disturbance in depressed patients with insomnia (Potter et al. 1991). An incidental benefit of antihistaminic potency of the TCAs has been the antiallergic and antiulcer activities noted in Table 1–3, especially for amitriptyline, doxepin, and trimipramine.

Weight Gain

Use of TCAs is often associated with a degree of weight gain, which more than compensates for any prior weight loss associated with depression-related anorexia. This effect is believed to result from the antihistaminic and possibly α-receptor blocking actions of the TCAs, as well as a TCA-induced carbohydrate craving and slowing of metabolism. In one survey of clinical practice (Berken et al. 1984), outpatients treated with amitriptyline—possibly the worst offender among the TCAs—gained an average of more than 7 kg (with craving for sweets) during 6 months of treatment. This side effect does appear to vary among the TCAs (Fernstrom et al. 1986) and is minimal or absent with the most stimulatory members of the class (e.g., protriptyline and desipramine).

DRUG-DRUG INTERACTIONS

TCAs interact, pharmacodynamically and pharmacokinetically, with a variety of other compounds. The well-established adverse cognitive and psychomotor consequences of combining 3° amine TCAs with alcohol (Shoaf and Linnoila 1991) are primarily of a pharmacodynamic nature. Most adverse TCA pharmacodynamic interactions with other medications involve additive sedative or anticholinergic effects (e.g., with hypnotics or neuroleptics).

Tricyclics have pharmacokinetic interactions with drugs that induce or impair the liver cytochrome P450 microsomal enzyme system (Rudorfer and Potter 1987). Barbiturates and carbamazepine, for example, induce hepatic enzymes, accelerating tricyclic metabolism and reducing steady-state blood levels. On the other hand, valproate reduces TCA clearance (Wong et al. 1996). Concomitant neuroleptics are associated with elevated TCA levels, apparently by interfering with the hydroxylation pathway of tricyclic metabolism (Rudorfer et al. 1994).

Of particular interest is the competitive inhibition of CYP2D6 by all of the currently marketed SSRIs except fluvoxamine (Bergstrom et al. 1992; Kurtz et al. 1997; Nemeroff et al. 1996; Preskorn et al. 1994). These TCA-SSRI interactions are associated with often-dramatic elevations of steady-state TCA plasma concentrations and with reduced clearance via hydroxylation. Nonetheless, such combinations may be safe and effective, provided that tricyclic dosages are adjusted downward (Bergstrom et al. 1992; Nelson et al. 1991; Rudorfer et al. 1994).

Potentially Hazardous Interactions

The following listing is a distillation of warnings provided in the USPDI (1997) and/or *Therapeutic Drugs* (Dollery 1991, 1992).

MAOIs.   Giving TCAs to individuals taking MAOIs may produce stroke, hyperpyrexia, convulsions, and death through a variety of mechanisms. Nonetheless, safely combining most TCAs with MAOIs is possible. The one exception is clomipramine, which (because of its potent serotonin-uptake-inhibiting action) can

produce a potentially fatal "serotonin syndrome" when combined with MAOIs.

Norepinephrine and epinephrine.   Following administration of the biogenic amines norepinephrine and epinephrine for other medical conditions, unexpectedly large increases in blood pressure and a greater incidence of arrhythmias may occur in individuals taking TCAs.

Phenothiazines.   Additive anticholinergic effects may occur with phenothiazines, which may be manifested as psychosis and/or agitation, especially in elderly subjects. Nonetheless, combinations of phenothiazines with TCAs are appropriate and necessary for the treatment of delusional depression (Spiker et al. 1985).

Other Significant Reactions

Barbiturates.   Barbiturates can increase the metabolism of TCAs, requiring higher than usual doses of the antidepressant to achieve a therapeutic effect.

Cimetidine.   The use of cimetidine can block the metabolism of both 3° and 2° amine TCAs. Lower doses may therefore be appropriate in patients taking this H_2-receptor antagonist. Other H_2-receptor antagonists are not reported to decrease the metabolism of TCAs.

Clonidine.   The effects of clonidine are reduced or blocked by desipramine, presumably secondary to its ability to increase norepinephrine in the synapse. Other TCAs can be expected to have a similar effect.

Guanethidine.   All TCAs can be expected to block the antihypertensive effects of guanethidine by inhibiting its uptake into nerve endings.

Haloperidol.   Haloperidol can block the metabolism of TCAs, depending on the dose and sequence of administration.

Methylphenidate. The use of methylphenidate has been reported to block the metabolism of TCAs but not to the same extent as do antipsychotic drugs.

Phenothiazines. The phenothiazines—in particular, chlorpromazine—can block the metabolism of TCAs.

Phenytoin. The concentrations of phenytoin may be elevated to a toxic range by administration of TCAs.

Warfarin. The activity of the anticoagulant warfarin may be increased by administration of TCAs, which are competitive inhibitors of warfarin metabolism.

CONCLUSION

After several decades as the standard medication for treatment of major depression, the TCAs today occupy a narrower role in the psychopharmacological armamentarium. They remain a first-line and, more commonly, second-line intervention for moderate to severe depression, particularly in the presence of melancholic symptoms. In psychotic depression, TCAs are commonly combined with antipsychotic medications. Additionally, one or more tricyclics are used as an effective treatment for a variety of nonaffective disorders, including obsessive-compulsive disorder, enuresis, panic disorder, ADHD, and chronic pain syndromes. TCAs also have a current role in combination with SSRIs and other newer antidepressant compounds in treatment-refractory depression. Pharmacokinetic interactions resulting from such combinations have furthered understanding of the metabolism of TCAs and the inducing and inhibiting effects of newer antidepressants on isoenzymes of the hepatic cytochrome P450 system.

REFERENCES

Aberg-Wistedt A, Ross SB, Jostell KG, et al: A double-blind study of zimelidine, a serotonin uptake inhibitor, and desipramine, a noradrenaline uptake inhibitor, in endogenous depression, II: biochemical findings. Acta Psychiatr Scand 66: 66–82, 1982

Abernethy DR, Greenblatt DJ, Shader RI: Trimipramine kinetics and absolute bioavailability: use of gas-liquid chromatography with nitrogen-phosphorus detection. Clin Pharmacol Ther 35:348–353, 1984

Aizenberg D, Zemishlany Z, Hermesh H, et al: Painful ejaculation associated with antidepressants in four patients. J Clin Psychiatry 52: 461–463, 1991

Altshuler LL, Hendrick VC: Pregnancy and psychotropic medication: changes in blood levels. J Clin Psychopharmacol 16:78–80, 1996

American Psychiatric Association: Diagnostic and Statistical Manual of Mental Disorders, 4th Edition. Washington, DC, American Psychiatric Association, 1994

American Psychiatric Association Task Force: Task Force on the Use of Laboratory Tests in Psychiatry: tricyclic antidepressants—blood level measurements and clinical outcome. Am J Psychiatry 142:155–162, 1985

Amitai Y, Erikson T, Kennedy EJ, et al: Tricyclic antidepressants in red cells and plasma: correlation with impaired intraventricular conduction in acute overdose. Clin Pharmacol Ther 54:219–227, 1993

Amsterdam J, Brunswick D, Mendels J: The clinical application of tricyclic antidepressant pharmacokinetics and plasma levels. Am J Psychiatry 137:653–662, 1981

Ananth J, Pecknold JC, Van der Steen N: Double blind comparable study of clomipramine and amitriptyline in obsessive neurosis. Prog Neuropsychopharmacol Biol Psychiatry 5: 257–262, 1981

Anton RF, Ressner EL, Hitri A, et al: Efficacy of amoxapine in psychotic depression: relationship to serum prolactin and neuroleptic activity (monograph). J Clin Psychiatry 3:8–13, 1985

Asberg M, Cronholm B, Sjoqvist F, et al: Relationship between plasma levels and therapeutic effect of nortriptyline. BMJ 3:331–334, 1971

Baldessarini RJ: Drugs and the treatment of psychiatric disorders, in The Pharmacological Basis of Therapeutics, 4th Edition. Edited by Gilman AG, Goodman IS, Rall TW, et al. New York, Macmillan, 1985, pp 387–445

Balon R, Yeragani VK, Pohl R, et al: Sexual dysfunction during antidepressant treatment. J Clin Psychiatry 54:209–212, 1993

Barden N: Modulation of glucocorticoid receptor gene expression by antidepressant drugs. Pharmacopsychiatry 29:12–22, 1996

Bech P: A review of the antidepressant properties of serotonin reuptake inhibitors. Adv Biol Psychiatry 17:58–69, 1988

Beckmann H, Goodwin FK: Antidepressant response to tricyclics and urinary MHPG in unipolar patients. Arch Gen Psychiatry 32:17–22, 1975

Bergstrom RF, Peyton AL, Lemberger L: Quantification and mechanism of the fluoxetine and tricyclic antidepressant interaction. Clin Pharmacol Ther 51:239–248, 1992

Berken GN, Weinstein DO, Stern WC: Weight gain: a side effect of tricyclic antidepressants. J Affect Disord 7:133–138, 1984

Bertilsson L, Mellstrom B, Sjoqvist F: Pronounced inhibition of noradrenaline uptake by 10-hydroxy-metabolites of nortriptyline. Life Sci 25:1285–1291, 1979

Biederman J, Baldessarini RJ, Wright V, et al: A double-blind placebo controlled study of desipramine in the treatment of ADD, I: efficacy. J Am Acad Child Adolesc Psychiatry 28:777–784, 1989

Biederman J, Baldessarini RJ, Goldblatt A, et al: A naturalistic study of 24-hour electrocardiographic recording and echocardiographic findings in children and adolescents treated with desipramine. J Am Acad Child Adolesc Psychiatry 32:805–813, 1993

Brosen K, Skjelbo E: Fluoxetine and norfluoxetine are potent inhibitors of $P_{450}IID6$—the source of the sparteine/debrisoquine oxidation polymorphism. Br J Clin Pharmacol 31:136–137, 1991

Brosen K, Otton SV, Gram LF: Sparteine oxidation polymorphism in Denmark. Acta Pharmacol Toxicol 57:357–360, 1985

Brosen K, Zeugin T, Myer UA: Role of $P_{450}IID6$, the target of the sparteine/debrisoquin oxidation polymorphism, in the metabolism of imipramine. Clin Pharmacol Ther 49:609–617, 1991

Bunney WE, Davis JM: Norepinephrine in depressive reactions: a review. Arch Gen Psychiatry 13:483–494, 1965

Calvo B, Garcia MJ, Pedraz JL, et al: Pharmacokinetics of amoxapine and its active metabolites. Int J Clin Pharmacol Ther Toxicol 23:180–185, 1985

Charney DS, Delgado PL, Southwick SM, et al: Current hypotheses of the mechanism of antidepressant treatments: implications for the treatment of refractory depression, in Advances in Neuropsychiatry and Psychopharmacology, Vol 2. Edited by Amsterdam JD. New York, Raven, 1991, pp 23–41

Chen J, Rasenick MM: Chronic treatment of C6 glioma cells with antidepressant increases functional coupling between a G protein (Gs) and adenylyl cyclase. J Neurochem 64:724–732, 1995

Collins GH: The use of parenteral and oral clomipramine (Anafranil) in the treatment of depressive states. Br J Psychiatry 122:189–190, 1973

Coryell W, Turner R: Outcome with desipramine therapy in subtypes of nonpsychotic major depression. J Affect Disord 9:149–154, 1985

Coupet I, Rauh CE, Szucs-Myers VA, et al: 2-chloro-11(piperazinyl)[b,f][1,4]oxazepine (amoxepine), an antidepressant with antipsychotic properties—a possible role for 7-hydroxy-amoxapine. Biochem Pharmacol 28:2514–2515, 1979

Cutler NR, Zavadil AP III, Eisdorfer C, et al: Concentration of desipramine in elderly women. Am J Psychiatry 138:1235–1237, 1981

Daly AK, Brockmoller J, Broly F, et al: Nomenclature for human CYP2D6 alleles. Pharmacogenetics 6:193–201, 1996

Danish University Antidepressant Group: Paroxetine: a selective serotonin reuptake inhibitor showing better tolerance, but weaker antidepressant effect than clomipramine in a controlled multicenter study. J Affect Disord 18:289–299, 1990

Dollery C (ed): Therapeutic Drugs. Edinburgh, Churchill Livingstone, 1991, 1992

Donnelly M, Zametkin AJ, Rapoport JL, et al: Treatment of childhood hyperactivity with desipramine: plasma drug concentration, cardiovascular effects, plasma and urinary catecholamine levels, and clinical response. Clin Pharmacol Ther 39:72–81, 1986

Duman RS, Heninger GR, Nestler EJ: A molecular and cellular theory of depression. Arch Gen Psychiatry 54:597–606, 1997

Evans DAP, Mahgoub A, Sloan TP, et al: A family and population study of the genetic polymorphism of debrisoquine oxidation in a white British population. J Med Genet 17:102–105, 1980

Fairchild CJ, Rush AJ, Vasavada N, et al: Which depressions respond to placebo? Psychiatry Res 18:217–226, 1986

Fernstrom MD, Krowinski RL, Kupfer DJ: Chronic imipramine treatment and weight gain. Psychiatry Res 17:269–273, 1986

Ferris RM, White HL, Cooper BR, et al: Some neurochemical properties of a new antidepressant, bupropion hydrochloride (Wellbutrin). Drug Development Research 1:21–35, 1981

Forsythe WI, Merrett JD: A controlled trial of imipramine and nortriptyline in the treatment of enuresis. Br J Clin Pract 23:210–215, 1969

Geller B: Psychopharmacology of children and adolescents: pharmacokinetics and relationships of plasma/serum levels to response. Psychopharmacol Bull 27:401–409, 1991

Glassman A, Perel J, Shostak M, et al: Clinical implication of imipramine plasma levels for depressive illness. Arch Gen Psychiatry 34: 197–204, 1977

Glassman AH, Bigger JT Jr, Giardina EV, et al: Clinical characteristics of imipramine induced orthostatic hypotension. Lancet 1:468–472, 1979

Glassman AH, Roose SP, Giardina EGV, et al: Cardiovascular effects of tricyclic antidepressants, in Psychopharmacology: The Third Generation of Progress. Edited by Meltzer HY. New York, Raven, 1987, pp 1437–1442

Glassman AH, Roose SP, Bigger JT Jr: The safety of tricyclic antidepressants in cardiac patients: risk-benefit reconsidered. JAMA 269:2673–2675, 1993

Golden RN, Markey SP, Risby ED, et al: Antidepressants reduce whole-body norepinephrine turnover while maintaining 6-hydroxymelatonin output. Arch Gen Psychiatry 45:144–149, 1988

Gram LF: Inadequate dosing and pharmacokinetic variability as confounding factors in assessment of efficacy of antidepressants. Clin Neuropharmacol 13 (suppl 1):S35–S44, 1990

Gram LF, Overo KF, Kirk L: Influence of neuroleptics and benzodiazepines on metabolism of tricyclic antidepressants in man. Am J Psychiatry 131:863–866, 1974

Green AR, Deakin JFW: Brain noradrenaline depletion prevents ECS-induced enhancement of serotonin and dopamine-mediated behavior. Nature 285:232–233, 1980

Hall H, Ogren SO: Effects of antidepressant drugs on different receptors in the brain. Eur J Pharmacol 70:393–407, 1981

Hauger RL, Paul SM: Neurotransmitter receptor plasticity: alterations by antidepressants and antipsychotics. Psychiatric Annals 13:399–407, 1983

Heninger GR, Charney DS: Mechanism of action of antidepressant treatments: implications for the etiology and treatment of depressive disorders, in Psychopharmacology: The Third Generation of Progress. Edited by Meltzer HY. New York, Raven, 1987, pp 535–545

Hsiao JK, Agren H, Rudorfer MV, et al: Monoamine neurotransmitter interactions and the prediction of antidepressant response. Arch Gen Psychiatry 44:1078–1083, 1987

Hyman SE, Nestler EJ: Initiation and adaptation: a paradigm for understanding psychotropic drug action. Am J Psychiatry 153:151–162, 1996

Insel TR, Mueller EA, Alterman I, et al: Obsessive-compulsive disorder and serotonin: is there a connection? Biol Psychiatry 20:1174–1188, 1985

Jandhyala B, Steenberg M, Perel JM, et al: Effects of several tricyclic antidepressants on the hemodynamics and myocardial contractility of anesthetized dogs. Eur J Pharmacol 42:403–410, 1977

Jarvis MR: Clinical pharmacokinetics of tricyclic antidepressant overdose. Psychopharmacol Bull 27:541–550, 1991

Jobson K, Linnoila M, Gillam J, et al: Successful treatment of severe anxiety attacks with tricyclic antidepressants: a possible mechanism of action. Am J Psychiatry 135:863–864, 1978

Joyce PR, Paykel ES: Predictors of drug response in depression. Arch Gen Psychiatry 46:89–99, 1989

Kitanaka I, Ross RI, Cutler NR, et al: Altered hydroxydesipramine concentrations in elderly depressed patients. Clin Pharmacol Ther 31: 51–55, 1982

Kroessler D: Relative efficacy rates for therapies of delusional depression. Convuls Ther 1:173–182, 1985

Kuhn R: The treatment of depressive states with G22355 (imipramine hydrochloride). Am J Psychiatry 115:459–464, 1958

Kurtz DL, Bergstrom RF, Goldberg MJ, et al: The effect of sertraline on the pharmacokinetics of desipramine and imipramine. Clin Pharmacol Ther 62:145–156, 1997

Laborit H, Huguenard P, Alluaume R: Un nouveau stabilisateur végétatif: le 4560 RP [A new vegetative stabilizer: 4560 RP]. Presse Med 60: 206–208, 1952

Laird LK, Lydiard RB, Morton WA, et al: Cardiovascular effects of imipramine, fluvoxamine and placebo in depressed outpatients. J Clin Psychiatry 54:224–228, 1993

Lake B: Controlled trial of nortriptyline in childhood enuresis. Med J Aust 5 (suppl 14):582–585, 1968

Leonard HL, Swedo S, Rapoport JL, et al: Treatment of obsessive compulsive disorder in children and adolescents with clomipramine and desipramine: a double-blind crossover comparison. Arch Gen Psychiatry 46:1088–1092, 1989

Lesch KP, Manji HK: Signal-transducing G proteins and antidepressant drugs: evidence for modulation of alpha subunit gene expression in rat brain. Biol Psychiatry 32:549–579, 1992

Li Q, Hrdina PD: GAP-43 phosphorylation by PKC in rat cerebrocortical synaptosomes: effect of antidepressants. Res Commun Mol Pathol Pharmacol 96:3–13, 1997

Liebowitz MR, Quitkin FM, Stewart JW, et al: Antidepressant specificity in atypical depression. Arch Gen Psychiatry 45:129–137, 1988

Linnoila M, George L, Guthrie S, et al: Effect of alcohol consumption and cigarette smoking on antidepressant levels of depressed patients. Am J Psychiatry 138:841–842, 1981

Maas JW, Fawcett JA, Dekirmenjian H: Catecholamine metabolism, depressive illness, and drug response. Arch Gen Psychiatry 26:353–363, 1972

Madsen H, Rasmussen BB, Brosen K, et al: Imipramine demethylation in vivo: impact of CYP1A2, CYP2C19, and CYP3A4. Clin Pharmacol Ther 61:319–324, 1997

Manji HK, Lenox RH: Long-term action of lithium: a role for transcriptional and posttranscriptional factors regulated by protein kinase C. Synapse 16:11–28, 1994

Manji HK, Potter WZ: Emerging strategies in affective disorders, in Emerging Strategies in Neurotherapeutics. Edited by Pullan L, Patel J. Totowa, NJ, Humana Press, 1995, pp 35–83

Manji HK, Chen G, Bitran JA, et al: Down-regulation of beta receptors by desipramine in vitro involves PKC/phospholipase A_2. Psychopharmacol Bull 27:247–253, 1991

Manji HK, Potter WZ, Lenox RH: Signal transduction pathways: molecular targets for lithium's actions. Arch Gen Psychiatry 52: 531–543, 1995

Mogilnicka E, Arbilla S, Depoortere H, et al: Rapid-eye-movement sleep deprivation decreases the density of ^{3}H-dihydroalprenolol and ^{3}H-imipramine binding sites in the rat cerebral cortex. Eur J Pharmacol 65:289–292, 1980

Moody JP, Whyte SF, MacDonald AJ, et al: Pharmacokinetic aspects of protriptyline plasma levels. Eur J Clin Pharmacol 11:51–56, 1977

Morishita S, Watanabe S: Effect of the tricyclic antidepressant desipramine on protein kinase C in rat brain and rabbit platelets in vitro. Psychiatry and Clinical Neuroscience 51:249–252, 1997

Munjack DJ, Usigli R, Zulueta A, et al: Nortriptyline in the treatment of panic disorder and agoraphobia with panic attacks. J Clin Psychopharmacol 8:204–207, 1988

Nakamura S: Effects of phospholipase A2 inhibitors on the antidepressant-induced axonal regeneration of noradrenergic locus coeruleus neurons. Microsc Res Tech 29:204–210, 1994

Nalepa I, Vetulani J: Modulation of electro-convulsive treatment induced beta-adrenergic down-regulation by previous chronic imipramine administration: the involvement of protein kinase C. Pol J Pharmacol 48:489–494, 1996

Nelson JC, Mazure CM, Bowers MB Jr, et al: A preliminary open study of the combination of fluoxetine and desipramine for rapid treatment of major depression. Arch Gen Psychiatry 48:303–307, 1991

Nemeroff CB, DeVane CL, Pollock BG: Newer antidepressants and the cytochrome P450 system. Am J Psychiatry 153:311–320, 1996

Nibuya M, Nestler EJ, Duman RS: Chronic antidepressant administration increases the expression of cAMP response element-binding protein (CREB) in rat hippocampus. J Neurosci 16:2365–2372, 1996

Nierenberg AA, Cole JO: Antidepressant adverse drug reactions. J Clin Psychiatry 52(suppl): 40–47, 1991

Nies A, Robinson DS, Friedman DS, et al: Relationship between age and tricyclic antidepressant plasma levels. Am J Psychiatry 134:790–793, 1977

Orsulak PJ: Therapeutic monitoring of antidepressant drugs: guidelines updated. Ther Drug Monit 11:497–507, 1989

Owens MJ: Molecular and cellular mechanisms of antidepressant drugs. Depression and Anxiety 4:153–159, 1996

Pandey SC, Davis JM, Schwertz DW, et al: Effect of antidepressants and neuroleptics on phosphoinositide metabolism in human platelets. J Pharmacol Exp Ther 256:1010–1018, 1991

Paykel ES: Depressive typologies and response to amitriptyline. Br J Psychiatry 120:147–156, 1972

Paykel ES: Treatment of depression: the relevance of research for clinical practice. Br J Psychiatry 155:754–763, 1989

Paykel ES, Rowan PR, Parker RR, et al: Response to phenelzine and amitriptyline in subtypes of outpatient depression. Arch Gen Psychiatry 39:1041–1049, 1982

Peroutka SJ, Snyder SH: Long term antidepressant treatment decreases spiroperidol-labeled serotonin receptor binding. Science 210:88–90, 1980

Perry PJ, Morgan DE, Smith RE, et al: Treatment of unipolar depression accompanied by delusions. J Affect Disord 4:195–200, 1982

Perry PJ, Pfohl BM, Holstad SG: The relationship between antidepressant response and tricyclic antidepressant plasma concentrations. Clin Pharmacokinet 13:381–392, 1987

Pinder RM, Brogden RN, Speight TM, et al: Doxepin up-to-date: a review of its pharmacological properties and therapeutic efficacy with particular reference to depression. Drugs 13:161–218, 1977

Pollock BG, Perel JM: Tricyclic antidepressants: contemporary issues for therapeutic practice. Can J Psychiatry 34:609–617, 1989

Pollock BG, Everett G, Perel JM: Comparative cardiotoxicity of nortriptyline and its isomeric 10-hydroxymetabolites. Neuropsychopharmacology 6:1–10, 1992a

Pollock BG, Perel JM, Altieri LP, et al: Debrisoquine hydroxylation phenotyping in geriatric psychopharmacology. Psychopharmacol Bull 28:163–168, 1992b

Potter WZ: Psychotherapeutic drugs and biogenic amines: current concepts and therapeutic implications. Drugs 28:127–143, 1984

Potter WZ, Calil NM, Manian AA, et al: Hydroxylated metabolites of tricyclic antidepressants: preclinical assessment of activity. Biol Psychiatry 14:601–613, 1979

Potter WZ, Bertilsson L, Sjoqvist F: Clinical pharmacokinetics of psychotropic drugs: fundamental and practical aspects, in The Handbook of Biological Psychiatry. Edited by Van Praag NM, Rafaelson O, Lader O, et al. New York, Marcel Dekker, 1980, pp 71–134

Potter WZ, Scheinin M, Golden RN, et al: Selective antidepressants and cerebrospinal fluid: lack of specificity on norepinephrine and serotonin metabolites. Arch Gen Psychiatry 42:1171–1177, 1985

Potter WZ, Rudorfer MV, Manji HK: The pharmacologic treatment of depression: an update. N Engl J Med 523:633–642, 1991

Prange AI: The pharmacology and biochemistry of depression. Diseases of the Nervous System 25:217–221, 1965

Preskorn SH, Fast GA: Therapeutic drug monitoring for antidepressants: efficacy, safety, and cost effectiveness. J Clin Psychiatry 52 (6, suppl): 23–33, 1991

Preskorn SH, Irwin HA: Toxicity of tricyclic antidepressants: kinetics, mechanism, intervention: a review. J Clin Psychiatry 43:151–156, 1982

Preskorn SH, Alderman J, Chung M, et al: Pharmacokinetics of desipramine coadministered with sertraline or fluoxetine. J Clin Psychopharmacol 14:90–98, 1994

Psychoyos S: Antidepressant inhibition of H_1-H_2-histamine-receptor-mediated adenylate cyclase in [2-^{3}H]adenine-prelabeled vesicular preparations from guinea pig brain. Biochem Pharmacol 30:2182–2185, 1981

Quitkin FM, Harrison W, Stewart JW, et al: Response to phenelzine and imipramine in placebo nonresponders with atypical depression. Arch Gen Psychiatry 48:319–323, 1991

Rahman MK, Akhtar MJ, Savla NC, et al: A double-blind randomized comparison of fluvoxamine with dothiepin in the treatment of depression in elderly patients. Br J Clin Pract 45:255–258, 1991

Randrup A, Braestrup C: Uptake inhibition of biogenic amines by newer antidepressant drugs: relevance to the dopamine hypothesis of depression. Psychopharmacology (Berl) 53:309–314, 1977

Rapoport J, Potter WZ: Tricyclic antidepressants: use in pediatric psychopharmacology, in Pharmacokinetics: Youth and Age. Edited by Raskin A, Robinson D. Amsterdam, Elsevier, 1981, pp 105–123

Rapoport JL, Quinn PO, Bradbard G, et al: A double-blind comparison of imipramine and methylphenidate treatments of hyperactive boys. Arch Gen Psychiatry 30:789–793, 1974

Rapoport JL, Mikkelson EJ, Zavadil AP, et al: Childhood enuresis II: psychopathology, tricyclic concentration in plasma and anti-enuretic effect. Arch Gen Psychiatry 37:1146–1152, 1980

Rasenick MM, Chaney KA, Chen J: G protein-mediated signal transduction as a target of antidepressant and antibipolar drug action: evidence from model systems. J Clin Psychiatry 57 (suppl 13):49–55, 1996

Raskin A, Crook TA: The endogenous-neurotic distinction as a predictor of response to antidepressant drugs. Psychol Med 6:59–70, 1976

Ravaris CL, Robinson DS, Ives JO, et al: Phenelzine and amitriptyline in the treatment of depression: a comparison of present and past studies. Arch Gen Psychiatry 37:1075–1080, 1980

Ray WA: Psychotropic drugs and injuries among the elderly: a review. J Clin Psychopharmacol 12: 386–396, 1992

Richelson E, Nelson A: Antagonism by antidepressants of neurotransmitter receptors of normal human brain in vitro. J Pharmacol Exp Ther 230:94–102, 1984

Richelson E, Pfenning M: Blockade by antidepressants and related compounds of biogenic amine uptake into rat brain synaptosomes: most antidepressants selectively block norepinephrine uptake. Eur J Pharmacol 130:277–286, 1984

Riddle MA, Geller B, Ryan N: Another sudden death in a child treated with desipramine. J Am Acad Child Adolesc Psychiatry 32:792–797, 1993

Rosen J, Pollock BG, Altieri LP, et al: Treatment of nortriptyline's side effects in elderly patients: a double-blind study of bethanechol. Am J Psychiatry 150:1249–1251, 1993

Ross RI, Zavadil AP, Calil NM, et al: The effects of desmethylimipramine on plasma norepinephrine, pulse and blood pressure in volunteers. Clin Pharmacol Ther 33:429–437, 1983

Rudorfer MV, Potter WZ: Pharmacokinetics of antidepressants, in Psychopharmacology: The Third Generation of Progress. Edited by Meltzer HY. New York, Raven, 1987, pp 1353–1364

Rudorfer MV, Potter WZ: The role of metabolites of antidepressants in the treatment of depression. CNS Drugs 7:273–312, 1997

Rudorfer MV, Robins E: Amitriptyline overdose: clinical effects of tricyclic antidepressant plasma levels. J Clin Psychiatry 43:457–460, 1982

Rudorfer MV, Young RC: Desipramine: cardiovascular effects and plasma levels. Am J Psychiatry 137:984–986, 1980

Rudorfer MV, Manji HK, Potter WZ: Comparative tolerability profiles of the newer versus older antidepressants. Drug Saf 10:18–46, 1994

Schildkraut JJ: The catecholamine hypothesis of affective disorders: a review of supporting evidence. Am J Psychiatry 122:509–522, 1965

Schwaninger M, Schofl C, Blume R, et al: Inhibition by antidepressant drugs of cyclic AMP response element-binding protein/cyclic AMP response element-directed gene transcription. Mol Pharmacol 47:1112–1118, 1995

Shen WW: The metabolism of psychoactive drugs: a review of enzymatic biotransformation and inhibition. Biol Psychiatry 41:814–826, 1997

Shoaf SE, Linnoila M: Interaction of ethanol and smoking on the pharmacokinetics and pharmacodynamics of psychotropic medications. Psychopharmacol Bull 27:577–594, 1991

Smith MA, Makino S, Altemus M, et al: Stress and antidepressants differentially regulate neurotrophin 3 mRNA expression in the locus coeruleus. Proc Natl Acad Sci U S A 92: 8788–8792, 1995

Spencer T, Biederman J, Wilens T, et al: Pharmacotherapy of attention-deficit hyperactivity disorder across the life cycle. J Am Acad Child Adolesc Psychiatry 35:409–432, 1996

Spiker D, Weiss A, Chang S, et al: Tricyclic antidepressant overdose: clinical presentation and plasma levels. Clin Pharmacol Ther 18: 539–546, 1975

Spiker DG, Weiss JC, Dealy RS, et al: The pharmacologic treatment of delusional depression. Am J Psychiatry 142:430–436, 1985

Stewart JW, Quitkin FM, Liebowitz MR, et al: Efficacy of desipramine in depressed outpatients: response according to Research Diagnostic Criteria and severity of illness. Arch Gen Psychiatry 40:202–207, 1989

Sugrue MF: Chronic antidepressant therapy and associated changes in central monoaminergic function. Pharmacol Ther 21:1–37, 1983

Sulser F: Antidepressant treatments and regulation of norepinephrine-receptor-coupled adenylate cyclase systems in brain. Adv Biochem Psychopharmacol 39:249–261, 1984

Sulser F, Vetulani J, Mobley PL: Mode of action of antidepressant drugs. Biochem Pharmacol 27: 257–261, 1978

Sunderland T, Tariot PN, Cohen RM, et al: Anticholinergic sensitivity in patients with dementia of the Alzheimer type and age-matched controls: a dose-response study. Arch Gen Psychiatry 44:418–426, 1987

Thoren P, Asberg M, Cronholm B, et al: Clomipramine treatment of obsessive compulsive disorder: a controlled clinical trial. Arch Gen Psychiatry 37:1281–1289, 1980

Traskman L, Asberg M, Bertilsson L, et al: Plasma levels of clomipramine and its dimethyl metabolite during treatment of depression. Clin Pharmacol Ther 26:600–610, 1979

Turner P, Ehsanullah RSB: Clomipramine and maprotiline on human platelet uptake of 5-hydroxytryptamine and dopamine in vitro: relevance to their antidepressive and other central actions? Postgrad Med J 53 (suppl 4):14–18, 1977

Uhde TW, Nemiah JC: Panic and generalized anxiety disorders, in Comprehensive Textbook of Psychiatry, 5th Edition. Edited by Sadock BJ. Baltimore, MD, Williams & Wilkins, 1989, pp 952–972

United States Pharmacopeia Dispensing Information: Drug Information for the Health Care Professional, 17th Edition. Rockville, MD, United States Pharmacopeial Convention, 1997

Wells BG, Gelenberg AJ: Chemistry, pharmacology, pharmacokinetics, adverse effects and efficacy of the antidepressant maprotiline hydrochloride. Pharmacotherapy 1:121–139, 1981

Wilens TE, Biederman J, Prince J, et al: Six-week, double-blind, placebo-controlled study of desipramine for adult attention deficit hyperactivity disorder. Am J Psychiatry 153:1147–1153, 1996

Wisner KL, Perel JM, Findling RL, et al: Nortriptyline and its hydroxymetabolites in breastfeeding mothers and newborns. Psychopharmacol Bull 33:249–251, 1997

Wong SL, Cavanaugh J, Shi H, et al: Effects of divalproex sodium on amitriptyline and nortriptyline pharmacokinetics. Clin Pharmacol Ther 60:48–53, 1996

Young RC, Alexopoulos GS, Shamoian CA, et al: Plasma 10-hydroxynortriptyline in elderly depressed patients. Clin Pharmacol Ther 35: 540–544, 1984

Young RC, Alexopoulous GS, Shindledeker R, et al: Plasma 10-hydroxynortriptyline and therapeutic response in geriatric depression. Neuropsychopharmacology 1:213–215, 1988

Ziegler VE, Biggs JT: Tricyclic plasma levels: effect of age, race, sex, and smoking. JAMA 238: 2167–2169, 1977

Ziegler VE, Biggs JT, Wylie LT, et al: Protriptyline kinetics. Clin Pharmacol Ther 23:580–584, 1978

Zis AP, Goodwin FK: Novel antidepressants and the biogenic amine hypothesis of depression: the case of iprindole and mianserin. Arch Gen Psychiatry 36:1097–1107, 1979

Zitrin CM, Klein DF, Woerner MG: Treatment of agoraphobia with group exposure in vivo and imipramine. Arch Gen Psychiatry 37:63–72, 1980

TWO

Selective Serotonin Reuptake Inhibitors

Gary D. Tollefson, M.D., Ph.D., and
Jerrold F. Rosenbaum, M.D.

The class of selective serotonin reuptake inhibitors (SSRIs) represents an important advance in pharmacotherapy and has been the catalyst for substantial serotonin-oriented basic and clinical research. Considerable evidence demonstrates that this drug class has a broad spectrum of clinical indications. In general, an advantageous safety profile has propelled these agents to their current level of popularity. Although the members of this category share several common features, we also highlight some of their unique differences.

HISTORY AND DISCOVERY

Serotonin is an indoleamine with wide distribution in plants, animals, and humans. Pioneering histochemistry by Falck and colleagues (1962) found that serotonin was localized within specific neuronal pathways and cell bodies. These originate principally from two discrete nuclei—the medial and dorsal raphe. Across animal species, serotonin innervation is widespread. Although regional variations exist, several limbic structures manifest especially high levels of serotonin (Amin et al. 1954).

However, serotonin levels in the central nervous system (CNS) represent only a small fraction of that found in the body (Bradley 1989). Because serotonin does not cross the blood-brain barrier, it must be synthesized locally. Serotonin is released into the synapse from the cytoplasmic and vesicular reservoirs (Elks et al. 1979). Following release, serotonin is principally inactivated by reuptake into nerve terminals through a sodium/potassium (Na^+/K^+) adenosine triphosphatase (ATPase)-dependent carrier (Shaskan and Snyder 1970). The transmitter is subsequently subject to either degradation by monoamine oxidase (MAO) or vesicular restorage. Abnormalities in central serotonin function have been hypothesized to underlie disturbances in mood, anxiety, satiety, cognition, aggression, and sexual drives, to highlight a few. As described by Fuller (1985), there are several loci at which therapeutic drugs might alter serotonin neurotransmission (see Figure 2–1). The recent explosion of knowledge regarding the serotonin system can largely be traced to the develop-

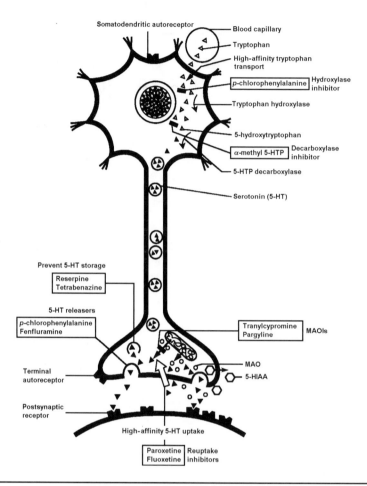

Figure 2–1.   Serotonin neuron showing the main steps in the life cycle of serotonin and the sites at which drugs act. For clarity, drugs acting at serotonin (5-HT) receptors have been omitted.
MAOI = monoamine oxidase inhibitor; 5-HIAA = 5-hydroxyindoleacetic acid.
Source.   Reprinted from Marsden CA: "The Neuropharmacology of Serotonin in the Central Nervous System," in *Selective Serotonin Re-Uptake Inhibitors.* Edited by Feighner JP, Boyer WF. Chichester, England, Wiley, 1991, pp. 11–35. Copyright 1991, John Wiley & Sons Limited. Used with permission.

ment of compounds that block the reuptake of this neurotransmitter.

STRUCTURE-ACTIVITY RELATIONS

Drugs that inhibit serotonin reuptake vary in their selectivity (see Table 2–1). Despite the tendency to lump the contemporary SSRIs into the same class designation, significant structural and activity differences exist. Their structural formulas help illustrate this diversity (see Figure 2–2). Both paroxetine and sertraline exist as single isomers; in contrast, fluoxetine and citalopram are racemic. Fluvoxamine has no optically active forms. Structural differences bestow both pharmacokinetic and pharmacodynamic heterogeneity.

The family of SSRIs manifests diverse structural and activity relations. Such data are in vitro

Table 2–1. Inhibition of [^{3}H]-monoamine uptake into rat brain synaptosomes in vitro

Compound	K_1 (nM)		
	[^{3}H]-5-HT	[^{3}H]-NE	[^{3}H]-DA
Paroxetine	1.1	350	2,000
Citalopram	1.8	8,800	>10,000
Fluvoxamine	6.2	1,100	>10,000
Sertraline	7.3	1,400	230
Clomipramine	7.4	96	9,100
Fluoxetine	25	500	4,200
Amitriptyline	87	79	4,300

Note. Relative values from a series of related trials from Boyer and Feighner 1991.
5-HT = serotonin; NE = norepinephrine; DA = dopamine.

and thus subject to methodological variability (Thomas et al. 1987). Paroxetine appears to be the most potent in vitro SSRI, whereas citalopram may be the most selective. However, note that in vitro potency does not necessarily equate with in vivo dosing experience, clinical efficacy, adverse-event profile, and so on. Of the SSRIs, sertraline is the only class member that is a more potent inhibitor of dopamine than norepinephrine reuptake (Richelson 1996).

The tricyclic antidepressants (TCAs) have been characterized by their inhibitory activity at other receptor targets mediating their adverse-event profile (Hall and Ogren 1981; Snyder and Yamamura 1977; U'Prichard et al. 1978). These include histaminergic, α_1-adrenergic, and muscarinic receptors. For most of the SSRIs, inhibitory activity (IC$_{50}$) at histaminergic or adrenergic sites is in the micromolar range and thus unlikely to be of clinical significance. Sertraline is an exception at the α_1-adrenergic receptor (Stockmeier et al. 1987). This affinity is approximately one-fourth that of imipramine. SSRI activity at the muscarinic receptor is negligible for fluoxetine, fluvoxamine, citalopram, and sertraline; however, paroxetine has an IC$_{50}$ of 89 nM, which suggests some increased chance for anticholinergic effects. Sertraline also has a high affinity for the sigma binding site in vitro, but the clinical relevance of this property is unknown. In contrast, neither paroxetine nor fluoxetine is sig-

nificantly active at this site (Schmidt et al. 1989). The sigma binding site is of theoretical interest in schizophrenia and related psychoses. Stauderman and colleagues (1992) reported that fluoxetine and paroxetine inhibited the binding of ^{3}H-nitrendipine to L-type calcium channels. However, this was at concentrations that were probably in excess of those achieved during in vivo treatment of depression.

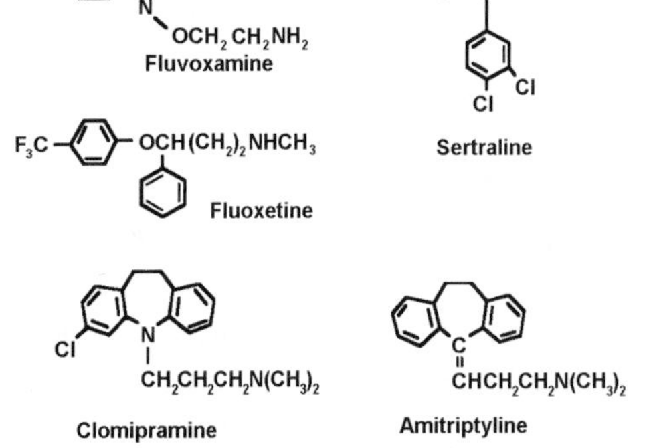

Figure 2–2. Chemical structures for selective serotonin reuptake inhibitors (SSRIs) and some tricyclic antidepressants (TCAs).

In summary, in vitro radioligand-binding techniques show that SSRIs have a lower probability of many of the troublesome side effects associated with TCAs and are relatively selective in their serotonin reuptake inhibition yet retain an individual variability in their receptor pharmacology. (For a general review of synaptic effects of several SSRIs compared with other antidepressants, see Richelson 1996.)

PHARMACOLOGICAL PROFILE

Serotonin

The action of an SSRI extends beyond the inhibition of serotonin reuptake. At least 14 different serotonin (5-HT) receptor subtypes reside at pre- and postsynaptic locations (Fuller 1996). $5-HT_{1A}$ binding sites include both somatodendritic and presynaptic autoreceptors (which inhibit serotonin firing) and postsynaptic receptors. The latter are predominantly hippocampal, and their sensitivity is increased after chronic antidepressant exposure (Aghajanian et al. 1988). Antidepressant-induced changes at the $5-HT_{1B}$ binding site are not definitive (Sleight et al. 1988). Reduced sensitivity of $5-HT_{1B}$ sites may uniquely characterize the SSRIs. The R enantiomer of fluoxetine antagonizes the $5-HT_{1C}$ receptor at near-micromolar concentrations in vitro (Wong et al. 1991); however, the clinical relevance of this observation to other models and the extent to which other SSRIs share this interaction are unknown.

$5-HT_2$ receptors are located postsynaptically throughout the hippocampus, cortex, and spinal cord. Functionally, they inhibit postsynaptic propagation of a nerve impulse. The upregulation of $5-HT_2$ binding sites has been implicated in major depression (Pandey et al. 1990). Although receptor studies are not conclusive, $5-HT_2$ animal behavioral models (e.g., 5-hydroxytryptophan [5-HTP] head twitch response) show that sensitivity diminishes after chronic SSRI exposure consistent with $5-HT_2$ receptor adaptation (Marshall et al. 1988). After chronic administration, many contemporary antidepressants downregulate or reduce the density of $5-HT_2$ binding sites in rat frontal cortex (Peroutka and Snyder 1980). Some, but not all, SSRIs have been associated with this effect (Fraser et al. 1988). These adaptive changes have been cited as necessary for an antidepressant response (Cowen 1991). However, the apparent absence of such activity by some antidepressants calls into question how essential this effect is.

The specific receptor effects, however, may not be independent. For example, an interaction between $5-HT_{1A}$ and $5-HT_2$ binding sites seems quite plausible. $5-HT_2$ antagonists attenuate a $5-HT_{1A}$ agonist's (8-hydroxydipropylaminotetralin [8-OH-DPAT]) ability to release serotonin (Backus et al. 1990). SSRIs, as a drug class, have been reported to normalize both $5-HT_{1A}$ and $5-HT_2$ receptor density among depressed patients (Leonard 1992).

Studies of fluoxetine (Blier et al. 1988), citalopram (Chaput et al. 1986), paroxetine (deMontigny et al. 1989), fluvoxamine (Dresse and Scuvee-Moreau 1984), and sertraline (Heym and Koe 1988) found that SSRIs transiently inhibit dorsal raphe firing, decrease terminal autoreceptor function, and ultimately increase net serotonin synaptic transmission within CA_3 pyramidal cells in the hippocampus. Blier and colleagues (1990) concluded that electrophysiological studies indicate that most antidepressants enhance net serotonin transmission after chronic administration, albeit at different loci—the TCAs via enhanced sensitivity of postsynaptic $5-HT_{1A}$ receptors and the SSRIs (and MAO inhibitors [MAOIs]) via reduced sensitivity of somatodendritic ($5-HT_{1A}$) and terminal autoreceptors ($5-HT_{1D}$). These observations of different mechanisms may help explain why certain depressive symptoms that do not respond to one class of antidepressant will respond to another and may explain the enhanced response reported when combinations of antidepressant agents are used.

Norepinephrine

Chronic administration of most somatic treatments for depression downregulates or reduces the density of β-norepinephrine binding sites in the brain (Bergstrom and Kellar 1979). These include traditional norepinephrine-specific and mixed uptake inhibitors (Charney et al. 1981). However, results with the SSRIs have been less consistent (Johnson 1991). Despite their in vitro serotonin selectivity, several of these agents (e.g., fluoxetine by autoradiography and sertraline by autoradiography or membrane binding) have been observed to induce β-norepinephrine receptor downregulation.

Most studies with the SSRIs have not shown a consistent change in β-norepinephrine binding or β-norepinephrine-stimulated cyclic adenosine monophosphate (cAMP) production. However, Baron et al. (1988) reported that fluoxetine coadministered with desipramine augmented the reduction in cortical β-norepinephrine receptors expected with desipramine alone. Asakura and colleagues (1987) noted that coadministration with mianserin or maprotiline also increased the duration of downregulation. Sertraline induced downregulation of the β receptor and reduced production at the β receptor of the second messenger cAMP (Koe et al. 1987). In contrast, investigations with fluvoxamine, paroxetine, and citalopram have not yielded consistent results. In general, the greater the serotonin selectivity of a compound, the less in vitro evidence for β-norepinephrine downregulation has been seen. Thus, β-norepinephrine downregulation may not be essential for clinical efficacy.

Current data do not support a significant effect on α-norepinephrine receptor affinity or density by the SSRIs. Studies using several different radiolabels to investigate paroxetine (Nelson et al. 1989), fluoxetine (Wong et al. 1985), and citalopram (Nowak 1989) have shown a relative inactivity at this site. Studies with sertraline or fluvoxamine are limited. Fluoxetine has been reported to reduce

desipramine-induced release of growth hormone after 4 weeks of treatment (O'Flynn et al. 1991). This effect suggests a possible indirect activity at the α_2-norepinephrine receptor.

In summary, most SSRIs do not manifest significant norepinephrine activity. However, relative differences in adrenoceptor affinity exist across the class; the clinical significance of these differences is negligible based on present information.

Dopamine

Animal studies provide evidence that the serotonin system may exert tonic inhibition on the central dopaminergic system. Thus, SSRIs might diminish dopaminergic transmission consistent with anecdotes of extrapyramidal side effects (EPS) during fluoxetine therapy (Bouchard et al. 1989). Serotonin agonists, however, also exert a facilitory influence on dopamine release (Benloucif and Galloway 1991), which can be antagonized by the 5-HT$_1$ blocker pindolol, and evidence suggests that SSRIs may actually sensitize mesolimbic dopamine receptors (Arnt et al. 1984a, 1984b). Many structurally diverse antidepressants are associated with a net enhancement of mesolimbic dopamine (Klimek and Maj 1990). The benefits of antidepressants in an animal model of depression can be antagonized by a dopamine D$_1$ (SCH-23390) or D$_2$ blocker (sulpiride) (Sampson et al. 1991). Repeated administration of several SSRIs increased the hypermotility response to several dopaminergic agents, including amphetamine, methylphenidate (Arnt et al. 1984b), quinpirole (Maj et al. 1984), and apomorphine (Plaznik and Kostowski 1987).

The induction of catalepsy or inhibition of apomorphine-induced catalepsy is not a property of the SSRIs. Within the family of SSRIs, citalopram reportedly downregulated rat striatolimbic D$_1$ receptors (Klimek and Nielsen 1987). Both citalopram and fluoxetine have been inactive in displacing D$_2$ blockers (Peroutka and Snyder 1980). Baldessarini and co-workers (1992) reported that fluoxetine "even at high doses or with repeated treatment" demonstrated "no significant inhibition of the DA [dopamine]-metabolism—increasing actions of haloperidol" (p. 191).

In summary, the SSRIs do not appear to exert a significant effect on the dopamine system. However, in clinical use, a multitude of variables makes simple conclusions regarding dopamine-mediated events unreliable.

Miscellaneous

Neuroendocrine and neurotransmitter dysfunction in major depression has been linked to corticotropin-releasing factor (CRF) in locus coeruleus neurons. Antidepressants have been hypothesized to reverse CRF-related increases in locus coeruleus discharge. Sertraline has been proposed as an acute functional CRF antagonist (Valentino and Curtis 1991). However, net serotonin enhancement by an SSRI would be expected to promote the release of CRF (Fuller 1985). Activity through $5-HT_{1A}$ receptors has been proposed by Lorens and Van der Kar (1987); the role for SSRIs, however, as CRF antagonists awaits further clarification.

In summary, the SSRIs enhance central serotonin transmission through increased output and/or increased postsynaptic receptor sensitivity (Blier et al. 1987). However, such changes alone do not guarantee a clinically meaningful response (Charney et al. 1984). A change in baseline serotonin function or a "permissive" set of interactions with other colocalized neurotransmitter receptors is likely involved in the highly individualized responses in depressed patients.

PHARMACOKINETICS AND DISPOSITION

Pharmacokinetic variability exists within the SSRI class (Leonard 1992) (Table 2–2). Discussion of drug half-life must also include consideration of the presence or absence of active metab-

olites. Fluoxetine is principally metabolized to norfluoxetine, which has similar activity to fluoxetine on serotonin reuptake. The elimination half-life of norfluoxetine is longer (4–16 days) than that of fluoxetine (1–3 days). The desmethyl metabolite of sertraline manifests uptake inhibition of serotonin, albeit of a magnitude approximately one-tenth that of the parent (Heym and Koe 1988). The elimination half-life of desmethyl sertraline also exceeds that of its parent (66 vs. 24–26 hours) (Doogan and Caillard 1988). The principal desmethyl metabolite of citalopram is approximately 4 times less potent as an SSRI than its parent and 11 times more potent as a norepinephrine uptake inhibitor (Hyttel 1982). However, this metabolite's concentration is typically less than that of citalopram and weakly crosses the blood-brain barrier. Thus, an antidepressant contribution from the metabolite is probably negligible.

In contrast, paroxetine (Haddock et al. 1989) and fluvoxamine (Claassen 1983) have metabolites with minimal or no activity. An SSRI with a relatively long half-life offers greater protection from the discontinuation syndrome associated with abrupt discontinuation or noncompliance related to interruption of treatment. Conversely, those drugs require a more prolonged vigilance for drug-drug interactions following their discontinuation; for example, a 5-week washout from fluoxetine is recommended before initiating an MAOI (Ciraulo and Shader 1990). Variability in drug half-life is associated with a range in time to steady-state plasma concentrations, which does not predict or correlate with onset of antidepressant activity. The time to onset of antidepressant effect is the same for all SSRIs.

MECHANISM OF ACTION

In the absence of pharmacological manipulation, the reuptake of serotonin into the presynaptic nerve terminal typically leads to its inactivation. The SSRIs, through blockade of

Table 2–2. **A comparison of several selective serotonin reuptake inhibitors**

	Fluoxetine	Paroxetine	Sertraline	Citalopram	Fluvoxamine
Volume of distribution (L/kg)	3–40	17	20	12–16	>5
Percent protein bound	94	95	99	80	77
Peak plasma level (hours)	6–8	2–8	6–8	1–6	2–8
Parent half-life (hours)	24–72	20	24–26	33	15
Major metabolite half-life	4–16 days	N/A	66 hours	N/A	N/A
Standard dose range (mg)	20–80	10–50	50–200	10–40	50–300
Absorption altered by a fast or fed status	No	No	Yes	No	No
Altered half-life in the geriatric patient	No	Yes	Yes	Yes	No
Reduced clearance in renal patients	±	+	±	±	±

Note. N/A = not applicable.

the reuptake process, acutely enhance serotonergic neurotransmission by permitting serotonin to act for an extended time at synaptic binding sites. A net result is an acute increase in synaptic serotonin. One difference separating the SSRIs from the direct-acting agonists is that the SSRIs are dependent on neuronal release of serotonin for their action. That is, SSRIs can be considered as augmentors of basal physiological signals, but they are not direct stimulators of postsynaptic receptor function and are dependent on presynaptic neuronal integrity; these pharmacodynamic features might explain SSRI nonresponse. If the release of serotonin from presynaptic neuronal storage sites was substantially compromised, and in turn their net synaptic serotonin concentration was negligible, a clinically meaningful response to an SSRI would not be expected.

Serotonin receptors also include a family of presynaptic autoreceptors that suppress the further release of serotonin, thus limiting the degree of postsynaptic receptor stimulation that can be achieved. DeMontigny and colleagues (1989) investigated the mechanism of action of several SSRIs and suggested that the enhanced efficacy of serotonergic synaptic transmission is not the result of increased postsynaptic sensitivity. Rather, longer-term SSRI treatment induced a desensitization of somatodendritic and terminal serotonin autoreceptors. Such a desensitization would permit serotonin neurons to reestablish a normal rate of firing despite sustained reuptake blockade. These neurons could then release a greater amount of serotonin per impulse into the synaptic cleft. This modification reportedly occurs over a time course compatible with the antidepressant response.

INDICATIONS

SSRIs are approved for use in major depression, obsessive-compulsive disorder, bulimia nervosa, panic disorder, social phobia, posttraumatic stress disorder, and premenstrual dysphoric disorder. They also appear to be effective in dysthymia and chronic depression. Uses of SSRIs are discussed in Chapters 18, 21, 23, 25–27, 30, and 31.

SIDE EFFECTS AND TOXICOLOGY

Safety and a favorable side-effect profile, as well as lack of multiple receptor affinity that mediates adverse events associated with TCAs, distinguish SSRIs from TCAs. SSRIs as a class have a similar side-effect profile.

For most patients, SSRIs are better tolerated, based on the number of early trial discontinuations attributable to an adverse event, than TCAs (see Boyer and Feighner 1991). In general, for three-arm trials, a 5%–10% incidence of early discontinuations because of an adverse event occurred for the placebo group, 10%–20% for the SSRI group, and 30%–35% for the TCA group. The SSRIs, presumably by enhancement of serotonin within the CNS, may induce agitation, anxiety, sleep disturbance, tremor, sexual dysfunction (primarily anorgasmia), or headache. Baseline clinical features do not appear to predispose to these adverse events (Montgomery 1989). Although CNS adverse events may occur with the SSRIs, Kerr and colleagues (1991) suggested that these drugs have a more favorable profile of behavioral toxicity overall than do the conventional TCAs.

Because the enteric nervous system is richly innervated by serotonin, adverse events may include altered gastrointestinal motility and nausea. Certain autonomic adverse events, including dry mouth, sweating, and weight change, also occur.

As was discussed earlier in this chapter, SSRIs are unlikely to alter dopamine function. Anecdotal reports of EPS (Meltzer et al. 1979) associated with the SSRIs are not more frequent than has been reported historically with TCAs (Fann et al. 1976; Zubenko et al. 1987), MAOIs (Teusink et al. 1984), or trazodone (Papini et al. 1982). Very rare events, including arthralgia, lymphadenopathy, inappropriate antidiuretic syndrome, agranulocytosis, and hypoglycemia, have been reported during clinical trials or postmarketing surveillance; however, causality typically is uncertain.

One additional rare and life-threatening idiosyncratic event associated with the SSRIs (and, more prominently, their interaction with MAOIs or other serotonin enhancers) is the central serotonin syndrome. This phenomenon appears to represent an overactivation of central serotonin receptors and may manifest with features such as abdominal pain, diarrhea, sweating, fever, tachycardia, elevated blood pressure, altered mental state (e.g., delirium), myoclonus, increased motor activity, irritability, hostility, and mood change. Severe manifestations of this syndrome can induce hyperpyrexia, cardiovascular shock, or death. Realistically, data are inadequate to rate one MAOI or SSRI as more or less likely to be associated with serotonin syndrome. The risk of serotonin syndrome seems to be increased when an SSRI is administered temporally with a second serotonin-enhancing agent (e.g., an MAOI) (Marley and Wozniak 1984a, 1984b). When following an SSRI with an MAOI, drug half-life (and that of any active metabolite, where applicable) should serve as a guide to the length of the washout period. A standard recommendation would be to wait at least five times the half-life of the SSRI or its metabolite, whichever is longer, before administering the next serotonergic agent. (For a review, see Lane and Baldwin 1997.)

Although some variability in adverse event frequency has been reported among the SSRIs, all are characterized by the above-mentioned features. Tolerance to an adverse event may change with dose and/or length of exposure; higher doses are typically associated with higher rates of adverse events (Bressa et al. 1989). Many events such as activation are transient, usually beginning early in the course of therapy and then remitting (Beasley et al. 1991). Comparisons between A.M. and P.M. administration did not identify differences in efficacy (Usher et al. 1991); however, the P.M. dosing was associated with fewer intolerable side effects in a fluvoxamine trial (Siddiqui et al. 1985). Individual patient differences suggest the need for some flexibility in dosing schedules.

TCAs behave like type IA antiarrhythmics and, thus, in a dose-dependent fashion may retard His-Purkinje conduction. SSRIs are essentially devoid of this property. In clinical trials, the incidence of increased heart rate or conduction disturbance has been very uncommon across several of the SSRIs (Edwards et al. 1989; Fisch 1985; Guy and Silke 1990). However, very high doses of citalopram reportedly mimicked TCA-like cardiovascular effects only in a specific animal model (Boeck et al. 1984). SSRIs are not associated with α-adrenergic antagonism and thus rarely have been associated with orthostatic hypotension. The above-mentioned properties of the SSRIs translate into a wider safety profile than that of TCAs.

Sleep

Fluoxetine decreases rapid eye movement (REM) and increases nonrapid eye movement (NREM) sleep at dose ranges of 5–40 mg/kg in rodent models (Gao et al. 1992). Citalopram (Hilakivi et al. 1987) and fluvoxamine (Scherschlicht et al. 1982) also shorten REM sleep in laboratory animal models. This is a common property of many antidepressant medications. Interestingly, both fluoxetine and sertraline induce higher rates of sedation as dosages are increased. In contrast, paroxetine causes a dose-dependent increase in arousal, wakening, reduced slow-wave sleep, and REM suppression (Kleinlogel and Burki 1987).

Suicidality

Evidence implicating serotonin in suicide or violence is compelling. Reduced cerebrospinal fluid 5-hydroxyindoleacetic acid (5-HIAA) concentrations correlate highly with completed suicides in depressed patients (Edman et al. 1986; Ninan et al. 1984). In vitro binding assays have shown an increased density (B_{max}) of 5-HT$_2$ receptors in depressed and suicidal individuals (Pandey et al. 1990). Both observations are consistent with a relative state of serotonin depletion among suicidal subjects. The American College of Neuropsychopharmacology (1992) reviewed evidence that antidepressants result in substantial improvement or remission of suicidal ideation and impulses in the vast majority

of patients. SSRIs were thought to potentially "carry a lower risk for suicide than older tricyclic antidepressants" (p. 181) when taken in overdose. Furthermore, this task force stated that no evidence indicated that SSRIs triggered emergent suicidal ideation above base rates associated with depression. Also, Warshaw and Keller (1996) determined that fluoxetine use did not increase the rate of suicide in a group of 654 patients with anxiety disorders. In a large retrospective review of patients receiving one or more of 10 antidepressants (including fluoxetine), Jick and colleagues (1995) concluded that the risk for suicide was similar among all agents.

Pregnancy and Lactation

Given the widespread use of SSRIs and the high prevalence of mood disorders during the childbearing years, these agents probably will be used during pregnancy and breast-feeding. Except for fluoxetine, published information about the use and safety of SSRIs in this special population is very limited. Goldstein and colleagues (1997) evaluated the outcomes of 796 prospectively identified pregnancies with confirmed first-trimester exposure to fluoxetine. Historical reports of newborn surveys were used for comparison. Abnormalities were observed in 5% of the fluoxetine-exposed newborns, which was consistent with historical controls.

Pregnancy outcomes and follow-up cognitive and behavioral assessments of 135 children exposed in utero to a TCA or fluoxetine (55 infants) were compared with a control group of infant-mother pairs (Nulman et al. 1997). The incidence of major malformations and perinatal complications was similar among the three groups. No statistically significant differences in mean global intelligence quotient (IQ) scores or language development were found in the children of mothers who received a TCA or fluoxetine or were in the control group. There were also no differences among the groups on several behavioral assessments. The results of children exposed during the first trimester were not different from those of children exposed throughout the pregnancy. Prospectively derived data are not available for paroxetine, sertraline, fluvoxamine, or citalopram.

Fluoxetine is secreted into breast milk. One naturalistic study (Taddio et al. 1996) and two case reports (Burch and Wells 1992; Isenberg 1990) with a total of 13 infants noted no adverse effects in these infants during the short-term study periods. One case report described adverse events in a breast-fed infant whose mother was taking fluoxetine (Lester et al. 1993). In addition, two cases reported no adverse effects and plasma levels that were very low or nondetectable (<2 ng/mL) in 4 breast-fed infants whose mothers were taking sertraline (Altshuler et al. 1995; Mammen et al. 1997).

SSRI Discontinuation Syndrome

Discontinuation symptoms have been described with several antidepressants, including TCAs and MAOIs. SSRI discontinuation symptoms have been reported most frequently with paroxetine (short elimination half-life and no active metabolite) and least frequently with fluoxetine (long elimination half-lives of parent and active metabolite). SSRIs are not drugs of abuse; when these agents are discontinued, patients show neither the characteristic abstinence syndrome of CNS-depressant withdrawal nor drug-seeking behavior. The most common physical symptoms are dizziness, nausea and vomiting, fatigue, lethargy, flulike symptoms (aches and chills), and sensory and sleep disturbances. Psychological symptoms most commonly reported are anxiety, irritability, and crying spells. For most patients, the discontinuation symptoms are different from the adverse effects they may have had while taking an SSRI. Discontinuation symptoms most often emerge within 1–3 days (Schatzberg et al. 1997).

SSRIs with short half-lives (paroxetine and fluvoxamine) and related drugs such as venlafaxine should be tapered. Fluoxetine does not require tapering because of its extended half-life.

Drug Overdosage

A major advantage of SSRIs relative to other antidepressants has been their superior therapeutic index (Cooper 1988; Pedersen et al. 1982). The number of deaths per 1 million prescriptions across several SSRIs (0–6) is substantially lower than that of the conventional TCAs (8–53) or the MAOIs (0–61) (Leonard 1992).

Borys and colleagues (1992) reported on 234 cases of fluoxetine overdose (232–1,390 ng/mL) obtained in a prospective multicenter study. Fluoxetine was the sole ingestant in 87 cases and was taken in combination with alcohol and/or other drugs in the remaining 147 cases. Common symptoms included tachycardia, sedation, tremor, nausea, and emesis. These authors concluded that the emergent symptoms were minor and of short duration; thus, aggressive supportive care "is the only intervention necessary" (p. 115).

The SSRIs represent an important addition to the therapeutic armamentarium for the depressed patient at risk for a drug overdose.

DRUG-DRUG INTERACTIONS

Although the potential for significant interactions exists, SSRIs are unlikely to be associated with many of the conventional problems seen with the earlier antidepressants. These problems include cumulative CNS-depressant effects with alcohol, anticholinergic agents, or antihistaminic compounds. The structural differences (see Figure 2–2) among the SSRIs offer a basis for some intraclass differences. Paroxetine and fluvoxamine have been associated with increased bleeding time when given with warfarin. Lithium concentrations are generally unaffected.

One potential for clinically relevant antidepressant pharmacokinetic interactions is based on drug effect on the cytochrome P450 (CYP) family of isoenzymes (Brosen and Gram 1989). For example, SSRIs are both substrates and inhibitors for oxidation via CYP2D6. Crewe and colleagues (1992) ranked the potency of CYP2D6 inhibition for serotonin antidepressants from most potent to least: paroxetine, fluoxetine, sertraline, fluvoxamine, citalopram, clomipramine, and amitriptyline.

By inhibition of CYP2D6, the SSRIs may elevate the concentration of concomitantly administered drugs that rely on this isoenzyme for metabolism. This has particular clinical relevance when the second agent has a narrow therapeutic index. Examples of such agents include flecainide, quinidine, carbamazepine, propafenone, TCAs, and several antipsychotics (Rudorfer and Potter 1989). The clinical consequence of such an interaction may either enhance or impair efficacy and/or heighten the adverse-event profile.

SSRIs vary in their effect on the other cytochromes including 1A2, 3A3/4, 2C9, and 2C19.

CONCLUSION

The SSRIs have been shown to be a safe and effective drug class. They are frequently better tolerated than conventional TCAs and have a superior safety profile in overdosage for patients with comorbid medical illness. Preliminary evidence suggests a broad utilitarian role for SSRIs across a spectrum of psychopathology. As experience with these compounds broadens, continued advances in scientific knowledge about the serotonin system and its role with human pathophysiology can be expected.

REFERENCES

Aghajanian JK, Sprouse JS, Rasmussen K: Electrophysiology of central serotonin receptor subtypes, in The Serotonin Receptors. Edited by Sanders-Bush E. Clifton, NJ, Humana Press, 1988, pp 225–252

Altshuler LL, Burt VK, McMullen M, et al: Breastfeeding and sertraline: a 24-hour analysis. J Clin Psychiatry 56:243–245, 1995

American College of Neuropsychopharmacology: Suicidal behavior and psychotropic medication (consensus statement). Neuropsychopharmacology 8:177–183, 1992

Amin AH, Crawford TBB, Gaddum JH: The distribution of substance P and 5-hydroxytryptamine in the central nervous system of the dog. J Physiol (Lond) 126:596–618, 1954

Arnt J, Hyttel J, Overo FK: Prolonged treatment with the specific 5-HT uptake inhibitor citalopram: effect on dopaminergic and serotonergic functions. Pol J Pharmacol Pharm 36:221–230, 1984a

Arnt J, Overo KF, Hyttel J, et al: Changes in rat dopamine and serotonin function in vivo after prolonged administration of the specific 5-HT uptake inhibitor citalopram. Psychopharmacology (Berl) 84:457–465, 1984b

Asakura M, Tsukamoto T, Kubota H, et al: Role of serotonin in regulation of β-adrenoceptors by antidepressants. Eur J Pharmacol 141:95–100, 1987

Backus LI, Sharp T, Grahame-Smith DJ: Behavioral evidence for a functional interaction between central 5-HT$_2$ and 5-HT$_{1A}$ receptors. Journal of Pharmacology 100:793–799, 1990

Baldessarini RJ, Marsh ER, Kula NS: Interactions of fluoxetine with metabolism of dopamine and serotonin in rat brain regions. Brain Res 579:152–156, 1992

Baron BM, Ogden AM, Siegel BW, et al: Rapid down-regulation of β-adrenoceptors by coadministration of desipramine and fluoxetine. Eur J Pharmacol 154:125–134, 1988

Beasley CM, Sayler ME, Bosomworth JC, et al: High-dose fluoxetine: efficacy and activating-sedating effects in agitated and retarded depression. J Clin Psychopharmacol 11:166–174, 1991

Benloucif S, Galloway MP: Facilitation of dopamine release in vivo by serotonin agonists: studied with microdialysis. Eur J Pharmacol 200:1–8, 1991

Bergstrom DA, Kellar JK: Adrenergic and serotonergic receptor binding in rat brain after chronic desmethyl imipramine treatment. J Pharmacol Exp Ther 209:256–261, 1979

Blier P, deMontigny C, Chaput Y: Modifications of the serotonin system by antidepressant treatments: implications for the therapeutic response in major depression. J Clin Psychopharmacol 7:24S–35S, 1987

Blier P, Chaput Y, deMontigny C: Long-term 5-HT reuptake blockade, but not monoamine oxidase inhibition, decreases the function of terminal 5-HT autoreceptors; an electrophysiological study in the rat brain. Naunyn Schmiedebergs Arch Pharmacol 337:246–254, 1988

Blier P, deMontigny C, Chaput Y: A role for the serotonin system in the mechanism of action of antidepressants. J Clin Psychiatry 51 (suppl 4): 14–20, 1990

Boeck V, Jorgensen A, Overo KF: Comparative animal studies on cardiovascular toxicity of tri- and tetracyclic antidepressants and citalopram; relation to drug plasma levels. Psychopharmacology (Berl) 82:275–281, 1984

Borys DJ, Setzer SC, Ling LJ, et al: Acute fluoxetine overdose: a report of 234 cases. Am J Emerg Med 10:115–120, 1992

Bouchard RH, Pourcher E, Vincent P: Fluoxetine and extrapyramidal side effects. Am J Psychiatry 146:1352–1353, 1989

Boyer WF, Feighner JP: The efficacy of selective serotonin uptake inhibitors in depression, in Selective Serotonin Uptake Inhibitors. Edited by Feighner JP, Boyer WF. Chichester, England, Wiley, 1991, pp 89–108

Bradley PB: Introduction to Neuropharmacology. Boston, MA, Wright, 1989

Bressa GM, Brugnoli R, Pancheri P: A double-blind study of fluoxetine and imipramine in major depression. Int Clin Psychopharmacol 4 (suppl 1): 69–73, 1989

Brosen K, Gram LF: Clinical significance of the sparteine/debrisoquine oxidation polymorphism. Eur J Clin Pharmacol 36:537–547, 1989

Burch KJ, Wells BG: Fluoxetine/norfluoxetine concentrations in human milk. Pediatrics 89: 676–677, 1992

Chaput Y, deMontigny C, Blier P: Effects of a selective 5-HT reuptake blocker citalopram on the sensitivity of 5-HT autoreceptors, electrophysiological studies in the rat. Naunyn Schmiedebergs Arch Pharmacol 333:342–348, 1986

Charney DS, Menkes DB, Heninger GR: Receptor sensitivity and the mechanism of action of antidepressant treatment. Arch Gen Psychiatry 38:1160–1180, 1981

Charney DS, Heninger GR, Sternberg DE: Serotonin function and mechanism of action of antidepressant treatment. Arch Gen Psychiatry 41: 359–365, 1984

Ciraulo DA, Shader RI: Fluoxetine drug-drug interactions, I: antidepressants and antipsychotics. J Clin Psychopharmacol 10:48–50, 1990

Claassen V: Review of the animal pharmacology and pharmacokinetics of fluvoxamine. Br J Clin Pharmacol 15:349S–355S, 1983

Cooper GL: The safety of fluoxetine—an update. Br J Psychiatry 153:77–86, 1988

Cowen PJ: Serotonin receptor subtypes: implications for psychopharmacology. Br J Psychiatry 159 (suppl 12):7–14, 1991

Crewe HK, Lennard MS, Tucker GT, et al: The effect of selective serotonin reuptake inhibitors on the cytochrome P450IID6 activity in human liver microsomes. Br J Clin Pharmacol 34: 262–265, 1992

deMontigny C, Chaput Y, Blier P: Long-term tricyclic and electroconvulsive treatment increases responsiveness of dorsal hippocampus 5-HT$_{1A}$ receptors: an electrophysiological study. Society for Neuroscience Abstracts 15:854, 1989

Doogan DP, Caillard V: Sertraline: a new antidepressant. J Clin Psychiatry 49 (suppl):46–51, 1988

Dresse A, Scuvee-Moreau J: The effects of various antidepressants on the spontaneous firing rates of noradrenergic and serotonergic neurons. Clin Neuropharmacol 7 (suppl 1):572–573, 1984

Edman G, Asberg M, Levander S, et al: Skin conductance habituation and cerebrospinal fluid 5-hydroxyindoleacetic acid in suicidal patients. Arch Gen Psychiatry 43:586–592, 1986

Edwards JG, Goldie A, Papayanni-Papasthatis S: Effect of paroxetine on the electrocardiogram. Psychopharmacology (Berl) 97:96–98, 1989

Elks ML, Youngblood WW, Kizer JS: Serotonin synthesis and release in brain slices, independence of tryptophan. Brain Res 172:471–486, 1979

Falck B, Hillarp N-A, Thieme G, et al: Fluorescence of catecholamines and related compounds condensed with formaldehyde. J Histochem Cytochem 10:348–354, 1962

Fann WE, Sullivan JL, Richman BW: Dyskinesias associated with tricyclic antidepressants. Br J Psychiatry 128:490–493, 1976

Fisch C: Effect of fluoxetine on the electrocardiogram. J Clin Psychiatry 46:42–44, 1985

Fraser A, Offord SJ, Lucki I: Regulation of serotonin receptors and responsiveness in the brain, in The Serotonin Receptors. Edited by Sanders-Bush E. Clifton, NJ, Humana Press, 1988, pp 319–362

Fuller RW: Drugs altering serotonin synthesis and metabolism, in Neuropharmacology of Serotonin. Edited by Green AR. New York, Oxford University Press, 1985, pp 1–20

Fuller RW: Mechanisms and functions of serotonin neuronal systems: opportunities for neuropeptide interactions. Ann N Y Acad Sci 780: 176–184, 1996

Gao B, Duncan WC Jr, Wehr ATA: Fluoxetine decreases brain temperature and REM sleep in Syrian hamsters. Psychopharmacology (Berl) 106:321–329, 1992

Goldstein DJ, Corbin LA, Sundell KL: Effects of first-trimester fluoxetine exposure on the newborn. Obstet General 89 (5 pt 1):713–718, 1997

Guy S, Silke B: The electrocardiogram as a tool for therapeutic monitoring: a critical analysis. J Clin Psychiatry 51 (12, suppl B):37–39, 1990

Haddock RE, Johnson AM, Langley PE, et al: Metabolic pathway of paroxetine in animals and man and the comparative pharmacological properties of its metabolites. Acta Psychiatr Scand 80 (suppl 350):24–26, 1989

Hall H, Ogren SO: Effects of antidepressant drugs on different receptors in rat brain. Eur J Pharmacol 70:393–407, 1981

Heym J, Koe BK: Pharmacology of sertraline: a review. J Clin Psychiatry 49 (suppl):40–45, 1988

Hilakivi I, Kovala T, Leppavuori A, et al: Effects of serotonin and noradrenaline uptake blockers on wakefulness and sleep in cats. Pharmacol Toxicol 60:161–166, 1987

Hyttel J: Citalopram—pharmacological profile of a specific serotonin uptake inhibitor with antidepressant activity. Prog Neuropsychopharmacol Biol Psychiatry 6:277–295, 1982

Isenberg KE: Excretion of fluoxetine in human breast milk (letter). J Clin Psychiatry 51:169, 1990

Jick SS, Dean AD, Jick H: Antidepressants and suicide. BMJ 310:215–218, 1995

Johnson AM: The comparative pharmacological properties of selective serotonin re-uptake inhibitors in animals, in Selective Serotonin Uptake Inhibitors. Edited by Feighner JP, Boyer WF. Chichester, England, Wiley, 1991, pp 37–70

Kerr JS, Sherwood N, Hindmarch I: The comparative psychopharmacology of 5-HT reuptake inhibitors. Human Psychopharmacology 6: 313–317, 1991

Kleinlogel H, Burki HR: Effects of the selective 5-hydroxytryptamine uptake inhibitors, paroxetine and zimeldine, on EEG sleep and waking changes in the rat. Neuropsychobiology 17: 206–212, 1987

Klimek V, Maj J: Repeated administration of antidepressant drugs enhanced agonist affinity for mesolimbic D-2 receptors. J Pharm Pharmacol 41:555–558, 1990

Klimek V, Nielsen M: Chronic treatment with antidepressants decreases the number of [^{3}H]-SCH 23390 binding sites in rat striatum and limbic system. Eur J Pharmacol 139:163–169, 1987

Koe BK, Koch SW, Lebel LA, et al: Sertraline, a selective inhibitor of serotonin uptake, induces subsensitivity of β-adrenoceptor of rat brain. Eur J Pharmacol 141:187–194, 1987

Lane R, Baldwin D: Selective serotonin reuptake inhibitor–induced serotonin syndrome: review. J Clin Psychopharmacol 17:208–221, 1997

Leonard BE: Pharmacological differences of serotonin reuptake inhibitors and possible clinical relevance. Drugs 43 (suppl 2):3–10, 1992

Lester BM, Cucca J, Andreozzi BA, et al: Possible association between fluoxetine hydrochloride and colic in an infant. J Am Acad Child Adolesc Psychiatry 32:1253–1255, 1993

Lorens SA, Van der Kar LD: Differential effects of serotonin (5-HT$_{1A}$ and 5-HT$_2$) agonists and antagonists on renin and corticosterone secretion. Neuroendocrinology 45:305–310, 1987

Maj J, Rogoz Z, Skuza G, et al: Repeated treatment with antidepressant drugs potentiates the locomotor response to (+)-amphetamine. J Pharm Pharmacol 36:127–130, 1984

Mammen OK, Perel JM, Rudolph G, et al: Sertraline and norsertraline levels in three breastfed infants. J Clin Psychiatry 58:100–103, 1997

Marley E, Wozniak KM: Interactions of a nonselective monoamine oxidase inhibitor, phenelzine, with inhibitors of 5-hydroxytryptamine, dopamine or noradrenaline re-uptake. J Psychiatr Res 18:173–189, 1984a

Marley E, Wozniak KM: Interactions of non-selective monoamine oxidase inhibitors, tranylcypromine and nialamide, with inhibitors of 5-hydroxytryptamine, dopamine or noradrenaline re-uptake. J Psychiatr Res 18:191–203, 1984b

Marsden CA: The neuropharmacology of serotonin in the central nervous system, in Selective Serotonin Re-Uptake Inhibitors. Edited by Feighner JP, Boyer WF. Chichester, England, Wiley, 1991, pp 11–35

Marshall EF, Nelson DR, Johnson AM, et al: Desensitisation of central 5-HT$_2$ receptor mechanisms after repeated administration of the antidepressant paroxetine (abstract). Journal of Psychopharmacology (Oxf) 2:194, 1988

Meltzer HY, Young M, Metz J, et al: Extrapyramidal side effects and increased serum prolactin following fluoxetine, a new antidepressant. J Neural Transm 45:165–175, 1979

Montgomery SA: New antidepressants and 5-HT uptake inhibitors. Acta Psychiatr Scand 80 (suppl 350):107–116, 1989

Nelson DR, Thomas DR, Johnson AM: Pharmacological effects of paroxetine after repeated administration to animals. Acta Psychiatr Scand 80 (suppl 350):21–23, 1989

Ninan PT, van-Kammen DP, Scheinin M, et al: CSF 5-hydroxyindoleacetic acid levels in suicidal schizophrenic patients. Am J Psychiatry 141:566–569, 1984

Nowak G: Long term effect of antidepressant drugs and electroconvulsive shock (ECS) on cortical α_1-adrenoceptors following destruction of dopaminergic nerve terminals. Pharmacol Toxicol 64:469–470, 1989

Nulman I, Rovet J, Stewart DE, et al: Neurodevelopment of children exposed in utero to antidepressant drugs. N Engl J Med 336:258–262, 1997

O'Flynn K, O'Keane V, Lucey JV, et al: Effect of fluoxetine on noradrenergic mediated growth hormone release: a double-blind, placebo-controlled study. Biol Psychiatry 30:377–382, 1991

Pandey GN, Pandey SC, Janicak PG, et al: Platelet serotonin-2 receptor binding sites in depression and suicide. Biol Psychiatry 28:215–222, 1990

Papini M, Martinetti MJ, Pasquinelli A: Trazodone symptomatic extrapyramidal disorders of infancy and childhood. Ital J Neurol Sci 3:161–162, 1982

Pedersen OL, Kragh-Sorensen P, Bjerre M, et al: Citalopram, a selective serotonin reuptake inhibitor: clinical antidepressive and long-term effect—a phase II study. Psychopharmacology (Berl) 77:199–204, 1982

Peroutka SJ, Snyder SH: Long-term antidepressant treatment decreases spiroperidol-labelled serotonin receptor binding. Science 210:88–90, 1980

Plaznik A, Kostowski W: The effects of antidepressants and electroconvulsive shocks on the functioning of the mesolimbic dopaminergic system: a behavioural study. Eur J Pharmacol 135:389–396, 1987

Richelson E: Synaptic effects of antidepressants. J Clin Psychopharmacol 16 (suppl 2):1S–9S, 1996

Rudorfer MV, Potter WZ: Combined fluoxetine and tricyclic antidepressants. Am J Psychiatry 146:562–564, 1989

Sampson D, Willner P, Muscat R: Reversal of antidepressant action by dopamine antagonists in an animal model of depression. Psychopharmacology (Berl) 104:491–495, 1991

Schatzberg AF, Haddad P, Kaplan EM, et al: Serotonin reuptake discontinuation syndrome: a hypothetical definition (discontinuation consensus panel). J Clin Psychiatry 58 (suppl 7):5–10, 1997

Scherschlicht R, Polc P, Schneeberger J, et al: Selective suppression of rapid eye movement sleep in cats by typical and atypical antidepressants. Adv Biochem Psychopharmacol 31:359–364, 1982

Schmidt A, Lebel L, Koe BK, et al: Sertraline patently displaces (+)-[³H]-3-PPP binding to α sites in rat brain. Eur J Pharmacol 165:335–336, 1989

Shaskan EG, Snyder SH: Kinetics of serotonin accumulation into slices from rat brain: relationship to catecholamine uptake. J Pharmacol Exp Ther 175:404–418, 1970

Siddiqui UA, Chakravarti SK, Jesinger DK: The tolerance and antidepressive activity of fluvoxamine as a single dose compared to a twice-daily dose. Curr Med Res Opin 9:681–690, 1985

Sleight AJ, Marsden CA, Martin KF, et al: Relationship between extracellular 5-hydroxytryptamine and behaviour following monoamine oxidase inhibition and L-tryptophan. Br J Pharmacol 93:303–310, 1988

Snyder SH, Yamamura HI: Antidepressants and the muscarinic acetylcholine receptor. Arch Gen Psychiatry 34:236–239, 1977

Stauderman KA, Gandhi DC, Jones DJ: Fluoxetine-induced inhibition of synaptosomal [³H] 5-HT release: possible calcium-channel inhibition. Life Sci 50:2125–2138, 1992

Stockmeier CA, McLeskey SW, Blendy JA, et al: Electroconvulsive shock but not antidepressant drugs increase α_1-adrenoceptor binding sites in rat brain. Eur J Pharmacol 139:259–266, 1987

Taddio A, Ito S, Koren G: Excretion of fluoxetine and its metabolite, norfluoxetine, in human breast milk. J Clin Pharmacol 36:42–47, 1996

Teusink JP, Alexopoulos GS, Shamoian CA: Parkinsonian side effects induced by a monoamine oxidase inhibitor. Am J Psychiatry 141:118–119, 1984

Thomas DR, Nelson DR, Johnson AM: Biochemical effects of the antidepressant paroxetine, a specific 5-hydroxytryptamine uptake inhibitor. Psychopharmacology (Berl) 93:193–200, 1987

U'Prichard DC, Greenberg DA, Sheehan PB, et al: Tricyclic antidepressants: therapeutic properties and affinity for α-noradrenergic receptor binding sites in the brain. Science 199:197–198, 1978

Usher RW, Beasley CM, Bosomworth JC: Efficacy and safety of morning versus evening fluoxetine administration. J Clin Psychiatry 52:134–136, 1991

Valentino RJ, Curtis AL: Pharmacology of locus coeruleus spontaneous and sensory evoked activity. Prog Brain Res 88:249–256, 1991

Warshaw MG, Keller MB: The relationship between fluoxetine use and suicidal behavior in 654 subjects with anxiety disorders. J Clin Psychiatry 57:158–166, 1996

Wong DT, Reid LR, Bymaster FP, et al: Chronic effects of fluoxetine, a selective inhibitor of serotonin uptake, on neurotransmitter receptors. J Neural Transm 64:251–269, 1985

Wong DT, Threlkeld PG, Robertson DW: Affinities of fluoxetine, its enantiomers, and other inhibitors of serotonin uptake for subtypes of serotonin receptors. Neuropsychopharmacology 5:43–47, 1991

Zubenko GS, Cohen BM, Lipinski JF: Antidepressant-related akathisia. J Clin Psychopharmacol 7:254–257, 1987

THREE

Monoamine Oxidase Inhibitors

K. Ranga Rama Krishnan, M.D.

Monoamine oxidase inhibitors (MAOIs) were first identified as effective antidepressants in the late 1950s. An early report suggested that iproniazid, an antituberculosis agent, had mood-elevating properties in patients who had been treated for tuberculosis (Bloch et al. 1954). Following these observations, two studies confirmed that iproniazid did indeed have antidepressant properties (Crane 1957; Kline 1958). Zeller (1963) reported that iproniazid caused potent inhibition of MAO enzymes both in vivo and in vitro in the brain.

The use of iproniazid soon fell into disfavor because of its significant hepatotoxicity. Other MAOIs, both hydrazine derivatives (e.g., isocarboxazid and phenylhydrazine) and nonhydrazine derivatives (e.g., tranylcypromine), were introduced. These MAOIs were not specific for any subtype of MAO enzyme and were irreversible inhibitors of MAO (see next section). Their use has been rather limited, because hypertensive crisis by the MAOIs may occur in some patients from potentiation of the pressor effects of amines (such as tyramine) in food (Blackwell et al. 1967).

In the last few years, there has been a resurgence of interest in the development of new MAOIs—those that are more specific subtypes of MAO enzyme and those that are reversible in

nature. Newer MAOIs, such as L-deprenyl (selegiline hydrochloride), an MAO β-inhibitor, have been introduced.

MONOAMINE OXIDASE ISOENZYMES

MAO is widely distributed in mammals. Two isoenzymes— monoamine oxidase A (MAO-A) and monoamine oxidase B (MAO-B)—are of special interest to psychiatry (Cesura and Pletscher 1992). Both are present in the central nervous system (CNS) and in some peripheral organs. Both MAO-A and MAO-B are present in discrete cell populations within the CNS. MAO-A is present in both dopamine and norepinephrine neurons, whereas MAO-B is present to a greater extent in serotonin-containing neurons. They are also present in non-aminergic neurons in various subcortical regions of the brain (Cesura and Pletscher 1992). The main substrates for MAO-A are epinephrine, norepinephrine, and serotonin. The main substrates for MAO-B are phenylethylamine, phenylethanolamine, tyramine, and benzylamine. Dopamine and tryptamine are metabolized by both isoenzymes.

The primary structures of both MAO-A and MAO-B have been fully described. MAO-A has

527 amino acids to MAO-B's 520. About 70% of the amino acid sequence of the two forms are homologous. The genes for both are located on the short arm of the human X chromosome. Both are linked and have been located in the XP11.23-P11 and XP22.1 regions, respectively (Cesura and Pletscher 1992). A rare inherited disorder, Norrie's disease, is characterized by deletion of both genes. Patients with this disorder have very severe mental retardation and blindness.

MONOAMINE OXIDASE INHIBITORS

Mechanism of Action

The target function of MAOIs is regulation of the monoamine content within the nervous system. Because MAO is bound to the outer site of plasma membrane of the mitochondria, in neurons MAO is unable to deaminate amines that are present inside stored vesicles and can metabolize only amines that are present in the cytoplasm. As a result, MAO maintains a low cytoplasmic concentration of amines within the cells. Inhibition of neuronal MAO produces an increase in the MAO content in the cytoplasm. It was initially believed that the therapeutic action of the MAOIs was a result of this amine accumulation (Finberg and Youdim 1984; Murphy et al. 1984, 1987). More recently, it was suggested that secondary adaptive mechanisms may be important for their antidepressant action.

After several weeks of treatment, MAOIs produce effects such as a reduction in the number of β-adrenoceptors, α_1- and α_2-adrenoceptors, and serotonin-1 (5-HT$_1$) and serotonin-2 (5-HT$_2$) receptors. These changes are similar to those produced by chronic use of tricyclic antidepressants (TCAs) and other antidepressant treatment (DaPrada et al. 1984, 1989).

MAOIs can be subdivided not only on the basis of the particular type of enzyme inhibition but also by whether the inhibition they produce is reversible or irreversible. The reversible MAOIs are basically chemically inert substrate analogues. MAOIs are recognized by the enzyme as substrates and are converted into intermediates by the normal mechanism. These converted compounds react to the inactive site of the enzyme and form a stable bound enzyme. This effect occurs gradually, and a correlation usually exists between the plasma concentration of the reversible inhibitors and pharmacological action.

The classic MAOIs inhibit both forms of the enzyme and are divided into two main subtypes: hydrazine and nonhydrazine derivatives. The hydrazine derivatives, two of which are currently available—phenelzine and isocarboxazid—are related to iproniazid. The nonhydrazine irreversible MAOI is tranylcypromine. Tranylcypromine is chemically similar to amphetamine. Clorgiline is an example of an irreversible inhibitor of MAO-A, whereas selegiline is an irreversible inhibitor of MAO-B. Reversible inhibitors of MAO-A include brofaromine and moclobemide, but these are not available in the United States and will not be discussed in detail in this chapter.

Three classic MAOIs (i.e., tranylcypromine, phenelzine, and isocarboxazid) are of clinical interest.

Efficacy

Many studies have examined the efficacy of MAOIs in the treatment of different types of depression (Table 3–1). MAOIs have been effective in the treatment of major depression or atypical depression (Davidson et al. 1987a; Himmelhoch et al. 1982, 1991; Johnstone 1975; Johnstone and Marsh 1973; McGrath et al. 1986; Paykel et al. 1982; Quitkin et al. 1979, 1990, 1991; Rowan et al. 1981; Thase et al. 1992; Vallejo et al. 1987; White et al. 1984; Zisook et al. 1985). Although early studies of relatively low-dose regimens suggested that MAOI efficacy was lower than that of TCAs, more recent studies have documented that their efficacy is comparable.

Quitkin and colleagues (1979, 1991) reviewed both phenelzine and tranylcypromine studies in patients with either atypical and neurotic depression or melancholic depression. They reported that phenelzine appeared to be effective for treatment of atypical depression.

Relatively few studies of endogenous depression in patients have been done. It is difficult to conclude from the limited number of patient studies initially done that phenelzine is effective in treatment of these patients. Also, very few well-controlled studies of tranylcypromine compared with placebo have been done. Three of the four studies of tranylcypromine compared with placebo showed that tranylcypromine was more effective. In one study, a nonsignificant trend was found favoring tranylcypromine. More recently, studies have documented the efficacy of tranylcypromine in treating anergic depression and in high doses for patients with treatment-resistant depression (Himmelhoch et al. 1982, 1991; Thase et al. 1992; White et al. 1984).

The heterogeneity of acetylation rate may account for some of the variance in response to phenelzine (Johnstone 1975; Johnstone and Marsh 1973; Paykel et al. 1982; Rowan et al. 1981).

Table 3–1. Indications for use of MAOIs

Definitely effective	Other possible uses
Atypical depression	Obsessive-compulsive
Major depression	disorder
Dysthymia	Narcolepsy
Melancholia	Headache
Panic disorder	Chronic pain
Bulimia	syndrome
Atypical facial pain	Generalized anxiety
Anergic depression	disorder
Treatment-resistant depression	
Parkinson's disease[a]	

Note. MAOIs = monoamine oxidase inhibitors.
[a]Selegiline is the only MAOI that is useful in the treatment of Parkinson's disease.

MAOIs are used in a wide range of psychiatric disorders. Early studies suggested that MAOIs are particularly effective in patients who have atypical depression originally defined as depression with anxiety or chronic pain, reversed vegetative symptoms, and rejection sensitivity (Quitkin et al. 1990).

The concept of atypical depression remains controversial and has not been completely validated. In general, patients with atypical depression have an earlier age at onset than do patients with melancholic depression, and the prevalence of dysthymia, alcohol abuse, sociopathy, and atypical depression is increased in relatives of patients with atypical depression. The best differentiating criterion appears to be that phenelzine and other irreversible MAOIs are more effective than TCAs in treating these patients (Cesura and Pletscher 1992; Quitkin et al. 1990; Zisook et al. 1985).

Some studies have also suggested that MAOIs are effective in treating typical major depression and melancholic depression (Davidson et al. 1987a; McGrath et al. 1986; Vallejo et al. 1987).

Treatment of Various Psychiatric Disorders

Panic disorder. Both single-blind and double-blind studies have found that phenelzine and iproniazid are effective in treating panic disorder (Lydiard et al. 1989; Quitkin et al. 1990; Tyrer et al. 1973). About 50%–60% of patients with panic disorder respond to MAOIs. In the early stages of treatment, patients may have a worsening of symptoms. This is reduced in clinical practice by combining the MAOI with a benzodiazepine for the initial phase of the study. The time-course of effect and the dose used are similar to that for major depression.

Social phobia. Liebowitz and colleagues (1992) reported that phenelzine is effective in treating social phobia. In an open-label study, Versiani and colleagues (1988) suggested that tranylcypromine is effective and also demonstrated the efficacy of moclobemide in a double-blind study (Versiani et al. 1992). In clinical experience, about 50% of patients' conditions respond to MAOIs. The onset of response is gradual (usually about 2–3 weeks).

Obsessive-compulsive disorder.   Although initial case reports suggested that MAOIs may be effective in the treatment of obsessive-compulsive disorder (Jenike 1981), no double-blind studies indicate efficacy.

Posttraumatic stress disorder.   The classic MAOI phenelzine has been proven effective for treatment of posttraumatic stress disorder (PTSD) in both single-blind trials (Davidson et al. 1987b) and a double-blind crossover trial (Kosten et al. 1991).

Generalized anxiety disorder.   MAOIs are not usually used to treat generalized anxiety disorder because the risk-benefit ratio favors the use of azaspirones or benzodiazepines. MAOIs are used primarily in treatment-resistant patients with generalized anxiety disorder.

Bulimia nervosa.   Both phenelzine and isocarboxazid have been shown to be effective in treating some symptoms of bulimia nervosa (Kennedy et al. 1988; McElroy et al. 1989; Walsh et al. 1985, 1987).

Premenstrual dysphoria.   Preliminary studies and clinical experience suggest that MAOIs may be effective in treatment of premenstrual dysphoria (Glick et al. 1991).

Chronic pain.   MAOIs are believed to be effective in the treatment of atypical facial pain and other chronic pain syndromes. However, only limited data on these conditions are available.

Neurological diseases.   The classic MAOIs have not been found to be effective for treating neurological disorders such as Parkinson's disease and Alzheimer's dementia. However, the MAOI-B selegiline has been shown to be effective in slowing the progression of Parkinson's disease (Cesura and Pletscher 1992), but the mechanism underlying this effect is unknown.

Side Effects of Monoamine Oxidase Inhibitors

Side effects of MAOIs are generally more severe or frequent than for other antidepressants (Zisook 1984). The most frequent side effects include dizziness, headache, dry mouth, insomnia, constipation, blurred vision, nausea, peripheral edema, forgetfulness, fainting spells, trauma, hesitancy of urination, weakness, and myoclonic jerks. Loss of weight and appetite may occur with isocarboxazid use (Davidson and Turnbull 1982). Hepatotoxicity is rarer with the currently available MAOIs compared with iproniazid. However, liver enzymes such as serum glutamic-oxaloacetic transaminase (SGOT) and serum glutamic-pyruvic transaminase (SGPT) are elevated in 3%–5% of patients. Liver function tests must be done only when patients have symptoms such as malaise, jaundice, and excessive fatigue.

Some side effects first emerge during maintenance treatment (Evans et al. 1982). These side effects include weight gain (which occurs in almost half of the patients), edema, muscle cramps, carbohydrate craving, sexual dysfunction (usually anorgasmia), pyridoxine deficiency (Goodheart et al. 1991), hypoglycemia, hypomania, urinary retention, and disorientation. Peripheral neuropathy (Goodheart et al. 1991) and speech blockage (Goldstein and Goldberg 1986) are rare side effects of MAOIs. Weight gain is more of a problem with the hydrazine compounds such as phenelzine than with tranylcypromine. Therefore, weight gain caused by the hydrazine derivatives is an indication to switch to tranylcypromine. Edema is also more common with phenelzine than with tranylcypromine.

The management of some of these side effects can be problematic. Orthostatic hypotension is common with MAOIs. Addition of salt and salt-retaining steroids such as flurohydrocortisol is sometimes effective in treating orthostatic hypotension. Elastic support stockings are also helpful. Small amounts of coffee or tea taken during the day also keep the blood pressure elevated. The dose of flurohydrocortisol should be adjusted carefully, because in elderly patients, it could provoke cardiac failure resulting from fluid retention.

Sexual dysfunction that occurs with these compounds is also difficult to treat. Common problems include anorgasmia, decreased libido, impotence, and delayed ejaculation (Harrison et al. 1985; Jacobson 1987).

Insomnia occasionally occurs as an intermediate or late side effect of these compounds. Myoclonic jerks, peripheral neuropathy, and paresthesia, when present, are also difficult to treat. When a patient has paresthesia, the clinician should evaluate for peripheral neuropathy and pyridoxine deficiency. In general, patients taking MAOIs should also take concomitant pyridoxine therapy.

MAOIs also have the potential to suppress anginal pain; therefore, coronary artery disease could be overlooked or underestimated. Patients with hyperthyroidism are more sensitive to MAOIs because of their overall sensitivity to pressor amines. MAOIs can also worsen hypoglycemia in patients taking hypoglycemic agents such as insulin.

Dietary Interactions of Monoamine Oxidase Inhibitors

After the MAOIs were introduced, several reports of severe headaches in patients who were taking these compounds were published (Anonymous 1970; Cronin 1965; Hedberg et al. 1966; Simpson and Gratz 1992). These headaches were caused by a drug-food interaction. The risk of such an interaction is highest for tranylcypromine and lower for phenelzine, providing the dose of the latter remains low. The interaction of MAOIs with food has been attributed to increased tyramine levels. Tyramine, which has a pressor action, is present in a number of foodstuffs. It is normally broken down by the MAO enzymes and has both direct and indirect sympathomimetic actions.

The tyramine effect is potentiated by MAOIs 10- to 20-fold. A mild tyramine interaction occurs with about 6 mg of tyramine; 10 mg can produce a moderate episode, and 25 mg can produce a severe episode, characterized by hypertension, occipital headache, palpitations, nausea, vomiting, apprehension, occasional chills, sweating, and restlessness. On examination, neck stiffness, pallor, mild pyrexia, dilated pupils, and motor agitation may be seen. The reaction usually develops within 20 minutes to 1 hour after ingestion of the food. Occasionally, the reaction can be very severe and may lead to alteration of consciousness, hyperpyrexia, cerebral hemorrhage, and death. Death is exceedingly rare and has been calculated to be about 0.01%–0.02% for tranylcypromine.

The classic treatment of the hypertensive reaction is 5 mg of phentolamine administered intravenously (Youdim et al. 1987; Zisook 1984). More recently, nifedipine, a calcium channel blocker, has been shown to be effective. Nifedipine has an onset of action in about 5 minutes, and it lasts approximately 3–5 hours.

Because of the drug interaction of the classic MAOIs with food, clinicians usually make several dietary recommendations (see Table 3–2). These recommendations are quite varied.

All the MAOI diets recommend restriction of cheese (except for cream cheese and cottage cheese), wine, beer, sherry, liquors (except vodka and occasional white wine), pickled fish, overripe aged fruit, brewer's yeast, fava beans, beef and chicken liver, and fermented products. Other diets also recommend restriction of all alcoholic beverages, coffee, chocolate, colas, tea, yogurt, soy sauce, avocados, and bananas. The more restrictive the diet, the greater the risk of patient noncompliance.

Table 3–2. Food restrictions for MAOIs

To be avoided	To be used in moderation
Cheese (except for cream cheese, cottage cheese)	Coffee
	Chocolate
	Colas
Overripe aged fruit (banana peel)	Tea
	Soy sauce
Fava beans	White wine, vodka
Sausage, salami	Yogurt
Sherry, liquors	Avocados
Sauerkraut	Bananas
Monosodium glutamate	
Pickled fish	
Brewer's yeast	
Beef and chicken liver	
Fermented products	
Red wine	

Note. MAOIs = monoamine oxidase inhibitors.

In evaluating patients who have had a drug-food reaction, it is also important to evaluate the hypertensive reaction and differentiate it from histamine headache, which can occur with an MAOI. Histamine headaches are usually accompanied by hypotension, colic, loose stools, salivation, and lacrimation (Cooper 1967). The clinician should provide oral instructions as well as printed cards outlining these instructions to patients who are taking classic MAOIs.

In addition to the food interaction, drug interactions are extremely important (see next section). Each patient should be given a card indicating that he or she is taking an MAOI and should be instructed to carry it at all times. A medical bracelet indicating that the wearer takes an MAOI is also a good idea.

Drug Interactions

The extensive inhibition of MAO by MAOI enzymes raises the potential for a number of drug interactions (Table 3–3). These interactions are particularly important because many over-the-counter medications can interact with the MAOIs. These medications include cough syrups containing sympathomimetic agents, which, in the presence of an MAOI, can precipitate a hypertensive crisis.

Another area of caution is the use of MAOIs in patients who need surgery. In this situation, interactions include those with narcotic drugs, especially meperidine. Meperidine administered with MAOIs can produce a syndrome characterized by coma, hyperpyrexia, and hypertension. This syndrome has been reported primarily with phenelzine but also with tranylcypromine (Mendelson 1979; Stack et al. 1988). Stack and colleagues (1988) noted that this syndrome is most likely to occur with meperidine and may be related to its serotonergic properties.

The issue of whether directly acting sympathomimetic amines interact with MAOIs is more controversial. Intravenous administration of sympathomimetic amines to patients receiving MAOIs does not provoke hypertension (Wells 1989).

Caution should be exercised when using MAOIs in patients with pheochromocytoma and cardiovascular, cerebrovascular, and hepatic disease. Because phenelzine tablets contain gluten, they should not be given to patients with coeliac disease.

PHENELZINE

Phenelzine, a hydrazine derivative, is a potent MAOI and the best studied among the MAOIs. Phenelzine undergoes acetylation. Thus, the levels are lower in fast acetylators than in slow acetylators. However, because it is an irreversible inhibitor, plasma concentrations are not relevant.

Efficacy

Phenelzine is useful in the treatment of major depression, atypical depression, panic disorder, social phobia, and atypical facial pain. (See gen-

Table 3–3. Drug interactions with MAOIs

Drug	Interaction	Comment
Other MAOIs (e.g., furazolidone, pargyline, and procarbazine)	Potentiation of side effects; convulsions possible	Allow at least 1 week before changing MAOI
Tricyclic antidepressants (TCAs) (e.g., maprotiline, bupropion)	Severe side effects possible, such as hypertension and convulsions	Allow at least 2 weeks before changing MAOI; combinations have been used occasionally for refractory depression
Carbamazepine	Low possibility of interaction; similar to TCAs	Same as for TCAs
Cyclobenzaprine	Low possibility of interaction; similar to TCAs	Same as for TCAs
Selective serotonin reuptake inhibitors	Serotonin syndrome	Avoid combinations; allow at least 2 weeks before changing MAOI and 5 weeks if switching from fluoxetine to MAOI
Stimulants (e.g., methylphenidate, dextroamphetamine)	Potential for increased blood pressure (hypertension)	Avoid combination
Buspirone	Potential for increased blood pressure (hypertension)	Avoid; if used, monitor blood pressure
Meperidine	Severe, potentially fatal interaction possible (see text)	Avoid combination
Dextromethorphan	Reports of brief psychosis	Avoid high doses
Direct sympathomimetics (e.g., L-dopa)	Increased blood pressure	Avoid, if possible; use with caution
Indirect sympathomimetics	Hypertensive crisis possible	Avoid use
Oral hypoglycemics (e.g., insulin)	May worsen hypoglycemia	Monitor blood sugar levels and adjust medications
Fenfluramine	Serotonin syndrome possible	Avoid use
L-Tryptophan	Serotonin syndrome possible	Avoid use

Note. MAOIs = monoamine oxidase inhibitors.

eral discussion of efficacy in "Monoamine Oxidase Inhibitors" earlier in this chapter.)

Side Effects

The primary side effects of phenelzine are similar to those of other MAOIs. Hepatitis secondary to phenelzine may occur. This effect is quite rare (<1 in 30,000). The most difficult side effect often leading to discontinuation is postural hypotension.

Contraindications

The contraindications to phenelzine include known sensitivity to the drug, pheochromocytoma, congestive heart failure, and history of liver disease (see also sections "Dietary Interactions of Monoamine Oxidase Inhibitors" and "Drug Interactions" earlier in this chapter).

ISOCARBOXAZID

Isocarboxazid is a hydrazine type of MAOI. Isocarboxazid is rapidly absorbed from the gastrointestinal tract and metabolized in the liver. It is primarily excreted as hippuric acid. Its half-life is of little interest because it is an irreversible MAOI.

Efficacy

Isocarboxazid is the least studied of the MAOIs. Its indications are similar to those of the other MAOIs.

Side Effects

The side effects of isocarboxazid are similar to those of phenelzine. Postural hypotension is the most common problem.

Contraindications

The contraindications to isocarboxazid are similar to those of phenelzine.

TRANYLCYPROMINE

Tranylcypromine, a nonhydrazine reversible MAOI, increases the concentration of norepinephrine, epinephrine, and serotonin in the CNS. When tranylcypromine is discontinued, about 5 days are needed for recovery of MAO function. Tranylcypromine has a mild stimulant effect.

Efficacy

See the general discussion of efficacy in "Monoamine Oxidase Inhibitors" earlier in this chapter.

Side Effects

Tranylcypromine's side effects are similar to those of other MAOIs. In addition, problems with physical dependence on tranylcypromine have been reported. Thus, withdrawal symptoms such as anxiety, restlessness, depression, and headache may occur. Syndrome of inappropriate antidiuretic hormone (SIADH) has been reported with tranylcypromine. Rare cases of toxic hepatitis have been reported. Tranylcypromine can lead to increased agitation, insomnia, and restlessness compared with phenelzine.

Contraindications

The contraindications to tranylcypromine are the same as those for phenelzine.

SELEGILINE HYDROCHLORIDE

Selegiline hydrochloride is an irreversible MAO-B inhibitor (Cesura and Pletscher 1992). Its primary use is in treatment of Parkinson's disease as an adjunct to L-dopa and carbidopa. The average daily dose for Parkinson's disease is 5–10 mg/day. The exact mechanism of action of MAO-B in Parkinson's disease is unknown (Gerlach et al. 1996; Hagan et al. 1997; Lyytinen et al. 1997). Selegiline is metabolized to levoamphetamine, methamphetamine, and N-desmethylselegiline.

Efficacy

The efficacy of selegiline in treating depression has not been well studied. The few studies that have examined its utility have been equivocal. The dose required for treating depression may be much higher than that required to treat Parkinson's disease. Clinical experience suggests that doses of 20–40 mg/day are needed. At these doses, dietary interactions could occur. Early studies have reported that selegiline is of modest benefit in patients with Alzheimer's disease (Lawlor et al. 1997).

Side Effects

Selegiline has been found to have no adverse effects when combined with other antidepressants during treatment of depression in patients with Parkinson's disease. The few side effects that have been noted with selegiline include nausea, dizziness, and light-headedness. When the drug is abruptly discontinued, nausea, hallucinations, and confusion have been reported.

Food and Drug Interactions

Because MAO-B is not involved in the intestinal tyramine interaction, at low doses of 5–10 mg/day, dietary interaction with selegiline would probably be minimal; therefore, no drug interactions have been reported. An interaction between selegiline and narcotics has been reported and should be kept in mind. A transdermal formulation to allow for higher doses without risk of foodstuff interactions is being developed.

SUMMARY

Various MAOIs have been shown to be effective in treating a wide variety of psychiatric disorders, including depression, panic disorder, social phobia, and PTSD. The classic MAOIs are currently used only rarely as first-line medication because of potential dietary interaction and other long-term side effects. Reversible inhibitors of MAO-A enzyme, such as moclobemide and brofaromine, have fewer side effects and no dietary restrictions compared with classic MAOIs. This could make them first-line agents, although they are not likely to appear soon in the United States. They are available in Europe and Canada. In fact, the risk-benefit ratio for these compounds is highly favorable compared with other antidepressants. The MAO-B inhibitor selegiline is used to reduce the progression of Parkinson's disease. Its utility in treating other degenerative disorders is currently being assessed. New applications and wider use of these compounds may be found in the near future.

REFERENCES

Anonymous: Cheese and tranylcypromine (letter). BMJ 3(718):354, 1970

Blackwell B, Marley E, Price J, et al: Hypertensive interactions between monoamine oxidase inhibitors and food stuffs. Br J Psychiatry 113: 349–365, 1967

Bloch RG, Doonief AS, Buchberg AS, et al: The clinical effect of isoniazid and iproniazid in the treatment of pulmonary tuberculosis. Ann Intern Med 40:881–900, 1954

Cesura AM, Pletscher A: The new generation of monoamine oxidase inhibitors. Prog Drug Res 38:171–297, 1992

Cooper AJ: MAO inhibitors and headache (letter). BMJ 2:420, 1967

Crane GE: Iproniazid (Marsilid) phosphate, a therapeutic agent for mental disorders and debilitating disease. Psychiatry Research Reports 8: 142–152, 1957

Cronin D: Monoamine-oxidase inhibitors and cheese (letter). BMJ 5469:1065, 1965

DaPrada M, Kettler R, Burkard WP, et al: Moclobemide, an antidepressant with short-lasting MAO-A inhibition: brain catecholamines and tyramine pressor effects in rats, in Monoamine Oxidase and Disease: Prospects for Therapy With Reversible Inhibitors. Edited by Tipton KF, Dostert P, Strolin Benedetti M. New York, Academic Press, 1984, pp 137–154

DaPrada M, Kettler R, Keller HH, et al: Neurochemical profile of moclobemide, a short-acting and reversible inhibitor of monoamine oxidase type A. J Pharmacol Exp Ther 248:400–414, 1989

Davidson J, Turnbull C: Loss of appetite and weight associated with the monoamine oxidase inhibitor isocarboxazid. J Clin Psychopharmacol 2: 263–266, 1982

Davidson J, Raft D, Pelton S: An outpatient evaluation of phenelzine and imipramine. J Clin Psychiatry 48:143–146, 1987a

Davidson J, Walker JI, Kilts C: A pilot study of phenelzine in the treatment of post-traumatic stress disorder. Br J Psychiatry 150:252–255, 1987b

Evans DL, Davidson J, Raft D: Early and late side effects of phenelzine. J Clin Psychopharmacol 2:208–210, 1982

Finberg JPM, Youdim MBH: Reversible monoamine oxidase inhibitors and the cheese effect,
in Monoamine Oxidase and Disease: Prospects
for Therapy With Reversible Inhibitors. Edited
by Tipton KF, Dostert P, Strolin Benedetti M.
New York, Academic Press, 1984, pp 479–485

Gerlach M, Youdim MB, Riederer P: Pharmacology
of selegiline. Neurology 47 (6 suppl 3):
S137–S145, 1996

Glick R, Harrison W, Endicott J, et al: Treatment of
premenstrual dysphoric symptoms in depressed
women. J Am Med Wom Assoc 46:182–185,
1991

Goldstein DM, Goldberg RL: Monoamine oxidase
inhibitor-induced speech blockage (case report).
J Clin Psychiatry 47:604, 1986

Goodheart RS, Dunne JW, Edis RH: Phenelzine associated peripheral neuropathy clinical and
electrophysiologic findings. Aust N Z J Med
21:339–340, 1991

Hagan JJ, Middlemiss DN, Sharpe PC, et al: Parkinson's disease: prospects for improved drug
therapy. Trends Pharmacol Sci 18:156–163,
1997

Harrison WM, Stewart J, Ehrhardt AA, et al: A controlled study of the effects of antidepressants on
sexual function. Psychopharmacol Bull 21:
85–88, 1985

Hedberg DL, Gordon MW, Glueck BC Jr: Six cases
of hypertensive crisis in patients on tranylcypromine after eating chicken livers. Am J Psychiatry 122:933–937, 1966

Himmelhoch JM, Fuchs CZ, Symons BJ: A double-
blind study of tranylcypromine treatment of
major anergic depression. J Nerv Ment Dis 170:
628–634, 1982

Himmelhoch JM, Thase ME, Mallinger AG, et al:
Tranylcypromine versus imipramine in anergic
bipolar depression. Am J Psychiatry 148:
910–916, 1991

Jacobson JN: Anorgasmia caused by an MAOI (letter). Am J Psychiatry 144:527, 1987

Jenike MA: Rapid response of severe obsessive-compulsive disorder to tranylcypromine. Am J Psychiatry 138:1249–1250, 1981

Johnstone EC: Relationship between acetylator
status and response to phenelzine. Mod Probl
Pharmacopsychiatry 10:30–37, 1975

Johnstone EC, Marsh W: The relationship between
response to phenelzine and acetylator status in
depressed patients. Proc R Soc Lond B Biol Sci
66:947–949, 1973

Kennedy SH, Warsh JJ, Mainprize E, et al: A trial of
isocarboxazid in the treatment of bulimia. J Clin
Psychopharmacol 8:391–396, 1988

Kline NS: Clinical experience with iproniazid
(Marsilid). Journal of Clinical and Experimental
Psychopathology 19 (suppl 1):72–78, 1958

Kosten TR, Frank JB, Dan E, et al: Pharmacotherapy for posttraumatic stress disorder using
phenelzine or imipramine. J Nerv Ment Dis
179:366–370, 1991

Lawlor BA, Aisen PS, Green C, et al: Selegiline in
the treatment of behavioural disturbance in Alzheimer's disease. Int J Geriatr Psychiatry 12:
319–322, 1997

Liebowitz MR, Schneier F, Campeas R, et al:
Phenelzine vs atenolol in social phobia: a placebo-controlled comparison. Arch Gen Psychiatry 49:290–300, 1992

Lydiard RB, Laraia MT, Howell EF, et al:
Phenelzine treatment of panic disorder: lack of
effect on pyridoxal phosphate levels. J Clin
Psychopharmacol 9:428–431, 1989

Lyytinen J, Kaakkola S, Ahtila S, et al: Simultaneous
MAO-B and COMT inhibition in L-dopa-
treated patients with Parkinson's disease. Mov
Disord 12:497–505, 1997

McElroy SL, Keck PE Jr, Pope HG Jr, et al: Pharmacological treatment of kleptomania and
bulimia nervosa. J Clin Psychopharmacol 9:
358–360, 1989

McGrath PJ, Stewart JW, Harrison W, et al:
Phenelzine treatment of melancholia. J Clin
Psychiatry 47:420–422, 1986

Mendelson G: Narcotics and monoamine
oxidase-inhibitors (letter). Med J Aust 1:400,
1979

Murphy DL, Garrick NA, Aulakh CS, et al: New
contribution from basic science of understanding the effects of monoamine oxidase inhibiting
antidepressants. J Clin Psychiatry 45:37–43,
1984

Murphy DL, Sunderland T, Garrick NA, et al: Selective amine oxidase inhibitors: basic to clinical
studies and back, in Clinical Pharmacology in
Psychiatry. Edited by Dahl SG, Gram A, Potter
W. Berlin, Springer Verlag, 1987, pp 135–146

Paykel ES, West PS, Rowan PR, et al: Influence of acetylator phenotype on antidepressant effects of phenelzine. Br J Psychiatry 141:243–248, 1982

Quitkin F, Rifkin A, Klein DF: Monoamine oxidase inhibitors: a review of antidepressant effectiveness. Arch Gen Psychiatry 36:749–760, 1979

Quitkin FM, McGrath PJ, Stewart JW, et al: Atypical depression, panic attacks, and response to imipramine and phenelzine: a replication. Arch Gen Psychiatry 47:935–941, 1990

Quitkin FM, Harrison W, Stewart JW, et al: Response to phenelzine and imipramine in placebo nonresponders with atypical depression: a new application of the crossover design. Arch Gen Psychiatry 48:319–323, 1991

Rowan PR, Paykel ES, West PS, et al: Effects of phenelzine and acetylator phenotype. Neuropharmacology 20(12B):1353–1354, 1981

Simpson GM, Gratz SS: Comparison of the pressor effect of tyramine after treatment with phenelzine and moclobemide in healthy male volunteers. J Clin Pharm Ther 52:286–291, 1992

Stack CG, Rogers P, Linter SPK: Monoamine oxidase inhibitors and anaesthesia: a review. Br J Anaesth 60:222–227, 1988

Thase ME, Mallinger AG, McKnight D, et al: Treatment of imipramine-resistant recurrent depression, IV: a double-blind crossover study of tranylcypromine for anergic bipolar depression. Am J Psychiatry 149:195–198, 1992

Tyrer PJ, Candy J, Kelly D: A study of the clinical effects of phenelzine and placebo in the treatment of phobic anxiety. Psychopharmacologia 32:237–254, 1973

Vallejo J, Gasto C, Catalan R, et al: Double-blind study of imipramine versus phenelzine in melancholias and dysthymic disorders. Br J Psychiatry 151:639–642, 1987

Versiani M, Mundim FD, Nardi AE, et al: Tranylcypromine in social phobia. J Clin Psychopharmacol 8:279–283, 1988

Versiani M, Nardi AE, Mundim FD, et al: Pharmacotherapy of social phobia: a controlled study with moclobemide and phenelzine. Br J Psychiatry 161:353–360, 1992

Walsh BT, Stewart JW, Roose SP, et al: A double-blind trial of phenelzine in bulimia. J Psychiatr Res 19(2–3):485–489, 1985

Walsh BT, Gladis M, Roose SP, et al: A controlled trial of phenelzine in bulimia. Psychopharmacol Bull 23:49–51, 1987

Wells DG: MAOI revisited. Can J Anaesth 36:64–74, 1989

White K, Razani J, Cadow B, et al: Tranylcypromine vs nortriptyline vs placebo in depressed outpatients: a controlled trial. Psychopharmacology (Berl) 82:258–262, 1984

Youdim MBH, DaPrada M, Amrein R (eds): The cheese effect and new reversible MAO-A inhibitors. Proceedings of the Round Table of the International Conference on New Directions in Affective Disorders, Jerusalem, Israel, 5–9 April 1987

Zeller EA: Diamine oxidase, in The Enzymes, Vol 8, 2nd Edition. Edited by Boyer PD, Lardy H, Myrback K. London, Academic Press, 1963, pp 313–335

Zisook S: Side effects of isocarboxazid. J Clin Psychiatry 45(7 part 2):53–58, 1984

Zisook S, Braff DL, Click MA: Monoamine oxidase inhibitors in the treatment of atypical depression. J Clin Psychopharmacol 5:131–137, 1985

FOUR

Trazodone, Nefazodone, Bupropion, and Mirtazapine

Robert N. Golden, M.D.,
Karon Dawkins, M.D.,
Linda Nicholas, M.D., and
Joseph M. Bebchuk, M.D., F.R.C.P.C.

Beginning in the early 1980s, and continuing through the 1990s, several novel agents that do not readily fit into the classic categories of antidepressants became available for clinical use in the United States. These medications are often relegated to the unassuming label of "other" or "miscellaneous" antidepressants. In this chapter, we review the basic and clinical pharmacology of the four currently available "other" antidepressants: trazodone, nefazodone, bupropion, and mirtazapine.

TRAZODONE

History and Discovery

Trazodone was first synthesized in Italy nearly three decades ago. This drug differed from the conventional antidepressants that were available at that time in several ways. First, it was the first triazolopyridine derivative to be developed as an antidepressant. Second, it was developed as an outgrowth of a specific hypothesis (i.e., that depression is caused by an imbalance in the brain mechanisms responsible for the emotional integration of adverse, unpleasant experiences). For this reason, new animal models that measured the response to noxious stimuli or situations (rather than the usual models) were used as screening tests for developing the drug (Silvestrini 1980). In fact, trazodone is inactive in classic antidepressant screening tests, such as the reserpine model, the potentiation of yohimbine toxicity, and the behavioral despair/forced swim paradigm (Rudorfer et al. 1984), yet it inhibits painful and conditioned emotional responses (Silvestrini and Lisciani 1973). In sharp contrast to most other antidepressants available at the time of its development, trazodone showed minimal effects on muscarinic cholinergic receptors (Taylor et al. 1980).

In 1982, trazodone was introduced for clinical use in the United States under the brand name Desyrel. It quickly became a widely prescribed medication, capturing up to one-third of the American market. More recently, the availability of the extremely popular selective serotonin reuptake inhibitors (SSRIs) has led to a decline in trazodone use. The medication is now available in generic formulation.

Structure-Activity Relations

Trazodone is chemically unrelated to other antidepressant drugs, although it does resemble some of the side-chain components of tricyclic antidepressants (TCAs) and the phenothiazines (Figure 4–1).

Pharmacological Profile

Trazodone itself is a relatively weak SSRI compared with the more potent SSRIs such as fluoxetine and sertraline (Hyttel 1982). In addition, trazodone has some serotonin (5-HT) receptor antagonist activity, particularly at 5-HT_{1A}, 5-HT_{1C}, and 5-HT_2 receptor subtypes (Haria et al. 1994). Furthermore, its active metabolite, m-chlorophenylpiperazine (mCPP), is a potent direct serotonin agonist. Thus, trazodone can be viewed as a mixed serotonergic agonist/antagonist, with the relative amount of mCPP accumulation affecting the relative degree of the predominant agonist activity.

In vivo, trazodone is virtually devoid of anticholinergic activity, and in clinical studies, the incidence of anticholinergic side effects is similar to that seen with placebo (Boschsmans 1987; Schuckit 1987). Trazodone is a relatively weak blocker of presynaptic α_2-adrenergic receptors and a relatively potent antagonist of postsynaptic α_1-adrenergic receptors (Brogden et al. 1981). The latter property probably accounts for trazodone's propensity to cause orthostatic hypotension, as discussed in the section "Indications" later in this chapter. Trazo-

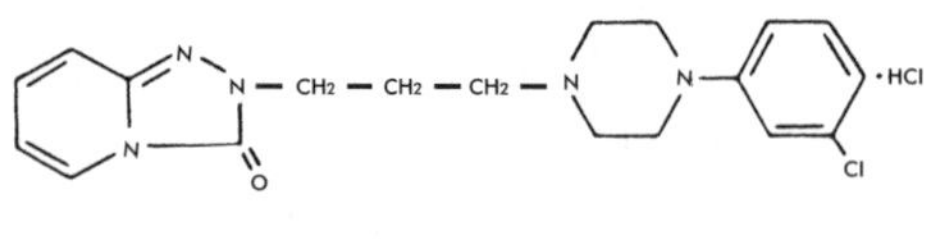

Figure 4–1. Chemical structure for trazodone.

done has moderate antihistaminergic (H_1) activity (Marek et al. 1992).

Pharmacokinetics and Disposition

Trazodone is well absorbed after oral administration, with peak blood levels occurring about 1 hour after dosing when the drug is taken on an empty stomach and about 2 hours after dosing when the drug is taken with food. Trazodone is 89%–95% bound to protein in plasma. Elimination appears to be biphasic, consisting of an initial alpha phase followed by a slower beta phase, with half-lives of 3–6 and 5–9 hours, respectively.

Trazodone undergoes extensive hepatic metabolism, including hydroxylation, splitting at the pyridine ring, oxidation, and N-oxidation (Garattini 1974). The active metabolite, mCPP (see "Pharmacological Profile" above), is cleared more slowly than the parent compound (4- to 14-hour half-life), and it reaches higher concentrations in the brain than in plasma (Caccia et al. 1981). The cytochrome P450 (CYP) 2D6 isoenzyme appears to be involved in the metabolism of trazodone, suggesting the potential for interaction with other drugs that compete as a substrate for this isoenzyme (Yasui et al. 1995).

Mechanism of Action

The ultimate mechanism of action of trazodone remains unclear. The mixed agonist/antagonist profile for its effects on serotonin is interesting. Although the drug is often referred to as a serotonin reuptake inhibitor, such labeling overlooks the complexity of its effects on this neurotransmitter system. For example, binding studies confirm that trazodone has relative selectivity for serotonin reuptake sites (Hyttel 1982); however, in vivo, it blocks the head twitch response induced by classic serotonin agonists in animals (Brogden et al. 1981). In addition, the potent serotonin agonist properties of trazodone's major metabolite, mCPP, probably play a role in the mechanism of action of the parent compound. It is also interesting that trazodone, unlike the vast majority of antidepressants, does not produce downregulation of β-adrenergic receptors in rat cortex (Sulser 1983).

Indications

The primary indication for trazodone is the treatment of major depression. In more than two dozen double-blind, placebo-controlled studies in Europe and the United States, trazodone's efficacy has been consistently superior to that of placebo and equivalent to that of conventional TCAs (Golden et al. 1988a). In a review of the double-blind studies published after trazodone's release in the United States, Schatzberg (1987) found trazodone's therapeutic efficacy to be similar to that of TCAs in patients with either endogenous or non-endogenous depression. Furthermore, the accumulated data suggest that trazodone may have a more pronounced, earlier onset of anxiolytic action compared with conventional antidepressants—perhaps reflecting its potent sedative properties (Schatzberg 1987). Lader's (1987) review of the European literature yielded similar findings: data from open and double-blind trials suggest that trazodone's antidepressant efficacy is comparable to that of amitriptyline, doxepin, and mianserin.

Questions have been raised about trazodone's effectiveness in treating severely ill patients, especially those with prominent psychomotor retardation (Klein and Muller 1985). Shopsin et al. (1981) pointed out that in several unpublished, double-blind, controlled studies, independent groups at different institutions found extremely low rates of response to trazodone (i.e., 10%–20%) in depressed patients. Lader (1987) acknowledged that the actual numbers of depressed patients with severe psychomotor retardation that have been reported in individual studies are too small to resolve the continued impression among many clinicians that trazodone's efficacy is limited in this population.

In relatively recent direct comparisons with other second-generation antidepressants, trazodone's performance has been mixed. In a double-blind, placebo-controlled trial, both trazodone and venlafaxine were significantly superior to placebo in terms of mean change from baseline in Hamilton Rating Scale for Depression (Hamilton 1960) scores, yet the final response rates were 55% for placebo, 60% for trazodone, and 72% for venlafaxine. It is not surprising that trazodone was more effective than venlafaxine in ameliorating sleep disturbances and was associated with the most dizziness and somnolence (Cunningham et al. 1994). In a double-blind comparison, trazodone and bupropion response rates were 46% and 58%, respectively. Trazodone was more likely to be associated with somnolence, appetite increase, and edema (Weisler et al. 1994).

Because trazodone has minimal anticholinergic activity, it was especially welcomed as a treatment for depressed geriatric patients when it first became available in 1982. Three double-blind studies reported that trazodone has antidepressant efficacy similar to that of other antidepressants in geriatric patients (Gerner 1987). However, a side effect of trazodone, orthostatic hypotension, which causes dizziness and the risk of falling, can have devastating consequences in elderly patients; thus, this side effect, along with sedation, often makes trazodone less acceptable in this population compared with newer compounds that share its lack of anticholinergic activity but not the rest of its side-effect profile. Still, trazodone is often helpful for depressed geriatric patients with severe agitation and insomnia.

Trazodone has been reported to have antianxiety properties as well. In a randomized, double-blind, placebo-controlled trial, trazodone's anxiolytic efficacy was comparable to that of diazepam in weeks 3 through 8 of treatment for generalized anxiety disorder, although patients treated with diazepam had greater improvement during the first 2 weeks of treatment (Rickels et al. 1993).

Many clinicians use low-dose trazodone as a sleep-promoting agent, especially in patients for whom benzodiazepines may be risky (e.g., patients with sleep apnea or histories of sedative-hypnotic abuse). In a double-blind, placebo-controlled trial of 17 depressed patients with insomnia related to fluoxetine or bupropion pharmacotherapy, trazodone was an effective hypnotic agent at doses of 50–100 mg (Nierenberg et al. 1994). Several case series reported trazodone (25–150 mg) response rates to antidepressant-associated insomnia ranging from 31% to 92% (Jacobsen 1990; Metz and Shader 1990; Nierenberg and Keck 1989).

Side Effects and Toxicology

As mentioned earlier in this chapter, trazodone lacks the anticholinergic side effects of TCAs; thus, trazodone is especially useful in those situations in which antimuscarinic effects would be particularly problematic (e.g., patients with prostatic hypertrophy, closed-angle glaucoma, severe constipation). Its propensity to cause sedation is a dual-edged sword. For many patients, the relief from agitation, anxiety, and insomnia can be rapid; for others, including those with considerable psychomotor retardation and feelings of low energy, therapeutic doses of trazodone may not be tolerable because of sedation.

Trazodone elicits orthostatic hypotension in some patients, probably as a consequence of α_1-adrenergic receptor blockade. Trazodone-related syncope in the elderly has been described (Nambudiri et al. 1989). At therapeutic doses, it has no negative inotropic effect on the heart and, therefore, no tendency to cause heart failure. However, case reports have noted cardiac arrhythmias emerging in apparent relation to trazodone treatment, both in patients with preexisting mitral valve prolapse and in patients with negative personal and family histories of cardiac disease (Janowsky et al. 1983; Lippman et al. 1983).

A relatively rare, but dramatic, side effect associated with trazodone is priapism. More than

200 cases have been reported (Thompson et al. 1990), and the manufacturer estimates the incidence of any abnormal erectile function to be approximately 1 in 6,000 male patients treated with trazodone. The risk for this side effect appears to be greatest during the first month of treatment at low doses (i.e., <150 mg/day). Early recognition of any abnormal erectile function, including prolonged or inappropriate erections, is important and should prompt discontinuation of trazodone treatment.

Mania has been observed in association with trazodone treatment, as with nearly all antidepressants. The switch to mania has been described in bipolar patients as well as in patients with previous diagnoses of unipolar depression (Arana and Kaplan 1985; Knobler 1986; Lennhoff 1987; Zmitek 1987). In a literature review, Terao (1993) found that the switch process occurs more rapidly in trazodone-treated patients than in fluoxetine-treated patients (average time to onset of mania: 16 days vs. 59 days, respectively).

Trazodone has an important advantage—a wider therapeutic margin—in comparison with tricyclics, monoamine oxidase inhibitors (MAOIs), and a few other second-generation antidepressants. Trazodone appears to be *relatively* safer than other antidepressants in overdose situations, especially when it is the only agent taken. Fatalities are rare, even with large overdoses; uneventful recoveries have been reported after ingestion of doses as high as 6,000–9,200 mg (Ayd 1984). In one report, 9 of 294 overdose cases were fatal, and all 9 patients had taken other central nervous system (CNS) depressants with trazodone (Gamble and Peterson 1986). When trazodone overdoses occur, clinicians should carefully monitor for hypotension, a potentially serious toxic effect.

Drug-Drug Interactions

Trazodone can potentiate the effects of other CNS depressants. Patients should be warned about increased drowsiness and sedation when trazodone is combined with other CNS depressants, including alcohol.

In theory, the combination of trazodone with other pro-serotonergic agents could result in the development of the *serotonin syndrome* (Sternbach 1991); this toxic syndrome has been reported after the combined use of trazodone and buspirone (Goldberg and Huk 1992), trazodone and an MAOI plus methylphenidate (Bodner et al. 1995), and trazodone and paroxetine (Reeves and Bullen 1995). The combination of trazodone with an MAOI, as with other antidepressants, should be handled with great caution. However, there are case reports of the successful combination of trazodone with an MAOI in treatment-resistant depressed patients (Zimmer et al. 1984).

Trazodone can cause hypotension, especially orthostatic hypotension, and the manufacturer states in the package insert that concomitant administration of Desyrel with antihypertensive therapy may require a reduction in the dose of the antihypertensive agent.

NEFAZODONE

History and Discovery

Nefazodone has selective and unique effects on the serotonin system. Its analogue, trazodone, was found to be an effective second-generation antidepressant. Unfortunately, as discussed earlier in this chapter, trazodone is also very sedating and has a propensity to cause postural hypotension. A deliberate effort to improve the pharmacological profile of trazodone with receptor-binding techniques led to the discovery of nefazodone (Taylor et al. 1986). It became available for clinical use in the United States in the latter part of 1994.

Structure-Activity Relations

Nefazodone's chemical structure, which is similar to that of trazodone, is depicted in Figure 4–2.

Pharmacological Profile

In vitro studies have found that nefazodone is a 5-HT_2 receptor antagonist, but it has little affinity for α_2, β-adrenergic, or 5-HT_{1A} receptors (Eison et al. 1990). Nefazodone's inhibition of serotonin reuptake and norepinephrine reuptake is limited (Bolden-Watson and Richelson 1993). Its affinity for the α_1-adrenergic receptor is less than that of trazodone (Eison et al. 1990). Nefazodone is inactive at most other receptor-binding sites, including muscarinic, H_1, dopamine, benzodiazepine, γ-aminobutyric acid, μ-opiate, and calcium channel receptors (Taylor et al. 1986).

Nefazodone has two principal active metabolites—hydroxynefazodone and mCPP. Hydroxynefazodone has similar affinities for 5-HT_2 receptors and serotonin reuptake sites compared with nefazodone, whereas mCPP has modest activity at serotonin reuptake sites (Eison et al. 1990) and is a potent direct serotonin agonist. Another human metabolite, triazoledione, has been identified and appears to have pharmacological activity similar to that of nefazodone (Mayol et al. 1994).

Nefazodone's activity in animal models is suggestive of antidepressant activity. For example, it prevents reserpine-induced ptosis in mice and reverses learned helplessness in rats (Eison et al. 1990).

Pharmacokinetics and Disposition

Nefazodone is rapidly and completely absorbed from the gastrointestinal tract and has an absolute bioavailability of 15%–23% because of extensive first-pass hepatic metabolism. Peak

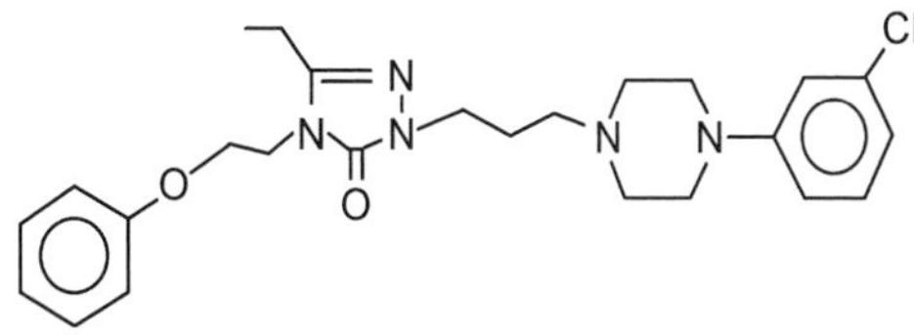

Figure 4–2. Chemical structure for nefazodone.

plasma levels occur between 1 and 3 hours, and steady state is achieved in 3–4 days with a twice-daily dosing regimen. Nefazodone has nonlinear kinetics, which result in greater than proportional mean plasma concentrations with higher doses. The elimination half-life is 2–4 hours for the parent compound and hydroxynefazodone, 18–33 hours for desmethylhydroxynefazodone, and 4–9 hours for mCPP. Nefazodone is extensively (99%) but loosely protein bound. In patients with hepatic cirrhosis, single-dose nefazodone and hydroxynefazodone levels are about twice as high as in healthy volunteers, but the difference decreases to approximately 25% at steady state (Barbhaiya et al. 1995).

Mechanism of Action

The most likely means by which nefazodone acts as an antidepressant is through its effects on serotonin neurotransmission, but these effects are complex. Nefazodone blocks serotonin reuptake, thereby increasing serotonin availability in the synapse while functioning as a 5-HT_2 receptor antagonist. In addition, mCPP, nefazodone's active metabolite, functions as a serotonin agonist. Nefazodone's effects on electrophysiological measures of serotonergic systems are similar to those of many other effective antidepressants (Blier et al. 1990).

Indications

Eight double-blind, placebo-controlled trials found that nefazodone is an effective antidepressant. Patients with symptoms meeting DSM-III-R (American Psychiatric Association 1987) criteria for major depression had a 72% response rate when treated with nefazodone in doses of 300–500 mg/day. The response rate dropped to 56% with doses of 200–300 mg/day and to 48% with a dose of 600 mg/day (placebo response rates did not differ significantly from those of the low- or high-dose ranges; Rickels et al. 1995). These findings suggest that nefazo-

done may have a "therapeutic window" similar to that of nortriptyline.

Nefazodone is effective in both first-episode and recurrent major depression, and several studies have shown that its efficacy is comparable to that of imipramine (Feighner et al. 1989; Fontaine et al. 1994). In one published multicenter comparison, nefazodone and imipramine were significantly superior to placebo in treating major depression. However, the response to the lower dose range of nefazodone (50–250 mg/day) was suboptimal, whereas the higher dose range (100–500 mg/day) produced more robust clinical response. In both nefazodone dose-range groups, fewer side effects were reported than in the imipramine group, and more nefazodone-treated patients completed 6 weeks of therapy than did the imipramine or placebo groups (Fontaine et al. 1994). The lower response rate at lower nefazodone doses has been confirmed by others (Mendels et al. 1995).

In a European study of patients with moderate to severe major depression, the efficacy of amitriptyline (50–200 mg/day) was clearly superior to that of nefazodone (100–400 mg/day) (Ansseau et al. 1994). In another study, both nefazodone and the comparison tricyclic imipramine were superior to placebo during long-term (1 year or longer) continuation therapy (Anton et al. 1994).

Side Effects and Toxicology

Nefazodone has been found to be safe and well tolerated in clinical trials that included approximately 2,250 patients (Fontaine 1993). It has a relatively benign side-effect profile, as expected based on its lack of affinity for muscarinic and histaminic receptors. Its lower affinity, compared with that of trazodone, for α_1-adrenergic receptors suggests that it should have a lower propensity to cause orthostatic hypotension. Side effects that occur more frequently in patients who receive nefazodone, compared with placebo, include dizziness, asthenia, dry mouth, nausea, and constipation (Fontaine 1993).

There was no evidence of cardiac dysfunction or cardiotoxicity in a careful review of more than 2,000 patients. Nefazodone modestly reduced the resting pulse and supine blood pressure, but orthostatic hypotension was rare (Fontaine 1993).

Preskorn (1995) recently compared reported treatment-emergent adverse effects in patients receiving nefazodone and other antidepressants. The total cumulative incidence of treatment-emergent adverse effects for nefazodone was lower than that for imipramine or fluoxetine. The most common placebo-adjusted adverse effects associated with nefazodone were dry mouth (7.5%), somnolence (5.8%), dizziness (5.6%), nausea (5.5%), constipation (3.3%), blurred vision (3.2%), and postural hypotension (2.6%) (Preskorn 1995).

In two published case reports of suicide attempts by overdose with nefazodone, involving 3,400 mg and 3,600 mg, life-threatening symptoms did not occur, and both patients recovered without any sequelae (Fontaine 1993). A published case report of nefazodone-induced mania suggested that the popular clinical opinion that probably all effective antidepressants can stimulate the switch process may be correct (Jeffries and Al-Jeshi 1995).

Drug-Drug Interactions

There are some reports on interactions between nefazodone and other drugs. In Phase 2 and 3 trials, the kinetics of alprazolam and triazolam, but not nefazodone, changed when these medications were given together. The manufacturer of triazolam issued a statement warning that its concurrent use with nefazodone was contraindicated because of nefazodone's significant inhibition of oxidative metabolism mediated by CYP3A. In the Phase 2 and 3 trials, some small increases in the plasma concentration of digoxin occurred with concurrent nefazodone administration. Although the observed increases in plasma digoxin concentrations were modest, the combined administration of the two drugs should be avoided, in light of the narrow thera-

peutic index for digoxin. There is some concern that nefazodone should not be administered with protease inhibitors used by HIV-positive patients, but clinical studies have not borne this out. Also, nefazodone's effects on H_2 antagonists appear minimal. Nefazodone does not appear to potentiate the sedative-hypnotic effects of alcohol and causes less disruption of human performance on psychomotor and memory tasks in combination with alcohol when compared with the coadministration of imipramine and alcohol (Frewer and Lader 1993).

BUPROPION

History and Discovery

Nearly three decades ago, a group of pharmacologists decided to search for a new antidepressant compound that was active in conventional antidepressant screening models yet was 1) different chemically, pharmacologically, and biochemically from TCAs; 2) not an inhibitor of monoamine oxidase; 3) not sympathomimetic; 4) not anticholinergic; and 5) not a cardiac depressant (Soroko and Maxwell 1983). The culmination of this intensive research program resulted in the development of bupropion.

Early studies confirmed that bupropion has efficacy comparable to that of conventional antidepressants but a side-effect profile that was generally viewed as milder and safer, with notable lack of substantial anticholinergic toxicity and relatively innocuous effects on cardiovascular function. Then, just as the drug was about to be released in 1986, seizures were reported in a few nondepressed bulimic study patients treated with bupropion. The manufacturer voluntarily withdrew the drug pending further, extensive clinical investigations. Finally, in 1989, bupropion was released for clinical use in the United States.

Structure-Activity Relations

Bupropion's chemical structure is unique among the antidepressants (Figure 4–3). It is a unicyclic aminoketone. The lack of complex heterocyclic fused rings, as well as the more common functional groups (e.g., *N*-methyl-piperazine) often found in neuroleptics, is thought to contribute to bupropion's lack of the side effects usually seen in polycyclic antidepressants (Mehta 1983). Bupropion's chemical structure does resemble, in some aspects, that of certain psychostimulants, including amphetamine and the diet pill diethylpropion (Tenuate) (Mehta 1983), which may account for certain shared characteristics (Golden 1988). In fact, bupropion metabolites produced false-positive results on urine amphetamine toxicology screens (Nixon et al. 1995).

Pharmacological Profile

Bupropion is a relatively weak inhibitor of dopamine reuptake, with modest effects on norepinephrine reuptake and no effect on serotonin reuptake (Richelson 1991). It does not appear to be associated with downregulation of postsynaptic β-adrenergic receptors, nor does it have significant effects on 5-HT$_2$, α$_2$-adrenergic, imipramine, or dopaminergic receptors in brain tissue (Ferris and Beaman 1983). It lacks anticholinergic activity and is at least 10-fold weaker than TCAs in terms of cardiac depressant effects (Soroko and Maxwell 1983).

Bupropion is active in the classic animal

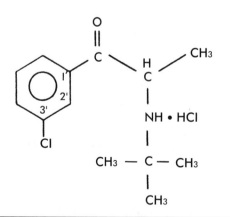

Figure 4–3. Chemical structure for bupropion.

models for predicting antidepressant activity (Soroko and Maxwell 1983). Furthermore, its active metabolites, especially hydroxybupropion, have been shown to possess antidepressant profiles in mice (Martin et al. 1990). This finding may be relevant to preliminary observations from human studies exploring the roles these metabolites might play in determining clinical outcome (see next section) (Golden 1991).

Pharmacokinetics and Disposition

Bupropion is rapidly absorbed after oral administration, with peak blood levels occurring within 2 hours (Lai and Schroeder 1983). Mean protein binding in healthy subjects is 85% (Findlay et al. 1981). The elimination is biphasic, with an initial phase of approximately 1.5 hours and a second phase of about 14 hours.

Bupropion undergoes extensive hepatic metabolism, including a pronounced first-pass effect. Three active metabolites—hydroxybupropion, threo-hydrobupropion, and erythyro-hydrobupropion—predominate over the parent compound in both plasma and cerebrospinal fluid at steady state and may play an important role in determining clinical response (Golden et al. 1988b).

There does not appear to be a consistent, clear relation between steady-state bupropion plasma concentrations and clinical response (Goodnick 1991). Preskorn (1983) found a curvilinear relationship between antidepressant efficacy and trough bupropion plasma concentrations, with greatest efficacy associated with bupropion plasma concentrations greater than 25 ng/mL but less than 100 ng/mL. On the other hand, Goodnick (1992) reported better response with trough levels of less than 30 ng/mL. In another study, no relation was found between plasma bupropion concentrations and clinical response; however, higher concentrations of each of the three active metabolites, especially hydroxybupropion, were significantly related to poor clinical outcome (Golden et al. 1988b).

Bupropion is now available in both immediate- and extended-release formulations. Data on the extended-release product suggest that 300 mg/day provides efficacy similar to that of higher doses of the immediate-release formulation.

Mechanism of Action

The mechanism of action for bupropion remains unclear (Ascher et al. 1995). From the start, its effects on dopaminergic function have been a focus of investigation. Some of the behavioral effects of bupropion, including stimulation of locomotor activity and effects on the Porsolt forced swim test, are abolished after dopaminergic neurons are destroyed by 6-hydroxydopamine (Cooper et al. 1980). Bupropion-induced behavioral sensitization in the rat is accompanied by a selective potentiation of the effects of this compound on interstitial dopamine concentrations in the nucleus accumbens (Nomikos et al. 1992). In humans, plasma concentrations of homovanillic acid, a major metabolite of dopamine, increased in patients who did not respond to bupropion treatment but not in clinical responders (Golden et al. 1988d).

Noradrenergic systems may also play a critical role in the mechanism of action of bupropion. In a study investigating the effects of antidepressants on noradrenergic function in hospitalized depressed patients, bupropion, along with the norepinephrine reuptake inhibitor desipramine and MAOIs, increased 24-hour excretion of 6-hydroxymelatonin, a physiological gauge of noradrenergic activity, and simultaneously reduced "whole-body norepinephrine turnover," (i.e., the 24-hour excretion of norepinephrine and its metabolites) (Golden et al. 1988c). Bupropion's active metabolites, especially hydroxybupropion, inhibit the reuptake of norepinephrine into rat cortical tissue (Perumal et al. 1986).

Bupropion's metabolites may be quite important in determining clinical response. In animal models, hydroxybupropion has more potent antidepressant properties than does the parent compound, and threo-hydrobupropion also has some antidepressant activity (Martin et al. 1990). In depressed patients, metabolite concentrations predominate over bupropion concentrations in both plasma and cerebrospinal fluid (Golden et al. 1988b). Hydroxybupropion may be responsible for bupropion's therapeutic effects, and a curvilinear plasma level–response relationship (similar to that seen with nortriptyline) may exist.

Indications

Bupropion has been shown to be as effective as standard TCAs and SSRIs and superior to placebo in treating hospitalized, as well as ambulatory, depressed patients (Chouinard 1983; Davidson et al. 1983; Feighner et al. 1986, 1991; Mendels et al. 1983; Merideth and Feighner 1983; Pitts et al. 1983). Under double-blind conditions, bupropion was superior to placebo in treating hospitalized patients who were refractory to tricyclics, and in an open-label study, outpatients with a history of either nonresponse or nonresponse plus intolerance to tricyclics had a marked improvement in their conditions after taking bupropion (Stern et al. 1983). In an open study of 41 depressed patients who did not respond to well-documented tricyclic treatment, about half responded to bupropion (Ferguson et al. 1994).

One report suggested that bupropion may be particularly promising in treating rapid-cycling bipolar II disorder (Haykal and Akiskal 1990). In that case series, all 6 patients' conditions improved, and 4 had "dramatic" improvement that was sustained after an average of 2 years of treatment. In addition, none of the patients developed hypomania or rapid cycling, in contrast to the experience with conventional antidepressants (Haykal and Akiskal 1990). Although there are case reports of possible bupropion precipitation of mania and a mixed affective state (Masand and Stern 1993; Zubieta and Demitrack 1991), a prospective, double-blind trial found that bupropion was less likely to induce hypomania or mania in bipolar depressed patients than was desipramine (Sachs et al. 1994). In contrast, in a series of 11 consecutive bipolar patients, 6 experienced hypomanic or manic symptoms when bupropion was added to their treatment regimen (Fogelson et al. 1992).

Bupropion has been found to be effective in the treatment of attention-deficit/hyperactivity disorder in double-blind studies in children (Barrickman et al. 1995; Casat et al. 1989) and in an open trial in adults (Wender and Reimherr 1990). However, it may exacerbate tics in children with attention-deficit/hyperactivity disorder and comorbid Tourette's disorder (Spencer et al. 1993). Bupropion's activating properties have led to explorations of its potential use in the treatment of chronic fatigue syndrome (Goodnick 1990; Goodnick et al. 1992) and in the treatment of fatigue associated with multiple sclerosis (Duffy and Campbell 1994).

In a placebo-controlled, double-blind trial in patients with bulimia, bupropion was superior to placebo in reducing episodes of binge eating and purging (Horne et al. 1988). However, because four subjects experienced grand mal seizures during treatment, the use of bupropion in the treatment of bulimia should be avoided (Horne et al. 1988).

Bupropion is approved for use in smoking cessation. In a double-blind study of nondepressed smokers, bupropion was significantly more effective than placebo in promoting abstinence, although the vast majority of subjects relapsed (Hurt et al. 1997). In another trial, bupropion and bupropion plus nicotine patch were significantly more effective than placebo and produced higher abstinence rates than those in the other trial (Jorenby et al. 1999).

Side Effects and Toxicology

Bupropion's side-effect profile is clearly different from that of conventional TCAs. It lacks anticholinergic effects, is clearly not sedating, and suppresses appetite in some patients (Rudorfer and Potter 1989). Unlike several other second-generation antidepressants, bupropion does not cause psychosexual dysfunction (Gardner and Johnston 1985). Patients who experience psychosexual dysfunction in conjunction with fluoxetine treatment report substantially greater satisfaction with their sexual function while taking bupropion (Walker et al. 1993).

Bupropion's cardiovascular profile is especially favorable. It does not cause electrocardiogram changes and does not trigger orthostatic hypotension, even in patients with preexisting heart disease (Roose et al. 1987). Bupropion has been shown to be safer than nortriptyline in regard to cardiovascular side effects (Kiev et al. 1994).

Bupropion appears to be relatively less lethal following overdose than tricyclics and certain other antidepressants (Hayes and Kristoff 1986). In a review of 58 cases of bupropion overdose and 9 cases of combined bupropion/benzodiazepine ingestion, bupropion seemed to lack major cardiovascular toxicity. Neurological toxicity was found, including lethargy, tremors, and seizures (which responded well to either benzodiazepines or phenytoin) (Spiller et al. 1994). Two fatal overdoses that were reported were associated with peripheral blood levels of 4.0–4.2 mg/L of bupropion and total metabolite levels of 15 and 16.6 mg/L. By history, the estimated lethal doses were less than 10 g (Friel et al. 1993).

Bupropion can have activating effects, which are often helpful in patients with psychomotor retardation but can be experienced as agitation or insomnia in others. Appetite suppression is also perceived as an advantage in some patients but a disadvantage in others. Psychotic symptoms, including hallucinations and delusions, can emerge in association with bupropion treatment (Golden et al. 1985). Since the initial description of bupropion-related psychoses, numerous case reports have described similar toxic reactions, including organic mental disorders (Ames et al. 1992), delirium (Dager and Heritch 1990), and catatonia (Jackson et al. 1992).

A rare but serious side effect of bupropion is seizure induction. A careful review by Davidson (1989) found the incidence of seizures in patients receiving bupropion at doses of 450 mg/day or less ranged from 0.33% to 0.44%, depending on the method used to make the calculation. The cumulative 2-year risk in patients receiving 450 mg/day or less was 0.48%. To place these observations in the proper context, clinicians should be aware that the estimated frequency of seizures in outpatients with no predisposing factors who are receiving TCAs at modest doses (e.g., 150 mg/day or less) is 0.1% (Jick et al. 1983); at higher doses (e.g., 200 mg/day or greater), it rises to 0.6%–0.9% (Peck et al. 1983). Careful evaluation for risk factors (e.g., history of seizures, recent withdrawal from alcohol or anxiolytic drugs, concomitant therapy with drugs that lower the seizure threshold, history of organic brain disease or abnormal electroencephalogram), conservative dose titration with a maximum dose of 450 mg/day, and use of divided dose schedules (three times a day) should minimize the risk for bupropion-related seizures (Davidson 1989).

Drug-Drug Interactions

As with most antidepressants, the combined use of bupropion with MAOIs should be approached with caution because of the risk of a hypertensive reaction if bupropion is added to ongoing monoamine oxidase inhibition. Because bupropion provides dopaminergic activation, clinicians treating patients with coexisting Parkinson's disease and depression can often decrease the dose of antiparkinsonian medication when bupropion is added. The combination of bupropion and antiparkinsonian medication should be administered with care. Goetz et al. (1984) reported the emergence of hallucina-

tions, confusion, and dyskinesia following the addition of bupropion to previously therapeutic doses of L-dopa.

The addition of bupropion to fluoxetine treatment has coincided with the onset of delirium (Van Putten and Shaffer 1990) and a grand mal seizure (Ciraulo and Shader 1990). Still, the combination has been commonly used for patients who have not responded to fluoxetine or have experienced sexual dysfunction. Conservative titration with bupropion when used in combination is generally recommended. Recent studies suggest the combination is minimally superior to monotherapy (Fischer et al. 1998). The combination of bupropion and lithium may affect lithium serum levels and has been linked to seizures in three patients (Goodnick 1991), although this combination generally has been safe and well tolerated in a few published studies (Apter and Woolfolk 1990; Goodnick, in press; Haykal and Akiskal 1990). A report of two cases suggests that carbamazepine may decrease bupropion blood levels and increase hydroxybupropion levels, whereas bupropion may increase sodium valproate levels (Popli et al. 1995).

MIRTAZAPINE

History and Discovery

Mirtazapine was introduced in the United States in August 1996. Mirtazapine is structurally similar to mianserin, which has been prescribed in several European countries for many years.

Structure-Activity Relations

Mirtazapine is a tetracyclic member of the piperazinoazepine class of compounds. The chemical structure for mirtazapine is shown in Figure 4–4.

Pharmacological Profile

Mirtazapine has a pharmacological profile that is different from those of the currently available

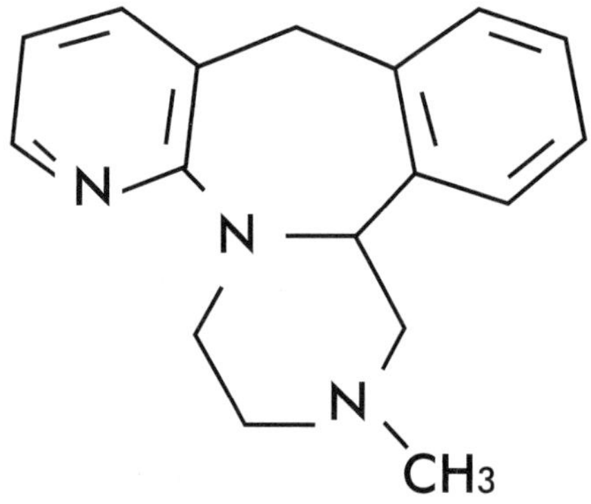

Figure 4–4. Chemical structure for mirtazapine.

antidepressants. Mirtazapine has a unique pattern of effects on monoamine neurotransmission compared with other available antidepressants. It is a potent antagonist of central α_2-adrenergic auto- and heteroreceptors, is an antagonist of both 5-HT$_2$ and 5-HT$_3$ receptors, and has minimal effects on monoamine reuptake (de Boer 1996).

Mirtazapine enhances noradrenergic transmission but not via reuptake inhibition. Blockade of presynaptic α_2 noradrenergic autoreceptors leads to increased norepinephrine release (de Boer et al. 1988). In addition, it preferentially blocks α_2 heteroreceptors on serotonin neurons, which affects serotonin release (de Boer 1995). Mirtazapine's affinity for central presynaptic noradrenergic α_2 autoreceptors is approximately 10-fold higher than for central postsynaptic and peripheral presynaptic α_2 autoreceptors. In addition, its affinity for central presynaptic α_2 autoreceptors is about 30-fold greater than its affinity for central and peripheral α_1 adrenoceptors (de Boer 1995). Thus, this profile suggests that mirtazapine has selective α_2-adrenergic antagonist properties with a preference for central presynaptic α_2-adrenergic auto- and heteroreceptors.

Blockade of the α_2 heteroreceptors leads to enhanced serotonin release. At the same time, mirtazapine blocks 5-HT$_2$ and 5-HT$_3$ receptors. The net effect is selective enhancement of 5-HT$_1$-mediated neurotransmission (de Boer

1995). Mirtazapine has low affinity for muscarinic, cholinergic, and dopaminergic receptors. It does have a high affinity for H$_1$ receptors (de Boer 1995). This combination of potent antihistaminic activity and enhanced noradrenergic neurotransmission may explain the clinical observation that mirtazapine is *more* sedating at low doses than at higher doses; antihistaminergic side effects emerge at the lower doses but are somewhat counteracted by activation via noradrenergic stimulation at higher doses.

Pharmacokinetics and Disposition

Bioavailability following single and multiple doses of mirtazapine is approximately 50% (Voortman and Paanakker 1995). Peak plasma concentrations are reached within 2 hours after oral administration (Sitsen and Zikov 1995). The average elimination half-life is 21.5 hours, with a range of 20–40 hours (Sitsen and Zikov 1995). The parent compound is eliminated via hepatic metabolism, with demethylation and oxidation and subsequent conjugation of the metabolites. Desmethyl-mirtazapine is approximately three- to fourfold less active than the parent drug. Mirtazapine has linear pharmacokinetics over clinically relevant dose ranges. It is approximately 85% bound to protein in plasma (Kehoe and Schorr 1996).

Mechanism of Action

The putative mechanism of action of mirtazapine is unique among currently available antidepressant drugs in the United States. Blockade of presynaptic central α_2-adrenergic autoreceptors leads to enhanced noradrenergic neurotransmission via increased noradrenergic cell firing and norepinephrine release. In turn, norepinephrine stimulates α_1 adrenoreceptors on the cell bodies of serotonergic neurons, which leads to increased serotonin cell firing. In addition, mirtazapine blocks α_2-adrenergic heteroreceptors on the synaptic terminals of serotonin neurons, which leads to a further increase in serotonin release (de Boer 1995). Thus, by increasing the serotonergic firing rate and blocking the α_2-adrenergic heteroreceptors on serotonin terminals, mirtazapine increases intracellular serotonin levels. Coupled with its antagonistic properties at 5-HT_{2A}, 5-HT_{2C}, and 5-HT_3 receptors, mirtazapine's stimulation of serotonin release leads to functional enhancement of 5-HT_{1A} neurotransmission (de Boer 1995). The overall effect of these pharmacological actions is increased noradrenergic and 5-HT_{1A} activity.

Indications

Mirtazapine is superior to placebo and comparable to standard antidepressants in the treatment of major depression (Davis and Wilde 1996; Kasper 1995; Zikov et al. 1995). Hamilton Rating Scale for Depression scores begin to improve significantly during the first week of mirtazapine treatment (and during the first week of amitriptyline treatment) compared with placebo (Bremner 1995), probably because of early effects on sleep and anxiety symptoms. When depressed patients are classified on the basis of symptom severity, those with severe depression (i.e., 17-item Hamilton Rating Scale for Depression scores > 24) have the same response to mirtazapine as those with moderate depression, whereas the placebo response rate is lower in the more severely ill patients (Claghorn and Lesem 1995). In a 20-week extension trial, mirtazapine was superior to placebo and amitriptyline in endpoint analyses of symptom severity (Bremner and Smith 1996). In a double-blind, controlled study of elderly depressed patients, mirtazapine and trazodone both had superior efficacy compared with placebo. The trend, which failed to reach statistical significance, was toward greater efficacy in the mirtazapine than in the trazodone treatment group (Halikas 1995).

Recent trials have indicated that mirtaza-

pine has comparable but slightly greater or faster efficacy than the SSRIs in outpatients or venlafaxine in inpatients (Guelfi et al. 2000; Leinonen et al. 1999; Montgomery et al. 2000).

Side Effects and Toxicology

A meta-analysis that included all of the patients participating in the mirtazapine clinical trial development program who had received at least one dose of medication compared mirtazapine- and placebo-related side effects. In this sample of 359 mirtazapine- and 328 placebo-treated patients, the following side effects occurred more frequently in association with mirtazapine than with placebo: drowsiness (23% vs. 14%), excessive sedation (19% vs. 5%), dry mouth (25% vs. 16%), increased appetite (11% vs. 2%), and weight gain (10% vs. 2%). Usually, these side effects were mild and transient and often decreased over time despite increases in mirtazapine dosages. No significant increases in cardiovascular side effects (e.g., blood pressure changes, tachycardia) or in psychosexual side effects were associated with mirtazapine compared with placebo (Montgomery 1995). Thus, mirtazapine has antihistaminic side effects, without the cardiovascular side effects or gastrointestinal/psychosexual side effects that are associated with TCAs and SSRIs, respectively.

In a comparative trial in elderly patients, dry mouth and somnolence occurred more frequently with both mirtazapine and trazodone treatment than with placebo. Compared with placebo, trazodone treatment was linked to a higher incidence of dizziness and amblyopia, whereas mirtazapine was associated with increased appetite and a modest weight gain (Davis and Wilde 1996).

Clinicians may start treatment with many psychoactive medications at rather low doses to allow for accommodation to mild side effects and then gradually increase the dosage as tolerated. Because of the unique pharmacological profile of mirtazapine, this practice should be avoided. Mirtazapine's affinity for histaminergic receptors is greater than its affinity for α_2-adrenergic receptors. Thus, at doses lower than the recommended 15-mg starting dose, maximum sedation caused by substantial antihistaminergic activity occurs. At 15 mg and higher doses, the enhancement of noradrenergic neurotransmission via α_2-adrenergic receptor blockade leads to activating effects that, at least in part, counteract the antihistaminergic sedation.

A few abnormal laboratory parameters have been rarely associated with mirtazapine treatment. Transient elevations in liver alanine aminotransferase (ALT) levels to greater than three times the upper limit of normal range were reported in about 2% of patients (Davis and Wilde 1996). These enzyme elevations returned to normal after treatment was discontinued. Random plasma total cholesterol levels have been reported to increase by an average of 3%–4% in depressed patients receiving mirtazapine (Davis and Wilde 1996). However, it is very difficult to interpret the meaning of random (i.e., nonfasting) cholesterol levels, which would be expected to increase in relation to improved appetite and increased food intake.

To date, the available data suggest that mirtazapine is relatively safe in overdose situations compared with conventional TCAs. In the 10 overdose cases that have been reported, transient excessive somnolence was the only observed symptom.

Drug-Drug Interactions

Few drug-drug interactions involving mirtazapine have been described at this point. Mirtazapine can have additive subjective and objective effects on motor and cognitive performance when taken in conjunction with alcohol or diazepam (Kuitunen 1994; Sitsen and Zikov 1995). Mirtazapine is metabolized by several subfamilies of the cytochrome P450 enzyme system, including CYP2DG, CYP1A2, CYP3A4, and CYP2C9.

SUMMARY

We reviewed the pharmacological properties of four antidepressants that are not readily cataloged within the conventional classifications of antidepressants. Do any common themes link these medications, other than their relegation to the category of miscellaneous antidepressants?

In a way, trazodone, nefazodone, and bupropion all serve to remind us of the potential importance of metabolites on the clinical profile of pharmacological agents. In the case of trazodone and nefazodone, the active metabolite mCPP may play a role in the mechanism of action, in light of its potent activity as a serotonin agonist. For bupropion, several active metabolites may influence clinical response and/or side effects.

Another important theme that has emerged from our review is the important advantage that an understanding of a drug's basic pharmacology provides for clinicians. Many side effects can be understood, or even predicted, based on the pharmacological profiles of the newer agents. Thus, trazodone's propensity to evoke orthostatic hypotension makes sense in light of its effects on α-adrenergic receptors, and many of the side effects associated with bupropion could be anticipated based on its effects on dopaminergic neurotransmission.

Finally, each novel antidepressant adds to our available tools for the treatment of depression. Although we do not have a "perfect" antidepressant therapy that is safe and effective for all patients, all of the compounds, with their various side-effect profiles, provide clinicians with additional options and flexibility in selecting the best available approach for each patient.

REFERENCES

American Psychiatric Association: Diagnostic and Statistical Manual of Mental Disorders, 3rd Edition, Revised. Washington, DC, American Psychiatric Association, 1987

Ames D, Wirshing WC, Szuba MP: Organic mental disorders associated with bupropion in three patients. J Clin Psychiatry 53:53–55, 1992

Ansseau M, Darimont P, Lecoq A, et al: Controlled comparison of nefazodone and amitriptyline in major depressive inpatients. Psychopharmacology (Berl) 115:254–260, 1994

Anton SF, Robinson DS, Roberts DL, et al: Long-term treatment of depression with nefazodone. Psychopharmacol Bull 30:165–169, 1994

Apter JT, Woolfolk RL: Lithium augmentation of bupropion in refractory depression. Ann Clin Psychiatry 2:7–10, 1990

Arana GW, Kaplan GB: Trazodone-induced mania following desipramine-induced mania in major depressive disorders (letter). Am J Psychiatry 142:386, 1985

Ascher JA, Cole JO, Colin JN, et al: Bupropion: a review of its mechanism of antidepressant activity. J Clin Psychiatry 56:395–401, 1995

Ayd FJ Jr: Pharmacology update: which antidepressant to choose, II: the overdose factor. Psychiatric Annals 14:212–214, 1984

Barbhaiya RJ, Sukla UA, Matarakam CS, et al: Single- and multiple-dose pharmacokinetics of nefazodone in patients with hepatic cirrhosis. Clin Pharmacol Ther 58:390–398, 1995

Barrickman LL, Perry PJ, Allen AJ, et al: Bupropion versus methylphenidate in the treatment of attention-deficit hyperactivity disorder. J Am Acad Child Adolesc Psychiatry 34:649–657, 1995

Blier P, de Montigny C, Chaput Y: A role for the serotonin system in the mechanism of action of antidepressant treatments: preclinical evidence. J Clin Psychiatry 51 (suppl 4):14–20, 1990

Bodner RA, Lynch T, Lewis L, et al: Serotonin syndrome. Neurology 45:219–223, 1995

Bolden-Watson C, Richelson E: Blockade by newly developed antidepressants of biogenic amine uptake into rat brain synaptosomes. Life Sci 52:1023–1029, 1993

Boschmans SA, Perkin MF, Terblanche SE: Antidepressant drugs: imipramine, mianserin and trazodone. Comp Biochem Physiol 86:225–232, 1987

Bremner JD: A double-blind comparison of Org 3770, amitriptyline, and placebo in major depression. J Clin Psychiatry 56:519–525, 1995

Bremner JD, Smith WT: Org 3770 vs amitriptyline in the continuation treatment of depression: a placebo controlled trial. European Journal of Psychiatry 10:5–15, 1996

Brogden RN, Heel RC, Speight TM, et al: Trazodone: a review of its pharmacological properties and therapeutic uses in depression and anxiety. Drugs 21:401–429, 1981

Caccia S, Ballabio M, Fanelli R, et al: Determination of plasma and brain concentrations of trazodone and its metabolite, 1-m-chlorophenylpiperazine, by gas-liquid chromatography. J Chromatogr 210:311–318, 1981

Casat CD, Pleasants DZ, Schroeder DH, et al: Bupropion in children with attention deficit disorder. Psychopharmacol Bull 25:198–201, 1989

Chouinard G: Bupropion and amitriptyline in the treatment of depressed patients. J Clin Psychiatry 44 (sec 2):121–129, 1983

Ciraulo DA, Shader RI: Fluoxetine drug-drug interactions II. J Clin Psychopharmacol 10:213–217, 1990

Claghorn JL, Lesem MD: A double-blind placebo-controlled study of Org 3770 in depressed outpatients. J Affect Disord 34:165–171, 1995

Cooper BR, Hester TJ, Maxwell RA: Behavioral and biochemical effects of the antidepressant bupropion (Wellbutrin): evidence for selective blockade of dopamine uptake *in vivo*. J Pharmacol Exp Ther 215:127–134, 1980

Cunningham LA, Borison RL, Carman JS, et al: A comparison of venlafaxine, trazodone, and placebo in major depression. J Clin Psychopharmacol 14:99–106, 1994

Dager SR, Heritch AJ: A case of bupropion-associated delirium. J Clin Psychiatry 51:307–308, 1990

Davidson J: Seizures and bupropion: a review. J Clin Psychiatry 50:256–261, 1989

Davidson J, Miller R, Fleet JVW, et al: A double-blind comparison of bupropion and amitriptyline in depressed patients. J Clin Psychiatry 44 (sec 2):115–117, 1983

Davis R, Wilde MI: Mirtazapine: a review of its pharmacology and therapeutic potential in the management of major depression. CNS Drugs 5:389–402, 1996 de Boer T: The effects of mirtazapine on central noradrenergic and serotonergic neurotransmission. Int Clin Psychopharmacol 10 (suppl 4): 19–23, 1995

de Boer T: The pharmacological profile of mirtazapine. J Clin Psychiatry 57 (suppl 4): 19–25, 1996

de Boer T, Maura G, Raiteri M, et al: Neurochemical and autonomic pharmacological profiles of the 6-aza-analogue of mianserin, mirtazapine and its enantiomers. Neuropharmacology 27:399–408, 1988

Duffy JD, Campbell J: Bupropion for the treatment of fatigue associated with multiple sclerosis (letter). Psychosomatics 35:170–171, 1994

Eison AS, Eison MS, Torrente JR, et al: Nefazodone: preclinical pharmacology of a new antidepressant. Psychopharmacol Bull 26:311–315, 1990

Feighner J, Hendrickson G, Miller L, et al: Double-blind comparison of doxepin versus bupropion in outpatients with a major depressive disorder. J Clin Psychopharmacol 6:27–32, 1986

Feighner JP, Pambakian R, Fowler RC, et al: A comparison of nefazodone, imipramine, and placebo in patients with moderate to severe depression. Psychopharmacol Bull 25:219–221, 1989

Feighner JP, Gardner EA, Johnston JA, et al: Double-blind comparison of bupropion and fluoxetine in depressed outpatients. J Clin Psychiatry 52:329–335, 1991

Ferguson J, Cunningham L, Merideth C, et al: Bupropion in tricyclic antidepressant nonresponders with unipolar major depressive disorder. Ann Clin Psychiatry 6:153–160, 1994

Ferris RM, Beaman OJ: Bupropion: a new antidepressant drug, the mechanism of action of which is not associated with down-regulation of postsynaptic β-adrenergic, serotonergic (5-HT$_2$), α_2-adrenergic, imipramine and dopaminergic receptors in brain. Neuropharmacology 22: 1257–1267, 1983

Findlay JWA, Van Wyck Fleet J, Smith PG, et al: Pharmacokinetics of bupropion, a novel antidepressant agent, following oral administration to healthy subjects. Eur J Clin Pharmacol 21: 127–135, 1981

Fischer P, Tauscher J, Kufferle B, et al: Weak antidepressant response after buspirone augmentation of serotonin reuptake inhibitors in refractory severe depression. Int Clin Psychopharmacol 13: 83–86, 1998

Fogelson DL, Bystritsky A, Pasnau R: Bupropion in the treatment of bipolar disorders: the same old story? J Clin Psychiatry 53:443–446, 1992

Fontaine R: Novel serotonergic mechanisms and clinical experience with nefazodone. Clin Neuropharmacol 16 (suppl 3):S45–S50, 1993

Fontaine R, Ontiveros A, Elie R, et al: A double-blind comparison of nefazodone, imipramine, and placebo in major depression. J Clin Psychiatry 55:234–241, 1994

Frewer LJ, Lader M: The effects of nefazodone, imipramine and placebo, alone and combined with alcohol, in normal subjects. Int Clin Psychopharmacol 8:13–20, 1993

Friel PN, Logan BK, Fligner CL: Three fatal drug overdoses involving bupropion. J Anal Toxicol 17:436–438, 1993

Gamble DE, Peterson LG: Trazodone overdose: four years of experience from voluntary reports. J Clin Psychiatry 47:544–546, 1986

Garattini S: Biochemical studies with trazodone, in Trazodone: Modern Problems of Pharmacopsychiatry, Vol 9. Edited by Ban TA, Silvestrini B. Basel, Karger, 1974, pp 29–46

Gardner EA, Johnston A: Bupropion: an antidepressant without sexual pathophysiological action. J Clin Psychopharmacol 5:24–29, 1985

Gerner RH: Geriatric depression and treatment with trazodone. Psychopathology 20:82–91, 1987

Goetz CG, Tanner CM, Klawans HL: Bupropion in Parkinson's disease. Neurology 34:1092–1094, 1984

Goldberg RJ, Huk M: Serotonin syndrome from trazodone and buspirone (letter). Psychosomatics 33:235–236, 1992

Golden RN: Diethylpropion, bupropion, and psychoses (letter). Br J Psychiatry 153:265–266, 1988

Golden RN: Antidepressant profile of bupropion and three metabolites: clinical and pre-clinical studies (letter). Pharmacopsychiatry 24:68, 1991

Golden RN, James S, Sherer M, et al: Psychoses associated with bupropion treatment. Am J Psychiatry 142:1459–1462, 1985

Golden RN, Brown DO, Miller H, et al: The new antidepressants. N C Med J 49:549–554, 1988a

Golden RN, DeVane L, Laizure SC, et al: Bupropion in depression: the role of metabolites in clinical outcome. Arch Gen Psychiatry 45:145–149, 1988b

Golden RN, Markey SP, Risby ED, et al: Antidepressants reduce whole-body norepinephrine turnover while enhancing 6-hydroxymelatonin output. Arch Gen Psychiatry 45:150–154, 1988c

Golden RN, Rudorfer MV, Sherer M, et al: Bupropion in depression: biochemical effects and clinical response. Arch Gen Psychiatry 45:139–143, 1988d

Goodnick PJ: Bupropion in chronic fatigue syndrome (letter). Am J Psychiatry 147:1091, 1990

Goodnick PJ: Pharmacokinetics of second generation antidepressants: bupropion. Psychopharmacol Bull 27:513–519, 1991

Goodnick PJ: Blood levels and acute response to bupropion. Am J Psychiatry 149:399–400, 1992

Goodnick PJ: Adjunctive lithium treatment with bupropion and fluoxetine: a naturalistic report. Lithium (in press)

Goodnick PJ, Sandoval R, Brickman A, et al: Bupropion treatment of fluoxetine-resistant chronic fatigue syndrome. Biol Psychiatry 32:834–838, 1992

Guelfi JD, Van Hensbeek M, Ansseau M, et al: Efficacy and tolerability of mirtazapine versus venlafaxine in hospitalized severely depressed patients with melancholia, in Abstracts of the 13th ECNP Congress, 2000, p 266

Halikas JA: Org 3770 (mirtazapine) versus trazodone: a placebo controlled trial in depressed elderly patients. Human Psychopharmacology 10 (suppl):S125–S133, 1995

Hamilton M: A rating scale for depression. J Neurol Neurosurg Psychiatry 23:56–62, 1960

Haria M, Fitton A, McTavish D: Trazodone: a review of its pharmacology, therapeutic use in depression and therapeutic potential in other disorders. Drugs Aging 4:331–335, 1994

Hayes PE, Kristoff CA: Adverse reactions to five new antidepressants. Clinical Pharmacology 5:471–480, 1986

Haykal RF, Akiskal HS: Bupropion as a promising approach to rapid cycling bipolar II patients. J Clin Psychiatry 51:450–455, 1990

Horne RL, Rerguson JM, Pope HG Jr, et al: Treatment of bulimia with bupropion: a multicenter controlled trial. J Clin Psychiatry 49:262–266, 1988

Hurt RD, Sachs DPL, Glover ED, et al: A comparison of sustained-release bupropion and placebo for smoking cessation. N Engl J Med 337:1195–1202, 1997

Hyttel J: Citalopram-pharmacologic profile of a specific serotonin uptake inhibitor with antidepressant activity. Prog Neuropsychopharmacol Biol Psychiatry 6:277–295, 1982

Jackson CW, Head LA, Kellner CH: Catatonia associated with bupropion treatment (letter). J Clin Psychiatry 53:210, 1992

Jacobsen FM: Low-dose trazodone as a hypnotic in patients treated with MAOIs and other psychotropics: a pilot study. J Clin Psychiatry 51:298–302, 1990

Janowsky D, Curtis G, Zisook S, et al: Ventricular arrhythmias possibly aggravated by trazodone. Am J Psychiatry 140:796–797, 1983

Jeffries JJ, Al-Jeshi A: Nefazodone-induced mania (letter). Can J Psychiatry 40:218, 1995

Jick H, Binan B, Hunter JR, et al: Tricyclic antidepressants and convulsions. J Clin Psychopharmacol 3:128–185, 1983

Jorenby DE, Leischow SJ, Nides MA, et al: A controlled trial of sustained-release bupropion, a nicotine patch, or both for smoking cessation. N Engl J Med 340:685–691, 1999

Kasper S: Clinical efficacy of mirtazapine: a review of meta-analyses of pooled data. Int Clin Psychopharmacol 10 (suppl 4):25–35, 1995

Kehoe WA, Schorr RB: Focus on mirtazapine: a new antidepressant with noradrenergic and specific serotonergic activity. Formulary 31:455–469, 1996

Kiev A, Masco HL, Wenger TL, et al: The cardiovascular effects of bupropion and nortriptyline in depressed outpatients. Ann Clin Psychiatry 6:107–115, 1994

Klein HE, Muller N: Trazodone in endogenous depressed patients: a negative report and a critical evaluation of the pertaining literature. Prog Neuropsychopharmacol Biol Psychiatry 9:173–186, 1985

Knobler H: Trazodone-induced mania. Br J Psychiatry 149:787–789, 1986

Kuitunen T: Drug and ethanol effects on the clinical test for drunkenness: single doses of ethanol, hypnotic drugs and antidepressant drugs. Pharmacol Toxicol 75:91–98, 1994

Lader M: Recent experience with trazodone. Psychopathology 20 (suppl 1):39–47, 1987

Lai AA, Schroeder DH: Clinical pharmacokinetics of bupropion: a review. J Clin Psychiatry 44 (sec 2):82–84, 1983

Leinonen E, Skarstein J, Behnke K, et al: Efficacy and tolerability of mirtazapine versus citalopram: a double-blind, randomized study in patients with major depressive disorder. Int Clin Psychopharmacol 14:329–337, 1999

Lennhoff M: Trazodone-induced mania. J Clin Psychiatry 48:423–424, 1987

Lippman S, Bedford P, Manshadi M, et al: Trazodone cardiotoxicity (letter). Am J Psychiatry 140:1383, 1983

Marek GJ, McDougle CJ, Price LH, et al: A comparison of trazodone and fluoxetine: implications for serotonergic mechanism of antidepressant action. Psychopharmacol 109:2–11, 1992

Martin P, Massol J, Colin JN, et al: Antidepressant profile of bupropion and three metabolites in mice. Pharmacopsychiatry 23:187–194, 1990

Masand P, Stern TA: Bupropion and secondary mania: is there a relationship? Ann Clin Psychiatry 5:271–274, 1993

Mayol RF, Cole CA, Luke GM, et al: Characterization of the metabolites of the antidepressant drug nefazodone in human urine and plasma. Drug Metab Dispos 22:304–311, 1994

Mehta NB: The chemistry of bupropion. J Clin Psychiatry 44 (sec 2):56–59, 1983

Mendels J, Amin MM, Chouinard G, et al: A comparative study of bupropion and amitriptyline in depressed outpatients. J Clin Psychiatry 44 (sec 2):118–120, 1983

Mendels J, Reimherr F, Marcus RN, et al: A double-blind, placebo-controlled trial of two dose ranges of nefazodone in the treatment of depressed outpatients. J Clin Psychiatry 56 (suppl 6):30–36, 1995

Merideth CH, Feighner JP: The use of bupropion in hospitalized depressed patients. J Clin Psychiatry 44 (sec 2): 85–87, 1983

Metz A, Shader RI: Adverse interactions encountered when using trazodone to treat insomnia associated with fluoxetine. Int Clin Psychopharmacol 5:191–194, 1990

Montgomery SA: Safety of mirtazapine: a review. Int Clin Psychopharmacol 10 (suppl 4):37–45, 1995

Montgomery SA, Schutte AJ, Reimitz P: Mirtazapine and onset of action of antidepressant activity, in Abstracts of the 13th ECNP Congress, 2000, p 266

Nambudiri DE, Mirchandani IC, Young RC: Two more cases of trazodone-related syncope in the elderly (letter). J Geriatr Psychiatry Neurol 2: 225, 1989

Nierenberg A, Keck PE: Management of monoamine oxidase inhibitor-associated insomnia with trazodone. J Clin Psychopharmacol 9: 42–45, 1989

Nierenberg A, Adler LA, Peselow E, et al: Trazodone for antidepressant-associated insomnia. Am J Psychiatry 151:1069–1072, 1994

Nixon AL, Long WH, Puopolo PR, et al: Bupropion metabolites produce false-positive urine amphetamine results (letter). Am J Psychiatry 152:813, 1995

Nomikos GG, Damsma G, Wenkstern D, et al: Effects of chronic bupropion on interstitial concentrations of dopamine in rat nucleus accumbens and striatum. Neuropsychopharmacology 7:7–14, 1992

Peck AW, Stern WC, Watkinson C: Incidence of seizures during treatment with tricyclic antidepressant drugs and bupropion. J Clin Psychiatry 44 (sec 2):197–201, 1983

Perumal AS, Smith TM, Suckow RF, et al: Effect of plasma from patients containing bupropion and its metabolites on the uptake of norepinephrine. Neuropharmacology 25:199–202, 1986

Pitts WM, Fann WE, Halaris AE, et al: Bupropion in depression: a tri-center placebo-controlled study. J Clin Psychiatry 44 (sec 2):95–100, 1983

Popli AP, Tanquary J, Lamparella V, et al: Bupropion and anticonvulsant drug interactions. Ann Clin Psychiatry 7:99–101, 1995

Preskorn SH: Antidepressant response and plasma concentrations of bupropion. J Clin Psychiatry 44 (sec 2):137–139, 1983

Preskorn SH: Comparison of the tolerability of bupropion, fluoxetine, imipramine, nefazodone, paroxetine, sertraline, and venlafaxine. J Clin Psychiatry 56 (suppl):12–21, 1995

Reeves RR, Bullen JA: Serotonin syndrome produced by paroxetine and low-dose trazodone (letter). Psychosomatics 36:159–160, 1995

Richelson E: Biological basis of depression and therapeutic relevance. J Clin Psychiatry 52 (suppl): 4–10, 1991

Rickels K, Downing R, Schweizer E, et al: Antidepressants for the treatment of generalized anxiety disorder: a placebo-controlled comparison of imipramine, trazodone, and diazepam. Arch Gen Psychiatry 50:884–895, 1993

Rickels K, Robinson DS, Schweizer E, et al: Nefazodone: aspects of efficacy. J Clin Psychiatry 56 (suppl 6):43–46, 1995

Roose SP, Glassman AH, Giardina EGV, et al: Cardiovascular effects of imipramine and bupropion in depressed patients with congestive heart failure. J Clin Psychopharmacol 7: 247–251, 1987

Rudorfer MV, Potter WZ: Antidepressants: a comparative review of the clinical pharmacology and therapeutic use of the "newer" versus the "older" drugs. Drugs 37:713–738, 1989

Rudorfer MV, Golden RN, Potter WZ: Second generation antidepressants. Psychiatr Clin North Am 7:519–534, 1984

Sachs GS, Lafer B, Stoll AL, et al: A double-blind trial of bupropion versus desipramine for bipolar depression. J Clin Psychiatry 55:391–393, 1994

Schatzberg AF: Trazodone: a 5-year review of antidepressant efficacy. Psychopathology 20 (suppl 1):48–56, 1987

Schuckit MA: United States experience with trazodone: a literature review. Psychopathology 20 (suppl 1):32–38, 1987

Shopsin B, Cassano GB, Conti L: An overview of new "second generation" antidepressant compounds: research and treatment implications, in Antidepressants: Neurochemical, Behavioral and Clinical Perspectives. Edited by Enna SJ, Molick J, Richelson E. New York, Raven, 1981, pp 219–251

Silvestrini B: Introductory remarks on trazodone and its position in treatment of psychiatric diseases, in Trazodone: A New Broad-Spectrum Antidepressant (Proceedings of the Symposium of the 11th Congress of the Collegium Internationale Neuro-Psychopharmacologicum, Vienna 1978). Edited by Gershon ES, Rickels K, Silvestrini G. Amsterdam, Excerpta Medica, 1980, pp 34–38

Silvestrini B, Lisciani R: Pharmacology of trazodone, round table discussion—trazodone: a new psychotropic agent. Current Therapeutic Research 15:749–754, 1973

Sitsen JMA, Zikov M: Mirtazapine: clinical profile. CNS Drugs 4 (suppl 1):39–48, 1995

Soroko FE, Maxwell RA: The pharmacologic basis for therapeutic interest in bupropion. J Clin Psychiatry 44 (sec 2): 67–73, 1983

Spencer T, Biederman J, Steingard T, et al: Bupropion exacerbates tics in children with attention-deficit hyperactivity disorder and Tourette's syndrome. J Am Acad Child Adolesc Psychiatry 32:211–214, 1993

Spiller HA, Ramoska EA, Krenzelok EP: Bupropion overdose: a 3-year multi-center retrospective analysis. Am J Emerg Med 12:43–45, 1994

Stern WC, Harto-Truax N, Bauer N: Efficacy of bupropion in tricyclic-resistant or intolerant patients. J Clin Psychiatry 44 (sec 2):148–152, 1983

Sternbach H: The serotonin syndrome. Am J Psychiatry 148:705–713, 1991

Sulser F: Mode of action of antidepressant drugs. J Clin Psychiatry 44 (sec 2):14–20, 1983

Taylor DP, Hyslop DK, Riblet A: Trazodone, a new non-tricyclic antidepressant without anticholinergic activity. Biochem Pharmacol 29: 2149–2150, 1980

Taylor DP, Smith DW, Hyslop DK, et al: Receptor binding and atypical antidepressant drug discovery, in Receptor Binding in Drug Research. Edited by O'Brien RA. New York, Marcel Dekker, 1986, pp 151–165

Terao T: Comparison of manic switch onset during fluoxetine and trazodone treatment (letter). Biol Psychiatry 33:477–478, 1993

Thompson JW Jr, Ware MR, Blashfield RK: Psychotropic medication and priapism: a comprehensive review. J Clin Psychiatry 51: 430–433, 1990

Van Putten T, Shaffer I: Delirium associated with bupropion (letter). J Clin Psychopharmacol 10:234, 1990

Voortman G, Paanakker JE: Bioavailability of mirtazapine from Remeron tablets after single and multiple oral dosing. Human Psychopharmacology 10 (suppl):S83–S96, 1995

Walker PW, Cole JO, Gardner EA, et al: Improvement in fluoxetine-associated sexual dysfunction in patients switched to bupropion. J Clin Psychiatry 54:459–465, 1993

Weisler RH, Johnston JA, Lineberry CG, et al: Comparison of bupropion and trazodone for the treatment of major depression. J Clin Psychopharmacol 14:170–179, 1994

Wender PH, Reimherr FW: Bupropion treatment of attention-deficit hyperactivity disorder in adults. Am J Psychiatry 147:1018–1020, 1990

Yasui N, Otani K, Keneko S, et al: Inhibition of trazodone metabolism by thioridazine in humans. Ther Drug Monit 17:333–335, 1995

Zikov M, Roes KCR, Pols AG: Efficacy of Org 3770 (mirtazapine) vs amitriptyline in patients with major depressive disorder: a meta-analysis. Human Psychopharmacology 10 (suppl):S135–S145, 1995

Zimmer B, Daly F, Benjamin L: More on combination antidepressant therapy. Arch Gen Psychiatry 41:527–528, 1984

Zmitek A: Trazodone-induced mania. Br J Psychiatry 151:274–275, 1987

Zubieta JK, Demitrack MA: Possible bupropion precipitation of mania and a mixed affective state (letter). J Clin Psychopharmacol 11:327–328, 1991

FIVE

Benzodiazepines

James C. Ballenger, M.D.

HISTORY AND DISCOVERY

The development of the benzodiazepines began in the mid-1950s when Roche Laboratories began to investigate the potential therapeutic properties of myanesin. Myanesin had demonstrated sedative and muscle relaxant features when tested on animals, but when administered to humans, its effects were weak and only brief in duration (Randall 1982). However, this finding stimulated interest and subsequent investigation of two compounds that had been initially developed in 1955 by Roche chemists Leo Sternbach and Earl Reeder. In May 1957, when these compounds were submitted for pharmacological evaluation, laboratory tests indicated their superiority to meprobamate on all measures used and to chlorpromazine on some.

The first benzodiazepine was patented in 1959 and introduced as Librium in 1960. Known generically as methaminodiazepoxide, Librium's generic name was later changed to chlordiazepoxide (Sternbach 1982). Continued testing of related compounds led to the development and introduction in 1963 of diazepam, an antianxiety agent 3–10 times more potent than chlordiazepoxide, with a broader spectrum of activity and greater muscle relaxant properties. The study of benzodiazepine derivatives has continued, and now more than three dozen benzodiazepines are available on the market (Smith and Wesson 1985) derived from or related to these early compounds (Sternbach 1982). Alprazolam, a triazolobenzodiazepine, has received the most recent attention. In 1992, it was given the first U.S. Food and Drug Administration (FDA) approval for treatment of panic disorder.

STRUCTURE-ACTIVITY RELATIONS

Chemically, the benzodiazepines are made up of 2-amino-benzodiazepine 4-oxides (Sternbach 1982). The first benzodiazepine developed, chlordiazepoxide, was the result of a compound created by treating the quinazoline N-oxide with methylamine, a primary amine (Sternbach 1982). Investigation revealed that the development of chlordiazepoxide resulted from the expansion of an atypical ring in the benzodiazepine derivative, and the compound contained a seven-member diazepine ring rather than a six-member pyrimidine ring (Sternbach and Reeder 1961).

Continued laboratory study and attempts to develop other related but improved compounds led to the discovery that the features shared by these compounds were the 1,4-benzodiazepine ring system, a chlorine in the 7 position, and the phenyl group in the 5 position (Sternbach 1982) (Figure 5–1). This discovery ultimately led to the development of several related compounds, including diazepam. Most benzodiazepines have a 5-aryl and a 1,4-diazepine ring, and modification of the ring systems produces benzodiazepines with somewhat different properties. Also, increasing the electron-attracting ability of the attachment at the R_1 position (occupied by chlorine in Figure 5–1) increases the potency of the resultant benzodiazepine (e.g., NO_2 for the potent benzodiazepine nitrazepam) (Malizia and Nutt 1995). The benzodiazepine currently most often prescribed for the treatment of anxiety— alprazolam—is a triazolobenzodiazepine, formed by the addition of a heterocyclic ring that joins the 1 and 2 positions of the benzodiazepine ring system (Sternbach 1982).

PHARMACOLOGICAL PROFILE

Animal Studies

Numerous hypotheses regarding the mechanism by which the benzodiazepines reduce anxiety have undergone rigorous scientific investi-

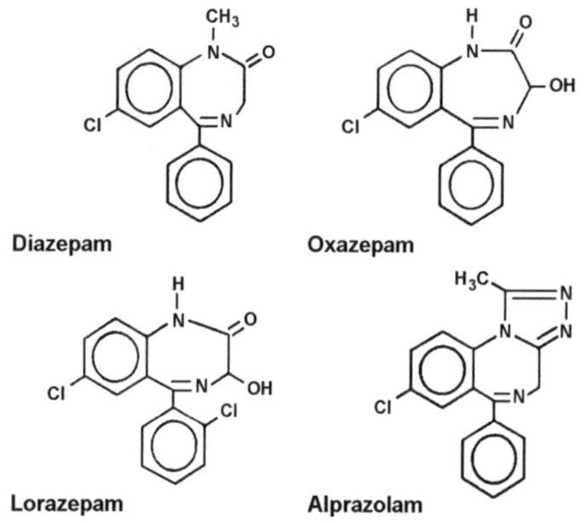

Figure 5–1. Chemical structures for benzodiazepines.
Source. Reprinted from Bernstein JG: *Handbook of Drug Therapy in Psychiatry,* 2nd Edition. Littleton, MA, PSG Publishing, 1988. Copyright 1988, Mosby-Year Book. Used with permission.

gation with animal experimentation. Most of the animal studies conducted to predict the ability of the benzodiazepines to reduce anxiety use an anticonflict or antipunishment effect, also known as a behavioral disinhibitory or behavioral antisuppressant action (Dantzer 1977; Gray 1982; Haefely 1978; Kilts et al. 1981; Sepinwall and Cook 1978; Simon and Soubrie 1979; Thiébot and Soubrié 1983).

The Geller-Seifter test (Geller and Seifter 1960) and the Vogel punished drinking test (Vogel et al. 1971), two of the most frequently used conflict tests, predict antianxiety efficacy of benzodiazepines (or other drugs) by their ability to increase responsivity in a conflict or punishment situation. In the Geller-Seifter test, the rat is rewarded with food for pressing a lever. However, the rat is alternately and variably given shocks when pressing the lever, thereby decreasing its willingness to depress the lever. In the Vogel punished drinking test, thirsty rats are allowed to drink water but are given shocks through either the water spout or the bars on the floor of the cage. In both of these tests, when rats were administered benzodiazepines, their response rate during the potential shock situation increased, but the benzodiazepine had no effect on their responsivity in a nonshock situation (Cook and Sepinwall 1975; File and Hyde 1978; Margules and Stein 1968).

The punished locomotion test, which was developed more recently than the other two tests, administers shock to the rat as it moves from one metal plate to another, alternating shock with no shock on a variable schedule (File 1990).

Other predictive tests have been developed that assess animal responses in social situations. Rats are placed in settings that are either unfamiliar or extremely well lit, and then the setting is alternated on a variable basis. Antianxiety potency is predicted by the amount of time rats spend engaged socially in these settings. Benzodiazepines have been shown to be effective in increasing the amount of time spent in social interaction in the unfamiliar or bright conditions.

These tests have been validated behaviorally and by measuring changes in adrenocorticotropic hormone (ACTH), hypothalamic noradrenaline, and corticosterone (File 1980, 1985, 1990; File and Hyde 1978, 1979).

Anxiety in the social situation has also been assessed with the elevated plus-maze, a device shaped like a plus sign with two closed and two open arms. The benzodiazepines or other anxiolytics lead the rat to spend increased amounts of time on the open arms of the maze. This measure has also been validated physiologically and behaviorally with regard to anxiety (Pellow and File 1986; Pellow et al. 1985).

Pharmacological Properties

Almost all of the benzodiazepines have similar pharmacological profiles. All are sedating; in fact, it is difficult to separate the anxiety-reducing properties of the benzodiazepines from their sedating properties. Therefore, they have prominent hypnotic activity, and all have anticonvulsant and muscle relaxant activity.

Muscle relaxation is thought to be mediated at the spinal cord level and antianxiety effects in cortical or, perhaps, limbic areas (Lader 1987). Anticonvulsant activity appears to occur through inhibition of seizure activity by potentiation of γ-aminobutyric acid (GABA)–ergic neuronal circuits (see "Mechanism of Action" section) at multiple levels of the central nervous system (CNS), including the brain stem. Ataxic side effects presumably are secondary to benzodiazepine actions in the cerebellum, hypnotic effects in the reticular formation, and amnestic effects in the hippocampus.

At routine doses, benzodiazepines have little effect on the cardiovascular and respiratory systems, which probably explains their wide margin of safety. Even in overdose situations, patients who have taken only a benzodiazepine rarely experience respiratory depression severe enough to require attention. More commonly, serious overdoses are the result of combining a benzodiazepine with another depressant drug, usually alcohol (Finkle et al. 1979; Greenblatt et al. 1977).

The effects of benzodiazepines on sleep have been well studied and include increases in total time asleep, reduction in sleep latency, decreased awakenings, and decreases in Stages 1, 2, 3, and 4 sleep (Greenblatt and Shader 1974; Mendelson et al. 1977). Benzodiazepines generally decrease time spent in rapid eye movement (REM) sleep but increase the number of REM cycles and, therefore, the number of dreams. When benzodiazepines are discontinued after chronic use, rebound increases in REM sleep often occur, and patients often report increases in nightmares or bizarre dreams.

PHARMACOKINETICS AND DISPOSITION

Administered orally, benzodiazepines are generally well absorbed from the gastrointestinal tract and reach peak levels within 30 minutes to 6–8 hours. Clorazepate is metabolized in the stomach to its active metabolite before absorption. Only lorazepam and midazolam are predictably absorbed after intramuscular injection. The high lipid solubility of most of the benzodiazepines (e.g., diazepam) allows for easy passage into the brain (DeVane et al. 1991). This also means, however, that activity of the benzodiazepines may be prolonged in extremely overweight people, who tend to have a higher ratio of fat to lean tissue (Bernstein 1988; Harvey 1985).

The benzodiazepines are metabolized primarily through the liver, and most are biotransformed by oxidation (Phase I metabolism). A few benzodiazepines, including lorazepam, temazepam, and lormetazepam, are biotransformed by conjugation to inactive glucuronides, sulfates, and acetylated substances (Phase II metabolism) (Greenblatt et al. 1983). Some benzodiazepines, including diazepam, chlordiazepoxide, and flurazepam, are metabolized through both Phase I and II processes (Lader 1987).

The mechanism by which these drugs are metabolized (i.e., through the liver) is of significance in prescribing the benzodiazepines for certain groups of patients. Benzodiazepines that are metabolized by Phase II alone are better tolerated in patients with impaired liver function. Patients affected include elderly people, alcoholic individuals with cirrhotic livers, and people who smoke (Lader 1987).

Duration of benzodiazepine action is, in part, related to lipid solubility, in that how quickly a benzodiazepine gets into the brain and how quickly it leaves the brain defines its duration of therapeutic action. Half-life is almost as important, and the benzodiazepines have widely divergent half-lives with different clinical effects (Table 5–1). Obviously, the shorter half-life benzodiazepines require multiple daily dosing. This clinical feature can be positive and reassuring for some patients but may have negative connotations for others. Specifically, the recurrence of anxiety symptoms with a rapid decline in blood level in those agents with short half-lives (e.g., alprazolam) can be a concern for some patients (e.g., those with panic disorder).

The duration of action of many of the benzodiazepines is much more dependent on the half-lives of the active metabolites than of the parent compounds. Perhaps the most clinically important example is the hypnotic flurazepam. Although its half-life is only 2–3 hours, the half-life of its primary metabolite, N-desalkylflurazepam, is more than 50 hours. In the case of flurazepam, this feature is often negative because it can cause unwanted daytime drowsiness.

Other factors that affect elimination rate and half-life include the length of time that the drug is prescribed and the number of doses administered each day (Bernstein 1988).

There are conflicting reports regarding the correlation between dose and plasma levels. Four early studies using benzodiazepines to treat anxiety, sleep difficulties, or a combination of symptoms showed no correlation between plasma concentrations and patient responsivity (Bond et al. 1977; Kangas et al. 1979; Tansella et al. 1975, 1978). However, other studies in which patients were treated for anxiety found a positive correlation between benzodiazepine plasma levels and patient improvement (Bellantuono et al. 1980; Curry 1974; Dasberg et al. 1974).

Lesser and colleagues (1992) reported a significant correlation between plasma level of alprazolam and reduction in panic and phobic symptomatology and in side effects. Plasma level was definitely correlated with reduction in panic attacks. Greenblatt and colleagues (1993) also reported a greater reduction in spontaneous panic attacks in patients with higher plasma levels of alprazolam at week 3.

MECHANISM OF ACTION

The GABA Role

The elucidation of the mechanism of action for the benzodiazepines began with the discovery that GABA serves as the major inhibitory neurotransmitter in the CNS, with receptors located on approximately 30% of cortical and thalamic neurons (Costa et al. 1975; Haefely 1985; Olsen and Tobin 1990). Considerable evidence now indicates that the major pharmacological effects of the benzodiazepines are produced secondary to the binding of the benzodiazepines to $GABA_A$ receptors in the CNS. Extensive research has confirmed the critical interrelatedness of benzodiazepine actions and GABAergic mechanisms (Costa et al. 1975; Haefely et al. 1975; Polc et al. 1974).

Knowledge of how benzodiazepines produce anxiolytic effects is evolving rapidly. GABA increases the propensity of the benzodiazepines to bind to specific receptor sites on the GABA-benzodiazepine receptor complex, and the converse is also true (i.e., both mutually enhance the binding of the other) (Paul and Skolnick 1982; Tallman et al. 1978, 1980). The principal action of GABA is to open the chloride ionophore on this complex. Although benzodiazepines appear to have no effect themselves

Table 5–1. Benzodiazepines and their metabolites (including half-life)

Drug	Half-life	Active metabolites	Half-life
Triazolam	Short (<6 hours)	None	
Alprazolam	Intermediate (6–20 hours)	Not clinically important	
Lorazepam	Intermediate (6–20 hours)	None	
Oxazepam	Intermediate (6–20 hours)	None	
Temazepam	Intermediate (6–20 hours)	None	
Chlordiazepoxide	Intermediate (6–20 hours)	Desmethylchlordiazepoxide	Intermediate (6–20 hours)
		Demoxepam	Long (>20 hours)
		Nordiazepam	Long (>20 hours)
Diazepam	Long (>20 hours)	Nordiazepam	Long (>20 hours)
Clorazepate	Short (<6 hours)	Nordiazepam	Long (>20 hours)
Halazepam	Short (<6 hours)	Nordiazepam	Long (>20 hours)
Prazepam	Short (<6 hours)	Nordiazepam	Long (>20 hours)
Flurazepam	Short (<6 hours)	N-hydroxyethyl-flurazepam	Short (<6 hours)
		N-desalkylflurazepam	Long (>20 hours)

Source. Adapted from Harvey SC: "Hypnotics and Sedatives," in *Goodman and Gilman's The Pharmacological Basis of Therapeutics,* 7th Edition. Edited by Gilman AG, Goodman LS, Rall TW. New York, Macmillan, 1985, pp. 339–371. Copyright 1985, the McGraw-Hill Companies. Used with permission.

on the $GABA_A$ complex or the ionophore, in the presence of GABA, benzodiazepines increase GABA's effects on the chloride ionophore. That is, they increase the number of openings of the chloride channel, which causes decreased cellular excitability (Bernstein 1988; Hsiao and Potter 1990; Study and Barker 1981).

Benzodiazepine Receptors

In the 1970s, several groups of researchers identified specific benzodiazepine binding sites in the brain (Bossman et al. 1977; Braestrup and Squires 1977; Möhler and Okada 1977a, 1977b; Squires and Braestrup 1977). The important discovery of high affinity, saturable, and stereospecific binding of benzodiazepine in the CNS provided the basis for the diverse actions of benzodiazepines. Evidence that these benzodiazepine receptors are localized on neurons in the CNS and mediate the pharmacological actions of the benzodiazepines is principally provided by the strong correlation between anxio-

lytic potencies of various benzodiazepines and their ability to displace tritiated benzodiazepines from benzodiazepine receptors in vitro. This mediation is also shown by the benzodiazepines' potencies as anticonvulsants, anxiolytics, and muscle relaxants and in various animal models of inhibited behaviors (Young and Kuhar 1980). By convention, these receptors have been called the *benzodiazepine receptor* or the *benzodiazepine-GABA receptor.* However, it is important to remember that other substances also bind to this receptor complex (e.g., picrotoxin, alcohol, barbiturates, muscimol, penicillin, neurosteroids).

The $GABA_A$ receptor complex is an oligomeric glycoprotein. It was originally thought to have two subunits (α and β), each with 4 segments with 20 amino acids (Barnard et al. 1988). The GABA site is apparently associated with the β subunit and the benzodiazepine receptor with the α subunit (Thomas and Tallman 1981). It also appears that there are 4 membrane-spanning regions of approximately

20–30 hydrophobic amino acids in each subunit (Figure 5–2) (Zorumski and Isenberg 1991). However, cloning studies have defined 15 different proteins in this receptor in the mammalian CNS (Lüddens and Korpi 1995; Lüddens et al. 1995; Seeburg et al. 1990), and at least 5 subunits have multiple (1–6) variants within each. Although the possible number of variations in the benzodiazepine receptor probably exceeds 500, currently 6α, 3β, 2 (or 3) σ, and 1δ subunits are known (Lüddens and Wisden 1991). Other studies suggest 5 subunits: 6α, 4β, 2γ, 2δ, and a retinal (rho) (Malizia and Nutt 1995). It is now known that the pharmacology of the benzodiazepine receptor varies principally according to the α subunit expressed. Expression of the σ_2 subunit is required for the $GABA_A$-chloride channels formed to respond consistently and robustly to benzodiazepines. If the σ_2 subunit is replaced by an σ_1 subunit, the benzodiazepine receptors are more reminiscent of the peripheral-type benzodiazepine receptors (Ymer et al. 1990).

Although most benzodiazepines bind to $GABA_A$-benzodiazepine receptors with similar affinities throughout the brain, there are some differences for certain benzodiazepines. Although controversy in this area remains (Malizia and Nutt 1995), benzodiazepine receptors have been characterized as either type I (with high affinity for triazolopyridazines and β-carbolines) (Nielsen and Braestrup 1980; Sieghart et al. 1985) or type II (with lower affinities for these compounds). Type I receptors are the most common $GABA_A$ receptor class in the CNS. The number of type II receptors is high in the hippocampus, striatum, and spinal cord (Lo et al. 1983; Sieghart et al. 1985), whereas the number of type I receptors is high in the cerebellum and low in the hippocampus. Numbers of both subtypes are equally high in cortical layers (Faull and Villiger 1988; Faull et al. 1987; Olsen et al. 1990). A third class of benzodiazepine receptor is primarily located in cerebellar granule cells, involves the α_6 subunit, and is relatively insensitive to benzodiazepines (Lüddens et al. 1990).

The functions of the β, σ, and δ subunits are less well known, but they do seem to be involved in agonist (GABA) binding (Lüddens and Wisden 1991). The $GABA_A$-benzodiazepine receptor complex is presumably a pentamer composed of α, β, and σ glycoprotein subunits, each with four regions that span the membrane (Figure 5–3) (Zorumski and Isenberg 1991). The actual functional characteristics of the receptor in terms of GABA or benzodiazepine binding would presumably result from whatever subunits were involved in the unit. Given the apparent and probably tremendous heterogeneity of these subunits, there appears to be a strong possibility that new and potentially more selective therapeutic agents can be synthesized because of this heterogeneity.

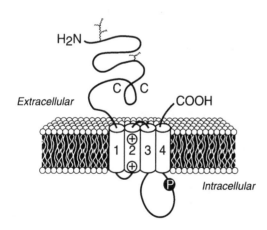

Figure 5–2.   Model for γ-aminobutyric acid A (GABA_A) receptor subunits.
Source.   Reprinted from Zorumski CF, Isenberg KE: "Insights Into the Structure and Function of GABA-Benzodiazepine Receptors: Ion Channels and Psychiatry." *American Journal of Psychiatry* 148:162–173, 1991. Used with permission.

Ligands of the Benzodiazepine Receptor: Agonists, Antagonists, and Inverse Agonists

The benzodiazepines' action on the GABA receptor complex is mediated through the benzodiazepine receptor on this complex but in what

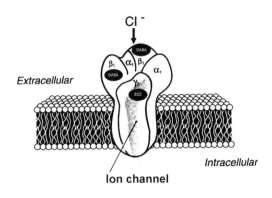

Extracellular

Intracellular

Ion channel

Figure 5–3. Model of the γ-aminobutyric acid (GABA)–benzodiazepine (BDZ) receptor complex.
Source. Reprinted from Zorumski CF, Isenberg KE: "Insights Into the Structure and Function of GABA-Benzodiazepine Receptors: Ion Channels and Psychiatry." *American Journal of Psychiatry* 148:162–173, 1991. Used with permission.

appears to be a unique mechanism described as *positive allosteric modulation* (Haefely 1990). The binding site for the benzodiazepines operates differently from that for other neurotransmitter receptors; that is, the benzodiazepine receptor mediates the effects of different drugs that have directly opposing effects (i.e., either increasing or decreasing anxiety). Differing agents that have agonist, antagonist, and inverse agonist actions have been studied (for review, see Doble and Martin 1992; Gardner et al. 1993; Nutt 1989).

In addition to the benzodiazepines, zopiclone, triazolopyridazines, pyrazoloquinolinone derivatives, zolpidem, and some β-carboline derivatives have benzodiazepine agonist activity, reduce anxiety, and are sedating in a manner similar, but not identical, to the benzodiazepines. They do so by acting synergistically with GABA to increase the openings of the chloride channel (Blanchard et al. 1979; Klepner et al. 1979; Stephens et al. 1984; Yokoyama et al. 1982).

Benzodiazepine antagonists block the ability of benzodiazepine agonists to amplify the effects of GABA but have no intrinsic activity themselves. The imidazobenzodiazepine deriv-

ative Ro 15-1788 is one of the best studied. In both animal and human studies, this antagonist has been found to have properties that enable it to totally negate all anxiety-reducing actions of benzodiazepines (Bonetti et al. 1982; Darragh et al. 1981a, 1981b, 1982a, 1982b; Haefely 1985; Hunkeler et al. 1981; Möhler et al. 1981; Polc et al. 1981) by inhibiting benzodiazepine binding to CNS neuronal binding sites (Möhler and Richards 1981; Richards et al. 1982).

The important discovery of an anxiogenic (i.e., anxiety-increasing) ligand utilized the social interaction test and found that ethyl-β-carboxylate (β-CCE) increased anxiety (File et al. 1982). The anxiogenic property attributed to β-CCE in animals was replicated in humans (Dorow et al. 1983) and was confirmed in animal experiments (Corda et al. 1983; File and Pellow 1984; File et al. 1984; Hindley et al. 1985; Pellow and File 1986; Petersen et al. 1982, 1983; Stephens and Kehr 1985). Although most β-carbolines are anxiogenic, others have been developed that have anxiolytic properties instead (File 1990).

Inverse agonists act directly to decrease the number of times that the chloride channel opens (Costa and Guidotti 1985; Zorumski and Isenberg 1991); thus, they have anxiogenic properties. These inverse agonists include β-carboline derivatives and the diazepam-binding inhibitor peptide (Breier and Paul 1988).

Partial agonists. Partial agonists are compounds that have less functional effect after occupying the receptor than do full agonists, and, therefore, a higher fraction of receptors must be occupied to match the action of a full agonist. A full response might not occur even with 100% receptor occupancy. The discovery that certain compounds can function as partial agonists at one receptor and full agonists at another complicated the issue (Knoflach et al. 1993; Wafford et al. 1993). Partial agonists along the entire spectrum of agonist, antagonist, and inverse agonist have now been synthesized (Cole et al. 1995).

There is considerable clinical research under way based on the theoretical possibility that partial agonists have anxiolytic properties but would not be as sedating as or as prone to cause withdrawal symptoms as full agonists (Feely et al. 1989; Martin et al. 1990). The agent under most vigorous clinical study has been abecarnil (Ballenger 1991; Potokar and Nutt 1994).

Endogenous ligands. The presence of the benzodiazepine receptor argues for the existence of an endogenous ligand for this receptor (Paul et al. 1980). In theory, it could be an anxiolytic agonist or, in fact, an anxiogenic inverse agonist (see Haefely 1988 for review). However, no ligand in living humans has been found (Costa 1989). Perhaps the most likely candidate at this time is the diazepam-binding inhibitor, which is thought to have anxiogenic properties (DeRobertis et al. 1988).

Note that DeBlas and Sangameswaran (1986) isolated *N*-desmethyldiazepam (a metabolite of several benzodiazepines, including diazepam, chlordiazepoxide, and medazepam) from the brains of rats never exposed to benzodiazepines. Benzodiazepine metabolites were also found in human brains that were stored in the 1940s (long before development of the first benzodiazepine in the early 1960s) (File 1988). Investigators have hypothesized that the source of these naturally occurring benzodiazepine-like substances may come from the diet, based on evidence that benzodiazepine biosynthesis exists in fungi (Luckner 1984), and diazepam and lorazepam have been found in various foods (Unseld et al. 1988; Wildmann 1988).

INDICATIONS

Benzodiazepines are generally well tolerated, with minimal side effects, and are efficacious for several conditions, most notably the treatment of anxiety and anxiety-related disorders. Indications for which benzodiazepines are used are similar to those for which barbiturates were once prescribed. However, the greater tolerability and safety profile of benzodiazepines have been responsible in large part for virtually eliminating barbiturates from being prescribed for anxiety conditions (Hollister 1982). In addition to their use as effective antianxiety agents, benzodiazepines have been proven to be effective hypnotics.

Flurazepam has been one of the most frequently prescribed hypnotics in the United States. It is effective in helping patients achieve and maintain sleep and does so with fewer of the troublesome side effects attributed to most other nonbenzodiazepine hypnotics and without the tolerance that develops to other drugs with long-term use (Kales et al. 1975). The short half-life benzodiazepine triazolam reached widespread popularity as a hypnotic largely because it was cleared from the system before morning and therefore was not associated with daytime drowsiness. However, concern and controversy surrounding triazolam's potential serious side effects (particularly at higher doses) have dampened enthusiasm and significantly reduced its use.

Benzodiazepines are also effective when used as muscle relaxants or as anticonvulsants, during alcohol withdrawal, and as intravenous anesthetics (Hollister 1982). Clonazepam is labeled as an anticonvulsant and is widely used for that indication, but it is also popular for treating anxiety conditions.

Benzodiazepines have become one of the most frequently used treatments for alcohol withdrawal. They are quite effective because of their cross-reactivity with alcohol as well as their anticonvulsant properties and anxiety-reducing efficacy. Benzodiazepines are traditionally given in a loading fashion and then rapidly tapered over the first 3–7 days of alcohol withdrawal.

The primary indications for benzodiazepines are certainly in the treatment of anxiety disorders. Eight benzodiazepines are labeled for anxiety (generalized anxiety disorder [GAD]), alprazolam is designated for panic disorder, and clonazepam is also widely used for these indications. Although benzodiazepines are used as ancillary medications in the management of obsessive-compulsive disorder, social phobia, and posttraumatic stress disorder (PTSD), their primary use has been in the treatment of GAD and more recently for panic disorder. Benzodiazepines have become the primary pharmacological treatment for GAD. Although certain psychotherapeutic techniques (e.g., support, meditation, relaxation) are effective and widely used, they are often relatively unavailable or unacceptable for various reasons.

GAD is characterized by excessive anxiety and worry, accompanied by motoric symptoms of anxiety (e.g., tension, autonomic hyperactivity, and vigilance). Despite the seemingly simple nature of this disorder, GAD is often chronic (Angst and Vollrath 1991) and associated with considerable impairment and distress (Croft-Jeffreys and Wilkinson 1989).

Panic disorder is characterized by recurrent severe panic attacks and persistent worry that the panic attacks will recur or that they indicate serious medical or psychiatric consequences (Ballenger and Fyer 1993). Panic disorder is also a chronic condition in most clinical cases and is associated with even more morbidity than GAD. This includes frequent visits to the emergency room, family and occupational difficulties, financial dependency, abuse of alcohol, and even increased suicide attempts (Cowley 1992; Klerman et al. 1991; Markowitz et al. 1989; Weissman et al. 1989).

Because all benzodiazepines are apparently equally efficacious (Greenblatt and Shader 1974), the choice of a specific benzodiazepine is often influenced by physician or patient preference, side-effect differences (there are actually few), and marketplace issues. Diazepam was the most popular anxiolytic through the 1970s and early 1980s, when it was supplanted by alprazolam. In part, this change reflected a shift from one type of benzodiazepine to another. Diazepam has a long half-life and therefore has considerable accumulation over time. This feature results in the advantages of not needing multiple daily dosing and having less potential for withdrawal symptomatology when the drug is abruptly discontinued. However, these same characteristics can result in excess sedation and interference with optimal functioning. Alprazolam has a shorter half-life (6–20 hours), and its effective half-life is even shorter and therefore is associated with less accumulation, a multiple daily dosing requirement, and more potential for withdrawal symptoms when abruptly discontinued. More recently, clonazepam has become increasingly popular as a potent benzodiazepine with a longer half-life.

Early work with alprazolam in treating patients with panic disorder suggested it might have unique efficacy. Considerable research has established its efficacy for patients with panic disorder (Ballenger et al. 1988; Cross National Collaborative Panic Study, Second Phase Investigators 1992), leading to FDA approval for this indication. However, other benzodiazepines (e.g., diazepam, lorazepam, clonazepam) clearly are also effective when taken in sufficient doses (Charney and Woods 1989; Howell et al. 1987; Noyes et al. 1984; Schweizer et al. 1988).

Benzodiazepine treatment of GAD or panic disorder frequently proves to be long term, in keeping with the chronic nature of these disorders (Ballenger 1991; Romach et al. 1992; Schatzberg and Ballenger 1991). Most research experience with the benzodiazepines is short term, although longer-term treatment efficacy (i.e., up to 6 months) has been established in some trials (Cohn and Wilcox 1984; Fabre et al. 1981). In trials in which the benzodiazepine is discontinued blindly, original anxiety symptoms return in many patients (i.e., relapse), but this is not true for all patients (Rickels et al. 1980, 1983, 1990, 1991). Clinicians must periodically reassess the need for continued benzodiazepine therapy by tapering and discontinuing benzodiazepines if symptoms do not recur.

Benzodiazepines are also used to treat a number of conditions other than those previously described (Wesson 1985). Because of clonazepam's rapid onset of action, it has been used as an adjunctive treatment with lithium to control the agitation seen during the acute manic phase of bipolar disorder (Chouinard et al. 1983). Benzodiazepines have also been used to treat night terrors as well as sleep or dream disturbances in patients with PTSD because benzodiazepines can decrease Stage 4 sleep (Friedman 1981; Kramer 1979). Clonazepam has also been used to treat nocturnal myoclonus (Boghew 1980; Matthews 1979) and tic douloureux when carbamazepine is ineffective (Court and Kase 1976).

Finally, the benzodiazepines have been used successfully in Third-World countries to treat tetanus, cerebral malaria, chloroquine toxicity, and maternal eclampsia (Ward 1985).

SIDE EFFECTS AND TOXICOLOGY

Benzodiazepines have proven efficacy for many conditions. Benzodiazepines that are used to treat anxiety disorders generally have a more favorable side-effect profile than many of the other pharmacological agents used for this indication (i.e., monoamine oxidase inhibitors and tricyclic antidepressants). Also, benzodiazepines begin to exert their therapeutic effects rapidly, with improvement generally seen in the first week of treatment.

As a class, benzodiazepines have remarkably few side effects; the principal one is sedation. Patients report feeling sedated, drowsy, and slowed down and may fall asleep during daytime activities or have ataxia or slurred speech (Lader 1995; Linnoila et al. 1983). In laboratory settings, slowed psychomotor function has been observed (Hindmarch et al. 1991). Amnesia (anterograde) occurs with intravenous administration, and this effect is used widely in anesthesia induction (King 1992). However, amnesia has also been reported with oral dosing, especially with the hypnotic triazolam (Greenblatt et al. 1991). Amnesia is also present in less dramatic fashion in routine use, with some patients reporting relatively minor but demonstrable difficulties in learning new material (Barbee 1993;

Ghoneim and Mewaldt 1990; Greenblatt et al. 1991; Hindmarch et al. 1991; King 1992; Lader 1995; Linnoila et al. 1983; L. G. Miller et al. 1988; Roth et al. 1984; Shader et al. 1986; Tönne et al. 1995). However, these side effects are generally transient and disappear quickly (usually within days) as tolerance to these effects develops in most patients (L. G. Miller et al. 1988).

Perhaps the greatest concern with the use of benzodiazepines is in elderly patients, in whom adverse events including falls from ataxia, hip fractures, and confusion are more common than in younger patients (Aiden et al. 1995; Lader 1995; Ray et al. 1987). In younger individuals, caution has always been suggested around benzodiazepine use and operation of heavy machinery. This advice is probably most important around the driving of automobiles (O'Hanlon et al. 1995).

The controversy surrounding benzodiazepine administration and potential abuse or addiction in routine patient use is generally not supported by the available scientific evidence. (See Shader and Greenblatt 1993 for an excellent review of this complex area.) In a large community study of long-term alprazolam users, Romach and colleagues (1992) found that dosage did not escalate over prolonged use and that most patients used the benzodiazepines as prescribed. In fact, if deviations occurred, it was generally that a patient took less than the prescribed dosage. This area has been more controversial than warranted in part because of confusion over the meanings of addiction, dependence, and abuse. Efforts have been made to clear up this confusion, especially differentiating abuse from withdrawal symptom liability (Ballenger et al. 1993; Linsen et al. 1995; N. S. Miller 1995; N. S. Miller et al. 1995).

Evidence regarding the use of benzodiazepines during pregnancy is inconclusive. For this reason, pregnancy should be postponed until benzodiazepine treatment has been discontinued. In addition, because benzodiazepines are excreted through breast milk and place the nursing infant at risk for lethargy and inadequate temperature regulation, nursing mothers should also be cautioned against the use of benzodiazepines (Bernstein 1988).

Discontinuation

For the sake of thoroughness, a statement about discontinuation of the benzodiazepines is in order (see Ballenger et al. 1993; Shader and Greenblatt 1993). Numerous groups, including some medical professionals, have perpetuated the idea that if benzodiazepines are used long term, patients become "addicted" to the benzodiazepines, implying that they will abuse them or have an extreme withdrawal syndrome when the medication is discontinued. Actually, what occurs with benzodiazepines is similar to the effects of other medications used for long-term treatment of a medical and/or psychiatric condition and can be compared to what happens when a patient's cardiovascular medicine (e.g., propranolol, methyldopa) is suddenly discontinued (Garbus et al. 1979). In essence, the body goes through an adaptational process to the drug, and if medication is discontinued too abruptly, the patient can have withdrawal symptoms. The patient may also experience a transient recurrence of anxiety symptoms at levels more intense than those experienced before treatment; this is called *rebound*. The patient may also experience a return of symptoms that were present before treatment (relapse). However, if dosage is adjusted and gradually titrated downward, and if patients and their families are educated about what to expect during the discontinuation process, most patients can manage the transient withdrawal symptoms without much difficulty (see Ballenger et al. 1993 and Shader and Greenblatt 1993 for review), although this area remains somewhat controversial (Ashton 1995; Lader 1995).

DRUG-DRUG INTERACTIONS

Because benzodiazepines are frequently used for long-term treatment of conditions such as

anxiety, the chances are high that at some point during treatment, the patient will receive another medication, either a prescription or an over-the-counter drug. It was originally believed that benzodiazepines did not interact with other drugs; however, it is now known that this is not the case. Cimetidine and disulfiram both slow the metabolism of benzodiazepines, particularly the longer-acting benzodiazepines, including chlordiazepoxide and diazepam (Bernstein 1988; Glassman and Salzman 1987; Ruffalo and Thompson 1980). If a patient taking diazepam is also prescribed gallamine or succinylcholine, paralysis can result (Hansten 1985). Other drugs that can exacerbate the effects of benzodiazepines include isoniazid and estrogens, an effect produced by enzyme inhibition. Fluvoxamine inhibits the cytochrome P450 (CYP) 3A4 enzyme and can be associated with increased levels of alprazolam.

Other drugs act to reduce benzodiazepine effects. These drugs include antacids, which affect benzodiazepine metabolism by reduced gastrointestinal absorption, and tobacco and rifampin, which interfere with enzyme induction (Bernstein 1988). When digoxin is given to a patient taking benzodiazepines, the digoxin half-life increases; however, the mechanism by which this occurs is not known (Bernstein 1988).

At times, benzodiazepines, along with other sedative and anxiety-reducing medications, can cause significant sedation and CNS depression. When these drugs are taken at doses that are too high or when they are combined with alcohol or other sedating medications, they can cause significant sedation and occasionally respiratory depression as well (Bernstein 1988).

SUMMARY

Although the benzodiazepines continue to generate some controversy in the lay press and public, they are widely utilized because of their overall effectiveness in many common conditions (e.g., anxiety, alcoholism, stress, insomnia) and their favorable side-effect spectrum. Advances in the molecular neurobiology of the CNS benzodiazepine receptors hold considerable promise for better understanding of brain mechanisms underlying anxiety and for the possible development of even more specific and effective antianxiety agents.

REFERENCES

Aiden F, O'Connell D, Henry D, et al: Benzodiazepine use as a cause of cognitive impairment in elderly hospital inpatients. J Gerontol 50A (2): M99–M106, 1995

Angst J, Vollrath M: The natural history of anxiety disorders. Acta Psychiatr Scand 84:446–452, 1991

Ashton H: Protracted withdrawal from benzodiazepines: the post-withdrawal syndrome. Psychiatric Annals 25:174–179, 1995

Ballenger JC: Long-term pharmacologic treatment of panic disorder. J Clin Psychiatry 52:18–23, 1991

Ballenger JC, Fyer AJ: Examining criteria for panic disorder. Hosp Community Psychiatry 44: 226–228, 1993

Ballenger JC, Burrows G, DuPont R, et al: Alprazolam in panic disorder and agoraphobia: results from a multicenter trial, I: efficacy in short-term treatment. Arch Gen Psychiatry 455:413–422, 1988

Ballenger JC, Pecknold J, Rickels K, et al: Medication discontinuation in panic disorder. J Clin Psychiatry 54 (10 suppl):15–21, 1993

Barbee JG: Memory, benzodiazepines, and anxiety: integration of theoretical and clinical perspectives. J Clin Psychiatry 54 (10 suppl):86–97, 1993

Barnard EA, Darlison MG, Fujita N, et al: Molecular biology of the GABA$_A$ receptor. Adv Exp Med Biol 236:31–45, 1988

Bellantuono C, Reggi V, Tognoni G, et al: Benzodiazepines: clinical pharmacology and therapeutic use. Drugs 19:195–219, 1980

Bernstein JG: Handbook of Drug Therapy in Psychiatry, 2nd Edition. Littleton, MA, PSG Publishing, 1988

Blanchard JC, Boireau A, Garret C, et al: In vitro and in vivo inhibition by zopiclone of benzodiazepine binding to rodent brain receptors. Life Sci 24:2417–2420, 1979

Boghew D: Successful treatment of restless legs with clonazepam (letter). Ann Neurol 8:341, 1980

Bond AJ, Hally DM, Lader MH: Plasma concentrations of benzodiazepines. British Journal of Clinical Psychopharmacology 4:51–56, 1977

Bonetti EP, Pieri L, Cumin R, et al: Benzodiazepine antagonist Ro 15-1788: neurological and behavioral effects. Psychopharmacology (Berl) 78: 8–18, 1982

Bossman HB, Case KR, DiStefano P: Diazepam receptor characterization: specific binding of a benzodiazepine to macromolecules in various areas of rat brain. FEBS Lett 82:368–372, 1977

Braestrup C, Squires RF: Specific benzodiazepine receptors in rat brain characterized by high-affinity ^{3}H diazepam binding. Proc Natl Acad Sci U S A 74:3805–3809, 1977

Breier A, Paul SM: Anxiety and the benzodiazepine-GABA receptor complex, in Handbook of Anxiety, Vol 1. Edited by Roth M, Noyes R, Burrows GD. Amsterdam, Elsevier, 1988, pp 193–212

Charney DS, Woods SW: Benzodiazepine treatment of panic disorder: a comparison of alprazolam and lorazepam. J Clin Psychiatry 50:418–423, 1989

Chouinard G, Young SN, Annable L: Antimanic effects of clonazepam. Biol Psychiatry 18: 451–466, 1983

Cohn JB, Wilcox CS: Long-term comparison of alprazolam, lorazepam and placebo in patients with an anxiety disorder. Pharmacotherapy 4: 93–98, 1984

Cole BJ, Hellmann M, Seidelmann D, et al: Effects of benzodiazepine receptor partial inverse agonists in the elevated plus maze test of anxiety in the rat. Psychopharmacology (Berl) 12: 118–126, 1995

Cook L, Sepinwall J: Behavioral analysis of the effects of and mechanisms of action of benzodiazepines, in Mechanism of Action of Benzodiazepines. Edited by Costa E, Grengard P. New York, Raven, 1975, pp 1–28

Corda MG, Blaker WD, Mendelson WB, et al: Beta-carbolines enhance shock-induced suppression of drinking rats. Proc Natl Acad Sci U S A 80:2072–2076, 1983

Costa E: Allosteric modulating centers of transmitter amino and receptors. Neuropsychopharmacology 2:167–174, 1989

Costa E, Guidotti A: Endogenous ligands for benzodiazepine recognition sites. Biochem Pharmacol 34:3399–3403, 1985

Costa E, Guidotti A, Mao CC, et al: New concepts in the mechanism of activity of BZs. Life Sci 17:167–185, 1975

Court JE, Kase CS: Treatment of tic douloureux with a new anticonvulsant (clonazepam). J Neurol Neurosurg Psychiatry 39:297–299, 1976

Cowley DS: Alcohol abuse, substance abuse, and panic disorder. Am J Med 92 (suppl 1A): 41S–48S, 1992

Croft-Jeffreys C, Wilkinson G: Estimated costs of neurotic disorder in UK general practice 1985. Psychol Med 19:549–558, 1989

Cross National Collaborative Panic Study, Second Phase Investigators: Drug treatment of panic disorder: comparative efficacy of alprazolam, imipramine, and placebo. Br J Psychiatry 160:191–202, 1992

Curry SH: Concentration-effect relationship with major and minor tranquilizers. Clin Pharmacol Ther 16:192–197, 1974

Dantzer R: Behavioral effects of benzodiazepines: a review. Biobehavioral Reviews 1:71–86, 1977

Darragh A, Lambe R, Brick I, et al: Reversal of benzodiazepine-induced sedation by intravenous Ro 15-1788 (letter). Lancet 2:1042, 1981a

Darragh A, Lambe R, Scully M, et al: Investigation in man of the efficacy of a benzodiazepine antagonist, Ro 15-1788. Lancet 2:8–10, 1981b

Darragh A, Lambe R, Brick I, et al: Antagonism of the central effects of 3-methyl-clonazepam. Br J Clin Pharmacol 14:871–872, 1982a

Darragh A, Lambe R, Kenny M, et al: Ro 15-1788 antagonizes the central effects of diazepam in man without altering diazepam bioavailability. Br J Clin Pharmacol 14:677–682, 1982b

Dasberg HH, van der Klijn E, Guelen PJR, et al: Plasma concentrations of diazepam and its metabolite N-desmethyldiazepam in relation to anxiolytic effect. Clin Pharmacol Ther 15: 473–483, 1974

DeBlas A, Sangameswaran L: Demonstration and purification of an endogenous benzodiazepine from the mammalian brain with a monoclonal antibody to benzodiazepines. Life Sci 39: 1927–1936, 1986

DeRobertis E, Pena C, Paladini AC, et al: New developments in the search for the endogenous ligand(s) of central benzodiazepine receptors. Neurochem Int 13:1–11, 1988

DeVane CL, Ware MR, Lydiard RB: Pharmacokinetics, pharmacodynamics, and treatment issues of benzodiazepines: alprazolam, adinazolam, and clonazepam. Psychopharmacol Bull 27:463–473, 1991

Doble A, Martin IL: Multiple benzodiazepine receptors: no reason for anxiety. Trends Pharmacol Sc 13:76–81, 1992

Dorow R, Horowski R, Paschelke G, et al: Severe anxiety induced by FG 7142, a beta-carboline ligand for benzodiazepine receptor function. Lancet 2:98–99, 1983

Fabre LF, McLendon DM, Stephens AG: Comparison of the therapeutic effect, tolerance and safety of ketazolam and diazepam administered for six months to outpatients with chronic anxiety neurosis. J Int Med Res 9:191–198, 1981

Faull RL, Villiger JW: Benzodiazepine receptors in the human hippocampal formation: a pharmacological and quantitative autoradiographic study. Neuroscience 26:783–790, 1988

Faull RL, Villiger JW, Holford NH: Benzodiazepine receptors in the human cerebellar cortex: a quantitative autoradiographic and pharmacological study demonstrating the predominance of type I receptors. Brain Res 411:379–385, 1987

Feely M, Boyland P, Picardo A, et al: Lack of anticonvulsant tolerance with RU 32698 and Ro 17-1812. Eur J Pharmacol 164:377–380, 1989

File SE: The use of social interaction as a method for detecting anxiolytic activity of chlordiazepoxide-like drugs. J Neurosci Methods 2: 219–238, 1980

File SE: Animal models for predicting clinical efficacy of anxiolytic drugs: social behaviour. Neuropsychobiology 13:55–62, 1985

File SE: The benzodiazepine receptor and its role in anxiety. Br J Psychiatry 152:599–600, 1988

File SE: Preclinical studies of the mechanisms of anxiety and its treatment, in Neurobiology of Anxiety Disorders. Edited by Ballenger JC. New York, Wiley-Liss, 1990, pp 31–48

File SE, Hyde JRG: Can social interaction be used to measure anxiety? Br J Pharmacol 62:19–24, 1978

File SE, Hyde JRG: A test of anxiety that distinguishes between the actions of benzodiazepines and those of other minor tranquilizers and of stimulants. Pharmacol Biochem Behav 11: 65–69, 1979

File SE, Pellow S: The anxiogenic action of PG 7142 in the social interaction test is reversed by chlordiazepoxide and Ro 15-1788 but not by CGS 8216. Arch Int Pharmacodyn Ther 271: 198–205, 1984

File SE, Lister RG, Nutt DG: The anxiogenic action of benzodiazepine antagonists. Neuropharmacology 21:1033–1037, 1982

File SE, Lister RG, Maninov R, et al: Intrinsic behavioural actions of propyl beta-carboline-3-carboxylate. Neuropharmacology 23:463–466, 1984

Finkle BS, McCloskey KL, Goodman LS: Diazepam and drug associated deaths. JAMA 242: 429–434, 1979

Friedman MJ: Post-Vietnam syndrome. Psychosomatics 22:931–941, 1981

Garbus SB, Weber MS, Priest RT, et al: The abrupt discontinuation of antihypertensive treatment. J Clin Pharmacol 19:476–486, 1979

Gardner CR, Tully WR, Hedgecock CJ: The rapidly expanding range of neuronal benzodiazepine receptor ligands. Prog Neurobiol 40: 1–61, 1993

Geller I, Seifter J: The effects of meprobamate, barbiturates, D-amphetamine, and promazine on experimentally induced conflict in the rat. Psychopharmacologia 1:482–492, 1960

Ghoneim MM, Mewaldt SP: Benzodiazepines and human memory: a review. Anesthesiology 72: 926–938, 1990

Glassman R, Salzman C: Interactions between psychotropic and other drugs: an update. Hosp Community Psychiatry 38:236–242, 1987

Gray JA: The Neuropsychology of Anxiety: An Enquiry into the Functions of the Septo-Hippocampal System. Oxford, England, Clarendon, 1982

Greenblatt DJ, Shader RI: Benzodiazepines in Clinical Practice. New York, Raven, 1974

Greenblatt DJ, Allen MD, Noel BJ, et al: Acute overdose with benzodiazepine derivatives. Clin Pharmacol Ther 21:497–514, 1977

Greenblatt DJ, Divoll M, Abernethy DR, et al: Clinical pharmacokinetics of the newer benzodiazepines. Clin Pharmacokinet 8: 233–253, 1983

Greenblatt DJ, Harmatz JS, Shapiro L, et al: Sensitivity to triazolam in the elderly. N Engl J Med 324:1691–1698, 1991

Greenblatt DJ, Harmatz JS, Shader RI: Plasma alprazolam concentrations: relation to efficacy and side effects in the treatment of panic disorder. Arch Gen Psychiatry 50:715–722, 1993

Haefely W: Behavioral and neuropharmacological aspects of drugs used in anxiety and related states, in Psychopharmacology: A Generation of Progress. Edited by Lipton MA, DiMascio A, Killam KF. New York, Raven, 1978, pp 1359–1374

Haefely W: The biological basis of benzodiazepine actions, in The Benzodiazepines: Current Standards for Medical Practice. Edited by Smith DE, Wesson DR. Hingham, MA, MTP Press, 1985, pp 7–42

Haefely W: Endogenous ligands of the benzodiazepine receptor. Pharmacopsychiatry 21 (suppl 1): 43–46, 1988

Haefely W: The GABA$_A$-benzodiazepine receptor: biology and pharmacology, in Handbook of Anxiety, Vol 3: The Neurobiology of Anxiety. Edited by Burrows GD, Roth M, Noyes R. Amsterdam, Elsevier Science, 1990, pp 165–188

Haefely W, Kuksar A, Möhler H, et al: Possible involvement of GABA in the central action of BZ derivatives. Adv Biochem Psychopharmacol 14:131–151, 1975

Hansten PD: Drug Interactions, 5th Edition. Philadelphia, PA, Lea & Febiger, 1985

Harvey SC: Hypnotics and sedatives, in Goodman and Gilman's The Pharmacological Basis of Therapeutics, 7th Edition. Edited by Gilman AG, Goodman LS, Rall TW. New York, Macmillan, 1985, pp 339–371

Hindley SW, Hobbs A, Paterson IA, et al: Microinjection of methyl-beta-carboline-3-carboxylate into nucleus raphe dorsalis reduces social interaction in the rat. Br J Pharmacol 86:753–761, 1985

Hindmarch I, Kerr JS, Sherwood N: The effects of alcohol and other drugs on psychomotor performance and cognitive function. Alcohol 26: 71–79, 1991

Hollister LE: Pharmacology and clinical use of benzodiazepines, in Pharmacology of Benzodiazepines. Edited by Usdin E, Skolnick P, Tallman JF Jr, et al. London, Macmillan Press, 1982, pp 29–36

Howell EF, Laraia M, Ballenger JC, et al: Lorazepam treatment of panic disorder. Paper presented at the 140th annual meeting of the American Psychiatric Association, Chicago, IL, May 1987

Hsiao JK, Potter WZ: Mechanism of action of antipanic drugs, in Clinical Aspects of Panic Disorder. Edited by Ballenger JC. New York, Wiley-Liss, 1990, pp 297–317

Hunkeler W, Möhler H, Pieri L, et al: Selective antagonists of benzodiazepines. Nature 290: 514–516, 1981

Kales A, Kales JD, Bixler EO, et al: Effectiveness of hypnotic drugs with prolonged use: flurazepam and pentobarbital. Clin Pharmacol Ther 18:356–364, 1975

Kangas L, Kanto J, Lehtinen V, et al: Long-term nitrazepam treatment in psychiatric outpatients with insomnia. Psychopharmacology (Berl) 63: 63–66, 1979

Kilts CD, Commissaris RL, Rech RH: Comparison of anti-conflict drug effects in three experimental animal models of anxiety. Psychopharmacology (Berl) 74:290–296, 1981

King DJ: Benzodiazepines, amnesia, and sedation: theoretical and clinical issues and controversies. Human Psychopharmacology 7:79–87, 1992

Klepner CA, Lippa AS, Benson DI, et al: Resolution of two biochemically and pharmacologically distinct benzodiazepine receptors. Pharmacol Biochem Behav 11:457–462, 1979

Klerman GL, Weissman MM, Ouellette R, et al: Panic attacks in the community: social morbidity and health care utilization. JAMA 265: 742–746, 1991

Knoflach F, Drescher U, Scheurer L, et al: Full and partial agonism displayed by benzodiazepine receptor ligands at recombinant γ-aminobutyric acid$_A$ receptor subtypes. J Pharmacol Exp Ther 266:385–391, 1993

Kramer M: Dream disturbances. Psychiatric Annals 9:50–68, 1979

Lader M: Clinical pharmacology of benzodiazepines. Annu Rev Med 38:19–28, 1987

Lader M: Clinical pharmacology of anxiolytic drugs: past, present and future, in GABA Receptors and Anxiety: From Neurobiology to Treatment. Edited by Biggio G, Sanna E, Costa E. New York, Raven, 1995, pp 135–153

Lesser IM, Lydiard RB, Antal E, et al: Alprazolam plasma concentrations and treatment response in panic disorder and agoraphobia. Am J Psychiatry 149:1556–1562, 1992

Linnoila M, Erwin CW, Brendle A, et al: Psychomotor effects of diazepam in anxious patients and healthy volunteers. J Clin Psychopharmacol 3:988–996, 1983

Linsen SM, Zitman FG, Breteler MHM: Defining benzodiazepine dependence: the confusion persists. European Psychiatry 10:306–311, 1995

Lo MM, Niehoff DL, Kuhar MJ, et al: Differential localization of type I and type II benzodiazepine binding sites in substantia nigra. Nature 306:57–60, 1983

Luckner M: Secondary Metabolism in Microorganisms, Plants and Animals. Berlin, Springer-Verlag, 1984, pp 272–276

Lüddens H, Korpi ER: Biological functions of GABA$_A$ benzodiazepine receptor heterogeneity. J Psychiatr Res 29:77–94, 1995

Lüddens H, Wisden W: Function and pharmacology of multiple GABA$_A$ receptor subunits. Trends Pharmacol Sci 12:49–51, 1991

Lüddens H, Pritchett DB, Kohler M, et al: Cerebellar GABA$_A$ receptor selective for a behavioural alcohol antagonist. Nature 346:648–651, 1990

Lüddens H, Korpi ER, Seeburg PH: GABA$_A$/benzodiazepine receptor heterogeneity: neurophysiological implications. Neuropharmacology 34:245–254, 1995

Malizia A, Nutt DJ: Psychopharmacology of benzodiazepines—an update. Human Psychopharmacology 10:S1–S14, 1995

Margules DL, Stein L: Increase of antianxiety activity and tolerance to behavioural depression during chronic administration of oxazepam. Psychopharmacology (Berl) 13:74–80, 1968

Markowitz JS, Weissman MM, Ouellette R, et al: Quality of life in panic disorder. Arch Gen Psychiatry 46:984–992, 1989

Martin JR, Kuwahara A, Horii I, et al: Evidence that benzodiazepine receptor partial agonist Ro 16-6028 has minimal abuse and physical dependence liability. Society for Neuroscience Abstracts 16:1104, 1990

Matthews WB: Treatment of restless legs syndrome with clonazepam (letter). BMJ 1:751, 1979

Mendelson WB, Gillin JC, Wyatt RJ: Human Sleep and Its Disorders. New York, Plenum, 1977

Miller LG, Greenblatt DJ, Barnhill JG, et al: Chronic benzodiazepine administration, I: tolerance is associated with benzodiazepine receptor down regulation and decreased γ-aminobutyric acid$_A$ receptor function. J Pharmacol Exp Ther 246:170–176, 1988

Miller NS: Liability and efficacy from long-term use of benzodiazepines: documentation and interpretation. Psychiatric Annals 25:166–173, 1995

Miller NS, Gold MS, Stennie K: Benzodiazepines: the dissociation of addiction from pharmacological dependence/withdrawal. Psychiatric Annals 25:149–152, 1995

Möhler H, Okada T: Benzodiazepine receptors: demonstration in the central nervous system. Science 198:849–851, 1977a

Möhler H, Okada T: Properties of ^{3}H diazepam binding to benzodiazepine receptors in rat cerebral cortex. Life Sci 20:2101–2110, 1977b

Möhler H, Richards JG: Agonist and antagonist benzodiazepine receptor interaction in vitro. Nature 294:763–764, 1981

Möhler H, Wu JY, Richards JG: Benzodiazepine receptors: autoradiographical and immunocytochemical evidence for their localization in regions of GABAergic synaptic contacts, in GABA and Benzodiazepine Receptors. Edited by Costa E, DiChaira G, Gessa GL. New York, Raven, 1981, pp 139–146

Nielsen M, Braestrup C: Ethyl β-carboline 3-carboxylate shows differential benzodiazepine receptor interaction. Nature 286:606–607, 1980

Noyes R, Anderson DJ, Clancy J, et al: Diazepam and propranolol in panic disorder and agoraphobia. Arch Gen Psychiatry 41:287–292, 1984

Nutt D: Selective ligands for benzodiazepine receptors: recent developments, in Current Aspects of the Neurosciences. Edited by Osborne NN. New York, Macmillan, 1989, pp 259–293

O'Hanlon JF, Vermeeren A, Uiterwijk MMC, et al: Anxiolytics' effects on the actual driving performance of patients and healthy volunteers in a standardized test: an integration of three studies. Neuropsychobiology 31:81–88, 1995

Olsen RW, Tobin AJ: Molecular biology of GABA$_A$ receptors. FASEB J 4:1469–1480, 1990

Olsen RW, McCabe RT, Wamsley JK: GABA$_A$ receptor subtypes: autoradiographic comparison of GABA, benzodiazepine, and convulsant binding sites in the rat central nervous system. J Chem Neuroanat 3:59–76, 1990

Paul SM, Skolnick P: Comparative neuropharmacology of antianxiety drugs. Pharmacol Biochem Behav 17 (suppl 1):37–41, 1982

Paul SM, Zatz M, Skolnick P: Demonstration of brain-specific benzodiazepine receptors in rat retina. Brain Res 187:243–246, 1980

Pellow S, File SE: Anxiolytic and anxiogenic drug effects in exploratory activity in an elevated plus-maze: a novel test of anxiety in the rat. Pharmacol Biochem Behav 24:525–529, 1986

Pellow S, Chopin P, File SE, et al: The validation of open/closed arm entries in an elevated plus-maze as a measure of anxiety in the rat. J Neurosci Methods 14:149–167, 1985

Petersen EN, Paschelke G, Kehr W, et al: Does the reversal of the anticonflict effect of phenobarbital by beta-CCE and FG 7142 indicate benzodiazepine receptor-mediated anxiogenic properties? Eur J Pharmacol 82:217–221, 1982

Petersen EN, Jensen LH, Honore T, et al: Differential pharmacological effects of benzodiazepine receptor inverse agonists, in Benzodiazepine Recognition Site Ligands: Biochemistry and Pharmacology. Edited by Biggio G, Costa E. New York, Raven, 1983, pp 57–64

Polc P, Möhler H, Haefely W: The effect of diazepam on spinal cord activities: possible sites and mechanisms of action. Naunyn Schmiedebergs Arch Pharmacol 284:319–337, 1974

Polc P, Laurent JP, Scherschlicht R, et al: Electrophysiological studies on the specific benzodiazepine antagonist Ro 15-1788. Naunyn Schmiedebergs Arch Pharmacol 316: 317–325, 1981

Potokar J, Nutt DJ: Anxiolytic potential of benzodiazepine receptor partial agonists. CNS Drugs 1:305–315, 1994

Randall LO: Discovery of benzodiazepines, in Pharmacology of Benzodiazepines. Edited by Usdin E, Skolnick P, Tallman JF Jr, et al. London, Macmillan Press, 1982, pp 15–22

Ray WA, Griffin MR, Schaffner W, et al: Psychotropic drug use and the risk of hip fracture. N Engl J Med 316:363–369, 1987

Richards JG, Möhler H, Haefely W: Benzodiazepine binding sites: receptors or acceptors? Trends Pharmacol Sci 3:233–235, 1982

Rickels K, Case WG, Diamond L: Relapse after short-term drug therapy in neurotic outpatients. International Pharmacopsychiatry 15:186–192, 1980

Rickels K, Case WG, Downing RW, et al: Long-term diazepam therapy and clinical outcome. JAMA 250:767–771, 1983

Rickels K, Schweizer E, Case WG, et al: Long-term therapeutic use of benzodiazepines, I: effects of abrupt discontinuation. Arch Gen Psychiatry 47:899–907, 1990

Rickels K, Case WG, Schweizer E, et al: Long-term benzodiazepine users 3 years after participation in a discontinuation program. Am J Psychiatry 148:757–761, 1991

Romach MK, Somer GR, Sobell LC, et al: Characteristics of long-term alprazolam users in the community. J Clin Psychopharmacol 12: 316–332, 1992

Roth T, Roehrs T, Wittig R, et al: Benzodiazepines and memory. Br J Clin Pharmacol 18:45S–49S, 1984

Ruffalo RL, Thompson JF: Effect of cimetidine on the clearance of benzodiazepines. N Engl J Med 303:753–754, 1980

Schatzberg AF, Ballenger JC: Decisions for the clinician in the treatment of panic disorder: when to treat, which treatment to use, and how long to treat. J Clin Psychiatry 52:26–31, 1991

Schweizer E, Fox I, Case G, et al: Lorazepam vs alprazolam in the treatment of panic disorder. Psychopharmacol Bull 24:224–227, 1988

Seeburg PH, Wisden W, Verdoorn TA, et al: The $GABA_A$ receptor family: molecular and functional diversity. Cold Spring Harb Symp Quant Biol 55:29–44, 1990

Sepinwall J, Cook L: Behavioral pharmacology of anti-anxiety drugs, in Handbook of Psychopharmacology, Vol 13. Edited by Iversen LL, Iversen SD, Snyder SH. New York, Plenum, 1978, pp 345–393

Shader RI, Greenblatt DJ: Use of benzodiazepines in anxiety disorders. N Engl J Med 328: 1398–1405, 1993

Shader RI, Dreyfuss D, Gerrein JR, et al: Sedative effects and impaired learning and recall following single oral doses of lorazepam. Clin Pharmacol Ther 39:526–529, 1986

Sieghart W, Eichinger A, Riederer P, et al: Comparison of benzodiazepine receptor binding in membranes from human or rat brain. Neuropharmacology 24:751–759, 1985

Simon P, Soubrie P: Behavioral studies to differentiate anxiolytic and sedative activity of the tranquilizing drugs, in Modern Problems in Pharmacopsychiatry, Vol 14. Edited by Boissier JR. Basel, Karger, 1979, pp 99–142

Smith DE, Wesson DR (eds): The Benzodiazepines: Current Standards for Medical Practice. Boston, MA, MTP Press Limited, 1985, pp 289–292

Squires RF, Braestrup CL: Benzodiazepine receptors in rat brain. Nature 266:732–734, 1977

Stephens DN, Kehr W: Beta-carbolines can enhance or antagonize the effects of punishment in mice. Psychopharmacology (Berl) 85:143–147, 1985

Stephens DN, Shearman GT, Kehr W: Discriminative stimulus properties of beta-carbolines characterized as agonists and inverse agonists at central benzodiazepine receptors. Psychopharmacology (Berl) 83:233–239, 1984

Sternbach LH: The discovery of CNS active 1,4-benzodiazepines (chemistry), in Pharmacology of Benzodiazepines. Edited by Usdin E, Skolnick P, Tallman JR Jr, et al. London, Macmillan Press, 1982, pp 7–14

Sternbach LH, Reeder E: Quinazolines and 1,4-benzodiazepines, II: the rearrangement of 6-chloro-5-2-chloromethyl-4-phenylquinazoline 3-oxide into 2-amino-derivatives of 7-chloro-5-phenyl-³H-1,4-benzodiazepine 4-oxide. Journal of Organic Chemistry 26:1111–1118, 1961

Study RE, Barker JL: Diazepam and pentobarbital: fluctuation analysis reveals different mechanisms for potentiation of gamma-aminobutyric acid responses in cultured central neurons. Proc Natl Acad Sci U S A 78:7180–7184, 1981

Tallman JF, Thomas JW, Gallager DW: GABAergic modulation of benzodiazepine binding site sensitivity. Nature 274:383–385, 1978

Tallman JF, Paul SM, Skolnick P, et al: Receptors for the age of anxiety: the pharmacology of benzodiazepines. Science 207:274–281, 1980

Tansella M, Siciliani O, Burti L, et al: N-Desmethyldiazepam and amylobarbitone sodium as hypnotics in anxious patients: plasma levels, clinical efficacy and residual effects. Psychopharmacologia 41:81–85, 1975

Tansella M, Zimmermann-Tansella CH, Ferrario L, et al: Plasma concentrations of diazepam, nordiazepam and amylobarbitone after short-term treatment of anxious patients. Pharmacopsychiatrie Neuropsychopharmakologie 11:68–75, 1978

Thiébot MH, Soubrié P: Behavioral pharmacology of the benzodiazepines, in Benzodiazepines—Molecular Biology to Clinical Practice. Edited by Costa E. New York, Raven, 1983, pp 67–92

Thomas JW, Tallman JF: Characterization of photoaffinity labeling of benzodiazepine binding sites. J Biol Chem 156:9839–9842, 1981

Tönne U, Hiltunen AJ, Vikander B, et al: Neuropsychological changes during steady-state drug use, withdrawal and abstinence in primary benzodiazepine-dependent patients. Acta Psychiatr Scand 91:299–304, 1995

Unseld E, Krishna DR, Fischer C, et al: Endogenous benzodiazepines in brain right or wrong? Trends Neurosci 11:490–497, 1988

Vogel JR, Beer B, Clody DE: A simple and reliable conflict procedure for testing antianxiety agents. Psychopharmacologia 21:1–7, 1971

Wafford KA, Whiting PJ, Kemp JA: Differences in affinity and efficacy of benzodiazepine receptor ligands at recombinant γ-aminobutyric acid_A receptor subtypes. Mol Pharmacol 43:240–244, 1993

Ward J: Vital uses of diazepam in third world countries, in The Benzodiazepines: Current Standards for Medical Practice. Edited by Smith DE, Wesson DR. Boston, MA, MTP Press Limited, 1985, pp 167–175

Weissman MM, Klerman GL, Markowitz JS, et al: Suicidal ideation and suicide attempts in panic disorder and attacks. N Engl J Med 321: 1209–1214, 1989

Wesson DR: Additional clinical uses of benzodiazepines, in The Benzodiazepines: Current Standards for Medical Practice. Edited by Smith DE, Wesson DR. Boston, MA, MTP Press Limited, 1985, pp 163–166

Wildmann J: Increase of natural benzodiazepines in wheat and potato during germination. Biochem Biophys Res Commun 157:1436–1443, 1988

Ymer S, Draguhn A, Wisden W, et al: Structural and functional characterization of the γ_1-subunit of GABA_A benzodiazepine receptors. European Molecular Biology Organization Journal 9: 3261–3267, 1990

Yokoyama N, Ritter B, Neubert AD: 2-Arylpyrazolo(4,30c)quinolin-3-ones: novel agonists, partial agonists and antagonists of benzodiazepines. J Med Chem 25:337–339, 1982

Young WS, Kuhar MJ: Radiohistochemical localization of benzodiazepine receptors in rat brain. J Pharmacol Exp Ther 212:337–346, 1980

Zorumski CF, Isenberg KE: Insights into the structure and function of GABA-benzodiazepine receptors: ion channels and psychiatry. Am J Psychiatry 148:162–173, 1991

SIX

Nonbenzodiazepine Anxiolytics

Philip T. Ninan, M.D.,
Jonathan O. Cole, M.D., and
Kimberly A. Yonkers, M.D.

Anxiety can present as a *symptom* in a variety of situations and psychopathological conditions such as depression, hypomania, and psychosis. Anxiety can also manifest as a *syndrome*—an anxiety disorder with anxiety as the core component. Several terms—*worry, nervousness, fear, apprehension, agitation, restlessness,* and *jitteriness*—are used interchangeably to denote symptomatic anxiety or some overlapping component of it. Anxiety has different dimensions, including the emotional state of anxiety with concomitant cognitive and somatic components. DSM-IV (American Psychiatric Association 1994) emphasizes the difficulty in controlling worry as a necessary cognitive component of generalized anxiety disorder. Somatic symptoms of anxiety include muscle tension, trembling, cold clammy hands, dry mouth, sweating, gastrointestinal upset, urinary frequency, dysphagia, and an exaggerated startle response.

Clinical therapeutic research is largely driven by the U.S. Food and Drug Administration (FDA) regulatory requirements for documenting safety and efficacy. Because efficacy was only a recent requirement, studies of older agents have focused on safety, and efficacy data from randomized controlled trials may not have been documented.

BARBITURATES

Barbiturates are infrequently used in psychiatry today, although many barbiturates are available. They are well described in earlier editions of *Goodman and Gilman's The Pharmacological Basis of Therapeutics* (e.g., Goodman and Gilman 1970).

Barbiturates, in a dose-dependent manner, appear to calm psychomotor activity and induce drowsiness, which leads to sleep. The anxiolytic effects occur within a narrow dose range close to the hypnotic dose. Daytime central nervous system (CNS) effects, including subtle impairment of fine motor skills and judgment as well as changes in mood, are often present at hypnotic doses. Phenobarbital and mephobarbital, which substitute a phenyl group at the 5 position, have anticonvulsant effects at doses that are not hypnotic. At increasingly higher doses, barbiturates induce anesthesia, coma, and ultimately death because the neurogenic- and hypoxic-driven respiratory drives are depressed. Simultaneous alcohol consumption reduces the lethal dose of barbiturates.

Tolerance and Dependence

With continued use, barbiturates result in the development of tolerance and dependence. Thus, sedative effects of barbiturates are largely lost by the third week of continuous fixed-dose treatment. The development of tolerance leads to the risk that the dose will be increased to obtain the same pharmacological effect. In addition, withdrawal symptoms can occur with abrupt discontinuation. Barbiturates have a higher abuse potential than other anxiolytics because of their powerful reinforcing effects and possible euphoriant effects. Alcohol and other sedative-hypnotics have additive CNS depressant effects when used with barbiturates.

Pharmacokinetics

Barbiturates are metabolized by the 2C19 family of the cytochrome P450 system. Barbiturates induce their own metabolism, which results in a faster metabolism of the dose ingested and a reduced pharmacological effect. This is clinically relevant, because at maximal induction, the rate of metabolism is approximately doubled. Metabolism of barbiturates is slower in the elderly and infants.

Mechanism of Action

Barbiturates allosterically modulate the γ-aminobutyric acid (GABA$_A$) receptor complex at a site different from the benzodiazepine site. Barbiturates increase the potency of GABA on the chloride ion channel (Haefely and Polc 1986). Electrophysiologically, barbiturates prolong the open configuration of the chloride channel, resulting in presynaptic (e.g., in the spinal cord) and postsynaptic (e.g., in the cortical and cerebellar pyramidal cells) inhibition. At higher concentrations, barbiturates increase chloride conductance even in the absence of GABA, an effect that contributes to their lethal potential. Phenobarbital and pentobarbital are weak in this respect and, therefore, have a higher therapeutic index.

Indications

The use of barbiturates today in psychiatry is limited because their effects are not selective, and they have a low therapeutic index. Thus, they are used rarely to control anxiety, particularly given the availability of safer anxiolytics such as benzodiazepines (Koch-Weser and Greenblatt 1974). Likewise, the availability of safer sedative-hypnotics makes the use of barbiturates unnecessary. Barbiturates are used mainly in medicine as anticonvulsants and for intravenous anesthesia.

ANTIHISTAMINES

Antihistamines have not been adequately studied as anxiolytic agents and are probably less effective than appropriate benzodiazepines. Their antianxiety effects may be an aspect of their sedative effects. Hydroxyzine hydrochloride and hydroxyzine pamoate are both available by prescription. The disadvantages of antihistamines include their unpredictable effects, use in subtherapeutic doses, paradoxical agitation, rapid development of tolerance, and residual daytime sedation.

MEPROBAMATE

Meprobamate was the first nonbarbiturate antianxiety drug to become extensively used. It was synthesized in 1950 and initially drew attention because of its muscle relaxant properties (Berger 1970).

The original approval of meprobamate by the FDA in 1955 was based on two positive open clinical trials in heterogeneous groups of anxious outpatients. In those days, the FDA, by law, required only proof of safety, not of efficacy. Meprobamate was marketed under the trade names of Miltown and Equanil. Meprobamate continued in wide general use through 1972, when the benzodiazepines generally replaced it.

Pharmacological Profile

Meprobamate falls pharmacologically between the barbiturates and the benzodiazepines. It causes CNS depression but does not produce anesthesia. In animals, it releases behaviors suppressed by past adverse experiences, a property it shares with all other antianxiety drugs.

Pharmacokinetics and Disposition

Meprobamate taken orally in humans reaches a peak blood concentration in 1–3 hours. It is not bound much to plasma proteins. Meprobamate is metabolized in the liver by hydroxylation and glucuronide formation, and a small proportion is excreted unchanged. Its half-life is 6–17 hours in studies of acute administration; with chronic administration, the half-life may increase to 24–48 hours. The exact hepatic microsomal enzymes involved and the degree to which meprobamate induces their activity are unclear.

In suicidal overdose, meprobamate tablets can form a lump (bezoar) in the stomach. As the patient emerges from coma, gastric activity will break up the bezoar and reinduce the coma if gastroscopy has not been used to identify and remove the undissolved tablet mass (Rall 1993). Otherwise, suicide attempts with meprobamate are treated as one would treat a barbiturate overdose. The lethal dose can be as low as 30 tablets (12,000 mg), but the average lethal dose is approximately 28,000 mg.

Proposed Mechanisms of Action

There is a presumption that meprobamate, because of its pharmacological effects, *should* work like the barbiturates or the benzodiazepines, through GABA; however, meprobamate does not bind to any of the relevant receptors (Paul et

al. 1981; Rall 1993; Squires and Braestrup 1977).

Abuse Liability

The human abuse liability of meprobamate (compared with lorazepam and placebo) was studied on a research ward by Roache and Griffiths (1987) with drug-free persons who had formerly been addicted to sedatives. These investigators found, surprisingly, that subjects preferred meprobamate to lorazepam based on well-tested measures of abuse liability. Meprobamate resembled a barbiturate more than a benzodiazepine in that subjects taking high single doses of meprobamate (or barbiturates) were aware of their deficits in psychomotor performance, whereas those taking lorazepam believed they were doing well when their performance was in fact impaired.

Indications

Meprobamate is available in 200-mg, 400-mg, and 600-mg tablets and in a sustained-release capsule form called Meprospan. The only FDA-approved indication for meprobamate is as an anxiolytic, but the drug was also widely used in the past, and even studied, as a hypnotic.

A review of efficacy studies of meprobamate concluded that its efficacy had not been adequately proven (Greenblatt and Shader 1971). However, many of those studies were done in the 1950s and 1960s before the methodology for such studies was well established. A well-done study with an adequate sample size would likely show meprobamate's efficacy in generalized anxiety disorder (GAD) to be comparable to that of a standard benzodiazepine.

The appropriate initial dose of meprobamate, if used as a hypnotic, is 400 mg at bedtime, increasing to 600 mg or decreasing to 200 mg if the 400-mg dose is too weak or too sedating, respectively. In studies of meprobamate in the treatment of chronic anxiety, typical initial dosages were 400 mg orally three times a day, but starting with 200 mg orally three times a day might be adequate. Physical dependence on meprobamate has been observed after doses as low as 3,200 mg/day. The equivalent dose in diazepam units is probably 1 mg of diazepam to 50–60 mg of meprobamate. In the past, a number of patients found 400 mg of meprobamate at bedtime useful as a hypnotic. Studies in the 1970s reported it to be as effective as flurazepam in insomnia (Vogel et al. 1990).

Conclusion

Meprobamate deserves to remain in the armamentarium of the clinical psychopharmacologist, although it has no clear advantages over benzodiazepines. It may be abusable, but it is not abused in the current drug culture. Occasional patients find meprobamate more effective or better tolerated than newer drugs. However, it is clearly, on the basis of present knowledge, a third- or fourth-line drug to be tried only when more obviously effective drugs have failed.

BUSPIRONE

History and Discovery

Buspirone was the first nonsedative, non-benzodiazepine antianxiety drug to be developed and marketed. Buspirone blocks the conditioned avoidance response in rats. It does not cause catalepsy in animals; instead, it reverses neuroleptic-induced catalepsy.

Buspirone did show efficacy on some animal tests predictive of antianxiety drug actions (Riblet et al. 1982, 1984), such as inhibition of footshock-induced fighting in mice, decrease in aggression in rhesus monkeys, and attenuation of conflict behavior. It had no sedative-hypnotic or anticonvulsant effects.

The earliest study in patients with DSM-II (American Psychiatric Association 1968) anxiety disorder had clearly positive results (Goldberg and Finnerty 1979). A series of double-blind, placebo-controlled studies compared buspirone with several benzodiazepines and placebo and documented efficacy in anxiety without any suggestion of neuroleptic side effects or of abuse liability. On this basis, the drug received FDA approval and was marketed in 1986.

Pharmacological Profile

Buspirone is believed to exert its antianxiety effect through serotonin-1A (5-HT$_{1A}$) presynaptic and postsynaptic receptors. Lesions in the brain serotonergic system will block the antianxiety effects of both benzodiazepines and buspirone (Eison and Eison 1994). Buspirone is a full agonist at presynaptic (dorsal raphe) 5-HT$_{1A}$ receptors, with resulting inhibition of neuronal firing and a decrease in serotonin synthesis. Buspirone is also a partial agonist at postsynaptic (hippocampus, cortex) 5-HT$_{1A}$ receptors. In the presence of functional serotonin excess, buspirone acts as an antagonist, but in serotonin deficit states, it functions as an agonist.

Buspirone "passes" antianxiety drug tests in animals by reversing conditioned suppression of behavior, reversing learned helplessness, and being effective in the Porsolt behavioral despair model. It reverses inhibition of conflict behavior (antianxiety) but also blocks conditioned avoidance responding (antipsychotic) (Eison et al. 1991).

Buspirone has no major effects on the benzodiazepine-GABA-chloride ionophore complex, the major site of benzodiazepine action. Buspirone lacks the benzodiazepines' sedative, muscle relaxant, or anticonvulsant actions. Buspirone does not affect benzodiazepine withdrawal symptoms (Schweizer and Rickels 1986).

Buspirone lacks abuse potential as judged by relevant animal and human studies (Cole et al. 1982; Griffith et al. 1986). In humans, it does not impair psychomotor performance or potentiate the performance-impairing effects of alcohol. Benzodiazepines tend to impair performance in the above paradigms (Smiley 1987); buspirone not only does not impair performance but also improves the subject's awareness of any alcohol-induced decrements in performance (Sussman and Chou 1988).

Pharmacokinetics

Buspirone, taken orally at usual doses, has a short half-life ranging from 1 to 10 hours in healthy volunteers. If the drug is taken with food, first-pass metabolism is decreased, and higher "area-under-the-curve" values for buspirone blood levels are achieved (Jann 1988).

Buspirone has multiple metabolites, mainly hydroxylated derivatives. The major metabolite is 1-pyrimidinylpiperazine (1-PP); brain levels of 1-PP can be several times higher than blood levels. 1-PP lacks buspirone's serotonergic effects but may block α_2-noradrenergic receptors and cause an increase in 3-methoxy-4-hydroxyphenylglycol (MHPG) production. This effect is of interest because one study found a strong correlation between 1-PP blood levels and buspirone's efficacy in alcoholic patients (Tollefson et al. 1991).

Buspirone's pharmacokinetics are not altered in elderly persons, in whom buspirone is probably effective both in depression and in GAD (Bohm et al. 1990; Napoliello 1986). Buspirone has favorable effects in agitated patients with dementia but may have a slow (up to 7 weeks) onset of action (Gelenberg 1994).

Indications

Anxiety disorders. In a meta-analysis of 8 placebo-controlled studies in 520 patients with GAD, buspirone was significantly effective over placebo (Gammans et al. 1992). Buspirone is superior to placebo in the treatment of GAD even when depressive symptoms are present (Gammans et al. 1992; Sramek et al. 1996). Buspirone also is likely to be more effective in relieving coexisting depressive symptoms than are the benzodiazepines, except perhaps for alprazolam. At doses in the range of 30–90 mg/day, buspirone is effective in major depres-

sive disorder and even in melancholic depression. Buspirone has even been suggested to induce mania (Liegghio and Yeragani 1988; McDaniel et al. 1990), a sign that it may really be an antidepressant.

Buspirone has been shown to have efficacy in GAD and has been available for use in that condition in the United States since 1986. Most large-scale (i.e., $N > 60$) double-blind, random-assignment clinical studies have shown that buspirone is equal in efficacy to that of standard benzodiazepines in GAD or in less clearly specified chronic anxiety states.

Buspirone's efficacy may increase over time. In one large open study of patients with GAD, improvement rates increased from about 50% at 3 months to about 70% over 6 months (Feighner 1987). These numbers may be slightly deceptive because dropouts were fairly numerous in this study.

Buspirone seems in most ways to be the ideal antianxiety drug. It lacks the benzodiazepines' sedation, ataxia, tolerance, and withdrawal symptoms; abuse liability; and propensity to interfere with complex psychomotor tasks on driving simulators and related tests. In addition, benzodiazepines are linked by association to driving accidents and to falls and injuries in the elderly (Hemmelgarn et al. 1997; Smiley 1987; Sussman 1987; Sussman and Chou 1988). Buspirone does not impair performance; furthermore, it leaves the subject more aware of impairment resulting from alcohol ingestion than do the benzodiazepines (Sussman 1987).

Buspirone appears to improve respiratory functions and partial arterial carbon dioxide (Pa_{CO2}) pressure in patients with anxiety and severe lung disease (Sussman and Chou 1988). Buspirone lacks the ability of benzodiazepines to depress respiration, making it potentially the preferred drug in anxious patients with pulmonary disease.

Several pilot studies have suggested that buspirone may decrease alcohol consumption in both animals and humans and may have a role in the detoxification and postdetoxification treatment of anxious alcoholic patients (Bruno 1989; Kranzler and Myers 1989; Schuckit 1993; Tollefson et al. 1991).

Buspirone was found to be helpful in some injection drug users with anxiety who were receiving methadone maintenance and who had developed acquired immunodeficiency syndrome (AIDS) or AIDS-related complex (ARC) (Batki 1990). In this sample, no evidence of abuse of buspirone was found, and some evidence indicated that abuse of other drugs decreased. Unfortunately, the positive effects of buspirone faded after a few months in one-third of the patients.

Buspirone has few side effects, both absolutely and compared with placebo. The rates reported are 12% for dizziness, 6% for headache, 8% for nausea, 5% for nervousness, 3% for light-headedness, and 2% for agitation (Gelenberg 1994). Tolerance to these side effects probably develops. They may be handled by dosage reduction. If the dose is increased slowly, side effects may be minimized.

Buspirone dosage should be started at 5 mg three times a day for 1 week and then increased by 5 mg every 2–4 days as tolerated until the patient is receiving 10 mg orally three times a day. The patient should be encouraged to continue taking that dose for at least 6 weeks before deciding that the drug is ineffective. The drug customarily has been given three times per day because of its short half-life, but it is not known whether giving all or two-thirds of the dose at bedtime might work as well with better patient acceptance.

Buspirone has never been used clinically to the extent that its apparent safety and efficacy would support. Why? Observing the reduction in anxiety symptoms over weeks in reports of double-blind studies of buspirone compared with a benzodiazepine leaves one doubting that most patients' conditions improve much faster with a benzodiazepine. Patients taking both drugs show some improvement (on the average) after 1 week, a bit more after 2 weeks, and the most by 4 weeks. Although benzodiazepine-pla-

cebo differences are often statistically significant at week 1 or 2, and benzodiazepines and buspirone both achieve significance by weeks 3 and 4, buspirone-benzodiazepine differences are not significant early in these studies.

Buspirone is presumably ineffective when given as a single dose to relieve anxiety, whereas benzodiazepines may be effective in such circumstances. However, one suspects that benzodiazepines are better for insomnia early in treatment, whereas buspirone relieves insomnia later as part of a general improvement; benzodiazepines, as a group, are good hypnotics independent of their other effects.

Another part of the problem may be that psychiatrists, who can handle complicated drug regimens, rarely see drug-free patients with GAD or the medical patients with secondary anxiety who are the ideal candidates for buspirone, whereas primary care physicians may not have the time or motivation to explain buspirone's delayed response to their patients and then to adjust the dose carefully over several weeks until the patient's condition is clearly improved.

In other anxiety disorders, matters are less clear. In panic disorder, buspirone (mean dose, 61 mg) was no different from placebo and inferior to alprazolam in a double-blind study (Sheehan et al. 1993). However, in a 16-week placebo-controlled trial of buspirone in panic disorder with agoraphobia, in which all patients received cognitive-behavior therapy, buspirone had beneficial effects on generalized anxiety and agoraphobia (Cottraux et al. 1995). Two open trials of buspirone in treatment of social phobia at dosages generally in the 30- to 60-mg/day range showed substantial improvement rates (Bruns et al. 1989; Schneier et al. 1993). An open trial of buspirone reported significantly reduced posttraumatic stress disorder symptoms in 7 of 8 patients (Duffy and Malloy 1994).

In obsessive-compulsive disorder, one crossover study comparing buspirone and clomipramine seemed to show equal efficacy for obsessive-compulsive disorder, a condition with a low rate of placebo response (Murphy et al. 1990); however, subsequent open and blind studies did not support efficacy of buspirone in obsessive-compulsive disorder (Grady et al. 1993; Jenike and Baer 1988; McDougle et al. 1993). Pigott and colleagues (1992) reported that buspirone, as an augmenting agent, is not statistically better than placebo, although a subgroup of patients (29%) did obtain an additional greater than 25% benefit. None of the previous studies were properly statistically powered to be able to detect such an effect.

Thus, buspirone has advantages over benzodiazepines in GAD, especially among the elderly, in whom the cognitive and psychomotor impairment of benzodiazepines can be particularly problematic. It might also have a role in the management of alcoholism.

Depression. The assessment of buspirone's efficacy in depression began when multisite, controlled trials comparing buspirone with a benzodiazepine showed that buspirone was superior in relieving (or preventing the emergence of) depressive symptoms in patients selected initially as having an anxiety disorder. Then, Schweizer and colleagues (1986) conducted an open study of buspirone at doses between 30 and 60 mg/day in outpatients with nonmelancholic depression with favorable results. This was followed by a placebo-controlled, double-blind 8-week trial (Rickels et al. 1990), in which buspirone doses were permitted to increase to as high as 90 mg/day. The average dose by week 8 was, in fact, 57 mg/day. The study involved 143 evaluable patients. Side effects were similar in frequency and type to those attributed to buspirone in anxiety studies. Patients who completed the study had a 65% improvement after taking buspirone and a 28% improvement with placebo.

Because buspirone is available in pharmacies, physicians can prescribe it as an antidepressant. Because no comparative studies are available contrasting buspirone with more widely used antidepressants, it is difficult to guess its ul-timate place in a psychopharmacologist's armamentarium compared with the now-ubiquitous selective serotonin reuptake inhibitors (SSRIs), the older tricyclic antidepressants, or the monoamine oxidase inhibitors (MAOIs). Buspirone is certainly worth a trial in patients whose symptoms have not responded to two or three prior antidepressants, although the clinician should keep in mind the need to increase the dose, the relative expense of the drug, and the relatively benign side-effect profile. The recent availability of the 15-mg unit dose is helpful.

A few open trials suggested that adding buspirone to an antidepressant, including an SSRI, will often produce a better antidepressant response (Bakish 1991; Jacobsen 1991; Joffe and Schuller 1993). More systematic and controlled studies are needed.

Drug-Drug Interactions

When buspirone was first released, it was said to have caused hypertensive states when added to MAOIs. These symptoms now appear to have been mild to moderate elevations in blood pressure rather than serious hypertensive or serotonergic crises of the sort elicited by SSRI-MAOI combinations. However, it is too early to say that buspirone can be added to MAOIs with impunity. Ciraulo and Shader (1990), after reviewing all data available to Bristol-Myers on buspirone-MAOI interactions, found insufficient evidence for a total prohibition of combined buspirone-MAOI therapy; we concur.

Gelenberg (1994) noted that buspirone may reverse sexual dysfunction caused by SSRIs. An earlier report by Othmer and Othmer (1987) found that buspirone improved sexual function in patients with GAD. One drug-drug interaction that fortunately does not exist is between SSRIs and buspirone. The combination of two serotonergic drugs could cause a serotonergic syndrome but in this case does not.

Conclusion

Buspirone is a novel drug with unique probable mechanisms of action that, somehow, has never been as widely used as it probably deserves. It is effective in GAD and almost certainly in major depression. It seems likely that this drug may have efficacy in social phobia and in anxiety disorders accompanying various chronic medical disorders. Buspirone's side effects are mainly mildly bothersome, and its drug-drug interactions are benign. It is relatively safe in overdose and free from abuse liability and performance impairment. If the drug is started cautiously, with the dose raised as needed up to 60–90 mg in major disorders, it should be a major addition to the psychopharmacological armamentarium.

Researchers now should develop a drug—perhaps a buspirone analogue with some improvements (faster onset of action and better customer acceptance but no physical or psychic dependence)—or attain a better understanding of how to best use buspirone. It is clear that many patients with symptoms that meet DSM-IV criteria for GAD either have relatively lifelong anxiety symptoms of GAD or have waxing and waning symptoms that could be helped by prolonged intermittent pharmacotherapy (Feighner 1987). Anxiety associated with chronic medical conditions may be similarly prolonged, recurrent, episodic, or fully chronic. Social phobia can be equally chronic, as can dysthymia, with an admixture of anxiety symptoms (Dubovsky 1990; Rickels 1987).

Benzodiazepines do work, and tolerance to their antianxiety effects does not develop over weeks or months (Rickels 1987); however, in patients with chronic anxiety, it can prove difficult to test the patient's need for longer benzodiazepine therapy because withdrawal symptoms are likely to resemble or to reactivate the symptoms of the patient's original condition (Lader 1987). Buspirone—or our hypothetical "super-buspirone"—could be tapered and stopped periodically without the complication of anxiety-like withdrawal symptoms.

In this chapter, we considered various ideas as to why buspirone is less widely used than it might be. More research is needed on how to optimize physician and patient response to buspirone until an even better anxiolytic drug emerges. The relative paucity of clinical articles on newer anxiolytics makes one suspect that none of these agents is close to release in the United States or Europe.

REFERENCES

American Psychiatric Association: Diagnostic and Statistical Manual of Mental Disorders, 2nd Edition. Washington, DC, American Psychiatric Association, 1968

American Psychiatric Association: Diagnostic and Statistical Manual of Mental Disorders, 4th Edition. Washington, DC, American Psychiatric Association, 1994

Bakish D: Fluoxetine potentiation by buspirone: three case histories. Can J Psychiatry 36: 749–750, 1991

Batki SL: Buspirone in drug users with AIDS or AIDS-related complex. J Clin Psychopharmacol 10 (suppl 3):111S–115S, 1990

Berger FM: The discovery of meprobamate, in Discoveries in Biological Psychiatry. Edited by Ayd F, Blackwell B. Philadelphia, PA, JB Lippincott, 1970, pp 115–129

Bohm C, Robinson DS, Gammans RE, et al: Buspirone therapy in anxious elderly patients: a controlled clinical trial. J Clin Psychopharmacol 10 (suppl 3):47S–51S, 1990

Bruno F: Buspirone in the treatment of alcoholic patients. Psychopathology 22 (suppl 1):49–50, 1989

Bruns JR, Munjack DJ, Baltazar PL, et al: Buspirone for the treatment of social phobia. Family Practice Recertification (Cl. 22 Selective Therapeutic Index) 11 (No 9, suppl): 46–52, 1989

Ciraulo DA, Shader RL: Question the experts: safety of buspirone with an MAOI. J Clin Psychopharmacol 10:306, 1990

Cole JO, Orzack MH, Beake B, et al: Assessment of the abuse liability of buspirone in recreational sedative users. J Clin Psychiatry 43:69–74, 1982

Cottraux J, Note ID, Cungi C, et al: A controlled study of cognitive behavior therapy with buspirone or placebo in panic disorder with agoraphobia. Br J Psychiatry 167:635–641, 1995

Dubovsky SL: Generalized anxiety disorder: new concepts and psychopharmacologic therapies. J Clin Psychiatry 51 (suppl l):3–10, 1990

Duffy JD, Malloy PF: Efficacy of buspirone in the treatment of posttraumatic stress disorder: an open trial. Ann Clin Psychiatry 6:33–37, 1994

Eison AS, Eison MS: Serotonergic mechanisms in anxiety. Prog Neuropsychopharmacol Biol Psychiatry 18:47–62, 1994

Eison AS, Yocca FD, Taylor DP: Mechanism of Action of Buspirone: Current Perspectives. New York, Academic Press, 1991, pp 279–326

Feighner JP: Buspirone in the long-term treatment of generalized anxiety disorder. J Clin Psychiatry 48 (No 12, suppl):3–6, 1987

Gammans RE, Stringfellow JC, Hvizdos AJ, et al: Use of buspirone in patients with generalized anxiety disorder and coexisting depressive symptoms: a meta-analysis of eight randomized, controlled trials. Neuropsychobiology 25:193–201, 1992

Gelenberg AJ: Academic highlights—buspirone: seven year update. J Clin Psychiatry 55:222–229, 1994

Goldberg HL, Finnerty RJ: The comparative efficacy of buspirone and diazepam in the treatment of anxiety. Am J Psychiatry 136:1184–1187, 1979

Goodman LS, Gilman A (eds): The Pharmacologic Basis of Therapeutics, 4th Edition. New York, Macmillan, 1970

Grady TA, Pigott TA, L'Heureux F, et al: Double-blind study of adjuvant buspirone for fluoxetine-treated patients with obsessive-compulsive disorder. Am J Psychiatry 150:819–821, 1993

Greenblatt D, Shader R: Meprobamate: a study of irrational drug use. Am J Psychiatry 127:1297–1303, 1971

Griffith JD, Jasinaski DR, Casten GP, et al: Investigation of the abuse liability of buspirone in alcohol-dependent patients. Am J Med 80:30–35, 1986

Haefely W, Polc P: Physiology of GABA enhancement by benzodiazepines and barbiturates, in Benzodiazepine-GABA Receptors and Chloride Channels: Structural and Functional Properties. Edited by Olsen RW, Venter JC. New York, Alan R Liss, 1986, pp 97–133

Hemmelgarn B, Suissa S, Huang A, et al: Benzodiazepine use and the risk of motor vehicle crash in the elderly. JAMA 278:27–31, 1997

Jacobsen FM: Possible augmentation of antidepressant response by buspirone. J Clin Psychiatry 52:217–220, 1991

Jann MW: Buspirone: an update on a unique anxiolytic agent. Pharmacotherapy 8:100–116, 1988

Jenike MA, Baer L: An open trial of buspirone in obsessive-compulsive disorder. Am J Psychiatry 145:1285–1286, 1988

Joffe RT, Schuller DR: An open study of buspirone augmentation of serotonin reuptake inhibitors in refractory depression. J Clin Psychiatry 54:269–271, 1993

Koch-Weser J, Greenblatt DJ: The archaic barbiturate hypnotics. N Engl J Med 291:790–791, 1974

Kranzler HR, Myers RE: An open trial of buspirone in alcoholics. J Clin Psychopharmacol 9:379–380, 1989

Lader M: Long-term anxiolytic therapy: the issue of drug withdrawal. J Clin Psychiatry 48 (No 12, suppl):12–16, 1987

Liegghio NE, Yeragani VK: Buspirone-induced hypomania: a case report. J Clin Psychopharmacol 8:226–227, 1988

McDaniel JS, Ninan PT, Magnuson JV: Possible induction of mania by buspirone (letter). Am J Psychiatry 147:125–126, 1990

McDougle CJ, Goodman WK, Leckman JF, et al: Limited therapeutic effect of addition of buspirone in fluvoxamine-refractory obsessive-compulsive disorder. Am J Psychiatry 150:647–649, 1993

Murphy DL, Pato MT, Pigott TA: Obsessive compulsive disorder: treatment with serotonin-selective uptake inhibitors, azapirones, and other agents. J Clin Psychopharmacol 10 (suppl 3):91S–100S, 1990

Napoliello MJ: An interim multicentre report on 677 anxious geriatric outpatients treated with buspirone. Br J Clin Pract 2:71–73, 1986

Othmer E, Othmer SC: Effect of buspirone on sexual dysfunction in patients with generalized anxiety disorder. J Clin Psychiatry 48:201–203, 1987

Paul S, Marangos P, Skolnick P: The benzodiazepine-GABA-chloride ionophore receptor complex: common site of minor tranquilizer action. Biol Psychiatry 16:213–229, 1981

Pigott TA, L'Heureux F, Hill JL, et al: A double-blind study of adjuvant buspirone hydrochloride in clomipramine-treated patients with obsessive-compulsive disorder. J Clin Psychopharmacol 12:11–18, 1992

Rall TW: Hypnotics and sedatives, in Goodman and Gilman's The Pharmacological Basis of Therapeutics, 8th Edition. Edited by Gilman AG, Rall TW, Nies AS, et al. New York, McGraw-Hill, 1993, pp 345–382

Riblet LA, Taylor DP, Eison MS, et al: Pharmacology and neurochemistry of buspirone. J Clin Psychiatry 43:11–16, 1982

Riblet LA, Eison AS, Eison MS, et al: Neuropharmacology of buspirone. Psychopathology 17:69–78, 1984

Rickels K: Antianxiety therapy: potential value of long-term treatment. J Clin Psychiatry 48 (No 12, suppl):7–11, 1987

Rickels K, Amsterdam J, Clary C, et al: Buspirone in depressed outpatients: a controlled study. Psychopharmacol Bull 26:163–167, 1990

Roache J, Griffiths RR: Lorazepam and meprobamate dose effects in humans: behavioral effects and abuse liability. J Pharmacol Exp Ther 243:978–988, 1987

Schneier FR, Saoud JB, Campeas R, et al: Buspirone in social phobia. J Clin Psychopharmacol 18:251–256, 1993

Schuckit MA: Buspirone: is it an effective drug for alcohol rehabilitation? Drug Abuse and Alcoholism Newsletter 22(2), April 1993

Schweizer E, Rickels K: Failure of buspirone to manage benzodiazepine withdrawal. Am J Psychiatry 143:1590–1592, 1986

Schweizer E, Rickels K, Lucki I: Resistance to the antianxiety effect of buspirone in patients with a history of benzodiazepine use. N Engl J Med 314:719–720, 1986

Sheehan DV, Harnett-Sheehan K, Soto S, et al: The relative efficacy of high-dose buspirone and alprazolam in the treatment of panic disorder: a double-blind placebo-controlled study. Acta Psychiatr Scand 88:1–11, 1993

Smiley A: Effects of minor tranquilizers and antidepressants on psychomotor performance. J Clin Psychiatry 48 (suppl 12):22–28, 1987

Squires R, Braestrup C: Benzodiazepine receptors in rat brain. Nature 266:732–734, 1977

Sramek JJ, Tansman M, Suri A, et al: Efficacy of buspirone in generalized anxiety disorder with coexisting mild depressive symptoms. J Clin Psychiatry 57:287–291, 1996

Sussman N: Treatment of anxiety with buspirone. Psychiatric Annals 17:114–118, 1987

Sussman N, Chou JCY: Current issues in benzodiazepine use of anxiety disorders. Psychiatric Annals 18:139–145, 1988

Tollefson GD, Lancaster SP, Montagne-Clouse J: The association of buspirone and its metabolic 1-pyrimidinylpiperazine in the remission of co-morbid anxiety with depressive features and alcohol dependency. Psychopharmacol Bull 27:163–170, 1991

Vogel GW, Buffenstein A, Hennessey M, et al: Drug effects on REM sleep and on endogenous depression. Neurosci Biobehav Rev 14:49–63, 1990

SEVEN

Venlafaxine

Justine M. Kent, M.D., and
Jack M. Gorman, M.D.

HISTORY AND DISCOVERY

Venlafaxine is a bicyclic phenylethylamine derivative with a structure and chemical profile that distinguish it from the tricyclic antidepressants and the selective serotonin reuptake inhibitors (SSRIs). In vitro, it was found to block the reuptake of both norepinephrine and serotonin, leading to its description as a serotonin-norepinephrine reuptake inhibitor (SNRI). Clinical trials confirmed venlafaxine's antidepressant properties along with a benign side-effect profile. Venlafaxine was released for the treatment of depression in the United States in spring 1994.

STRUCTURE-ACTIVITY RELATIONS

Venlafaxine is a bicyclic compound (Figure 7–1). It has a novel biochemical structure that is unrelated to any of the heterocyclic antidepressants or SSRIs.

PHARMACOLOGICAL PROFILE

Venlafaxine and its active metabolite, *O*-desmethylvenlafaxine (ODV), are potent inhibitors of neuronal reuptake of serotonin, norepinephrine, and, more weakly, of dopamine in in vitro preparations (Bolden-Watson and Richelson 1993; Muth et al. 1986). Venlafaxine and ODV have no substantial affinity for muscarinic, cholinergic, histamine-H_1, or α-adrenergic receptors in vitro; they also have no monoamine oxidase A (MAO-A) or monoamine oxidase B (MAO-B) inhibitory activity (Muth et al. 1986).

PHARMACOKINETICS AND DISPOSITION

After oral administration, venlafaxine is well absorbed from the gastrointestinal tract and undergoes extensive first-pass metabolism in the liver to its active metabolite, ODV. The primary route of excretion for venlafaxine, ODV, and its other minor metabolites is via the kidney (Howell et al. 1993). ODV's clearance (half-life = 10 hours) is slower than that of venlafaxine (half-life = 4 hours); therefore, steady-state ODV concentrations in plasma are higher than those of venlafaxine in most patients (Klamerus et al. 1992).

Venlafaxine and its major metabolite, ODV, are 27% and 30%, respectively, bound to pro-

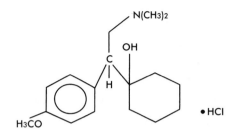

Figure 7–1. Chemical structure for venlafaxine.

tein in human plasma (package insert). This relatively low degree of binding suggests that the probability of drug-drug interactions based on protein binding is remote.

Venlafaxine is available in immediate-release (IR) and extended-release (XR) formulations. The XR preparation is available in 37.5-, 75-, and 150-mg doses. Once-daily dosing with the XR formulation achieves bioavailability equivalent to that of twice-daily dosing with the IR formulation. The XR preparation may be taken in the morning or evening, and bioavailability is not affected by coadministration with a meal (Troy et al. 1997).

Clearance of venlafaxine and its metabolites may be significantly reduced in patients with cirrhosis and in patients with severe renal disease; therefore, dosing should be adjusted accordingly. In otherwise healthy elderly depressed patients, adjustments in dosing do not appear to be necessary. However, beginning with a low starting dose and increasing the dose slowly is a sensible approach in elderly patients.

INDICATIONS

Venlafaxine is currently approved by the U.S. Food and Drug Administration (FDA) for the treatment of depression and for generalized anxiety disorder (GAD). In comparative studies for the treatment of depression, venlafaxine has been at least as effective as imipramine, clomipramine, fluoxetine, and trazodone (Clerc

et al. 1994; Cunningham et al. 1994; Dierick et al. 1996; Samuelian et al. 1992; Schweizer et al. 1994). In dosages up to 225 mg/day, venlafaxine's side-effect profile was superior to that of imipramine and clomipramine and comparable to that of trazodone and fluoxetine.

In two studies of severely depressed inpatients with melancholia, venlafaxine was shown to be an effective antidepressant when compared with placebo (Guelfi et al. 1995) and to be comparable or superior to fluoxetine (Clerc et al. 1994).

Venlafaxine has the unique ability to induce a rapid desensitization of β-adrenoreceptors in the rat pineal gland, unlike other antidepressants that require repeated administration to induce noradrenergic subsensitivity (down-regulation of receptors). This finding raised the question of whether venlafaxine's effects correlate with a shorter latency to clinical antidepressant efficacy compared with other available antidepressants (Moyer et al. 1984, 1992). Most clinical studies to date appear to support the potential advantage of venlafaxine having a more rapid onset of action than do reference antidepressants. Several studies (Guelfi et al. 1995; Khan et al. 1991; Rudolph et al. 1991; Schweizer et al. 1991; Shrivastava et al. 1994) found an earlier onset of action when compared with placebo in the first 2 weeks of treatment. However, none of these studies were designed as comparative trials to examine specifically latency of onset of clinical antidepressant effect. In support of an early onset of activity, two placebo-controlled clinical studies were reviewed in which the venlafaxine dose was rapidly escalated, and efficacy was measured frequently early in treatment of depressed outpatient populations. Three different statistical approaches were used to assess the onset of activity, and all three methodologies indicated that venlafaxine was superior to placebo by the time of the first efficacy measurements at day 7 of treatment. This superiority was maintained throughout the length of the clinical trials (Derivan et al. 1995). This supports the idea that aggressive dosing of venlafaxine may result in more rapid clinical improvement. However, rapid escalation of dose may also be associated with increased incidence of adverse effects (see section "Side Effects and Toxicology" later in this chapter) and therefore may be best reserved for those patients requiring rapid treatment because of severe morbidity and mortality risks.

Long-term open-label trials of venlafaxine in the treatment of depression originally suggested that venlafaxine's efficacy is maintained over a 12-month period (Magni and Hackett 1992; Tiller et al. 1992). A meta-analysis of three double-blind, placebo-controlled extension studies confirmed that the 1-year relapse rate was significantly lower in the venlafaxine-treated group than in the placebo group (Mendlewicz 1995).

The efficacy of venlafaxine in the treatment of GAD has been demonstrated in two placebo-controlled trials (Sheehan 1999). In a comparative study with buspirone, venlafaxine at fixed doses of 75 mg and 150 mg showed superior efficacy to placebo on most measures (Davidson et al. 1999). Although venlafaxine demonstrated statistical superiority to buspirone on some measures, dosing of buspirone (30 mg) may have been suboptimal for some patients.

In a 6-month study, venlafaxine produced significant responses in 67% of patients compared with 33% of patients taking placebo (Gelenberg et al. 2000).

SIDE EFFECTS AND TOXICOLOGY

The most frequently reported adverse effect associated with venlafaxine is nausea. Absorption of venlafaxine is not affected by administration with food (package insert).

Other common side effects reported (>10% of subjects) in published pooled data include headache, insomnia, somnolence, dry mouth, dizziness, constipation, asthenia, sweating, and nervousness. Although venlafaxine has not been associated with adverse cardiovascular effects,

modest increases in blood pressure have been reported in association with venlafaxine treatment (Cunningham et al. 1994; Fabre and Putman 1987; Schweizer et al. 1991). Sustained hypertension, manifest as an increase in supine diastolic blood pressure, has been reported in 3%–13% of patients taking venlafaxine and appears to be dose related (package insert). The manufacturer recommends regular monitoring of blood pressure for all patients taking venlafaxine.

During premarketing evaluation, there were 14 reports of acute overdose with venlafaxine, either alone or in combination with other drugs and/or alcohol. The dose ingested in all cases was estimated to be only several times the usual therapeutic dose. All 14 patients recovered without sequelae (data on file, Wyeth-Ayerst Laboratories, April 1994).

Because of venlafaxine's short half-life, rapid discontinuation has been associated with serotonin rebound syndromes (Schatzberg et al. 1997).

DRUG-DRUG INTERACTIONS

In vitro and in vivo studies suggest that venlafaxine is a significantly weaker CYP2D6 inhibitor compared with fluoxetine and paroxetine (Amchin et al. 1996; Lam et al. 1997). Furthermore, in vitro and in vivo studies have shown venlafaxine to cause little or no inhibition of other cytochrome P450 isoenzymes, including CYP1A2, CYP2C9, CYP2C19, and CYP3A4 (Ball et al. 1997; data on file, Wyeth-Ayerst Laboratories, December 1997).

Cimetidine inhibits the first-pass hepatic metabolism of venlafaxine. However, because cimetidine causes only a minimal increase in overall pharmacological activity of venlafaxine and ODV, close monitoring and dose adjustment may only be necessary in cases of preexisting hypertension or hepatic disease or in elderly patients. Venlafaxine is not highly protein bound, so interactions resulting from displacement of a highly bound drug are not expected.

Venlafaxine is contraindicated in patients taking monoamine oxidase inhibitors (MAOIs) because of the risk of neuroleptic malignant-like syndrome, hypertensive crisis, or a serotonin-like syndrome. As with cyclic antidepressants and SSRIs, venlafaxine treatment should not be initiated until 2 weeks after discontinuation of an MAOI, and MAOI therapy should not be initiated until at least 7 days after discontinuation of venlafaxine. Venlafaxine appears to have no clinically significant interactions with lithium (Troy et al. 1996), diazepam (Troy et al. 1995), or alcohol (Troy et al. 1992).

SUMMARY

In summary, venlafaxine's clinical profile is similar to that of the SSRIs in terms of safety and tolerability, and its efficacy appears to be comparable to that of the heterocyclic antidepressants and the SSRIs. The XR preparation allows a once-daily dosing schedule, like the SSRIs, which increases medication compliance. Venlafaxine offers an advantage over other antidepressants in having a low potential for cytochrome P450–mediated drug-drug interactions, making it a good choice in patients taking other drugs utilizing the P450 system for metabolism. It is also the only antidepressant currently approved for the treatment of GAD.

REFERENCES

Amchin JD, Ereshefsky L, Zaryaranski WM: Effect of venlafaxine versus fluoxetine on the metabolism of dextromethorphan, a CYP2D6 marker. American Psychiatric Association 1996 Annual Meeting New Research Program and Abstracts (NR362). Washington, DC, American Psychiatric Association, 1996, p 165

Ball SE, Ahern D, Scatina J, et al: Venlafaxine: *in vitro* inhibition of CYP2D6 dependent imipramine and desipramine metabolism; comparative studies with selected SSRIs, and effects on human hepatic CYP3A4, CYP2C9 and CYP1A2. Br J Clin Pharmacol 43:619–626, 1997

Bolden-Watson C, Richelson E: Blockade by newly developed antidepressants of biogenic amine uptake into rat brain synaptosomes. Life Sci 52: 1023–1029, 1993

Clerc GE, Ruimy P, Verdeau-Palles J: A double-blind comparison of venlafaxine and fluoxetine in patients hospitalized for major depression and melancholia. Int Clin Psychopharmacol 9:139–143, 1994

Cunningham LA, Borison RL, Carman JS, et al: A comparison of venlafaxine, trazodone, and placebo in major depression. J Clin Psychopharmacol 14:99–106, 1994

Davidson JRT, DuPont RL, Hedges D, et al: Efficacy, safety, and tolerability of venlafaxine extended release and buspirone in outpatients with generalized anxiety disorder. J Clin Psychiatry 60:528–535, 1999

Derivan A, Entsuah AR, Kikta D: Venlafaxine: measuring the onset of antidepressant action. Psychopharmacol Bull 31:439–447, 1995

Dierick M, Ravizza L, Realini R, et al: A double-blind comparison of venlafaxine and fluoxetine for treatment of major depression in outpatients. Prog Neuropsychopharmacol Biol Psychiatry 20:57–71, 1996

Fabre LF, Putman HP: An ascending single-dose tolerance study of Wy-45,030, a bicyclic antidepressant in healthy men. Current Therapeutic Research 42:901–909, 1987

Gelenberg AJ, Lydiard RB, Rudolph RL, et al: Efficacy of venlafaxine extended-release capsules in nondepressed outpatients with generalized anxiety disorder: a 6-month randomized controlled trial. JAMA 283:3082–3088, 2000

Guelfi JD, White C, Hackett D, et al: Effectiveness of venlafaxine in patients hospitalized for major depression and melancholia. J Clin Psychiatry 56:450–458, 1995

Howell SR, Husbands GE, Scatina JA, et al: Metabolic disposition of 14C-venlafaxine in mouse, rat, dog, rhesus monkey and man. Xenobiotica 23:349–359, 1993

Khan A, Fabre LF, Rudolph R: Venlafaxine in depressed outpatients. Psychopharmacol Bull 27: 141–144, 1991

Klamerus KJ, Maloney K, Rudoph RL, et al: Introduction of a composite parameter to the pharmacokinetics of venlafaxine and its active *O*-desmethyl metabolite. J Clin Pharmacol 32:716–724, 1992

Lam YWF, Alfaro CL, Ereshefsky L, et al: Cross-over comparison of CYP2D6 inhibition: insignificant effect of venlafaxine compared to sertraline, paroxetine and fluoxetine. American Psychiatric Association 1997 Annual Meeting New Research Program and Abstracts (NR267). Washington, DC, American Psychiatric Association, 1997, p 139

Magni G, Hackett D: An open-label evaluation of the long-term safety and clinical acceptability of venlafaxine in depressed patients (abstract). Clin Neuropharmacol 15 (suppl 1):323, 1992

Mendlewicz J: Pharmacologic profile and efficacy of venlafaxine. Int Clin Psychopharmacol 10 (suppl 2):5–13, 1995

Moyer JA, Muth EA, Haskins JT, et al: *In vivo* antidepressant profiles of the novel bicyclic compounds Wy-45,030 and Wy-45,881 (abstract no 76.12). Society for Neuroscience Abstracts 10:261, 1984

Moyer JA, Andree TH, Haskins JT, et al: The preclinical pharmacological profile of venlafaxine: a novel antidepressant agent (abstract). Clin Neuropharmacol 15 (suppl 1):435B, 1992

Muth EA, Haskins JT, Moyer JA, et al: Antidepressant biochemical profile of the novel bicyclic compound Wy-45,030, an ethyl cyclohexanol derivative. Biochem Pharmacol 35:4493–4497, 1986

Rudolph R, Entsuah R, Derivan A: Early clinical response in depression to venlafaxine hydrochloride (abstract no P-26–12). Biol Psychiatry 29:630S, 1991

Samuelian JC, Tatossian A, Hackett D: A randomized, double-blind, parallel group comparison of venlafaxine and clomipramine in outpatients with major depression (abstract). Clin Neuropharmacol 15 (suppl 1):324B, 1992

Schatzberg AF, Haddad P, Kaplan ER, et al: Possible biological mechanisms of the serotonin reuptake inhibitor discontinuation syndrome. J Clin Psychiatry 57 (suppl 7):23–27, 1997

Schweizer E, Weise C, Clary C, et al: Placebo-controlled trial of venlafaxine for the treatment of major depression. J Clin Psychopharmacol 11:233–236, 1991

Schweizer E, Feighner J, Mandos LA, et al: Comparison of venlafaxine and imipramine in the acute treatment of major depression in outpatients. J Clin Psychiatry 55:104–108, 1994

Sheehan DV: Venlafaxine extended release (XR) in the treatment of generalized anxiety disorder. J Clin Psychiatry 60 (suppl 22):23–28, 1999

Shrivastava R, Patrick R, Scherer N, et al: A dose-response study of venlafaxine (abstract). Neuropharmacology 10 (suppl 3):221, 1994

Tiller J, Johnson G, O'Sullivan B, et al: Venlafaxine: a long term study (abstract). Clin Neuropharmacol 14 (suppl):342B, 1992

Troy S, Piergies A, Lucki I, et al: Venlafaxine pharmacokinetics and pharmacodynamics (abstract). Clin Neuropharmacol 15 (suppl 1): 324B, 1992

Troy SM, Lucki I, Peirgies AA, et al: Pharmacokinetic and pharmacodynamic evaluation of the potential drug interaction between venlafaxine and diazepam. J Clin Pharmacol 35:410–419, 1995

Troy SM, Parker VD, Hicks DR, et al: Pharmacokinetic interaction between multiple-dose venlafaxine and single-dose lithium. J Clin Pharmacol 36:175–181, 1996

Troy SM, DiLea C, Martin PT, et al: Pharmacokinetics of once daily venlafaxine extended release (XR) in healthy volunteers. Current Therapeutic Research 58:504–514, 1997

Antipsychotics

EIGHT

Antipsychotic Medications

Stephen R. Marder, M.D.

Antipsychotic drugs are used to treat nearly all forms of psychosis, including schizophrenia, schizoaffective disorder, affective disorders with psychosis, and psychoses associated with organic mental disorders. Although these drugs have become standard treatments in psychiatry and medicine, they have important limitations: they are not effective for all patients, they have several serious adverse effects, and even patients who respond well often continue to have serious signs and symptoms of illness. These limitations have led to a search for newer drugs that have fewer adverse effects and similar or improved effectiveness. In this chapter, I discuss the conventional antipsychotics that were discovered during the early 1950s and that have defined antipsychotic treatment until recently. Owens and Risch, in Chapter 9 of this volume, focus on newer antipsychotics, including clozapine, risperidone, olanzapine, and quetiapine.

All of the conventional antipsychotics produce significant neurological side effects and, for this reason, are often referred to as neuroleptics. However, the discovery of newer drugs with fewer motor side effects indicates that defining this group by a particular side effect is probably inaccurate. Thus, the term *antipsychotic* is preferable for describing these drugs. In this chapter, I use the terms *traditional* or *conventional*

antipsychotic to describe drugs that were previously termed *neuroleptic*. Table 8–1 summarizes information about representatives of each of the major classes of conventional antipsychotic drugs, including structure, dose, and major side effects.

PHARMACOLOGICAL PROFILE

Behavioral Effects

Antipsychotic drugs produce a wide spectrum of physiological actions, only some of which are essential to their antipsychotic action. Some of these effects differ among the various classes of antipsychotics. For example, aliphatic phenothiazines have potent antimuscarinic and autonomic effects, whereas others have more potent effects on dopaminergic or serotonergic systems. The effect that is common to all conventional antipsychotic agents is a high affinity for dopamine receptors, particularly D_2 receptors. These effects are useful for defining this class of compounds.

Chlorpromazine has the unusual property of inducing a state of relative indifference to stressful situations. All of the traditional antipsychotics share this property, which has been called *ataraxia*. The effect differs from sedation in that the individual may not be drowsy but is instead calm and relatively uninterested in

Table 8–1.   **Selected antipsychotic drugs**

Drug	Routes of administration	Usual daily oral dose (mg)	Sedation	Autonomic effects	Extra-pyramidal side effects	Structure
Phenothiazines						
Chlorpromazine	Oral, intra-muscular, depot	200–600	+++	+++	++	
Fluphenazine	Oral, intra-muscular, depot	2–20	+	+	+++	
Trifluoperazine	Oral, intra-muscular	5–30	++	+	+++	
Perphenazine	Oral, intra-muscular	8–64	++	+	+++	
Thioridazine	Oral	200–600	+++	+++	++	
Butyrophenones						
Haloperidol	Oral, intra-muscular, depot	5–20	+	+	+++	
Thioxanthenes						
Thiothixene	Oral, intra-muscular	5–30	+	+	+++	
Dihydroindolones						
Molindone	Oral	20–100	++	+	++	
Dibenzoxazepines						
Loxapine	Oral, intra-muscular	20–100	++	+	++	

Note.   + = mild; ++ = moderate; +++ = severe.
Source.   Adapted from Silver et al. 1994, pp. 901–903.

the environment. Individuals who are taking antipsychotics appear to have a decrease in their emotional responsiveness and have been described as lacking initiative. When patients are agitated or excited, these drugs may calm them without causing excessive sedation.

In rodents, traditional antipsychotics also block responses such as stereotypies and hyperactivity, which are induced by dopamine agonists such as apomorphine. This effect has been found to be a reasonably reliable predictor of antipsychotic activity in patients. Moreover, the dose-response relationship in animals provides information about the likely clinical dose range for patients. It is commonly used as a screening device to identify compounds that are likely to have clinical efficacy as antipsychotics (Gerlach 1991).

Motor Effects

When animals are administered a traditional antipsychotic in relatively high doses, they develop a syndrome with immobility, increased muscle tone, and abnormal postures called *catalepsy*. In addition, these agents decrease spontaneous motor activity. These motor effects in animals and humans are caused by dopamine-receptor blockade in the striatum and inactivation of dopamine neurons in the substantia nigra (Gerlach 1991).

In humans, all of the traditional antipsychotic medications produce extrapyramidal side effects (EPS), including parkinsonism (i.e., stiffness, tremor, and shuffling gait), dystonia (i.e., abrupt onset, sometimes bizarre muscular spasms affecting mainly the musculature of the head and neck), and akathisia (with objective and subjective restlessness). These effects are described in greater detail in the section "Side Effects and Toxicology."

Endocrine Effects

Antipsychotic drugs influence the secretion of hormones in the pituitary and elsewhere mainly as a result of their blockade of dopamine receptors. All traditional antipsychotics increase serum prolactin concentration in the usual clinical dose range (Meltzer 1985). This increase occurs because prolactin secretion by the anterior pituitary is tonically inhibited by dopamine. Therefore, blockade of dopamine receptors in the tuberoinfundibular pathway results in prolactin elevation. This sometimes produces gynecomastia and galactorrhea. Antipsychotics also suppress levels of luteinizing hormone (LH) and follicle-stimulating hormone (FSH) (Reichlin 1992). These changes can lead to amenorrhea and inhibition of orgasm in women. Other changes in sexual functioning are described in the section "Side Effects and Toxicology."

PHARMACOKINETICS AND DISPOSITION

All of the antipsychotics are well absorbed when they are administered orally or parenterally. Oral administration leads to less predictable absorption than parenteral administration. Liquid concentrates are absorbed slightly more rapidly than pills. In general, intramuscular preparations reach their peak concentrations sooner than oral drugs and, as a result, have an earlier onset of action. For example, intramuscular administration of most antipsychotics results in peak plasma levels in about 30 minutes, with clinical effects emerging within 15–30 minutes. Oral administration of most antipsychotics results in peak plasma levels 1–4 hours after administration. Steady-state levels are reached in 4–7 days. However, an optimal clinical response to these agents may emerge within the first week or may be delayed for 6 weeks or longer.

The bioavailability (i.e., the amount of drug reaching the site of action in the brain) is substantially greater when antipsychotics are administered parenterally than when they are administered orally. This difference may result from the incomplete absorption of the drug in the gastrointestinal tract and from extensive metabolism of oral drugs during the first pass through liver and gut. Several factors can interfere with the gastrointestinal absorption of these drugs, including antacids, coffee, smoking, and food. The metabolism of antipsychotic drugs is largely hepatic and occurs through conjugation with glucuronic acid, hydroxylation, oxidation, demethylation, and sulfoxide formation. The metabolism of the phenothiazines and thioxanthenes is particularly complex. For example, chlorpromazine has more than 100 different potential metabolites, with some metabolites having significant amounts of pharmacological activity. Although most phenothiazine metabolites are inactive, some such as 7-hydroxychlorpromazine and 7-hydroxyfluphenazine may contribute to the therapeutic activity of the parent drug (Midha et al. 1993).

In the case of thioridazine, a substantial amount of the drug's activity is from metabolites that may be more active than thioridazine itself. One metabolite, mesoridazine, is also marketed as an antipsychotic. On the other hand, haloperidol has only one major metabolite, reduced haloperidol, which has substantially less antidopaminergic activity than the parent compound. However, a study found that reduced haloperidol is converted back to the parent compound and may contribute to antipsychotic activity (Chakraborty et al. 1989).

Most antipsychotics are metabolized by the cytochrome P450 (CYP) 2D6 and CYP3A subfamilies (Preskorn 1996). These isoenzymes also metabolize a number of drugs that are commonly combined with antipsychotics, resulting in important drug-drug interactions. These interactions are discussed in a later section (see "Drug-Drug Interactions") and in Table 8–2.

The systemic clearance of antipsychotics is high as the result of a high hepatic extraction ratio. As a result, only negligible amounts of the unchanged drug are excreted by the kidneys. Most antipsychotics have elimination half-lives of about 10–30 hours, partially because of the high lipid solubility of antipsychotics, which results in large amounts of drug being stored in tis-

Table 8–2. Antipsychotic drugs and cytochrome P450 (CYP) isoenzymes

Isoenzyme	Antipsychotic drugs	Other drugs
CYP1A2	Clozapine	**Substrates:** amitriptyline, clomipramine, imipramine, propranolol, theophylline, warfarin, caffeine **Inhibitors:** fluvoxamine, paroxetine
CYP2D6	Haloperidol, perphenazine, risperidone, thioridazine, sertindole, olanzapine, clozapine	**Substrates:** fluoxetine, paroxetine, sertraline, venlafaxine, amitriptyline, clomipramine, desipramine, imipramine, nortriptyline, propranolol, metoprolol, timolol, codeine, encainide, flecainide, propafenone **Inhibitors:** paroxetine, sertraline, fluoxetine
CYP3A3/4	Clozapine, sertindole, quetiapine	**Substrates:** amitriptyline, clomipramine, imipramine, nefazodone, sertraline, carbamazepine, ethosuximide, terfenadine, alprazolam, clonazepam, diazepam, midazolam, triazolam, diltiazem, nifedipine, verapamil, erythromycin, cyclosporine, lidocaine, acetaminophen, quinidine, cisapride **Inhibitors:** ketoconazole, nefazodone, fluvoxamine, fluoxetine

Source. Adapted from Preskorn 1996 and Ereshefsky et al. 1996.

sues such as fat, lung, and brain. This may explain the high concentrations of antipsychotic drugs—about twice the plasma concentration—that have been found in human and animal brain. Note that the biological activity of antipsychotics may persist for periods of time that would not be predicted from their terminal half-lives. The pharmacokinetics of antipsychotics in plasma may not accurately reflect the kinetics at receptor sites in the brain (Campbell and Baldessarini 1985; Hubbard et al. 1987).

The pharmacokinetics of long-acting injectable antipsychotics differ markedly from those of short-acting oral and injectable drugs. Long-acting fluphenazine and haloperidol are administered as esters dissolved in sesame oil. The oil is injected into a muscle, and the drug gradually diffuses from the oily vehicle into the surrounding tissues. The rate-limiting step appears to be the rate of diffusion, because once the drug enters the tissue, it is rapidly hydrolyzed, and the parent compound is released. Plasma concentrations of short-acting drugs rise rather rapidly during the absorption phase and then decline during a distribution and elimination phase. Long-acting compounds, on the other hand, are absorbed continually during the interval between injections. Moreover, for patients who have received multiple injections, the drug will be absorbed from multiple injection sites simultaneously. As a result, long-acting compounds need a much longer time to reach steady state, and they are eliminated much more slowly than short-acting compounds. For example, the decanoate forms of haloperidol and fluphenazine require about 3 months to reach steady state, and substantial plasma concentrations can be detected months after therapy has been discontinued (Marder et al. 1989).

MECHANISM OF ACTION

The discovery of drugs that were effective against psychosis was an important event in biological psychiatry; understanding the mechanism of action of these drugs could provide valuable information about the biology of psychosis. The important breakthrough came in 1963 when Carlsson and Lindqvist reported that administering chlorpromazine or haloperidol to mice resulted in an accumulation of dopamine metabolites in dopamine-rich brain areas. They hypothesized that the drugs blocked receptors for dopamine and that feedback mechanisms resulted in an increase in dopamine release. Since that time, others have found that all of the effective antipsychotics bind to dopamine receptors. In 1976, Seeman and colleagues and Creese and colleagues reported that the affinity of the traditional antipsychotics for D_2 receptors is highly correlated with their effective clinical dose. In contrast, a similar relationship does not exist between affinity for other receptors (e.g., muscarinic or adrenergic) and clinical effectiveness. This observation has led to the conclusion that the traditional antipsychotic drugs exert their effects against psychosis by blocking D_2 receptors.

Others have proposed that schizophrenia and other psychotic illnesses are related to an overactive dopamine system. This dopamine hypothesis of schizophrenia has resulted in an exhaustive search for abnormalities in the dopamine systems of schizophrenic individuals. For the most part, this search has had mixed results and remains unproven (Marder et al. 1991). The fact that antipsychotic medications relieve schizophrenic psychosis by decreasing dopamine activity does not mean that schizophrenia is caused by increased dopamine activity. It is common in medicine for illnesses to be treated through mechanisms that are unrelated to the actual cause of the illness. For example, hypertension can be treated by drugs with different biological activities that are far removed from the actual cause of hypertension. In a similar manner, schizophrenic psychosis—or any psychosis—may be attenuated by methods that are unrelated to the cause of schizophrenia.

Studies using positron emission tomography have improved the understanding of the importance of D_2 receptors in the clinical effects of traditional antipsychotics. Investigators used highly selective D_2 receptor ligands and found that EPS tend to occur when a drug occupies a high proportion of D_2 receptor sites, usually more than 80%. Occupancy rates that were somewhat lower resulted in antipsychotic responses without obvious EPS (Farde et al. 1992). Clozapine, a nontraditional antipsychotic, was effective when D_2 occupancy was 20%–60%; thus, other transmitters, particularly serotonin, may contribute to clozapine's effectiveness (Sedvall 1996).

Research results indicate that the theory that antipsychotic drugs work by blocking D_2 receptors is an oversimplification. An antipsychotic will occupy dopamine receptor sites within hours after a patient receives an adequate dose of drug (Farde et al. 1992). However, the clinical response to the medication may require days or weeks. Studies monitoring plasma homovanillic acid (HVA), a metabolite of dopamine, are consistent with the hypothesis that the delayed response may be caused by a decrease in dopamine turnover. When drug-free patients receive an antipsychotic, plasma HVA levels increase during the first few days and then decline in some patients (Bowers 1984). Some (but not all) studies indicate that the decline in HVA levels is correlated with the amount of reduction in psychosis. Furthermore, patients who have high plasma HVA levels prior to treatment appear to be more likely to respond to antipsychotics. These observations are supported by studies on the firing rates of midbrain dopamine neurons of rats. Treatment with haloperidol results in a short-term increase in the firing of these neurons followed by a prolonged decrease in firing that has been referred to as *depolarization inactivation* (Chiodo and Bunney 1987). It has been proposed that the antipsychotic effects of these drugs are associated with the decrease in firing. Taken together, these findings suggest that for an antipsychotic response to occur, the blockade of D_2 receptors is an initial response that must be followed by a decrease in dopamine activity.

INDICATIONS

Antipsychotic medications are effective in the treatment of psychoses associated with a variety of medical and psychiatric conditions. In this regard, this group of drugs is antipsychotic rather than antischizophrenic. The effectiveness of these conventional antipsychotic drugs is often limited by their neurological side effects. For this reason, clinicians may choose not to treat certain psychotic conditions with these agents if the conditions are either mild or transitory.

Acute Schizophrenia and Schizoaffective Disorder

Numerous clinical studies have found that antipsychotic medications are effective for reducing psychotic symptoms in acute schizophrenia and schizoaffective disorder. The effectiveness of these agents was confirmed by a systematic review carried out by a Schizophrenia Patient Outcome Research Team (Dixon et al. 1995).

Antipsychotic medications are effective for treating nearly all of the symptoms associated with schizophrenia, although the extent of their effectiveness is highly variable in specific patients. Symptoms such as hallucinations, delusions, and disorganized thoughts—also called *positive symptoms* because they were attributed to reflect abnormal function—are more likely to decrease with drugs than are symptoms such as blunted affect, emotional withdrawal, and lack of social interest—also called *negative symptoms* because they were attributed to the absence of normal brain function. For many patients, antipsychotics will result in substantial reduction, or even remission, of positive symptoms, but negative symptoms will be minimally affected and will continue to impair the patient's social recovery.

Antipsychotics may also cause what has been referred to as *secondary negative symptoms* (Buchanan and Gold 1996). That is, both EPS and sedation from antipsychotics can either worsen negative symptoms or cause new symptoms to arise. Akinesia, a manifestation of antipsychotic-induced parkinsonism, can lead to decreased gestures, masked facies, decreased speech, and reduced interest in social activities. These symptoms may decline if EPS are adequately treated.

All of the traditional antipsychotic medications are equally effective. Clinicians and researchers who prescribed these drugs during the years immediately following their discovery reported that certain forms or subtypes of schizophrenia improved more with particular antipsychotics. These observations have not withstood careful study. In other words, all of the traditional antipsychotic drugs are equally effective for all subtypes of schizophrenia.

In certain conditions, antipsychotic drug treatment becomes problematic, and the risk-benefit ratio shifts. Antipsychotics should be prescribed cautiously for patients with seriously impaired hepatic function because these drugs are primarily metabolized in the liver. Patients with Parkinson's disease may have difficulty tolerating traditional antipsychotics because of EPS.

In the past, some senior psychotherapists reported that patients who were able to engage in intensive psychotherapy appeared to do better without antipsychotic medications. Clinicians are often impressed by an occasional patient who does extremely well without antipsychotics and sustains a complete or nearly complete recovery while receiving skilled psychotherapy. It is important not to generalize from experience with these rather rare individuals to the vastly greater number of patients with schizophrenia who will be helped to a substantial degree by medication. Moreover, an extensive literature indicates that psychosocial treatments are most effective when they are administered to patients who are also receiving antipsychotics.

A review by Wyatt (1991) concluded that early intervention with antipsychotics reduced long-term morbidity and decreased the number of rehospitalizations. In other words, even if a patient eventually recovers without drugs, the amount of time spent in a psychotic state may be related to a worse long-term outcome.

Maintenance Therapy in Schizophrenia

Antipsychotics have been reliably shown to decrease the frequency of relapse in schizophrenic patients who have recovered from a psychotic episode (Dixon et al. 1995). Kissling (1992) used placebo-controlled studies to estimate that approximately 72% of patients will have a relapse in a year without an antipsychotic, whereas treated patients are likely to have relapse rates of approximately 23%. These findings support the practice of continuing antipsychotic treatment in patients after they have recovered from a psychotic episode. Some clinicians are often tempted to discontinue medications in patients who have been well and stable for a prolonged period. Unfortunately, these patients also have high relapse rates when their medications are discontinued (Hogarty et al. 1976).

The value of long-term antipsychotic drug treatment for well-stabilized patients has also been clarified by a series of studies by Johnson and colleagues (1983). Patients who relapsed while receiving antipsychotic medications had episodes that were less severe than those in patients who discontinued their drugs. Drug-maintained patients were less likely to have episodes with self-destructive behavior, violence, and antisocial acts. In addition, patients who relapsed while not taking medications were more likely to require involuntary hospitalization. Patients who discontinued their medications actually ended up, on average, receiving more total medication, because the drug dose needed to treat relapses was much higher than the dose for relapse prevention.

In 1989, an international group of experts reached a consensus on the indications for neuroleptic relapse prevention: 1–2 years of maintenance antipsychotic therapy was recommended for patients following a first episode.

Although this may be somewhat longer than current practice in many settings, this recommendation was made because individuals at this stage of their illness often have the most to lose. Patients may be working or involved in educational programs, both of which can be jeopardized by a second psychotic episode. Moreover, the self-image of patients and their personal relationships may be permanently altered by their illness. The experts at the consensus conference also recommended that patients who have had multiple episodes receive maintenance neuroleptic treatment for at least 5 years. For patients with a history of serious suicide attempts or violent, aggressive behavior, maintenance treatment with neuroleptics may be indicated for longer periods—perhaps indefinitely (Kissling et al. 1991).

Mania

All of the traditional antipsychotic drugs are effective in reducing symptoms of acute mania. In comparison with lithium, valproic acid, and carbamazepine, antipsychotic drugs often have a more rapid onset of action. Therefore, an antipsychotic may be combined with an antimanic drug during the first days of treatment of severe excited states, before the antimanic compound has begun to exert its therapeutic effects. Once lithium or another antimanic compound becomes effective, the dose of antipsychotic may be reduced and eventually discontinued. In most cases, antimanic drugs are more effective and are associated with fewer side effects than antipsychotic drugs for mania, though this may not be true for atypical antipsychotic agents. Some studies indicate that patients with mood disorders are more vulnerable to developing tardive dyskinesia than are patients with schizophrenia; thus, these drugs should be used for as short a time as possible.

Depression With Psychotic Features

Patients with major depressive episodes with psychotic features require a combination of antipsychotic and antidepressant medications. The added benefits of antipsychotic medications are most apparent for those patients with severe delusions. When the psychotic component of the episode has responded to treatment, the antipsychotic medications should be withdrawn.

Other Indications

Antipsychotic drugs are effective for reducing psychotic symptoms in a number of organic mental syndromes, including dementia, and psychotic states due to stimulant drugs. They can be useful for controlling agitation and chorea in Huntington's disease. Both haloperidol and pimozide have been shown to be helpful in treating symptoms of Tourette's disorder. Antipsychotics are occasionally useful for patients with pervasive developmental disorder and mental retardation, but there is some concern that these drugs are overprescribed for these conditions. Prochlorperazine is commonly prescribed for nausea and vomiting. Chlorpromazine is sometimes useful for intractable hiccups.

SIDE EFFECTS AND TOXICOLOGY

Acute Extrapyramidal Side Effects

EPS, including akathisia, dystonia, tremor, akinesia, bradykinesia, and rigidity, are the major problems in prescribing traditional antipsychotics. The most common extrapyramidal side effect is akathisia, which is a subjective feeling of restlessness. Patients who experience severe akathisia will often pace continuously or move their feet restlessly while sitting. Some patients complain that they are unable to feel comfortable, regardless of what they do. Severe akathisia can cause patients to feel anxious or irritable, and some reports suggest that severe akathisia can result in aggressive or suicidal acts. One study found that as many as 75% of patients treated with a conventional dose of haloperidol will experience some degree of akathisia (Van Putten et al. 1984). Other studies reported that 25% of patients experience akathisia (Braude et al. 1983). Akathisia can be difficult to assess and is frequently misdiagnosed as anxiety or agitation (Weiden et al. 1987).

Acute dystonic reactions are abrupt-onset, sometimes bizarre muscular spasms affecting mainly the musculature of the head and neck. Sometimes, however, dystonias of the trunk and lower extremities lead to gait disturbances that may be confused with hysteria. Dystonia usually appears within the first few days of therapy, particularly when patients are treated with large doses of high-potency neuroleptics such as haloperidol or fluphenazine. Dystonia almost always responds rapidly to antiparkinsonian medications and can usually be prevented by either pretreating with these drugs or limiting the neuroleptic dosage prescribed. Younger patients and males are more prone than other patients to develop acute dystonias (Lavin and Rifkin 1992). One study found that 21% of male subjects younger than 30 developed acute dystonic reactions (Swett 1975).

Parkinsonism, which includes symptoms such as stiffness, tremor, and shuffling gait, affects about 30% of patients who receive chronic treatment with traditional antipsychotics. Patients with parkinsonism may also experience akinesia, a side effect that causes difficulty in initiating movement. In some cases, drug-induced parkinsonism can be nearly identical to Parkinson's disease (Lavin and Rifkin 1992).

For most patients, EPS are treatable. The anticholinergic antiparkinsonian drugs such as benztropine or trihexyphenidyl are by far the most commonly used drugs for EPS. Many clinicians prescribe these drugs routinely for patients who are taking antipsychotics, particularly potent antipsychotics. Several studies indicate that prescribing antiparkinsonian medications before patients have EPS can prevent dystonias (Lavin and Rifkin 1992; Winslow et al. 1986). Unfortunately, these drugs also have their own side effects, including dry mouth, constipation, urinary retention, and blurry vision. Other studies indicate that anticholinergic antiparkinsonian drugs can also cause some loss of memory (Gelenberg et al. 1989). This side effect is dose dependent and remits when the drug is stopped.

Other drugs for treating EPS include amantadine (which is effective against parkinsonism) and propranolol (which is effective in managing akathisia). Both of these drugs can be added to anticholinergic antiparkinsonian drugs.

Some people are highly sensitive to EPS—particularly akathisia—at the dose that is necessary to control their psychoses. Some of these patients may agree to tolerate these side effects, at least temporarily, while their most troublesome psychotic symptoms are being treated. For others, the discomfort brought on by medication side effects may seem worse than the illness itself. These patients may be good candidates for newer agents such as clozapine, ziprasidone, olanzapine, or risperidone.

Tardive Dyskinesia

Tardive dyskinesia is a movement disorder that may occur after chronic treatment with antipsychotic medications. Patients with tardive dyskinesia may have any or all of a number of abnormal movements, such as mouth and tongue movements (e.g., lip smacking, sucking, and puckering) and facial grimacing. Other movements may include irregular movements of the limbs, particularly choreoathetoid-like movements of the fingers and toes, and slow, writhing movements of the trunk. Younger patients tend to develop slower athetoid movements of the trunk, extremities, and neck. The movements from tardive dyskinesia tend to increase when a patient is aroused and tend to decrease when he or she is relaxed. They are typically absent during sleep. Diagnostic criteria for tardive dyskinesia developed by Schooler and Kane (1982) require that patients have at least 3 months of antipsychotic drug exposure and that the movements persist for at least 4 weeks. Seriously disabling dyskinesia is uncommon, but a small proportion of patients may have tardive dyskinesia that affects walking, breathing, eating, and talking.

At least 10%–20% of patients treated with antipsychotics for more than 1 year develop tardive dyskinesia. In chronically institutionalized patients, the prevalence is 15%–20% (Kane et al. 1986). Prospective studies indicate that the cumulative incidence of tardive dyskinesia is 5% at 1 year, 10% at 2 years, 15% at 3 years, and 19% at 4 years (Kane et al. 1986). Certain populations are at greater risk than others for developing tardive dyskinesia. Older patients are at increased risk, and elderly women are particularly vulnerable. Moreover, tardive dyskinesia in elderly patients is less likely to remit when antipsychotics are discontinued. Patients with affective disorders may also be at a greater risk for developing tardive dyskinesia when they are treated with antipsychotics. Other possible risk factors for tardive dyskinesia are the dose of antipsychotic medications and the length of time taking these drugs (Kane and Lieberman 1992).

Early observations of the course of tardive dyskinesia suggested that the disorder was inevitably progressive and irreversible. In other words, once patients developed even mild dyskinesia, they would likely progress toward severe tardive dyskinesia. More recent evidence indicates otherwise. Tardive dyskinesia does not appear to be a progressive disorder for most patients. It seems to develop rapidly and then to stabilize and often to improve. Several studies have followed the course of tardive dyskinesia in patients who continued taking antipsychotic drugs for several years. The consensus was that most patients had a reduction in the severity of tardive dyskinesia, even if their antipsychotic drugs were continued. Moreover, this reduction can be clinically meaningful in some patients.

The American Psychiatric Association Task Force on Tardive Dyskinesia (1992) issued a report that included many recommendations for preventing and managing tardive dyskinesia. These recommendations include the following:

1. Establishing objective evidence that antipsychotic medications are effective for an individual
2. Using the lowest effective dose of antipsychotic
3. Prescribing cautiously to children, elderly people, and individuals with mood disorders
4. Examining patients on a regular basis for evidence of tardive dyskinesia
5. When tardive dyskinesia is diagnosed, considering alternatives to antipsychotics, obtaining informed consent, and also considering dosage reduction
6. If the tardive dyskinesia worsens, considering a number of options, including discontinuing the antipsychotic, switching to a different drug, or considering a trial of clozapine

Neuroleptic Malignant Syndrome

The clinical characteristics of neuroleptic malignant syndrome (NMS) include 1) severe muscular rigidity; 2) autonomic instability, including hyperthermia, tachycardia, increased blood pressure, tachypnea, and diaphoresis; and 3) changing levels of consciousness. A patient with NMS usually presents with muscular rigidity, and the condition progresses to elevated temperature, fluctuating consciousness, and unstable vital signs. These symptoms are often associated with elevations in creatine phosphokinase (CPK). Elevations in liver transaminases, leukocytosis, myoglobinemia, and myoglobinuria are less frequent. Acute renal failure may also occur. Mortality in well-developed cases has been reported to range from 20% to 30% and may be higher when depot forms are used, but more recent studies indicate that mortality from NMS has been reduced (Shalev et al. 1989).

NMS is more common when high-potency

antipsychotics are prescribed in high doses and when dose is escalated rapidly. The syndrome is twice as common in males as in females and is more likely to be present in younger patients. Clinicians should be concerned about any patient who has severe muscular rigidity and a rising body temperature because early diagnosis and treatment can be life-saving. The most effective means for preventing NMS probably involves the early diagnosis and management of severe muscular rigidity.

When NMS is diagnosed or suspected, antipsychotics should be discontinued and supportive and symptomatic treatment begun. This treatment may include reducing EPS with antiparkinsonian medications, correcting fluid and electrolyte imbalances, reducing fevers, and managing cardiovascular symptoms such as hyper- or hypotension. Gratz and colleagues (1992) suggested that when patients have fevers higher than 101°F, antipsychotics and anticholinergics should be discontinued. At that time, treatment with dopamine agonists such as bromocriptine should be considered, along with intensive medical monitoring if the fever exceeds 103°F. If these treatments are inadequate, dantrolene or benzodiazepines should be considered. After patients recover from NMS, they can usually be treated with a different antipsychotic drug or even with the same drug that caused NMS.

Neuroendocrine Side Effects

The most significant and consistent neuroendocrine effect of antipsychotics is hyperprolactinemia. Some patients develop tolerance to the prolactin-elevating effects of these drugs after several weeks (Meltzer 1985). In women, elevated prolactin can lead to menstrual abnormalities, including anovulatory cycles and infertility, menses with abnormal luteal phases, or frank amenorrhea and hypoestrogenemia (Reichlin 1992). Galactorrhea is a relatively common side effect that results from the direct effect of prolactin on the breast tissue. It may be uncomfortable but is seldom of any medical significance. Female patients have also reported decreased libido and anorgasmia.

In men, elevated prolactin levels can lower testosterone levels and result in impotence. Male patients frequently report ejaculatory and erectile disturbances that are probably related to the autonomic effects of the antipsychotic. These problems tend to be most prominent with low-potency drugs and are usually dose related.

Cardiovascular Side Effects

Low-potency antipsychotic medications such as chlorpromazine or thioridazine can cause orthostatic hypotension through α_1-adrenergic blockade. The more potent dopamine blockers such as haloperidol or fluphenazine are less likely to cause autonomic effects. Chlorpromazine may cause prolongation of the Q-T and P-R intervals, ST depression, and T-wave blunting, and thioridazine may cause Q-T and T-wave changes. Both should be used cautiously in patients with increases in their Q-T intervals.

Other Side Effects

Low-potency antipsychotics, particularly chlorpromazine, may cause photosensitivity reactions consisting of severe sunburn or rash. As a result, patients should be instructed to use sunscreens. These drugs may also be associated with an uncommon discoloration of the skin. Skin areas that are exposed to sunlight, particularly the face and neck, develop blue-gray metallic discoloration. This skin reaction is usually associated with long-term treatment involving high drug doses.

Patients receiving long-term treatment with chlorpromazine may develop granular deposits in the anterior lens and posterior cornea. These deposits (visualized on slit lamp examination) seldom affect the patient's vision. Changing the drug given to the patient will usually result in a gradual improvement in the condition.

High dosages of thioridazine (i.e., >1,000 mg/day) can result in retinal pigmentation. This condition can lead to serious visual impairment or blindness. Moreover, the condition may not remit when thioridazine is discontinued. Therefore, thioridazine should not be prescribed in doses higher than 800 mg/day.

Coexisting Medical Conditions

Pregnancy.   No clear evidence indicates that antipsychotic drugs are associated with congenital malformations. These drugs do cross the placenta, and there are suggestions from animal studies that prenatal exposure may affect the development of the dopamine system. Altshuler et al. (1996) performed a meta-analysis on the effects of first-trimester exposure to low-potency antipsychotics and found that these agents resulted in a very small increase in the relative risk for congenital anomalies. (The baseline incidence was 2.0%, and the incidence with antipsychotics was 2.4%.) No evidence suggests that high-potency drugs increase the risk to the fetus.

Clinicians should attempt to discontinue antipsychotic drugs during the first trimester if this is feasible and should consider carefully whether the risks of prescribing these drugs during the remainder of a patient's pregnancy are justified by the likely benefits. If patients have a history of relapse when antipsychotics are discontinued, the drugs are relatively safe. When an antipsychotic is prescribed, high-potency compounds are probably safer than low-potency compounds.

Antipsychotics are secreted in breast milk and therefore mothers who are being treated with these drugs should not breast-feed.

Seizure disorders.   Antipsychotics lower seizure thresholds and should be prescribed with caution to patients with seizure disorders. This adverse effect is more likely to occur with low-potency drugs than with high-potency drugs.

DRUG-DRUG INTERACTIONS

Several drugs, including certain heterocyclic antidepressants, selective serotonin reuptake inhibitors (SSRIs), β-blockers, and anticonvulsants, can affect the metabolism of antipsychotics. As noted in Table 8–2, a number of traditional antipsychotics are metabolized by the CYP2D6 isoenzyme. Thus, drugs such as fluoxetine can lead to an increase in plasma levels and a resultant worsening of EPS. This also explains the observation that chlorpromazine and thioridazine levels are increased when propranolol is added. Conversely, barbiturates and carbamazepine may decrease plasma levels by enhancing metabolism of the antipsychotic. Many studies have found that anticholinergic antiparkinsonian medications decrease antipsychotic blood levels, but more recent and better controlled studies have concluded that antipsychotic levels are unaffected (Leipzig and Mendelowitz 1992). Antacids can decrease the absorption of antipsychotic.

Antipsychotic drugs antagonize the effects of dopamine agonists or L-dopa when these drugs are used to treat parkinsonism. Chlorpromazine, haloperidol, and thiothixene can block the antihypertensive effects of guanethidine (Janowsky et al. 1973). Antipsychotics may also enhance the effects of central nervous system depressants such as analgesics, anxiolytics, and hypnotics (Leipzig and Mendelowitz 1992).

CONCLUSION

Antipsychotic drugs are effective agents for treating psychosis that results from schizophrenia or other illnesses. In treating schizophrenia, these agents are also effective in preventing relapse in stabilized individuals. However, antipsychotic medications have some important limitations. They have serious side effects (particularly neurological effects) that can result in severe discomfort on the one hand and prolonged abnormal movement disorders on the other. In addition, not every patient's psychosis responds well to these agents. Newer atypical antipsychotic drugs such as clozapine, olanzapine, ziprasidone, and risperidone have milder side effects without compromising effectiveness. These drugs have largely replaced the traditional antipsychotic agents.

REFERENCES

Altshuler LL, Cohen L, Szuba MP, et al: Pharmacologic management of psychiatric illness during pregnancy: dilemmas and guidelines. Am J Psychiatry 153:592–606, 1966

American Psychiatric Association Task Force on Tardive Dyskinesia: Tardive Dyskinesia: A Task Force Report of the American Psychiatric Association. Washington, DC, American Psychiatric Press, 1992

Bowers MB Jr: Homovanillic acid in caudate and prefrontal cortex following neuroleptics. Eur J Pharmacol 99:103–105, 1984

Braude WM, Barnes TRE, Gore SM, et al: Clinical characteristics of akathisia: a systematic investigation of acute psychiatric inpatient admissions. Br J Psychiatry 143:139–150, 1983

Buchanan RW, Gold JM: Negative symptoms: diagnosis, treatment and prognosis. Int Clin Psychopharmacol 11 (suppl 2):3–11, 1996

Campbell A, Baldessarini RJ: Prolonged pharmacologic activity of neuroleptics (letter). Arch Gen Psychiatry 42:637, 1985

Carlsson A, Lindquist M: Effect of chlorpromazine or haloperidol on the formation of 3-methoxytyramine and normetanephrine in mouse brain. Acta Pharmacologica et Toxicologica 20:140–144, 1963

Chakraborty BS, Hubbard JW, Hawes EM, et al: Interconversion between haloperidol and reduced haloperidol in healthy volunteers. Eur J Clin Pharmacol 37:45–48, 1989

Chiodo LA, Bunney BS: Population response of midbrain dopaminergic neurons to neuroleptics: further studies on time course and nondopaminergic neuronal influences. J Neurosci 7:629–633, 1987

Creese I, Burt DR, Snyder SH: Dopamine receptor binding predicts clinical and pharmacologic potencies of antischizophrenic drugs. Science 192:481–483, 1976

Dixon LB, Lehman AF, Levine J: Conventional antipsychotic medications for schizophrenia. Schizophr Bull 21:567–577, 1995

Ereshefsky L, Riesenman C, Lam YWF: Serotonin selective reuptake inhibitor drug interactions and cytochrome P450 system. J Clin Psychiatry 57 (suppl 8):17–25, 1996

Farde L, Nordstrom AL, Wiesel FA, et al: Positron emission tomographic analysis of central D_1 and D_2 dopamine receptor occupancy in patients treated with classical neuroleptics and clozapine. Arch Gen Psychiatry 49:538–544, 1992

Gelenberg AJ, Van Putten T, Lavori PW, et al: Anticholinergic effects on memory: benztropine versus amantadine. J Clin Psychiatry 9:180–185, 1989

Gerlach J: New antipsychotics classification, efficacy, and adverse effects. Schizophr Bull 17:289–309, 1991

Gratz SS, Levinson DF, Simpson GM: Neuroleptic malignant syndrome, in Adverse Effects of Psychotropic Drugs. Edited by Kane JM, Lieberman JA. New York, Guilford, 1992, pp 266–284

Hogarty GE, Ulrich RF, Mussare F, et al: Drug discontinuation among long term, successfully maintained schizophrenic outpatients. Disorders of the Nervous System 37:494–500, 1976

Hubbard JW, Ganes DA, Midha KK: Prolonged pharmacologic activity of neuroleptic drugs. Arch Gen Psychiatry 44:99–100, 1987

Janowsky DS, El-Yousef MK, Davis JM, et al: Antagonism of guanethidine by chlorpromazine. Am J Psychiatry 130:808–812, 1973

Johnson DAW, Pasterski JM, Ludlow JM, et al: The discontinuance of maintenance neuroleptic therapy in chronic schizophrenic patients: drug and social consequences. Acta Psychiatr Scand 67:339–352, 1983

Kane JM, Lieberman J: Tardive dyskinesia, in Adverse Effects of Psychotropic Drugs. Edited by Kane JM, Lieberman JA. New York, Guilford, 1992, pp 235–245

Kane JM, Woerner M, Borenstein M: Integrating incidence and prevalence of tardive dyskinesia. Psychopharmacol Bull 22:254–258, 1986

Kissling W: Ideal and reality of neuroleptic relapse prevention. Br J Psychiatry 161 (suppl):133–139, 1992

Kissling W, Kane JM, Barnes TRE, et al: Guidelines for neuroleptic relapse prevention in schizophrenia: towards a consensus view, in Guidelines for Neuroleptic Relapse Prevention in Schizophrenia. Edited by Kissling W. Berlin, Springer-Verlag, 1991, pp 155–163

Lavin MR, Rifkin A: Neuroleptic-induced parkinsonism, in Adverse Effects of Psychotropic Drugs. Edited by Kane JM, Lieberman JA. New York, Guilford, 1992, pp 175–188

Leipzig RM, Mendelowitz A: Adverse psychotropic drug-drug interactions, in Adverse Effects of Psychotropic Drugs. Edited by Kane JM, Lieberman JA. New York, Guilford, 1992, pp 13–76

Marder SR, Hubbard JW, Van Putten T, et al: The pharmacokinetics of long-acting injectable neuroleptic drugs: clinical implications. Psychopharmacology (Berl) 98:433–439, 1989

Marder SR, Wirshing W, Van Putten T: Drug treatment of schizophrenia: overview of recent research. Schizophr Res 4:81–90, 1991

Meltzer HY: Long-term effects of neuroleptic drugs on the neuroendocrine system. Biochem Psychopharmacol 40:50–68, 1985

Midha KK, Marder SR, Jaworski TJ, et al: Clinical perspectives of some neuroleptics through development and application of their assays. Ther Drug Monit 15:179–189, 1993

Preskorn SH: Clinical Pharmacology of Selective Serotonin Reuptake Inhibitors. Caddo, OK, Professional Communications, 1996, p 158

Reichlin S: Neuroendocrinology, in Williams Textbook of Endocrinology, 8th Edition. Edited by Williams RH. Orlando, FL, WB Saunders, 1992, pp 135–219

Schooler NR, Kane JM: Research diagnoses for tardive dyskinesia. Arch Gen Psychiatry 39:486–487, 1982

Sedvall GC: Neurobiological correlates of acute neuroleptic treatment. Int Clin Psychopharmacol 11 (suppl 2):41–46, 1996

Seeman P, Lee T, Chau-Wong M, et al: Antipsychotic drug doses and neuroleptic/dopamine receptors. Nature 261:717–719, 1976

Shalev A, Hermesh H, Munitz H: Mortality from neuroleptic malignant syndrome. J Clin Psychiatry 51:18–25, 1989

Silver JM, Yudofsky SC, Hurowitz GI: Psychopharmacology and electroconvulsive therapy, in The American Psychiatric Press Textbook of Psychiatry, 2nd Edition. Edited by Hales RE, Yudofsky SC, Talbott JA. Washington, DC, American Psychiatric Press, 1994, pp 897–1007

Swett C: Drug-induced dystonia. Am J Psychiatry 132:532–534, 1975

Van Putten T, May PRA, Marder SR: Akathisia with haloperidol and thiothixene. Arch Gen Psychiatry 41:1036–1039, 1984

Weiden PJ, Mann JJ, Haas G, et al: Clinical nonrecognition of neuroleptic-induced movement disorders: a cautionary study. Am J Psychiatry 144:1148–1153, 1987

Winslow RS, Stiller V, Coons DJ, et al: Prevention of acute dystonic reactions in patients beginning high potency neuroleptics. Am J Psychiatry 143:707–710, 1986

Wyatt RJ: Neuroleptics and the natural course of schizophrenia. Schizophr Bull 17:325–351, 1991

NINE

Atypical Antipsychotics

Michael J. Owens, Ph.D., and
S. Craig Risch, M.D.

The widely held dopamine hypothesis regarding the pathophysiology of schizophrenia is based on two main lines of evidence. First, almost all clinically useful antipsychotic drugs are dopamine receptor antagonists. Second, dopamine agonists (i.e., drugs such as dextroamphetamine that increase the synaptic availability of dopamine) can produce positive symptoms of psychosis (i.e., hallucinations, delusions, and thought disorders) that are indistinguishable from those produced by paranoid schizophrenia. Indeed, the ability of antipsychotic drugs to produce an antipsychotic action, as well as extrapyramidal side effects (EPS), has been primarily attributed to their ability to block the dopamine, subtype 2 (D_2), receptor in the mesolimbocortical and nigrostriatal dopamine systems, respectively. Although the inhibitory effects of these antipsychotics on classical D_2 receptors appear to correlate superbly with their clinical antipsychotic potency, this neurochemical effect alone cannot explain all of the clinically relevant differences between these drugs.

Since the advent of antipsychotic use in the treatment of schizophrenia, there has been a search for superior drugs because the "typical,"

"classical," or "traditional" D_2 blocking antipsychotics often do not result in a full remission of symptoms or, in many cases, even a significant reduction. This search has focused on compounds with an improved therapeutic profile (i.e., improved efficacy on both positive and negative symptoms and decreased side effects). These compounds, of which clozapine is considered the prototypical agent, have been termed *atypical antipsychotics*. Indeed, clozapine differs from typical antipsychotics (i.e., haloperidol and chlorpromazine) in producing minimal or no EPS in humans or catalepsy in rodents at therapeutic doses. Perhaps more important is that clozapine, unlike typical antipsychotics, reduces both the positive and the negative symptoms of schizophrenia. The fact that clozapine differs clinically from typical antipsychotics, together with the data showing that clozapine is a relatively weak D_2 antagonist and that the efficacy of all antipsychotics increases over time, has made up the dominant impetus suggesting that the original dopamine hypothesis of schizophrenia needs revising.

Only clozapine, risperidone, olanzapine, and quetiapine are routinely used as atypical antipsychotics at this time. Therefore, we begin this chapter by reviewing several hypotheses, based primarily on animal studies of clozapine and recent advances in molecular neuropharmacology (i.e., the cloning of a number of receptors that bind antipsychotic drugs), that have been promulgated to explain the differences between typical and atypical antipsychotics. This portion of the chapter summarizing preclinical data falls under the categories "Mechanism of Action" and "Pharmacological Profile." It is beyond the scope of this chapter to review in detail all the atypical antipsychotics currently under clinical investigation. Therefore, we focus primarily on the clinical pharmacology and therapeutics of clozapine, risperidone, olanzapine, and quetiapine, the only atypical antipsychotics currently approved for use in the United States.

MECHANISM OF ACTION

On the basis of clozapine's activity, the mechanism of action of atypical antipsychotics is thought to be based on either the drugs' differential actions in various subpopulations of dopamine neurons, their binding to different dopamine receptor subtypes, or additional binding to other neurotransmitter receptors. First, we compare and contrast the neurophysiological effects of clozapine with those of typical antipsychotics. Some of these differences possibly give clozapine an atypical profile. Second, we describe the receptor binding profile of several putative atypical antipsychotic agents. Note that these differences in receptor binding are probably responsible for the neurophysiological differences between clozapine and other typical antipsychotics.

It has been suggested that clozapine, unlike other typical antipsychotics, has mesolimbic dopaminergic specificity relative to its actions on nigrostriatal dopamine neurons and that this may underlie its relative lack of EPS and tardive dyskinesia liability. Much of this evidence has come from electrophysiological studies of midbrain dopamine neurons. In general, dopa-

mine neurons originating in the ventral tegmental area (VTA; A10 cell group) project to the nucleus accumbens, amygdala, and neocortex and make up the mesolimbocortical dopamine system. These projections are thought to be responsible for most symptoms associated with schizophrenia, although data to confirm this are limited. In contrast, the dopamine cells of the substantia nigra (SN; A9 cell group) project primarily to the caudate-putamen and make up the nigrostriatal dopamine system. This pathway is thought to be involved in the motor disturbances associated with EPS and tardive dyskinesia, although recent evidence suggests that this pathway also may be involved in the behavioral manifestations of schizophrenia.

The pioneering work of Bunney et al. (1987, 1991) showed that acute administration of haloperidol increases the firing rate of VTA and SN dopamine neurons. This response is probably the result of a lack of local and distant negative feedback on dopamine cells after D_2 receptor blockade. In contrast, acute clozapine administration only increases the firing rate of VTA neurons.

Of more physiological significance are the changes observed after chronic administration of these compounds. On a time scale similar to that in which antipsychotics exert their clinical effects, typical antipsychotics such as haloperidol significantly decrease the number of spontaneously active dopamine neurons encountered in the VTA and SN. Subsequent examination reveals that these cells enter into a state of depolarization-induced block (inactivation) and decreased dopaminergic function. Clozapine differs from typical antipsychotics in that chronic administration does not induce depolarization block of SN dopamine neurons but does induce inactivation in dopamine neurons of the VTA (Chiodo and Bunney 1983, 1985; Hand et al. 1987). The delayed onset of depolarization block in the VTA is thought to be related to the increased efficacy observed over time with all antipsychotic drugs, including clozapine, whereas the lack of EPS with clozapine is hypothesized to be the result of preservation of the activity of the SN neurons.

In addition to the differential effects of typical and atypical antipsychotics on dopamine neuronal firing, clozapine and haloperidol produce different patterns of electrotonic coupling (i.e., passive flow of current between neurons) that can occur in the absence of an action potential in neurons of the striatum or nucleus accumbens (Onn and Grace 1995). Excellent reviews on the actions of antipsychotics on dopamine neuronal activity and the neurophysiology of dopaminergic terminal fields can be found in O'Donnell and Grace (1996) and Grace et al. (1997).

The electrophysiological actions just described are thought to result in neurochemical differences as well. Studies have shown that acute administration of typical antipsychotic drugs results in more prominent effects on dopamine metabolism in the striatum than in mesolimbocortical areas; in contrast, clozapine appears to augment dopamine turnover to a relatively greater degree in mesolimbic areas (Deutch et al. 1991). Based on the electrophysiological findings suggesting that increased firing of dopamine neurons after acute antipsychotic drug administration is secondary to a lack of negative feedback caused by D_2 receptor blockade, the data suggest that clozapine preferentially alters mesolimbocortical dopamine neurons.

Additional studies have been reported using in vivo microdialysis, another technique that can measure local dopamine release in specific brain regions. Ichikawa and Meltzer (1991) found evidence that chronically administered clozapine does not interfere with either mesolimbic (nucleus accumbens) or nigrostriatal dopamine metabolism. These findings also suggest that dopamine release from nerve terminals may not be significantly affected by the presence of depolarization block.

There is also evidence that clozapine may preferentially increase dopamine release in the prefrontal cortex (Moghaddam 1994; Moghaddam and Bunney 1990). This finding, together with the relatively weaker D_2 receptor blockade produced by clozapine in relation to that produced by typical antipsychotics, may lead to a net increase in mesocortical dopamine activity. Indeed, the "hypofrontality" theory states that the negative symptoms of schizophrenia may be the result of a cortical dopamine deficit. Thus, one could speculate that clozapine may reduce both the negative and the positive symptoms of schizophrenia because of its ability to increase cortical and decrease nucleus accumbens dopamine activity, respectively. Moreover, the relative lack of effect on nigrostriatal dopamine systems may be responsible for the lack of EPS associated with clozapine.

PHARMACOLOGICAL PROFILE

D_2, D_3, and D_4 Receptors

Although, as we stated at the outset of this chapter, recent findings have suggested that the dopamine hypothesis of schizophrenia needs revision, findings from positron-emission tomography (PET) studies have provided further proof that the D_2 receptor is involved in the pathophysiology of schizophrenia and the mechanism of action of antipsychotics. Seeman and colleagues have reported that drug-naive schizophrenic patients have increased numbers of D_2 receptors in the putamen (Seeman 1987, 1992b; Seeman et al. 1989a). These increases in D_2 receptor binding may actually represent increases in D_4 receptors and not D_2 receptors. Moreover, chemically distinct antipsychotic agents occupy from 65% to—in the case of haloperidol—upward of 90% of D_2 receptors in the putamen at clinically relevant doses (Farde et al. 1986, 1988, 1993). Of special significance is the finding that, unlike typical antipsychotics, clozapine occupies only 40%–50% of D_2 receptors in the striatum, whereas 80%–90% occupancy is observed in limbic areas (Farde et al. 1989).

Although it is generally thought that the

high affinity for D_2 receptors in the striatum is responsible for the EPS associated with typical antipsychotics, selective D_2 antagonists may possess some atypical antipsychotic activity. Before describing some of these findings, it is helpful to briefly characterize some properties of the D_2 receptor.

The cloning of the D_2 receptor (Bunzow et al. 1988; Grandy et al. 1989) has enabled the simultaneous visualization and distribution of D_2 receptors and messenger ribonucleic acid (mRNA) in the brains of rats (Mansour et al. 1990; Meador-Woodruff et al. 1989; Mengod et al. 1989), primates (Lidow et al. 1989; Meador-Woodruff et al. 1991), and humans (Meador-Woodruff et al. 1996) (Figure 9–1). Along with the anterior pituitary, the highest concentrations are observed in the nigrostriatal and mesolimbic dopamine systems, and somewhat less is observed in primate cortex. D_2 receptors are located both postsynaptically and presynaptically, where they probably act as autoreceptors. Increases in D_2 receptor binding are observed after antipsychotic treatment through unclear mechanisms that are thought to include both transcriptional (i.e., increased mRNA synthesis) and posttranscriptional (i.e., not related to changes in receptor synthesis) processes (Seeman 1992b; Srivastava et al. 1990; Van Tol et al. 1990; Xu et al. 1992).

Shortly after the initial cloning of the D_2 receptor, it was found that different isoforms of the same receptor are synthesized through alternative RNA splicing (Chio et al. 1990; Giros et al. 1989; Monsma et al. 1989). The two different isoforms vary by 29 amino acids in the third cytoplasmic loop near the guanine nucleotide binding protein (G protein) recognition site. Although this difference does not appear to result in binding differences between D_2 ligands, its location near the G protein regulatory site may result in differences in intracellular transduction mechanisms and receptor regulation (L.-J. Zhang et al. 1994).

As mentioned earlier in this chapter, D_2 receptors can act presynaptically as autoreceptors

located either on the somatodendritic portion of the neuron or on presynaptic terminals. Those located on presynaptic terminals inhibit the release of dopamine into the synaptic cleft when activated. Utilizing low doses of the dopamine agonist apomorphine, Tamminga and others have investigated its antipsychotic potential (Tamminga and Gerlach 1987). The main effect of apomorphine at low doses is stimulation of presynaptic dopamine autoreceptors and diminishment of dopaminergic function, whereas at higher doses postsynaptic agonistic actions predominate. Pursuing this line of research, medicinal chemists and pharmacologists have synthesized compounds purported to have higher affinity for autoreceptors than apomorphine does and reduced postsynaptic affinity. These compounds have been reported in preclinical studies to produce fewer EPS than do typical antipsychotic agents (Carlsson 1988a, 1988b; Heffner et al. 1992; Wiedemann et al. 1992). Although these compounds are hoped to primarily decrease transmission in the mesolimbic dopamine system, it is not clear whether this can be achieved, because some dopaminergic neurons do not have autoreceptors (Kilts et al. 1987).

A somewhat similar, related strategy is represented by partial dopamine agonists. These compounds, by definition, have a high affinity for the D_2 receptor but limited intrinsic activity to produce a full agonist effect. Thus, in the presence of normal or increased dopaminergic stimulation (mesolimbic system; positive symptoms), such compounds would compete with endogenous dopamine and act as functional antagonists. Conversely, under conditions of low dopaminergic tone (mesocortical system; negative symptoms), partial agonists would be expected to augment dopaminergic function. For example, the $S(+)$-N-n-propylnoraporphines act as functional dopamine antagonists and also show an apparent limbic selectivity (Baldessarini et al. 1991; Campbell et al. 1991). Partial agonists with relatively high intrinsic activity, such as B-HT-920, do not induce catalepsy in laboratory studies. Partial agonists such as SDZ

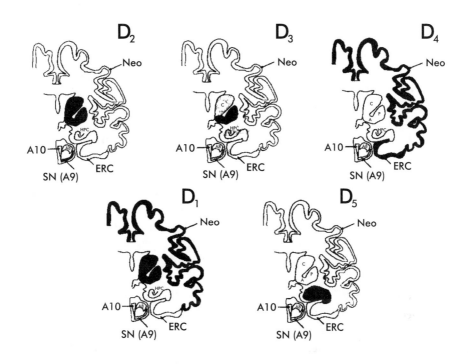

Figure 9–1. Brain region location of mRNA for human dopamine receptors (grey stippled regions). Abbreviations: 3 = third ventricle; AC = nucleus accumbens; AM = amygdala; C = caudate nucleus; Cx = cerebral cortex; G = globus pallidus; H = hypothalamus; Hipp = hippocampus; ICJ = islands of Calleja; L = lateral ventricle; O = olfactory tubercle; P = putamen; SN = substantia nigra; VTA = ventral tegmental area.

Source. Reprinted from Meador-Woodruff JH, Mansour A, Civelli O, et al: "Dopamine Receptor mRNA Expression in Human Striatum and Neocortex." *Neuropsychopharmacology* 15:17–29, 1996. Copyright 1996, the American College of Neuropsychopharmacology; and Seeman P: "Dopamine Receptor Sequences: Therapeutic Levels of Neuroleptics Occupy D_2 Receptors, Clozapine Occupies D_4." *Neuropsychopharmacology* 7:261–284, 1992. Copyright 1992, the American College of Neuropsychopharmacology. Used with permission of Elsevier Science Publishing Co., Inc.

208-912 display a clear separation of doses between those producing catalepsy and those antagonizing dopamine-mediated behaviors (Coward et al. 1990; Meltzer 1991; Naber et al. 1992), although SDZ 208-912 was removed from clinical trials because it produced EPS.

The D_3 receptor has also been cloned and studied (Sokoloff et al. 1990, 1992a). This receptor has considerable homology with the D_2 receptor but has 10–100 times higher affinity for dopamine than do D_2 receptors. Thus, the effects of dopaminergic agonists and autoreceptor-selective agonists may be attributable to their actions primarily on D_3 receptors. The D_3 receptor appears to be expressed predominantly in the mesolimbic dopaminergic system and substantially less in the nigrostriatal system, hippocampus, and entorhinal cortex (Bouthenet et al. 1991; Buckland et al. 1992; Diaz et al. 1994; Meador-Woodruff et al. 1996; Sokoloff et al. 1990) (Figure 9–1). A small amount of D_3 mRNA is expressed in human cortex, as Schmauss et al. (1993) reported an absence of D_3 mRNA in postmortem motor and parietal cortex from 16 of 18 schizophrenic patients compared with control subjects. The diagnostic specificity—and relationship to schizophrenia compared with antipsychotic drug treatment—

of this finding is unclear because similar alterations were observed in samples from long-term hospitalized patients with affective disorders.

Like the D_2 receptor, the D_3 receptor has a high affinity for antipsychotic drugs in vitro. Typical antipsychotics such as haloperidol are 10–20 times more potent at D_2 receptors than at D_3 receptors. However, atypical antipsychotics such as clozapine and several substituted benzamides are only 2–3 times more potent at the D_2 receptor (Schwartz et al. 1992; Sokoloff et al. 1990, 1992b). Thus, the ratio of binding in vitro to the D_3 receptor compared with the D_2 receptor is higher for several atypical antipsychotics compared with typical antipsychotics. This, combined with the localization of D_3 receptors primarily in the mesolimbic system, might represent the ability of atypical antipsychotics such as clozapine to treat schizophrenia while sparing the nigrostriatal dopamine system (Snyder 1990).

There are shortcomings, however, of relying on drug affinities derived from in vitro binding studies. Only free drug in the extracellular water compartment is available in vivo for binding to a given receptor. This fraction of total drug is dependent on several bioavailability and pharmacokinetic considerations. Therefore, selectivity based on in vitro binding affinities may not be apparent in vivo. For example, at commonly used clinical doses, the D_2 receptors are blocked by about 80%, whereas D_3 receptors would be blocked by only 2%–40% (Seeman 1992a, 1992b). As Seeman has pointed out, no neuroleptics block D_3 receptors more readily than D_2. Moreover, no agonists discriminate between these receptors because the affinities of agonists at the D_3 receptor are similar to those at the high-affinity state of the D_2 receptor.

Although a selective D_3 antagonist would be of considerable interest as an antipsychotic, preliminary genetic linkage studies have not found evidence for a link between D_3 receptor abnormalities and schizophrenia (Sokoloff et al. 1992c). Indeed, numerous linkage studies have led to consistent and incontrovertible results

that there is no significant linkage between schizophrenia and D_1, D_2, D_3, D_4, or D_5 receptors.

The D_4 receptor is the latest receptor in the D_2 receptor family to be cloned (Van Tol et al. 1991). The D_4 receptor has homology similar to both the D_2 and the D_3 receptor. In general, the D_4 receptor has less or equal affinity for dopamine agonists and antagonists as does the D_2 receptor. The finding that clozapine has greater than 10-fold higher affinity for the D_4 receptor than for the D_2 receptor is of considerable interest. Moreover, the affinity constant of clozapine for the D_4 receptor is similar to the free concentration of clozapine observed during antipsychotic treatment (Figure 9–2) (Seeman 1992a, 1992b; Van Tol et al. 1991). However, Roth et al. (1995) examined a series of typical and atypical antipsychotics and determined that the ratio of D_4 to D_2 binding could not be used to differentiate the two classes of antipsychotics.

Several variants of the D_4 receptor have been found in the human population and have different antipsychotic binding properties, although the importance of this finding is not known (Van Tol et al. 1992). Seeman et al. (1993, 1995) and others (Murray et al. 1995; Sumiyoshi et al. 1995) have reported increases in D_4 receptors in schizophrenic striatal and nucleus accumbens tissue. D_4 receptors were determined by a somewhat controversial method wherein binding of radioligands that label D_2 and D_3 receptors was subtracted from binding of radioligands that label D_2, D_3, and D_4 receptors. This increase in D_4 receptors may actually represent the increases in D_2 receptors reported in the past. Reynolds and Mason (1994) were unable to discriminate D_4 from D_2 and D_3 receptors using raclopride (D_2 and D_3) to competitively inhibit [^{3}H]nemonapride (D_2, D_3, and D_4) binding in schizophrenic tissue; however, Seeman and Van Tol (1995) presented evidence to suggest that this is a methodological issue. It is not known whether this apparent increase in D_4 receptors is related to the pathophysiology of schizophrenia or is a consequence of antipsychotic treatment, be-

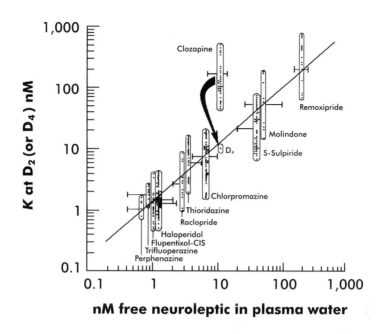

Figure 9–2. The neuroleptic dissociation constants (*K*) at the D_2 receptor closely match the free neuroleptic concentrations in the patients' plasma water. Each point indicates a *K* value. Clozapine is the only drug that does not fit the D_2 correlate, but its affinity at D_4 (arrow) does. The plasma molarities for *cis*-flupentixol and for *S*-sulpiride are half those published for the racemates that are used clinically.

Source. Reprinted from Seeman P: "Dopamine Receptor Sequences: Therapeutic Levels of Neuroleptics Occupy D_2 Receptors, Clozapine Occupies D_4." *Neuropsychopharmacology* 7:261–284, 1992. Copyright 1992, the American College of Neuropsychopharmacology. Used with permission of Elsevier Science Publishing Co., Inc.

cause chronic haloperidol administration increases striatal D_4 mRNA expression and receptor protein concentrations in laboratory animals (Schoots et al. 1995).

Areas of high D_4 receptor mRNA expression include the frontal and entorhinal cortex and hippocampus (Figure 9–1). However, D_4 receptor binding, using the subtraction method, is observed in cortex, striatum, and nucleus accumbens (Lahti et al. 1995; Murray et al. 1995). This distribution differs from the D_2 and D_3 receptors and may partly explain the lack of EPS with clozapine. Additionally, the D_4 receptor may represent frontal cortical labeling observed with ^{11}C-clozapine in a PET study reported by Lundberg et al. (1989).

D_1 and D_5 Receptors

Although the existence of the D_1 receptor has been known since the late 1970s, it was not until 1990 that the receptor was cloned from rat and human tissue by four groups simultaneously (Dearry et al. 1990; Monsma et al. 1990; Sunahara et al. 1990; Zhou et al. 1990). D_1 mRNA expression is highest in caudate, putamen, and nucleus accumbens and is somewhat lower in neocortex (Meador-Woodruff et al. 1996) (Figure 9–1). The D_1 receptor, unlike the D_2 receptor, stimulates the production of cyclic adenosine monophosphate (cAMP) and is distributed similarly to D_2 receptors (Clark and White 1987; Cortés et al. 1989; Mansour et al. 1991) (Figure 9–1). Of particular interest to this review is the finding that selective D_1 antagonists are effective in preclinical tests predictive of antipsychotic activity just like D_2 antagonists (Clark and White 1987; Waddington and Daly 1992). It has since been shown that these two receptors can interact either synergistically or antagonistically through G proteins and/or second-messenger generation (Bertorello et al. 1990; Piomelli et al. 1991; Seeman et al. 1989b, 1994; Wachtel et al. 1989). Indeed, Seeman et al. (1989b) found this link uncoupled in the brains of schizophrenic patients. These authors have suggested that a consequence of this might be excessive D_2 activity and the possible inability of antipsychotics to bind efficiently to their receptors. These investigators reported that this uncoupling is not the result of an altered amino acid sequence of the D_1 receptor, as deduced from the D_1 gene (Ohara et al. 1993).

In general, most antipsychotics currently in use bind to both D_2 and D_1 receptors. No correlation has been found between the atypical nature of an antipsychotic and its D_1 affinity, although as a group, atypical antipsychotics are less potent at the D_1 receptor (Meltzer et al. 1989). However, Farde et al. (1989) reported that clozapine displaces the D_1 PET ligand ^{11}C-SCH-23390 more efficiently than do typical antipsychotic drugs.

In addition to preclinical antipsychotic activity, D_1 antagonists can produce catalepsy in rodents and EPS in primates. Therefore, an atypical nature assigned to these compounds is certainly not due to D_1 selectivity alone but may be the result of the combination of low subclinical doses of a D_1 antagonist and a D_2 antagonist, which may potentiate each other, resulting in an antipsychotic effect without producing EPS.

The D_5 receptor, a second member of the D_1 receptor subfamily that has homology similar to the D_1 receptor, has been isolated and cloned from human (Sunahara et al. 1991) and rat (Tiberi et al. 1991) tissue. Like the D_1 receptor, the D_5 receptor is linked to adenylate cyclase and cAMP production and has affinities for various

agonists and antagonists—much like the D_1 receptor—with the notable exception of dopamine itself, which is about 10 times more potent at the D_5 receptor. This suggests that the D_5 receptor may be important in maintaining dopaminergic tone. The D_5 receptor is expressed at much lower concentrations than the D_1 receptor, and its highest expression is observed in the hippocampus and entorhinal cortex (Meador-Woodruff et al. 1996) (Figure 9–1). Until a selective antagonist can be found, the clinical utility of D_5 ligands as antipsychotics remains unknown.

Serotonin Receptors

It has been hypothesized that clozapine's atypical actions may at least partly result from its actions at other neurotransmitter receptors, such as certain serotonin (5-hydroxytryptamine [5-HT]) receptor subtypes. The involvement of serotonin neural circuits in the mechanism of action of atypical antipsychotic drugs was postulated partly because serotonin is known to exert a regulatory action on dopamine neurons. Neurochemical studies suggest that serotonin projections tonically inhibit mesolimbic and nigrostriatal dopaminergic activity. Moreover, serotonin may directly inhibit dopamine release from striatal nerve terminals (Dray et al. 1976; Soubrie et al. 1984). These findings led to the hypothesis that 5-HT_{2A} antagonists might decrease the inhibition of dopamine activity produced by chronic antipsychotics (i.e., depolarization block, postsynaptic D_2 antagonism), functionally increasing dopaminergic activity in certain areas. This hypothesis is supported by PET studies examining the effects of 5-HT_{2A} antagonists on ^{11}C]raclopride binding (Dewey et al. 1995). This also suggests that there may be relative differences in the optimal magnitude of dopaminergic blockade needed in different brain areas. Moreover, complete dopaminergic blockade may not be beneficial for negative symptoms and may result in EPS.

Much of the data suggesting the involvement of the 5-HT_{2A} receptor has come from

Meltzer and colleagues (Meltzer 1995; Meltzer et al. 1989), who examined the receptor-binding profile of a large series of antipsychotic drugs. They noted that typical and atypical antipsychotics can be distinguished by lower D_2 and higher 5-HT_{2A} pK_i values (a logarithmic measure of drug affinity for its receptor) of atypical compounds. Absolute potency at the 5-HT_{2A} receptor alone is not the determining factor, but atypical antipsychotics appear to have 5-HT_{2A}-to-D_2 pK_i ratios of at least 1.1 (>13-fold higher affinity). Likewise, Seeman (1992a) reported that those antipsychotics with less propensity to cause rigidity have higher 5-HT_{2A}-to-D_2 ratios. 5-HT_{2A} blockade, however, cannot account for the atypical actions of all purported atypical antipsychotics, such as remoxipride and raclopride, because their $5\text{-HT}_{2A}/D_2$ blocking profile is similar to that of classical antipsychotics.

The suggestion has been made to co-administer 5-HT_{2A} antagonists with a typical antipsychotic to determine whether this would produce a clozapine-like profile. Even low doses of typical antipsychotics, however, produce 80%–90% D_2 receptor blockade, which makes it difficult to produce the relatively greater 5-HT_{2A}-to-D_2 receptor occupancy rates as are observed with clozapine (40%–50% D_2 occupancy [Farde et al. 1989, 1993] and 80%–90% frontal cortical 5-HT_{2A} receptor occupancy [Nordstrom et al. 1993]) determined by PET studies.

In addition to the 5-HT_{2A} receptor, there is evidence that other serotonin receptor subtypes may play a role in the action of atypical antipsychotics. The 5-HT_{2C} receptor has been implicated in the mechanism of action of atypical antipsychotics because clozapine has a higher affinity for 5-HT_{2C} receptors than for D_2 receptors (Canton et al. 1990). Also, in situ hybridization studies have shown that there are high densities of 5-HT_{2C} mRNA in the SN and nucleus accumbens, whereas the striatum and VTA have lower densities (Molineaux et al. 1989). However, chlorpromazine has a higher affinity for 5-HT_{2C} receptors than for D_2 receptors. Indeed, most typical and atypical antipsychotics bind weakly to 5-HT_{2C} receptors labeled with ^{3}H-mesulergine.

5-HT_3 antagonists have also been proposed to be potential antipsychotics. Unlike other serotonin receptors, the 5-HT_3 receptor is a component of a ligand-gated cation channel. After binding, serotonin rapidly increases membrane sodium and potassium conductance, resulting in depolarization. 5-HT_3 receptors are found in the area postrema, where they are probably responsible for the antiemetic properties of these compounds. Receptors are also found in the nucleus of the solitary tract, entorhinal cortex, and limbic regions (Kilpatrick et al. 1987). Activation of these receptors leads to an increase in dopamine release in the mesolimbic and perhaps the nigrostriatal pathway. It is also known that clozapine binds with moderate affinity (dissociation constant [K_d] ≈ 100 nmol/L) to the 5-HT_3 receptor, whereas the typical antipsychotics spiperone, haloperidol, fluphenazine, and (−)sulpiride are inactive (Bolanos et al. 1990; Watling et al. 1990). However, loxapine, also a typical antipsychotic, binds to 5-HT_3 receptors with the same affinity as clozapine (Hoyer et al. 1989).

Conflicting evidence has also been generated from electrophysiological studies examining the effect of 5-HT_3 antagonists on dopamine neuron firing rates. In a study by Sorensen et al. (1989) comparing MDL 73,147EF (dolasetron) (a 5-HT_3 antagonist) and haloperidol, acute haloperidol administration increased dopamine firing rates in the SN and the VTA, whereas acute MDL 73,147EF had no effect. However, chronic treatment with both haloperidol and MDL 73,147EF decreased the firing rate of neurons in both the SN and the VTA, results consistent with evidence of depolarization block and likely antipsychotic efficacy. But in vivo studies (Ashby et al. 1990) using the 5-HT_3 antagonist BRL 43694 (granisetron) showed no effect on the firing rate of dopamine neurons acutely or chronically in either brain region. In contrast, the potent and selective 5-HT$_3$ antagonist BRL 46470A selectively reduced the number of spontaneously active dopamine neurons in the VTA of the rat brain while having no effect on the SN region, an action shared by clozapine. This finding suggests that BRL 46470A may possess an atypical antipsychotic profile.

Similar selective inhibition of VTA dopamine neurons has been reported for the 5-HT$_3$ antagonists zatosetron (Rasmussen et al. 1991) and granisetron (Minabe et al. 1992). However, based on the clinical findings or lack thereof (see next paragraph), the model of selective VTA inactivation may produce false-positive results.

In a review by Reynolds (1992), consistent with the lack of data since then, he concluded that in several clinical trials the 5-HT$_3$ antagonist ondansetron was not clinically effective in the treatment of schizophrenia. However, this finding may have resulted from the nature of the experimental design of these studies and the pharmacokinetic properties of the drug more than a lack of intrinsic efficacy.

Monsma et al. (1993) reported the cloning of a novel serotonin receptor linked to the stimulation of adenylate cyclase, tentatively identified as the 5-HT$_6$ receptor. This receptor is localized exclusively in the central nervous system, predominantly in the striatum, limbic, and cortical regions (Monsma et al. 1993; Ward et al. 1995). The pharmacological profile of this receptor is of interest because clozapine, olanzapine, and some other atypical antipsychotics display relatively high affinity for this site (K_i < 20 nmol/L), unlike dopamine or spiperone (both > 10 μmol/L). However, some typical antipsychotics, such as loxapine, chlorpromazine, and fluphenazine, also display relative high affinity for this site (Monsma et al. 1993; Roth et al. 1994). The more recently cloned 5-HT$_7$ receptor also binds several antipsychotic drugs (Roth et al. 1994; Shen et al. 1993) but does not discriminate atypical from typical antipsychotics.

Sigma (σ) receptors have been implicated in schizophrenia because a stereoisomer of certain related benzomorphans (opiates) possesses profound psychotomimetic properties and antagonists might therefore possess antipsychotic properties. Indeed, several drugs possessing preclinical antipsychotic activity, including haloperidol, bind to the receptor. These drugs (it is unclear whether they are agonists or antagonists), some of which bind only weakly to the D$_2$ receptor, can also alter dopaminergic firing rates (Largent et al. 1988; Snyder and Largent 1989; Steinfels et al. 1989; Taylor and Schlemmer 1992; Wachtel and White 1988).

Critical review of the literature has shown that the psychotomimetic and dysphoric effects of these opiates have been attributed to the wrong stereoisomer—that is, the psychotomimetic effects are produced by the levoenantiomer, but the dextro-enantiomer is what is defined as the site (Itzhak and Stein 1990; Musacchio 1990; Walker et al. 1990). Additionally, classic ligands, such as pentazocine, dextromethorphan, (+)3-PPP [(+)-3-(3-hydroxyphenyl)-N-propylpiperidine hydrochloride], and 1,3-di-o-tolylguanidine, do not block or cause psychotomimetic behaviors. Finally, clozapine is essentially devoid of activity at the receptor, and ligands possessing preclinical antipsychotic activity may cause motor disturbances (see Walker et al. 1990).

There is increasing evidence that cortical glutamatergic neurons can regulate dopaminergic function, particularly in projection fields of the mesolimbocortical and nigrostriatal systems. Although there are both ionotropic and metabotropic glutamate receptors, we focus on the ionotropic class.

The ionotropic glutamate receptors (N-methyl-D-aspartate [NMDA], α-amino-3-hydroxy-5-methylisoxazole-4-propionic acid [AMPA], and kainate) are oligomers composed of individual subunits: NMDA (NMDAR1 and NMDAR2A–D); AMPA (GluR1–GluR4); and kainate (GluR5–GluR7, KA1, and KA2). This important new development in neuropsychopharmacology (i.e., glutamate receptors; excitatory amino acid receptors) has been reviewed in various detail by Hyman and Nestler (1993), Hollmann and Heinemann (1994), and Owens et al. (1997). Phencyclidine acts as an antagonist at the NMDA subtype of the glutamate receptor and can cause profound schizophrenia-like symptoms. This implies that mechanisms that decrease NMDA receptor (glutamatergic) function may produce psychosis and that the glutamatergic system might be hypofunctional in schizophrenia. Based on known glutamatergic neurobiology (see reviews above), this is not inconsistent with the dopamine hypothesis of schizophrenia (Olney and Farber 1995), although there is little pharmacological evidence of effective antipsychotic actions of glutamate agonists (Kalivas et al. 1989; Olney 1992; Tamminga et al. 1992). However, Goff and colleagues (1995) recently reported that D-cycloserine, a partial agonist at the glycine recognition site of the NMDA receptor, at a dose of 50 mg/day produced a significant reduction in negative symptoms when added to conventional antipsychotic therapy in patients who have schizophrenia with prominent negative symptoms.

This observation, coupled with increasingly compelling data for glutamatergic abnormalities in schizophrenia (Tsai et al. 1995), has led to increasing interest in the glutamatergic properties of atypical antipsychotic medications. For example, preclinical studies have found that chronic antipsychotic treatment can alter glutamatergic activity. Both chronic haloperidol and raclopride administration increase NMDAR1 subunit immunoreactivity in the striatum. This effect is not observed for clozapine (Fitzgerald et al. 1995). In this study, both haloperidol and clozapine increased GluR1 immunoreactivity in the prefrontal cortex, and clozapine alone increased GluR2 immunoreactivity in the frontal/parietal cortex, nucleus accumbens, and hippocampus.

In the last 15 years, there has been an explosion of information about the neurotransmitter role of neuropeptides. Indeed, opioid peptides,

cholecystokinin, and neurotensin can regulate dopaminergic activity in laboratory animals. For example, haloperidol increases neurotensin and neurotensin mRNA concentrations in the mesolimbic (nucleus accumbens) and nigrostriatal (dorsolateral striatum) dopamine systems, whereas the atypical antipsychotics clozapine and sertindole only increase neurotensin activity in the mesolimbic system (Kinkead et al. 1993). Interestingly, Diaz et al. (1994) observed that in the nucleus accumbens, antipsychotic blockade of D_2 receptors increases neurotensin expression, whereas D_3 blockade decreases it. These actions occur in distinct subnuclei of the nucleus accumbens, but the effects of D_2 blockade predominate. Thus, there is ample evidence that neuropeptide-based drugs would alter dopaminergic activity. Unfortunately, few peptidergic ligands are available for detailed preclinical studies predictive of antipsychotic activity, although peptide-based drugs may hold great promise in the future.

Neuronal expression of Fos, a nuclear transcription factor and the protein product of the immediate-early gene *c-fos*, is increased by several physiological and pharmacological treatments that activate neuronal function. As such, Fos immunoreactivity or *c-fos* mRNA expression has been used to map functional pathways in the central nervous system. Of interest is the finding that clozapine and haloperidol produce different induction patterns after acute administration; haloperidol increases expression in the striatum, nucleus accumbens, and septum, and clozapine increases it in the nucleus accumbens, septum, and prefrontal cortex. Moreover, all antipsychotics referred to as atypical produce a greater increase in expression in the nucleus accumbens than in the dorsolateral striatum (Guo et al. 1995; Robertson and Fibiger 1996; Robertson et al. 1994). Deutch et al. (1995) observed that clozapine, but not risperidone, induces Fos expression in the paraventricular nucleus of the thalamus. Although the functional significance of these findings is unclear, they further support a neuroanatomically selective or different pattern of effects produced by clozapine. Because transcription factors such as Fos are required for alterations in gene transcription, it can be assumed that clozapine and haloperidol, for example, do produce distinct differences in the expression of various genes in the striatum. It will be of great interest to determine what these gene products are.

To summarize, we use the known pharmacology of clozapine to review those biological characteristics that may confer an atypical nature on an antipsychotic. Clozapine may be able to decrease mesolimbic dopamine activity while sparing nigrostriatal function and possibly even increasing cortical dopamine activity. The mechanisms as to how this selectivity occurs are unknown but are certainly based on preferential binding to certain populations of dopamine receptors (i.e., mesolimbic) and/or dopamine receptor subtypes (i.e., D_4), perhaps along with relatively greater $5\text{-HT}_{2A}/D_2$ blockade than that observed with typical antipsychotics. Although these types of mechanisms are certain to exist, the ultimate therapeutic efficacy almost certainly derives from adaptive changes in neuronal structure (e.g., synaptic arborization patterns) and function (e.g., persistent changes in the levels of neurotransmitter, receptors, and/or intracellular signaling messengers) induced by chronic exposure to antipsychotics. Indeed, for most classes of psychotherapeutic agents, understanding this neuronal plasticity is what will define the mechanism of action of a given drug.

CLOZAPINE

History and Discovery

As elaborated above, over the past several decades animal and molecular studies have begun to further elucidate the neuroanatomical and neurotransmitter circuits involved in cognition and behavior. This increased understanding of brain neurobiology has led to the development of newer hypotheses regarding the pathophysiology of psychosis and innovative approaches to psychopharmacological treatments. Specifically, putative medications exploiting differential potencies on D_1, D_2, D_3, and D_4 receptors; partial dopamine receptor agonists; sigma receptor antagonists; NMDA receptor antagonists; serotonin receptor antagonists (5-HT_{2A}, 5-HT_3, 5-HT_6, and 5-HT_7); muscarinic receptor antagonists; and α-adrenergic agonists and antagonists have been developed and are being studied in clinical trials. Excellent reviews of ongoing research on a wide variety of novel atypical antipsychotic medications have been produced by Gerlach (1991), Meltzer (1992a), Lieberman (1993), Pickar (1995), Jibson and Tandon (1996), Arnt and Skarsfeldt (1998), Tamminga (1998), and W. Zhang and Bymaster (1999).

Clozapine received approval from the U.S. Food and Drug Administration (FDA) for clinical use in the United States in 1990; however, it has been extensively used outside of the United States since the 1970s.

As reviewed by Hippius (1989), clozapine was first reported to be an effective antipsychotic medication by Austrian and German clinicians in the mid-1960s. Its use was controversial even then because it was dogma that EPS were "necessary" for antipsychotic efficacy. Although clozapine was clearly an effective antipsychotic, it lacked EPS, causing some clinicians to questions its inclusion as a "real neuroleptic." Unfortunately, in 1974, as clozapine's popularity was growing in Europe, eight patients in Finland died from clozapine-associated agranulocytosis, and the routine use of clozapine was discontinued in many parts of the world. However, clozapine remained available in some countries, and its remarkable efficacy in otherwise refractory patients eventuated in its reemergence in the late 1980s for use in selected (treatment-resistant or medication-intolerant) patients with the current laboratory monitoring system.

Structure-Activity Relations

As reviewed in detail by Baldessarini and Frankenburg (1991), clozapine is 8-chloro-

11-(4-methyl-1-piperazinyl)-5*H*-dibenzo[*b,e*] [1,4]diazepine. It was originally developed in 1960 by Hünziker et al. (1963). Clozapine's principal metabolites are believed to be *N*-desmethyl and *N*-oxide metabolites with low pharmacological activity (Baldessarini and Frankenburg 1991).

Indications and Pharmacotherapeutics

Clozapine is currently approved for use in 1) "treatment-refractory" schizophrenic patients (i.e., those in whom adequate trials of several different classes of typical D_2-blocking antipsychotic medications have failed), 2) patients with unmanageable EPS from typical D_2-blocking antipsychotic medications, and/or 3) patients with tardive dyskinesia. However, ongoing clinical research investigations suggest the clinical utility of clozapine, alone or in combination with other psychotropics, in patients with schizoaffective disorder and refractory bipolar disorder (manic or depressed), as well as during the early stages (i.e., first and second episodes) of schizophrenia.

The major reason for the current restrictions on clozapine's clinical indications has been the occurrence of clozapine-induced agranulocytosis in approximately 1%–2% of patients, with reports of occasional fatalities. Because clozapine-induced agranulocytosis occurs in approximately 1%–2% of patients, weekly laboratory monitoring of a patient's complete and differential blood count is required for the pharmaceutical dispensing of clozapine in the United States. Several ongoing studies are attempting to elucidate both the mechanisms and the predictors of clozapine-associated agranulocytosis in attempts to reduce or eliminate this potentially fatal side effect.

Clozapine has received approval for use in human subjects, despite its infrequent but potentially fatal adverse side effects, because 1) an increasing number of studies has suggested its antipsychotic efficacy in otherwise treatment-refractory or unresponsive schizophrenic patients, and 2) it has a markedly reduced incidence of EPS and tardive dyskinesia as compared with typical antipsychotic medications.

Many open studies, and several randomized, parallel-design, short-term (4–6 weeks) studies (Kane et al. 1988) and crossover studies (Pickar et al. 1992b), have shown the superior antipsychotic efficacy of clozapine over standard D_2-blocking antipsychotic reductions (i.e., chlorpromazine and fluphenazine) in approximately one-third of treatment-refractory schizophrenic patients. The superior antipsychotic efficacy of clozapine in these studies has been confirmed for both the positive symptoms of psychosis (i.e., hallucinations, delusions, thought disorder) and the negative symptoms of psychosis (i.e., anhedonia, asociality, blunted affect). Other preliminary studies suggest that an additional 15%–30% of patients who are unresponsive to clozapine in the first few months may show significant improvement after 6 months to 2 years of continued clozapine pharmacotherapy (Meltzer 1992b).

Chronic treatment with clozapine has also been associated with improvement in "functionality," including increased vocational, social, and interpersonal adaptation in otherwise chronically impaired, treatment-refractory patients. This improvement has resulted in diminished frequency and duration of hospitalizations and an increased ability of disabled patients to increase their educational level and to reenter the workplace. Consequently, several studies throughout the world have indicated that clozapine therapy, despite a higher cost of medication to the individual, has resulted in significant savings to society, as evidenced by reduced hospital costs (Meltzer et al. 1993), and in potentially improved economic productivity of otherwise chronically ill patients. In addition to significant clinical improvement in a large minority of otherwise treatment-resistant schizophrenic patients, an apparent complete remission of illness has been noted in a smaller subset of patients.

Unlike traditional antipsychotic medications, clozapine monotherapy is only rarely associated with EPS or tardive dyskinesia (Lieberman et al. 1991). Furthermore, some investigators have observed a marked attenuation or complete elimination of EPS and tardive dyskinesia in affected patients. Although it is not yet known whether these findings are the result of withdrawal from traditional antipsychotics or a specific therapeutic effect, we have noted the disappearance of tardive dyskinesia with clozapine treatment and its reappearance with the withdrawal of clozapine prior to reinstitution of other pharmacotherapy. Finally, although a few cases of neuroleptic malignant syndrome have been reported to be associated with clozapine monotherapy, the incidence of clozapine-associated neuroleptic malignant syndrome would be expected to be less than that occurring with typical antipsychotics. It is of interest that clozapine has been used successfully in the antipsychotic treatment of patients who have experienced neuroleptic malignant syndrome associated with typical antipsychotic pharmacotherapy.

Despite its increasingly widespread clinical use, there is still a great deal of disparity in clinical practice in the administration of clozapine pharmacotherapy. When clozapine was first introduced, it was recommended that candidates for clozapine pharmacotherapy have antipsychotic medication "washouts" for up to 1 week prior to the initiation of clozapine. However, the withdrawal of typical antipsychotic medication prior to the initiation of clozapine may sometimes be associated with significant clinical deterioration. Withdrawal should therefore be individualized. Starting clozapine in drug-withdrawn patients is preferable, but if necessary, low doses of a high-potency agent may be used until clozapine pharmacotherapy is established. Typically, clozapine is begun at 12.5–25 mg/day and increased in 25-mg increments each day, as tolerated (see the next section, "Side Effects and Toxicology"). When patients begin to show appreciable clinical improvement, their previous D_2-blocking, typical antipsychotic therapy may then be titrated

downward and discontinued. Rarely, patients need or benefit from continued combined treatment with clozapine and a high-potency typical antipsychotic medication (e.g., haloperidol, fluphenazine). The continued use of "combination therapy," however, puts the patient at increased and continued risk for EPS, tardive dyskinesia, and neuroleptic malignant syndrome.

As noted earlier in this section, in addition to the antipsychotic efficacy of clozapine, preliminary studies suggest that it has significant antimanic and antidepressant effects in patients with schizoaffective and bipolar disorders in whom traditional psychopharmacological regimens have failed. Conversely, patients with schizoaffective or bipolar disorder unresponsive to clozapine monotherapy may benefit from the addition of lithium, valproic acid, or antidepressants when clozapine monotherapy does not adequately control the affective symptoms. Lithium plus clozapine has been associated with a higher rate of neurological side effects, including neuroleptic malignant syndrome. Although any antidepressant may be used, the serotonin-specific reuptake inhibitors have fewer synergistic side effects (i.e., decreased anticholinergic, hypotensive, sedative, and cardiac conduction effects). Fluoxetine administration has been reported to increase clozapine plasma levels markedly and produce toxicity via pharmacokinetic interactions (displacing serum-bound proteins and competing for hepatic microsomal enzyme metabolism). These same pharmacokinetic interactions may also occur with tricyclic and other antidepressant agents metabolized by the hepatic P450 microsomal system. The antidepressant bupropion probably should not be used in patients receiving clozapine because both medications are associated with a significantly increased incidence of seizures. Although benzodiazepines have been used concurrently with clozapine, there have been occasional reports of severe respiratory depression or arrests with their combined use. Thus their concomitant use is discouraged, especially, but not exclusively, with their concurrent initiation.

There is no universal agreement as to the "optimal" daily dose of clozapine pharmacotherapy. Although doses in the range of 200–400 mg/day have occasionally been associated with significant improvement and efficacy, greater improvement in otherwise unresponsive or partially responsive patients may occur with doses in the range of 500–900 mg/day. Seizures occur with an increased incidence in clozapine-treated patients. The occurrence of seizures appears to be dose related, possibly occurring at a rate of 0.7% per 100-mg dose. Patients experiencing seizures may be treated with concurrent anticonvulsants, but carbamazepine should be avoided because of its occasional propensity to suppress bone marrow (aplastic anemia). Although both agents (carbamazepine and clozapine) can cause bone marrow toxicity, carbamazepine is thought to be directly toxic to bone marrow, and clozapine may represent an immunological mechanism. Valproate may be the safest and best tolerated anticonvulsant in clozapine-treated patients who experience seizures. It is emphasized that clozapine-associated seizures do not necessarily contradict its continued use. If a patient experiences a clozapine-associated seizure, the clozapine dose may be temporarily reduced or stopped and anticonvulsants initiated. When therapeutic levels of anticonvulsants are achieved, the clozapine dose may be titrated upward to its previous therapeutic levels.

Confounding the determination of a particular patients' most effective daily dose is the observation that some patients appear to need increased time taking medication, rather than increased doses of medication, for an optimal therapeutic response. Thus, some patients who experience little or no improvement during the first 3–4 months of therapy will go on to improve significantly after 6 months to 2 years of continued pharmacotherapy.

There is currently no consensus as to the optimal daily dose or adequacy of duration of a trial of clozapine pharmacotherapy. Some centers recommend the titration of a patient's dose up to approximately 450–650 mg/day during the first few months unless significant improvement occurs at lower doses. If a patient has had no appreciable improvement at 450–650 mg/day for 6 months, then titration up to a maximum of 900 mg/day with concurrent anticonvulsant administration may be considered, with a continued trial for an additional 6 months to 1 year. Other clinicians are less or more aggressive in dose titration. However, it does appear that approximately one-third of patients will not experience significant benefits from clozapine pharmacotherapy, regardless of the dose or the duration of the trial.

Side Effects and Toxicology

In addition to an approximately 1%–2% incidence of potentially life-threatening agranulocytosis and the above-described dose-related seizures, clozapine has a few other undesirable but usually manageable side effects. Clozapine may frequently produce profound and often prolonged sedation, hypersalivation, enuresis (daytime and nighttime), and anticholinergic side effects (i.e., dry mouth, blurred vision, urinary retention, and constipation). Elderly patients and patients taking other medications with significant anticholinergic properties may rarely experience anticholinergic delirium. These side effects are usually time limited, although they may persist for months. They are often dose related and may respond to a temporary reduction in dose or to treatment with other medications with pharmacological properties opposite to the problematic side effects (i.e., caffeine for sedation, bulk-increasing agents for constipation, cholinomimetic drugs for anticholinergic side effects, and anticholinergic medications for hypersalivation). Occasional patients may also experience urinary incontinence, either nighttime or daytime, which may also respond to anticholinergic agents. In almost all cases, these side effects eventually remit or are manageable with continued clozapine administration.

Orthostatic hypotension and tachycardia, not necessarily interrelated, occur frequently during clozapine pharmacotherapy and may respond to a temporary dose reduction or adjunctive pharmacological interventions. Both of these side effects are potentially dangerous and need careful clinical monitoring and attention to the side effects of concurrently administered medications that may be synergistic in toxicity.

During the first few months of clozapine pharmacotherapy, some patients experience high "benign" fevers (100–103°F). These temperature elevations are usually not related to neuroleptic malignant syndrome or sepsis, nor are they anticholinergically mediated, although these etiologies must be ruled out. These temperature elevations usually remit with continued clozapine administration. When they occur, they may be managed with antipyretic agents.

As discussed earlier in this chapter, 1%–2% of clozapine-treated patients develop clinically significant suppression of bone marrow blood precursors, particularly the granulocyte series, but rarely also the erythroid and platelet progenitors. Consequently, weekly monitoring of complete blood count and differential is recommended throughout the duration of clozapine pharmacotherapy. Although agranulocytosis can occur at any time, its incidence peaks between 2 and 6 months of pharmacotherapy. In some cases, even more frequent monitoring may be indicated during this time in high-risk patients (i.e., those who are older, medically ill, receiving potentially toxic concurrent medications, or experiencing large fluctuations in white blood cell count). It is important to note, however, that significant fluctuations—both increases and decreases—in white blood cell count occur frequently early in clozapine pharmacotherapy and do not necessarily indicate agranulocytosis or sepsis. Current laboratory monitoring recommendations include temporarily discontinuing clozapine if the white blood cell count drops to $3,000/\text{mm}^3$ or the granulocyte count falls to $1,500/\text{mm}^3$. Subsequently, clozapine may be carefully reinstituted after complete recovery of white blood cell and granulocyte counts. Clozapine should be permanently discontinued if the white blood cell count drops to $2,000/\text{mm}^3$ or the granulocyte count falls to $1,000/\text{mm}^3$. Patients experiencing agranulocytosis should be seen and monitored by a hematologist and usually need immediate hospital admission to a medical service for reverse isolation and aggressive monitoring and treatment.

Because clozapine most frequently suppresses the granulocyte series of white blood cells, a differential cell count is recommended. Theoretically, the total white blood cell count could remain within normal limits despite the presence of agranulocytosis. Clozapine, like any medication, may also affect other organ systems, and other laboratory indices, including liver function tests, should also be monitored, although less frequently if they remain normal. More in-depth, comprehensive reviews of the clinical use of clozapine have been produced by Kane et al. (1988), Lieberman et al. (1989), and Baldessarini and Frankenburg (1991).

Mechanism of Action

As reviewed in the beginning of this chapter, several hypotheses have been generated to explain the increased efficacy of certain atypical antipsychotics. Clozapine appears to have many of these properties, including an increased ratio of D_1 to D_2 blockade, greater D_3 and D_4 antagonism, 5-HT_{2A} and 5-HT_{2C} antagonistic properties, anticholinergic and antiadrenergic properties, and increased mesolimbic specificity with relative sparing of nigrostriatal dopaminergic neurons.

In addition to its greater effectiveness in the treatment of positive symptoms, clozapine has also been associated with relatively greater effectiveness in the treatment of the negative, or deficit, symptoms of psychosis. Many investigators have noted the association of prominent negative symptoms with relative reductions in prefrontal cortical blood flow and glucose metabolism seen during PET or single photon emission computerized tomography (SPECT) scanning of schizophrenic patients (Andreasen et al. 1992; Berman et al. 1992; Buchsbaum et al. 1992; Wolkin et al. 1992). Several preliminary studies (Pickar et al. 1992a) have reported the ability of clozapine pharmacotherapy to improve, or at least not worsen, this relative "hypofrontality" as compared with traditional D_2-blocking antipsychotics. This effect, as shown in functional brain imaging, has been proffered as a possible explanation for clozapine's reduction of the negative symptoms of psychosis.

Current experience suggests that at least one-third of typical antipsychotic-refractory schizophrenic patients will not show appreciable benefit from clozapine pharmacotherapy. Given the considerable expense and adverse side effects associated with clozapine pharmacotherapy, it would be of considerable clinical utility to predict a priori potential responders and nonresponders to clozapine. In this regard, Pickar et al. (1992b) and Risch and Lewine (1993, 1995) have reported preliminary data suggesting that schizophrenic patients with relatively low ratios of homovanillic acid (HVA) to 5-hydroxyindoleacetic acid (5-HIAA) in cerebrospinal fluid may experience significantly greater benefit with clozapine pharmacotherapy than patients with relatively higher HVA-to-5-HIAA ratios. These observations have involved only a small number of subjects and require replications in larger groups of patients. They add support, however, to the theoretical hypotheses elaborated by Meltzer (1992a) and others of the potential importance of central nervous system dopaminergic and serotonergic interactions in the pathogenesis and pharmacotherapy of schizophrenia.

RISPERIDONE

Risperidone was introduced in 1993 in the United States. Chemically it is 3-[2-[4-(6-fluoro-1,2-benzisoxazol-3-yl)-1-piperidinyl]ethyl]-6,7,8,9-tetrahydro-2-methyl-4H-pyrido[1,2-a]pyrimidin-4-one.

Pharmacokinetics[1]

Risperidone is well absorbed. Total recovery of radioactivity at 1 week from a single 1-mg oral dose is 85%, including 70% in the urine and 15% in the feces. Risperidone is extensively metabolized in the liver by cytochrome P450 (CYP) 2D6, to a major active metabolite, 9-hydroxyrisperidone, which is the predominant circulating species, and appears approximately of equal efficacy with risperidone with respect to receptor-binding activity and some effects in animals (a second minor pathway is *N*-dealkylation). Consequently, the clinical effect of the drug probably results from the combined concentrations of risperidone plus 9-hydroxyrisperidone, which are dose proportional over the dosing range of 1–16 mg daily (0.5–8 mg twice daily).

The relative oral bioavailability of risperidone from a tablet is 94% (coefficient of variation [CV] = 10%) as compared with a solution. Because food does not affect either the rate or the extent of absorption of risperidone, the drug can be given with or without meals. The enzyme that catalyzes the hydroxylation of risperidone to 9-hydroxyrisperidone is CYP2D6, also called debrisoquin hydroxylase. It is also the enzyme responsible for the metabolism of many neuroleptics, antidepressants, antiarrhythmics, and other drugs. CYP2D6 is subject to genetic polymorphism (about 6%–8% of whites and a very low percentage of Asians have little or no activity and are "poor metabolizers") and to inhibition by a variety of substrates and some nonsubstrates,

---

[1] Information in this section was abstracted from the *Physicians' Desk Reference*, 1996, and package insert.

notably quinidine. Extensive metabolizers convert risperidone rapidly into 9-hydroxyrisperidone, whereas poor metabolizers convert it much more slowly. Extensive metabolizers, therefore, have lower risperidone and higher 9-hydroxyrisperidone concentrations than do poor metabolizers.

After oral administration of solution or tablet, mean peak plasma concentrations occur at about 1 hour. Peak 9-hydroxyrisperidone concentrations occur at about 3 hours in extensive metabolizers and 17 hours in poor metabolizers. The apparent half-life of risperidone is 3 hours (CV = 30%) in extensive metabolizers and 20 hours (CV = 40%) in poor metabolizers. The apparent half-life of 9-hydroxyrisperidone is about 21 hours (CV = 20%) in extensive metabolizers and 30 hours (CV = 25%) in poor metabolizers. Steady-state concentrations of risperidone are reached in 1 day in extensive metabolizers and would be expected to be reached in about 5 days in poor metabolizers. Steady-state concentrations of 9-hydroxyrisperidone are reached in 5–6 days (measured in extensive metabolizers).

Because risperidone and 9-hydroxyrisperidone are approximately of equal efficacy, the sum of their concentrations is pertinent. The pharmacokinetics of the sum of risperidone and 9-hydroxyrisperidone after single and multiple doses are similar in extensive and poor metabolizers; overall mean elimination half-life is about 20 hours. In analyses comparing adverse reaction rates in extensive and poor metabolizers in controlled and open studies, no important differences were seen.

Risperidone could be subject to two kinds of drug-drug interactions. First, inhibitors of CYP2D6 could interfere with the conversion of risperidone to 9-hydroxyrisperidone. This in fact occurs with quinidine, giving essentially all recipients a risperidone pharmacokinetic profile that is typical of poor metabolizers. The plasma protein binding of risperidone is about 90% over the in vitro concentration range of 0.5–200 ng/mL and increases with increasing concentra-

tions of α_1-acid glycoprotein. The plasma binding of 9-hydroxyrisperidone is about 77%. Neither the parent nor the metabolite displace each other from the plasma binding sites (Medical Economics Company 1996).

Clinical Studies

Multicenter clinical trials that led to the FDA approval of risperidone found that risperidone had an efficacy that was at least equal to that of haloperidol and produced significantly fewer EPS (Borison et al. 1987; Chouinard et al. 1993; Marder and Meibach 1994; Peuskens 1995). Combined results from several trials showed risperidone at 6 mg/day to have greater efficacy than haloperidol at 20 mg/day with respect to reduced positive and negative symptoms.

Since risperidone's introduction in 1993, there has been a great deal of clinical experience, which is summarized below. In fact, risperidone is currently the antipsychotic most frequently prescribed by psychiatrists in the United States.

Pharmacologically, risperidone is a D_2 antagonist that also has potent 5-HT_{2A}, as well as α_1 and α_2, antagonistic effects. It is essentially devoid of anticholinergic effects. As noted above, the parent compound risperidone has a pharmacologically active metabolite, 9-OH-risperidone, which is believed to be essentially equipotent with the parent drug. Risperidone itself has a half-life of approximately 4–6 hours, whereas its metabolite has a half-life of approximately 22 hours.

A United States multicenter study and an international multicenter study have indicated that risperidone can be given once daily with equal efficacy and with no significant increase in adverse side effects because of the long half-life of its active metabolite. Side effects accompanying risperidone that occur at a level of greater than 5% and twice that of placebo include somnolence, fatigue, orthostatic dizziness, tachycardia, nausea, dyspepsia, diarrhea, weight gain, sexual dysfunction (including ejaculatory problems, dysmenorrhea, priapism, erectile dysfunction, and diminished desire), and rhinitis. Many of these side effects also appear to occur with other atypical antipsychotics. However, in premarketing studies, discontinuation because of adverse side effects when placebo adjusted was remarkably low: discontinuation due to EPS was 2.1%, dizziness 0.7%, hypotension 0.6%, somnolence 0.5%, and nausea 0.3%. At present, no true estimate of the prevalence of tardive dyskinesia accompanying risperidone is known. However, case reports in the literature have described possible risperidone-induced tardive dyskinesia.

Risperidone has also been reported to be rarely associated with neuroleptic malignant syndrome (Tarsy 1996; Webster and Wijeratne 1994). However, for theoretical reasons, such as its 5-HT_{2A} blocking actions, which potentiate its nigrostriatal dopamine transmission, as well as the numbers of patients with 3–4 years of exposure, it would appear that the prevalence of tardive dyskinesia may be substantially lower with risperidone than with typical antipsychotics. Confirmation of this possibility awaits larger numbers of patients with longer periods of exposure to this medication.

In neuroleptic-naive patients, risperidone is typically begun at 1 mg twice a day and increased as tolerated to a target dose of 3–6 mg/day. Experience suggests that the initially recommended target dose of 6 mg/day is unnecessarily high and that at least 70% of patients can be optimally treated at daily doses of 3 mg/day or less and approximately 90% at doses below 6 mg/day. Of note is that at this dose the incidence of EPS produced by risperidone is indistinguishable from that of placebo.

When risperidone was first introduced into the United States market, it was suggested that risperidone could be given at 1 mg twice a day on day 1, 2 mg twice a day on day 2, and 3 mg twice a day on day 3. However, clinical experience suggests that this titration was too rapid for some patients. Consequently, patients should be monitored for tolerance of risperidone in relation to side effects (e.g., sedation, hypotension) and the titration performed as clinically tolerated.

For patients already taking other antipsychotics with risperidone, it is suggested, as previously described for clozapine in this chapter, that the medications be overlapped. Specifically, 1) for patients taking high doses of high-potency antipsychotics, the high-potency antipsychotic dose should be reduced by approximately one-third as risperidone is added at 1–2 mg/day and titrated upward; and 2) for patients taking relatively low doses of high-potency antipsychotics, a dose reduction of approximately two-thirds of the high-potency antipsychotics is recommended as risperidone is added in an identical manner. Typical antipsychotics should be tapered as the risperidone is adjusted upward, again to a target dose of 3–6 mg/day. In premarketing studies, a dosage of 6 mg/day was associated with the greatest efficacy with fewest EPS. However, in postmarketing studies, most patients' conditions can be managed at approximately 3 mg/day.

Some investigators believe that the onset of risperidone's efficacy may be delayed in a subgroup of patients, much like that of clozapine as described earlier in this chapter, and consequently, it is not clear what the optimal dose titration with respect to time should be in any given individual. However, our experience indicates that some patients may need several months of risperidone trial before an optimal response is achieved; therefore, it should not be discontinued before this time of exposure simply because of an apparent lack of efficacy. This is another reason for overlapping of the typical and atypical antipsychotics to allow the full benefit from the atypical profile. However, Meltzer and others argue that, optimally, the typical antipsychotics should be discontinued as soon as clinically appropriate because they may 1) predispose subjects to tardive dyskinesia, 2) complicate the pharmacokinetics and pharmacodynamics of dosage titration, and 3) potentially attenuate the full efficacy of the atypical medication.

A number of reports have emerged suggesting that risperidone, like clozapine, is associated with continued improvement over several years in quality-of-life scales, social functioning, reductions in length of hospital stays, and overall reductions in lifetime cost of illness (Addington et al. 1993; Bouchard et al. 1994; Chouinard et al. 1993; Lindstrom et al. 1994; Polsker 1994). Most recently, risperidone was compared with haloperidol in a randomized, double-blind study of 59 treatment-resistant schizophrenic patients (Green et al. 1997). Risperidone was shown to have significantly greater benefit than haloperidol on verbal working memory. The results of this study suggest that risperidone, in addition to reducing symptoms, may improve cognitive deficits in treatment-resistant schizophrenic patients and thus potentially further diminish disability.

Several studies, as reviewed by Mendelowitz and Lieberman (1995), have suggested risperidone's utility in patients whose symptoms are refractory to treatment with typical antipsychotics. Although clozapine remains the most studied of the antipsychotics in treatment-refractory patients, several studies have suggested that risperidone may sometimes be efficacious in true clozapine nonresponders. It is of particular note, however, that clozapine should not be discontinued in patients who are currently responding beneficially because severe withdrawal psychoses have emerged that may subsequently be treatment refractory to the reinitiation of clozapine.

Because of risperidone's relative safety and fewer adverse side effects as compared with typical antipsychotics, preliminary case reports and open studies, as reviewed by Mendelowitz and Lieberman (1995), have suggested its utility in the treatment of other psychotic disorders, including psychotic depression, mania, psychotic dementias, and psychosis in children and adolescents. Children, adolescents, and elderly patients have been successfully treated with as little as 0.5–1.5 mg/day. It has been reported (D. Jeste, personal communication, 1997) that risperidone may actually be cognitively enhancing in elderly patients with dementia, increasing Mini-Mental State Exam (Folstein et al. 1975) scores by an average of 3 points. Thus, given its lack of EPS at low doses, lack of anticholinergic side effects, and apparent cognitive enhancing effects, risperidone may be particularly useful in the treatment of delirium and dementia in elderly patients. However, these preliminary reports await confirmation in controlled studies of larger subject populations. In this regard, it is emphasized that there have been, at the time of this writing, no double-blind, placebo-controlled studies of risperidone's efficacy in patients with any of these syndromes and that there are currently no labeling indications in these areas.

OLANZAPINE

Olanzapine is of particular note because it is structurally related to clozapine. Chemically, olanzapine is 2-methyl-4-(4-methyl-1-piperazinyl)-10H-thieno[2,3-b][1,5]benzodiazepine. It is a potent antipsychotic agent with nanomolar receptor affinity in vitro at serotonin 5-$HT_{2A/2C}$, 5-HT_3, and 5-HT_6; $D_4/D_3/D_1/D_2$; and muscarinic cholinergic (M_1–M_5), α_1-adrenergic, and histamine H_1 receptors (Bymaster et al. 1996).

In preclinical pharmacological studies, olanzapine had a range of receptor affinities distinct from those of traditional drugs and generally comparable to those of clozapine (Bymaster et al. 1996). The compound shows a greater affinity for serotonin (5-HT_{2A}) than for dopamine (D_1, D_2) receptors. In addition, the compound has affinity at the binding sites of D_4, D_3, 5-HT_3, 5-HT_6, H_1, α_1-adrenergic, and muscarinic M_{1-5} receptors. There is no significant binding at 5-HT_{1A}, 5-HT_{1B}, 5-HT_{1D}, 5-HT_7, β-adrenoceptors, γ-aminobutyric acid (GABA)$_A$, GABA$_B$, sigma, opioid, or benzodiazepine receptors.

Electrophysiological studies corroborate the desirable property of olanzapine to selectively reduce dopamine activity in the meso-limbic (A_{10}) pathways thought to mediate psychosis while sparing striatal (A_9) pathways involved in extrapyramidal signs and symptoms. In addition, olanzapine blocks the NMDA receptor–mediated excitotoxicity induced by phencyclidine.

Behavioral studies with olanzapine have been consistent with the compound's receptor-binding profile. Olanzapine blocks 5-hydroxy-tryptophan–induced head twitches and increases quipazine-induced secretion of corticosterone, demonstrating 5-HT$_{2A}$ receptor antagonism in vivo. These actions occur at doses lower than those required to block dopamine-mediated behaviors. Inhibition of conditioned avoidance response has been widely used to predict the antipsychotic potential of a compound, whereas the induction of catalepsy is associated with the occurrence of EPS. The ratio of the dose required to interfere with conditioned avoidance to that required to induce catalepsy suggests antipsychotic activity with relatively low potential for EPS.

Olanzapine also increased punished responding in an animal conflict test predictive of a compound's anxiolytic potential. Similar to clozapine, olanzapine selectively antagonizes cocaine-induced hyperactivity compared with dextroamphetamine-induced hyperactivity in rats and also low-dose compared with high-dose *d*-amphetamine-induced hyperactivity. Olanzapine selectively antagonizes NMDA antagonist–induced activities, similar to clozapine.

Overall, the toxicological profile of olanzapine in animal studies has been quite unremarkable. Especially noteworthy has been the absence of evidence of bone marrow cytotoxicity in any of the species examined in these toxicology studies.

Both United States and international multicenter studies comparing olanzapine with haloperidol have suggested that olanzapine is effective in doses of 5.5–20 mg/day (Beasley et al. 1996; Tollefson et al. 1997). Its efficacy with respect to positive symptoms is equivalent to that of haloperidol, and its efficacy with respect to negative symptoms is superior to that of haloperidol (Tollefson and Sanger 1997). In addition, these studies suggest that long-term treatment with olanzapine is associated with fewer relapses and higher achievement on a quality-of-life scale. In the studies reported to date, olanzapine has few, if any, significant EPS, especially as compared in blinded studies with haloperidol (Tran et al. 1997). In this regard, however, an animal study (Robertson and Fibiger 1996) indicated that olanzapine may increase *c-fos* activity in striatal areas in a dose-dependent manner, which may be an indication of potential EPS activity. In addition, akathisia was observed in premarketing trials at an incidence of greater than 5% and at least twice that of placebo. Akathisia occurs in a dose-dependent manner. Of particular note is that there has been only rare evidence of leukopenia or agranulocytosis associated with olanzapine in either animal or human studies.

Although a 10-mg starting dose is recommended, current data suggest that approximately 25% of patients will respond to 5 mg/day, 25% will require up to 10 mg/day, 25% will require up to 15 mg/day, and approximately 25% will require 20 mg/day. Olanzapine has also been given to some patients in 25-mg doses; however, labeling suggests that doses of greater than 20 mg/day have not yet been studied.

QUETIAPINE

Chemically, quetiapine[2] is 2-[2-(4-dibenzo[*b,f*] [1,4]-thiazepin-11-yl-1-piperazinyl)ethoxy]-ethanol fumarate and is structurally related to clozapine and olanzapine. Quetiapine was previously referred to as ICI 204,636 and as

---

[2] The information in this section was abstracted from investigators' brochures and other literature of premarketing studies of quetiapine.

Seroquel, which has now become the trade name under which it is marketed.

Quetiapine is a novel antipsychotic agent that has high affinity for brain serotonin 5-HT$_{2A}$ receptors and markedly lower affinity for D$_2$ and D$_1$ receptors as compared with standard antipsychotic agents. Quetiapine also has considerably less muscarinic cholinergic and α$_1$-adrenergic receptor antagonist activity than standard antipsychotic agents.

Quetiapine is active orally in classical tests for antipsychotic activity (i.e., conditioned avoidance tests and behavioral or electrophysiological tests measuring the reversing actions of dopamine agonists) and has substantial selectivity for the limbic system. Additionally, quetiapine, unlike standard antipsychotic agents, has little or no depolarization inactivation of nigrostriatal dopamine neurons, paradigms considered predictive of EPS liability.

Quetiapine has been studied in healthy volunteers or subjects with schizophrenia at daily doses of 25–450 mg. Quetiapine was well tolerated in clinical pharmacology studies. After oral administration, the absorption of quetiapine is rapid (mean time to maximum concentration [T$_{max}$] = 1.2–1.8 hours) and complete. The steady-state pharmacokinetics are dose proportional when quetiapine is given three times daily over a dose range of 25–150 mg. Steady-state plasma concentrations are within the limits predicted from single-dose data. Food has a variable, clinically insignificant effect on the bioavailability of quetiapine. The largest fractions of quetiapine-related material circulating in plasma are unchanged quetiapine (11%) and the inactive sulfoxide metabolite (10%). The elimination of quetiapine is relatively rapid (mean half-life of 2.2–3.2 hours) and primarily by metabolism. Less than 1% of the administered oral dose is excreted unchanged in urine and feces. Approximately 73% and 21% of the dose are quetiapine-related material excreted in the urine and feces, respectively.

Quetiapine's half-life is approximately 3 hours, so that two- or three-times-a-day dosing may be initially indicated.

Quetiapine has been shown to be effective in the treatment of both positive and negative symptoms of schizophrenia in doses of 150–800 mg/day. It is comparable to typical neuroleptics in this regard (Jibson and Tandon 1996). Quetiapine is notable for having a very low incidence of EPS, no sustained elevations of plasma prolactin, and no anticholinergic side effects.

SUMMARY

The increasingly sophisticated understanding of neurobiology has led to significant advances in the understanding of the pathophysiology of schizophrenia. These insights have led to the development of new-generation atypical antipsychotic medications with potentially fewer adverse side effects and improved therapeutic efficacy. The prototype atypical antipsychotic agent, clozapine, has generated a new era of excitement and hope for the pharmacotherapy of treatment-resistant schizophrenic patients. An entire series of newer atypical antipsychotic agents, currently undergoing clinical trials, may further increase the understanding of the pathogenesis of schizophrenia and expand treatment alternatives.

REFERENCES

Addington DE, Jones B, Bloom D, et al: Reduction of hospital days in chronic schizophrenic patients with risperidone: a retrospective study. Clin Ther 15:917–926, 1993

Andreasen NC, Rezai K, Alliger R, et al: Hypofrontality in neuroleptic-naive patients and in patients with chronic schizophrenia: assessment with xenon 133 single-photon emission computed tomography and the Tower of London. Arch Gen Psychiatry 49:943–958, 1992

Arnt J, Skarsfeldt T: Do novel antipsychotics have similar pharmacological characteristics? A review of the evidence. Neuropsychopharmacology 18:63–101, 1998

Ashby CR, Jiang LH, Kasser RJ, et al: Electrophysiological characterization of 5-hydroxytryptamine$_3$ receptors in rat medial prefrontal cortex. J Pharmacol Exp Ther 251:171–178, 1990

Baldessarini RJ, Frankenburg FR: Clozapine—a novel antipsychotic agent. N Engl J Med 324:746–754, 1991

Baldessarini RJ, Campbell A, Yeghiayan S, et al: Limbic-selective antidopaminergic effects of S(+)-aporphines compared to typical and atypical antipsychotic agents in the rat, in Biological Psychiatry, Vol 2. Edited by Racagni G, Brunello N, Fukuda T. Amsterdam, Elsevier Science Publishers, 1991, pp 837–840

Beasley CM, Tollefson G, Tran P, et al: Olanzapine versus placebo and haloperidol: acute phase results of the North American double-blind olanzapine trial. Neuropsychopharmacology 14:111–124, 1996

Berman KF, Torrey EF, Daniel AG, et al: Regional cerebral blood flow in monozygotic twins discordant and concordant for schizophrenia. Arch Gen Psychiatry 49:927–934, 1992

Bertorello AM, Hopfield JF, Aperia A, et al: Inhibition by dopamine of (Na$^+$+K$^+$) ATPase activity in neostriatal neurons through D$_1$ and D$_2$ dopamine receptor synergism. Nature 347:386–388, 1990

Bolanos FJ, Schechter LE, Miquel MC, et al: Common pharmacological and physicochemical properties of 5-HT$_3$ binding sites in the rat cerebral cortex and NG 108-15 clonal cells. Biochem Pharmacol 40:1541–1550, 1990

Borison RL, Pathiraja AP, Diamond BL, et al. Risperidone: clinical safety and efficacy in schizophrenia. Psychopharmacol Bull 13:261–276, 1987

Bouchard RH, Pourcher E, et al: Multidimensional evaluation of risperidone efficacy in an institutional setting. Abstracts of the Annual Meeting of Collegium Internationale Neuro-Psychopharmacologicum, 1994, p 174

Bouthenet ML, Souil E, Martres MP, et al: Localization of dopamine D$_3$ receptor mRNA in the rat brain using in situ hybridization histochemistry: comparison with dopamine D$_2$ receptor mRNA. Brain Res 564:203–219, 1991

Buchsbaum MS, Haier RJ, Potkin SG, et al: Frontostriatal disorder of cerebral metabolism in never-medicated schizophrenics. Arch Gen Psychiatry 49:935–942, 1992

Buckland PR, O'Donovan MC, McGuffin P: Changes in dopamine D$_1$ and D$_3$ receptor mRNA levels in rat brain following antipsychotic treatment. Psychopharmacology 106:479–483, 1992

Bunney BS, Sesack SR, Silva NL: Midbrain dopamine systems: neurophysiology and electrophysiological pharmacology, in Psychopharmacology: The Third Generation of Progress. Edited by Meltzer HY. New York, Raven, 1987, pp 113–126

Bunney BS, Chiodo LA, Grace AA: Midbrain dopamine system electrophysiological functioning: a review and new hypothesis. Synapse 9:79–94, 1991

Bunzow JR, Van Tol HHM, Grandy DK: Cloning and expression of a rat D$_2$ dopamine receptor cDNA. Nature 336:783–787, 1988

Bymaster FP, Calligaro DO, Falcone JF, et al: Radioreceptor binding profile of the atypical antipsychotic olanzapine. Neuropsychopharmacology 14:87–96, 1996

Campbell A, Yeghiayan S, Baldessarini RJ, et al: Selective antidopaminergic effects of S(+)N-n-propylnoraporphine in limbic versus extrapyramidal sites in rat brain: comparisons with typical and atypical antipsychotic agents. Psychopharmacology 103:323–329, 1991

Canton H, Verriele L, Colpaert FC: Binding of typical and atypical antipsychotics to 5-HT$_{1C}$ and 5-HT$_2$ sites: clozapine potently interacts with 5-HT$_{1C}$ sites. Eur J Pharmacol 191:93–96, 1990

Carlsson A: The current status of the dopamine hypothesis of schizophrenia. Neuropsychopharmacology 1:179–186, 1988a

Carlsson A: Dopamine autoreceptors and schizophrenia, in Receptors and Ligands in Psychiatry. Edited by Sen AK, Lee T. Cambridge, England, Cambridge University Press, 1988b, pp 1–10

Chio CL, Hess GF, Graham RS, et al: A second molecular form of D$_2$ dopamine receptor in rat and bovine caudate nucleus. Nature 343:266–269, 1990

Chiodo LA, Bunney BS: Typical and atypical neuroleptics: differential effects of chronic administration on the activity of A9 and A10 midbrain
dopaminergic neurons. J Neurosci 3:1607–
1619, 1983

Chiodo LA, Bunney BS: Possible mechanisms by
which repeated clozapine administration differentially affects the activity of two subpopulations of midbrain dopamine neurons. J Neurosci
5:2539–2544, 1985

Chouinard G, Jones B, Remington G, et al: A Canadian multicenter placebo-controlled study of
fixed doses of risperidone and haloperidol in the
treatment of chronic schizophrenic patients.
J Clin Psychopharmacol 13:25–40, 1993

Clark D, White FJ: Review: D_1 dopamine receptor—the search for a function: a critical evaluation of the D_1/D_2 dopamine receptor classification and its functional implications. Synapse
1:347–388, 1987

Cortés R, Gueye B, Pazos A, et al: Dopamine receptors in human brain: autoradiographic distribution of D_1 sites. Neuroscience 28:263–273, 1989

Coward DM, Dixon AK, Urwyler S, et al: Partial
dopamine-agonistic and atypical neuroleptic
properties of the amino-erolines SDZ 208-911
and SDZ 208-912. J Pharmacol Exp Ther
252:279–285, 1990

Dearry A, Gingrich JA, Falardeau P, et al: Molecular
cloning and expression of the gene for a human
D_1 dopamine receptor. Nature 247:71–76, 1990

Deutch AY, Moghaddam B, Innis RB, et al: Mechanisms of action of atypical antipsychotic drugs:
implications for novel therapeutic strategies for
schizophrenia. Schizophr Res 4:121–156, 1991

Deutch AY, Öngür D, Duman RS: Antipsychotic
drugs induce fos protein in the thalamic
paraventricular nucleus: a novel locus of
antipsychotic action. Neuroscience 66:337–346,
1995

Dewey SL, Smith GS, Logan J, et al: Serotonergic
modulation of striatal dopamine measured with
positron emission tomography (PET) and in
vivo microdialysis. J Neurosci 15:821–829, 1995

Diaz J, Lévesque D, Griffon N, Lammers CH, et al:
Opposing roles for dopamine D_2 and D_3 receptors on neurotensin mRNA expression in nucleus accumbens. Eur J Neurosci 6:1384–1387,
1994

Dray A, Gonye TJ, Oakley NR, et al: Evidence for
the existence of a raphe projection to the substantia nigra in rat. Brain Res 113:45–57, 1976

Farde L, Hall H, Ehrin E, et al: Quantitative analysis of D_2 dopamine receptor binding in the living
human brain by PET. Science 231:258–260,
1986

Farde L, Wiesel FA, Halldin C, et al: Central D_2-
dopamine receptor occupancy in schizophrenic
patients treated with antipsychotic drugs. Arch
Gen Psychiatry 45:71–76, 1988

Farde L, Nordstrom AL, Weisel FA, et al: D_1 and D_2
dopamine occupancy during treatment with
conventional and atypical neuroleptics.
Psychopharmacology 99(suppl):S28–S31, 1989

Farde L, Nordstrom AL, Weisel FA, et al: Positron
emission tomographic analysis of central D_1 and
D_2 dopamine receptor occupancy in patients
treated with classical neuroleptics and clozapine:
relation to extrapyramidal side effects. Arch
Gen Psychiatry 49:538–544, 1993

Fitzgerald LW, Deutch AY, Gasic G, et al: Regulation of cortical and subcortical glutamate receptor subunit expression by antipsychotic drugs.
J Neurosci 15:2453–2464, 1995

Folstein MF, Folstein SE, McHugh PR: Mini-Mental State: a practical method for grading the cognitive state of patients for the clinician.
J Psychiatr Res 12:189–198, 1975

Gerlach J: New antipsychotics: classification, efficacy, and adverse effects. Schizophr Bull 17:
289–309, 1991

Giros B, Sokoloff P, Martres MP, et al: Alternative
splicing directs the expression of two D_2 dopamine receptor isoforms. Nature 342:923–926,
1989

Goff DC, Guschaun G, Manaach DS, et al:
Dose-finding study of D-cycloserine added to
neuroleptics for negative symptoms of schizophrenia. Am J Psychiatry 152:1213–1215, 1995

Grace AA, Bunney BS, Moore H, Todd CL: Dopamine cell depolarization block as a model for the
actions of antipsychotic drugs. Trends Neurosci
20:31–37, 1997

Grandy DK, Marchionni MA, Makam H, et al:
Cloning of the cDNA and gene for a human D_2
dopamine receptor. Proc Natl Acad Sci U S A
86:9762–9766, 1989

Green MF, Marshall BD, Wirshing WC, et al: Does risperidone improve verbal working memory in treatment resistant schizophrenia? Am J Psychiatry 154:797–804, 1997

Guo N, Klitenick MA, Tham C-S, Fibiger HC: Receptor mechanisms mediating clozapine-induced *c-fos* expression in the forebrain. Neuroscience 65:747–756, 1995

Hand TH, Hu XT, Wang RY: Differential effects of acute clozapine and haloperidol in the activity of ventral tegmental (A10) and nigrostriatal (A9) dopamine neurons. Brain Res 415:257–269, 1987

Heffner TG, Caprathe B, Davis M, et al: Effects of PD 128482, a novel dopamine autoreceptor agonist in preclinical antipsychotic tests, in Novel Antipsychotic Drugs. Edited by Meltzer HY. New York, Raven, 1992, pp 79–90

Hippius H: The history of clozapine. Psychopharmacology (Berl) 99:53–55, 1989

Hollmann M, Heinemann S: Cloned glutamate receptors. Annu Rev Neurosci 17:31–108, 1994

Hoyer D, Gozlan H, Bolanos F, et al: Interaction of psychotropic drugs with central 5-HT$_3$ recognition sites: fact or fiction? Eur J Pharmacol 171:137–139, 1989

Hünziker F, Künzle F, Schmutz J: Uber ein 5-Stellung basisch substituierte 5-H Dibenzo [b,e]-1,4-diazepine. Helv Chir Acta 46:2337–2346, 1963

Hyman SE, Nestler EJ: The Molecular Foundations of Psychiatry. Washington, DC, American Psychiatric Press, 1993

Ichikawa J, Meltzer HY: Differential effects of repeated treatment with haloperidol and clozapine on dopamine release and metabolism in the striatum and the nucleus accumbens. J Pharmacol Exp Ther 256:248–357, 1991

Itzhak Y, Stein I: Sigma binding sites in the brain: an emerging concept for multiple sites and their relevance for psychiatric disorders. Life Sci 47:1073–1081, 1990

Jibson MD, Tandon R: A summary of research findings on the new antipsychotic drugs. Essential Psychopharmacology 1:27–37, 1996

Kalivas PW, Duffy P, Barrow J: Regulation of the mesocorticolimbic dopamine system by glutamic acid receptor subtypes. J Pharmacol Exp Ther 251:378–387, 1989

Kane J, Honigfeld G, Singer J, et al: Collaborative study group: clozapine for the treatment-resistant schizophrenic: a double-blind comparison with chlorpromazine. Arch Gen Psychiatry 45:789–796, 1988

Kilpatrick GJ, Jones BJ, Tyers MB: Identification and distribution of 5-HT$_3$ receptors in rat brain using radioligand binding. Nature 330:746–748, 1987

Kilts CD, Anderson CM, Ely TD, et al: Absence of synthesis-modulating nerve terminal autoreceptors on mesamygdaloid and other mesolimbic dopamine neuronal populations. J Neurosci 7:3961–3975, 1987

Kinkead BL, Owens MJ, Nemeroff CB: Serotonin antagonists as antipsychotics, in Serotonin: From Cell Biology to Pharmacology and Therapeutics. Edited by Vanhooutte PM, Saxena PR, Paoletti R, et al. Dordrecht, The Netherlands, Kluwer, 1993, pp 289–296

Lahti RA, Roberts RC, Tamminga CA: D$_2$-family receptor distribution in human postmortem tissue: an autoradiographic study. NeuroReport 6:2505–2512, 1995

Largent BL, Wikström H, Snowman AM, et al: Novel antipsychotic drugs share high affinity for receptors. Eur J Pharmacol 155:345–347, 1988

Lidow MS, Goldman-Rakic PS, Rakic P, et al: Dopamine D$_2$ receptors in the cerebral cortex: distribution and pharmacological characterization with [^{3}H]raclopride. Proc Natl Acad Sci U S A 86:6412–6416, 1989

Lieberman JA: Understanding the mechanism of action of atypical antipsychotic drugs. Br J Psychiatry 163 (suppl 22):7–18, 1993

Lieberman JA, Kane JM, Johns CA: Clozapine: guidelines for clinical management. J Clin Psychiatry 50:329–338, 1989

Lieberman JA, Saltz BL, Johns CA, et al: The effects of clozapine on tardive dyskinesia. Br J Psychiatry 158:503–510, 1991

Lindstrom E, Knorring L, Eberhard G: Studies of selected outcome-related clinical parameters following short-term and long-term treatment with risperidone. Annual Meeting of Collegium International, NeuroPsychopharmacologicum P-58-223, 1994

Lundberg T, Lindström LH, Hartvig P, et al: Striatal and frontal cortex binding of 11-C-labelled clozapine visualized by positron emission tomography (PET) in drug-free schizophrenics and healthy volunteers. Psychopharmacology 99:8–12, 1989

Mansour A, Meador-Woodruff JH, Bunzow JR, et al: Localization of dopamine D_2 receptor mRNA and D_1 and D_2 receptor binding in the rat brain and pituitary: an in situ hybridization-receptor autoradiographic analysis. J Neurosci 10:2587–2600, 1990

Mansour A, Meador-Woodruff JH, Zhou QY, et al: A comparison of D_1 receptor binding and mRNA in rat brain using receptor autoradiographic and in situ hybridization techniques. Neuroscience 45:359–371, 1991

Marder SR, Meibach RC: Risperidone in the treatment of schizophrenia. Am J Psychiatry 151:825–835, 1994

Meador-Woodruff JH, Mansour A, Bunzow JR, et al: Distribution of D_2 dopamine receptor mRNA in rat brain. Proc Natl Acad Sci U S A 86:7625–7628, 1989

Meador-Woodruff JH, Mansour A, Civelli O, et al: Distribution of D_2 dopamine receptor mRNA in the primate brain. Prog Neuropsychopharmacol Biol Psychiatry 15:885–893, 1991

Meador-Woodruff JH, Damask SP, Wang J, et al: Dopamine receptor mRNA expression in human striatum and neocortex. Neuropsychopharmacology 15:17–29, 1996

Medical Economics Company: Physicians' Desk Reference, 50th Edition. Montvale, NJ, Medical Economics, 1996

Meltzer HY: The mechanism of action of novel antipsychotic drugs. Schizophr Bull 17:263–287, 1991

Meltzer HY: Novel Antipsychotic Drugs. New York, Raven, 1992a

Meltzer HY: Dimensions of outcome with clozapine. Br J Psychiatry 160 (suppl 17):46–53, 1992b

Meltzer HY: Role of serotonin in the action of atypical antipsychotic drugs. Clin Neurosci 3:64–75, 1995

Meltzer HY, Matsubara S, Lee JC: Classification of typical and atypical drugs on the basis of dopamine D_1, D_2 and serotonin$_2$ pK$_i$ values. J Pharmacol Exp Ther 251:238–246, 1989

Meltzer HY, Cole P, Way L, et al: Cost-effectiveness of clozapine in neuroleptic resistant schizophrenia. Am J Psychiatry 150:1630–1638, 1993

Mendelowitz AJ, Lieberman SA: New findings in the use of atypical antipsychotics: focus on risperidone. J Clin Psychiatry Case Comment Series 2:1–12, 1995

Mengod G, Martinez-Mir MI, Vilaró MT, et al: Localization of the mRNA for the dopamine D_2 receptor in the rat brain by in situ hybridization histochemistry. Proc Natl Acad Sci U S A 86:8560–8564, 1989

Minabe Y, Ashby CR, Wang RY: Effects produced by acute and chronic treatment with granisetron alone or in combination with haloperidol on midbrain dopamine neurons. Eur Neuropsychopharmacol 2:127–133, 1992

Moghaddam B: Preferential activation of cortical dopamine neurotransmission by clozapine: functional significance. J Clin Psychiatry 55 (suppl B):27–29, 1994

Moghaddam B, Bunney BS: Acute effects of typical and atypical antipsychotic drugs on the release of dopamine from prefrontal cortex, nucleus accumbens, and striatum of the rat: an in vivo microdialysis study. J Neurochem 54:1755–1760, 1990

Molineaux SM, Jessell TM, Axel R, et al: 5-HT$_{1C}$ receptor is a prominent serotonin receptor subtype in the central nervous system. Proc Natl Acad Sci U S A 86:6793–6797, 1989

Monsma FJ, McVittie LD, Gerfen CR, et al: Multiple D_2 dopamine receptors produced by alternative RNA splicing. Nature 342:926–929, 1989

Monsma FJ, Mahan LC, McVittie LD, et al: Molecular cloning and expression of a D_1 dopamine receptor linked to adenylyl cyclase activation. Proc Natl Acad Sci U S A 87:6723–6727, 1990

Monsma FJ, Shen Y, Ward RP, et al: Cloning and expression of a novel serotonin receptor with high affinity for tricyclic psychotropic drugs. Mol Pharmacol 43:320–327, 1993

Murray AM, Hyde TM, Knable MB, et al: Distribution of putative D_4 dopamine receptors in postmortem striatum from patients with schizophrenia. J Neurosci 15:2186–2191, 1995

Musacchio JM: The psychotomimetic effects of opiates and the receptor. Neuropsychopharmacology 3:191–199, 1990

Naber D, Gaussares C, Moeglen JM, et al: Efficacy and tolerability of SDZ HDC 912, a partial dopamine D_2 agonist, in the treatment of schizophrenia, in Novel Antipsychotic Drugs. Edited by Meltzer HY. New York, Raven, 1992, pp 99–107

Nordstrom AL, Farde L, Halldin C: High 5-HT$_2$ receptor occupancy in clozapine treated patients demonstrated by PET. Psychopharmacology 110:365–367, 1993

O'Donnell PO, Grace AA: Basic neurophysiology of antipsychotic drug action, in Handbook of Experimental Pharmacology: Antipsychotics. Edited by Csernansky JC. New York, Springer-Verlag, 1996, pp 163–202

Ohara K, Ulpian C, Seeman P, et al: Schizophrenia: dopamine D_1 receptor sequence is normal, but has DNA polymorphisms. Neuropsychopharmacology 8:131–135, 1993

Olney JW: Glutamatergic mechanisms in neuropsychiatry, in Novel Antipsychotic Drugs. Edited by Meltzer HY. New York, Raven, 1992, pp 155–169

Olney JW, Farber NB: Glutamate receptor dysfunction and schizophrenia. Arch Gen Psychiatry 52:998–1007, 1995

Onn S-P, Grace AA: Repeated treatment with haloperidol and clozapine exerts differential effects on dye coupling between neurons in subregions of striatum and nucleus accumbens. J Neurosci 15:7024–7036, 1995

Owens MJ, Mulchahey JJ, Stout SC, et al: Molecular and neurobiological mechanisms in the treatment of psychiatric disorders, in Psychiatry. Edited by Tasman A, Kay J, Lieberman JA. Philadelphia, PA, WB Saunders, 1997, pp 210–257

Peuskens J, Risperidone Study Group: Risperidone in the treatment of chronic schizophrenic patients: a multi-national, multi-centre, double-blind, parallel-group study versus haloperidol. Br J Psychiatry 166:712–726, 1995

Pickar D: Prospects for the pharmacotherapy of schizophrenia. Lancet 345:557–562, 1995

Pickar D, Litman RE, Owen RR, et al: Response to clozapine predictors. Abstracts of the 31st Annual Meeting of the American College of Neuropsychopharmacology, San Juan, Puerto Rico, December 1992a, p 48

Pickar D, Woen RR, Litman RE, et al: Clinical and biologic response to clozapine in patients with schizophrenia. Arch Gen Psychiatry 49:345–353, 1992b

Piomelli D, Pilon C, Giros B, et al: Dopamine activation of the arachidonic acid cascade as a basis for D_1/D_2 receptor synergism. Nature 353:164–167, 1991

Polsker GL: Risperidone: does it give "enough bang for the buck"? Inpharma 16:7–8, 1994

Rasmussen K, Stockton ME, Czachura JF: The 5-HT$_3$ receptor antagonist zatosetron decreases the number of spontaneously active A10 dopamine neurons. Eur J Pharmacol 205:113–116, 1991

Reynolds GP: Developments in the drug treatment of schizophrenia. Trends Pharmacol Sci 13:116–121, 1992

Reynolds GP, Mason SL: Are striatal dopamine D_4 receptors increased in schizophrenia? J Neurochem 63:1576–1577, 1994

Risch SC, Lewine RJ: Low cerebrospinal fluid homovanillic acid/5-hydroxyindoleacetic acid ratio predicts clozapine efficacy: a replication (letter). Arch Gen Psychiatry 50:670, 1993

Risch SC, Lewine RRJ: CSF HVA:5-HIAA ratio increases accompanying clozapine efficacy (letter). Arch Gen Psychiatry 52:244, 1995

Robertson GS, Fibiger HC: Effects of olanzapine on regional *c-fos* expression in rat forebrain. Neuropsychopharmacology 14:105–110, 1996

Robertson GS, Matsumura H, Fibiger HC: Induction patterns of fos-like immunoreactivity in the forebrain as predictors of atypical antipsychotic activity. J Pharmacol Exp Ther 271:1058–1066, 1994

Roth BL, Craigo SC, Choudhary MS, et al: Binding of typical and atypical antipsychotic agents to 5-hydroxytryptamine-6 and 5-hydroxytryptamine-7 receptors. J Pharmacol Exp Ther 268:1403–1410, 1994

Roth BL, Tandra S, Burgess LH, et al: D_4 dopamine receptor binding affinity does not distinguish between typical and atypical antipsychotic drugs. Psychopharmacology 120:365–368, 1995

Schmauss C, Haroutunian V, Davis KL, et al: Selective loss of dopamine D_3-type receptor mRNA expression in parietal and motor cortices of patients with chronic schizophrenia. Proc Natl Acad Sci U S A 90:8942–8946, 1993

Schoots O, Seeman P, Guan H-C, et al: Long-term haloperidol elevates dopamine D_4 receptors by 2-fold in rats. Eur J Pharmacol 289:67–72, 1995

Schwartz JC, Sokoloff P, Giros B, et al: The dopamine D_3 receptor as a target for antipsychotics, in Novel Antipsychotic Drugs. Edited by Meltzer HY. New York, Raven, 1992, pp 135–144

Seeman P: Dopamine receptors and the dopamine hypothesis of schizophrenia. Synapse 1:133–152, 1987

Seeman P: Receptor selectivities of atypical neuroleptics, in Novel Antipsychotic Drugs. Edited by Meltzer HY. New York, Raven, 1992a, pp 145–154

Seeman P: Dopamine receptor sequences: therapeutic levels of neuroleptics occupy D_2 receptors, clozapine occupies D_4. Neuropsychopharmacology 7:261–284, 1992b

Seeman P, Van Tol HHM: Dopamine D_4-like receptor elevation in schizophrenia: cloned D_2 and D_4 receptors cannot be discriminated by raclopride competition against [^{3}H] nemonapride. J Neurochem 64:1413–1415, 1995

Seeman P, Guan HC, Niznik HB: Endogenous dopamine lowers the dopamine D_2 receptor density as measured by [^{3}H]raclopride: implications for positron emission tomography of the human brain. Synapse 3:96–97, 1989a

Seeman P, Niznik HB, Guan HC, et al: Link between D_1 and D_2 dopamine receptors is reduced in schizophrenia and Huntington diseased brain. Proc Natl Acad Sci U S A 86:10156–10160, 1989b

Seeman P, Hong-Chang G, Van Tol HHM: Dopamine D_4 receptors elevated in schizophrenia. Nature 365:441–445, 1993

Seeman P, Sunahara RK, Niznik HB: Receptor-receptor link in membranes revealed by ligand competition: example for dopamine D_1 and D_2 receptors. Synapse 17:62–64, 1994

Seeman P, Guan H-C, Van Tol HHM: Schizophrenia: elevation of dopamine D_4-like sites, using [^{3}H]nemonapride and [^{125}I]epidepride. Eur J Pharmacol 286:R3–R5, 1995

Shen Y, Monsma FJ, Metcalf MA, et al: Molecular cloning and expression of a 5-hydroxytryptamine$_7$ serotonin receptor subtype. J Biol Chem 268:18200–18204, 1993

Snyder SH: The dopamine connection. Nature 247:121–122, 1990

Snyder SH, Largent BL: Receptor mechanisms in antipsychotic drugs action: focus on sigma receptors. J Neuropsychiatry 1:7–15, 1989

Sokoloff P, Giros B, Martres MP, et al: Molecular cloning and characterization of a novel dopamine receptor (D_3) as a target for neuroleptics. Nature 247:146–151, 1990

Sokoloff P, Martres MP, Giros B, et al: The third dopamine receptor (D_3) as a novel target for antipsychotics. Biochem Pharmacol 43:656–666, 1992a

Sokoloff P, Andrieux M, Besancon R, et al: Pharmacology of human dopamine D_3 receptor expressed in a mammalian cell line: comparison with D_2 receptor. Eur J Pharmacol 225:331–337, 1992b

Sokoloff P, Levesque D, Martres MP, et al: The dopamine D_3 receptor as a key target for antipsychotics. Clin Neuropharmacol 15 (suppl 1): 456A–457A, 1992c

Sorensen SM, Humphreys TM, Palfreyman MF: Effects of acute and chronic MDL 73,147, a 5-HT$_3$ receptor antagonist, on A9 and A10 dopamine neurons. Eur J Pharmacol 163:115–120, 1989

Soubrie P, Reisine TD, Glowinski J: Functional aspects of serotonin transmission in the basal ganglia: a review and an in vivo approach using the push-pull cannula technique. Neuroscience 131:615–624, 1984

Srivastava LK, Morency MA, Bajwa SB, et al: Effect of haloperidol on expression of dopamine D_2 receptor mRNAs in rat brain. J Mol Neurosci 2:155–161, 1990

Steinfels GF, Tam SW, Cook L: Electrophysiological effects of selective σ-receptor agonists, antagonists, and the selective phencyclidine receptor agonist MK-801 on midbrain dopamine neurons. Neuropsychopharmacology 2:201–207, 1989

Sumiyoshi T, Stockmeier CA, Overholser JC, et al: Dopamine D_4 receptors and effects of guanine nucleotides on [^{3}H]raclopride binding in postmortem caudate nucleus of subjects with schizophrenia or major depression. Brain Res 681: 109–116, 1995

Sunahara RK, Niznik HB, Weiner DM, et al: Human dopamine D_1 receptor encoded by an intronless gene on chromosome 5. Nature 247:80–83, 1990

Sunahara RK, Guan HC, O'Dowd BF, et al: Cloning of the gene for a human dopamine D_5 receptor with higher affinity for dopamine than D_1. Nature 350:614–619, 1991

Tamminga CA: Schizophrenia and glutamatergic transmission. Crit Rev Neurobiol 12:21–36, 1998

Tamminga CA, Gerlach J: New neuroleptics and experimental antipsychotics in schizophrenia, in Psychopharmacology: The Third Generation of Progress. Edited by Meltzer HY. New York, Raven, 1987, pp 1129–1140

Tamminga CA, Cascella N, Fakouhi TD, et al: Enhancement of NMDA-mediated transmission in schizophrenia: effects of milacemide, in Novel Antipsychotic Drugs. Edited by Meltzer HY. New York, Raven, 1992, pp 171–177

Tarsy D: Risperidone and neuroleptic malignant syndrome (letter). JAMA 275:446, 1996

Taylor DP, Schlemmer RF: Sigma "antagonists": potential antipsychotics? in Novel Antipsychotic Drugs. Edited by Meltzer HY. New York, Raven, 1992, pp 189–201

Tiberi M, Jarvie KR, Silvia C, et al: Cloning, molecular characterization, and chromosomal assignment of a gene encoding a second D_1 dopamine receptor subtype: differential expression pattern in rat brain compared with the D_{1A} receptor. Proc Natl Acad Sci U S A 88:7491–7495, 1991

Tollefson GD, Sanger JR: Negative symptoms: a path analytic approach to a double-blind placebo and haloperidol-controlled clinical trial with olanzapine. Am J Psychiatry 154:466–474, 1997

Tollefson GD, Beasley CM, Tran PV, et al: Olanzapine versus haloperidol in the treatment of schizophrenia and schizoaffective and schizophreniform disorders: results of an international collaborative study. Am J Psychiatry 154:457–465, 1997

Tran PV, Dellva MA, Tollefson GD, et al: Extrapyramidal symptoms and tolerability of olanzapine versus haloperidol in the acute treatment of schizophrenia. J Clin Psychiatry 58: 205–211, 1997

Tsai G, Passani LA, Slusher BS, et al: Abnormal excitatory neurotransmitter metabolism in schizophrenic brain. Arch Gen Psychiatry 52: 829–836, 1995

Van Tol HHM, Riva M, Civelli O, et al: Lack of effect of chronic dopamine receptor blockade on D_2 dopamine receptor mRNA level. Neurosci Lett 111:303–308, 1990

Van Tol HHM, Bunzow JR, Guan H, et al: Cloning of the gene for a human dopamine D_4 receptor with high affinity for the antipsychotic clozapine. Nature 350:610–614, 1991

Van Tol HH, Wu CM, Guan HC, et al: Multiple dopamine D_4 receptor variants in the human population. Nature 358:149–152, 1992

Wachtel SR, White FJ: Electrophysiological effects of BMY 14802, a new potential antipsychotic drug, on midbrain dopamine neurons in the rat: acute and chronic studies. J Pharmacol Exp Ther 244:410–416, 1988

Wachtel SR, Hu XT, Gallaway MP, et al: D_1 dopamine receptor stimulation enables the postsynaptic, but not autoreceptor, effects of D_2 dopamine agonists in nigrostriatal and mesoaccumbens dopamine systems. Synapse 4: 327–346, 1989

Waddington JL, Daly SA: The status of "second generation" selective D_1 dopamine receptor antagonists as putative atypical antipsychotic agents, in Novel Antipsychotic Drugs. Edited by Meltzer HY. New York, Raven, 1992, pp 109–115

Walker JM, Bowen WD, Walker FD, et al: Sigma receptors: biology and function. Pharmacol Rev 42:355–402, 1990

Ward RP, Hamblin MW, Lachowicz JE, et al: Localization of serotonin subtype 6 receptor messenger RNA in the rat brain by in situ hybridization histochemistry. Neuroscience 64:1105–1111, 1995

Watling KJ, Beer MS, Stanton JA, et al: Interaction of the atypical neuroleptic clozapine with 5-HT_3 receptors in the cerebral cortex and superior ganglion of the rat. Eur J Pharmacol 182: 465–472, 1990

Webster P, Wijeratne C: Risperidone-induced neuroleptic malignant syndrome. Lancet 334: 1228–1229, 1994

Wiedemann K, Krieg JC, Loycke A: Novel dopamine autoreceptor agonists B-HT 920 and EMD 49980 in the treatment of patients with schizophrenia, in Novel Antipsychotic Drugs. Edited by Meltzer HY. New York, Raven, 1992, pp 91–98

Wolkin A, Sanfilipo M, Wolf AP, et al: Negative symptoms and hypofrontality in chronic schizophrenia. Arch Gen Psychiatry 49:959–965, 1992

Xu S, Monsma FJ, Sibley DR, et al: Regulation of D_{1A} and D_2 dopamine receptor mRNA during ontogenesis, lesion and chronin antagonist treatment. Life Sci 50:383–396, 1992

Zhang L-J, Lachowicz JE, Sibley DR: The D_{2S} and D_{2L} dopamine receptor isoforms are differentially regulated in Chinese hamster ovary cells. Mol Pharmacol 45:878–889, 1994

Zhang W, Bymaster FP: Effects of olanzapine and other antipsychotics in receptor occupancy and antagonism of dopamine D_1, D_2, D_3, $5HT_{2A}$ and muscarinic receptors. Psychopharmacology (Berl) 141:267–278, 1999

Zhou QY, Grandy DK, Thambi L, et al: Cloning and expression of human and rat D_1 dopamine receptors. Nature 347:76–80, 1990

TEN

Treatment of Extrapyramidal Side Effects

Joseph K. Stanilla, M.D., and
George M. Simpson, M.D.

HISTORY OF EXTRAPYRAMIDAL SIDE EFFECTS

The description of chlorpromazine's therapeutic properties (Delay and Deniker 1952; Laborit et al. 1952) was soon followed by the description of its tendency to produce extrapyramidal side effects (EPS), which were indistinguishable from classic Parkinson's disease. A debate soon arose regarding the relationship between EPS and therapeutic efficacy. Flügel (1953) suggested that a therapeutic response from chlorpromazine required the development of EPS. Haase (1954) postulated that the dose of antipsychotic medication that produced minimal subclinical rigidity and hypokinesia—the "neuroleptic threshold"—was the minimal dose necessary for therapeutic antipsychotic effect and was manifested by micrographic handwriting changes.

Brooks (1956), though, suggested that "signs of parkinsonism heralded the particular effect being sought" (p. 1122), but "the therapeutic effects were not dependent on extrapyramidal dysfunction. On the contrary, alleviation of such dysfunction, as soon as it oc-

curred, sped the progress of recovery" (p. 1122).

Subsequent investigation demonstrated that patients treated with doses beyond the neuroleptic threshold received significantly larger doses of medication without further therapeutic benefit (Angus and Simpson 1970a; G. M. Simpson et al. 1970). This finding has been discussed more fully (Baldessarini et al. 1988) and replicated (McEvoy et al. 1991).

Clozapine's efficacy demonstrated that a drug could provide antipsychotic effect without producing EPS. The current goal in the development of new antipsychotic medications is to replicate the EPS profile of clozapine and to develop antipsychotics that do not produce EPS. This situation essentially brings the story of EPS full circle (Hippius 1989).

The terms used to name and characterize antipsychotic medications have also evolved. The term *tranquilizer* was initially introduced to characterize the psychic effects of reserpine. The term *neuroleptic*, derived from Greek and meaning *to clasp the neuron*, was introduced to describe chlorpromazine and the extrapyramidal effects it produced (Delay et al. 1952). Until clozapine was approved for use, all commercially available drugs with antipsychotic properties had the *neuroleptic* properties of 1) blocking apomorphine- and amphetamine-induced stereotypy; 2) antagonizing the conditioned avoidance response; and 3) producing catalepsy, elevated serum prolactin levels, and EPS. For that reason, all antipsychotic drugs were referred to as *neuroleptics*.

With the subsequent development of clozapine and other atypical antipsychotic drugs that have reduced EPS profiles, the term *neuroleptic* no longer correctly categorizes all drugs with antipsychotic effects, so that the term *antipsychotic* is more accurate and preferable.

Severe EPS can have a significantly negative effect on treatment outcome by contributing to poor compliance and exacerbation of psychiatric symptoms (Van Putten et al. 1981). Akathisia, in particular, is associated with a poor clinical outcome (Levinson et al. 1990; Van Putten et al. 1984), increased violence (Keckich 1978), and even suicide (Shear et al. 1983). The presence of EPS early in treatment may place a patient at increased risk for developing tardive dyskinesia (Saltz et al. 1991). Orofacial tardive dyskinesia may have a negative effect on the social acceptability of patients, even though they are often unaware of the movements (Boumans et al. 1994). Laryngeal dystonia can adversely affect speech, breathing, and swallowing (Feve et al. 1995; Khan et al. 1994) and potentially can be life-threatening (Koek and Pi 1989). Clearly, EPS are significant, need to be assessed, and should be minimized so that the overall treatment and health of patients may be optimized.

TYPES OF EXTRAPYRAMIDAL SIDE EFFECTS

Four types of EPS have been delineated. The treatment of each should be individualized.

Acute dystonic reactions (ADRs) generally are the first EPS to appear and are often the most dramatic (Angus and Simpson 1970b). Dystonias are involuntary sustained or spasmodic muscle contractions that cause abnormal twist-ing or rhythmical movements and/or postures. ADRs tend to occur suddenly and generally involve muscles of the head and neck (e.g., torticollis, facial grimacing, oculogyric crisis). Almost 90% of all ADRs occur within 4 days of antipsychotic initiation or dosage increase, and virtually 100% occur by day 10 (Singh et al. 1990; Sramek et al. 1986). Although tardive dystonia can occur, movements beyond this time frame are much less likely to be ADRs, and other conditions, including seizures, should be considered.

Akathisia is the next type of EPS to appear. Akathisia, meaning "inability to sit," comprises both an objective, restless movement and a subjective feeling of restlessness that the patient experiences as the need to move. Because it may be difficult for a patient to explain the sensation of akathisia, the diagnosis can be overlooked. At times, patients may show the classic movements of akathisia but not have the subjective distress. This condition has been termed *pseudoakathisia* and may be a type of tardive syndrome (Barnes 1990).

The third type of EPS, *(pseudo)parkinsonism*, is virtually indistinguishable from classic Parkinson's disease. The symptoms include a generalized slowing of movement (akinesia), masked facies, cogwheeling, rigidity, resting tremor, and hypersalivation. Parkinsonism generally occurs after a few weeks or more of antipsychotic treatment. Akinesia must be differentiated from primary depression and the blunted affect of schizophrenia (Rifkin et al. 1975).

Tardive syndromes constitute the fourth type of EPS; tardive dyskinesia and tardive dystonia are the two most common tardive syndromes. Tardive dyskinesia consists of irregular, stereotypical movements of the mouth, face, and tongue and choreoathetoid movements of the fingers, arms, legs, and trunk. Patients frequently have no awareness of the abnormal movements, which may be related to frontal-lobe dysfunction (Sandyk et al. 1993).

PREVALENCE OF EXTRAPYRAMIDAL SIDE EFFECTS

Ayd (1961) first reported the prevalence of EPS: the overall prevalence was 39%, and 21% had akathisia, 15% had parkinsonism, and only 2% had ADRs. Varying rates of occurrence have been reported since then, including much more frequent rates for ADRs. A prospective study found the prevalence of ADR to range from 17% to 38%, with the higher rate occurring with haloperidol (Sramek et al. 1986). In general, higher prevalence rates for all types of EPS occur with higher doses and higher-potency antipsychotics.

ETIOLOGY OF EXTRAPYRAMIDAL SIDE EFFECTS

The exact mechanisms involved in the production of EPS are not known. Control of motor activity appears to involve an interaction between nigrostriatal dopaminergic, intrastriatal cholinergic, and γ-aminobutyric acid (GABA)–ergic neurons (Côté and Crutcher 1991).

Extrapyramidal movements classically have been thought to result from blockade of nigrostriatal dopaminergic tracts by antipsychotic medications, resulting in a relative increase in cholinergic activity (Snyder et al. 1974). Drugs that decrease cholinergic activity or increase dopaminergic activity reduce EPS, presumably by restoring the two systems to their previous equilibrium. This effect has been observed in ADRs in monkeys (Casey et al. 1980).

ANTICHOLINERGIC MEDICATIONS

Antiparkinsonian medications, including anticholinergic, antihistaminic, and dopaminergic agents, primarily have been used to treat EPS (Table 10–1).

Trihexyphenidyl

History and Discovery

Trihexyphenidyl, a synthetic analogue of atropine, was introduced in 1949 (as benzhexol hydrochloride) and was found to be effective in the treatment of Parkinson's disease in a study of 411 patients (Doshay et al. 1954). Thereafter, it was also used to treat neuroleptic-induced parkinsonism (NIP) (Rashkis and Smarr 1957).

Structure-Activity Relations

Trihexyphenidyl, a tertiary amine analogue of atropine, is a competitive antagonist of acetylcholine and other muscarinic agonists that competes for a common binding site on muscarinic receptors (Yamamura and Snyder 1974). It exerts little blockade at nicotinic receptors (Timberlake et al. 1961). Trihexyphenidyl and all drugs in this class are referred to as anticholinergic, antimuscarinic, or atropine-like drugs.

Pharmacological Profile

The pharmacological properties of trihexyphenidyl are qualitatively similar to those of atropine and other anticholinergic drugs, although trihexyphenidyl acts primarily centrally with few peripheral effects and little sedation. In the eye, anticholinergic drugs block both the sphincter muscle of the iris, which leads to pupil dilation (mydriasis), and the ciliary muscle of the lens, which prevents accommodation and causes cycloplegia. In the heart, anticholinergics usually produce a mild tachycardia through vagal blockade at the sinoatrial (S-A) node pacemaker, although a mild slowing can occur. In the gastrointestinal tract, anticholinergics reduce gut motility and salivary and gastric secretions. Salivary secretion is particularly sensitive and can be completely abolished. In the respiratory system, anticholinergics reduce secretions and can produce mild bronchodilatation. Anticholinergics inhibit the activity of sweat glands and mildly decrease contractions in the urinary and biliary tracts (Brown and Taylor 1996).

Table 10–1. Pharmacological agents used for the treatment of neuroleptic-induced parkinsonism and acute dystonic reactions

Compound	Type	Relative equivalence (mg)[a]	Route	Availability	Dosing	Therapeutic dosage used in studies (mg)
Trihexyphenidyl (Artane)	Anticholinergic	2.5	Oral	Tablets (2 or 5 mg) Elixir (2 mg/mL) Sequels (5 mg [sustained release])	Once to twice a day	2–30
Benztropine (Cogentin)	Anticholinergic	1	Oral Injectable	Tablets (0.5, 1, 2 mg) Ampules (1 mg/mL [2 mL])	Once to twice a day Every 30 minutes until symptom relief	1–12 2–8
Biperiden (Akineton)	Anticholinergic	1	Oral Injectable	Tablets (2 mg) Ampules (5 mg/mL [1 mL])	Two to three times a day Every 30 minutes until symptom relief	2–24 2–8
Procyclidine (Kemadrin)	Anticholinergic	2[b]	Oral	Tablets (5 mg, scored)	Two to three times a day	5–55
Diphenhydramine (Benadryl)	Antihistaminic	50	Oral Injectable	Tablets (25 or 50 mg) Ampules (10 mg/mL [10 or 30 mL] or 50 mg/mL [10 mL])	Two to four times a day Every 30 minutes until symptom relief	50–400
Amantadine (Symmetrel)	Dopaminergic	N/A	Oral	Tablets (100 mg)	Once to twice a day	100–300

Source. [a]de Leon et al. 1994; [b]Timberlake et al. 1961.

Pharmacokinetics and Disposition

Peak concentration for trihexyphenidyl is reached 1–2 hours after oral administration, and its half-life is 10–12 hours (Cedarbaum and McDowell 1987). As a tertiary amine, it readily crosses the blood-brain barrier to enter the central nervous system (CNS) (Brown and Taylor 1996).

Mechanism of Action

The presumed mechanism of action of trihexyphenidyl for treatment of EPS is the blockade of intrastriatal cholinergic activity, which is relatively increased compared with nigrostriatal dopaminergic activity, which is decreased by antipsychotic blockade. The blockade of cholinergic activity returns the system to its previous equilibrium.

Indications

Anticholinergic agents were reported to be effective treatment for NIP from open empiric trials (Medina et al. 1962; Rashkis and Smarr 1957). Eventually, controlled trials were conducted, but most only involved comparisons with other anticholinergics and not with placebo. Despite the limited evidence of efficacy compared with placebo, anticholinergic agents became the mainstay of treatment for NIP and remain so today.

Trihexyphenidyl has U.S. Food and Drug Administration (FDA) approval for the treatment of all forms of parkinsonism, including NIP. Daily doses of 2–30 mg have been used in studies of trihexyphenidyl in treatment of Parkinson's disease and NIP. The individual therapeutic dose must be determined empirically, though, and can vary widely.

Side Effects and Toxicology

Peripheral side effects.   Peripheral effects of trihexyphenidyl result from parasympathetic muscarinic blockade and occur in a consistent hierarchy among different organs. They are qualitatively similar to the side effects of atropine and other anticholinergic drugs but are quantitatively fewer because of trihexyphenidyl's reduced peripheral activity (Brown 1990).

Anticholinergic drugs initially reduce salivary and bronchial secretions and sweat production. Reduced salivation produces dry mouth and contributes to the high incidence of dental caries among chronically ill psychiatric patients (Winer and Bahn 1967). Treatment for this condition is basically nonexistent. Activities that stimulate salivation, such as chewing sugar-free gum or sucking hard candy, are limited by the need for constant use. Reduced sweating can contribute to heat prostration and heat stroke, particularly in warmer ambient temperatures.

The next physiological effects occur in the eyes and heart. Pupillary dilation and inhibition of accommodation in the eye lead to photophobia and blurred vision. Attacks of acute glaucoma can occur in susceptible subjects with narrow-angle glaucoma, although this is relatively uncommon. The next effect, vagus nerve blockade, leads to increased heart rate and is more apparent in patients with high vagal tone (usually younger males). Subsequent effects are inhibition of urinary bladder function and bowel motility, which can produce urinary retention, constipation, and obstipation. Sufficiently high doses of anticholinergics will inhibit gastric secretion and motility (Brown 1990).

Central side effects.   Memory disturbance is the most common central side effect of anticholinergic medications because memory is dependent on the integrity of the cholinergic system (Drachman 1977). Patients with underlying brain disorders are more susceptible to memory disturbance (Fayen et al. 1988). Patients with chronic psychiatric disorders often have a decreased ability to express themselves, so evaluation of memory is more difficult, and subtle memory changes may be overlooked or attributed to the underlying illness. Memory disturbances were identified in patients with Parkinson's disease treated with anticholinergics (Yahr and Duvoisin 1968), even in some patients receiving only small doses (Stephens 1967).

Anticholinergic toxicity produces restlessness, irritability, disorientation, hallucinations, and delirium. Elderly patients are at increased risk for both memory loss and toxic delirium, even at very low anticholinergic doses, because of the natural loss of cholinergic neurons with aging (Perry et al. 1977). Toxic levels can produce a clinical situation identical to that of atropine poisoning, including fixed, dilated pupils; flushed face; sinus tachycardia; urinary retention; dry mouth; and fever. This condition can proceed to coma, cardiorespiratory collapse, and death.

Drug-Drug Interactions

Anticholinergic effects, including side effects, may increase when trihexyphenidyl or any anticholinergic is combined with amantadine.

Anticholinergic effect on antipsychotic blood levels. Some investigators have suggested that anticholinergic medications can affect antipsychotic blood levels. A review of this subject indicated that the available data were too limited to reach a definite conclusion on this matter (McEvoy 1983). The best studies indicate that anticholinergic drugs do not affect antipsychotic blood levels or, at most, lower levels only transiently.

Anticholinergic effect on antipsychotic activity. Haase and Janssen (1965) reported from open studies that if anticholinergic drugs were added to antipsychotic drugs given at the neuroleptic threshold, rigidity, hypokinesia, and therapeutic effects would disappear. Other studies have found no change or an improvement in scores of psychopathology with the addition of anticholinergics (Hanlon et al. 1966; G. M. Simpson et al. 1980).

Anticholinergic Abuse

Anticholinergic drugs may be abused for their euphoriant and hallucinogenic effects and may be combined with street drugs for enhanced effect. Trihexyphenidyl reportedly is the anticholinergic most likely to be abused (MacVicar 1977). Theoretically, one anticholinergic should be as effective as another, although idiosyncratic responses are possible. The potential for abuse must be considered, particularly in patients with a history of substance abuse.

Benztropine

History and Discovery

Benztropine was found to be effective in the treatment of 302 patients with Parkinson's disease (Doshay 1956). The best results in the control of rigidity, contracture, and tremor were obtained at dosages of 1–4 mg/day for older patients and 2–8 mg/day for younger ones. Dosages of 15–30 mg/day caused excessive flaccidity in some patients, who became unable to lift their arms or raise their heads off the bed. Subsequently, benztropine was found to be effective for treatment of NIP (Karn and Kasper 1959).

Structure-Activity Relations

Benztropine was synthesized by uniting the tropine portion of atropine with the benzohydryl portion of diphenhydramine hydrochloride. Benztropine is a tertiary amine with activity similar to that of trihexyphenidyl. As a tertiary amine, it enters the CNS.

Pharmacological Profile

Benztropine has the pharmacological properties of an anticholinergic and an antihistaminic. It produces less sedation (in experimental animals) than does diphenhydramine, however.

Pharmacokinetics and Disposition

Little is known about the pharmacokinetics of benztropine. A correlation between serum anticholinergic levels and the presence of EPS has been found (Tune and Coyle 1980). There is little correlation between the total daily dose of benztropine and the serum anticholinergic level, with the serum activity for a given dose varying 100-fold among subjects. When treated with increased doses of benztropine, patients with EPS had increased serum anticholinergic activity and decreased EPS. Relatively small increments in the oral dose of all anticholinergic drugs can result in significant nonlinear increases in serum anticholinergic activity levels. Benztropine has a long-acting effect and can be given once or twice a day.

Indications

Benztropine has FDA approval for the treatment of all forms of parkinsonism, including NIP. Daily doses of 1–8 mg have generally been used to treat NIP.

Mechanism of Action, Side Effects, and Drug Interactions

The mechanism of action, side effects, and drug interactions of benztropine are similar to those of trihexyphenidyl. Benztropine was reported to be less stimulating and more sedating than trihexyphenidyl and other anticholinergic agents when used to treat patients with Parkinson's disease (Doshay 1956; England and Schwab 1959). Although this finding has not been tested in double-blind studies, these properties might account for the fact that trihexyphenidyl is reportedly the anticholinergic drug more likely to be abused.

Biperiden

Biperiden is an analogue of trihexyphenidyl. It has greater peripheral anticholinergic activity than trihexyphenidyl and greater activity against nicotinic receptors (Timberlake et al. 1961). Biperiden is well absorbed from the gastrointestinal tract. Its metabolism is not completely understood but involves hydroxylation in the liver. Its activity, pharmacological profile, and side effects are similar to those of other anticholinergics. It has FDA approval for the treatment of all forms of parkinsonism, including NIP. Daily doses of 2–24 mg have been used

in studies of biperiden for treatment of parkinsonism and NIP.

Procyclidine

Procyclidine is an analogue of trihexyphenidyl (Schwab and Chafetz 1955). Its activity, pharmacology, and side effects are similar to those of other anticholinergics. Little information is available on its pharmacokinetics. It has FDA approval for the treatment of all forms of parkinsonism, including NIP. Daily doses of 5–55 mg have been used in studies of procyclidine for treatment of parkinsonism and NIP (Timberlake et al. 1961).

ANTIHISTAMINIC MEDICATIONS

Diphenhydramine

History and Discovery

Antihistaminic agents have been used to treat Parkinson's disease. Diphenhydramine, one of the first antihistamines developed and used clinically (Bovet 1950), has been the primary antihistamine studied in the treatment of EPS. Other antihistamines have not been systematically studied for the treatment of EPS, but those with central anticholinergic activity may be effective for the treatment of EPS.

Structure-Activity Relations

All drugs referred to as antihistamines are reversible, competitive inhibitors of histamine at the H_1 receptor. Some antihistamines also inhibit the action of acetylcholine at the muscarinic receptor. Central muscarinic blockade rather than histaminic blockade is believed to be responsible for the therapeutic effect of antihistamines for EPS. Ethanolamine antihistamines (diphenhydramine, dimenhydrinate, carbinoxamine maleate) have the greatest anticholinergic activity, and ethylenediamines have the least. Antihistamines, such as terfenadine and astemizole, have no anticholinergic activity, whereas many of the remaining antihistamines have very mild anticholinergic activity (Babe and Serafin 1996).

Pharmacological Profile

Antihistamines inhibit the constrictor action of histamine on respiratory smooth muscle. They restrict the vasoconstrictor and vasodilatory effects of histamine on vascular smooth muscle and block histamine-induced capillary permeability. Antihistamines with CNS activity are depressants, producing diminished alertness, slowed reaction times, and somnolence. They can also block motion sickness. Antihistaminic drugs with anticholinergic activity also have mild antimuscarinic pharmacological properties similar to other atropine-like drugs (Babe and Serafin 1996).

Pharmacokinetics and Disposition

Diphenhydramine is well absorbed from the gastrointestinal tract. Peak concentrations occur 2–3 hours after oral administration. Its therapeutic effects usually last 4–6 hours, and it has a half-life of 3–9 hours. Diphenhydramine is widely distributed throughout the body, and as a tertiary amine, it enters the CNS. Age does not affect its pharmacokinetics. It undergoes demethylations in the liver and is then oxidized to carboxylic acid (Paton and Webster 1985).

Mechanism of Action

Diphenhydramine has some anticholinergic activity. Central anticholinergic activity is believed to be the basis for its effect in diminishing EPS.

Indications

Diphenhydramine has FDA approval for the treatment of all forms of parkinsonism, including NIP, in the elderly and for mild cases in other age groups. It is probably not as efficacious for treating EPS as pure anticholinergic drugs, but it may be better tolerated in patients bothered by anticholinergic side effects, such as geriatric patients. Diphenhydramine also tends to be more sedating than anticholinergics, which can also be beneficial for some patients. Dosages generally range from 50 to 400 mg/day given in divided doses.

Diphenhydramine also has indications for multiple other conditions unrelated to EPS.

Side Effects and Toxicology

The primary side effect of diphenhydramine is sedation. Although other antihistamines may cause gastrointestinal distress, diphenhydramine has a low incidence of this effect. Dry mouth and dry respiratory passages may occur. In general, the toxic effects are similar to those of trihexyphenidyl and other anticholinergics.

Drug-Drug Interactions

Diphenhydramine has no reported interactions with other drugs. It has an additive depressant effect when used in combination with alcohol or other CNS depressants.

DOPAMINERGIC MEDICATIONS

Anticholinergic side effects and inadequate treatment response eventually led to the investigation of other agents to treat EPS. Initially, both methylphenidate and intravenous caffeine were investigated as treatments of NIP. Neither achieved general use despite apparent efficacy (Brooks 1956; Freyhan 1959).

Amantadine

History and Discovery

Amantadine is an antiviral agent that is effective against A2 (Asian) influenza (Wingfield et al. 1969). It was unexpectedly found to reduce symptoms in patients with Parkinson's disease (Parkes et al. 1970; Schwab et al. 1969). Soon after, amantadine was reported to be effective for NIP (Kelly and Abuzzahab 1971).

Structure-Activity Relations

Amantadine is a water-soluble tricyclic amine. It binds to the M2 protein, a membrane protein that functions as an ion channel on the influenza

A virus (Hay 1992). Its activity in reducing EPS is not known.

Pharmacological Profile

Amantadine is effective in preventing and treating illness from influenza A virus. It also reduces the symptoms of parkinsonism.

Pharmacokinetics and Disposition

In young, healthy subjects, amantadine is slowly and well absorbed from the gastrointestinal tract, with unchanged oral bioavailability over the dose range of 50–300 mg. It reaches steady state in 4–7 days. Plasma concentrations (0.12–1.12 μg/mL) appear to correlate with decline in EPS (Greenblatt et al. 1977; Pacifici et al. 1976). It has relatively constant blood levels, has a long duration of action (Aoki et al. 1979), and is excreted unchanged by the kidneys. Its elimination half-life is about 16 hours, which is prolonged in elderly patients and those with impaired renal function (Hayden et al. 1985).

Mechanism of Action

Amantadine produces antiviral activity by binding to the M2 protein on the viral membrane and inhibiting replication (Hay 1992). Its mechanism of action as an antiparkinsonian agent is less clear. It has no anticholinergic activity in tests on animals and is only 1/209,000th as potent as atropine (Grelak et al. 1970). It appears to cause the release of dopamine and other catecholamines from intraneuronal storage sites in an amphetamine-like mechanism. It also has activity at glutamate receptors, which may contribute to its antiparkinsonian effect (Stoof et al. 1992). Amantadine has preferential selectivity for central catecholamine neurons (Grelak et al. 1970; Strömberg et al. 1970).

Indications

Amantadine was investigated more extensively than anticholinergic agents with respect to efficacy for EPS. Most, but not all, studies found that amantadine was effective and equivalent to benztropine for treatment of parkinsonism (DiMascio et al. 1976; Fann and Lake 1976; Stenson et al. 1976). Some found that amantadine was more effective than benztropine (Merrick and Schmitt 1973) or effective in EPS refractory to benztropine (Gelenberg 1978). Some studies, though, found that amantadine was inferior to benztropine (Kelly et al. 1974), no more effective than placebo (Mindham et al. 1972), or unable to control EPS when used to replace an anticholinergic agent (McEvoy et al. 1987). The different results can be attributed to inconsistent methodologies and patient populations. The conclusion that can be drawn from these studies is that amantadine is an effective drug for treating parkinsonism, but no clear data support its use prior to using anticholinergic agents.

Most of the studies of treatment of EPS have been of short duration. In patients who have Parkinson's disease, amantadine appears to lose efficacy after several weeks (Mawdsley et al. 1972; Schwab et al. 1972). Similar studies evaluating the long-term efficacy of amantadine for EPS have not been conducted.

Amantadine has also been evaluated for the specific treatment of akathisia but in only a small number of patients. The conclusion from these studies was that amantadine is probably not effective for the specific treatment of akathisia (Fleischhacker et al. 1990).

Amantadine has FDA approval for the treatment of NIP and Parkinson's disease as well as for the treatment and prophylaxis of influenza A respiratory illness. Dosages of 100–300 mg/day are used for treatment of NIP, and plasma concentrations appear to correlate with improvement.

Side Effects and Toxicology

At 100–300 mg/day, amantadine does not produce adverse effects as readily as anticholinergic medications do. Side effects result from CNS stimulation, with symptoms including irritability, tremor, dysarthria, ataxia, vertigo, agitation, reduced concentration, hallucinations, and delirium (Postma and Tilburg 1975). Hallucinations often are visual. Side effects are more likely to occur in elderly patients and those with reduced renal function (Borison 1979; Ing et al. 1979). Toxic effects are directly related to elevated amantadine serum levels (>1.5 µg/mL). Resolution of toxic symptoms is dependent on renal clearance and may require dialysis in extreme cases, although less than 5% of amantadine is removed by dialysis.

Patients with congestive heart failure or peripheral edema should be monitored because of amantadine's ability to increase availability of catecholamines. Long-term use of amantadine may produce livedo reticularis in the lower extremities from the local release of catecholamines and resulting vasoconstriction (Cedarbaum and Schleifer 1990). Amantadine should be used with caution in patients with seizures because of possible increased seizure activity. Amantadine is embryotoxic and teratogenic in animals, but no well-controlled studies of teratogenicity have been done in women.

Drug-Drug Interactions

Amantadine has no reported interactions with other drugs. Anticholinergic side effects may be increased when amantadine is used in combination with an anticholinergic agent.

β-Adrenergic Receptor Antagonists

History and Discovery

Propranolol was reported to be effective for the treatment of restless legs syndrome (Ekbom's syndrome; Ekbom 1965), which resembles the physical movements of akathisia (Strang 1967). Later it was reported to be effective in treatment of neuroleptic-induced akathisia (Kulik and Wilbur 1983; Lipinski et al. 1983). Subsequently, other β-blockers have been investigated for treatment of akathisia (Table 10–2).

Structure-Activity Relations

Competitive β-adrenergic receptor antagonism is the property common to all β-blockers. β-Blockers are distinguished by the additional

properties of their relative affinity for β_1 and β_2 receptors (selectivity), lipid solubility, intrinsic β-adrenergic receptor *agonist* activity, blockade of α-receptors, capacity to induce vasodilation, and general pharmacokinetic properties (Hoffman and Lefkowitz 1996). β-Blockers with high lipid solubility readily cross the blood-brain barrier.

Pharmacological Profile

The major pharmacological effects of β-blockers involve the cardiovascular system. They slow the heart rate and decrease cardiac contractility, although these effects are modest in a normal heart. In the lung, they can cause bronchospasm, but, again, there is little effect in normal lungs. They block glycogenolysis, which prevents production of glucose during hypoglycemia (Hoffman and Lefkowitz 1996). They affect lipid metabolism by preventing release of free fatty acids while elevating triglyceride levels (Miller 1987). In the CNS, they produce fatigue, sleep disturbance (insomnia and nightmares), and CNS depression (Drayer 1987; Gengo et al. 1987).

Pharmacokinetics and Disposition

All β-blockers, except atenolol and nadolol, are well absorbed from the gastrointestinal tract. All are metabolized in the liver. Propranolol and metoprolol undergo significant first-pass effect with bioavailability as low as 25%. Large interindividual variation (as much as 20-fold) leads to wide variation in clinically therapeutic doses (Hoffman and Lefkowitz 1996). Metabolites appear to have limited β-receptor antagonistic activity. The degree to which a particular β-blocker enters the CNS is related directly to its lipid solubility (see Table 10–2).

Mechanism of Action

The exact mechanism of action of β-blockers in the treatment of EPS is unclear. The existence of a noradrenergic pathway from the locus coeruleus to the limbic system has been proposed as a modulator involved in symptoms of tardive

Table 10–2. β-Blockers investigated in the treatment of akathisia

Compound	Relative lipid solubility[a]	Relative potency of β-receptor blockade[b]	Bio-availability (% of dose)	Selectivity of β-receptor blockade	Effective for akathisia?	Therapeutic dosage used in studies (mg)
Propranolol (Inderal)	20.2	1	~30	$\beta_1 = \beta_2$	Yes	20–120
Betaxolol (Kerlone)	3.89	4	~80–90	β_1	Yes	5–20
Metoprolol (Lopressor)	0.98	1	~40–50	$\beta_1 > \beta_2$	Yes	~300
Pindolol (Visken)	0.82	6	~90	$\beta_1 = \beta_2$	Yes	5
Nadolol (Corgard)	0.066	2.9	~30	$\beta_1 = \beta_2$	Yes	40–80
Sotalol (Betapace)	0.039	0.3	~100	$\beta_1 = \beta_2$	No	40–80
Atenolol (Tenormin)	0.015	1	~40–50	β_1	No	50–100

[a]Relative extent to which the drug partitions between an organic solvent and an aqueous buffer; in this case, η-octanol/aqueous phosphate.
[b]Extent of inhibition of isoprenaline-induced tachycardia.
Source. Pharmacological properties from Drayer 1987; McDevitt 1987.

dyskinesia, akathisia, and tremor (Wilbur et al. 1988). Lipid solubility and the corresponding ability to enter the CNS appear to be the most important factors determining the efficacy of a β-blocker in treating akathisia and perhaps other types of EPS (Adler et al. 1991).

Indications

β-Blockers have FDA approval primarily for cardiovascular indications, and propranolol is also indicated for familial essential tremor, but there are no FDA-approved indications for the treatment of any type of EPS.

β-Blockers primarily have been studied for the treatment of akathisia. Both nonselective (β_1 and β_2 antagonism) and selective (β_1 antagonism) β-blockers have been reported to be efficacious. The studies generally have been done for short periods and have involved small numbers of patients who were often receiving varying combinations of additional antiparkinsonian agents or benzodiazepines to which β-blockers were added (Fleischhacker et al. 1990). Based on these studies, it is difficult to draw any firm conclusions, but β-blockers probably have some efficacy in the treatment of akathisia.

The maximum benefit for propranolol occurred at 5 days (Fleischhacker et al. 1990). Betaxolol may be the β-blocker of choice in patients with lung disease and smokers because of its β1 selectivity at lower dosages (5–10 mg/day).

β-Blockers have been reported to be beneficial for tremor of Parkinson's disease (Foster et al. 1984) and lithium-induced tremor (Gelenberg and Jefferson 1995) in addition to essential tremor. However, for neuroleptic-induced tremor, propranolol was no better than placebo (Metzer et al. 1993), which could indicate a difference in etiologies for the different tremors.

Side Effects and Toxicology

Side effects of β-blockers result from β-receptor blockade. β_2 blockade of bronchial smooth muscle causes bronchospasm. Individuals with normal lung function are unlikely to be affected, but smokers and patients with lung disease can develop serious breathing difficulties. β-Blockers can contribute to heart failure in susceptible individuals, such as those with compensated heart failure, acute myocardial infarction, or cardiomegaly. Abrupt cessation of β-blockers can also exacerbate coronary heart disease in susceptible patients and produce angina or, potentially, myocardial infarction (Hoffman and Lefkowitz 1996).

In individuals with normal heart function, bradycardia produced by β-blockers is insignificant. However, in patients with conduction defects or when β-blockers are combined with other drugs that impair cardiac conduction, β-blockers can contribute to serious conduction problems.

β-Blockers can block the tachycardia associated with hypoglycemia, eliminating this warning sign in diabetic patients. β_2 blockade also can inhibit glycogenolysis and glucose mobilization, interfering with recovery from hypoglycemia (Hoffman and Lefkowitz 1996).

β-Blockers can impair exercise performance and produce fatigue, insomnia, and major depression. The development of major depression probably only occurs in individuals with a predisposition to developing depression, though.

Drug-Drug Interactions

β-Blockers can have significant interactions with other drugs. Chlorpromazine in combination with propranolol may increase blood levels of both drugs. Additive effects on cardiac conduction and blood pressure may occur when β-blockers are combined with drugs with similar effects (e.g., calcium channel blockers). Phenytoin, phenobarbital, and rifampin increase the clearance of propranolol. Cimetidine increases propranolol blood levels by decreasing hepatic metabolism. Propranolol reduces theophylline clearance. Aluminum salts (antacids), cholestyramine, and colestipol may decrease absorption of β-blockers (Hoffman and Lefkowitz 1996). Plasma levels of β-blockers can be increased by coadministration of SSRIs that inhibit the cytochrome P450 2D6 isoenzyme.

BENZODIAZEPINES

History and Discovery

Diazepam was initially shown to be effective in the treatment of restless legs syndrome (Ekbom 1965). Subsequently, diazepam, lorazepam, and clonazepam were reported to be beneficial for neuroleptic-induced akathisia (Adler et al. 1985; Donlon 1973; Kutcher et al. 1987). Clonazepam has also been reported to be beneficial for drug-induced dystonia (O'Flanagan 1975).

Structure-Activity Relations

The benzodiazepines have a benzene ring fused to a seven-membered diazepine ring. All benzodiazepines promote the binding of GABA to GABA receptors, magnifying the effects of GABA. Benzodiazepines require the presence of GABA to exert their effects, unlike barbiturates, which can directly affect the GABA receptor (Hobbs et al. 1996).

Pharmacological Profile

All benzodiazepines have similar effects qualitatively but differ quantitatively. Nearly all the effects occur in the CNS, including sedation, hypnosis, decreased anxiety, anterograde amnesia, and anticonvulsant activity. Two peripheral effects are coronary vasodilatation after intravenous administration of certain benzodiazepines and neuromuscular blockade, which occurs only with very high doses (Hobbs et al. 1996).

Benzodiazepines are not general neuronal depressants, unlike barbiturates. Increasing doses produce sedation, hypnosis, and then stupor. At standard doses, benzodiazepines cause only muscle relaxation in animals but not in humans, except for clonazepam, but at only very high doses. Benzodiazepines inhibit seizures but do not stop the seizure focus. Clonazepam is a more selective anticonvulsant than most benzodiazepines, but tolerance develops to the anticonvulsant effect. All benzodiazepines decrease sleep latency, decrease rapid eye movement (REM) and Stage 4 sleep, and increase total sleep time. During chronic use, the effect on various stages of sleep usually declines. Cardiac effects are minor except in severe intoxication. No direct gastrointestinal effects are apparent (Hobbs et al. 1996).

Pharmacokinetics and Disposition

All benzodiazepines are rapidly absorbed orally, except for clorazepate, which is first decarboxylated in gastric juice and then absorbed. Benzodiazepines are characterized by their elimination half-lives as ultrashort-, short-, intermediate-, and long-acting. They are bound to protein in direct proportion to their lipid solubility.

Benzodiazepines have an initial rapid uptake into the brain, directly correlated with the degree of lipid solubility, followed by a redistribution into other organs. The duration of CNS effects is probably affected more by the rate of redistribution than by any other property (Dettli 1986). This contributes to the fact that the clinical duration of action is frequently much shorter than the half-life.

All benzodiazepines but three are extensively metabolized to produce active by-products, which generally have half-lives much longer than the parent compound. The active metabolites are generally of little therapeutic benefit and frequently are responsible for side effects and toxicity. Only temazepam, oxazepam, and lorazepam have no active metabolites and instead directly undergo glucuronic acid conjugation and then renal elimination.

Mechanism of Action

Benzodiazepines are thought to enhance GABA-induced increases in conductance of the chloride ion (Cl$^-$) at the GABA receptor, augmenting the inhibitory effects of GABAergic pathways. The mechanism of action of reduction in EPS is unknown, but it may be related to augmentation of inhibitory GABAergic effects (Hobbs et al. 1996).

Indications

Benzodiazepines have FDA approval for the treatment of anxiety disorders, agoraphobia, insomnia, and seizure disorders; the management of alcohol withdrawal; anesthetic premedication; and skeletal muscle relaxation; however, they have not been approved for any type of EPS. As noted above, a few initial reports indicated that benzodiazepines were beneficial for the treatment of akathisia. Other studies have also reported similar benefit (Bartels et al. 1987; Braude et al. 1983; Director and Muniz 1982; Gagrat et al. 1978; Horiguchi and Nishimatsu 1992; Kutcher et al. 1989; Pujalte et al. 1994).

Clonazepam has been reported to be effective in the treatment of tardive dyskinesia (Bobruff et al. 1981; Thaker et al. 1990). Doses of 1–10 mg were used in the first study; the optimal dosage was reported to be 4 mg/day, and many patients were unable to tolerate higher doses. In the second study, 2–4.5 mg/day were used, and tolerance developed after 5–8 months.

Although some of the studies were limited by short duration and small numbers of subjects who were also receiving other antiparkinsonian agents, the overall conclusion was that benzodiazepines probably have some efficacy in the treatment of akathisia and tardive dyskinesia. The potential problems associated with chronic use of benzodiazepines—tolerance and abuse—must be kept in mind, however.

Lorazepam (intermediate-acting) and clonazepam (long-acting) are the two primary benzodiazepines that have been studied in the treatment of EPS. Because clonazepam has a long duration of action, it can often be given once a day. Lorazepam has the advantage of no active metabolites, so potential side effects and toxicity are avoided.

Side Effects and Toxicology

The side effects of benzodiazepines at low doses are relatively mild. As dosages increase, benzodiazepines cause increased reaction time, motor incoordination, impairment of mental and motor function, somnolence, lethargy, confusion, and anterograde amnesia. Cognition appears to be less affected than motor performance, and patients are often unaware of these effects (Hobbs et al. 1996).

Hypnotic doses of benzodiazepines do not affect respiration in healthy adults. At higher doses, alveolar respiration is suppressed from depression of the hypoxic drive, which is exaggerated in patients with chronic obstructive pulmonary disease. Benzodiazepines can cause apnea when given with anesthesia or opiates. Apnea can also occur when benzodiazepine intoxication occurs in combination with another CNS depressant, such as alcohol (Hobbs et al. 1996).

Dizziness, ataxia, vomiting, and slurred speech have also been reported (Bobruff et al. 1981). The incidence of side effects increases with age (Meyer 1982; Monane 1992).

Benzodiazepine withdrawal is a potential serious occurrence, with symptoms generally beginning 1–3 days after the last dose. Symptoms are similar to those of acute alcohol withdrawal and include anxiety, tremulousness, autonomic irregularities (including blood pressure and heart rate fluctuations), gastrointestinal symptoms, agitation, hallucinations (particularly visual), delirium, and seizures. Withdrawal seizures can occur without the appearance of any other significant withdrawal symptoms. Withdrawal symptoms are more likely to occur with higher doses, although we have witnessed grand mal seizures and acute persecutory delusions following withdrawal of daily doses of only 1–2 mg of clonazepam.

Although not an actual side effect, benzodiazepine abuse should always be considered, particularly in patients with a history of abuse of drugs and other medications.

Drug-Drug Interactions

Benzodiazepines produce increased CNS depression when administered with other CNS depressants, but otherwise there are few known drug interactions. Because many benzodiazepines are metabolized by the cytochrome P450 3A4 isoenzyme, drugs that inhibit this enzyme, such as nefazodone, will increase plasma levels of benzodiazepines.

BOTULINUM TOXIN

History and Discovery

Botulinum toxin, produced by *Clostridium botulinum*, causes botulism when ingested. The first clinical use of the toxin was to treat childhood strabismus (Scott 1980). The first focal dystonia treated was blepharospasm (Elston 1988). Since then, botulinum toxin has been used to treat several other conditions associated with excessive muscle activity, including neuroleptic-induced dystonias (Hughes 1994).

Structure-Activity Relations

There are seven immunologically distinct botulinum toxins (L. L. Simpson 1981). Type A is the primary type used clinically (Hambleton 1992). Type F and possibly B also have clinical utility but have much shorter durations of action—3 weeks or fewer compared with 3 months or more (Borodic et al. 1996). The toxin is quantified by bioassay, expressed as mouse units, which refers to the dose that is lethal to 50% of animals following intraperitoneal injection (Quinn and Hallet 1989).

Pharmacological Profile

Botulinum toxin binds to cholinergic motor nerve terminals, preventing release of acetylcholine and producing a functionally denervated muscle. The prevention of acetylcholine release occurs within a few hours, but the clinical effect does not occur for 1–3 days. The innervation gradually becomes restored, although the number or size of active muscle fibers is reduced (Odergren et al. 1994).

Pharmacokinetics and Disposition

After binding to the presynaptic nerve terminal, the toxin is taken into the nerve cell and metabolized. When antibodies are present, the toxin is metabolized by immunological processes.

Mechanism of Action

Botulinum toxin acts presynaptically to block the release of acetylcholine at the neuromuscular junction. This produces a functional chemical denervation and paralysis of the muscle. Clinical use of the toxin aims to reduce the excessive muscle activity without producing significant weakness (Hughes 1994).

Indications

The FDA has approved the use of botulinum toxin for strabismus, blepharospasm, and other facial nerve disorders (Jankovic and Brin 1991). Botulinum toxin has also been used to treat focal neuroleptic-induced dystonias that may occur as part of tardive dyskinesia, including laryngeal dystonia (Blitzer and Brin 1991) and refractory torticollis (Kaufman 1994). For laryngeal dystonia, toxin is injected percutaneously through the cricothyroid membrane into the thyroarytenoid muscle bilaterally. Eighty percent to 90% of patients respond, and the effect lasts 3–4 months and sometimes longer.

Side Effects and Toxicology

The major potential side effect is focal weakness in the muscle group injected, which is usually dose dependent. This effect generally is temporary, given the mechanism of action. Transient weakness can occur through diffusion of the toxin into surrounding noninjected muscles (Hughes 1994).

Antibodies to the toxin can develop, which can prevent a therapeutic response, particularly during subsequent treatments. The two main factors that apparently contribute to the development of antibodies are an early age at first receiving toxin and total cumulative dose (Jankovic and Schwartz 1995). Some patients with antibodies will respond to other botulin serotypes, such as type F (Greene and Fahn 1993). Local skin reactions can also occur. Some degree of muscle atrophy can occur in injected muscles (Hughes 1994). Reinnervation usually takes place over 3–4 months (Odergren et al. 1994).

No contraindications are known. The effect on the fetus is unknown, so its use is not recommended during pregnancy. When neuromuscular junction disorders, such as myasthenia gravis, are present, patients could theoretically experience increased weakness. The long-term effects are unknown (Hughes 1994).

Drug-Drug Interactions

Botulinum toxin has no reported interactions with other drugs.

TREATMENT OF EXTRAPYRAMIDAL SIDE EFFECTS

Treatment of Acute Dystonic Reactions

Intramuscular anticholinergics are the treatment of choice for ADRs. Benztropine (2 mg) or diphenhydramine (50–100 mg) generally will produce complete resolution within 20–30 minutes. The dose should be repeated after 30 minutes if complete recovery does not occur. Starting a standing dose of an antiparkinsonian agent afterward is generally not necessary. ADRs do not recur unless large doses of high-potency antipsychotics are being used or the dose is increased. Prophylaxis is discussed more completely later in this chapter (see section, "Prophylaxis of EPS").

Treatment of Akathisia and Parkinsonism

The initial treatment of akathisia and parkinsonism (referred to here as EPS) is identical—evaluating the dose and type of antipsychotic (Table 10–3). An increase in dose beyond the neuroleptic threshold will *not* produce any greater therapeutic benefit but will increase EPS (Angus and Simpson 1970a; Baldessarini et al. 1988; McEvoy et al. 1991). Studies have found that EPS frequently can be eliminated with a reduction in dose or change to a lower-potency antipsychotic (Braude et al. 1983; Stratas et al. 1963).

If the steps listed above do not resolve EPS or cannot be accomplished, the addition of an anticholinergic drug would be the next step. Maximum therapeutic response occurs in 3–10 days; more severe EPS take a longer time to respond (DiMascio et al. 1976; Fann and Lake 1976). The anticholinergic dose should be increased until EPS are alleviated or an unacceptable degree of anticholinergic side effects is obtained.

Akathisia frequently does not respond as well to anticholinergic medications as do parkinsonism and ADRs (DiMascio et al. 1976).

Table 10–3.   **Treatment of akathisia and parkinsonism**

Step	Action
1	Reduce dose of antipsychotic, if clinically possible
2	Substitute lower-potency antipsychotic
3	Add anticholinergic agent
4	Titrate anticholinergic to maximum dose tolerable
5	Add amantadine in combination with anticholinergic or substitute as a single agent
6	Add benzodiazepine or β-blocker
7	In cases of severe extrapyramidal side effects, stop antipsychotic temporarily and repeat process, beginning with Step 3
8	Substitute antipsychotic with clozapine or another atypical antipsychotic

Akathisia is more likely to respond if symptoms of parkinsonism are also present (Fleischhacker et al. 1990).

If EPS remain uncontrolled, amantadine can be either added to the regimen or substituted as a single agent. The next step would be the addition of a benzodiazepine or a β-blocker, although fewer data support both of these treatments.

In cases of severe EPS, the antipsychotic should be stopped temporarily because severe EPS may be a risk factor for development of neuroleptic malignant syndrome (Levinson and Simpson 1986).

For patients who have severe, refractory EPS that have not responded to standard treatments, the use of clozapine specifically to treat the EPS is indicated (Casey 1989). This can even be true for patients who do not have any psychotic symptoms, if the EPS are judged to be severe enough to be disabling or potentially life-threatening, such as a laryngeal dystonia (laryngospasm).

Olanzapine, quetiapine, ziprasidone, and risperidone are also less likely to produce EPS than are typical antipsychotics. Their use in the prevention and treatment of EPS is discussed later in this chapter (see section, "Atypical Antipsychotics").

Treatment of Tardive Dyskinesia

Historically, tardive dyskinesia has been refractory to treatment, which helps explain the large number of drugs that have been used in attempts to alleviate the condition. Treatments investigated have included, but are not limited to, noradrenergic receptor antagonists (propranolol, clonidine), dopamine antagonists, dopaminergic agonists, catecholamine-depleting drugs (reserpine, tetrabenazine), GABAergic drugs, cholinergic drugs (deanol, choline, lecithin), catecholaminergic drugs (Kane et al. 1992), calcium channel blockers (Cates et al. 1993), and selective monoamine oxidase inhibitors (selegiline; Goff et al. 1993). Based on the investigations of the above drugs, the American Psychiatric Association Task Force on Tardive Dyskinesia concluded that no consistently effective treatment for tardive dyskinesia was available (Kane et al. 1992).

The variability of clinical raters (Bergen et al. 1984), the placebo response of patients (Sommer et al. 1994), and the diurnal and longitudinal variability of tardive dyskinesia (Hyde et al. 1995; Stanilla et al. 1996) contribute to difficulty in evaluating the effects of any treatment of tardive dyskinesia. The degree of improvement would need to be greater than the sum of the above variations to show an actual benefit.

Several drugs have been shown or have been suggested to have some benefit for treatment of tardive dyskinesia, although most have limitations. These drugs include botulinum toxin, clonazepam, vitamin E, and clozapine. Other atypical antipsychotics may also have a benefit in the prevention and treatment of tardive dyskinesia and are discussed below.

Botulinum toxin is beneficial for treating specific tardive dystonias, and laryngeal dystonia is probably the one that is most commonly associated with tardive dyskinesia (Hughes 1994). The injections must be repeated every 3–6 months, and botulinum toxin is not a general treatment for all movements of tardive dyskinesia.

Clonazepam was reported to reduce the movements of tardive dyskinesia for up to 9 months, although tolerance developed to the benefits. Thaker et al. (1990) reported that when the drug was weaned and stopped for 2 weeks and then resumed, the benefits returned. Potential limitations are the inherent problems associated with chronic use of a benzodiazepine.

Vitamin E was proposed as a treatment for tardive dyskinesia after it was noted that a neurotoxin in rats induced an irreversible movement disorder and axonal damage similar to that caused by vitamin E deficiency. Investigators proposed that chronic antipsychotic use might produce free radicals, which would contribute

to neurological damage and tardive dyskinesia, and that the antioxidant effect of vitamin E could attenuate the damage (Cadet et al. 1986).

Studies of vitamin E treatment of tardive dyskinesia have reported a range of results from general benefit (Adler et al. 1993; Dabiri et al. 1994; Lohr et al. 1988), to benefit only in subjects with tardive dyskinesia of less than 5 years (Egan et al. 1992; Lohr and Caligiuri 1996), to no benefit (Schmidt et al. 1991; Shriqui et al. 1992). Although definite conclusions regarding the efficacy of vitamin E in the treatment of tardive dyskinesia cannot yet be drawn, a recently completed long-term, randomized trial of vitamin E versus placebo demonstrated no evidence for such efficacy (Adler et al. 1999).

Clozapine decreases symptoms of tardive dyskinesia (G. M. Simpson et al. 1978), with the greatest reduction occurring in cases of severe tardive dyskinesia and tardive dystonia (Lieberman et al. 1991). Unlike studies of the other drugs described above, these findings have been replicated in large studies and suggest that clozapine does not cause tardive dyskinesia (Chengappa et al. 1994; Kane et al. 1993). The disadvantages of clozapine are the potential side effects of agranulocytosis and seizures and the need for blood monitoring every 2 weeks.

Three possible mechanisms for clozapine's benefit have been proposed. First, clozapine may suppress the tardive dyskinesia movements in a fashion similar to that of typical antipsychotics. Second, tardive dyskinesia may improve spontaneously because the typical antipsychotics are no longer present to cause or sustain tardive dyskinesia. This result occurs in a percentage of patients when antipsychotics are withdrawn. Third, clozapine may have an active therapeutic effect on tardive dyskinesia (Lieberman et al. 1991). This issue remains to be clarified. In some patients, tardive dyskinesia movements have recurred on withdrawal of clozapine, but long-term follow-up studies have not been reported.

Based on the above information, clozapine is the only drug that could be considered a definite treatment of tardive dyskinesia, with the potential for complete resolution. Before changing to clozapine for the purpose of treating tardive dyskinesia, however, a trial of clonazepam, risperidone, quetiapine, ziprasidone, or olanzapine should be considered, keeping in mind that the current data regarding their benefit in tardive dyskinesia are limited or inconsistent.

Atypical Antipsychotics

Risperidone has an antipsychotic effect at doses that do not produce parkinsonism. Unlike clozapine, though, higher doses are associated with EPS (Chouinard et al. 1993).

The mean changes in the Extrapyramidal Symptom Rating Scale (ESRS) scores from baseline to worst score were significantly lower for all doses of risperidone (2–16 mg/day) than for haloperidol (20 mg/day). At 6 mg/day, there was no difference in the mean change score between risperidone and placebo. There was a linear relationship between the mean change scores and the dose of risperidone on 4 of 12 ESRS scores and between the dose of risperidone and the use of antiparkinsonian medication. Both risperidone and haloperidol caused acute dystonic reactions. Patients with severe EPS at baseline were more likely to develop EPS while taking risperidone (Simpson and Lindermayer 1997).

Fewer data are available regarding risperidone's production of akathisia or effect on tardive dyskinesia. One study found that the occurrence of akathisia was the same for risperidone as it was for haloperidol (Marder and Meibach 1994). There have been anecdotal reports of risperidone's improvement of tardive dyskinesia in some patients, but controlled data regarding its effectiveness in the treatment of tardive dyskinesia are limited (Chouinard 1995; Meco et al. 1989).

Olanzapine, a thienobenzodiazepine with pharmacological properties of an "atypical" antipsychotic, has been shown to have antipsychotic effects comparable to those of haloperidol while producing less dystonia,

parkinsonism, and akathisia (Beasley et al. 1996; Tollefson et al. 1997a). The reduction in EPS occurred across the entire therapeutic range of 5–24 mg/day.

A prospective study of patients treated with olanzapine for up to 3 years found a statistically significant lower incidence of newly emergent tardive dyskinesia in olanzapine-treated patients than in haloperidol-treated patients (Tollefson et al. 1997b).

Quetiapine, a dibenzothiazepine derivative and a structural analogue of clozapine, has antipsychotic activity comparable to that of haloperidol at dosages ranging from 150 to 750 mg/day (Arvanitis et al. 1997; Small et al. 1997). The incidence of parkinsonism was similar to that of placebo across the entire dose range. For most patients, no significant changes were found in Abnormal Involuntary Movement Scale (AIMS; Guy 1976) scores at baseline and at the end of a 6-week period of treatment.

Prophylaxis of EPS

Prophylactic use of antiparkinsonian agents to prevent EPS is a common, but not completely accepted, practice. Most controlled prospective studies of prophylactic use of antiparkinsonian medication have shown that prophylaxis can be beneficial for certain high-risk patients, but it is *not* beneficial in routine use across all patient groups (Hanlon et al. 1966; Sramek et al. 1986). Studies that have shown a general benefit across all groups have involved the use of very high doses of antipsychotics. Several retrospective studies have also found that there is a limited need for prophylaxis of EPS (Swett et al. 1977). Those retrospective studies that have shown a greater benefit from prophylaxis have also involved the use of high antipsychotic doses (Keepers et al. 1983; Stern and Anderson 1979). The prophylactic use of antiparkinsonian medication is not routinely indicated for all patients but should be reserved for those patients at high risk for developing ADRs.

The risk factors for developing ADRs (Table

10–4) include higher potency of antipsychotic, higher doses of antipsychotic, younger age (under 35 years), intramuscular route of delivery, a history of ADRs from a similar antipsychotic (Keepers and Casey 1991), and (possibly) male gender (Sramek et al. 1986).

Dosages that have been used for prophylaxis are 1–4 mg/day for benztropine, 5–15 mg/day for trihexyphenidyl, and 75–150 mg/day for diphenhydramine, though the dose required to achieve prophylaxis for an individual is highly variable and can only be determined by trial and error (Moleman et al. 1982; Sramek et al. 1986). Serious anticholinergic side effects, such as acute urinary retention or paralytic ileus, can occur even in a young patient, so high doses of anticholinergics should not be used with impunity, even for brief periods.

Prophylactic anticholinergics for ADRs need to be used only for a limited time because 85%–90% of ADRs occur within the first 4 days of treatment, and the incidence drops to nearly 0% after 10 days (Keepers et al. 1983; Singh et al. 1990; Sramek et al. 1986). After this time, anticholinergics can be weaned slowly while the patient is being observed for development of parkinsonism or akathisia.

Depot Antipsychotics

In patients receiving depot antipsychotics, prophylactic anticholinergics need to be used only

Table 10–4. Risk factors leading to acute dystonic reactions

High-potency antipsychotics
  Haloperidol
  Fluphenazine
  Trifluoperazine
High doses
Younger age (under age 35)
  Approaches 100% under age 20
Intramuscular route of delivery
Previous dystonic reaction to similar
  neuroleptic and dose
Male gender

in patients at high risk for developing ADRs (Idzorek 1976). The onset and characterization of EPS may be different, however, including more bizarre dystonic reactions (G. M. Simpson 1970). The buildup of serum antipsychotic drug levels with depot antipsychotic medications can lead to the onset of EPS at later stages of treatment, so that ongoing evaluation is necessary. Some patients receiving fluphenazine decanoate experienced EPS only between days 3 and 10 following injection (McClelland et al. 1974).

Duration of Treatment

Withdrawal Studies

Studies investigating the withdrawal of antiparkinsonian agents have reported that not all subjects redevelop EPS, a serendipitous finding noted when only 20% of patients withdrawn from benztropine in preparation for a trial of a new antiparkinsonian agent developed recurrent parkinsonian symptoms. This finding led to the suggestion that antiparkinsonian agents should be withdrawn after 2 months and their use resumed only in those patients who redevelop EPS (Cahan and Parrish 1960).

Other subsequent withdrawal studies reported wide-ranging rates of EPS recurrence. Differences in rates of recurrence are related to the varied methodologies used in the studies, including methods of rating, and the initial reason for treatment with anticholinergics—prophylaxis or active treatment (Ananth et al. 1970). The types, dosages, and combinations of antipsychotics used have also been major factors determining recurrence rates—the same factors that contribute to the initial development of EPS (Baker et al. 1983; McClelland et al. 1974).

The conclusion that can be drawn from the withdrawal studies is that patients are more likely to develop EPS on withdrawal of antiparkinsonian agents if the risk factors for developing EPS are present. If these risk factors are minimized, the rate of EPS recurrence is lowered.

In patients who develop recurrence, EPS generally reappear within 2 weeks, and control is easily reestablished (Klett and Caffey 1972). Patients respond rapidly and often require smaller doses of antiparkinsonian medications for control while taking the same dose of antipsychotic (McClelland et al. 1974).

Withdrawal Syndrome

Almost all anticholinergic withdrawal studies have involved abrupt withdrawal of the anticholinergic medications. In only one study was the withdrawal of anticholinergic agents gradual, but the use of high antipsychotic doses and combinations of antipsychotics makes it difficult to analyze the data from this study (Manos et al. 1981).

Specific studies to evaluate the effect of cholinergic sensitization by anticholinergic agents on the development of EPS after withdrawal of the anticholinergic agent have not been done. Evidence indicates that sensitization can take place and can contribute to EPS and other symptoms. Some patients with no EPS before treatment with anticholinergics did develop EPS on withdrawal of the anticholinergics (Klett and Caffey 1972). Withdrawal symptoms of nausea, vomiting, diaphoresis, sebaceous secretion, and restlessness may occur following withdrawal of any psychotropic drug with anticholinergic properties (Luchins et al. 1980). These symptoms are most likely caused by cholinergic rebound and perhaps sensitization following removal of the cholinergic blockade of the drug (G. M. Simpson et al. 1965). Abrupt clozapine withdrawal can produce agitation, delirium, and severe choreoathetoid movements, which are also probably the result of cholinergic rebound related to clozapine's very high antimuscarinic activity (Stanilla et al. 1997).

The potential for cholinergic sensitization with use of anticholinergic agents is significant because EPS following withdrawal may be severe initially but also may diminish over time without treatment. Potential cholinergic sensitization leading to subsequent EPS would be a reason to limit the routine use of prophylactic anticholinergic agents.

It needs to be emphasized that antiparkinsonian agents should be withdrawn slowly and gradually over weeks or months, not abruptly as has been done in the reported studies. Patients should be evaluated for recurrence of EPS following a partial dose reduction of the antiparkinsonian agent. This process should be continued until the antiparkinsonian agent is completely withdrawn or the lowest dose for maintenance control is achieved.

CONCLUSION

The unique properties of chlorpromazine and other similarly active agents to ameliorate psychotic symptoms and to produce parkinsonian-like side effects were described in the early 1950s by French psychiatrists. The recognition of the benefits of reducing parkinsonian side effects led to investigations of methods to reduce EPS. It appears that prophylactic antiparkinsonian agents need to be used in some situations but probably less frequently and for briefer periods than has generally been the practice. The trend toward the use of lower dosages of antipsychotics should also lead to decreased need for use of antiparkinsonian agents. Finally, the advent of atypical antipsychotic agents has opened a new chapter in both the treatment and the prevention of EPS and suggests that, in the future, EPS will be less of a problem than they have been in the past.

A summary of an American Psychiatric Association Task Force report on tardive dyskinesia suggested that "[a] deliberate and sustained effort must be made to maintain patients on the lowest effective amount of drug and to keep the treatment regimen as simple as possible" (Baldessarini et al. 1980, p. 1168) and to discontinue anticholinergic drugs as soon as possible. Apart from a greater emphasis on avoiding the initial use of antiparkinsonian agents, this statement remains valid.

REFERENCES

Adler L, Angrist B, Peselow E, et al: Efficacy of propranolol in neuroleptic-induced akathisia. J Clin Psychopharmacol 5:164–166, 1985

Adler LA, Angrist B, Weinreb H, et al: Studies on the time course and efficacy of β-blockers in neuroleptic-induced akathisia and the akathisia of idiopathic Parkinson's disease. Psychopharmacol Bull 27:107–111, 1991

Adler LA, Peselow E, Rotrosen J, et al: Vitamin E treatment of tardive dyskinesia. Am J Psychiatry 150:1405–1407, 1993

Adler LA, Rotrosen J, Edson R, et al: Vitamin E treatment for tardive dyskinesia. Arch Gen Psychiatry 56:836–841, 1999

Ananth JV, Horodesky S, Lehmann HE, et al: Effect of withdrawal of antiparkinsonian medication on chronically hospitalized psychiatric patients. Laval Médical 41:934–938, 1970

Angus JWS, Simpson GM: Handwriting changes and response to drugs—a controlled study. Acta Psychiatr Scand Suppl 21:28–37, 1970a

Angus JWS, Simpson GM: Hysteria and drug-induced dystonia. Acta Psychiatr Scand Suppl 21:52–58, 1970b

Aoki FY, Sitar DS, Ogilvie RI: Amantadine kinetics in healthy young subjects after long-term dosing. Clin Pharmacol Ther 26:729–736, 1979

Arvanitis LA, Miller BG, and the Seroquel Trial 13 Study Group: Multiple fixed doses of "Seroquel" (quetiapine) in patients with acute exacerbation of schizophrenia: a comparison with haloperidol and placebo. Biol Psychiatry 42:233–246, 1997

Ayd FJ: A survey of drug-induced extrapyramidal reactions. JAMA 175:1054–1060, 1961

Babe KS, Serafin WE: Histamine, bradykinin, and their antagonists, in Goodman and Gilman's The Pharmacological Basis of Therapeutics, 9th Edition. Edited by Hardman JG, Limbird LE, Molinoff PB, et al. New York, McGraw-Hill, 1996, pp 581–600

Baker LA, Cheng LY, Amara IB: The withdrawal of benztropine mesylate in chronic schizophrenic patients. Br J Psychiatry 143:584–590, 1983

Baldessarini RJ, Cole JO, Davis JM, et al: Tardive dyskinesia: summary of a task force report of the American Psychiatric Association. Am J Psychiatry 137:1163–1172, 1980

Baldessarini RJ, Cohen BM, Teicher MH: Significance of neuroleptic dose and plasma level in the pharmacological treatment of psychoses. Arch Gen Psychiatry 45:79–91, 1988

Barnes TR: Movement disorder associated with antipsychotic drugs: the tardive syndromes. International Review of Psychiatry 2:355–366, 1990

Bartels M, Heide K, Mann K, et al: Treatment of akathisia with lorazepam: an open clinical trial. Pharmacopsychiatry 20:51–53, 1987

Beasley CM Jr, Tollefson G, Tran P, et al: Olanzapine versus placebo and haloperidol: acute phase results of the North American double-blind olanzapine trial. Neuropsychopharmacology 14:111–123, 1996

Bergen JA, Griffiths DA, Rey JM, et al: Tardive dyskinesia: fluctuating patient or fluctuating rater. Br J Psychiatry 144:498–502, 1984

Blitzer A, Brin MF: Laryngeal dystonia: a series with botulinum toxin therapy. Ann Otol Rhinol Laryngol 100:85–89, 1991

Bobruff A, Gardos G, Tarsy D, et al: Clonazepam and phenobarbital in tardive dyskinesia. Am J Psychiatry 138:189–193, 1981

Borison RL: Amantadine-induced psychosis in a geriatric patient with renal disease. Am J Psychiatry 136:111–112, 1979

Borodic G, Johnson E, Goodnough M, et al: Botulinum toxin therapy, immunologic resistance, and problems with available materials. Neurology 46:26–29, 1996

Boumans CE, de Mooij KJ, Koch PA, et al: Is the social acceptability of psychiatric patients decreased by orofacial dyskinesia. Schizophr Bull 20:339–344, 1994

Bovet D: Introduction to antihistamine agents and antergan derivatives. Ann N Y Acad Sci 50:1089–1126, 1950

Braude WM, Barnes TR, Gore SM: Clinical characteristics of akathisia: a systematic investigation of acute psychiatric inpatient admissions. Br J Psychiatry 143:139–150, 1983

Brooks GW: Experience with use of chlor-promazine and reserpine in psychiatry with special reference to the significance and management of extrapyramidal dysfunction. N Engl J Med 254:1119–1123, 1956

Brown JH: Atropine, scopolamine, and related antimuscarinic drugs, in Goodman and Gilman's The Pharmacological Basis of Therapeutics, 8th Edition. Edited by Gilman AG, Rall TW, Nies AS, et al. New York, Pergamon, 1990, pp 150–165

Brown JH, Taylor P: Muscarinic receptor agonists and antagonists, in Goodman and Gilman's The Pharmacological Basis of Therapeutics, 9th Edition. Edited by Hardman JG, Limbird LE, Molinoff PB, et al. New York, McGraw-Hill, 1996, pp 141–160

Cadet JL, Lohr J, Jeste D: Free radicals and tardive dyskinesia (letter). Trends Neurosci 9:107–108, 1986

Cahan RB, Parrish DD: Reversibility of drug-induced parkinsonism. Am J Psychiatry 116:1022–1023, 1960

Casey DE: Clozapine: neuroleptic-induced EPS and tardive dyskinesia. Psychopharmacology (Berl) 99:S47–S53, 1989

Casey DE, Gerlach J, Christensson E: Dopamine, acetylcholine, and GABA effects in acute dystonia in primates. Psychopharmacologia 70:83–87, 1980

Cates M, Lusk K, Wells BG: Are calcium-channel blockers effective in the treatment of tardive dyskinesia? Ann Pharmacother 27:191–196, 1993

Cedarbaum JM, McDowell FH: Sixteen-year follow-up of 100 patients begun on levodopa in 1968: emerging problems, in Advances in Neurology, Vol 45: Parkinson's Disease. Edited by Yahr MD, Bergmann KJ. New York, Raven, 1987, pp 469–472

Cedarbaum JM, Schleifer LS: Drugs for Parkinson's disease, spasticity, and acute muscle spasms, in Goodman and Gilman's The Pharmacological Basis of Therapeutics, 8th Edition. Edited by Gilman AG, Rall TW, Nies AS, et al. New York, Pergamon, 1990, pp 463–484

Chengappa KN, Shelton MD, Baker RW, et al: The prevalence of akathisia in patients receiving stable doses of clozapine. J Clin Psychiatry 55:142–145, 1994

Chouinard G: Effects of risperidone in tardive dyskinesia: an analysis of the Canadian multicenter risperidone study. J Clin Psychopharmacol 15 (suppl):36S–44S, 1995

Chouinard G, Jones B, Remington G, et al: A Canadian multicenter placebo-controlled study of fixed doses of risperidone and haloperidol in the treatment of chronic schizophrenic patients (published erratum appears in J Clin Psychopharmacol 13:149, 1993). J Clin Psychopharmacol 13:25–40, 1993

Côté L, Crutcher MD: The basal ganglia, in Principles of Neural Science, 3rd Edition. Edited by Kandel ER, Schwartz JH, Jessell TM. New York, Elsevier, 1991, pp 647–659

Dabiri LM, Pasta D, Darby JK, et al: Effectiveness of vitamin E for treatment of long-term tardive dyskinesia. Am J Psychiatry 151:925–926, 1994

Delay J, Deniker P: Trente-huit cas de psychoses traitées par la cure prolongée et continue de 4560 RP. Léme Congrès des Alién. et Neurol de Langue Française, Luxembourg, 21–27 juillet 1952 [Thirty-eight cases of psychoses treated with a long and continued course of 4560 RP. The Congress of the French Language for Alienists and Neurologists, Luxembourg, 21–27 July 1952]. Paris, Masson et Cie, 1952, pp 503–513

Delay J, Deniker P, Harl JM: Traitement des états d'excitation et d'agitation par une méthode médicamenteuse dérivée de l'hibernothérapie [Therapeutic method derived from hibernotherapy in excitation and agitation states]. Annales Medico-Psychologiques (Paris) 110:267–273, 1952

de Leon J, Canuso C, White AO, et al: A pilot effort to determine benztropine equivalents of anticholinergic medications. Hosp Community Psychiatry 45:606–607, 1994

Dettli L: Benzodiazepines in the treatment of sleep disorders: pharmacokinetic aspects. Acta Psychiatr Scand Suppl 332:9–19, 1986

DiMascio A, Bernardo DL, Greenblatt DJ, et al: A controlled trial of amantadine in drug-induced extrapyramidal disorders. Arch Gen Psychiatry 33:599–602, 1976

Director KL, Muniz CE: Diazepam in the treatment of extrapyramidal symptoms: a case report. J Clin Psychiatry 43:160–161, 1982

Donlon PT: The therapeutic use of diazepam for akathisia. Psychosomatics 14:222–225, 1973

Doshay LJ: Five-year study of benztropine (Cogentin) methanesulfonate: outcome in three hundred two cases of paralysis agitans. JAMA 162:1031–1034, 1956

Doshay LJ, Constable K, Zier A: Five year follow-up of treatment with trihexyphenidyl (Artane): outcome in four hundred and eleven cases of paralysis agitans. JAMA 154:1334–1336, 1954

Drachman DA: Memory and cognitive function in man: does the cholinergic system have a specific role? Neurology 27:783–790, 1977

Drayer DE: Lipophilicity, hydrophilicity, and the central nervous system side effects of beta blocker. Pharmacotherapy 7:87–91, 1987

Egan MF, Hyde TM, Albers GW, et al: Treatment of tardive dyskinesia with vitamin E. Am J Psychiatry 149:773–777, 1992

Ekbom KA: Restless legs. Swedish Medical Journal 62: 2376–2378, 1965

Elston J: Botulinum toxin treatment of blepharospasm. Adv Neurol 50:579–581, 1988

England AC Jr, Schwab RS: Treatment in internal medicine: the management of Parkinson's disease. AMA Archives of Internal Medicine 104:439–468, 1959

Fann WE, Lake CR: Amantadine versus trihexyphenidyl in the treatment of neuroleptic-induced parkinsonism. Am J Psychiatry 133:940–943, 1976

Fayen M, Goldman MB, Moulthrop MA, et al: Differential memory function with dopaminergic versus anticholinergic treatment of drug-induced extrapyramidal symptoms. Am J Psychiatry 145:483–486, 1988

Feve A, Angelard B, Lacau St Guily J: Laryngeal tardive dyskinesia. J Neurol 242:455–459, 1995

Fleischhacker WW, Roth SD, Kane JM: The pharmacologic treatment of neuroleptic-induced akathisia. J Clin Psychopharmacol 10:12–21, 1990

Flügel F: Neue klinische Beobachtungen zur Wirkung des Phenothiazinkorpers Megaphen auf psychische Krankheitsbidler [Clinical observations on the effect of the phenothiazine derivative megaphen on psychic disorders in children]. Med Klin 48:1027–1029, 1953

Foster NL, Newman RP, LeWitt, et al: Peripheral beta-adrenergic blockade treatment of parkinsonian tremor. Ann Neurol 16:505–508, 1984

Freyhan FA: Therapeutic implications of differential effects of new phenothiazine compounds. Am J Psychiatry 115:577–585, 1959

Gagrat D, Hamilton J, Belmaker RH: Intravenous diazepam in the treatment of neuroleptic-induced acute dystonia and akathisia. Am J Psychiatry 135:1232–1233, 1978

Gelenberg AJ: Amantadine in the treatment of benztropine-refractory extrapyramidal disorders induced by antipsychotic drugs. Current Therapeutic Research, Clinical and Experimental 23:375–380, 1978

Gelenberg AJ, Jefferson JW: Lithium tremor. J Clin Psychiatry 56:283–287, 1995

Gengo FM, Huntoon L, McHugh WB: Lipid-soluble and water-soluble beta-blockers: comparison of the central nervous system depressant effect. Arch Intern Med 147:39–43, 1987

Gerlach J, Korsgaard S, Clemmesen P, et al: The St. Hans Rating Scale for Extrapyramidal Syndromes: reliability and validity. Acta Psychiatr Scand 87:244–252, 1993

Goff DC, Renshaw PF, Sarid-Segal O, et al: A placebo-controlled trial of selegiline (L-deprenyl) in the treatment of tardive dyskinesia. Biol Psychiatry 33:700–706, 1993

Greenblatt DJ, DiMascio A, Harmatz JS, et al: Pharmacokinetics and clinical effects of amantadine in drug-induced extrapyramidal symptoms. J Clin Pharmacol 17:704–708, 1977

Greene PE, Fahn S: Use of botulinum toxin type F injections to treat torticollis in patients with immunity to botulinum toxin type A. Mov Disord 8:479–483, 1993

Grelak RP, Clark R, Stump JM, et al: Amantadine-dopamine interaction: possible mode of action in parkinsonism. Science 169:203–204, 1970

Guy W: ECDEU Assessment Manual for Psychopharmacology, Revised Edition. Washington, DC, U.S. Department of Health, Education and Welfare, 1976

Haase HJ: Über Vorkommen und Deutung des psychomotorischen Parkinson-symdroms bei Megaphen-bzw, Largactil Dauer-behandlung [The presentation and meaning of the psychomotor Parkinson syndrome during long-term treatment with megaphen, also known as Largactil]. Nervenarzt 25:486–492, 1954

Haase HJ, Janssen PAJ: The Action of Neuroleptic Drugs. Chicago, IL, Year Book, 1965

Hambleton P: Clostridium botulinum toxins: a general review of involvement in disease, structure, mode of action and preparation for clinical use. J Neurol 239:16–20, 1992

Hanlon TE, Schoenrich C, Freinek W, et al: Perphenazine-benztropine mesylate treatment of newly admitted psychiatric patients. Psychopharmacologia 9:328–339, 1966

Hay AJ: The action of amantadine against influenza A viruses: inhibition of the M2 ion channel protein. Seminars in Virology 3:21–30, 1992

Hayden FG, Minocha A, Spyker DA, et al: Comparative single-dose pharmacokinetics of amantadine hydrochloride and rimantadine hydrochloride in young and elderly adults. Antimicrob Agents Chemother 28:216–221, 1985

Hippius H: The history of clozapine. Psychopharmacology (Berl) 99 (suppl):S3–S5, 1989

Hobbs WR, Rall TW, Verdoorn TA: Hypnotics and sedatives; ethanol, in Goodman and Gilman's The Pharmacological Basis of Therapeutics, 9th Edition. Edited by Hardman JG, Limbird LE, Molinoff PB, et al. New York, McGraw-Hill, 1996, pp 361–396

Hoffman BB, Lefkowitz RJ: Catecholamines, sympathomimetic drugs, and adrenergic receptor antagonists, in Goodman and Gilman's The Pharmacological Basis of Therapeutics, 9th Edition. Edited by Hardman JG, Limbird LE, Molinoff PB, et al. New York, McGraw-Hill, 1996, pp 199–248

Horiguchi J, Nishimatsu O: Usefulness of antiparkinsonian drugs during neuroleptic treatment and the effect of clonazepam on akathisia and parkinsonism occurred after antiparkinsonian drug withdrawal: a double-blind study. Jpn J Psychiatry Neurol 46: 733–739, 1992

Hughes AJ: Botulinum toxin in clinical practice. Drugs 48:888–893, 1994

Hyde TM, Egan MF, Brown RJ, et al: Diurnal variation in tardive dyskinesia. Psychiatry Res 56: 53–57, 1995

Idzorek S: Antiparkinsonian agents and fluphenazine decanoate. Am J Psychiatry 133:80–82, 1976

Ing TS, Daugirdas JT, Soung LS, et al: Toxic effects of amantadine in patients with renal failure. Can Med Assoc J 120: 695–698, 1979

Jankovic J, Brin MF: Therapeutic uses of botulinum toxin. N Engl J Med 324:1186–1194, 1991

Jankovic J, Schwartz K: Response and immunoresistance to botulinum toxin injections. Neurology 45:1743–1746, 1995

Kane JM, Jeste DV, Barnes TRE, et al: Treatment of tardive dyskinesia, in Tardive Dyskinesia: A Task Force Report of the American Psychiatric Association. Washington, DC, American Psychiatric Association, 1992, pp 103–120

Kane JM, Werner MG, Pollack S, et al: Does clozapine cause tardive dyskinesia? J Clin Psychiatry 54:327–330, 1993

Karn WN, Kasper S: Pharmacologically induced Parkinson-like signs as index of the therapeutic potential. Diseases of the Nervous System 20:119–122, 1959

Kaufman DM: Use of botulinum toxin injections for spasmodic torticollis of tardive dystonia. J Neuropsychiatry Clin Neurosci 6:50–53, 1994

Keckich WA: Violence as a manifestation of akathisia. JAMA 240:2185, 1978

Keepers GA, Casey DE: Use of neuroleptic-induced extrapyramidal symptoms to predict future vulnerability to side effects. Am J Psychiatry 148:85–89, 1991

Keepers GA, Clappison VJ, Casey DE: Initial anticholinergic prophylaxis for neuroleptic-induced extrapyramidal syndromes. Arch Gen Psychiatry 40:1113–1117, 1983

Kelly JT, Abuzzahab FS: The antiparkinson properties of amantadine in drug-induced parkinsonism. J Clin Pharmacol 11:211–214, 1971

Kelly JT, Zimmermann RL, Abuzzahab FS Sr, et al: A double-blind study of amantadine hydrochloride versus benztropine mesylate in drug-induced parkinsonism. Pharmacology 12: 65–73, 1974

Khan R, Jampala VC, Dong K, et al: Speech abnormalities in tardive dyskinesia. Am J Psychiatry 151:760–762, 1994

Klett CJ, Caffey E: Evaluating the long-term need for antiparkinson drugs by chronic schizophrenics. Arch Gen Psychiatry 26:374–379, 1972

Koek RJ, Pi EH: Acute laryngeal dystonic reactions to neuroleptics. Psychosomatics 30:359–364, 1989

Kulik AV, Wilbur R: Case report of propranolol (Inderal) pharmacotherapy for neuroleptic-induced akathisia and tremor. Prog Neuropsychopharmacol Biol Psychiatry 7:223–225, 1983

Kutcher SP, Mackenzie S, Galarraga W, et al: Clonazepam treatment of adolescents with neuroleptic-induced akathisia (letter). Am J Psychiatry 144:823–824, 1987

Kutcher S, Williamson P, MacKenzie S, et al: Successful clonazepam treatment of neuroleptic-induced akathisia in older adolescents and young adults: a double-blind, placebo-controlled study. J Clin Psychopharmacol 9:403–406, 1989

Laborit H, Huguenard P, Alluaume R: Un nouveau stabilisateur vegetatif (le 4560 RP) [A new vegetative stabilizer (4560 RP)]. Presse Med 60:206–208, 1952

Levinson DF, Simpson GM: Neuroleptic-induced extrapyramidal symptoms with fever: heterogeneity of the "neuroleptic malignant syndrome." Arch Gen Psychiatry 43:839–848, 1986

Levinson DF, Simpson GM, Singh H, et al: Fluphenazine dose, clinical response, and extrapyramidal symptoms during acute treatment. Arch Gen Psychiatry 47:761–768, 1990

Lieberman JA, Saltz BL, Johns CA, et al: The effects of clozapine on tardive dyskinesia. Br J Psychiatry 158:503–510, 1991

Lipinski JF, Zubenko GS, Barreira P, et al: Propranolol in the treatment of neuroleptic-induced akathisia. Lancet 1:685–686, 1983

Lohr JB, Caligiuri MP: A double-blind placebo-controlled study of vitamin E treatment of tardive dyskinesia. J Clin Psychiatry 57:167–173, 1996

Lohr JB, Cadet JL, Lohr MA, et al: Vitamin E in the treatment of tardive dyskinesia: the possible involvement of free radical mechanisms. Schizophr Bull 14:291–296, 1988

Luchins DJ, Freed WJ, Wyatt RJ: The role of cholinergic supersensitivity in the medical symptoms associated with the withdrawal of antipsychotic drugs. Am J Psychiatry 137:1395–1398, 1980

MacVicar K: Abuse of antiparkinsonian drugs by psychiatric patients. Am J Psychiatry 134:809–811, 1977

Manos N, Gkiouzepas J, Tzotzoras T, et al: Gradual withdrawal of antiparkinson medication in chronic schizophrenics: any better than the abrupt? J Nerv Ment Dis 169:659–661, 1981

Marder SR, Meibach RC: Risperidone in the treatment of schizophrenia. Am J Psychiatry 151:825–835, 1994

Mawdsley C, Williams IR, Pullar IA, et al: Treatment of parkinsonism by amantadine and levodopa. Clin Pharmacol Ther 13:575–583, 1972

McClelland HA, Blessed G, Bhate S, et al: The abrupt withdrawal of antiparkinsonian drugs in schizophrenic patients. Br J Psychiatry 124:151–159, 1974

McDevitt DG: Comparison of pharmacokinetic properties of beta-adrenoceptor blocking drugs. Eur Heart J 8 (suppl M):9–14, 1987

McEvoy JP: The clinical use of anticholinergic drugs as treatment for extrapyramidal side effects of neuroleptic drugs. J Clin Psychopharmacol 3:288–302, 1983

McEvoy JP, McCue M, Freter S: Replacement of chronically administered anticholinergic drugs by amantadine in outpatient management of chronic schizophrenia. Clin Ther 9:429–433, 1987

McEvoy JP, Hogarty GE, Steingard S: Optimal dose of neuroleptic in acute schizophrenia: a controlled study of the neuroleptic threshold and higher haloperidol dose. Arch Gen Psychiatry 48:739–745, 1991

Meco G, Bedini L, Bonifati V, et al: Risperidone in the treatment of chronic schizophrenia with tardive dyskinesia: a single-blind crossover study vs. placebo. Current Therapeutic Research 46:876–883, 1989

Medina C, Kramer MD, Kurland AA: Biperiden in the treatment of phenothiazine-induced extrapyramidal reactions. JAMA 182:1127–1129, 1962

Merrick EM, Schmitt P: A controlled study of the clinical effects of amantadine hydrochloride (Symmetrel). Current Therapeutic Research 15:552–558, 1973

Metzer WS, Paige SR, Newton JE: Inefficacy of propranolol in attenuation of drug-induced parkinsonian tremor. Mov Disord 8:43–46, 1993

Meyer BR: Benzodiazepines in the elderly. Med Clin North Am 66:1017–1035, 1982

Miller NE: Effects of adrenoceptor-blocking drugs on plasma lipoprotein concentrations. Am J Cardiol 60:17E–23E, 1987

Mindham RHS, Gaind R, Anstee BH, et al: Comparison of amantadine, orphenadrine, and placebo in the control of phenothiazine-induced parkinsonism. Psychol Med 2:406–413, 1972

Moleman P, Schmitz PJM, Ladee GA: Extrapyramidal side effects and oral haloperidol: an analysis of explanatory patient and treatment characteristics. J Clin Psychiatry 43:492–496, 1982

Monane M: Insomnia in the elderly. J Clin Psychiatry 53 (suppl 6):23–28, 1992

Odergren T, Tollback A, Borg J: Electromyographic single motor unit potentials after repeated botulinum toxin treatments in cervical dystonia. Electroencephalogr Clin Neurophysiol 93:325–329, 1994

O'Flanagan PM: Clonazepam in the treatment of drug-induced dyskinesia. BMJ 1(5952):269–270, 1975

Pacifici GM, Nardini M, Ferrari P, et al: Effect of amantadine on drug-induced parkinsonism: relationship between plasma levels and effect. Br J Clin Pharmacol 3:883–889, 1976

Parkes JD, Zilkha KJ, Calver DM, et al: Controlled trial of amantadine hydrochloride in Parkinson's disease. Lancet 1:259–262, 1970

Paton DM, Webster DR: Clinical pharmacokinetics of H_1-receptor antagonists (the antihistamines). Clin Pharmacokinet 10:477–497, 1985

Perry EK, Perry RH, Blessed G, et al: Necropsy evidence of central cholinergic deficits in senile dementia (letter). Lancet 1(8004):189, 1977

Postma JU, Tilburg VW: Visual hallucinations and delirium during treatment with amantadine (Symmetrel). J Am Geriatr Soc 23:212–215, 1975

Pujalte D, Bottaï T, Huë B, et al: A double-blind comparison of clonazepam and placebo in the treatment of neuroleptic-induced akathisia. Clin Neuropharmacol 17:236–242, 1994

Quinn N, Hallet M: Dose standardisation of botulinum toxin (letter) (published erratum appears in Lancet 1[8646]:1092, 1989). Lancet 1(8644):964, 1989

Rashkis HA, Smarr ER: Protection against reserpine-induced "parkinsonism." Am J Psychiatry 113:1116, 1957

Rifkin A, Quitkin F, Klein DF: Akinesia, a poorly recognized drug-induced extrapyramidal behavioral disorder. Arch Gen Psychiatry 32:672–674, 1975

Saltz BL, Woerner MG, Kane JM, et al: Prospective study of tardive dyskinesia incidence in the elderly. JAMA 266:2402–2406, 1991

Sandyk R, Kay SR, Awerbuch GI: Subjective awareness of abnormal involuntary movements in schizophrenia. Int J Neurosci 69:1–20, 1993

Schmidt M, Meister P, Baumann P: Treatment of tardive dyskinesias with vitamin E. European Psychiatry 6:201–207, 1991

Schwab RS, Chafetz ME: Kemadrin in the treatment of parkinsonism. Neurology 5:273–277, 1955

Schwab RS, England AC, Poskanzer DC, et al: Amantadine in the treatment of Parkinson's disease. JAMA 208:1160–1170, 1969

Schwab RS, Poskanzer DC, England AC Jr, et al: Amantadine in Parkinson's disease: review of more than two years' experience. JAMA 222:792–795, 1972

Scott AB: Botulinum toxin injections into extra ocular muscles as an alternative to strabismus surgery. Ophthalmology 87:1044–1049, 1980

Shear MK, Frances A, Weiden P: Suicide associated with akathisia and depot fluphenazine treatment. J Clin Psychopharmacol 3:235–236, 1983

Shriqui CL, Bradwejn J, Annable L, et al: Vitamin E in the treatment of tardive dyskinesia: a double-blind placebo-controlled study. Am J Psychiatry 149:391–393, 1992

Simpson GM: Long-acting, antipsychotic agents and extrapyramidal side effects. Diseases of the Nervous System 31 (suppl):12–14, 1970

Simpson GM, Lindermayer JP: Extrapyramidal symptoms in patients treated with risperidone. J Clin Psychopharmacol 17:194–201, 1997

Simpson GM, Amin M, Kunz E: Withdrawal effects of phenothiazines. Compr Psychiatry 6: 347–351, 1965

Simpson GM, Krakov L, Mattke D, et al: A controlled comparison of the treatment of schizophrenic patients when treated according to the neuroleptic threshold or by clinical judgement. Acta Psychiatr Scand Suppl 212:38–43, 1970

Simpson GM, Lee JH, Shrivastava RK: Clozapine in tardive dyskinesia. Psychopharmacologia 56:75–80, 1978

Simpson GM, Cooper TB, Bark N, et al: Effect of antiparkinsonian medications on plasma levels of chlorpromazine. Arch Gen Psychiatry 37:205–208, 1980

Simpson LL: The origin, structure, and pharmacologic activity of botulinum toxin. Pharmacol Rev 33:155–188, 1981

Singh H, Levinson DF, Simpson GM, et al: Acute dystonia during fixed-dose neuroleptic treatment. J Clin Psychopharmacol 10:389–396, 1990

Small JG, Hirsch SR, Arvanitis LA, et al: Quetiapine in patients with schizophrenia: a high- and low-dose double-blind comparison with placebo. Arch Gen Psychiatry 54:549–557, 1997

Snyder S, Greenberg D, Yamamura HI: Antischizophrenic drugs and brain cholinergic receptors. Arch Gen Psychiatry 31:58–61, 1974

Sommer BR, Cohen BM, Satlin A, et al: Changes in tardive dyskinesia symptoms in elderly patients treated with ganglioside GM1 or placebo. J Geriatr Psychiatry Neurol 7:234–237, 1994

Sramek JJ, Simpson GM, Morrison RL, et al: Anticholinergic agents for prophylaxis of neuroleptic-induced dystonic reactions: a prospective study. J Clin Psychiatry 47:305–309, 1986

Stanilla JK, Büchel C, Alarcon J, et al: Diurnal and weekly variation of tardive dyskinesia measured by digital image processing. Psychopharmacology (Berl) 124:373–376, 1996

Stanilla JK, de Leon J, Simpson GM: Clozapine withdrawal resulting in delirium with psychosis: a report of three cases. J Clin Psychiatry 58: 252–255, 1997

Stenson RL, Donlon PT, Meyer JE: Comparison of benztropine mesylate and amantadine HCL in neuroleptic-induced extrapyramidal symptoms. Compr Psychiatry 17:763–768, 1976

Stephens DA: Psychotoxic effects of benzhexol hydrochloride (Artane). Br J Psychiatry 113: 213–218, 1967

Stern TA, Anderson WH: Benztropine prophylaxis of dystonic reactions. Psychopharmacologia 61:261–262, 1979

Stoof JC, Booij J, Drukarch B: Amantadine as N-methyl-D-aspartic acid receptor antagonist: new possibilities for therapeutic applications? Clin Neurol Neurosurg 94: S4–S6, 1992

Strang RR: The syndrome of restless legs. Med J Aust 24:1211–1213, 1967

Stratas NE, Phillips RD, Walker PA, et al: A study of drug induced parkinsonism. Diseases of the Nervous System 24:180, 1963

Strömberg U, Svensson TH, Waldeck B: On the mode of action of amantadine. J Pharm Pharmacol 22:959–962, 1970

Swett C, Cole JO, Shapiro S, et al: Extrapyramidal side effects in chlorpromazine recipients. Arch Gen Psychiatry 34:942–943, 1977

Thaker GK, Nguyen JA, Strauss ME, et al: Clonazepam treatment of tardive dyskinesia: a practical GABAmimetic strategy. Am J Psychiatry 147:445–451, 1990

Timberlake WH, Schwab RS, England AC Jr: Biperiden (Akineton) in parkinsonism. Arch Neurol 5:560–564, 1961

Tollefson GD, Beasley CM Jr, Tamura RN, et al: Blind, controlled, long-term study of the comparative incidence of treatment-emergent tardive dyskinesia with olanzapine or haloperidol. Am J Psychiatry 154:1248–1254, 1997a

Tollefson GD, Beasley CM Jr, Tran PV, et al: Olanzapine versus haloperidol in the treatment of schizophrenia and schizoaffective and schizophreniform disorders: results of an international collaborative trial. Arch Gen Psychiatry 54:457–465, 1997b

Tune L, Coyle JT: Serum levels of anticholinergic drugs in treatment of acute extrapyramidal side effects. Arch Gen Psychiatry 37:293–297, 1980

Van Putten T, May PR, Marder SR, et al: Subjective response to antipsychotic drugs. Arch Gen Psychiatry 38:187–190, 1981

Van Putten TR, May PR, Marder SR: Response to antipsychotic medication: the doctor's and the consumer's view. Am J Psychiatry 141:16–19, 1984

Wilbur R, Kulik FA, Kulik AV: Noradrenergic effects in tardive dyskinesia, akathisia and pseudoparkinsonism via the limbic system and basal ganglia. Prog Neuropsychopharmacol Biol Psychiatry 12:849–864, 1988

Winer JA, Bahn S: Loss of teeth with antidepressant drug therapy. Arch Gen Psychiatry 16:239–240, 1967

Wingfield WL, Pollack D, Grunert RR: Therapeutic efficacy of amantadine HCl and rimantadine HCl in naturally occurring influenza A2 respiratory illness in man. N Engl J Med 281:579–584, 1969

Yahr MD, Duvoisin RC: Medical therapy of parkinsonism. Modern Treatment 5:283–300, 1968

Yamamura HI, Snyder SH: Muscarinic cholinergic receptor binding in the longitudinal muscle of the guinea pig ileum with [^{3}H] quinuclidinyl benzilate. Mol Pharmacol 10:861–867, 1974

Drugs for Treatment of Bipolar Disorder

ELEVEN

Lithium

Robert H. Lenox, M.D., and
Husseini K. Manji, M.D., F.R.C.P.C.

HISTORY AND DISCOVERY

Lithium is an element that was discovered in 1817. For more than 150 years, lithium has been used in various formulations as a remedy for a multitude of maladies afflicting the human body (F. N. Johnson 1984). Basing his work on that of Alexander Ure in the early 1840s, Sir Alfred Garrod 20 years later first introduced the oral use of lithia salts as a treatment for gout or "uric acid diathesis," which was described as encompassing symptoms of "gouty mania" and "complete mental derangement" (Garrod 1859; Ure 1844/1845). During this period, Professor A. Trousseau referred to both mania and depression as being associated with uric acid diathesis (Trousseau 1868).

Although lithia salts were clearly thought to be effective as a therapy for this gouty syndrome, it was the work by the American physician John Aulde and the Danish internist Carl Lange in the late 1880s that brought attention to the prophylactic efficacy of lithium in the treatment of recurrent symptoms of depression (Aulde 1887; Lange 1886). Subsequent use of lithium salts at low concentrations in popular remedies and mineral waters around the beginning of the

twentieth century, and their use as a salt substitute (resulting in cases of lithium toxicity in the 1940s), led to their fall into disrepute within the medical community. It was not until lithium's serendipitous rediscovery by Cade more than 50 years ago, and seminal clinical studies by Schou in the early 1950s, that lithium was seen by modern psychiatry as an effective antimanic treatment and a prophylactic therapy for manic-depressive disorder (Cade 1949; Schou 1979b). Although investigations over the years have served to further document the efficacy of lithium in the treatment of bipolar disorder (Davis 1976; Goodwin and Jamison 1990), in light of more recent data and a broadening of the diagnostic indications, the response rate has come under question, as we discuss later in this chapter (Grof et al. 1993).

PHYSICOCHEMICAL AND PHARMACOLOGICAL PROFILE

Lithium—A Monovalent Cation

Lithium shares many of the physicochemical properties of the Group IA elements in the periodic table (a group that includes sodium and po-

The authors thank the Dean Foundation for assistance with literature searches and Ms. Celia Knobelsdorf and Mr. David Morgan for outstanding editorial assistance.

tassium) and is the smallest member among these alkali metals. It has the highest electrical field density and largest energy of hydration—giving it ready access to sodium channel transport—yet it has an ionic radius that is similar to those of the divalent cations magnesium and calcium (G. Johnson et al. 1971). The interaction and potential competition of lithium with physiological events associated with the transport and cofactor activities of these monovalent and divalent cations in cells throughout the body, especially the brain, have provided fertile ground for research over the years.

In a study of 14 patients with bipolar disorder who underwent ^{7}Li nuclear magnetic resonance (NMR) spectroscopy 1 month after initiation of lithium treatment for acute mania, the reduction in manic symptoms correlated significantly ($r = 0.64$) with the lithium concentration in the brain but not with that in serum ($r = 0.33$) (Kato et al. 1994). In a more recent study using ^{7}Li NMR spectroscopy in psychiatric patients, long-term lithium treatment resulted in a brain-to-serum concentration ratio of 0.76, as well as a significant correlation between lithium brain concentration and both serum concentration and daily dose (Riedl et al. 1997). Other studies using ^{7}Li NMR spectroscopy suggest that lithium is eliminated more slowly from brain and that the brain-to-serum concentration ratio varies with the circadian cycle (Komoroski et al. 1993; Plenge et al. 1994).

Lithium and Membrane Transport

It has been known for at least 45 years that lithium undergoes active transport across cell membranes (Zerahn 1955). Both membrane transport systems and ion channels play roles in the regulation of intracellular lithium. Transport systems may be either adenosine triphosphate (ATP) driven, like the sodium potassium ATPase pump, or driven by the net free energy of transmembrane concentration gradients, like the sodium-calcium exchange pump. These transport systems are likely to be relevant to the

regulation of lithium in the cell body because they essentially regulate all steady-state intracellular ion concentration.

Early evidence suggested that, in excitable cells, lithium influx occurred primarily through the voltage-sensitive Na$^+$ channel (Carmiliet 1964; El-Mallakh 1990; Keynes and Swan 1959). Lithium entry has been shown to occur on activation of the channel, especially during the depolarization phase, wherein lithium rushes into the cells at the expense of Na$^+$. This property of lithium may be reflected in the increase in plasma levels of lithium that occur as a patient becomes euthymic after treatment for an acute manic episode (Degkwitz et al. 1979). Extrusion of lithium from the cell appears to depend on the gradient-dependent Na$^+$-Li$^+$ exchange process, wherein intracellular lithium substitutes for intracellular Na$^+$ (Hitzemann et al. 1989; Sarkadi et al. 1978). However, although evidence indicates that lithium enters the cell equally displacing Na$^+$ in excitable cells, lithium does have a tendency to accumulate in the cell because the removal of lithium is less efficient than that of Na$^+$ (Coppen and Shaw 1967; El-Mallakh 1990). Na,K-ATPase may play an indirect role because it establishes the Na$^+$ gradient in neurons: the greater is the Na$^+$ gradient, the greater is the rate of Na$^+$ efflux through the Na$^+$-Li$^+$ exchange.

Studies have suggested that an alteration in the activity of the Na,K-ATPase pump could result in significant changes in neuronal excitability and may represent a pathogenesis for mood disorders (El-Mallakh 1983; Hokin-Neaverson et al. 1974; Naylor and Smith 1981). However, clinical studies in RBCs over the years have reported conflicting data in patients with bipolar disorder, and a reduction in Na,K-ATPase activity has been noted predominantly in the depressed phase of both unipolar and bipolar patients (Akagawa et al. 1980; Alexander et al. 1986; Choi et al. 1977; Dagher et al. 1984; El-Mallakh 1983; Glen and Reading 1973; Hokin-Neaverson and Jefferson 1989; Hokin-Neaverson et al. 1974; Naylor et al. 1974a;

Nurnberger et al. 1982; Reddy et al. 1989; Sengupta et al. 1980; Strzyzewski et al. 1984). Multiple factors, such as psychotropic drugs, circulating hormones, and diet, have probably contributed to much of this variability (Swann 1984, 1988; A. J. Wood et al. 1989b).

Studies of RBC membranes in patients treated with lithium have revealed evidence for increased activity of Na,K-ATPase (Bunney and Garland-Bunney 1987; Dick et al. 1978; Hokin-Neaverson et al. 1976; B. B. Johnson et al. 1980; Mallinger et al. 1987; Naylor et al. 1974b, 1980; Reddy et al. 1989; Swann 1988; A. J. Wood et al. 1989a). These data have been accounted for in part by a concomitant lithium-induced inhibition, mediated through intracellular interaction with the Na^+ binding site, and activation, mediated through an extracellular K site (Collard 1986; Lazarus and Muston 1978). However, although the flux of lithium through voltage-dependent sodium channels may contribute to the regulation of steady-state lithium homeostasis within the cell, the gating of lithium via ion channels is likely to be more physiologically relevant at the synapse.

RBCs have served as a cell model for a series of clinical investigations over the years because they share lithium transport properties with neurons and are easily accessible (Bach and Gallicchio 1990; Mota de Freitas et al. 1991). Although early studies suggested that the RBC-to-plasma lithium concentration ratio was related to a history of bipolar disorder, and that a higher ratio was associated with a clinical response to lithium treatment, it was soon evident that a large interindividual variation precluded adequate replication of these findings (Mendels and Frazer 1973; Ramsey et al. 1979; Richelson et al. 1986; Szentistvanyi and Janka 1979).

Over the years, investigators have observed that chronic administration of lithium increases choline concentration in RBCs by more than 10-fold (Jope et al. 1978, 1980; Lee et al. 1974; Lingsch and Martin 1976; Meltzer et al. 1982; Rybakowski et al. 1978; Stoll et al. 1991; Uney et al. 1985). This appears to be the result of not

only an inhibition of choline transport but also an enhanced phospholipase D–mediated degradation of choline-containing phospholipids (Chapman et al. 1982; Miller et al. 1989, 1990). The latter effect of chronic lithium use may be mediated by its action on protein kinase C (PKC), which is discussed later in this chapter.

It is of interest that lithium efflux appears to be inhibited by approximately 50% in patients after treatment with lithium for at least 1 week and is associated with a threefold increase in the apparent K_m (a dissociation constant that provides a measure of the affinity of the substrate(s) for the enzyme) for the Na^+-Li^+ pathway, with no change in the countertransport rate V_{max} (the maximum rate of metabolism) (Ehrlich et al. 1981). NMR studies have found that the intracellular uptake of lithium is rather slow and have confirmed the increased accumulation of intra-RBC lithium after several days of chronic exposure to lithium (Riddell 1991). Similarly, as we have noted, chronic use of lithium results in a significantly elevated intracellular concentration of choline that persists long after lithium levels in both plasma and RBCs are no longer detectable (Lee et al. 1974; Lingsch and Martin 1976; Meltzer et al. 1982; Rybakowski et al. 1978). These effects of lithium appear to correspond to the time course of the clinical efficacy of lithium treatment and have led to suggestions that chronic lithium use may induce an evolving change in membrane structure or interaction with membrane-bound enzymes (Ehrlich et al. 1983).

Although these data are of considerable interest, caution must be used in direct extrapolation from a nonnucleated peripheral cell model to one involving excitable nucleated neuronal cells within the brain. Moreover, several studies, such as those on Na,K-ATPase, support the evolution of specific gene products expressed and posttranslationally regulated uniquely, not only to neurons but also among brain regions (Arystarkhoua and Sweadner 1996; Grillo et al. 1994; Lecuona et al. 1996; Malik et al. 1996; Munzer et al. 1994; Sahin-Erdemli et al. 1995).

Thus, although the RBC may be used as a peripheral model for lithium transport, extrapolations to lithium homeostasis in the brain or as a potential genetic marker for variations in ionic homeostatic processes in the brain underlying the pathophysiology of a disease such as bipolar disorder remain highly speculative.

MECHANISM OF ACTION

Unlike most psychotropic drugs, which primarily treat symptomatology, lithium is effective in prophylactically stabilizing the underlying disease process by reducing the frequency and severity of the profound mood cycling associated with bipolar disorder. Thus, identification of the molecular target(s) for the long-term action of lithium in the brain may lead to new psychopharmacological strategies and, in concert with the discovery of susceptibility genes, will improve the understanding of the pathophysiology of the disorder (Lenox and Watson 1994; Lenox et al., in press).

Lithium and Circadian Rhythms

Although studies of circadian rhythms in patients with affective disorders have often been limited by their cross-sectional design and heterogeneous patient populations and have been confounded by significant variability, disturbance in biological rhythms has remained a viable hypothesis underlying the (episodic) dysregulation observed in bipolar illness (Goodwin and Jamison 1990). The alteration in circadian rhythms appears to be manifested in an overall reduction in amplitude, possibly attributable to phase instability, and the tendency to phase advance that is observed in rapid eye movement (REM) sleep and core temperature relative to the sleep-wake cycle. Lithium has been shown to slow circadian oscillators in a wide variety of species ranging from plants to humans (Klemfuss and Kripke 1989).

It has been observed in various studies that lithium can phase-delay circadian rhythms in human subjects entrained to a 24-hour-day schedule, consistent with its ability to lengthen the intrinsic period of a circadian oscillator (Kripke et al. 1979; Kupfer et al. 1970; Mendels and Chernik 1973). Although few studies have examined the effects of lithium on circadian rhythms in bipolar patients, one study of a bipolar patient studied in depth revealed evidence for a significant and sustained lithium-induced delay in circadian core temperature and onset of REM, with a reduction in percentage of REM during total sleep time (Campbell et al. 1989). These data were consistent with earlier electroencephalographic findings in a series of patients with bipolar disorder (Kupfer et al. 1970, 1974). However, it has been difficult to indicate a clinical correlation of change in affective state with a lithium-induced resynchronization of circadian rhythms (Campbell et al. 1989; Kripke et al. 1978; Wehr and Goodwin 1979).

It is also of interest that data from earlier studies by Lewy et al. (1987) reported that bipolar patients appear to be supersensitive to light-induced reduction of nocturnal plasma melatonin levels. Wever (1979) suggested that a pacemaker with increased sensitivity to zeitgebers might become phase-advanced relative to the slower intrinsic period of the human circadian oscillator. This observation is also of interest because melatonin has been reported to promote internal and external synchronization in both animals and humans. An alteration in relative melatonin concentrations might therefore be instrumental in dissociation between different circadian rhythms (Arendt et al. 1986; Gwinner and Benzinger 1978; Rao and Mager 1987). Furthermore, studies by Seggie et al. (1989) examining dark adaptation threshold documented an increased sensitivity to light in bipolar patients that appears to be reduced in male patients receiving chronic lithium administration. Such a lithium-induced increase in dark adaptation threshold appears to be related to the effects of lithium on the adenylate cyclase second-messenger system (Carney et al. 1988; Kaschka et al. 1987).

It remains a working hypothesis that the therapeutic action of lithium can be attributed to its efficacy in correcting a putative phase advance and/or internal desynchronization of these biological rhythms in patients with bipolar disorder.

Lithium and Neurotransmission

Serotonin

Extensive research has been devoted to the effect of lithium on brain monoaminergic systems. A leading current theory hypothesizes that the antidepressant effects of lithium are the result of an augmentation of serotonin (5-hydroxytryptamine [5-HT]) function in the central nervous system (CNS) (de Montigny et al. 1983, 1988; Meltzer and Lowy 1987; Price et al. 1990). Preclinical studies show that lithium's effects on serotonin function may occur at a variety of levels, including precursor uptake, synthesis, storage, catabolism, release, receptors, and receptor-effector interaction (Bunney and Garland 1984; Bunney and Garland-Bunney 1987; Goodnick and Gershon 1985; Knapp and Mandell 1975; Price et al. 1990). Overall, reasonable evidence from preclinical studies suggests that lithium enhances serotonergic neurotransmission, though its effects on serotonin appear to vary depending on brain region, length of treatment, and serotonin receptor subtype (Bunney and Garland 1984; Bunney and Garland-Bunney 1987; Goodnick and Gershon 1985; Price et al. 1990; A. J. Wood and Goodwin 1987). Several preclinical studies show that tryptophan uptake and/or content are increased in synaptosomes and brain tissue after short-term and long-term treatment, whereas a single dose is without effect (Berggren 1987; Goodnick and Gershon 1985; Laakso and Oja 1979; Price et al. 1990; Swann et al. 1981; Tagliamonte et al. 1971).

Studies of the effects of short-term lithium treatment on brain concentrations of serotonin or 5-hydroxyindoleacetic acid (5-HIAA) have yielded conflicting results, although most tend to show increases in one or both (Berggren 1987; Goodnick and Gershon 1985; Price et al. 1990; Swann et al. 1981; Tagliamonte et al. 1971). In contrast, most long-term studies tend to show that serotonin and 5-HIAA levels decrease with lithium treatment (Ahluwalia and Singhal 1980; Bunney and Garland 1984; Collard 1978; Collard and Roberts 1977; Shukla 1985; Treiser et al. 1981). Treiser et al. (1981) found that long-term lithium treatment increased basal and K^+-stimulated serotonin release in the hippocampus but not in the cortex. Another study also reported that lithium increased serotonin release in the parietal cortex, hypothalamus, and hippocampus after 2–3 weeks but not after a single injection or 1 week of treatment (Friedman and Wang 1988).

In a series of important preclinical investigations, Blier, de Montigny, and others (Blier and de Montigny 1985; Blier et al. 1987) used electrophysiological recordings to measure the effects of lithium on the serotonin system. Short-term lithium did not affect the responsiveness of the postsynaptic neuron to serotonin or the electrical activity of the serotonin neurons, but it enhanced the efficacy of the ascending (presynaptic) serotonin system (Blier and de Montigny 1985; Blier et al. 1987). These observations led the investigators to propose that lithium might increase the efficacy of other antidepressant treatments (Blier and de Montigny 1985; Blier et al. 1987). Several open and double-blind clinical investigations have reported that approximately 50% of nonresponders are converted to responders with lithium administration within 2 weeks (de Montigny et al. 1981, 1983; Heninger et al. 1983). Although these effects have been attributed to the net effect of presynaptic facilitation of serotonin release onto "sensitized" receptors, convincing direct evidence of enhanced serotonin function in humans has been difficult to obtain (Cowen et al. 1989; Manji et al. 1991b).

Overall, current evidence from both preclinical and clinical studies supports a role for lithium in enhancing presynaptic activity in the serotonergic system in the brain. Direct studies of lithium's effects on serotonergic neurotransmission in humans have previously been limited by several factors: the complexity of the widespread distribution of serotonergic fibers throughout the brain, the multiple receptor subtypes, the relative lack of serotonin-specific pharmacological agents and outcome variables reflecting selective serotonergic responses, and inadequate attention to effects dependent on duration of treatment and affective or physiological state of the patient. With the current understanding of the molecular neurobiology of both receptor subtypes and the transporter in the serotonergic system, we anticipate newer and more specific pharmacological probes for future preclinical and clinical investigations.

Dopamine

The effect of lithium on dopamine synthesis and transmission has been investigated extensively in preclinical studies by directly determining changes in dopamine or homovanillic acid and indirectly examining lithium-induced changes in dopamine-linked behaviors (Bunney and Garland 1984; Bunney and Garland-Bunney 1987; Goodnick and Gershon 1985).

Based on the heuristic hypothesis that supersensitive dopamine receptors underlie the development of manic episodes, it has been postulated that lithium would prevent dopamine receptor supersensitivity (Bunney and Garland 1984; Bunney and Garland-Bunney 1987; Goodnick and Gershon 1985). In a series of studies, lithium prevented haloperidol-induced dopamine receptor upregulation (Bunney 1981; Rosenblatt et al. 1980; Verimer et al. 1980) and supersensitivity to iontophoretically applied dopamine or intravenous apomorphine (Gallager et al. 1978). Lithium treatment also partially prevented the development of electrical intracranial self-stimulation usually produced by haloperidol in rats (Bunney and Garland-Bunney 1987; Goodnick and Gershon 1985; Staunton et al. 1982a, 1982b). Thus, lithium appears to be effective in blocking both the

behavioral and the biochemical manifestations of supersensitive dopamine receptors induced by receptor blockade. Interestingly, there is significantly less evidence that lithium is effective in blocking dopamine receptor supersensitivity induced by other methods (i.e., tyrosine hydroxylase inhibitors, reserpine, or lesions of the dopamine pathways) (Beckmann et al. 1975; Bloom et al. 1981; Bunney 1981; Pert et al. 1978; Rosenblatt et al. 1980; Tanimoto et al. 1983; Verimer et al. 1980).

A proposed site of action for lithium's ability to block behavioral supersensitivity is the postsynaptic receptor and the prevention of haloperidol-induced increases in dopamine receptors. Although this theory is consistent with the observation that lithium can decrease locomotor activity even in the absence of presynaptic dopamine terminals (Swerdlow et al. 1985), lithium treatment does not result in any consistent effects on the density of D_1 or D_2 receptors. Reports purporting to show its ability to block the increase in dopamine receptor density after receptor blockade are conflicting. However, a study designed to examine lithium's effects on both pre- and postsynaptic dopamine receptors using different doses of apomorphine suggested that the drug was equally effective at both sites (Verimer et al. 1980). Indeed, electrophysiological data examining the effects of lithium on presynaptic dopamine receptors in the substantia nigra are also compatible with a blockade of dopamine receptor supersensitivity (Gallager et al. 1978). Thus, despite significant functional evidence, dopamine receptor binding studies remain inconclusive, suggesting a possible postreceptor site of lithium action that may be related to receptor-effector coupling. Interestingly, some studies have reported a lack of effect when lithium is administered after the induction of dopamine supersensitivity (Bloom et al. 1983; Klawans et al. 1976; Staunton et al. 1982a, 1982b), suggesting that in this model lithium exerts its greatest effects prophylactically.

Among the numerous behavioral effects of

lithium in animals, perhaps the best studied are those on stimulant-induced activity. Lithium's ability to antagonize increases in locomotor activity produced by amphetamine has gained much attention, perhaps because this model has been postulated to be a better representation of lithium's effects on manic behavior (Allikmets et al. 1979; Bunney and Garland-Bunney 1987; Goodnick and Gershon 1985; Klawans et al. 1976; Pert et al. 1978; Staunton et al. 1982a). It is also of interest that lithium has been reported to attenuate the euphoriant and motor-activating effects of oral amphetamine in depressed patients, although equivocal results have been observed with methylphenidate challenge (Huey et al. 1981; van Kammen et al. 1985). Lithium has been shown to exert an inhibitory effect on intracranial self-stimulation subacutely. However, this effect does not persist with chronic administration, suggesting a possible lack of relevance to its long-term mood-stabilizing effects (Seeger et al. 1981).

Although data from human investigations are sparse, lithium's postulated ability to reduce both pre- and postsynaptic aspects of dopamine transmission represents an attractive mechanism for its antimanic therapeutic action.

Norepinephrine

Lithium's effects on norepinephrine have been reported to be specific for both time points and brain regions (Ahluwalia and Singhal 1981; Bliss and Ailion 1970; Cameron and Smith 1980; Colburn et al. 1967; Goodnick and Gershon 1985; Katz and Kopin 1969; Katz et al. 1968; Kuriyama and Speken 1970; Poitou and Bohuon 1975; Schildkraut et al. 1969; Stern et al. 1969; K. Wood et al. 1985).

As is the case with the other neurotransmitters, the effects of lithium on norepinephrine receptor binding studies in rodent brain have been generally inconclusive (Maggi and Enna 1980; Schultz et al. 1981; Treiser and Kellar 1979). However, significant effects have been consistently observed on β-adrenergic receptor-mediated cyclic adenosine monophosphate (cAMP) accumulation, lithium inhibiting the response both in vivo and in vitro (discussed in detail later in this chapter). Studies have also investigated the effects of chronic lithium on drug-induced changes in β receptor sensitivity. Lithium was unable to block antidepressant-induced downregulation (Rosenblatt et al. 1979) and in fact produced a greater subsensitivity (i.e., cAMP response) (Mork et al. 1990), but it prevented reserpine or 6-hydroxydopamine-induced β-adrenergic receptor supersensitivity (Hermoni et al. 1980; Pert et al. 1979; Treiser and Kellar 1979). Additional data from preclinical and clinical studies suggest that lithium treatment results in subsensitive α_2 receptors (Catalano et al. 1984; Goodnick and Meltzer 1984a; Goodwin et al. 1986; Huey et al. 1981; Murphy et al. 1974). In preclinical studies, long-term lithium attenuates α_2-adrenergic-mediated behavioral effects (Goodwin et al. 1986; Smith 1988) and presynaptic α_2 inhibition of norepinephrine release (Spengler et al. 1986) while enhancing K^+-evoked norepinephrine release (Ebstein et al. 1983).

In clinical investigations, both increases and decreases in plasma and urinary norepinephrine metabolite levels have been reported after lithium treatment (Beckmann et al. 1975; Corona et al. 1982; Goodnick 1990; Greenspan et al. 1970; Grof et al. 1986; Linnoila et al. 1983; Murphy et al. 1979; Schildkraut 1973, 1974; Swann et al. 1987). Lithium has been reported to reduce the excretion of norepinephrine and its metabolites in manic patients while increasing its excretion in depressed patients, an effect associated with higher plasma norepinephrine concentrations in some patients (Beckmann et al. 1975; Bowers and Heninger 1977; Greenspan et al. 1970; Schildkraut 1973). However, there is also evidence that urinary excretion of 3-methoxy-4-hydroxyphenylglycol is low during bipolar depression and elevated during mania-hypomania (Bond et al. 1972; Jones et al. 1973; Post et al. 1977; Schildkraut et al. 1973; Wehr 1977). In part, these inconsistencies may be related to the inability to control adequately for state-dependent changes in affective states, with associated changes in activity level, arousal, and sympathetic outflow.

Studies have found that 2 weeks of lithium administration in control subjects resulted in increases in urinary norepinephrine and normetanephrine, and an increase in fractional norepinephrine release, and a trend toward significantly increased plasma norepinephrine, suggesting an enhanced neuronal release of norepinephrine (Manji et al. 1991a). These data are compatible with similar observations of increased plasma levels of dihydroxyphenylglycol, a major extraneuronal norepinephrine metabolite (Poirier-Littre et al. 1993). Thus, current evidence supports an action of lithium in facilitating the release of norepinephrine, possibly through effects on the presynaptic α_2 "autoreceptor," and reducing the β-adrenergic–stimulated adenylate cyclase response, which may contribute to lithium's attenuation of the euphorigenic effects of amphetamine.

Acetylcholine

Neurochemical, behavioral, and physiological studies suggest that the cholinergic system is involved in affective illness (Dilsaver and Coffman 1989) and that lithium alters the synaptic processing of acetylcholine in rat brain. Early studies reporting an inhibitory effect on cholinergic activity utilized toxic concentrations of lithium (Krell and Goldberg 1973; Marchbanks 1982; Miyauchi et al. 1980), which replaced sodium and interfered with the high-affinity transport of choline into cholinergic terminals that is required for the synthesis of acetylcholine (Jope 1979; Simon and Kuhar 1976). The addition of up to 1 mM lithium in vitro has no effect on acetylcholine synthesis or release, but chronic in vivo lithium treatment appears to increase acetylcholine synthesis, choline transport, and acetylcholine release in rat brain (Jope 1979; Simon and Kuhar 1976). Although some investigators have reported reductions in acetylcholine levels in rat brain after subchronic administration (Ho and Tsai 1975; Krell and Goldberg 1973; Ronai

and Vizi 1975), Jope (1979) reported increased synthesis of acetylcholine in cortex, hippocampus, and striatum after 10 days of lithium administration.

Several laboratories have investigated lithium's effects on the density of muscarinic receptors, with conflicting results (Kafka et al. 1982; Lerer and Stanley 1985; Levy et al. 1983; Maggi and Enna 1980; Tollefson and Senogles 1982). Chronic lithium has been reported to increase (Kafka et al. 1982; Lerer and Stanley 1985; Levy et al. 1983), decrease (Tollefson and Senogles 1982), or have no effect on (Maggi and Enna 1980) the binding of [^{3}H]quinuclidinyl benzilate in various areas of rat brain, whereas in human caudate nucleus, lithium is reported to reduce the affinity of [^{3}H]quinuclidinyl benzilate binding. The effects of lithium on both up- and downregulation of muscarinic receptors in the brain have also been investigated. Although there have been reports that lithium can abolish the increase in [^{3}H]quinuclidinyl benzilate binding produced by atropine but is without effect on the downregulation induced by the cholinesterase inhibitor diisopropylfluorophosphonate, these data vary and are inconclusive (Lerer and Stanley 1985; Levy et al. 1983).

We examined both receptor binding and muscarinic receptor-coupled phosphoinositide (PI) response in rat hippocampus during atropine-induced upregulation (Ellis and Lenox 1990) and found that chronic treatment with atropine results in an upregulation of muscarinic receptors and a supersensitivity of the PI response in the hippocampus. Coadministration of chronic lithium prevented the development of the supersensitivity of the muscarinic receptor PI response without significantly affecting the extent of upregulation of receptor binding sites. These findings are consistent with an effect of chronic lithium on upregulation of neuronal muscarinic receptors observed by Liles and Nathanson (1988) in neuroblastoma cells. Those authors suggested that lithium's actions are exerted at a point beyond the receptor binding site, possibly affecting the coupling of the newly upregulated receptors at the level of the signal-transducing G proteins. Thus, similar to the case for dopaminergic and β-adrenergic receptors, it has been suggested that lithium can block the development of cholinergic receptor supersensitivity.

Perhaps the most striking example of lithium's ability to potentiate muscarinic responses comes from the lithium-pilocarpine seizure model (Hirvonen et al. 1990; Honchar et al. 1983; Jope et al. 1986; Ormandy and Jope 1991; Persinger et al. 1988; Terry et al. 1990). In large doses, pilocarpine and other muscarinic agonists cause prolonged and usually lethal seizures in rats. Although lithium alone is not a convulsant, pretreatment with lithium increases the sensitivity of pilocarpine by almost 20-fold (Hirvonen et al. 1990; Honchar et al. 1983; Jope et al. 1986; Ormandy and Jope 1991; Persinger et al. 1988; Terry et al. 1990). Significantly, this behavioral effect of lithium is markedly attenuated by intracerebroventricular administration of myoinositol in both rats and mice (Kofman et al. 1991; Tricklebank et al. 1991), representing perhaps the best correlation between a biochemical and a behavioral effect of lithium (see subsection "Phosphoinositide Turnover" under "Lithium and Signal Transduction" later in this chapter).

A synergism with the cholinergic system also occurs in electrophysiological studies in hippocampal slices, in which pilocarpine and lithium together (but neither alone) produce spontaneous epileptiform bursting (Jope et al. 1986; Ormandy and Jope 1991). Elegant studies of rat hippocampus have shown that lithium can reverse muscarinic agonist–induced desensitization, an effect that is mediated through PI hydrolysis and can be reversed by inositol (Pontzer and Crews 1990). Studies by Evans et al. (1990) have suggested that lithium's role in lithium-pilocarpine seizures is to increase excitatory transmission through a presynaptic facilitatory effect. Lithium alone also augmented synaptic responses, and this effect of lithium could be blocked by a PKC inhibitor.

These results suggest that lithium's effects in this model may occur through a PKC-mediated presynaptic facilitation of neurotransmitter release. Biochemical, electrophysiological, and behavioral data suggest that chronic lithium administration stimulates acetylcholine synthesis and release in rat brain and potentiates some cholinergic-mediated physiological events. Interestingly, similar to the situation observed with the catecholaminergic system, pharmacological studies indicate that chronic lithium prevents muscarinic receptor supersensitivity, most likely through postreceptor mechanisms.

γ-*Aminobutyric Acid*

In contrast with the abundant literature on lithium's effects on monoamine neurotransmitters, much less work has been conducted on γ-aminobutyric acid (GABA) (Bernasconi 1982; Lloyd et al. 1987; Nemeroff 1991). Studies have suggested that previously low levels of GABA in plasma and cerebrospinal fluid (CSF) are normalized in bipolar patients treated with lithium (Berrettini et al. 1983, 1986), paralleling reported GABA changes observed in several regions of rat brain (Ahluwalia et al. 1981; Gottesfeld et al. 1971; Maggi and Enna 1980). It is worth noting that, after withdrawal of chronic lithium, GABA levels return to normal in the striatum and the midbrain but remain elevated in the pons-medulla (Ahluwalia et al. 1981), possibly because of reportedly elevated levels of the GABA-synthesizing enzyme glutamic acid decarboxylase. Lithium has also been postulated to prevent GABA uptake, and chronic lithium administration was shown to significantly decrease low-affinity [^{3}H]GABA sites in the corpus striatum and the hypothalamus (Maggi and Enna 1980). Because lithium has no effect on in vitro [^{3}H]GABA binding, these receptor changes have been interpreted as downregulation secondary to activation of the GABAergic system (Maggi and Enna 1980). Although the clinical relevance of these findings remains unclear, it is significant that decreases in GABA levels in CSF have been reported in depressed patients (Berrettini et al. 1982; Post et al. 1980a).

Similarly to carbamazepine and valproic acid, lithium may facilitate certain aspects of GABAergic neurotransmission through several mechanisms. The clinical relevance of these findings at this point remains largely unknown. However, as one of the few systems likewise affected by the other commonly used mood stabilizers, the GABAergic system is worthy of more carefully controlled investigation.

Lithium and Signal Transduction

Phosphoinositide Turnover

Research on the molecular mechanisms underlying the therapeutic effects of lithium has focused on intracellular second-messenger generating systems and in particular on receptor-coupled hydrolysis of phosphatidylinositol-4,5-bisphosphate (PIP$_2$) (Baraban et al. 1989; Manji et al. 1995b). At therapeutically relevant concentrations in humans, lithium is a potent inhibitor of the intracellular enzyme inositol monophosphatase (the concentration at which 50% of the enzyme's activity was inhibited [K_i] = 0.8 mM) within the hydrolytic pathway of PIP$_2$, which results in an accumulation of inositol monophosphate (IP) and a reduction in the generation of free inositol (Allison and Stewart 1971; Hallcher and Sherman 1980; Sherman et al. 1986). Lithium has also been shown to have additional potential sites of action in the PI cycle, where it has been reported to inhibit the inositol polyphosphatase that dephosphorylates certain forms of inositol triphosphate [I(1,3,4)P] and inositol bisphosphate[I(1,4)P].

Because the brain has limited access to inositol other than that derived from the recycling of inositol phosphates, the ability of a cell to maintain sufficient supplies of myoinositol can be crucial to the resynthesis of the PIs and the maintenance and efficiency of signaling (Sherman 1991). Furthermore, because the mode of enzyme inhibition is uncompetitive,

lithium's effects have been postulated to be most pronounced in systems undergoing the highest rate of PIP$_2$ hydrolysis (see reviews in Nahorski et al. 1991, 1992).

Thus, Berridge et al. (1982) first proposed that the physiological consequence of lithium's action is derived through the relative depletion of free inositol. Its selectivity could be attributed to its preferential action in the brain, resulting in suppression of PI hydrolysis in the most overactive receptor-mediated neuronal pathways (Berridge 1989; Berridge et al. 1989). Because several subtypes of adrenergic (e.g., α_1), cholinergic (e.g., m$_1$, m$_3$, m$_5$), serotonergic (e.g., 5-HT$_2$, 5-HT$_1$), and dopaminergic (e.g., D$_1$) receptors are coupled to PIP$_2$ turnover in the CNS (Fisher et al. 1992; Mahan et al. 1990; Rana and Hokin 1990; Vallar et al. 1990), this hypothesis offers a plausible explanation for lithium's therapeutic efficacy in treating both poles of bipolar disorder by the compensatory stabilization of an inherent biogenic amine imbalance in critical regions of the brain (Lenox 1987).

Studies have examined the effects of lithium on receptor-mediated PI response in brain in a few neurotransmitter systems (e.g., cholinergic, serotonergic, noradrenergic, and histaminergic). Although some investigators have found a reduction in agonist-stimulated PIP$_2$ hydrolysis in brain slices from rats exposed acutely and chronically to lithium, these findings have often been small, inconsistent, and subject to methodological differences (Casebolt and Jope 1989; Ellis and Lenox 1990; Godfrey et al. 1989; Kendall and Nahorski 1987; Whitworth and Kendall 1989). Muscarinic receptor–mediated PIP$_2$ turnover appears to be a major site of action exerted by lithium in vivo. Early studies that were later replicated indicated that the increase in IP and the reduction in brain myoinositol content induced by lithium are significantly enhanced by the coadministration of the cholinergic agonist pilocarpine and are blocked by pretreatment with cholinergic antagonists (i.e., atropine and scopolamine) (Allison 1978; Allison et al. 1976; Sherman et al. 1986). In addition, studies of rat and mouse cerebral cortical slices have reported potent inhibitory effects of lithium on muscarinic-stimulated IP_3 and IP_4 accumulation (Kennedy et al. 1989, 1990; Whitworth and Kendall 1988). In these cases, the effects of lithium occur after a characteristic lag of 5–10 minutes, suggesting an indirect mechanism consistent with the inositol depletion hypothesis noted previously. Furthermore, as we have noted, studies from our laboratory have provided data supporting an indirect effect of chronic lithium in rat brain on the coupling of newly upregulated muscarinic receptor sites to the PI response (Ellis and Lenox 1990; Lenox and Ellis 1990; Lenox et al. 1991).

Several lines of evidence suggest that the action of chronic lithium may not simply be directly manifested in receptor-mediated activity coupled to this second-messenger pathway. Although investigators have observed that levels of inositol in brain remain reduced in rats receiving chronic lithium (Sherman et al. 1985), it has been difficult to confirm that the reduction in inositol levels results in a reduction in the resynthesis of PIP_2, which is the substrate for agonist-induced PI turnover. However, the inability to consistently demonstrate a lithium-induced reduction in levels of PIP_2 may be attributable to a small, rapidly turned over, signal-related pool of PIP_2 and/or evidence that the resynthesis of inositol phospholipids may also occur through base exchange reactions from other larger pools of phospholipids, such as phosphatidylcholine. Initial attempts to verify this hypothesis at this level of the PI cycle by examining the effects of lithium on muscarinic-stimulated accumulation of IP_1 in brain slices in the presence of exogenously added inositol were unsuccessful (Kendall and Nahorski 1987). More recently, studies examining the effects of chronic lithium on $I(1,4,5)P_3$ mass in cortical slices have shown a time-dependent decline that is attenuated in the presence of high concentrations of inositol (Kennedy et al. 1990; Varney et al. 1992). Further evidence in support of the inositol depletion hypothesis of lithium action

has been observed in studies examining the diacylglycerol (DAG) arm of the PIP_2 resynthesis pathway (see subsection "Protein Kinase C" later in this chapter).

Although pharmacological concentrations of extracellular inositol have been reported to attenuate some of lithium's biochemical, behavioral, and toxic effects, in animal studies, the addition of inositol appeared to prevent but did not reverse the effects of lithium on the PI system (Kennedy et al. 1990; Kofman and Belmaker 1993; Maslanski et al. 1992; Tricklebank et al. 1991). Furthermore, the therapeutic actions of lithium occur only after chronic treatment and remain in evidence long after discontinuation—actions that cannot be attributed only to inositol reductions evident in the presence of lithium. Indeed, in a study using proton magnetic resonance spectroscopy (^{1}H-labeled magnetic resonance spectroscopy), lithium administration to a small sample of bipolar depressed and manic patients produced a significant reduction in the levels of myoinositol in frontal (but not occipital) cortex. Although these changes persisted for at least 3–4 weeks, they were observed as early as after 5 days of treatment, when the clinical state was largely unchanged (Moore et al. 1997). Thus, overall, both the preclinical and the clinical data suggest that, although lithium causes a relative depletion of myoinositol in the brain, the effects of chronic lithium administration may be mediated via a secondary cascade of signaling changes (Jope and Williams 1994; Lenox and Manji 1995; Manji et al. 1995b). The possible role of G proteins and, in particular, the PKC signaling cascade as sites for the action of chronic lithium in brain is discussed later in this chapter.

Adenylate Cyclase

The other major receptor-coupled second-messenger system in which lithium has been shown to have significant effects is adenylate cyclase, which generates cAMP (Belmaker 1981). cAMP accumulation by various neurotransmitters and hormones is reported to be inhibited by lithium at therapeutic concentrations both in vivo and in vitro, but the sensitivity appears to be less than that observed in the PI system (Andersen and Geisler 1984; Ebstein et al. 1980; Forn and Valdecasas 1971; Geisler and Klysner 1985; Geisler et al. 1985; Mork and Geisler 1987, 1989a, 1989b, 1989c, 1995; Newman and Belmaker 1987). Norepinephrine- and adenosine-stimulated cAMP accumulation in rat cortical slices are inhibited significantly by 1–2 mM Li; in human brain tissue, the 50% inhibitory concentration (IC_{50}) for lithium inhibition of norepinephrine-stimulated cAMP accumulation is approximately 5 mM (Newman et al. 1983). Studies in humans have reported that lithium treatment at therapeutic levels results in an attenuation of the plasma cAMP increase in response to epinephrine (Ebstein et al. 1976; Friedman et al. 1979) and have produced evidence for an attenuation in adrenergic receptor coupling to adenylate cyclase in peripheral cells (Risby et al. 1991). In fact, lithium inhibition of vasopressin-sensitive or thyroid-stimulating hormone (TSH)–sensitive adenylate cyclase is thought to contribute to the commonly observed side effects of nephrogenic diabetes insipidus and hypothyroidism seen in patients being treated with lithium over an extended period (Dousa 1974; Wolff et al. 1970).

Lithium attenuation of β-adrenoceptor-stimulated adenylate cyclase activity has also been shown in membrane, slice, and synaptosomal preparations from rat brain both in vitro and ex vivo (Andersen and Geisler 1984; Ebstein et al. 1980; Geisler and Klysner 1985; Geisler et al. 1985; Mork and Geisler 1987, 1989a, 1989b, 1989c; Newman and Belmaker 1987). Mori et al. (1996) reported that lithium, but not rubidium, significantly decreased the cAMP-stimulated microtubule-associated protein (MAP2) endogenous phosphorylation in microtubule fraction, which appeared to be related to a direct inhibitory effect of lithium on cAMP-dependent phosphorylation (PKA).

Lithium in vitro inhibits the stimulation of adenylate cyclase by guanyl imidodiphosphate, or Gpp(NH)p (a poorly hydrolyzable analogue of guanosine triphosphate [GTP]), and calcium-calmodulin, both of which can be overcome by Mg^{2+} (Andersen and Geisler 1984; Mork and Geisler 1989c; Newman and Belmaker 1987). Lithium also competes with both Mg^{2+} and Ca^{2+} for membrane binding sites, and lithium's inhibition of the solubilized catalytic unit of adenylate cyclase can also be overcome by Mg^{2+}. These findings suggest that lithium's inhibition of adenylate cyclase in vitro may be caused by competition with Mg^{2+} on a site on the catalytic unit of adenylate cyclase (Andersen and Geisler 1984; Newman and Belmaker 1987). However, the inhibitory effects of chronic lithium treatment on adenylate cyclase in rat brain are not reversed by Mg^{2+}, and these effects persist after washing of the membranes but are reversed by increasing concentrations of GTP (Mork and Geisler 1989c). These results suggest that the physiologically relevant effects of lithium (i.e., those seen on chronic drug administration and not reversed immediately with drug discontinuation) may be exerted at the level of signal-transducing G proteins at a GTP-responsive step.

G Proteins

Because lithium has been shown to affect both PI turnover and adenylate cyclase activity, recent research has focused on mechanisms shared by these two major second-messenger-generating systems, namely the signal-transducing G proteins. Thus, neurotransmitter function might be modulated through alterations in intracellular signaling. Lithium might be effective because it alters the postsynaptic signal generated in response to several endogenous neurotransmitters (see review in Manji 1992). Multiple receptors converge onto a single G protein, but individual receptors may also "talk" to more than one G protein. Likewise, single G proteins may modulate more than one effector, and several G proteins may also converge on a single effector. Thus, the G proteins are in a position to coordinate receptor-effector activity that is critical to the regulation of neuronal function, thereby maintaining a functional balance between neurotransmitter systems in brain. In addition, these signaling proteins may represent attractive targets to explain lithium's efficacy in treating both poles of bipolar disorder.

As we have noted, experimental evidence has shown that lithium may alter receptor coupling to PI turnover in the absence of consistent changes in the density of the receptor sites themselves. Because fluoride ion will directly activate G-protein-coupled second-messenger response, efforts have been made to examine the effect of lithium on sodium fluoride–stimulated PI response in brain. Although Godfrey et al. (1989) reported a 21% reduction of fluoride-stimulated PI response in cortical membranes of rats treated with lithium for 3 days, no change in response was observed in cortical slices from rats that were given lithium for 30 days.

Investigations have also addressed the role of G proteins in the action of lithium-induced attenuation of receptor-mediated adenylate cyclase activity in both rodents and humans. In a series of studies in which in vivo microdialysis measurements of cAMP were used to assess lithium's effects on G proteins in the intact animal, chronic lithium treatment produced a significant increase in basal and postreceptor-stimulated (cholera toxin or forskolin) adenylate cyclase activity while attenuating the β-adrenergic-mediated effect in rat frontal cortex or hippocampus. In addition, pertussis toxin–catalyzed [^{32}P]adenosine 5'diphosphate (ADP)-ribosylation in membranes from these brain regions of lithium-treated animals was significantly increased (Manji et al. 1991b; Masana et al. 1992). Because pertussis toxin selectively catalyzes ADP ribosylation of the undissociated, inactive αβγ-heterotrimeric form of G_i, these results suggest that chronic lithium administration may reduce activation of G_i through a stabilization of the inactive conformation (Manji et

al. 1991b; Masana et al. 1992). If dissociation of G-protein subunits was inhibited by lithium, this could decrease β-adrenergic-stimulated adenylate cyclase activity while simultaneously producing a relative stabilization of the receptor in a high-affinity state.

Currently, the molecular mechanisms underlying lithium's effects on G proteins remain to be fully established. Although data indicate that competition with magnesium accounts for some of lithium's in vitro effects on G proteins, and investigators have speculated that an interaction with GTP binding might be relevant to the chronic effects of lithium (Avissar et al. 1988; Manji et al. 1995a, 1995b; Mork and Geisler 1989c), a direct effect of lithium on guanine nucleotide activation of G protein is unsubstantiated at this time.

Protein Kinase C

The accumulating evidence discussed here suggests that at least some of lithium's critical effects are mediated through long-term processes set in motion during the brain's exposure to lithium. In this context, it is noteworthy that, as a result of inositol depletion in the presence of lithium, metabolites within the phospholipid portion of the hydrolytic pathway that include DAG, phosphatidic acid, and cytidine monophosphate-phosphatidate (CMP-PA) have been shown to be significantly elevated in a variety of cell types, including brain. This effect can be prevented in the presence of high concentrations of inositol (Brami et al. 1991a, 1991b; Downes and Stone 1986; Drummond and Raeburn 1984; Godfrey et al. 1989; Watson et al. 1990). This might be expected, because the end metabolite in this pathway (i.e., CMP-PA) requires free myoinositol to resynthesize inositol phosphates for the regeneration of PIP_2. Thus, depletion of cellular inositol interferes with the recycling of the system, resulting in the consequent accumulation of CMP-PA and its metabolite DAG. The action(s) of both acute and chronic lithium (e.g., inhibition of agonist-mediated PI turnover) may therefore stem initially from its potent effect in inhibiting the recycling of inositol through the receptor-mediated hydrolysis of PIP_2. Ultimately, this may be explained by lithium's indirect action in accumulating DAG and subsequent changes in the activation of the family of PKC isozymes (Manji and Lenox 1994; Manji et al. 1995b).

PKC is a family of at least 12 phosphorylating isozymes with different tissue, intracellular, and regional distribution within the brain, second-messenger activators, and substrate affinities, indicating distinct cellular functions (K. P. Huang 1989; Nishizuka 1992, 1995; Stabel and Parker 1991; Tanaka and Nishizuka 1994). Postranslational phosphorylation of selective PKC protein substrates within the cell is responsible for regulation of processes critical to cell secretion, membrane trafficking, transcription, ion transport, receptor signaling, and transformation. Evidence accumulating from various laboratories, including our own, points to a role for PKC in mediating the effects of lithium in various cell systems, including the brain (see review in Manji and Lenox 1994; Manji et al. 1995b). Currently available data suggest that short-term lithium exposure often mimics the action of phorbol ester and facilitates several PKC-mediated responses. Longer-term exposure results in an attenuation of phorbol ester–mediated responses, which may be accompanied by a down-regulation of PKC (Anderson et al. 1988; Bitran et al. 1990, 1995; Evans et al. 1990; Lenox and Watson 1992; Lenox et al. 1992b; Manji et al. 1993; Reisine and Zatz 1987; Wang and Friedman 1989; Zatz and Reisine 1985). Biochemical studies have revealed biphasic effects of lithium on PKC-mediated events in rat hippocampus. Thus, short-term (i.e., 3-day) lithium exposure augments serotonin release, whereas chronic (i.e., 3-week) lithium exposure at "therapeutic" levels attenuates both the phorbol ester–induced cytosol to membrane PKC translocation and [^{3}H]serotonin release in the hippocampus (Anderson et al. 1988; Sharp et al. 1991; Wang and Friedman 1989).

Early reports provided evidence that exposure of neuroblastoma cells (Leli and Hauser 1992) or PC12 cells (Li and Jope 1995) to 1 mM lithium in vitro produced isozyme-selective decreases in PKC α and, in PC12 cells, the PKC ε isoforms. Studies of chronic valproate (an anticonvulsant with confirmed antimanic properties) in C-6 glioma cells revealed similar reductions in the levels of PKC α and ε isoforms (Chen et al. 1994). Other studies have reported that chronic lithium administration in rats results in a significant decrease in the membrane-associated PKC α and ε isoforms in the hippocampus (Manji et al. 1993, 1996b). Such PKC isoform selectivity may be attributable to the fact that individual PKC isozymes have subtle differences in their biochemical characteristics and intra- and intercellular locations and have different susceptibilities to degradation after activation (Borner et al. 1992; F. Huang et al. 1989; Isakov et al. 1990; Kuroda and Nishizuka 1989). Because PKC activation is often followed by its rapid proteolytic degradation (K. P. Huang 1989; Nishizuka 1992; Stabel and Parker 1991; Young et al. 1987), a prolonged increase in DAG levels by lithium may lead to an increased membrane translocation and subsequent degradation of PKC.

Coadministration (intracerebroventricularly) of myoinositol markedly attenuated lithium-induced decreases in PKC α and ε (Manji et al. 1996a), a finding consistent with the action of chronic lithium resulting in an inositol depletion, accumulation of DAG, and subsequent down-regulation of PKC isozymes. This finding is of particular interest in the light of a pilot clinical investigation that showed the efficacy of tamoxifen, an effective PKC inhibitor, in the treatment of acute mania in a small group of manic patients (Bebchuk et al. 1997). Although we do not yet fully understand the precise profile of PKC isozymes activated by lithium and the relative time course of downregulation, we have begun to identify critical protein substrates for PKC that may provide further insight into the mechanism of long-term action of lithium in the brain.

The activation of PKC results in the phosphorylation of numerous membrane-associated phosphoprotein substrates, the most prominent of which in brain is the myristoylated alanine-rich C kinase substrate (MARCKS). Direct activation of PKC by phorbol esters in immortalized hippocampal cells has been shown to effectively downregulate the MARCKS protein (Linder et al. 1992; Watson and Lenox 1996). Chronic lithium administered at a therapeutically relevant concentration (1 mEq/kg in brain) to rats over a 4-week period has been shown to result in a marked reduction in MARCKS in the hippocampus (Lenox et al. 1992b), which is not observed after acute treatment and persists beyond treatment discontinuation (Lenox et al. 1992b). The lithium-induced reduction in MARCKS has been replicated in immortalized hippocampal cells and has been shown to be prevented and reversible in the presence of elevated inositol concentrations (Watson and Lenox 1996). Furthermore, activation of muscarinic receptor–coupled PI signaling significantly potentiates the downregulation of MARCKS protein induced in the presence of 1 mM lithium, supporting the role of the PI signaling pathway and PKC isozymes in this long-term action of lithium (Watson and Lenox 1996).

MARCKS binds calmodulin in a calcium-dependent fashion and cross-links actin at the plasma membrane; both of these events are inhibited by PKC-mediated 12CA5, which serves to translocate MARCKS from the membrane to the cytosol (Aderem 1992; Blackshear 1993). MARCKS has been implicated in cellular processes associated with cytoskeletal restructuring and signaling that may be related to long-term 12CA5 changes in processes associated with receptor signal transduction and neurotransmitter release. Studies have indicated that this action of chronic lithium on MARCKS protein expression is not shared by psychotropic drugs in general but is a property of valproate at therapeutic concentrations relevant to the treatment of acute mania (Lenox et al. 1996). Thus, MARCKS may represent a clinically relevant target for the mood-stabilizing action of chronic lithium, which serves to regulate aberrant signaling in the brain in patients with bipolar disorder.

Although such data provide intriguing evidence for an action of chronic lithium on long-term cellular events through changes in PKC activation, the precise mechanism remains to be determined. Because PKC activation is often followed by a rapid proteolytic degradation of the enzyme, a prolonged increase in DAG levels by chronic lithium administration may lead to an increased membrane translocation and subsequent degradation and downregulation of PKC isozymes (K. P. Huang 1989; Kishimoto et al. 1989; Nishizuka 1992). Such a mechanism would be consistent with data indicating that lithium acutely activates PKC, whereas prolonged treatment is associated with reduced phorbol ester–mediated responses, including neurotransmitter release (Anderson et al. 1988; Bitran et al. 1990; Evans et al. 1990; Lenox et al. 1992b; Manji et al. 1993; Reisine and Zatz 1987; Sharp et al. 1991; Wang and Friedman 1989; Zatz and Reisine 1985). On the other hand, there is evidence that membrane translocation, degradation, and conversion of PKC to a constitutively active phorbol-insensitive form (i.e., PKM) may play a role in at least some of the PKC-mediated events observed after chronic lithium exposure (Manji and Lenox 1994). PKC isozymes involved in such a process may account for regulation of the expression of MARCKS observed in cells exposed to either long-term phorbol ester or chronic lithium, and they may ultimately play a role in the action of lithium at a nuclear level.

Glycogen Synthase Kinase-3 and Its Role in Development

It is well known that lithium ion can have a significant effect on the development of a variety of organisms (Stachel et al. 1993). In particular, in *Xenopus*, lithium significantly alters the ventral-dorsal axis of the developing embryo (Kao et al. 1986). One hypothesis regarding this action of lithium stemmed from its inhibition of inositol monophosphatase and alteration in the dorsal-ventral balance of PI signaling in the embryo (Ault et al. 1996; Berridge et al. 1989). Support for this hypothesis was derived by the observation that exposure to high concentrations of myoinositol could reverse the effect of lithium (Busa and Gimlich 1989). In an interesting series of studies in *Xenopus*, however, inhibition of inositol monophosphatase by another inhibitor did not result in similar alteration in morphogenesis, suggesting that lithium may be acting in an alternative pathway (Klein and Melton 1996). These studies revealed that lithium inhibits glycogen synthase kinase-3β activity (K_i = 2.1 mM), which antagonizes the *wnt* signaling pathway associated with normal dorsal-ventral axis development in the *Xenopus* embryo. Studies using an embryo expressing a dominant negative form of glycogen synthase kinase-3 suggest that myoinositol reversal of dorsalization of the embryonic axis by lithium may be mediated by events independent of inositol monophosphatase inhibition (Hedgepeth et al. 1997). It has yet to be determined to what extent this effect of lithium on glycogen synthase kinase-3β is relevant to its mood-stabilizing properties in the brain.

Lithium and Gene Expression

As discussed earlier in this chapter, it has become increasingly appreciated that any relevant biochemical models of lithium's actions must attempt to account for its special clinical profile (prophylactic efficacy against both mania and depression), which normally requires several weeks to develop, and the maximum benefit may not be even seen for several months (Goodwin and Jamison 1990; Schou 1991) and is not immediately reversible on drug discontinuation (Faedda et al. 1993; Suppes et al. 1991). Patterns of effects requiring such prolonged administration of the drug suggest alterations at the genomic level. Neuronal plasticity clearly de-

pends on making long-term adjustments to changing physiological and pharmacological stimuli and is mediated in large part by the activation and inactivation of the expression of subsets of genes with temporal specificity.

It has become clear that long-term changes in neuronal synaptic function are correlated with, and in some cases have been shown to be dependent on, the induction of new programs of gene expression (Sheng and Greenberg 1990). Substantial progress has been made both in identifying the genes responsive to trans-synaptic stimulation and in elucidating the processes that convert ephemeral second-messenger-mediated events into long-term cellular phenotypic alterations. This has been particularly important for neurobiology, wherein we attempt to understand the mechanism(s) by which short-lived events (e.g., stressors) can have profound, long-term (perhaps lifelong) behavioral consequences (Kandel 1983; Post 1992) and, more importantly for the present discussion, may help to unravel the processes by which a simple monovalent cation such as lithium may produce a long-term stabilization of mood in individuals vulnerable to bipolar illness.

Before the 1990s, little was known about the transcriptional and posttranscriptional factors regulated by chronic drug treatment, although it has long been appreciated that both the diversity of neuronal responses and the long-term changes in plasticity are dependent on the selective regulation of gene expression. As articulated by Morgan and Curran (1991), the nucleus can be viewed as a complex arena in which multiple signal transduction pathways converge and thus is a likely downstream target of drugs such as lithium and valproic acid, which require chronic administration to manifest clinical efficacy. Although gene expression can be regulated by a variety of processes, several lines of evidence suggest that phosphorylation is used most frequently to regulate long-term neuronal responsiveness. In view of the effects of lithium on PKC described above, we reviewed the effects of lithium on PKC-mediated gene expression. We found that this mood-stabilizing agent exerts major effects at the level of gene expression and that these effects are largely mediated via PKC-induced alterations in the nuclear transcription regulatory factors that are responsible for modulating the expression of specific genes of functional importance with the potential for long-term and enduring changes in the CNS.

Several studies have found that lithium alters *fos* expression in different cell systems, including the brain, through a PKC-mediated mechanism (Kalasapudi et al. 1990; Weiner et al. 1991). Thus, preincubation of cultured PC12 cells (a rat pheochromocytoma cell line) with lithium for 16 hours markedly potentiates *fos* expression in response to the muscarinic agonist carbachol. That lithium's effects are mediated via PKC is supported by the observation that lithium pretreatment also potentiates *fos* expression in response to phorbol esters (Kalasapudi et al. 1990). Moreover, lithium's effects appear be selective for the PKC signal transduction pathway and do not appear to be the result of a nonspecific alteration in messenger ribonucleic acid (mRNA) stability, because the *fos* expression in response to adenylate cyclase activation is unaffected under identical conditions (Divish et al. 1991).

Interestingly, paralleling the results observed in cell culture, a single intraperitoneal injection of lithium results in an augmentation of pilocarpine-induced *fos* gene expression in rat brain, which can be antagonized by the m_1/m_3 muscarinic antagonist pirenzepine (Weiner et al. 1991). Studies of chronic lithium in rats have also reported brain region–specific effects on both basal and inducible *fos* expression (Mathe et al. 1995). Studies in cloned cell lines have also reported that chronic lithium (1 mM) resulted in a significant increase in AP-1–binding activity (Chen et al. 1997). These results are similar to earlier findings from studies in which valproate was used. Using a luciferase reporter gene system and site-directed mutagenesis, the same

laboratory (Manji et al. 1996b; Yuan et al. 1997) confirmed the ability of lithium or valproate to alter the expression of genes driven by an AP-1–containing promoter. These lithium-induced effects on the expression of cfos mRNA and AP-1–binding activity, generally thought to mediate a "second wave" of specific neuronal genes of functional importance, suggest the potential for long-term and enduring changes in the CNS.

Long-term regulation of synaptic function could result from a modification in receptors, G proteins, effectors, proteins involved in neurotransmitter release, cytoskeletal remodeling, and enzymes involved in neurotransmitter biosynthesis. These complex effects on the gene expression of multiple neuromodulators and on various components of second-messenger-generating systems may serve to explain the role of lithium in the long-term restoration of the functional balance of neurotransmitter activity in the CNS and thereby to restabilize mood and dampen periodic neurobiological oscillations of mood in bipolar patients and depression in unipolar patients (Lenox and Manji 1995; Manji et al. 1995b).

Lithium and Neuroanatomical Site of Action

Although data related to the neuroanatomical localization of lesions in the brains of bipolar patients are only now being accumulated by using structural and functional neuroimaging strategies, alterations in the right hemisphere related to limbic and frontal association areas have been of particular interest (Manji et al., in press). Additional evidence implicating temporal-lobe dysfunction associated with epileptic disorders remains of considerable interest (Drezniak and Lenox, unpublished data). The premise that lithium exerts its therapeutic actions by acting at such specific neuroanatomical sites and/or their cells of projection is supported by several lines of evidence.

First, atomic absorption spectrophotometric, radiographic dielectric track registration, and NMR studies indicate that lithium does not distribute evenly throughout the brain after either acute or chronic administration. There is evidence for preferential accumulation in the forebrain diencephalon, that is, the hypothalamus, and telencephalon structures, namely, caudate and hippocampus (Bond et al. 1972; Ebadi et al. 1974; Edelfors 1975; Heurteaux et al. 1986; Lam and Christensen 1992; Mukherjee et al. 1976; Nelson et al. 1980; Ramaprasad et al. 1992; Sander et al. 1994; Savolainen et al. 1990; Smith and Amdisen 1981; Spirtes 1976; Thellier et al. 1980a, 1980b). Second, as noted previously, preclinical studies of lithium's effects on neurotransmitter systems have revealed changes, particularly in the serotonin system, that are brain region specific. Third, the relative regional and cell distribution of overactive ligand-gated ion channels in the brains of bipolar patients may be important in dictating relative rates of lithium transport. Fourth, studies in which PI turnover was assessed after lithium administration indicate regional differences in inositol depletion and agonist-stimulated [^{3}H]IP accumulation, primarily between forebrain structures and hindbrain structures (Allison et al. 1980; R. D. Johnson and Minneman 1985; Rooney and Nahorski 1986; Savolainen et al. 1990; Sherman et al. 1986; Song and Jope 1992). Moreover, the effects of lithium are most apparent in cells in which inositol is not only limiting but also undergoing the greatest activation of receptor-mediated PI hydrolysis (Gani et al. 1993; Heacock et al. 1993; Sarri et al. 1995; Watson and Lenox 1996). Finally, regional brain—namely, hippocampal—distribution of PKC isozymes and alterations in MARCKS expression after chronic lithium administration may confer even further specificity of action. Collectively, these studies indicate that the long-term therapeutic action of lithium may indeed possess cell and regional brain specificity that underlies its prophylactic efficacy in the treatment of bipolar disorder.

INDICATIONS

Psychiatric Indications

Affective Disorders

As discussed elsewhere in this book, lithium is the most widely used treatment for bipolar disorder. Although it is far from the perfect drug, it has clearly revolutionized treatment of this disorder. Lithium has proved useful in the treatment of acute episodes of mania and depression and, perhaps most important, in the long-term prophylaxis of the illness.

Acute mania.   Lithium was approved by the U.S. Food and Drug Administration (FDA) in 1970 for the treatment of acute mania. Results of early uncontrolled, single-blind studies, when combined, indicate that approximately 81% (334 of 413) of manic patients show at least a partial response to lithium monotherapy. Subsequently, controlled, double-blind studies similarly revealed a 70%–80% response rate of lithium monotherapy in the treatment of acute manic episodes (reviewed in Goodwin and Jamison 1990; Goodwin et al. 1969; Maggs 1963; Schou et al. 1954). Despite this impressive response rate and the evidence that lithium is the drug of choice for long-term prophylaxis (see below), its 5- to 10-day latency of response has limited its use as the sole agent in the treatment of acute manic episodes in everyday clinical practice.

In several double-blind studies (Goodnick and Meltzer 1984b; Post et al. 1980b; Prien et al. 1972; Shopsin et al. 1971), lithium was compared with neuroleptic drugs in the treatment of acute mania. The results suggested that the neuroleptics are superior only in the initial management of acutely manic patients. More recent clinical studies clearly verified the efficacy of benzodiazepines, such as lorazepam, as an adjunct to lithium in the acute manic phase of the illness to control hyperactivity, agitation, and insomnia (Lenox et al. 1992a). This strategy affords the practical advantage of parenteral administration and limits unnecessary exposure to neuroleptics in this patient population. Thus, most clinicians currently prescribe either a benzodiazepine or (when necessary) a neuroleptic in combination with lithium during the early stages of the treatment of mania, and then gradually taper the neuroleptic or benzodiazepine after stabilization of the patient's acute symptomatology. Moreover, clinicians frequently observe an increase in plasma lithium levels (which often necessitates a lowering of the lithium dose) after the manic episode has subsided. At present, it is unclear whether this is a result of increased uptake of lithium into excitable tissue during mania (as previously discussed), an increase in renal blood flow and glomerular filtration rate, or a combination thereof.

The use of anticonvulsants in the treatment of patients with bipolar disorder has increased significantly over the past decade, leading to FDA approval of valproate for the treatment of acute mania. In earlier observations and a more recent double-blind, placebo-controlled investigation in which valproate was compared with lithium in the 3-week treatment of acute mania, it was evident that lithium was particularly effective for a subpopulation of patients, whereas valproate appeared to have efficacy for a broader spectrum of patients (Bowden et al. 1994; Calabrese and Delucchi 1990; Gerner and Stanton 1992; McElroy et al. 1992). Carbamazepine has less consistent supporting data but remains actively used in clinical practice (Keck et al. 1992). With the enhanced clinical recognition of the anticonvulsants, treatment strategies have more readily shifted to combining lithium with an anticonvulsant when mood stabilization proves to be more refractory with monotherapy. Lithium remains the treatment of choice for adolescent or adult patients presenting for the first time with classical bipolar acute mania.

Long-term prophylaxis of bipolar disorder. Numerous placebo-controlled studies have unequivocally documented the efficacy of lithium in the long-term prophylactic treatment of bipolar disorder (reviewed in Goodwin and Jamison 1990). Lithium's beneficial effects appear to involve a reduction in both the number of episodes and their intensity; approximately 70%–80% of all bipolar patients have at least a partial response to lithium. The cumulative data from 10 major double-blind studies in which lithium prophylaxis was compared with placebo showed that approximately 34% of patients receiving lithium had relapses, whereas 81% of patients receiving placebo had relapses.

Additional evidence for lithium prophylaxis is found in studies in which successful lithium treatment was discontinued. In at least 14 studies, an average of 50% of patients relapsed within 5 months of abrupt termination of treatment (Suppes et al. 1991). It is of interest that the relative risk of mania appeared to be fivefold greater than that of depression. Additional reports have supported the appearance of an increased risk for precipitation of an affective episode during the period of discontinuation, but this risk is significantly reduced if the lithium is tapered slowly (Faedda et al. 1993). Although there is evidence that patients maintained at standard serum lithium concentrations (0.8–1.0 mM) not only significantly reduced the risk of relapse but also decreased the risk of subsyndromal symptomatology, the role of compliance has not been thoroughly addressed (Gelenberg et al. 1989; Keller et al. 1992; Solomon et al. 1996).

Adequate lithium treatment, particularly in the context of a lithium clinic, is also reported to reduce the excessive mortality observed in patients with the illness (Coppen and Abou-Saleh 1988; Coppen et al. 1991; Muller-Oerlinghausen et al. 1991; Vestergaard and Aagaard 1991). Debate continues as to the relative efficacy of lithium in preventing manic and depressive episodes. After careful analysis of the controlled studies, Goodwin and Jamison (1990) concluded that despite common clinical opinion, little support exists for the idea that lithium has greater prophylaxis against mania than against major depression. Nevertheless, patients do seem to report mild breakthrough depressive symptoms more commonly than hypomanic symptoms, although it is difficult to rule out the selective reporting of aversive symptoms by the patients. However, data are accumulating that perhaps as many as half of all bipolar patients show an inadequate long-term response to lithium monotherapy, necessitating the addition or substitution of another agent, most commonly an anticonvulsant or an antidepressant (see Bowden, Chapter 18, in this volume). Issues related to the widened spectrum of patients being treated with lithium, as well as lack of compliance and potential increased risk of relapse during lithium discontinuation (see below), may have contributed to this apparent reduction in the efficacy of the monotherapy (Grof et al. 1993). These questions deserve further attention in future investigations.

Reports over the past several years have suggested that certain features of bipolar disorder are predictive of a poor response to lithium. Patients who experience mixed states, severe stage III mania, and/or rapid cycling are all likely to show a poor response to lithium. In addition, the type and sequence of episodes may also be important—for example, patients with a sequence of mania-depression-normal intervals do better with lithium than do those with a sequence of depression-mania-normalcy. The greater the number of interepisode symptoms resulting from concomitant personality disorder or substance abuse, the less effective lithium response is likely to be. The potential phenomenon of "lithium discontinuation refractoriness" in certain individuals has been identified (Post et al. 1992), but more extensive study is required to assess the generalizability of the phenomenon. However, lithium is frequently discontinued for pregnant patients. Although controlled studies are lacking, refractoriness to lithium reinstitution does not appear to be a common occurrence in this population. It is more clear that abrupt lithium discontinuation after long-term maintenance treatment often results in the

emergence of a manic episode, and the rate of exacerbation can be modified by using a gradual discontinuation strategy (Faedda et al. 1993; Suppes et al. 1993).

Investigators studying the mechanism(s) of action of the drug and the neurobiology of bipolar affective disorder must be cognizant of the clinical features associated with lithium response and discontinuation. These may provide clues not only about the targets of lithium's actions but also about long-term homeostatic processes occurring during long-term lithium administration (Lenox et al., in press).

Acute treatment of bipolar depression. In addition to the well-established efficacy of lithium as a potentiating agent in the treatment of refractory depression (de Montigny et al. 1983; Heninger et al. 1983; Price 1989) (as discussed in the next section), there is now considerable evidence for the antidepressant efficacy of lithium monotherapy, particularly in the treatment of bipolar depression. However, the antidepressant effects (shown in placebo-controlled studies) often do not become evident until the third or fourth weeks of treatment, perhaps explaining the negative results noted in earlier studies of shorter duration (see Goodwin and Jamison 1990). Interestingly, an average of 79% of bipolar patients are reported to respond to the drug, compared with only 36% of unipolar patients. Also, in several controlled studies, the antidepressant efficacy of lithium has been compared with that of standard antidepressants. In four of five studies, lithium had efficacy equal to that of tricyclic antidepressants, albeit with a slower onset of action in two of the studies (Goodwin and Jamison 1990). The clinical observation of breakthrough depressions in bipolar patients despite maintenance of therapeutic lithium suggests that some patients may experience only modest antidepressant effects. Nevertheless, given the now well-documented ability of antidepressants to induce rapid cycling and precipitate manic episodes (Goodwin and Jamison 1990; Wehr and Goodwin 1987), lithium monotherapy is recommended for treatment of bipolar depression.

Potentiation of antidepressant response. One of the major advances in psychopharmacology in the past two decades has been the recognition of lithium augmentation as a strategy in treating depression that is refractory to monotherapy with conventional antidepressants (both tricyclic antidepressants and monoamine oxidase inhibitors). It has been established in open studies (and subsequently in controlled studies) that about half of all treatment-refractory depressed patients respond to the addition of lithium to their ongoing antidepressant regimen (with a higher response rate in bipolar subjects), usually within 1–2 weeks (de Montigny et al. 1983; Heninger et al. 1983; Price 1989). Although lithium potentiation is more efficacious in patients with bipolar disorder, it also has clear efficacy in the treatment of those with unipolar depression. The relative safety of this strategy and the short time needed to assess its efficacy suggest that a trial of lithium augmentation should be considered before switching antidepressants in patients with nonresponding depression. The lithium augmentation strategy derived from de Montigny's heuristic proposal that the enhancement of ascending presynaptic serotonergic function would translate into potentiation of antidepressant efficacy (de Montigny et al. 1983). However, considerable data have shown that lithium can affect PKC, which may regulate the function of multiple neurotransmitter systems (Manji and Lenox 1994). It is tempting to speculate that it is this effect on multiple interacting neurotransmitter systems that underlies its remarkable efficacy in treating refractory depression.

Schizophrenia

Given some degree of similarity in the acute symptomatology of mania and certain forms of schizophrenia (particularly paranoid schizophrenia), it is not surprising that the efficacy of lithium has been investigated in these disorders. The results of the double-blind studies of lithium in patients with schizophrenia have generally been disappointing; greater efficacy has been observed for neuroleptics. Lithium shows some efficacy in the treatment of the affective symptoms but is generally without benefit on the "core schizophrenic" symptoms (Atre-Vaidya and Taylor 1989; Collins et al. 1991). There is considerably more evidence for the efficacy of lithium in the treatment of schizoaffective disorder: a meta-analysis of published findings suggested an improvement in 77% of lithium-treated schizoaffective individuals (Delva and Letemendia 1982). Although lithium appears to be useful for patients with this condition, treatment with neuroleptics and other agents is usually necessary (Goodnick and Meltzer 1984b).

Aggression

The antiaggressive effect of lithium has been investigated in animal studies and in clinical studies over the past 25 years, and the preponderance of data has suggested that lithium reduces impulsive aggression (see Nilsson 1993 for an excellent review). Indeed, Schou (1987) described lithium's antiaggressive effects as one of its best-documented effects outside of the treatment of bipolar illness. At serum levels similar to those used in the treatment of bipolar illness, lithium has generally been reported to exert antiaggressive effects in psychiatric populations, in children with behavior problems, in individuals with mental retardation, and in prisoners with "uncontrolled rage outbursts" (Nilsson 1993). Note that most studies have been conducted in institutions, and there is little research on the antiaggressive effects of lithium in the outpatient setting. In view of the reported association between serotonergic function and aggressive and impulsive disorders, it is not surprising that the antiaggressive properties of lithium have generally been ascribed to an enhancement of serotonergic function (Coccaro et al. 1989). Although it is not approved by the FDA for treatment of aggression, it is clear that additional studies of lithium for this purpose are warranted, not only with respect to defining the range of clinically responsive conditions, but also regarding the neurobiological mechanisms underlying its efficacy.

Other Psychiatric Conditions

The efficacy of lithium has been investigated in the treatment of obsessive-compulsive disorder, attention-deficit/hyperactivity disorder, late luteal phase dysphoric disorder, borderline personality disorder, alcoholism, Tourette's disorder, anxiety disorders, and eating disorders. However, there is little convincing evidence for lithium's efficacy in treating these disorders (Jefferson et al. 1983; F. N. Johnson 1987).

Nonpsychiatric Indications

Cluster Headache

The best-established nonpsychiatric use of lithium is in the long-term prophylactic treatment of cluster headache (Bussone et al. 1990). The cyclic, recurrent nature of the illness was the original impetus for investigating lithium's efficacy. Indeed, there is general agreement that lithium not only is an effective treatment but also should be regarded as a first-line agent in this disorder. Interestingly, the therapeutic efficacy of lithium in cluster headache requires similar plasma levels and generally shows a 3-week latency to response (F. N. Johnson and Minnai 1993).

Effects of Lithium on Blood Cells and the Function of Granulocytes

After the administration of therapeutic doses of lithium, fairly reproducible hematopoietic effects have been documented, especially on granulocyte leukocytes. The observation that lithium stimulation of leukocytosis involves a true proliferative response, rather than just a shift of cell populations from the marginating to the circulatory pool of cells, led investigators to examine bone marrow for changes in miotic cell

proliferation. These studies showed that lithium increases the number of pluripotential hematopoietic stem cells (colony-forming unit [CFU]–stem cells), granulocyte-macrophage progenitors (CFU–granulocyte macrophages), and megakaryocyte progenitors (CFU-megakaryocytes) in several species, including humans. These now-well-documented effects of lithium on blood cell formation have led to an investigation of this monovalent cation in the treatment of various hematopoietic disorders (particularly after anticancer or anti-AIDS chemotherapy) to ameliorate the bone marrow toxicity associated with these treatments. Although Lyman and Williams (1991) concluded, after a detailed review of the literature, that lithium is clearly effective in reducing both the severity and the duration of chemotherapy- or radiotherapy-associated neutropenia, lithium is not routinely used as an adjunct in these conditions. Nevertheless, given the extensive clinical use of lithium worldwide and its lack of toxicity when administered at therapeutic doses, the use of lithium to ameliorate bone marrow suppression remains an area worthy of further long-term clinical investigation.

"Hematological" studies of lithium have highlighted its potential role in modulating the hematopoietic toxicity associated with zidovudine. Despite the reported efficacy of the drug in producing immunological improvement, decreasing the incidence of opportunistic infections, and reducing AIDS mortality, its use has been associated with hematopoietic suppression, manifested by anemia, neutropenia, and overall bone marrow suppression (Fischl et al. 1987). Studies have confirmed the efficacy of concentrations similar to those attained clinically (i.e., 1.0 mM) in attenuating the toxicity of zidovudine on CFU–granulocyte macrophages; CFU-megakaryocytes; and burst-forming unit, erythroid progenitor stem cells obtained from mice infected with Rauscher leukemia virus (Gallicchio and Hughes 1992; Gallicchio et al. 1992).

The clinical studies of lithium in HIV-infected patients are much more preliminary but offer promise. In a pilot study, Roberts et al. (1988) showed that three of five zidovudine-treated AIDS patients receiving doses of lithium sufficient to attain therapeutic plasma levels showed significant neutrophilia. Interestingly, three of five patients receiving lithium tolerated higher doses of zidovudine.

Antiviral Effects of Lithium

The use of lithium as an antiviral agent is receiving growing consideration following the demonstration about 15 years ago that lithium inhibited the replication of certain viruses under particular experimental conditions (Skinner et al. 1980). Several studies have since reported that lithium inhibits the replication of several DNA viruses (see Cernescu et al. 1988). There is less agreement on RNA viruses; two RNA virus groups are not inhibited by lithium, whereas inhibition of paramyxoviruses are reported. The mechanisms by which lithium inhibits DNA replication through DNA polymerase in herpesvirus are presently unknown but are thought to occur through modification of intracellular second-messenger systems.

In this context, it is noteworthy that the enhancement of tumor necrosis factor cytotoxicity by lithium has been shown to be mediated by alterations in the PI second-messenger system (Beyaert et al. 1993).

To date, virtually all of the relevant detailed clinical studies on the potential antiviral efficacy of lithium have been directed to the treatment of herpes simplex virus infections. A large study of 177 subjects found that chronic lithium administration resulted in a significant reduction in the recurrence rate of these infections, and most patients reported a reduction to less than half the pretreatment rate (Amsterdam et al. 1990a, 1990b). Other double-blind prospective studies have identified a similar beneficial effect of lithium, which appears to be independent of any modulation of affective symptoms.

SIDE EFFECTS AND TOXICOLOGY

General Considerations

Lithium has a narrow therapeutic index in humans; its currently recommended therapeutic serum concentration range is 0.8–1.2 mEq/L (Gelenberg et al. 1989; Schatzberg and Cole 1991). Side effects and toxicity become increasingly more evident at doses that result in higher serum levels (Jefferson et al. 1987). A review of the literature reveals that 35%–93% of patients complain about adverse side effects of lithium treatment. The most common side effects reported are noted in Table 11–1, which presents pooled data from 12 individual studies of 1,094 patients (Goodwin and Jamison 1990). It is of interest that when patients are asked about the most troublesome side effects that often lead to noncompliance with long-term lithium treatment, the most common are related to cognitive dysfunction (i.e., mental confusion, poor concentration, mental slowness, and memory problems).

The major physiological systems predisposed to lithium-induced symptomatology and toxicity include the gastrointestinal, renal, endocrine, and nervous systems, as well as the teratogenicity affecting the developing fetus. Most of the side effects appear to be dose related and transient in nature (Jefferson 1990; Schou 1989; Vestergaard et al. 1988). Although sustained-release formulations of lithium may be useful in ameliorating some lithium-induced side effects, enhanced gastrointestinal symptomatology may preclude this treatment strategy. Thus, risk factors that predispose to side effects and toxicity of lithium include reduced renal clearance with age or renal disease, organic brain disorder, physical illness with vomiting and/or diarrhea, diuretic and/or other concomitant pharmacotherapy, low sodium intake and/or high sodium excretion, and pregnancy.

The vulnerability of certain organ systems to lithium-induced effects may be due not only to a preferential accumulation of lithium but

Table 11–1. Lithium side effects

Side effect	Percentage with subjective complaint[a]	Relative importance in noncompliance[b]
Excessive thirst	35.9	
Polyuria	30.4	4
Memory problems	28.2	1
Tremor	26.6	3[c]
Weight gain	18.9	2
Drowsiness/tiredness	12.4	5
Diarrhea	8.7	
Any complaint	73.8	
No complaints	26.2	

[a]Pooled percentages from 12 studies including 1,094 patients.
[b]Relative ranking of importance of side effects for lithium noncompliance in 71 patients (Goodwin and Jamison 1990).
[c]Included incoordination.

also to its action on the various ion transport, second-messenger, and receptor-signaling systems shared in both the brain and periphery. The CNS, which is the apparent site of its therapeutic action, is particularly sensitive to side effects and toxicity. Studies have even reported that lithium distribution throughout brain regions can be nonuniform, resulting in relatively greater potential effects in selected regions of the brain (Sansone and Ziegler 1985). Clinical manifestations of a fine hand tremor is one of the most common reported side effects in 31%–65% of patients. This can be associated with reduced motor coordination, nystagmus, and muscular weakness most notable in the early phases of treatment (Goodwin and Jamison 1990). Evidence for cogwheel rigidity has been reported with long-term treatment with lithium alone and has been attributed to the antidopaminergic effects of lithium, although this observation has been most apparent during concomitant neuroleptic exposure (Asnis et al. 1979).

Central Nervous System

The cognitive effects of lithium appear to be some of the most problematic for patients, yet they remain the least studied. Clinical reports of noncompliance with lithium over the years have attributed difficulty with both creativity and productivity and a lack of drive to lithium treatment. Yet two noted studies carried out in artists, writers, and business executives ($N = 30$) being treated with lithium found that more than 75% of these patients believed that lithium either enhanced or did not change their creative productivity (Marshall et al. 1970; Schou 1979a). In addition, it has been difficult to find convincing evidence for cognitive effects of lithium in animal studies. Studies of lithium-induced effects on intellectual functioning such as memory, associative processing, semantic reasoning, and rate of psychomotor and cognitive performance in bipolar patients remain contradictory (see review in Goodwin and Jamison 1990). Judd et al. (1987) reported data demonstrating a "slowing of the rate of central information processing" (pp. 1467–1468) in a series of control subjects administered therapeutic doses of lithium, a finding that supported earlier observations by Schou (1968). However, these studies were relatively short term, and there is evidence that accommodation to some of the cognitive effects of lithium occurs. Further research in this area is warranted because lithium appears to have profound effects on PKC-mediated events in the brain (as noted previously), PKC has been implicated in long-term potentiation in the hippocampus (Manji and Lenox 1994), and the subjective effects of lithium on cognition remain such an important clinical issue in compliance.

The neurotoxic effects of lithium that generally occur at higher serum concentrations or in patients with the risk factors we have noted are associated with increasing signs of cognitive impairment, lassitude, restlessness, and irritability (Jefferson et al. 1987). Although this symptomatology is reversible within 5–10 days, neurotoxicity can progress to frank delirium, ataxia, coarse tremors, seizures, and ultimately to coma and death. It is of interest that behavioral models of lithium's action in the brain, as well as its neurotoxic effect on seizure threshold, have reported reversibility with inositol administration, thus implicating lithium's action on the PI signaling pathway in these neurobehavioral and neurotoxic events (Kofman and Belmaker 1993). Consistent with our earlier observations, these data may also implicate the PI system as a target for lithium action on a continuum from its therapeutic to its neurotoxic effects.

Endocrine Systems

Lithium has been shown to exert effects on various endocrine systems; interested readers are directed to excellent reviews of the subject (F. N. Johnson 1988; Lazarus 1986). In a study of 330 bipolar patients treated with lithium for 5 months to 3 years, Schou (1968) first reported that lithium therapy induced goiter at an overall rate of 3.6%. Lithium appears to exert antithyroid effects at different levels of thyroid function, including inhibition of hormone synthesis and release, inhibition of the action of TSH, and peripheral metabolism of thyroxine.

Although reports of lithium-induced hypothyroidism range from 5% to 35% because of variability in the criteria for diagnosis and the sensitivity of laboratory tests, the prevalence of clinical hypothyroidism is estimated more likely to be 5% and more common in women (Jefferson 1990). It is generally accepted that approximately 30% of patients have elevated levels of TSH, although most do not have statistically significant decreases in the levels of circulating thyroid hormones. This suggests that a compromised substrate may be necessary for the development of overt hypothyroidism (Amdisen and Andersen 1982; Lindstedt et al. 1977; Rogers and Whybrow 1971). Such a suggestion is supported by studies showing an increased likelihood of elevations in TSH and decreases in thyroid hormones during lithium therapy in individuals with serum antithyroid antibodies (Calabrese et al. 1985; Myers et al. 1985).

Patients taking lithium manifest a high prevalence of thyroid autoantibodies (15%–30%), suggesting a relative induction by lithium (Deniker et al. 1978; Lazarus 1986). Furthermore, low-normal thyronine levels have been associated with lethargy and cognitive impairment in patients treated with lithium for at least 6 months, and triiodothyronine was in the low-normal range in patients who relapsed (Hatterer et al. 1989). Because lithium has been shown to suppress the cAMP formation induced by TSH stimulation, lithium-induced hypothyroidism may occur by an "uncoupling" of the TSH receptor from adenylate cyclase, resulting in a compensatory increased secretion of TSH (McHenry et al. 1990; Mori et al. 1989; Tseng et al. 1989). Although this is an attractive hypothesis and is likely to play some role in the reduced sensitivity to the effects of TSH, lithium also inhibits forskolin-stimulated iodine uptake in thyroid cells, suggesting that additional effects distal to cAMP formation (e.g., protein kinase) are involved (Mori et al. 1989; Urabe et al. 1991). In this context, it is noteworthy that lithium's effects are mimicked by PKC activators and blocked by PKC inhibitors in cultured thyroid tissue, suggesting that lithium's action on both adenylate cyclase and PKC contributes to the observed thyroid dysfunction.

Another possible endocrine complication of lithium treatment, hyperparathyroidism, was first reported by Garfinkel et al. (1973) and is much less common (Nordenstrom et al. 1992; Taylor and Bell 1993). Although the clinical significance of lithium-induced primary hyperparathyroidism has remained controversial, studies have reported increased parathyroid hormone secretion in at least a subset of patients (Christiansen et al. 1978), and there is accompanying evidence for modest increases in serum calcium and parathyroid hyperplasia in several reports (Lazarus 1986; Mannisto 1980). Since then, hyperparathyroidism associated with lithium therapy has been reported in more than 20 cases. However, the effect of lithium on parathyroid hormone secretion during clinical treatment remains controversial, at least in part because of the lack of pretreatment parathyroid hormone levels in most of the cases and the inability to demonstrate an alteration in the set point for parathyroid hormone secretion in healthy subjects undergoing subacute lithium administration (Spiegel et al. 1984). Nevertheless, the longitudinal studies, together with the reports of parathyroid hyperplasia and elevations of serum calcium, suggest that abnormal parathyroid hormone secretion may occur in at least a subset of individuals treated with lithium.

Renal Function

Lithium is excreted from the body almost entirely from the kidney, and there is no evidence for any significant protein binding. Lithium reversibly reduces the kidney's ability to concentrate urine primarily through effects on renal tubular function, resulting in the clinical manifestation of polyuria (>3 L/24 hours) (E. Walker and Green 1982). This impairment of renal tubular concentrating ability has been associated with a reversible acute epithelial swelling and glycogen disposition in the distal nephron. It is related to both the dose and the duration of lithium treatment and occurs in

20%–30% of patients treated with lithium (Goodwin and Jamison 1990; R. G. Walker 1993). Studies have indicated that once-daily dosing of lithium may result in relatively less renal symptomatology than a multiple-dosing treatment strategy, but further confirmation is needed (Lauritsen et al. 1981; Schou et al. 1982). Lithium appears to inhibit vasopressin (V_2 receptor)-stimulated cAMP production, reducing water reabsorption in the distal tubules and collecting ducts and resulting in nephrogenic diabetes insipidus (Dousa and Hechter 1970a, 1970b; Jefferson 1990).

There is also evidence for a dipsogenic effect of lithium through interaction with the renin-angiotensin system in the brain (Jefferson 1990). The mechanism for the inhibition of cAMP generation probably involves an effect at the level of G proteins, and more recent studies have suggested additional mechanisms involving prostaglandin pathways and PKC (Anger et al. 1990; Yamaki et al. 1991). A more progressive development of impairment of urinary concentrating ability has been observed in patients taking long-term lithium treatment, especially in those exposed to periods of lithium toxicity or concomitant exposure treatment with neuroleptics (R. G. Walker 1993). Although such patients on renal biopsy may have chronic focal interstitial nephropathy, similar lesions have been noted in psychiatric patients with no exposure to lithium. There is little evidence for lithium-induced chronic glomerular toxicity, although there are case reports of a reversible minimal lesion nephrotic syndrome (R. G. Walker 1993). In a review, Gitlin (1993) cited evidence that up to 5% of lithium-treated patients may develop signs of renal insufficiency, and in two reported cases progressive renal failure was diagnosed. However, such data lack comparable statistics for rate of renal insufficiency in the general population or in untreated bipolar patients and may be related to an increased risk of renal effects of lithium observed in patients exposed to periods of acute toxicity (Schou et al. 1989; R. G. Walker 1993).

Less Common Side Effects

The cardiovascular effects of orally administered lithium are rather benign. Most commonly, electrocardiogram recordings show a flattening and inversion of the T wave (Tilkian et al. 1976). Lithium has been shown to prolong sinus node recovery time. Caution is recommended in patients with bradycardia or sinus node dysfunction, as well as in those being treated concomitantly with drugs affecting sinus node conduction (Jefferson 1991; Mitchell and MacKenzie 1982; Roose et al. 1979). Because weight gain can be a significant side effect of long-term lithium treatment, the action of lithium on glucose metabolism has been examined over the years with rather conflicting results (Garland et al. 1988; Mellerup et al. 1983; Peselow et al. 1980). Consistent with lithium's ability to inhibit cAMP formation, there appears to be more consistent evidence for an insulin-like action resulting in a relative hypoglycemia (Jefferson 1991). Other lesser side effects of lithium treatment include an exacerbation of existing psoriasis, hair loss, leukocytosis, decreased libido, and altered taste sensation (Schou 1989).

Teratogenic Effects

Lithium treatment in humans has been associated with teratogenic properties predominantly affecting the cardiovascular development during the first trimester of pregnancy. Earlier studies based on the original work of Schou et al. (1973), which led to the development of the International Register of Lithium Babies, revealed an increased rate of Ebstein's anomaly that was 400 times higher than that observed in the general population (Nora et al. 1974). More recent controlled epidemiological studies have reported an apparently reduced rate of Ebstein's anomaly in the range of 0.1%–0.7%, approximately 20–140 times greater than in the general population (Elia et al. 1987; Jacobson et al. 1992; Zalstein et al. 1990). The risk of major congenital malformations with lithium treatment in the first trimester is now thought to be in the range

of 4%–12%, whereas the prevalence in an untreated comparison cohort is in the range of 2%–4% (L. S. Cohen et al. 1994). Lithium is currently indicated as a category D drug in the current edition of *Drugs in Pregnancy and Lactation* (Briggs et al. 1990), which states that "there is positive evidence of human fetal risk, but benefits from use in pregnant women may be acceptable despite the risk" (pp. 357–358).

In a review, L. S. Cohen et al. (1994) recommended a reconsideration of the relative risks associated with discontinuation compared with maintenance of lithium treatment during pregnancy. They outlined new guidelines for patients continuing lithium during the first trimester of pregnancy, suggesting prenatal diagnosis by fetal echocardiogram and high-resolution ultrasound examination at 16–18 weeks of gestation. Lithium passes through the placental barrier in the latter months of pregnancy and is present in breast milk, which can result in toxicity to the neonate manifesting in lethargy, hypotonia, and cyanosis.

DRUG-DRUG INTERACTIONS

Psychotropic Drugs

Overall, lithium has surprisingly few clinically significant interactions with most routinely prescribed psychotropic drugs. This perhaps explains in part why (despite its relatively low therapeutic index) a trial of adjunctive lithium therapy has been investigated in the treatment of numerous psychiatric conditions (see section "Indications"; Table 11–2).

Benzodiazepines

Few clinically relevant interactions between lithium and benzodiazepines occur, although certain individuals may be at greater risk for CNS depressant effects when the combination of the two drugs is used. In this context, the lithium-benzodiazepine combination has been suggested to produce an idiosyncratic reaction

Table 11–2. **Potentially clinically significant drug interactions with lithium**

Drug	Potential manifestations
Diuretics	Affect lithium clearance
Thiazides	Alter (usually raise) plasma lithium levels
Aldosterone antagonists	
Xanthine derivatives	
Loop diuretics and potassium-sparing diuretics	Cause fewer problems than other diuretics
Nonsteroidal anti-inflammatory drugs (NSAIDs)	Decrease lithium clearance and raise plasma lithium levels
Diclofenac	
Indomethacin	
Ibuprofen	
Naproxen	
Phenylbutazone	
Sulindac	May cause fewer problems than other NSAIDs
Neuroleptics	Worsen extrapyramidal side effects
	May result in neurotoxicity (high-potency agents appear to carry greater risk)
Antiarrhythmics	May potentiate cardiac conduction effects

manifested by profound hypothermia in one individual (Naylor and McHarg 1977). Nevertheless, a combination of benzodiazepines and lithium has been used extensively in the clinical setting, and few major adverse effects have been noted (Jefferson et al. 1981; Lenox et al. 1992a). Indeed, in view of the potential for sleep deprivation to induce manic episodes (Wehr et al. 1987), the judicious use of a benzodiazepine is recommended in the treatment of bipolar patients experiencing sleep disruption.

Neuroleptics

The practice of combining neuroleptics with lithium is generally considered safe and efficacious (Goodwin and Jamison 1990), but caution is recommended, particularly with the high-potency neuroleptics. There are reports of pharmacokinetic interactions between lithium and neuroleptics, but these are generally regarded as not clinically significant (Jefferson et al. 1983). Although lithium-neuroleptic neurotoxicity is a relatively rare phenomenon, it has been most widely associated with haloperidol (W. J. Cohen and Cohen 1974), and more than 40 cases are reported in the literature (see Ross and Coffey 1987; Werstiuk and Steiner 1987). This syndrome is characterized by altered mental status, cerebellar signs and symptoms, tremor, and extrapyramidal symptoms. Some patients also have fever and elevations in serum liver enzymes, raising the possibility that these may represent atypical cases of neuroleptic malignant syndrome.

In contrast, a chart review of 425 patients treated with lithium and haloperidol revealed that side effects occurred with no greater incidence with the two drugs combined than with either drug alone (F. N. Johnson 1984). Similarly, a study examining the prevalence of electroencephalogram abnormalities in patients treated with a combination of lithium and haloperidol found that the incidence of such abnormalities was not greater with the two drugs combined than with either drug alone (or with no drug) (Abrams and Taylor 1979). Thus, overall, it appears that this potential interaction is relatively rare. Nevertheless, given the abundant preclinical data supporting an effect of lithium on the dopaminergic system and the severity of the neurotoxicity, it seems prudent for clinicians to be aware of this interaction and to discontinue both drugs if toxicity develops.

Clozapine, an atypical antipsychotic that has

been approved by the FDA for treatment-resistant schizophrenia (Baldessarini and Frankenburg 1991), has proven superior efficacy over traditional antipsychotics in patients with this condition (Baldessarini and Frankenburg 1991; Kane 1990; Kane et al. 1988). A growing body of literature suggests that clozapine may be a useful and well-tolerated agent in the treatment of excited manic-psychotic phases of bipolar and schizoaffective disorders, even in patients who have failed to respond to, or do not tolerate, conventional somatic therapies (reviewed in Tohen and Tollefson 2000). More recently, controlled studies have indicated that clozapine appears to be effective and well-tolerated in the short-term and maintenance treatment of severe or psychotic mood disorders, particularly in the manic-excited phases of schizoaffective and bipolar disorders, even in patients who have not responded well to conventional pharmacotherapies (Tohen and Tollefson 2000). Thus, it is not surprising that clinicians have coadministered clozapine and lithium. Seizures were reported in two patients shortly after the addition of lithium to clozapine (Guadalupe et al. 1994).

In addition, other adverse effects have been reported in the literature with the combination of clozapine and lithium; four patients developed reversible neurological symptoms (i.e., involuntary jerking of limbs, hand tremor, tongue twitching, agitation, confusion, and bizarre nihilistic delusions). Two of these patients were rechallenged, and only one had a recurrence of symptoms. Currently, the exact frequency with which the combination of lithium and clozapine (or the more recently introduced, structurally similar, atypical antipsychotic, olanzapine) lowers seizure threshold or results in other neurological sequelae remains unknown.

Also reported in the literature were two cases of diabetic ketoacidosis associated with concomitant clozapine and lithium treatment (Koval et al. 1994; Peterson and Byrd 1996). Although there were only two cases, some of the clinical similarities include the fact that both pa-

tients were African Americans who had been taking both clozapine and lithium at the time they first presented with diabetic ketoacidosis. Neither had a toxic level of lithium, and both had taken lithium for extended periods. Furthermore, in both cases, the complication occurred early (within 5–6 weeks) in the course of clozapine treatment. Interestingly, neither patient had a history of diabetes or hyperglycemia (although one patient had a family history of diabetes and continued to manifest insulin-dependent diabetes 2 years after clozapine treatment was discontinued). To date, the frequency of such a potential interaction is unknown and warrants further study.

Anticonvulsants

As noted earlier and more fully discussed in Chapter 18, several anticonvulsants—most notably, valproate and carbamazepine—are being extensively used in the treatment of bipolar disorder. Increasingly, these agents (in particular valproate) are being coadministered with lithium, and a study by Granneman et al. (1996) evaluated the pharmacokinetic effects and safety of coadministration of lithium and valproate in 16 healthy volunteers. In a randomized, placebo-controlled, two-period (12 days each), crossover trial, valproate or placebo was given twice daily. The investigators found that lithium pharmacokinetics were unchanged by valproate but that some of valproate's pharmacokinetic measures (maximum drug concentration in serum [C_{max}], minimum drug concentration in serum [C_{min}], and area under the concentration-time curve) rose slightly during lithium coadministration. Overall, however, adverse events did not change significantly, suggesting that the concomitant administration of lithium and valproate appears to be safe in patients with bipolar disorder.

Antidepressants

The combination of lithium and various classes of antidepressants has been used extensively in many patients. The preponderance of the data suggest that, although minor side effects are common, major adverse effects are relatively uncommon (Price 1987). There are reports of increased incidence of myoclonic jerks in patients receiving a combination of lithium and monoamine oxidase inhibitors, but this has not been extensively investigated. In view of the enhancement of serotonergic function by lithium, there is the potential for an increased risk of the so-called serotonin syndrome in individuals receiving a combination of lithium and selective serotonin reuptake inhibitors or monoamine oxidase inhibitors, but the clinical data to date are sparse.

Electroconvulsive Therapy

Although not a true drug-drug interaction, the use of lithium during a course of electroconvulsive therapy (ECT) warrants discussion. In recent years, ECT has emerged as a remarkably efficacious, potentially life-saving treatment for many psychiatric conditions for which lithium is also used, including severe depression and mania (Crowe 1984). There is thus a clear need to establish the safety and potential efficacy of lithium treatment during ECT. Despite this clinical need, however, there is a dearth of adequate studies addressing this important issue (Rudorfer and Linnoila 1987).

Several case reports have suggested that the combination of lithium and ECT may be associated with a neurotoxic syndrome characterized by confusion, disorientation, and decreased responsiveness (reviewed in Rudorfer and Linnoila 1987). However, a comprehensive retrospective review (Perry and Tsuang 1979) and a prospective, controlled, double-blind study (Coppen et al. 1981) both reported no increased morbidity for lithium-ECT. In fact, the well-known need to continue maintenance medication after ECT and lithium's latency of onset of action prompted Coppen et al. (1981) to suggest that lithium might be introduced early during the course of ECT to minimize the likelihood of relapse after ECT termination. This

suggestion has not been generally accepted in routine clinical practice. Despite the lack of clear-cut evidence of neurotoxicity in general, it does appear that some patients are more susceptible to neurotoxic manifestations. Additionally, given the lack of obvious benefit of combining lithium and ECT in most patients, it seems prudent to discontinue lithium during the course of ECT. In cases of established lack of adequate response to either treatment alone, or in cases of known rapid relapse after ECT discontinuation, the lithium-ECT combination treatment can be conducted judiciously, by using "low therapeutic" lithium levels, avoiding other medications, and monitoring for any symptoms that are suggestive of neurotoxicity.

Nonpsychotropic Drugs

The largest single class of drugs producing a clinically significant interaction with lithium are the diuretics, several types of which can elevate lithium levels and produce toxicity. It is now well established that diuretics decrease renal lithium clearance, which frequently necessitates a reduction of the lithium dose to avoid toxicity. Any drug capable of altering renal function should be used judiciously in patients receiving lithium, and more frequent plasma level determinations and a reduction of the dose should be performed if necessary. However, perhaps because of their more proximal site of action, thiazide diuretics are also sometimes used to treat lithium-induced nephrogenic diabetes insipidus (discussed previously). Other classes of diuretics have been less well studied, but loop diuretics and potassium-sparing diuretics appear to cause fewer problems than other diuretics. The present data suggest, however, that a careful monitoring of lithium levels is warranted when using osmotic diuretics, loop diuretics, aldosterone antagonists, or other potassium-sparing diuretics.

The effects of cardiac drugs that alter sinus node conduction (e.g., quinidine and digoxin) could be potentiated by lithium. It is clear that the combination of lithium with cardiac drugs requires careful monitoring, including regular electrocardiograms. Several nonsteroidal antiinflammatory drugs can also increase plasma lithium levels, perhaps by an inhibition of renal tubular prostaglandin synthesis. Almost all of the older nonsteroidal antiinflammatory drugs (including diclofenac, ibuprofen, indomethacin, naproxen, and phenylbutazone) have been shown to interact with lithium and often result in toxicity, although preliminary studies suggest that sulindac may be less frequently associated with toxicity. Lithium is also known to prolong the action of neuromuscular agents, necessitating a reduction in dose or, in the case of patients undergoing certain surgical procedures or ECT, complete cessation.

It has been recognized that methylxanthines (such as caffeine) may significantly interfere with the clearance of some psychotropic drugs, such as lithium, that are mainly excreted by the kidneys. Early studies (reviewed in Finley et al. 1995) found mixed effects of caffeine ingestion on lithium clearance. Jefferson (1988) described two case reports of enhanced lithium-induced tremor after elimination of caffeine from the diet and concluded that marked reduction in caffeine intake may cause lithium retention, increased lithium levels, and thus aggravation of lithium-induced tremor. Most recently, it has been shown that in lithium-maintained patients with high daily caffeine intake, abrupt cessation of caffeine results in a significant (24%) increase in lithium blood levels (Mester et al. 1995). Irrespective of the potential role of caffeine withdrawal in triggering affective episodes, this study suggests that the marked reduction of caffeine from the diet (as is frequently done in controlled inpatient settings) of lithium-treated patients should be done cautiously in patients with high baseline levels of lithium in blood.

CONCLUSION

Lithium is a monovalent cation with complex physiological and pharmacological effects within the brain. By virtue of the ionic properties it shares with other important monovalent and divalent cations, such as sodium, magnesium, and calcium, its transport into cells provides ready access to a host of intracellular enzymatic events affecting short- and long-term cell processes. It may be that, in part, the therapeutic efficacy of lithium in the treatment of both poles of bipolar disorder may rely on the "dirty" characteristics of its multiple sites of pharmacological interaction.

The ability of lithium to stabilize an underlying dysregulation of limbic and limbic-associated function is critical to understanding its mechanism of action. The biological processes in the brain that are responsible for the episodic clinical manifestation of mania and depression may be caused by an inability to mount the appropriate compensatory responses necessary to maintain homeostatic regulation, thereby resulting in sudden oscillations beyond immediate adaptive control (Depue et al. 1987; Goodwin and Jamison 1990; Mandell et al. 1984). The resultant clinical picture is reflected in disruptions of behavior, circadian rhythms, neurophysiology of sleep, and neuroendocrine and biochemical regulation within the brain. Regulation of signal transduction within critical regions of the brain remains an attractive target for psychopharmacological interventions. The behavioral and physiological manifestations of the illness are complex and are mediated by a network of interconnected neurotransmitter pathways. The biogenic amines have been strongly implicated in the regulation of these physiological processes by virtue of their pharmacological actions and predominant neuroanatomical distribution within limbic-related brain regions. Thus, lithium's ability to modulate the release of serotonin at presynaptic sites and modulate receptor-mediated supersensitivity in the brain remains a relevant line of investigation into the respective action of lithium in altering the clinical manifestation of depression and mania in patients with bipolar disorder.

Finally, it would appear that the current

studies of the long-term lithium-induced changes in PKC and potentially other kinase-mediated events in the brain offer a most promising avenue for future investigation. Critical phosphoprotein substrates that play a role in the neuroplastic processes involved in cytoskeletal restructuring provide an opportunity for long-term dynamic regulation of signaling involving ion transport, neurotransmitter release, and the receptor-response complex. Furthermore, downstream alterations in gene expression through phosphoproteins acting as transcription factors can have a significant long-term effect on the precise profile of proteins that are available for the regulation of signal transduction in specific regions of the brain. It remains to be determined whether forthcoming research identifying the molecular targets for lithium in the brain will lead to elucidation of the pathophysiology of bipolar disorder and the discovery of a new generation of mood stabilizers.

REFERENCES

Abrams R, Taylor MA: EEG observations during combined lithium and neuroleptic treatment. Am J Psychiatry 136:336–337, 1979

Aderem A: The MARCKS brothers: a family of protein kinase C substrates. Cell 71:713–716, 1992

Ahluwalia P, Singhal RL: Effect of low-dose lithium administration and subsequent withdrawal on biogenic amines in rat brain. Br J Pharmacol 71:601–607, 1980

Ahluwalia P, Singhal RL: Monoamine uptake into synaptosomes from various regions of rat brain following lithium administration and withdrawal. Neuropharmacology 20:483–487, 1981

Ahluwalia P, Grewaal DS, Singhal RL: Brain GABAergic and dopaminergic systems following lithium treatment and withdrawal. Progress in Neuro-Psychopharmacology 5:527–530, 1981

Akagawa K, Watanabe M, Tsukada Y: Activity of Na-K-ATPase in manic patients. J Neurochem 35:258–260, 1980

Alexander DR, Deeb M, Bitar F, et al: Sodium-potassium, magnesium, and calcium ATPase activities in erythrocyte membranes from manic-depressive patients responding to lithium. Biol Psychiatry 21:997–1007, 1986

Allikmets LH, Stanley M, Gershon S: The effect of lithium on chronic haloperidol enhanced apomorphine aggression in rats. Life Sci 25:165–170, 1979

Allison JH: Lithium and brain *myo*-inositol metabolism, in Cyclitols and Phosphoinositides. Edited by Wells WW, Eisenberg F Jr. New York, Academic Press, 1978, pp 507–519

Allison JH, Stewart MA: Reduced brain inositol in lithium treated rats. Nature: New Biology 233:267–268, 1971

Allison JH, Blisner MW, Holland WH, et al: Increased brain *myo*-inositol 1-phosphate in lithium-treated rats. Biochem Biophys Res Commun 71:664–670, 1976

Allison JH, Boshans RL, Hallcher LM, et al: The effects of lithium on myo-inositol levels in layers of frontal cerebral cortex, in cerebellum, and in corpus callosum of the rat. J Neurochem 34:456–458, 1980

Amdisen A, Andersen C: Lithium treatment of thyroid function: a survey of 237 patients in long term lithium treatment. Pharmacopsychiatria 15:149–155, 1982

Amsterdam JD, Maislin G, Potter L, et al: Reduced rate of recurrent genital herpes infections with lithium carbonate. Psychopharmacol Bull 26:343–347, 1990a

Amsterdam JD, Maislin G, Rybakowski J: A possible antiviral action of lithium carbonate in herpes simplex virus infections. Biol Psychiatry 27:447–453, 1990b

Andersen PH, Geisler A: Lithium inhibition of forskolin-stimulated adenylate cyclase. Neuropsychobiology 12:1–3, 1984

Anderson SMP, Godfrey PP, Grahame-Smith DG: The effects of phorbol esters and lithium on 5-HT release in rat hippocampal slices (abstract). Br J Pharmacol 93:96P, 1988

Anger MS, Shanley P, Mansour J, et al: Effects of lithium on cAMP generation in cultured rat inner medullary collecting tubule cells. Kidney Int 37:1211–1218, 1990

Arendt J, Aldhous M, Marks V: Alleviation of jet lag by melatonin: preliminary results of controlled double blind trial. BMJ 292:1170–1174, 1986

Arystarkhoua E, Sweadner KJ: Isoform-specific monoclonal antibodies to Na, K-ATPase alpha subunits: evidence for a tissue-specific post-translational modification of the alpha subunit. J Biol Chem 271:23407–23417, 1996

Asnis GM, Asnis D, Dunner DL, et al: Cogwheel rigidity during chronic lithium therapy. Am J Psychiatry 136:1225–1226, 1979

Atre-Vaidya N, Taylor MA: Effectiveness of lithium in schizophrenia: do we really have an answer? J Clin Psychiatry 50:170–173, 1989

Aulde J: The use of lithium bromide in combination with solution of potassium citrate. Medical Bulletin (Philadelphia) 9:35–39, 69–72, 228–233, 1887

Ault KT, Durmwicz G, Galione A, et al: Modulation of *Xenopus* embryo mesoderm-specific gene expression and dorsoanterior patterning by receptors that activate the phosphatidylinositol cycle signal transduction pathway. Development 122:2033–2041, 1996

Avissar S, Schreiber G, Danon A, et al: Lithium inhibits adrenergic and cholinergic increases in GTP binding in rat cortex. Nature 331:440–442, 1988

Bach RO, Gallicchio VS: Lithium and Cell Physiology. New York, Springer-Verlag, 1990

Baldessarini RJ, Frankenburg FR: Clozapine: a novel antipsychotic agent. N Engl J Med 324:746–754, 1991

Baraban JM, Worley PF, Snyder SH: Second messenger systems and psychoactive drug focus on the phosphoinositide system and lithium. Am J Psychiatry 146:1251–1260, 1989

Bebchuk JM, Arfken C, Dolan-Manji S, et al.: A preliminary investigation of a PKC inhibitor (tamoxifen) in the treatment of acute mania (abstract). Abstracts of the American College of Neuropsychopharmacology Annual Meeting, Hawaii, December 1997

Beckmann H, St-Laurent J, Goodwin FK: The effect of lithium on urinary MHPG in unipolar and bipolar depressed patients. Psychopharmacologia 42:277–282, 1975

Belmaker RH: Receptors, adenylate cyclase, depression, and lithium. Biol Psychiatry 16:333–350, 1981

Berggren U: Effects of short-term lithium administration on tryptophan levels and 5-hydroxytryptamine synthesis in whole brain and brain regions in rats. J Neural Transm 69:115–121, 1987

Bernasconi R: The GABA hypothesis of affective illness: influence of clinically effective antimanic drugs on GABA turnover, in Basic Mechanisms in the Action of Lithium. Edited by Emrich HM, Adenhoff JB, Lux HM. Amsterdam, Excerpta Medica, 1982, pp 183–192

Berrettini WH, Nurnberger JI Jr, Hare T, et al: Plasma and CSF GABA in affective illness. Br J Psychiatry 141:483–487, 1982

Berrettini WH, Nurnberger JI Jr, Hare TA, et al: Reduced plasma and CSF gamma-aminobutyric acid in affective illness. Biol Psychiatry 18:185–194, 1983

Berrettini WH, Nurnberger JI Jr, Hare TA, et al: CSF GABA in euthymic manic-depressive patients and controls. Biol Psychiatry 21:844–846, 1986

Berridge MJ: Inositol triphosphate, calcium, lithium, and cell signaling. JAMA 262:1834–1841, 1989

Berridge MJ, Downes CP, Hanley MR: Lithium amplifies agonist-dependent phosphatidylinositol responses in brain and salivary glands. Biochem J 206:587–595, 1982

Berridge MJ, Downes CP, Hanley MR: Neural and developmental actions of lithium: a unifying hypothesis. Cell 59:411–419, 1989

Beyaert R, Heyninck K, De Valck D, et al.: Enhancement of tumor necrosis factor cytotoxicity by lithium chloride is associated with increased inositol phosphate accumulation. J Immunol 151:291–300, 1993

Bitran JA, Potter WZ, Manji HK, et al: Chronic Li$^+$ attenuates agonist- and phorbol ester-mediated Na$^+$/Ha$^+$ antiporter activity in HL-60 cells. Eur J Pharmacol 188:193–202, 1990

Bitran JA, Manji HK, Potter WZ, et al: Down-regulation of PKC alpha by lithium in vitro. Psychopharmacol Bull 31:449–452, 1995

Blackshear PJ: The MARCKS family of cellular protein kinase C substrates. J Biol Chem 268:1501–1504, 1993

Blier P, de Montigny C: Short-term lithium administration enhances serotonergic neurotransmission: electrophysiological evidence in the rat CNS. Psychopharmacology (Berl) 113:69–77, 1985

Blier P, de Montigny C, Tardif D: Short-term lithium treatment enhances responsiveness of postsynaptic 5-HT$_{1A}$ receptors without altering 5-HT autoreceptor sensitivity: an electrophysiological study in the rat brain. Synapse 1: 225–232, 1987

Bliss EL, Ailion J: The effect of lithium upon brain neuroamines. Brain Res 24:305–310, 1970

Bloom FE, Rogers J, Schulman JA, et al: Receptor plasticity: inferential changes after chronic treatment with lithium desmethylimipramine or ethanol detected by electrophysiological correlates, in Neuroreceptors: Basic and Clinical Aspects. Edited by Usdin E, Bunney WE Jr, Davis JM. New York, Wiley, 1981, pp 37–53

Bloom FE, Baetge G, Deyo S, et al: Chemical and physiological aspects of the actions of lithium and antidepressant drugs. Neuropharmacology 22:359–365, 1983

Bond PA, Jenner JA, Sampson DA: Daily variation of the urine content of 3-methoxy-4-hydroxyphenylglycol in two manic-depressive patients. Psychol Med 2:81–85, 1972

Borner C, Guadagno SN, Fabbro D, et al: Expression of four protein kinase C isoforms in rat fibroblasts: distinct subcellular distribution and regulation by calcium and phorbol esters. J Biol Chem 267:12892–12899, 1992

Bowden CL, Brugger AM, Swann AC, et al: Efficacy of divalproex vs. lithium and placebo in the treatment of mania. JAMA 271:918–924, 1994

Bowers MB, Heninger GR: Lithium: clinical effects and cerebrospinal fluid acid monoamine metabolites. Communications in Psychopharmacology 1:135–145, 1977

Brami BA, Leli U, Hauser G: Influence of lithium on second messenger accumulation in NG108-15 cells. Biochem Biophys Res Commun 174:606–612, 1991a

Brami BA, Leli U, Hauser G: Origin of the diacylglycerol produced in excess of inositol phosphates by lithium in NG108-15 cells (abstract). J Neurochem 57 (suppl):S9, 1991b

Briggs GG, Freeman RK, Yaffe SJ: Drugs in Pregnancy and Lactation, 3rd Edition. Baltimore, MD, Williams & Wilkins, 1990

Bunney WE Jr: Neuronal receptor function in psychiatry: strategy and theory, in Neuroreceptors: Basic and Clinical Aspects. Edited by Usdin E, Bunney WE Jr, Davis JM. New York, Wiley, 1981, pp 241–255

Bunney WE, Garland BL: Lithium and its possible modes of action, in Neurobiology of Mood Disorders. Edited by Post RM, Ballenger J. Baltimore, MD, Williams & Wilkins, 1984, pp 731–743

Bunney WE, Garland-Bunney BL: Mechanism of action of lithium in affective illness: basic and clinical implications, in Psychopharmacology: The Third Generation of Progress. Edited by Meltzer HY. New York, Raven, 1987, pp 553–565

Busa WB, Gimlich RL: Lithium-induced teratogenesis in frog embryos prevented by a polyphosphoinositide cycle intermediate or a diacylglycerol analog. Dev Biol 132:315–324, 1989

Bussone G, Leone M, Peccarisi C, et al: Double blind comparison of lithium and verapamil in cluster headache prophylaxis. Headache 30: 411–417, 1990

Cade JFJ: Lithium salts in the treatment of psychotic excitement. Med J Aust 36:349–352, 1949

Calabrese JR, Delucchi GA: Spectrum of efficacy of valproate in 55 patients with rapid-cycling bipolar disorder. Am J Psychiatry 147:431–434, 1990

Calabrese JR, Gulledge AD, Hahn K, et al: Autoimmune thyroiditis in manic-depressive patients treated with lithium. Am J Psychiatry 142: 1318–1321, 1985

Cameron OG, Smith CB: Comparison of acute and chronic lithium treatment on ^{3}H-norepinephrine uptake by rat brain slices. Psychopharmacology (Berl) 67:81–85, 1980

Campbell SS, Gillin JC, Kripke DF, et al: Lithium delays circadian phase of temperature and REM sleep in a bipolar depressive: a case report. Psychiatry Res 27:23–29, 1989

Carmiliet EE: Influence of lithium ions on the transmembrane potential and cation content of cardiac cells. J Gen Physiol 47:501–530, 1964

Carney PA, Fitzgerald CT, Monaghan CE: Influence of climate on the prevalence of mania. Br J Psychiatry 152:820–823, 1988

Casebolt TL, Jope RS: Long-term lithium treatment selectively reduces receptor-coupled inositol phospholipid hydrolysis in rat brain. Biol Psychiatry 25:329–340, 1989

Catalano M, Bellodi L, Lucca A, et al: Lithium and alpha-2-adrenergic receptors: effects of lithium ion on clonidine-induced growth hormone release. Neuroendocrinology Letters 6:61–66, 1984

Cernescu C, Popescu L, Constantinescu S, et al: Antiviral effect of lithium chloride. Virologie 39:93–101, 1988

Chapman BE, Beilharz GR, York MJ, et al: Endogenous phospholipase and choline release in human erythrocytes: a study using ^{1}H NMR spectroscopy. Biochem Biophys Res Commun 105:1280–1287, 1982

Chen G, Manji HK, Hawver DB, et al: Chronic sodium valproate selectively decreases protein kinase C alpha and epsilon in vitro. J Neurochem 63:2361–2364, 1994

Chen G, Yuan P, Hawver DB, et al: Increase in AP-1 transcription factor DNA binding activity by valproic acid. Neuropsychopharmacology 16:238–245, 1997

Choi SJ, Taylor MA, Abrams R: Depression, ECT, and erythrocyte adenosine triphosphatase activity. Biol Psychiatry 12:75–81, 1977

Christiansen C, Baastrup PC, Lindgren P, et al: Endocrine effects of lithium, II: "primary" hyperparathyroidism. Acta Endocrinol (Copen) 88:528–534, 1978

Coccaro EF, Siever LJ, Klar HM, et al: Serotonergic studies in patients with affective and personality disorders: correlates with suicidal and impulsive aggressive behavior. Arch Gen Psychiatry 46:587–599, 1989

Cohen LS, Friedman JM, Jefferson JW, et al: A reevaluation of risk of in utero exposure to lithium. JAMA 271:146–150, 1994

Cohen WJ, Cohen NJ: Lithium carbonate, haloperidol and irreversible brain damage. JAMA 230:1283–1287, 1974

Colburn RW, Goodwin FK, Bunney WE Jr, et al: Effect of lithium on the uptake of noradrenaline by synaptosomes. Nature 215:1395–1397, 1967

Collard KJ: Lithium effects on brain 5-HT metabolism, in Lithium in Medical Practice. Edited by Johnson FN, Johnson S. Lancaster, England, MTP Press, 1978, pp 123–133

Collard KJ: Effects of lithium on brain metabolism, in Endocrine and Metabolic Effects of Lithium. Edited by Lazarus JH. New York, Plenum, 1986, pp 55–98

Collard KJ, Roberts MHT: Effects of lithium on the elevation of forebrain 5-hydroxyindoles by tryptophan. Neuropharmacology 16:671–673, 1977

Collins PJ, Larkin EP, Shubsachs AP: Lithium carbonate in chronic schizophrenia: a brief trial of lithium carbonate added to neuroleptics for treatment of resistant schizophrenic patients. Acta Psychiatr Scand 84:150–154, 1991

Coppen A, Abou-Saleh MT: Lithium therapy: from clinical trials to practical management. Acta Psychiatr Scand 78:754–762, 1988

Coppen A, Shaw DM: The distribution of electrolytes and water in patients after taking lithium carbonate. Lancet 2:805–806, 1967

Coppen A, Abou-Saleh MT, Milln P, et al: Lithium continuation therapy following electroconvulsive therapy. Br J Psychiatry 139:284–287, 1981

Coppen A, Standish-Barry H, Bailey J, et al: Does lithium reduce the mortality of recurrent mood disorders? J Affect Disord 23:1–7, 1991

Corona GL, Cucchi ML, Santagostino G, et al: Blood noradrenaline and 5-HT levels in depressed women during amitriptyline or lithium treatment. Psychopharmacology (Berl) 77:236–241, 1982

Cowen PJ, McCance SL, Cohen PR, et al: Lithium increases 5-HT-mediated neuroendocrine responses in tricyclic resistant depression. Psychopharmacology (Berl) 99:230–232, 1989

Crowe RR: Current concepts: electroconvulsive therapy—a current perspective. N Engl J Med 311:163–167, 1984

Dagher G, Gay C, Brossard M, et al: Lithium, sodium and potassium transport in erythrocytes of manic-depressive patients. Acta Psychiatr Scand 69:24–36, 1984

Davis JM: Overview: maintenance therapy in psychiatry, II: affective disorders. Am J Psychiatry 133:1–13, 1976

Degkwitz R, Koufen H, Consbruch U, et al: Untersuchungen zur lithiumbilanz wahrend der manie [Investigation on lithium levels during mania]. International Pharmacopsychiatry 14:199–212, 1979

Delva NJ, Letemendia FJ: Lithium treatment in schizophrenia and schizo-affective disorders. Br J Psychiatry 141:387–400, 1982

de Montigny C, Grunberg F, Mayer A, et al: Lithium induces rapid relief of depression in tricyclic antidepressant drug non-responders. Br J Psychiatry 138:252–256, 1981

de Montigny C, Cournoyer G, Morissette R, et al: Lithium carbonate addition in tricyclic antidepressant-resistant unipolar depression: correlations with the neurobiological actions of tricyclic antidepressant drugs and lithium ion on the serotonin system. Arch Gen Psychiatry 40:1327–1334, 1983

de Montigny C, Chaput Y, Blier P: Lithium augmentation of antidepressant treatments: evidence for the involvement of the 5-HT system?, in New Concepts in Depression. Edited by Briley M, Fillion G. Basingstoke, England, Macmillan, 1988, pp 144–160

Deniker P, Eygiem A, Bernheim R, et al: Thyroid antibody levels during lithium therapy. Neuropsychobiology 4:270–275, 1978

Depue RA, Karuss SP, Spoont MR: A two-dimensional threshold model of seasonal bipolar affective disorder, in Psychopathology: An Interactional Perspective. Edited by Magnusson D, Ohman A. Orlando, FL, Academic Press, 1987, pp 95–123

Dick DAT, Naylor GJ, Dick EG: Effects of lithium on sodium transport across membranes, in Lithium in Medical Practice. Edited by Johnson FN, Johnson S. Lancaster, England, MTP Press, 1978, pp 183–192

Dilsaver SC, Coffman JA: Cholinergic hypothesis of depression: a reappraisal. J Clin Psychopharmacol 9:173–179, 1989

Divish MM, Sheftel G, Boyle A, et al: Differential effect of lithium on fos protooncogene expression mediated by receptor and postreceptor activators of protein kinase C and cyclic adenosine monophosphate: model for its antimanic action. J Neurosci Res 28:40–48, 1991

Dousa TP: Interaction of lithium with vasopressin-sensitive cyclic AMP system of human renal medulla. Endocrinology 95:1359–1366, 1974

Dousa T, Hechter O: Lithium and brain adenylyl cyclase. Lancet 1:834–835, 1970a

Dousa T, Hechter O: The effect of NaCl and LiCl on vasopressin-sensitive adenyl cyclase. Life Sci 9:765–770, 1970b

Downes CP, Stone MA: Lithium-induced reduction in intracellular inositol supply in cholinergically stimulated parotid gland. Biochem J 234:199–204, 1986

Drummond AH, Raeburn CA: The interaction of lithium with thyrotropin releasing hormone-stimulated lipid metabolism in GH_3 pituitary tumor cells. Biochem J 224:129–136, 1984

Ebadi MS, Simmons VJ, Hendrickson MJ, et al: Pharmacokinetics of lithium and its regional distribution in rat brain. Eur J Pharmacol 27:324–329, 1974

Ebstein R, Belmaker R, Grunhaus L, et al: Lithium inhibition of adrenaline-stimulated adenylate cyclase in humans. Nature 259:411–413, 1976

Ebstein RP, Hermoni M, Belmaker RH: The effect of lithium on noradrenaline-induced cyclic AMP accumulation in rat brain: inhibition after chronic treatment and absence of supersensitivity. J Pharmacol Exp Ther 213:161–167, 1980

Ebstein RP, Lerer B, Shlaufman M, et al: The effect of repeated electroconvulsive shock treatment and chronic lithium feeding on the release of norepinephrine from rat cortical vesicular preparations. Cell Mol Neurobiol 3:191–201, 1983

Edelfors S: Distribution of sodium, potassium and lithium in the brain of lithium-treated rats. Acta Pharmacologica et Toxicologica 37:387–392, 1975

Ehrlich BE, Diamond JM, Gosenfeld L: Lithium-induced changes in sodium-lithium countertransport. Biochem Pharmacol 30:2539–2543, 1981

Ehrlich BE, Diamond JM, Fry V, et al: Lithium's inhibition of erythrocyte cation countertransport involves a slow process in the erythrocyte. J Membr Biol 75:233–240, 1983

Elia J, Katz IR, Simpson GM: Teratogenicity of psychotherapeutic medications. Psychopharmacol Bull 23:531–586, 1987

Ellis J, Lenox RH: Chronic lithium treatment prevents atropine-induced supersensitivity of the muscarinic phosphoinositide response in rat hippocampus. Biol Psychiatry 28:609–619, 1990

El-Mallakh RS: The Na,K-ATPase hypothesis for manic depression. Med Hypotheses 12:253–282, 1983

El-Mallakh RS: The ionic mechanism of lithium action. Lithium 1:87–92, 1990

Evans MS, Zorumski CF, Clifford DB: Lithium enhances neuronal muscarinic excitation by presynaptic facilitation. Neuroscience 38:457–468, 1990

Faedda GL, Tondo L, Baldessarini RJ: Outcome after rapid vs gradual discontinuation of lithium treatment in bipolar disorders. Arch Gen Psychiatry 50:448–455, 1993

Finley PR, Warner MD, Peabody CA: Clinical relevance of drug interactions with lithium. Clin Pharmacokinet 29:172–191, 1995

Fischl MA, Richman DD, Grieco MH, et al: The efficacy of azidothymidine (AZT) in the treatment of patients with AIDS and AIDS-related complex: a double-blind, placebo-controlled trial. N Engl J Med 317:185–191, 1987

Fisher SK, Heacock AM, Agranoff BW: Inositol lipids and signal transduction in the nervous system: an update. J Neurochem 58:18–38, 1992

Forn J, Valdecasas FG: Effects of lithium on brain adenylyl cyclase activity. Biochem Pharmacol 20:2773–2779, 1971

Friedman E, Wang HY: Effect of chronic lithium treatment on 5-hydroxytryptamine autoreceptors and release of 5-[³H]hydroxytryptamine from rat brain cortical, hippocampal, and hypothalamic slices. J Neurochem 50:195–201, 1988

Friedman E, Oleshansky MA, Moy P, et al: Lithium and catecholamine-induced plasma cyclic AMP elevation, in Lithium Controversies and Unresolved Issues. Edited by Cooper TB, Gershon S, Kline NS, et al. Amsterdam, Excerpta Medica, 1979, pp 730–736

Gallager DW, Pert A, Bunney WE Jr: Haloperidol-induced presynaptic dopamine supersensitivity is blocked by chronic lithium. Nature 273:309–312, 1978

Gallicchio VS, Hughes NK: Effective modulation of the haematopoietic toxicity associated with zidovudine exposure to murine and human haematopoietic progenitor stem cells in vitro with lithium chloride. J Intern Med 231:219–226, 1992

Gallicchio VS, Messino MJ, Hulette BC, et al: Lithium and hematopoiesis: effective experimental use of lithium as an agent to improve bone marrow transplantation. J Med 23:195–216, 1992

Gani D, Downes CP, Bramham J: Lithium and myo-inositol homeostasis. Biochemica Biophysica Acta 1177:253–269, 1993

Garfinkel PE, Ezrin C, Stancer HC: Hypothyroidism and hyperparathyroidism associated with lithium. Lancet 2:331–332, 1973

Garland EJ, Remick RA, Zis AP: Weight gain with antidepressants and lithium. J Clin Psychopharmacol 8:323–330, 1988

Garrod AB: The Nature and Treatment of Gout and Rheumatic Gout. London, Walton & Maberly, 1859

Geisler A, Klysner R: The effect of lithium in vitro and in vivo on dopamine-sensitive adenylate cyclase activity in dopaminergic areas of the rat brain. Acta Pharmacologica et Toxicologica (Copenhagen) 56:1–5, 1985

Geisler A, Klysner R, Andersen PH: Influence of lithium in vitro and in vivo on the catecholamine-sensitive cerebral adenylate cyclase systems. Acta Pharmacologica et Toxicologica (Copenhagen) 56:80–97, 1985

Gelenberg AJ, Kane JM, Keller MB, et al: Comparison of standard and low serum levels of lithium for maintenance treatment of bipolar disorder. N Engl J Med 321:1489–1493, 1989

Gerner RH, Stanton A: Algorithm for patient management of acute manic states: lithium, valproate or carbamazepine? J Clin Psychopharmacol 12:57S–63S, 1992

Gitlin MJ: Lithium-induced renal insufficiency. J Clin Psychopharmacol 13:276–279, 1993

Glen AIM, Reading HW: Regulatory action of lithium in manic-depressive illness. Lancet 2:1239–1241, 1973

Godfrey PP, McClue SJ, White AM, et al: Subacute and chronic in vivo lithium treatment inhibits agonist- and sodium fluoride-stimulated inositol phosphate production in rat cortex. J Neurochem 52:498–506, 1989

Goodnick P: Effects of lithium on indices of 5-HT and catecholamines in the clinical content: a review. Lithium 1:65–73, 1990

Goodnick PJ, Gershon ES: Lithium, in Handbook of Neurochemistry. Edited by Lajtha A. New York, Plenum, 1985, pp 103–149

Goodnick PJ, Meltzer HY: Neurochemical changes during discontinuation of lithium prophylaxis, I: increases in clonidine-induced hypotension. Biol Psychiatry 19:883–889, 1984a

Goodnick PJ, Meltzer HY: Treatment of schizoaffective disorders. Schizophr Bull 10: 30–48, 1984b

Goodwin FK, Jamison KR: Manic-Depressive Illness. New York, Oxford University Press, 1990

Goodwin FK, Murphy DL, Bunney WE: Lithium-carbonate treatment in depression and mania. Arch Gen Psychiatry 21:486–496, 1969

Goodwin GM, DeSouza RJ, Wood AJ, et al: Lithium decreases 5-HT1A and 5-HT2 receptor and alpha-2 adrenoceptor mediated function in mice. Psychopharmacology (Berl) 90:482–487, 1986

Gottesfeld Z, Ebstein BS, Samuel D: Effect of lithium on concentrations of glutamate and GABA levels in amygdala and hypothalamus of rat. Nature 234:124–125, 1971

Granneman GR, Schneck DW, Cavanaugh JH, et al: Pharmacokinetic interactions and side effects resulting from concomitant administration of lithium and divalproex sodium. J Clin Psychiatry 57:204–206, 1996

Greenspan K, Schildkraut JJ, Gordon EK, et al: Catecholamine metabolism in affective disorders, 3: MHPG and other catecholamine metabolites in patients treated with lithium carbonate. J Psychiatr Res 7:171–183, 1970

Grillo C, Piroli G, Gonzalez SL, et al: Glucocorticoid regulation of mRNA encoding (Na+K) ATPase alpha 3 and beta 1 subunits in rat brain measured by in situ hybridization. Brain Res 657:83–91, 1994

Grof E, Brown GM, Grof P, et al: Effects of lithium administration on plasma catecholamines. Psychiatry Res 19:87–92, 1986

Grof P, Alda M, Grof E, et al: The challenge of predicting response to stabilizing lithium treatment: the importance of patient selection. Br J Psychiatry 163 (suppl 21):16–19, 1993

Guadalupe G, Crismon ML, Dorson PG: Seizures in two patients after the addition of lithium to a clozapine regimen. J Clin Pharmacol 14: 426–428, 1994

Gwinner E, Benzinger J: Synchronization of a circadian rhythm in pinealectomized European starlings by daily injections of melatonin. J Comp Physiol [A] 127:209–213, 1978

Hallcher LM, Sherman WR: The effects of lithium ion and other agents on the activity of myo-inositol-1-phosphatase from bovine brain. J Biol Chem 255:10896–10901, 1980

Hatterer JA, Kocsis JH, Stokes PE: Thyroid function in patients maintained on lithium. Psychiatry Res 26:249–258, 1989

Heacock AM, Seguin EB, Agranoff BW: Measurement of receptor-activated phosphoinositide turnover in rat brain: nonequivalence of inositol phosphate and CDP-diacylglycerol formation. J Neurosci 60:1087–1092, 1993

Hedgepeth CM, Conrad LJ, Zhang J, et al: Activation of the Wnt signaling pathway: a molecular mechanism for lithium action. Dev Biol 185: 82–91, 1997

Heninger GR, Charney DS, Sternberg DE: Lithium carbonate augmentation of antidepressant treatment: an effective prescription for treatment-refractory depression. Arch Gen Psychiatry 40:1335–1342, 1983

Hermoni M, Lerer B, Ebstein RP, et al: Chronic lithium prevents reserpine-induced supersensitivity of adenylate cyclase. J Pharm Pharmacol 32:510–511, 1980

Heurteaux C, Baumann N, Lachapelle F, et al: Lithium distribution in the brain of normal mice and of "quaking" dysmelinating mutants. J Neurochem 46:1317–1321, 1986

Hirvonen MR, Paljarri L, Naukkarinen A, et al: Potentiation of malaoxon-induced convulsions by lithium: early neuronal injury, phosphoinositide signaling and calcium. Toxicol Appl Pharmacol 104:276–289, 1990

Hitzemann R, Mark C, Hirschowitz J, et al: RBC lithium transport in the psychoses. Biol Psychiatry 25:296–304, 1989

Ho AKS, Tsai CS: Lithium and ethanol preference. J Pharm Pharmacol 27:58–60, 1975

Hokin-Neaverson M, Jefferson JW: Erythrocyte sodium pump activity in bipolar affective disorder and other psychiatric disorders. Neuropsychobiology 22:1–7, 1989

Hokin-Neaverson M, Spiegel DA, Lewis WC: Deficiency of erythrocyte sodium pump activity in bipolar manic-depressive psychosis. Life Sci 15:1739–1748, 1974

Hokin-Neaverson M, Burckhardt WA, Jefferson JW: Increased erythrocyte Na^+ pump and NaK-ATPase activity during lithium therapy. Res Commun Mol Pathol Pharmacol 14:117–126, 1976

Honchar MP, Olney JW, Sherman WR: Systemic cholinergic agents induce seizures and brain damage in lithium-treated rats. Science 220:323–325, 1983

Huang F, Yoshida Y, Cunha-Melo JR, et al: Differential down-regulation of protein kinase C isozymes. J Biol Chem 264:4238–4243, 1989

Huang KP: The mechanism of protein kinase C activation. Trends Neurosci 12:425–432, 1989

Huey LY, Janowsky DS, Judd LL, et al: Effects of lithium carbonate on methylphenidate-induced mood, behaviour, and cognitive processes. Psychopharmacology (Berl) 73:161–164, 1981

Isakov N, McMahon P, Altman A: Selective post-transcriptional down-regulation of protein kinase C isoenzymes in leukemic T cells chronically treated with phorbol ester. J Biol Chem 265:2091–2097, 1990

Jacobson SJ, Jones K, Johnson K, et al: Prospective multicentre study of pregnancy outcome after lithium exposure during first trimester. Lancet 339:530–533, 1992

Jefferson JW: Lithium tremor and caffeine intake: two cases of drinking less and shaking more. J Clin Psychiatry 49:72–73, 1988

Jefferson JW: Lithium: the present and the future. J Clin Psychiatry 51 (suppl 8):4–19, 1990

Jefferson JW: Update on lithium in clinical practice: an interview with James W. Jefferson, M.D. Currents in Affective Illness 10:5–14, 1991

Jefferson JW, Greist JH, Baudhiun M: Lithium: interactions with other drugs. J Clin Psychopharmacol 1:124–134, 1981

Jefferson JW, Greist JH, Ackerman DL: Lithium Encyclopedia for Clinical Practice. Washington, DC, American Psychiatric Press, 1983

Jefferson JW, Greist JH, Ackerman DL, et al: Lithium Encyclopedia for Clinical Practice, 2nd Edition. Washington, DC, American Psychiatric Press, 1987

Johnson BB, Naylor GJ, Dick EG, et al: Prediction of clinical course of bipolar manic depressive illness treated with lithium. Psychol Med 10:329–334, 1980

Johnson FN: The History of Lithium Therapy. Basingstoke, England, Macmillan, 1984

Johnson FN: Depression and Mania: Modern Lithium Therapy. Oxford, England, IRL Press, 1987

Johnson FN: Lithium treatment of aggression, self-mutilation, and affective disorders in the context of mental handicap. Reviews in Contemporary Pharmacotherapy 1:9–18, 1988

Johnson FN, Minnai G: Potential alternative applications of oral lithium. Reviews in Contemporary Pharmacotherapy 4:237–250, 1993

Johnson G, Gershon S, Burdock EI, et al: Comparative effects of lithium and chlorpromazine in the treatment of acute manic states. Br J Psychiatry 119:267–276, 1971

Johnson RD, Minneman KP: Alpha 1-adrenergic receptors and stimulation of [3H] inositol metabolism in rat brain: regional distribution and parallel inactivation. Brain Res 341:7–15, 1985

Jones FD, Maas JW, Dekirmenjian M, et al: Urinary catecholamine metabolites during behavioural changes in a patient with manic-depressive cycles. Science 179:300–302, 1973

Jope RS: Effects of lithium treatment in vitro and in vivo on acetylcholine metabolism in rat brain. J Neurochem 33:487–495, 1979

Jope RS, Williams MB: Lithium and brain signal transduction systems. Biochem Pharmacol 47:429–434, 1994

Jope RS, Jenden DJ, Ehrlich BE, et al: Choline accumulates in erythrocytes during lithium therapy. N Engl J Med 299:833–834, 1978

Jope RS, Jenden DJ, Ehrlich BE, et al: Erythrocyte choline concentrations are elevated in manic patients. Proc Natl Acad Sci U S A 77:6144–6146, 1980

Jope RS, Morrisett RA, Snead OC: Characterization of lithium potentiation of pilocarpine induced status epilepticus in rats. Exp Neurol 91:471–480, 1986

Judd LL, Squire LR, Butters N, et al: Effects of psychotropic drugs on cognition and memory in normal humans and animals, in Psychopharmacology: The Third Generation of Progress. Edited by Meltzer HY. New York, Raven, 1987, pp 1467–1475

Kafka M, Wirz-Justice A, Naber D, et al: Effect of lithium on circadian neurotransmitter receptor rhythms. Neuropsychobiology 8:41–50, 1982

Kalasapudi VD, Sheftel G, Divish MM, et al: Lithium augments fos protoonocogene expression in PC12 pheochromocytoma cells: implications for therapeutic action of lithium. Brain Res 521:47–54, 1990

Kandel ER: From metapsychology to molecular biology: explorations into the nature of anxiety. Am J Psychiatry 140:1277–1293, 1983

Kane JM: The efficacy of clozapine in the treatment of schizophrenia: a long-term perspective. J Clin Psychiatry 8:9–14, 1990

Kane JM, Honigfeld G, Singer J, et al: Clozapine for the treatment-resistant schizophrenic: a double-blind comparison with chlorpromazine. Arch Gen Psychiatry 45:789–796, 1988

Kao KR, Masui U, Elinson RP, et al: Lithium-induced respecification of pattern in *Xenopus laevic* embryos. Nature 322:371–373, 1986

Kaschka WP, Mokrusch T, Korth M: Early physiological effects of lithium treatment: electrooculographic and adaptometric findings in patients with affective and schizoaffective psychoses. Pharmacopsychiatry 20:203–207, 1987

Kato T, Inubushi I, Takahashi S: Relationship of lithium concentrations in the brain measured by lithium-7 magnetic resonance spectroscopy to treatment response in mania. J Clin Psychopharmacol 14:330–335, 1994

Katz RI, Kopin KJ: Release of ^{3}H-norepinephrine and ^{3}H-serotonin evoked from brain slices by electric field stimulation: calcium dependence and the effects of lithium and tetrodotoxin. Biochem Pharmacol 18:1935–1939, 1969

Katz RI, Chase TN, Kopin IJ: Evoked release of norepinephrine and serotonin from brain slices: inhibition by lithium. Science 162:466–467, 1968

Keck PE, McElroy SL, Nemeroff CB: Anticonvulsants in the treatment of bipolar disorder. J Neuropsychiatry Clin Neurosci 4:395–405, 1992

Keller MB, Lavori PW, Kane JM, et al: Subsyndromal symptoms in bipolar disorder: a comparison of standard and low serum levels of lithium. Arch Gen Psychiatry 49:317–376, 1992

Kendall DA, Nahorski SR: Acute and chronic lithium treatments influence agonist- and depolarization-stimulated inositol phospholipid hydrolysis in rat cerebral cortex. J Pharmacol Exp Ther 241:1023–1027, 1987

Kennedy ED, Challiss RJ, Nahorski SR: Lithium reduces the accumulation of inositol polyphosphate second messengers following cholinergic stimulation of cerebral cortex slices. J Neurochem 53:1652–1655, 1989

Kennedy ED, Challiss RAJ, Ragan CI, et al: Reduced inositol polyphosphate accumulation and inositol supply induced by lithium in stimulated cerebral cortex slices. Biochem J 267:781–786, 1990

Keynes RS, Swan RC: The permeability of frog muscle fibers to lithium ions. J Physiol (Lond) 147:626–638, 1959

Kishimoto A, Mikawa K, Hashimoto K, et al: Limited proteolysis of protein kinase C subspecies by calcium-dependent neutral protease (calpain). J Biol Chem 264:4088–4092, 1989

Klawans HL, Weiner WJ, Nausieda PA: The effect of lithium on an animal model of tardive dyskinesia. Prog Neuropsychopharmacol Biol Psychiatry 1:53–60, 1976

Klein PS, Melton DA: A molecular mechanism for the effect of lithium on development. Proc Natl Acad Sci U S A 93:8455–8459, 1996

Klemfuss H, Kripke DF: Effects of lithium on circadian rhythms, in Chronopharmacology, Cellular and Biochemical Interactions. Edited by Lemmer B. New York, Marcel Dekker, 1989, pp 281–297

Knapp S, Mandell AJ: Effects of lithium chloride on parameters of biosynthetic capacity for 5-hydroxytryptamine in rat brain. J Pharmacol Exp Ther 193:812–823, 1975

Kofman O, Belmaker RH: Biochemical, behavioral and clinical studies of the role of inositol in lithium treatment and depression. Biol Psychiatry 34:839–852, 1993

Kofman O, Belmaker RH, Grisaru N, et al: Myo-inositol attenuates two specific behavioral effects of acute lithium in rats. Psychopharmacol Bull 27:185–190, 1991

Komoroski RA, Newton JEO, Sprigg JR, et al: In vivo [7] Li nuclear magnetic resonance study of lithium pharmacokinetics and chemical shift imaging in psychiatric patients. Psychiatry Res 50:67–76, 1993

Koval MS, Rames LJ, Christie S: Diabetic ketoacidosis associated with clozapine treatment (letter). Am J Psychiatry 151:1520–1521, 1994

Krell RD, Goldberg AM: Effect of acute and chronic administration of lithium on steady-state levels of mouse brain choline and acetylcholine. Biochem Pharmacol 22:3289–3291, 1973

Kripke DF, Mullaney DJ, Atkinson M, et al: Circadian rhythm disorders in manic-depressives. Biol Psychiatry 13:335–351, 1978

Kripke DF, Judd LL, Hubbard B, et al: The effect of lithium carbonate on the circadian rhythm of sleep in normal human subjects. Biol Psychiatry 14:545–548, 1979

Kupfer DJ, Wyatt RJ, Greenspan K, et al: Lithium carbonate and sleep in affective illness. Arch Gen Psychiatry 23:35–40, 1970

Kupfer DJ, Reynolds CF III, Weiss BL, et al: Lithium carbonate and sleep in affective disorders. Arch Gen Psychiatry 30:79–84, 1974

Kuriyama K, Speken R: Effect of lithium on content and uptake of norepinephrine and 5-hydroxytryptamine in mouse brain synaptosomes and mitochondria. Life Sci 9:1213–1220, 1970

Kuroda T, Nishizuka Y: Limited proteolysis of protein kinase C subspecies by calcium-dependent neural protease (calpain). J Biol Chem 264:4088–4092, 1989

Laakso ML, Oja SS: Transport of tryptophan and tyrosine in rat brain slices in the presence of lithium. Neurochem Res 4:411–423, 1979

Lam RH, Christensen S: Regional and subcellular localization of Li+ and other cations in the rat brain following long-term lithium administration. J Neurochem 59:1372–1380, 1992

Lange C: Om Periodiske Depressionstilstande og deres Patogenese [About periodic depression and its pathogenesis]. Copenhagen, Jacob Lunds Forlag, 1886

Lauritsen BJ, Mellerup ET, Plenge P, et al: Serum lithium concentrations around the clock with different treatment regimens and the diurnal variation of the renal lithium clearance. Acta Psychiatr Scand 64:314–319, 1981

Lazarus JH: Endocrine and Metabolic Effects of Lithium. New York, Plenum, 1986

Lazarus JH, Muston LJ: The effect of lithium on the iodide concentrating mechanism in mouse salivary gland. Acta Pharmacologica et Toxicologica (Copenhagen) 43:55–58, 1978

Lecuona E, Luquin S, Avila J, et al: Expression of the beta 1 and beta 2 (AMOG) subunits of the Na, K-ATPase in neural tissues: cellular and developmental distribution patterns. Brain Res Bull 40:167–174, 1996

Lee G, Lingsch C, Lyle PT, et al: Lithium treatment strongly inhibits choline transport in human erythrocytes. Br J Clin Pharmacol 1:365–370, 1974

Leli U, Hauser G: Lithium modifies diacylglycerol levels and protein kinase C in neuroblastoma cells. Abstract presented at the 8th International Conference on Second Messengers and Phosphoproteins, Z187F, Glasgow, Scotland, August 3–6, 1992

Lenox RH: Role of receptor coupling to phosphoinositide metabolism in the therapeutic action of lithium, in Molecular Mechanisms of Neuronal Responsiveness (Adv Exp Biol Med). Edited by Ehrlich YH. New York, Plenum, 1987, pp 515–530

Lenox RH, Ellis J: Potential targets for the action of lithium in the brain: muscarinic receptor regulation. Clin Neuropharmacol 13 (suppl):215–216, 1990

Lenox RH, Manji HK: Lithium, in American Psychiatric Press Textbook of Psychopharmacology. Edited by Nemeroff CB, Schatzberg AF. Washington, DC, American Psychiatric Press, 1995, pp 303–350

Lenox RH, Watson DG: Targets for lithium action in the brain: protein kinase C substrates and muscarinic receptor regulation. Clin Neuropharmacol 15:612A–614A, 1992

Lenox RH, Watson DG: Lithium and the brain: a psychopharmacological strategy to a molecular basis for manic depressive illness. Clin Chem 40:309–314, 1994

Lenox RH, Watson DG, Ellis J: Muscarinic receptor regulation and protein kinase C: sites for the action of chronic lithium in the hippocampus. Psychopharmacol Bull 27:191–199, 1991

Lenox RH, Newhouse PA, Creelman WL, et al: Adjunctive treatment of manic agitation with lorazepam versus haloperidol: a double-blind study. J Clin Psychiatry 53:47–52, 1992a

Lenox RH, Watson DG, Patel J, et al: Chronic lithium administration alters a prominent PKC substrate in rat hippocampus. Brain Res 570: 333–340, 1992b

Lenox RH, McNamara RK, Watterson JM, et al: Myristoylated Alanine-Rich C Kinase Substrate (MARCKS): a molecular target for the therapeutic action of mood stabilizers in the brain? J Clin Psychiatry 57 (suppl 13):23–31, 1996

Lenox RH, McNamara RK, Papke RL, et al: Neurobiology of lithium: an update. J Clin Psychiatry (in press)

Lerer B, Stanley M: Effect of chronic lithium on cholinergically mediated responses and [^{3}H] QNB binding in rat brain. Brain Res 344: 211–219, 1985

Levy A, Zohar J, Belmaker RH: The effect of chronic lithium pretreatment on rat brain muscarinic receptor regulation. Neuropharmacology 21:1199–1201, 1983

Lewy AJ, Sack RL, Miller LS, et al: Antidepressant and circadian phase-shifting effects of light. Science 235:352–354, 1987

Li X, Jope RS: Selective inhibition of the expression of signal transduction proteins by lithium in nerve growth factor-differentiated PC12 cells. J Neurochem 65:2500–2508, 1995

Liles WC, Nathanson NM: Alteration in the regulation of neuronal muscarinic acetylcholine receptor number induces by chronic lithium in neuroblastoma cells. Brain Res 439:88–94, 1988

Linder D, Gschwendt M, Marks F: Phorbol ester-induced down-regulation of the 80-kDa myristoylated alanine-rich C-kinase substrate-related protein in Swiss 3T3 fibroblasts. J Biol Chem 267:24–26, 1992

Lindstedt G, Nilsson L, Walinder J, et al: On the prevalence, diagnosis and management of lithium-induced hypothyroidism in psychiatric patients. Br J Psychiatry 130:452–458, 1977

Lingsch C, Martin K: An irreversible effect of lithium administration to patients. Br J Pharmacol 57:323–327, 1976

Linnoila M, Karoum F, Rosenthal N, et al: Electroconvulsive treatment and lithium carbonate. Arch Gen Psychiatry 40:677–680, 1983

Lloyd KG, Morselli PL, Bartholini G: GABA and affective disorders. Medical Biology (Helsinki) 65:159–165, 1987

Lyman GH, Williams CC: Lithium attenuation of leukopenia associated with cancer chemotherapy, in Lithium and the Blood. Edited by Gallicchio VS. Basel, Switzerland, Karger, 1991, pp 30–45

Maggi A, Enna SJ: Regional alterations in rat brain neurotransmitter systems following chronic lithium treatment. J Neurochem 34:888–892, 1980

Maggs R: Treatment of manic illness with lithium carbonate. Br J Psychiatry 109:56–65, 1963

Mahan LC, Burch RM, Monsma FJ Jr, et al: Expression of striatal D_1 dopamine receptors coupled to inositol phosphate production and Ca^{2+} mobilization in Xenopus oocytes. Proc Natl Acad Sci U S A 87:2196–2200, 1990

Malik N, Canfield VA, Beckers MC, et al: Identification of the mammalian Na,K-ATPase subunit. J Biol Chem 271:22754–22758, 1996

Mallinger AG, Hanin I, Himmelhoch JM, et al: Stimulation of cell membrane sodium transport activity by lithium: possible relationship to therapeutic action. Psychiatry Res 22:49–59, 1987

Mandell AJ, Knapp S, Ehlers C, et al: The stability of constrained randomness: lithium prophylaxis at several neurobiological levels, in Neurobiology of Mood Disorders. Edited by Post RM, Ballenger JC. Baltimore, MD, Williams & Wilkins, 1984, pp 744–776

Manji HK: G proteins: implications for psychiatry. Am J Psychiatry 149:746–760, 1992

Manji HK, Lenox RH: Long-term action of lithium: a role for transcriptional and posttranscriptional factors regulated by protein kinase C. Synapse 16:11–28, 1994

Manji HK, Bitran JA, Masana MI, et al: Signal transduction modulation by lithium: cell culture, cerebral microdialysis and human studies. Psychopharmacol Bull 27:199–208, 1991a

Manji HK, Hsiao JK, Risby ED, et al: The mechanisms of action of lithium. Arch Gen Psychiatry 48:505–512, 1991b

Manji HK, Etcheberrigaray R, Chen G, et al: Lithium dramatically decreases membrane-associated PKC in the hippocampus: selectivity for the alpha isozyme. J Neurochem 61:2303–2310, 1993

Manji HK, Chen G, Shimon H, et al: Guanine nucleotide-binding proteins in bipolar affective disorder: effects of long-term lithium treatment. Arch Gen Psychiatry 52:135–144, 1995a

Manji HK, Potter WZ, Lenox RH: Signal transduction pathways: molecular targets for lithium's actions. Arch Gen Psychiatry 52:531–543, 1995b

Manji HK, Bersudsky Y, Chen G, et al: Modulation of protein kinase C isozymes and substrates by lithium: the role of myo-inositol. Neuropsychopharmacology 15:370–381, 1996a

Manji HK, Chen G, Hsiao JK, et al: Regulation of signal transduction pathways by mood-stabilizing agents: implications for the delayed onset of therapeutic efficacy. J Clin Psychiatry 13 (suppl 57):34–46, 1996b

Manji HK, McNamara RK, Lenox RH: Mechanisms of action of lithium in bipolar illness, in Hormones, Neurotransmitters and Affective Disorders. Edited by Halbreich U. (in press)

Mannisto PT: Endocrine side-effects of lithium, in Handbook of Lithium Therapy. Edited by Johnson FN. Baltimore, MD, University Park Press, 1980, pp 310–322

Marchbanks RM: The activation of presynaptic choline uptake by acetylcholine release. J Physiol (Paris) 78:373–378, 1982

Marshall MH, Neumann CP, Robinson M: Lithium, creativity, and manic-depressive illness: review and prospectus. Psychosomatics 11:406–488, 1970

Masana MI, Bitran JA, Hsiao JK, et al: In vivo evidence that lithium inactivates G_i modulation of adenylate cyclase in brain. J Neurochem 59:200–205, 1992

Maslanski JA, Leshko L, Busa WB: Lithium-sensitive production of inositol phosphates during amphibian embryonic mesoderm induction. Science 256:243–245, 1992

Mathe AA, Miller JC, Stenfors C: Chronic dietary lithium inhibits basal c-fos mRNA expression in rat brain. Prog Neuropsychopharmacol Biol Psychiatry 19:1177–1187, 1995

McElroy SL, Keck PE, Pope HG, et al: Valproate in the treatment of bipolar disorder: literature review and clinical guidelines. J Clin Psychopharmacol 12:42S–52S, 1992

McHenry CR, Rosen IB, Rotstein LE, et al: Lithiumogenic disorders of the thyroid and parathyroid glands as surgical disease. Surgery 108:1001–1005, 1990

Mellerup ET, Dam H, Wildschiotz G, et al: Diurnal variation of blood glucose during lithium treatment. J Affect Disord 5:341–347, 1983

Meltzer HY, Lowy MT: The serotonin hypothesis of depression, in Psychopharmacology: The Third Generation of Progress. Edited by Meltzer HY. New York, Raven, 1987, pp 513–526

Meltzer HL, Kassir S, Dunner DL, et al: Repression of a lithium pump as a consequence of lithium ingestion by manic-depressive subjects. Psychopharmacology (Berl) 54:113–118, 1982

Mendels J, Chernik DA: The effect of lithium carbonate on the sleep of depressed patients. International Pharmacopsychiatry 8:184–192, 1973

Mendels J, Frazer A: Intracellular lithium concentration and clinical response: towards a membrane theory of depression. J Psychiatr Res 10:9–18, 1973

Mester R, Toren P, Mizrachi I, et al: Caffeine withdrawal increases lithium blood levels. Biol Psychiatry 37:348–350, 1995

Miller BL, Jenden DJ, Tang C, et al: Factors influencing erythrocyte choline concentrations. Life Sci 44:477–482, 1989

Miller BL, Lin KM, Djenderedjian A, et al: Changes in red blood cell choline and choline-bound lipids with oral lithium. Experientia 46:454–456, 1990

Mitchell JE, MacKenzie TB: Cardiac effects of lithium therapy in man: a review. J Clin Psychiatry 43:47–51, 1982

Miyauchi T, Okiawa S, Kitada Y: Effects of lithium chloride on the cholinergic system in different brain regions in mice. Biochem Pharmacol 29:654–657, 1980

Moore GJ, Bebchuk JM, Manji HK: Proton MRS in manic depressive illness: monitoring of lithium-induced brain myo-inositol (abstract). Abstracts of the Society of Neuroscience 27th Annual Meeting. New Orleans, LA, October 1997

Morgan JI, Curran T: Stimulus-transcription coupling in the nervous system: involvement of the inducible proto-oncogenes fos and jun. Annu Rev Neurosci 14:421–451, 1991

Mori M, Tajima K, Oda Y, et al: Inhibitory effect of lithium on the release of thyroid hormones from thyrotropin-stimulated mouse thyroids in a perifusion system. Endocrinology 124:1365–1369, 1989

Mori S, Zanardi R, Popoli M, et al: Inhibitory effect of lithium on cAMP dependent phosphorylation system. Life Sci 59:PL99–PL104, 1996

Mork A, Geisler A: Mode of action of lithium on the catalytic unit of adenylate cyclase from rat brain. Pharmacol Toxicol 60:241–248, 1987

Mork A, Geisler A: Effects of GTP on hormone-stimulated adenylate cyclase activity in cerebral cortex, striatum, and hippocampus from rats treated chronically with lithium. Biol Psychiatry 26:279–288, 1989a

Mork A, Geisler A: Effects of lithium ex vivo on the GTP-mediated inhibition of calcium-stimulated adenylate cyclase activity in rat brain. Eur J Pharmacol 168:347–354, 1989b

Mork A, Geisler A: The effects of lithium in vitro and ex vivo on adenylate cyclase in brain are exerted by distinct mechanisms. Neuropharmacology 28:307–311, 1989c

Mork A, Geisler A: Effects of chronic lithium treatment on agonist-enhanced extracellular concentrations of cyclic AMP in the dorsal hippocampus of freely moving rats. J Neurochem 65:134–139, 1995

Mork A, Klysner R, Geisler A: Effects of treatment with a lithium-imipramine combination on components of adenylate cyclase in the cerebral cortex of the rat. Neuropharmacology 29:261–267, 1990

Mota de Freitas DE, Espanol MT, Dorus E: Lithium transport in red blood cells of bipolar patients, in Lithium and the Blood. Edited by Gallicchio VS. Farmington, CT, Karger, 1991, pp 96–120

Mukherjee BP, Bailey PT, Pradhan SN: Temporal and regional differences in brain concentrations of lithium in rats. Psychopharmacology 48:119–121, 1976

Muller-Oerlinghausen B, Ahrens B, Volk J, et al: Reduced mortality of manic-depressive patients in long-term lithium treatment: an international collaborative study by IGSLI. Psychiatry Res 36:329–331, 1991

Munzer JS, Daly SE, Jewell-Motz EA, et al: Tissue- and isoform-specific kinetic behavior of the Na,K-ATPase. J Biol Chem 269:16668–16676, 1994

Murphy DL, Donnelly C, Moskowitz J: Inhibition by lithium of prostaglandin E1 and norepinephrine effects on cyclic adenosine monophosphate production in human platelets. Clin Pharmacol Ther 14:810–814, 1974

Murphy DL, Lake CR, Slater S, et al: Psychoactive drug effects on plasma norepinephrine and plasma dopamine beta-hydroxylase in man, in Catecholamines: Basic and Clinical Frontiers. Edited by Usdin E, Kopin IJ, Barchas J. New York, Pergamon, 1979, pp 918–920

Myers DH, Carter RA, Burns BH, et al: A prospective study of the effects of lithium on thyroid function and on the prevalence of antithyroid antibodies. Psychol Med 15:55–61, 1985

Nahorski SR, Ragan CI, Challiss RAJ: Lithium and the phosphoinositide cycle: an example of uncompetitive inhibition and its pharmacological consequences. Trends Pharmacol Sci 12:297–303, 1991

Nahorski SR, Jenkinson S, Challiss RA: Disruption of phosphoinositide signalling by lithium. Biochem Soc Trans 20:430–434, 1992

Naylor GJ, McHarg A: Profound hypothermia on combined lithium carbonate and diazepam treatment (letter). BMJ 2:22, 1977

Naylor GJ, Smith AHW: Defective genetic control of sodium-pump density in manic depressive psychosis. Psychol Med 11:257–263, 1981

Naylor GJ, Dick DAT, Dick EG, et al: Erythrocyte membrane cation carrier in mania. Psychol Med 6:659–663, 1974a

Naylor GJ, Dick DAT, Dick EG, et al: Lithium therapy and erythrocyte membrane cation carrier. Psychopharmacologia 37:81–86, 1974b

Naylor GJ, Smith AHW, Dick EG, et al: Erythrocyte membrane cation carrier in manic-depressive psychosis. Psychol Med 10:521–525, 1980

Nelson SC, Herman MM, Bensch KG, et al: Localization and quantitation of lithium in rat tissue following intraperitoneal injections of lithium chloride, II: brain. J Pharmacol Exp Ther 212:11–15, 1980

Nemeroff CB: Neuropeptides and Psychiatric Disorders. Washington, DC, American Psychiatric Press, 1991

Newman ME, Belmaker RH: Effects of lithium in vitro and ex vivo on components of the adenylate cyclase system in membranes from the cerebral cortex of the rat. Neuropharmacology 26:211–217, 1987

Newman M, Klein E, Birmaher B, et al: Lithium at therapeutic concentrations inhibits human brain noradrenaline sensitive cyclic AMP accumulation. Brain Res 278:380–381, 1983

Nilsson A: The anti-aggressive actions of lithium. Reviews in Contemporary Pharmacotherapy 4:269–285, 1993

Nishizuka Y: Intracellular signaling by hydrolysis of phospholipids and activation of protein kinase C. Science 258:607–614, 1992

Nishizuka Y: Protein kinase C and lipid signaling for sustained cellular responses. FASEB J 17:484–496, 1995

Nora JJ, Nora AH, Toews WH: Lithium, Ebstein's anomaly and other congenital heart defects. Lancet 1:594–595, 1974

Nordenstrom J, Strigard K, Perbeck L, et al: Hyperparathyroidism associated with treatment of manic-depressive disorders by lithium. Eur J Surg 158:207–211, 1992

Nurnberger J Jr, Jimerson DC, Allen JR, et al: Red cell ouabain-sensitive Na^+-K^+-adenosine triphosphatase: a state marker in affective disorder inversely related to plasma cortisol. Biol Psychiatry 17:981–992, 1982

Ormandy G, Jope RS: Analysis of the convulsant-potentiating effects of lithium in rats. Exp Neurol 111:356–361, 1991

Perry P, Tsuang MT: Treatment of unipolar depression following electroconvulsive therapy: relapse rate comparisons between lithium and tricyclics therapies following ECT. J Affect Disord 1:123–129, 1979

Persinger MA, Makarec K, Bradley JC: Characteristics of limbic seizures evoked by peripheral injections of lithium and pilocarpine. Physiol Behav 44:27–37, 1988

Pert A, Rosenblatt JE, Sivit C, et al: Long-term treatment with lithium prevents the development of dopamine receptor supersensitivity. Science 201:171–173, 1978

Pert CB, Pert A, Rosenblatt JE, et al: Catecholamine receptor stabilization: a possible mode of lithium's antimanic action, in Catecholamines: Basic and Clinical Frontiers. Edited by Usdin E, Kopin IJ, Barchas JD. New York, Pergamon, 1979, pp 583–585

Peselow ED, Dunner DL, Fieve RR, et al: Lithium carbonate and weight gain. J Affect Disord 2:303–310, 1980

Peterson GA, Byrd SL: Diabetic ketoacidosis from clozapine and lithium cotreatment (letter). Am J Psychiatry 153:737–738, 1996

Plenge P, Stensgaard A, Jensen HV, et al: 24-Hour lithium concentration in human brain studied by Li-7 magnetic resonance spectroscopy. Biol Psychiatry 36:511–516, 1994

Poirier-Littre MF, Loo H, Dennis T, et al: Lithium treatment increases norepinephrine turnover in the plasma of healthy subjects (letter). Arch Gen Psychiatry 50:72–73, 1993

Poitou P, Bohuon C: Catecholamine metabolism in the rat brain after short and long term lithium administration. J Neurochem 25:535–537, 1975

Pontzer NJ, Crews FT: Desensitization of muscarinic stimulated hippocampal cell firing is related to phosphoinositide hydrolysis and inhibited by lithium. J Pharmacol Exp Ther 253:921–929, 1990

Post RM: Transduction of psychosocial stress into the neurobiology of recurrent affective disorder. Am J Psychiatry 149:999–1010, 1992

Post RM, Stoddard FJ, Gillin JC, et al: Alterations in motor activity, sleep, and biochemistry in a cycling manic-depressive patient. Arch Gen Psychiatry 34:470–477, 1977

Post RM, Ballenger JC, Hare TA, et al: Cerebrospinal fluid GABA in normals and patients with affective disorders. Brain Res Bull 5 (suppl 2):755–759, 1980a

Post RM, Jimerson DC, Bunney WE Jr, et al: Dopamine and mania: behavioral and biochemical effects of the dopamine receptor blocker pimozide. Psychopharmacology (Berl) 67:297–305, 1980b

Post RM, Leverich GS, Altshuler L, et al: Lithium-discontinuation-induced refractoriness: preliminary observations. Am J Psychiatry 149:1727–1729, 1992

Price LH: Antidepressants, in Depression and Mania: Modern Lithium Therapy. Edited by Johnson FN. Oxford, England, IRL Press, 1987, pp 161–166

Price LH: Lithium augmentation in tricyclic-resistant depression, in Treatment of Tricyclic-Resistant Depression. Edited by Extein IL. Washington, DC, American Psychiatric Press, 1989, pp 49–79

Price LH, Charney DS, Delgado PL, et al: Lithium and serotonin function: implications for the serotonin hypothesis of depression. Psychopharmacology (Berl) 100:3–12, 1990

Prien RF, Caffey EM Jr, Klett CJ: Comparison of lithium carbonate and chlorpromazine in the treatment of mania: report of the Veterans Administration and National Institute of Mental Health Collaborative Study Group. Arch Gen Psychiatry 26:146–153, 1972

Ramaprasad S, Newton JE, Cardwell D, et al: In vivo ^{7}Li NMR imaging and localized spectroscopy of rat brain. Magn Reson Med 25:308–318, 1992

Ramsey TA, Frazer A, Mendels J, et al: The erythrocyte lithium-plasma lithium ratio in patients with primary affective disorder. Arch Gen Psychiatry 36:457–461, 1979

Rana RS, Hokin LE: Role of phosphoinositides in transmembrane signaling. Physiol Rev 70:115–164, 1990

Rao ML, Mager T: Influence of the pineal gland on the pituitary function in humans. Psychoendocrinology 12:141–147, 1987

Reddy PL, Khanna S, Subhash MN, et al: Erythrocyte membrane Na-K ATPase activity in affective disorder. Biol Psychiatry 26:533–537, 1989

Reisine T, Zatz M: Interactions between lithium, calcium, diacylglycerides and phorbol esters in the regulation of ACTH release from AtT-20 cells. J Neurochem 49:884–889, 1987

Richelson E, Snyder K, Carlson J, et al: Lithium ion transport in erythrocytes of randomly selected blood donors and manic-depressive patients: lack of association with affective illness. Am J Psychiatry 143:457–462, 1986

Riddell FG: Studies on Li$^+$ transport using ^{7}Li and ^{6}Li nuclear magnetic resonance, in Lithium and the Cell. Edited by Birch NJ. San Diego, CA, Academic Press, 1991, pp 85–98

Riedl U, Barocka A, Kolem H, et al: Duration of lithium treatment and brain lithium concentration in patients with unipolar and schizoaffective disorder—a study with magnetic resonance spectroscopy. Biol Psychiatry 41:844–850, 1997

Risby ED, Hsiao JK, Manji HK, et al: The mechanisms of action of lithium. Arch Gen Psychiatry 48:513–524, 1991

Roberts DE, Berman SM, Nakasato S, et al: Effect of lithium carbonate on zidovudine-associated neutropenia in the acquired immunodeficiency syndrome. Am J Med 85:428–431, 1988

Rogers M, Whybrow P: Clinical hypothyroidism occurring during lithium treatment: two case histories and a review of thyroid function in 19 patients. Am J Psychiatry 128:150–155, 1971

Ronai AZ, Vizi SE: The effect of lithium treatment on the acetylcholine content of rat brain. Biochem Pharmacol 24:1819–1820, 1975

Rooney TA, Nahorski SR: Regional characterization of agonist and depolarization-induced phosphoinositide hydrolysis in rat brain. J Pharmacol Exp Ther 239:873–880, 1986

Roose SP, Bone S, Haidorfer C, et al: Lithium treatment in older patients. Am J Psychiatry 136:843–844, 1979

Rosenblatt JE, Pert CB, Tallman JF, et al: The effect of imipramine and lithium on alpha- and beta-receptor binding in rat brain. Brain Res 160:186–191, 1979

Rosenblatt JE, Pert A, Layton B, et al: Chronic lithium reduced ^{3}H-spiroperidol binding in rat striatum. Eur J Pharmacol 67:321–322, 1980

Ross DR, Coffey CE: Neuroleptics and anxiolytics, in Depression and Mania: Modern Lithium Therapy. Edited by Johnson FN. Oxford, England, IRL Press, 1987, pp 167–171

Rudorfer MV, Linnoila M: Electroconvulsive therapy, in Lithium Combination Treatment. Edited by Johnson FN. Basel, Switzerland, Karger, 1987, pp 164–178

Rybakowski J, Frazer A, Mendels J: Lithium efflux from erythrocytes incubated in vitro during lithium carbonate administration. Communications in Psychopharmacology 2:105–112, 1978

Sahin-Erdemli I, Medford RM, Songu-Mize E: Regulation of Na⁺,K(+)-ATPase alpha-subunit isoforms in rat tissues during hypertension. Eur J Pharmacol 292:163–171, 1995

Sander G, Di Scala G, Oberling P, et al: Distribution of lithium in the rat brain after a single administration known to elicit aversive effects. Neurosci Lett 166:1–4, 1994

Sansone MEG, Ziegler DK: Lithium toxicity: a review of neurologic complications. Clin Neuropharmacol 8:242–248, 1985

Sarkadi B, Alifimoff JK, Gunn RB, et al: Kinetics and stoichiometry of Na-dependent Li transport in human red blood cells. J Gen Physiol 72:249–265, 1978

Sarri E, Picatoste F, Claro E: Neurotransmitter specific profiles of inositol phosphates in rat brain cortex: relation to the mode of receptor activation of phosphoinositide phospholipase C. J Pharmacol Exp Ther 272:77–84, 1995

Savolainen KM, Hirvonen MR, Tarhanen J, et al: Changes in cerebral inosito-1-phosphate concentrations in LiCl-treated rats: regional and strain differences. Neurochem Res 15:541–545, 1990

Schatzberg AF, Cole JO: Manual of Clinical Psychopharmacology, 2nd Edition. Washington, DC, American Psychiatric Press, 1991

Schildkraut JJ: The effects of lithium on norepinephrine turnover and metabolism: basic and clinical studies, in Lithium: Its Role in Psychiatric Research and Treatment. Edited by Gershon S, Shopsin B. New York, Plenum, 1973, pp 51–73

Schildkraut JJ: The effects of lithium on norepinephrine turnover and metabolism: basic and clinical studies. J Nerv Ment Dis 158:348–360, 1974

Schildkraut JJ, Logue MA, Dodge GA: The effect of lithium salts on the turnover and metabolism of norepinephrine in rat brain. Psychopharmacologia 14:135–141, 1969

Schildkraut JJ, Keeler BA, Grob EL, et al: MHPG excretion and clinical classification in depressive disorders. Lancet 1:1251–1252, 1973

Schou M: Lithium in psychiatric therapy and prophylaxis. J Psychiatr Res 6:67–95, 1968

Schou M: Artistic productivity and lithium prophylaxis in manic-depressive illness. Br J Psychiatry 135:97–103, 1979a

Schou M: Lithium research at the Psychopharmacology Research Unit, Risskov, Denmark: a historical account, in Origin, Prevention and Treatment of Affective Disorders. Edited by Schou M, Stromgren E. London, Academic Press, 1979b, pp 1–8

Schou M: Use in other psychiatric conditions, in Depression and Mania: Modern Lithium Therapy. Edited by Johnson FN. Oxford, England, IRL Press, 1987, pp 44–50

Schou M: Lithium Treatment of Manic-Depressive Illness, 4th Edition, Revised. Basel, Switzerland, Karger, 1989

Schou M: Clinical aspects of lithium in psychiatry, in Lithium and the Cell. Edited by Birch NJ. London, Academic Press, 1991, pp 1–6

Schou M, Juel-Neilsen N, Stromberg E, et al: The treatment of manic psychoses by the administration of lithium salts. J Neurol Neurosurg Psychiatry 17:250–260, 1954

Schou M, Goldfield MD, Weinstein MR, et al: Lithium and pregnancy, I: report from the Register of Lithium Babies. BMJ 2:135–136, 1973

Schou M, Amdisen A, Thomsen K, et al: Lithium treatment regimen and renal water handling: the significance of dosage pattern and tablet type examined through comparison of results from two clinics with different treatment regimens. Psychopharmacology (Berl) 77:387–390, 1982

Schou M, Hansen HE, Thomsen K, et al: Lithium treatment in Aarhus, 2: risk of renal failure and of intoxication. Pharmacopsychiatry 22:101–103, 1989

Schultz JE, Siggins GR, Schocker FW, et al: Effects of prolonged treatment with lithium and tricyclic antidepressants on discharge frequency, norepinephrine responses and beta receptor binding in rat cerebellum: electrophysiological and biochemical comparison. J Pharmacol Exp Ther 216:28–38, 1981

Seeger TF, Gardner EL, Bridger WF: Increase in mesolimbic electrical self-stimulation after chronic haloperidol: reversal by L-dopa or lithium. Brain Res 215:404–409, 1981

Seggie J, Carney PA, Parker J, et al: Effect of chronic lithium on sensitivity to light in male and female bipolar patients. Prog Neuropsychopharmacol Biol Psychiatry 13:543–549, 1989

Sengupta N, Datta SC, Sengupta D, et al: Platelet and erythrocyte membrane ATPase activity in depression and mania. Psychiatry Res 3: 337–344, 1980

Sharp T, Bramwell SR, Lambert P, et al: Effect of short- and long-term administration of lithium on the release of endogenous 5-HT in the hippocampus of the rat in vivo and in vitro. Neuropharmacology 30:977–984, 1991

Sheng M, Greenberg ME: The regulation and function of c-fos and other immediate early genes in the nervous system. Neuron 4:477–485, 1990

Sherman WR: Lithium and the phosphoinositide signalling system, in Lithium and the Cell. Edited by Birch NJ. London, Academic Press, 1991, pp 121–157

Sherman WR, Munsell LY, Gish BG, et al: Effects of systemically administered lithium on phosphoinositide metabolism in rat brain, kidney, and testis. J Neurochem 44:798–807, 1985

Sherman WR, Gish BG, Honchar MP, et al: Effects of lithium on phosphoinositide metabolism in vivo. Federation Proceedings 45:2639–2646, 1986

Shopsin B, Kim SS, Gershon S: A controlled study of lithium vs. chlorpromazine in acute schizophrenics. Br J Psychiatry 119:435–440, 1971

Shukla GS: Combined lithium and valproate treatment and subsequent withdrawal: serotonergic mechanism of their interaction in discrete brain regions. Prog Neuropsychopharmacol Biol Psychiatry 9:153–156, 1985

Simon JR, Kuhar MJ: High affinity choline uptake: ionic and energy requirement. J Neurochem 27:93–99, 1976

Skinner GR, Hartley C, Buchan A, et al: The effect of lithium chloride on the replication of herpes simplex virus. Med Microbiol Immunol (Berl) 168:139–148, 1980

Smith DF: Lithium attenuates clonidine-induced hypoactivity: further studies in inbred mouse strains. Psychopharmacology (Berl) 94: 428–430, 1988

Smith DF, Amdisen A: Lithium distribution in rat brain after long-term central administration by minipump. J Pharm Pharmacol 33:805–806, 1981

Solomon DA, Ristow WR, Keller MB, et al: Serum lithium levels and psychosocial function in patients with bipolar I disorder. Am J Psychiatry 153:1301–1307, 1996

Song L, Jope R: Chronic lithium treatment impairs phosphatidylinositol hydrolysis in membranes from rat brain regions. J Neurochem 58: 2200–2206, 1992

Spengler RN, Hollingsworth PJ, Smith CB: Effects of long-term lithium and desipramine treatment upon clonidine-induced inhibition of ^{3}H-norepinephrine release from rat hippocampal slices (abstract). Federation Proceedings 45:681, 1986

Spiegel AM, Rudorfer MV, Marx SJ, et al: The effect of short term lithium administration on suppressibility of parathyroid hormone secretion by calcium in vivo. J Clin Endocrinol Metab 59:354–357, 1984

Spirtes MA: Lithium levels in monkey and human brain after chronic, therapeutic oral dosage. Pharmacol Biochem Behav 5:143–147, 1976

Stabel S, Parker PJ: Protein kinase C. Pharmacol Ther 51:71–95, 1991

Stachel SE, Grunwald DJ, Myers PZ, et al: Lithium perturbation and goosecoid expression identify a dorsal specification pathway in the pregastrula zebrafish. Development 117:1261–1274, 1993

Staunton DA, Magistretti PJ, Shoemaker WJ, et al: Effects of chronic lithium treatment on dopamine receptors in the rat corpus striatum, I: locomotor activity and behavioral supersensitivity. Brain Res 232:391–400, 1982a

Staunton DA, Magistretti PJ, Shoemaker WJ, et al: Effects of chronic lithium treatment on dopamine receptors in the rat corpus striatum, II: no effect on denervation or neuroleptic-induced supersensitivity. Brain Res 232:401–412, 1982b

Stern DN, Fieve RR, Neff NH, et al: The effect of lithium chloride administration on brain and heart norepinephrine turnover rates. Psychopharmacologia 14:315–322, 1969

Stoll AL, Cohen BM, Snyder MB, et al: Erythrocyte choline concentration in bipolar disorder: a predictor of clinical course and medication response. Biol Psychiatry 29:1171–1180, 1991

Strzyzewski W, Rybakowski J, Potok E, et al: Erythrocyte cation transport in endogenous depression: clinical and psychophysiological correlates. Acta Psychiatr Scand 70:248–253, 1984

Suppes T, Baldessarini RJ, Faedda GL, et al: Risk of recurrence following discontinuation of lithium treatment in bipolar disorder. Arch Gen Psychiatry 48:1082–1088, 1991

Suppes T, Baldessarini RJ, Faedda GL, et al: Discontinuation of maintenance treatment in bipolar disorder: risks and implications. Harvard Reviews in Psychiatry 1:131–144, 1993

Swann AC: Caloric intake and (Na⁺,K⁺)-ATPase: differential regulation by alpha-1 and beta noradrenergic receptors. Am J Physiol 247:R449–R455, 1984

Swann AC: Norepinephrine and (Na⁺,K⁺)-ATPase: evidence for stabilization by lithium or imipramine. Neuropharmacology 27:261–267, 1988

Swann AC, Heninger GR, Roth RH, et al: Differential effects of short and long term lithium on tryptophan uptake and serotonergic function in cat brain. Life Sci 28:347–354, 1981

Swann AC, Koslow SH, Katz MM, et al: Lithium carbonate treatment of mania. Arch Gen Psychiatry 44:345–354, 1987

Swerdlow NR, Lee D, Koob GF, et al: Effects of chronic dietary lithium on behavioral indices of dopamine denervation supersensitivity in the rat. J Pharmacol Exp Ther 235:324–329, 1985

Szentistvanyi I, Janka Z: Correlation between lithium ratio and Na-dependent Li transport in red blood cells during lithium prophylaxis. Biol Psychiatry 14:973–977, 1979

Tagliamonte A, Tagliamonte P, Perez-Cruet J, et al: Effect of psychotropic drugs on tryptophan concentration in the rat brain. J Pharmacol Exp Ther 177:475–480, 1971

Tanaka C, Nishizuka Y: The protein kinase C family for neuronal signaling. Annu Rev Neurosci 17:551–567, 1994

Tanimoto K, Maeda K, Terada T: Inhibitory effect of lithium on neuroleptic and serotonin receptors in rat brain. Brain Res 265:148–151, 1983

Taylor JW, Bell AJ: Lithium-induced parathyroid dysfunction: a case report and review of the literature. Ann Pharmacother 27:1040–1043, 1993

Terry JB, Padzernik TL, Nelson SR: Effect of LiCl pretreatment on cholinomimetic-induced seizures and seizure-induced brain edema in rats. Neurosci Lett 114:123–127, 1990

Thellier M, Heurteaux C, Wissocq JC: Quantitative study of the distribution of lithium in the mouse brain for various doses of lithium given to the animal. Brain Res 199:175–197, 1980a

Thellier M, Wissocq JC, Heurteaux C: Quantitative microlocation of lithium in the brain by a (n,alpha) nuclear reaction. Nature 283:299–302, 1980b

Tilkian AG, Schroder JS, Kao J, et al: Effect of lithium on cardiovascular performance: report on extended ambulatory monitoring and exercise testing before and during lithium therapy. Am J Cardiol 38:701–708, 1976

Tohen M, Tollefson GD: Atypical antipsychotic agents in mania: clinical studies, in Bipolar Medications: Mechanisms of Action. Edited by Manji HK, Bowden CL, Belmaker RH. Washington, DC, American Psychiatric Press, 2000, pp 375–388

Tollefson GD, Senogles S: A cholinergic role in the mechanism of lithium in mania. Biol Psychiatry 18:467–479, 1982

Treiser S, Kellar KJ: Lithium effects on adrenergic receptor supersensitivity in rat brain. Eur J Pharmacol 58:85–86, 1979

Treiser SL, Cascio CS, O'Donohue TL, et al: Lithium increases serotonin release and decreases serotonin receptors in the hippocampus. Science 213:1529–1531, 1981

Tricklebank MD, Singh L, Jackson A, et al: Evidence that a proconvulsant action of lithium is mediated by inhibition of myo-inositol phosphatase in mouse brain. Brain Res 558:145–148, 1991

Trousseau A: Clinique Medicale de l'Hôtel-Dieu de Paris, 3rd Edition. Paris, France, JB Balliere et Fils, 1868

Tseng FY, Pasquali D, Field JB: Effects of lithium on stimulated metabolic parameters in dog thyroid slices. Acta Endocrinol (Copenh) 121:615–620, 1989

Uney JB, Marchbanks RM, Marsh A: The effect of lithium on choline transport in human erythrocytes. J Neurol Neurosurg Psychiatry 48:229–233, 1985

Urabe M, Hershman JM, Pang XP, et al: Effect of lithium on function and growth of thyroid cells in vitro. Endocrinology 129:807–814, 1991

Ure A: Researches on gout. Medical Times 11:145, 1844/1845

Vallar L, Muca C, Magni M, et al: Differential coupling of dopaminergic receptors expressed in different cell types: stimulation of phosphatidylinositol 4,5-bisphosphate hydrolysis in LtK-fibroblasts, hyperpolarization, and cytosolic-free Ca^{2+} concentration decrease in GH_4Cl cells. J Biol Chem 265:10320–10326, 1990

van Kammen DP, Docherty JP, Marder SR, et al: Lithium attenuates the activation-euphoria but not the psychosis induced by d-amphetamine in schizophrenia. Psychopharmacology (Berl) 87:111–115, 1985

Varney MA, Godfrey PP, Drummond AH, et al: Chronic lithium treatment inhibits basal and agonist-stimulated responses in rat cerebral cortex and GH_3 pituitary cells. Mol Pharmacol 4:671–678, 1992

Verimer T, Goodale DB, Long JP, et al: Lithium effects on haloperidol-induced pre- and postsynaptic dopamine receptor supersensitivity. J Pharm Pharmacol 32:665–666, 1980

Vestergaard P, Aagaard J: Five-year mortality in lithium-treated manic-depressive patients. J Affect Disord 21:33–38, 1991

Vestergaard P, Poulstrup I, Schou M: Prospective studies on a lithium cohort, 3: tremor, weight gain, diarrhea, psychological complaints. Acta Psychiatr Scand 78:434–441, 1988

Walker E, Green M: Soft signs of neurological dysfunction in schizophrenia: an investigation of lateral performance. Biol Psychiatry 17:381–386, 1982

Walker RG: Lithium nephrotoxicity. Kidney Int 44 (suppl 42):S93–S98, 1993

Wang HY, Friedman E: Lithium inhibition of protein kinase C activation-induced serotonin release. Psychopharmacology (Berl) 99:213–218, 1989

Watson DG, Lenox RH: Chronic lithium-induced down-regulation of MARCKS in immortalized hippocampal cells: potentiation by muscarinic receptor activation. J Neurochem 67:767–777, 1996

Watson SP, Shipman L, Godfrey PP: Lithium potentiates agonist formation of [^{3}H]CDP-diacylglycerol in human platelets. Eur J Pharmacol 188:273–276, 1990

Wehr TA: Phase and biorhythm studies in affective illness. Ann Intern Med 87:319–335, 1977

Wehr TA, Goodwin FK: Rapid cycling in manic-depressives induced by tricyclic antidepressants. Arch Gen Psychiatry 36:555–559, 1979

Wehr TA, Goodwin FK: Can antidepressants cause mania and worsen the course of affective illness? Am J Psychiatry 144:1403–1411, 1987

Wehr TA, Sack DA, Rosenthal NE: Sleep reduction as a final common pathway in the genesis of mania. Am J Psychiatry 144:201–204, 1987

Weiner ED, Kalaaspudi VD, Papolos DF, et al: Lithium augments pilocarpine-induced fos gene expression in brain. Brain Res 553:117–122, 1991

Werstiuk ES, Steiner M: Anti-psychotics, II: butyrophenones, in Lithium Combination Treatment. Edited by Johnson FN. Basel, Switzerland, Karger, 1987, pp 84–104

Wever RA: The Circadian System of Man. New York, Springer-Verlag, 1979

Whitworth P, Kendall DA: Lithium selectively inhibits muscarinic receptor-stimulated inositol tetrakisphosphate accumulation in mouse cerebral cortex slices. J Neurochem 51:258–265, 1988

Whitworth P, Kendall DA: Effects of lithium on inositol phospholipid hydrolysis and inhibition of dopamine D_1 receptor-mediated cyclic AMP formation by carbachol in rat brain slices. J Neurochem 53:536–541, 1989

Wolff J, Berens SC, Jones AB: Inhibition of thyrotropin-stimulated adenylyl cyclase activity of beef thyroid membranes by low concentration of lithium ion. Biochem Biophys Res Commun 39:77–82, 1970

Wood AJ, Goodwin GM: A review of the biochemical and neuropharmacological actions of lithium. Psychol Med 17:579–600, 1987

Wood AJ, Elphick M, Aronson JK, et al: The effect of lithium on cation transport measured in vivo in patients suffering from bipolar affective illness. Br J Psychiatry 155:504–510, 1989a

Wood AJ, Elphick M, Grahame-Smith DG: Effect of lithium and of other drugs used in the treatment of manic illness on the cation-transporting properties of Na⁺,K⁺-ATPase in mouse brain synaptosomes. J Neurochem 52:1042–1049, 1989b

Wood K, Swade C, Abou-Saleh MT, et al: Apparent supersensitivity of platelet 5-HT receptors in lithium-treated patients. J Affect Disord 8:69–72, 1985

Yamaki M, Kusano E, Tetsuka T, et al: Cellular mechanism of lithium-induced nephrogenic diabetes insipidus in rats. Am J Physiol 261:F505–F511, 1991

Young S, Parker PJ, Ullrich A, et al: Down-regulation of protein kinase C is due to an increased rate of degradation. Biochem J 24:775–779, 1987

Yuan PX, Chen G, Granneman GJ, et al: Increase in the expression of AP-1 regulated genes in brain by the mood stabilizing agents lithium and valproic acid (abstract). Abstracts of the Society of Neuroscience 27th Annual Meeting. New Orleans, LA, October 1997

Zalstein E, Koren G, Einarson T, et al: A case-control study on the association between first trimester exposure to lithium and Ebstein's anomaly. Am J Cardiol 65:817–818, 1990

Zatz M, Reisine TD: Lithium induces corticotropin secretion and desensitization in cultured anterior pituitary cells. Proc Natl Acad Sci U S A 82:1286–1290, 1985

Zerahn K: Studies on the active transport of lithium in the isolated frog skin. Acta Physiol Scand 33:347–358, 1955

TWELVE

Antiepileptic Drugs

Paul E. Keck Jr., M.D., and
Susan L. McElroy, M.D.

An increasing number of studies performed over the past several decades has shown that many drugs with antiepileptic properties are effective in the acute and prophylactic treatment of some patients with bipolar disorder, including those whose disorder inadequately responds to, and those who are intolerant of, treatment with lithium. These antiepileptic agents include a number of standard agents (e.g., carbamazepine and valproate), the investigational antiepileptic oxcarbazepine, and the benzodiazepines clonazepam and lorazepam (Keck et al. 1992; McElroy and Pope 1988; McElroy et al. 1992b; Post 1988, 1990; Post et al. 1991; Prien and Gelenberg 1989).

In this chapter, we review the pharmacology of carbamazepine and valproate and the research supporting their efficacy in the treatment of bipolar disorder. We also summarize research examining the efficacy of benzodiazepines and other antiepileptic agents in the treatment of bipolar disorder. In addition, we address issues such as predictors of response, use of these agents in combination with other psychotropics, and antiepileptic resistance.

CARBAMAZEPINE

History and Discovery

Carbamazepine was developed in the late 1950s in the laboratories of J. R. Geigy, AG, in Basel, Switzerland. Its synthesis was described by Schindler in 1961, its antiepileptic properties were first reported by Theobald and Kunz in 1963, and its efficacy in patients with epilepsy and paroxysmal pain syndromes was first demonstrated in Europe in the early 1960s (Kutt 1989; Levy et al. 1989; Loiseau and Duche 1989; Rall and Schleifer 1985). In the early 1960s, reports appeared indicating that carbamazepine had beneficial psychotropic effects in patients with epilepsy (Dalby 1971).

The first report of its therapeutic effects in patients with bipolar disorder appeared in Japan in 1971 (Takezaki and Hanaoka 1971). The association of carbamazepine with blood dyscrasias delayed its use in North America. However, once the rarity of this serious adverse effect became apparent, the U.S. Food and Drug Administration (FDA) approved carbamazepine in 1974 as an antiepileptic for adults, in 1978 as an antiepileptic for children older than 6 years, and in 1987 as an antiepileptic without age limitations.

Structure-Activity Relations

Carbamazepine (5-carbamyl-5*H*-dibenz[*b,f*] azepine or 5*H*-dibenz[*b,f*]azepine-5-carboxamide) is an iminostilbene derivative with a tricyclic structure similar to that of the tricyclic antidepressant (TCA) imipramine (Kutt 1989; Levy et al. 1989; Rall and Schleifer 1985).

Pharmacological Profile

Carbamazepine is effective against maximal electroshock seizures at nontoxic doses but is ineffective against pentylenetetrazol-induced seizures (Macdonald 1989). However, carbamazepine is more effective than phenytoin in reducing stimulus-induced discharges in the amygdala of kindled rats (Albright and Burnham 1980). In addition, it has antidiuretic effects that may be associated with reduced serum antidiuretic hormone (ADH) concentrations and (with chronic administration) is associated with decreases in peripheral thyroid function indices, increased urinary free cortisol secretion, and a high incidence of escape from dexamethasone suppression (Post et al. 1991).

In humans, carbamazepine has been shown to be effective in the treatment of simple-partial, complex-partial, and generalized tonic-clonic seizures. Carbamazepine is ineffective against and may even exacerbate absence seizures. It is also effective in the treatment of paroxysmal pain syndromes such as trigeminal neuralgia (Blom 1963).

Pharmacokinetics and Disposition

After oral ingestion, the absorption of carbamazepine is slow, erratic, and unpredictable, though absorption in patients with epilepsy may be more rapid than in healthy volunteer subjects, and first-pass metabolism is minimal (Morselli 1989). Peak plasma concentrations are generally attained 4–8 hours after ingestion, but peaks as late as 26 hours have been reported (Table 12–1). The time of administration may have a significant effect on the absorption rate; absorption is slower with evening than with morning doses. The irregular absorption of carbamazepine has been attributed to a very slow dissolution rate in gastrointestinal fluid and to modification of gastrointestinal transit time by the anticholinergic properties of the drug.

Precise data on the absolute bioavailability of carbamazepine do not exist (because of the lack of an injectable formulation), but ranges of 75%–85% have been estimated from studies in which the ^{14}C-labeled molecule has been used (Ketter and Post 1994). Solutions, suspensions, syrups, and the newly developed chewable and slow-release formulations of carbamazepine seem to have similar bioavailabilities. The slow-release formulations, however, produce more stable plasma concentrations. It is worth noting that, in cases of massive overdose, peak plasma carbamazepine concentrations have been reached during the second or third day after ingestion.

Table 12–1. Population data for carbamazepine and valproate

	Peak absorption (hours)	Elimination half-life (hours)	Time to steady state (days)	Protein binding (%)	Therapeutic range (μg/mL)
Carbamazepine	4–8	2–17	2–4	73–88	3–14
Valproate	1–4	5–20	2–4	70–95	50–150

Source. Adapted from Wilder BJ: "Pharmacokinetics of Valproate and Carbamazepine." *Journal of Clinical Psychopharmacology* 12:64S–68S, 1992. Used with permission.

Carbamazepine is distributed rapidly into all tissues; 73%–88% is bound to plasma proteins, including proteins other than albumin. Concentrations of carbamazepine in cerebrospinal fluid (CSF) correspond with concentrations of free drug in plasma and range from 17% to 31% of those in plasma.

Carbamazepine undergoes almost complete biotransformation in humans and is metabolized in the liver by the cytochrome P450 system to a wide number of metabolites, many of which have antiepileptic activity. The predominant pathway of metabolism in humans involves conversion to the 10,11-epoxide (Figure 12–1). This metabolite is as active as carbamazepine and has neurotoxic side effects. Its concentrations in plasma and brain may reach 50% of those of carbamazepine. The 10,11-epoxide is metabolized further to inactive compounds that are excreted in the urine, principally as glucuronides. Carbamazepine is also inactivated by conjugation and hydroxylation.

Carbamazepine's elimination half-life ranges from 18 to 55 hours. During long-term treatment, carbamazepine may induce its own metabolism (a phenomenon termed *autoinduction*), and its half-life may be decreased to 2–17 hours (Figure 12–2). The half-life of the 10,11-epoxide is much shorter than that of the parent compound (6–7 hours).

Treatment with carbamazepine for epilepsy, trigeminal neuralgia, and mania is usually started at a dose of 100–200 mg taken either once or twice daily. The dose is increased (usually by 100 or 200 mg every few days) according to the patient's response and side effects, usually to serum concentrations ranging from 4 to 15 µg/mL. Although there is no clear relationship between carbamazepine serum concentration and response, therapeutic concentrations for epilepsy, paroxysmal pain syndromes, and mania are reported to be in this range. Significantly, neurological side effects become more frequent at serum concentrations above 9 µg/mL. In one study in which low (15–25 µmol/L) and high (28–40 µmol/L) serum concentrations of carbamazepine were compared in the maintenance treatment of patients with bipolar disorder, no difference in efficacy was found between the two concentrations (Simhandl et al. 1993).

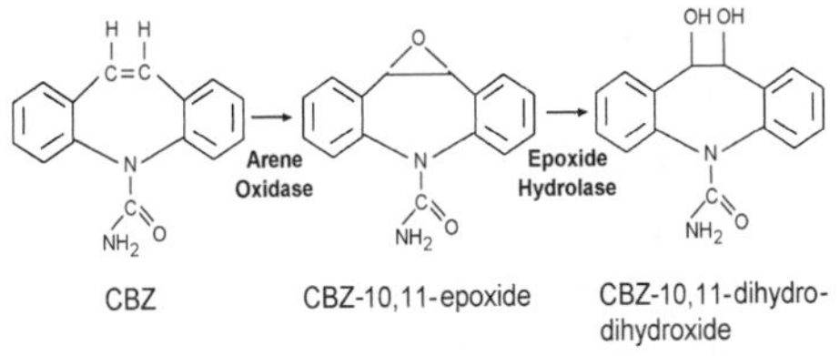

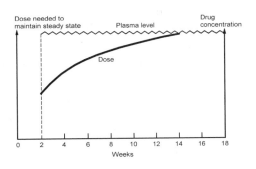

Figure 12–1. Major pathway of carbamazepine (CBZ) metabolism. This pathway of CBZ metabolism produces a CBZ-10,11-epoxide, a compound that has both anticonvulsant and toxic properties. The CBZ-10,11-epoxide is further metabolized by epoxide hydrolase. The action of epoxide hydrolase is blocked by valproate (VPA); therefore, when VPA is administered concurrently with CBZ, the CBZ-10,11-epoxide metabolite accumulates.
Source. Reprinted from Wilder BJ: "Pharmacokinetics of Valproate and Carbamazepine." *Journal of Clinical Psychopharmacology* 12:64S–68S, 1992. Used with permission.

Figure 12–2. Carbamazepine (CBZ) dosage adjustments versus time to compensate for autoinduction. The clearance of CBZ approximately doubles in the first 2–3 months of therapy. To maintain therapeutic plasma levels, the daily dose must be increased, often by 100%.
Source. Reprinted from Wilder BJ: "Pharmacokinetics of Valproate and Carbamazepine." *Journal of Clinical Psychopharmacology* 12:64S–68S, 1992. Used with permission.

Mechanism of Action

Carbamazepine's many actions can be divided into two basic mechanisms (reviewed in Levy et al. 1989; Macdonald 1989; Post et al. 1984a, 1991, 1992; Rall and Schleifer 1985): 1) effects on neuronal ion channels to reduce high-frequency repetitive firing of action potentials and 2) effects on synaptic and postsynaptic transmission. The weight of evidence suggests that carbamazepine's antiepileptic action can be attributed to the reduction of high-frequency neuronal discharge through binding to and inactivating voltage-sensitive sodium channels and decreasing sodium influx in a voltage-, frequency-, and use-dependent fashion (Macdonald 1989; Post et al. 1992). Because carbamazepine's effects on sodium channels are acute, and because its antiepileptic and antinociceptive effects are more rapid in onset than its antimanic or antidepressant effects, Post et al. (1992) speculated that the drug's sodium channel effects do not account for its mood-stabilizing properties. Noteworthy studies (Post et al. 1992; Zona et al. 1990) suggested that carbamazepine may also act on potassium channels to increase potassium conductance, thereby providing another possible mechanism for its antiepileptic effects.

Regarding synaptic and postsynaptic actions, carbamazepine has been reported to alter neurotransmitter concentrations, metabolism, receptors, and second-messenger systems. Indeed, the drug affects multiple neurotransmitter systems implicated in the pathophysiology of mood disorders (Macdonald 1989; Post et al. 1991, 1992). Carbamazepine binds to adenosine receptors and acts as an adenosine receptor antagonist. However, studies suggest that this property of carbamazepine is not responsible for its antiepileptic effects. Carbamazepine acutely increases locus coeruleus firing and decreases glutamate release; subchronic treatment decreases norepinephrine, dopamine, and γ-aminobutyric acid (GABA) turnover and blocks adenylate cyclase activity stimulated by norepinephrine, dopamine, and adenosine. Chronic carbamazepine administration is associated with increases in adenosine receptors, substance P sensitivity and levels, and plasma free tryptophan; decreases in CSF somatostatin; and greater decreases in GABA turnover (Post et al. 1991, 1992).

It is unclear whether carbamazepine's activities on these systems play a role in its antiepileptic properties. However, the ability of the drug to decrease release of the excitatory amino acid aspartate and its effects on α_2-adrenergic receptors have been implicated in its antiepileptic activity (Post et al. 1992). Additionally, although carbamazepine is not active at the central-type benzodiazepine receptor (which is linked to chloride channels and related to the antiepileptic effects of diazepam, clonazepam, and lorazepam), it may exert some of its antiepileptic effects by acutely binding to and acting as an antagonist at the "peripheral-type" benzodiazepine receptor, which appears to be linked to calcium channels (Post et al. 1992). Carbamazepine does not modify $GABA_A$ receptors, but it may have effects at the $GABA_B$ receptor. Although these effects probably do not contribute to the drug's antiepileptic properties, they may contribute to its antinociceptive effects. Finally, some of carbamazepine's effects on second-messenger systems include decreased activity of adenylate and guanylate cyclase and reductions of some aspects of phosphoinositide turnover (Post et al. 1992).

Thus far, none of these mechanisms has been linked to the psychotropic effects of carbamazepine, and it remains unknown whether the actions underlying the drug's antiepileptic effects are also responsible for its mood-stabilizing properties. It is noteworthy that carbamazepine does not block either stimulant-induced hyperactivity in animals or dopamine receptors in vitro. Thus, it exerts its antimanic effects through a mechanism other than dopamine receptor antagonism (Post et al. 1991).

Indications

Carbamazepine is currently approved in the United States for the treatment of complex-partial seizures, generalized tonic-clonic seizures, and other minor or partial seizure disorders (reviewed in Levy et al. 1989; Mattson et al. 1992). Carbamazepine is also approved for treatment of a variety of paroxysmal pain syndromes, including trigeminal neuralgia. Although not FDA approved for treatment of bipolar disorder, carbamazepine is frequently used as an alternative or adjunct to lithium in lithium-resistant or -intolerant patients. Research supporting its efficacy in patients with bipolar disorder is summarized later in this chapter.

Acute mania. At least 12 double-blind studies have shown that carbamazepine is superior to placebo and comparable to lithium and antipsychotics in the short-term treatment of acute mania; approximately two-thirds of patients in these studies have shown significant improvement (Ballenger and Post 1978; Brown et al. 1987; Desai et al. 1987; Grossi et al. 1984; Keck et al. 1992; Klein et al. 1984; Lenzi et al. 1986; Lerer et al. 1987; Lusznat et al. 1988; Möller et al. 1989; Müller and Stoll 1984; Okuma et al. 1979, 1990; Post 1990; Post et al. 1984a; Small 1990; Small et al. 1991) (Table 12–2). However, only 7 studies (Ballenger and Post 1978; Grossi et al. 1984; Hernandez-Avila et al. 1996; Lerer et al. 1987; Okuma et al. 1979; Post et al. 1984a; Small et al. 1991) are unconfounded by concurrent lithium and neuroleptic administration and thus allow for more meaningful interpretation.

Pooled data from the studies just mentioned reveal that the overall response rate to carbamazepine in patients with acute mania was 50%, compared with 56% for lithium monotherapy and 61% for neuroleptic monotherapy (differences that are not significant) (Keck et al. 1992). These studies further indicate that carbamazepine's onset of acute antimanic action is comparable to that of antipsychotics and is perhaps slightly more rapid than that of lithium

(significant antimanic effects are usually evident within 1–2 weeks of treatment). They also indicate that carbamazepine is generally better tolerated than conventional neuroleptics and lithium (with fewer extrapyramidal side effects [EPS]). In patients whose symptoms respond to carbamazepine, therapeutic serum concentrations are similar to those in epileptic patients, generally 4–15 µg/mL with carbamazepine dosages of 200–2,000 mg/day.

Acute major depression. Only three controlled studies have examined the efficacy of carbamazepine in the treatment of patients with unipolar or bipolar major depression. In the first study (Neumann et al. 1984), 10 patients (bipolar and unipolar) were randomly assigned to treatment with carbamazepine ($n = 5$) or trimipramine ($n = 5$). Both treatments were associated with significant antidepressant effects, and no significant differences were found between the two groups.

In the second study (Post et al. 1985), 12 (34%) of 35 bipolar and unipolar patients with treatment-resistant depression had a marked antidepressant response to treatment with carbamazepine alone. Fifty-four percent (19) of the patients had at least a mild degree of improvement. Substitution of carbamazepine with placebo was associated with loss of response in some patients whose depression had responded to carbamazepine.

In the third study (Small 1990), patients with treatment-resistant unipolar or bipolar depression were randomly assigned to a 4-week trial of lithium, carbamazepine, or a combination of both drugs. Of patients randomized to carbamazepine or to the combination, 32% had moderate or marked improvement, whereas 13% of the lithium-treated patients showed improvement.

Significantly, one small controlled study suggested that carbamazepine's acute antidepressant effects may be augmented by lithium. Of 15 patients with major depression refractory to carbamazepine alone, 8 (53%) had a rapid on-

Table 12–2. Controlled studies of carbamazepine in treatment of acute mania

Study	N	Design	Concomitant medications	Duration (days)	Outcome
Placebo-controlled					
Ballenger and Post 1978; Post et al. 1984a	19	B-A-B-A; CBZ v. P	None	11–56	63% response to CBZ; significant relapse on P
Placebo + neuroleptic					
Klein et al. 1984	14	CBZ + HAL v. P + HAL; CBZ + HAL	HAL, 15–45 mg/day; HAL	35	71% response to CBZ + HAL; 54% response to P + HAL; both groups improved, but CBZ + HAL group's improvement was greater
Müller and Stoll 1984	6	P + HAL		21	
Möller et al. 1989	11 CBZ; 9 P	CBZ + HAL v. P + HAL	HAL 24 mg/day; levomepromazine prn	21	No significant difference
Placebo + lithium					
Desai et al. 1987	5	CBZ + L v. P + L	L; ND	28	CBZ + L response > P + L response by 14
Lithium-controlled					
Lerer et al. 1987	14 CBZ; 14 L	CBZ v. L	None	28	79% response to L > 29% response to CBZ
Small et al. 1991	24 CBZ; 24 L	CBZ v. L	None	56	33% response for both groups
Neuroleptic-controlled					
Grossi et al. 1984	18 CBZ; 19 CPZ	CBZ v. CPZ	ND	21	67% response to CPZ; 59% response to CBZ

Okuma et al. 1979	32 CBZ; 28 CPZ	CBZ v. CPZ	None	21–35	66% response to CBZ; 54% response to CPZ
Hernandez-Avila et al. 1996	10 CBZ; 10 HAL	CBZ v. HAL	ND	35	71% response to CBZ; 67% response to HAL
Neuroleptic + neuroleptic					
Brown et al. 1987	8 CBZ; 9 HAL	CBZ + CPZ; HAL + CPZ	CPZ	28	HAL group had higher dropout rate because of EPS
Lithium + neuroleptic					
Lusznat et al. 1988	22	CBZ + CPZ; HAL v. L + CPZ, HAL	HAL, CPZ	42	No significant difference
Lenzi et al. 1986	22	CBZ + CPZ v. L + CPZ	CPZ	19	73% response for both groups
Okuma et al. 1990	101	CBZ + neuroleptics (80%); neuroleptics	Neuroleptics	28	62% response to CBZ; 59% response to mean level 0.46 mEq/L

Note.   CBZ = carbamazepine; P = placebo; HAL = haloperidol; L = lithium; ND = not documented; EPS = extrapyramidal side effects; CPZ = chlorpromazine.
Source.   Adapted from Keck PE Jr, McElroy SL, Nemeroff CB: "Anticonvulsants in the Treatment of Bipolar Disorder." *Journal of Neuropsychiatry and Clinical Neurosciences* 4:395–405, 1992. Used with permission.

set of antidepressant response (within a mean of 4 days) after the blind addition of lithium (Kramlinger and Post 1989).

Prophylactic treatment of bipolar disorder.   Six controlled studies have examined the efficacy of carbamazepine in the long-term treatment of patients with bipolar disorder. Approximately one-half to two-thirds of patients had a significant prophylactic response over 1–2 years (Bellaire et al. 1988; Denicoff et al. 1997; Lusznat et al. 1988; Okuma et al. 1981; Placidi et al. 1986; Watkins et al. 1987). In the only placebo-controlled study (Okuma et al. 1981), 60% of patients had not relapsed with carbamazepine treatment at 1-year follow-up, as compared with 22% of patients receiving placebo. In the other four controlled studies, carbamazepine appeared comparable to lithium in reducing affective episodes and prolonging euthymic intervals.

The prophylactic effects of carbamazepine, however, may be better for mania than for depression, are often incomplete even in responders, and may produce tachyphylaxis in some patients (Frankenburg et al. 1988; Post et al. 1990). For example, of 24 lithium-refractory, affectively ill patients who showed a marked acute response to carbamazepine and were followed up for a mean of 4 years, 50% had significant breakthrough episodes during the second or third year of treatment despite adequate serum concentrations (Post et al. 1990). This apparent loss of efficacy has been hypothesized to be due to the development of contingent tolerance or to the progression of the underlying illness. On the other hand, Murphy et al. (1989) suggested that the methodological limitations of the controlled trials cast doubt on the prophylactic efficacy of carbamazepine.

Predictors of treatment response.   Early studies suggested that certain factors associated with poor response to lithium might be associated with a favorable antimanic response to carbamazepine. These factors included more

severe mania, rapid cycling (the occurrence of four or more mood episodes within 1 year), greater dysphoria or depression during mania (so-called *mixed* or *dysphoric* mania), and a lower incidence of familial bipolar disorder (Goodwin 1990; Kishimoto et al. 1983; McElroy et al. 1992a; Post et al. 1987, 1991). However, studies indicate that decreasing or stable frequencies of episodes (Denicoff et al. 1997; Post et al. 1990), course of illness marked predominantly by manic episodes (Okuma 1993), and decreasing severity of mania (Small et al. 1991) correlate with a favorable response to carbamazepine. Factors not associated with antimanic response to carbamazepine include the presence of psychosensory symptoms and response to other antiepileptics (Post et al. 1991). For instance, patients whose mania did not respond to valproate and phenytoin have been reported to respond to carbamazepine (Post et al. 1984b).

Factors possibly associated with a favorable antidepressant response to carbamazepine in one study included more severe depression at the time of treatment, a history of more discrete episodes of depression, and a history of less chronicity (Post et al. 1985, 1991). In this study (Post et al. 1991), the patients with the greatest degree of thyroid hormone decrement (either thyroxine [T_4] or free T_4) while receiving carbamazepine had the best antidepressant response.

Side Effects and Toxicology

Carbamazepine has a favorable side-effect profile compared with lithium, antipsychotics, and other antiepileptics (Andrews et al. 1990; Gram and Jensen 1989; Levy et al. 1989; Mattson et al. 1992; Pellock 1987; Pellock and Willmore 1991; Post et al. 1991; Rall and Schleifer 1985; Smith and Bleck 1991). Notably, the drug rarely causes EPS or renal side effects. It is associated with less cognitive and neurological toxicity than are phenytoin and phenobarbital; was associated with less weight gain, hair changes, and tremor than was valproate in one study of a large group of patients with epilepsy (Mattson et al. 1992); and in another study was associated with less memory impairment than was lithium in a group of patients with mood disorders (Andrews et al. 1990). However, 33%–50% of patients receiving carbamazepine experience side effects. These most commonly include neurological symptoms such as diplopia, blurred vision, fatigue, nausea, vertigo, nystagmus, and ataxia. These neurological side effects are dose related, usually transient, and reversible with dose reduction. Elderly patients, however, may be more sensitive to them.

Less frequent side effects of carbamazepine include transient leukopenia, which occurs in approximately 10%–12% of patients with epilepsy and in approximately 2.1% of patients with major affective disorders (Tohen et al. 1995); transient thrombocytopenia; rash in up to 10%–12% of patients; hyponatremia and, less commonly, hypo-osmolality; liver enzyme elevations in 5%–15% of patients; and other central nervous system (CNS) toxicities, such as mild peripheral polyneuropathies and involuntary movement disorders.

The leukopenia associated with carbamazepine primarily involves granulocytes but does not predispose patients to infection, is not related to the serious idiopathic dyscrasias agranulocytosis and aplastic anemia, and usually resolves spontaneously despite continuation of medication. In the event of asymptomatic leukopenia, thrombocytopenia, or elevated liver enzymes, the carbamazepine dose can be reduced, or (in cases with severe changes) the drug can be discontinued. Once the abnormalities normalize, carbamazepine may be increased or restarted at a lower dose. If rash develops, carbamazepine may be continued as long as there is no associated fever, bleeding, exfoliative skin lesions, or other signs or symptoms of hypersensitivity. Carbamazepine-induced rash can be successfully treated with corticosteroids.

Hyponatremia is most likely the result of water retention resulting from carbamazepine's antidiuretic effect. It occurs in 6%–31% of patients, is rare in children but probably more common in elderly people, occasionally occurs many months after the initiation of carbamazepine treatment, and often necessitates withdrawal from the drug.

Rare, non-dose-related, idiosyncratic, and unpredictable but serious and potentially fatal side effects of carbamazepine include blood dyscrasias (agranulocytosis and aplastic anemia), hepatic failure, exfoliative dermatitis (e.g., Stevens-Johnson syndrome), and pancreatitis. Other rare side effects include systemic hypersensitivity reactions, conduction disturbances (sometimes resulting in bradycardia or Stokes-Adams syndrome), psychological disturbances (e.g., sporadic cases of psychosis and mania), and (very rarely) renal effects (e.g., renal failure, oliguria, hematuria, and proteinuria). The development of a severe blood dyscrasia caused by carbamazepine occurs in 2 of 575,000 treated patients per year, with a mortality of approximately 1 in 575,000 (Seetharam and Pellock 1991). Although most cases occur within the first 3–6 months of treatment, some have occurred after more extended periods of exposure. Note that transient leukopenia, thrombocytopenia, or hepatic enzyme elevations are not related to these life-threatening reactions. Routine blood monitoring does not permit anticipation of blood dyscrasias, hepatic failure, or exfoliative dermatitis (Pellock and Willmore 1991). Thus, educating the patient about the signs and symptoms of hepatic, hematological, or dermatological reactions and instructing him or her to report these signs and symptoms if they occur, along with careful monitoring of the patient's clinical status, are probably better than routine laboratory screening for detecting these serious side effects.

Carbamazepine has teratogenic effects (Jones et al. 1989; Levy et al. 1989; Rosa 1991). First-trimester exposure is associated with an increased risk of neural tube defects, craniofacial defects, fingernail hypoplasia, and developmental delay. Fortunately, the frequency of neural tube defects in general, as well as those associated with in utero antiepileptic exposure, may be reduced by prophylactic treatment with high doses of folate—ideally begun well before conception occurs (Centers for Disease Control 1991; Delcado-Escveta and Janz 1992).

Early signs of carbamazepine toxicity typically develop several hours after a given dose and include dizziness, ataxia, sedation, and diplopia. Higher concentrations are associated with nystagmus and obtundation. Acute intoxication can result in hyperirritability, stupor, or coma. Carbamazepine can be fatal in overdose: of 311 reported overdoses, 9 resulted in death, and the lethal doses of carbamazepine were 4–60 g (Gram and Jensen 1989). The most common symptoms of carbamazepine overdose are nystagmus, ophthalmoplegia, cerebellar signs and EPS, impaired consciousness, convulsions, and respiratory dysfunction. Cardiac symptoms include tachycardia, arrhythmia, conduction disturbances, and hypotension. Gastrointestinal and anticholinergic symptoms may also occur. Coma may develop with serum carbamazepine concentrations as low as 80 μmol/L.

In the presence of carbamazepine intoxication, the concentration of the 10,11-epoxide may exceed that of the parent compound. Treatment of carbamazepine intoxication includes symptomatic treatment, gastric lavage (which should be undertaken up to 12 hours after ingestion), and hemoperfusion, which may accelerate carbamazepine's elimination. Forced diuresis, peritoneal dialysis, and hemodialysis, however, are not recommended (Gram and Jensen 1989).

Drug-Drug Interactions

Carbamazepine has important interactions with a variety of other drugs (Ketter et al. 1991a, 1991b; Levy et al. 1989). First, because carbamazepine is a potent inducer of catabolic enzymes, it stimulates the metabolism and decreases the plasma levels of many other metabolized medications, including haloperidol and other antipsychotics, methadone, antiasthmatics (e.g., prednisone, methylpredni-

solone, and theophylline), warfarin, valproate, TCAs, benzodiazepines, and hormonal contraceptives. Indeed, although failure of oral contraceptives is more common in women using phenytoin and/or phenobarbital, instances in patients receiving carbamazepine have also been reported (Mattson et al. 1986).

Second, because the metabolism of carbamazepine is exclusively hepatic, certain enzyme inhibitors can inhibit carbamazepine metabolism, increase serum carbamazepine concentrations, and precipitate carbamazepine toxicity. These medications include acetazolamide, the calcium channel blockers diltiazem and verapamil (but not nifedipine), danazol, dextropropoxyphene, propoxyphene, erythromycin, isoniazid, and valproate.

Third, combinations of carbamazepine with other enzyme-inducing agents, including antiepileptics, can increase carbamazepine 10,11-epoxide concentrations and result in signs of toxicity at normally tolerable serum concentrations. Indeed, some studies indicate a connection between plasma 10,11-epoxide concentrations and side effects; neurological side effects are also more frequent in patients receiving carbamazepine with other antiepileptics (Gram and Jensen 1989).

Finally, the potential exists for pharmacodynamic interactions with other neurotoxic drugs. Thus, although most patients tolerate carbamazepine when it is given in conjunction with lithium or antipsychotics, cases of enhanced neurotoxicity have been reported with both combinations (Fogel 1988). In one study, the combination of carbamazepine and lithium caused greater memory impairment than either drug alone (Andrews et al. 1990).

VALPROATE

History and Discovery

Valproic acid was first synthesized by Burton in the United States in 1882 and subsequently was used as an organic solvent. The drug's antiepileptic properties were discovered seren-dipitously by Meunier in 1963 in France. Valproate was first introduced as an antiepileptic in France in 1967. It has been used in Holland and Germany since 1968 and in the United Kingdom since 1973, and it became available in the United States in 1978. An enteric-coated formulation, divalproex sodium, was introduced to the United States market in 1983, and a for-mulation consisting of a capsule containing coated particles of divalproex sodium was intro-duced in 1989. Interestingly, the first report of valproate having therapeutic effects in patients with bipolar disorder appeared in France in 1966 (Lambert et al. 1966). An extended release form was introduced in the United States in 2000.

Structure-Activity Relations

Valproic acid (dipropylacetic acid) is a simple branched-chain carboxylic acid that is structur-ally distinct from other antiepileptic and psychotropic compounds (Figure 12–3) (Levy et al. 1989; Rimmer and Richens 1985). The pri-mary amide of valproic acid (valpromide, which is available in Europe but not the United States) has been reported to be about twice as potent as the parent compound.

Pharmacological Profile

Valproate blocks pentylenetetrazole-induced and maximal electroshock seizures in a variety of

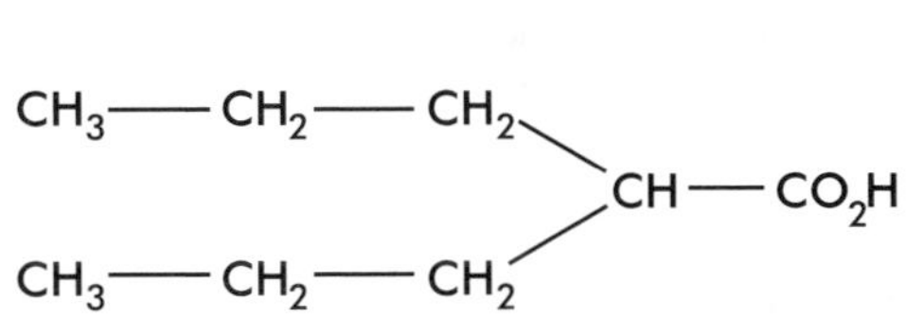

Figure 12–3. Chemical structure for valproic acid (2-propyl-pentanoic acid).
Source. Reprinted from Kupferberg AJ: "Valproate: Chemistry and Methods of Determi-nation," in *Antiepileptic Drugs*, 3rd Edition. Edited by Levy RH, Dreifuss FE, Mattson RH, et al. New York, Raven, 1989, pp. 577–582. Used with permission.

animals (with somewhat better efficacy in the former than in the latter) and suppresses sec-ondarily generalized seizures without affecting focal activity in cortical cobalt- and alumina-lesioned animals (Fariello and Smith 1989). Valproate also has antikindling properties—preventing the spread of epileptiform activity in cats without affecting focal seizures (Leveil and Nanquet 1977). In humans, valproate has activ-ity against a wide variety of epilepsy types while causing only minimal sedation and other CNS side effects.

Pharmacokinetics and Disposition

Valproate is commercially available in the United States in five oral preparations: dival-proex sodium, an enteric-coated, stable coordi-nation compound containing equal proportions of valproic acid and sodium valproate in a 1:1 molar ratio; valproic acid; sodium valproate; a new extended release form; and divalproex so-dium sprinkle capsules containing coated parti-cles of divalproex sodium that can be ingested intact or pulled apart and sprinkled on food. Valproate is also available in suppository form for rectal administration, and an intravenous preparation is now available. As mentioned, valpromide, the amide of valproic acid, is avail-able in Europe. There are only minor differ-ences in the pharmacokinetics of these prepara-tions, and valproic acid is the common compound in plasma (Table 12–1).

The bioavailability of valproate approaches 100% with all preparations (Levy et al. 1989; Penry and Dean 1989; Wilder 1992). All prepa-rations taken orally, except divalproex sodium, are rapidly absorbed after oral ingestion, attain-ing peak serum concentrations within 2 hours (see Table 12–1). Divalproex sodium reaches peak serum concentrations within 3–8 hours. The divalproex sodium sprinkle formulation has an earlier onset of absorption but a slower rate of absorption than divalproex sodium tab-lets (Figure 12–4). Absorption can also be de-layed if the drug is taken with food.

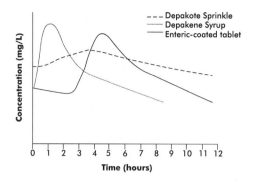

Figure 12–4. Absorption of three valproate (VPA) formulations after oral dosing in patients taking chronic VPA therapy: valproic acid (Depakene Syrup) versus enteric-coated divalproex sodium tablets versus divalproex sodium sprinkle capsules.
Source. Reprinted from Wilder BJ: "Pharmacokinetics of Valproate and Carbamazepine." *Journal of Clinical Psychopharmacology* 12:64S–68S, 1992. Used with permission.

Valproate is highly protein bound, predominantly to serum albumin and proportional to the albumin concentration. Although patients with low levels of albumin have a higher fraction of unbound drug, the steady-state level of total drug is not altered. Only the unbound drug crosses the blood-brain barrier and is bioactive. Thus, when valproate is displaced from protein-binding sites through drug interactions, the total drug concentration may not change; however, the pharmacologically active unbound drug does increase and may produce signs and symptoms of toxicity. Moreover, when the plasma concentration of valproate increases in response to increased dosing, the amount of unbound (active) valproate increases disproportionately and is metabolized with an apparent increase in clearance of total drug, yielding lower-than-expected total plasma concentrations (Levy et al. 1989; Wilder 1992). In addition, valproate protein binding is increased by low-fat diets and decreased by high-fat diets.

The correlation between valproate serum concentration and both its antiepileptic and its antimanic effects is poor, but the concentration range generally required for good clinical effect is approximately 50–125 or 150 µg/mL. There appears to be a response threshold at 50 µg/mL—the approximate valproate serum concentration at which plasma albumin sites begin to become saturated—because valproate concentrations equal to or greater than 50 µg/mL are more often associated with response than are lower concentrations (Rimmer and Richens 1985). However, some patients with epilepsy or mania have clinical response only with serum concentrations well above 100 µg/mL and, in some cases, with serum concentrations approaching 200 µg/mL (McElroy et al. 1992b). Conversely, patients with cyclothymia may respond to serum valproate concentrations of less than 50 µg/mL (Jacobsen 1993).

Valproate is metabolized primarily in the liver by two metabolic pathways to a large number of metabolites, some of which have antiepileptic and/or toxic effects (Levy et al. 1989; Penry and Dean 1989; Rimmer and Richens 1985; Wilder 1992) (Figure 12–5). These two metabolic pathways are 1) mitochondrial β-oxidation to 3-OH-valproate, 3-oxo-valproate, and 2-en-valproate; and 2) P450 microsomal metabolism to the toxic 4-en- and 2,4-en-metabolites and to a number of inactive metabolites that are conjugated with glucuronide. Of note, the 2-en-valproate metabolite is considered an active antiepileptic with a long half-life (Wilder 1992). Valproate's elimination half-life is typically 5–20 hours and can be altered by agents that affect the mitochondrial and/or microsomal enzyme systems responsible for its metabolism. Mitochondrial β-oxidation (the pathway used extensively for processing fatty acids) is the more important pathway for valproate's metabolism, especially when valproate is administered alone. However, P450 microsomal metabolism is increased (along with the toxic metabolites it generates) when valproate is administered with other drugs that induce the P450 system, thereby increasing chances of adverse effects, including (extremely rarely and primarily in children) liver necrosis.

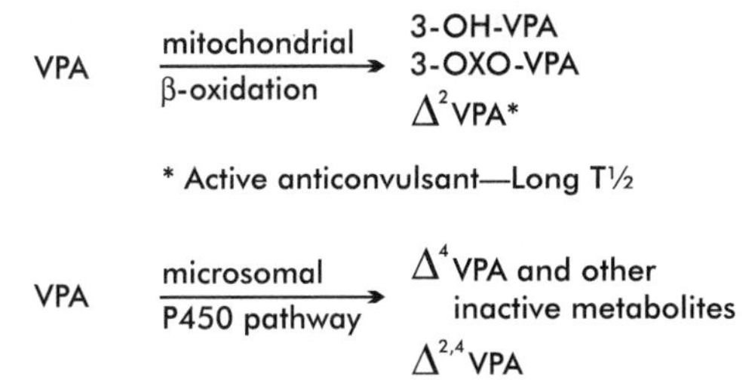

VPA $\xrightarrow[\beta\text{-oxidation}]{\text{mitochondrial}}$ 3-OH-VPA
3-OXO-VPA
Δ^2VPA*

* Active anticonvulsant—Long T½

VPA $\xrightarrow[\text{P450 pathway}]{\text{microsomal}}$ Δ^4VPA and other inactive metabolites
$\Delta^{2,4}$VPA

Figure 12–5. Two pathways for metabolism of valproate (VPA). VPA is metabolized within the mitochondria by the β-oxidative pathway, which metabolizes medium- and long-chain fatty acids. This is the major metabolic pathway used by patients taking VPA as monotherapy. VPA is also metabolized by the microsomal P450 pathway, which occurs outside the mitochondria and is increased when VPA is administered in combination with enzyme-inducing drugs (i.e., carbamazepine).
Source. Reprinted from Wilder BJ: "Pharmacokinetics of Valproate and Carbamazepine." *Journal of Clinical Psychopharmacology* 12:64S–68S, 1992. Used with permission.

Treatment with valproate for epilepsy or bipolar disorder is usually begun at a dosage of 15 mg/kg/day (usually 500–1,000 mg/day in two to four divided doses). The drug can be "orally loaded" at 20 mg/kg/day in patients with status epilepticus and acute mania to induce more rapid response. As with carbamazepine, the valproate dosage is increased according to the patient's response and side effects, usually by 250–500 mg/day every 1–3 days and to serum concentrations of 50–150 µg/mL. Of note, neurological side effects become more frequent at serum concentrations above 100 µg/mL. Once the patient is stabilized, the entire valproate dosage may be taken as one daily dose before sleep to enhance convenience and compliance.

Mechanism of Action

Valproate has many effects, and the mechanisms underlying its antiepileptic and mood-stabilizing actions are unknown. One theory is that valproate induces its antiepileptic and possibly its mood-stabilizing effects by changes in the metabolism of GABA, the major inhibitory neurotransmitter in the mammalian CNS (Emrich et al. 1981; Fariello and Smith 1989; Post et al. 1992; Rimmer and Richens 1985). Valproate inhibits the catabolism of GABA, increases its release, decreases GABA turnover, increases GABA$_B$ receptor density, and may also enhance neuronal responsiveness to GABA. Studies have suggested that valproate-induced increases in brain levels of GABA and improved neuronal responsiveness to GABA are associated with seizure control. Other research, however, suggests that valproate exerts its antiepileptic effects by direct neuronal effects (i.e., reducing sodium influx and increasing potassium efflux). Yet other effects of valproate include decreased dopamine turnover, decreased N-methyl-D-aspartate (NMDA)–mediated currents, decreased release of aspartate, and decreased CSF somatostatin concentrations.

Indications

The indications for valproate that are currently recognized by the FDA are for the treatment of the manic episodes associated with bipolar disorder, for sole and adjunctive therapy in the treatment of simple and complex absence seizures, and for adjunctive therapy in multiple seizure types that include absence seizures. Controlled studies have also shown that valproate is highly effective in other primarily generalized epilepsies, including generalized tonic-clonic and myoclonic seizures, as well as in secondarily generalized tonic-clonic seizures, infantile spasms, photosensitive epilepsy, and febrile seizures (Anonymous 1988; Bourgeois 1989; Rimmer and Richens 1985).

Acute mania. Numerous open studies and seven controlled trials (four placebo-controlled, one haloperidol-controlled, one lithium-controlled, and one placebo- and lithium-controlled) indicate that valproate is effective in the treatment of acute mania (Bowden et al. 1994;

McElroy et al. 1992b). In the controlled trials (Bowden et al. 1994; Brennan et al. 1984; Emrich et al. 1985; Freeman et al. 1992; McElroy et al. 1996; Pope et al. 1991; Post et al. 1984b), valproate was superior to placebo and comparable to lithium and haloperidol in the short-term treatment of acute mania; 71 (53%) of 134 patients who received valproate had a moderate or marked reduction in acute manic symptoms (Table 12–3). In these studies, the antimanic response to valproate occurred within several days to 2 weeks of achieving a serum valproate concentration equal to or greater than 50 µg/mL.

Indeed, in an open-label, rater-blind study of valproate administration via an oral loading dosage of 20 mg/kg/day to 19 patients with acute mania, 10 (53%) of the patients had a significant response within 5 days of treatment with minimal side effects (Keck et al. 1993). Similarly, in a controlled comparison study with haloperidol, divalproex administered at 20 mg/kg/day produced rapid antimanic and antipsychotic effects comparable to those of haloperidol (McElroy et al. 1996).

Acute major depression. No controlled studies of valproate in the treatment of acute unipolar or bipolar major depression have been done. Of 195 acutely depressed patients receiving valproate in four open trials, 58 (30%) had a significant acute antidepressant response (McElroy et al. 1992b). However, open data also suggest that valproate may be more effective in ameliorating depression when administered over longer periods (Hayes 1989); that its prophylactic antidepressant effects may be superior to its acute antidepressant effects (Calabrese and Delucchi 1990; Calabrese et al. 1992); and/or that it may be more likely to exert antidepressant effects in certain subtypes of bipolar patients—including, for example, those with bipolar II disorder (Puzynski and Klosiewicz 1984).

Prophylactic treatment of bipolar disorder. One controlled study has tested the effi-

Table 12–3. Controlled studies of valproate in treatment of acute mania

Study	N	Design	Concomitant medications	Duration (days)	Outcome
Brennan et al. 1984	8	A-B-A	None	14	6/8 marked response; 2/8 no response
Emrich et al. 1985	5	A-B-A	None	Variable	4/5 marked response; 1/5 no response
Post et al. 1984b	1	Crossover to P, CBZ, VPA; phenytoin	None	Variable	Marked response to CBZ only
Pope et al. 1991	36	VPA v. P	Lorazepam	21	VPA > P on all scales
Freeman et al. 1992	27	VPA v. L	None	21	92% response to L; 63% response to VPA
Bowden et al. 1994	179	VPA v. L v. P	Lorazepam, chloral hydrate	21	VPA > P, L > P, VPA = L
McElroy et al. 1996	36	VPA v. HAL	Lorazepam	6	VPA = HAL

Note.   VPA = valproate; P = placebo; CBZ = carbamazepine; L = lithium; HAL = haloperidol.
Source.   Adapted from Keck PE Jr, McElroy SL, Nemeroff CB: "Anticonvulsants in the Treatment of Bipolar Disorder." *Journal of Neuropsychiatry and Clinical Neurosciences* 4:395–405, 1992. Used with permission.

cacy of valproate in the long-term treatment of bipolar disorder. In this study, 83 patients with bipolar disorder (according to DSM-III criteria [American Psychiatric Association 1980]) were randomly assigned to treatment with lithium or valpromide (a formulation of valproate not available in the United States) and followed up for up to 2 years (Lambert and Venaud 1994). The mean number of recurrent affective episodes per patient during the maintenance period was comparable in the lithium-treated (0.61 per patient) and the valpromide-treated (0.51 per patient) groups. Other open studies suggested that the drug reduces the frequency and intensity of manic and depressive episodes over extended periods in some patients, including those with rapid cycling, mixed bipolar disorder, bipolar II disorder, and schizoaffective disorder (Calabrese and Delucchi 1990; Calabrese et al. 1992; Emrich and Wolf 1992; Guscott 1992; Hayes 1989; McElroy et al. 1992b; Puzynski and Klosiewicz 1984; Suppes et al. 1992). These studies also indicated that valproate may be more effective in the prevention of manic and mixed episodes than depressive episodes.

Predictors of treatment response. Although inconsistencies exist, various factors are emerging as possibly being associated with a favorable antimanic or mood-stabilizing response to valproate. These factors include rapid cycling, dysphoric or mixed mania, later age at onset and/or shorter duration of illness, and possibly mania due to or associated with medical or neurological illness (Calabrese et al. 1993; McElroy et al. 1988a, 1988b, 1992a, 1992b; Stoll et al. 1994). In a controlled comparison of valproate and lithium in 27 patients with bipolar disorder and acute mania, high depression scores during episodes of acute mania were associated with a favorable antimanic response to valproate (Clothier et al. 1992; Freeman et al. 1992). However, in a double-blind, placebo-controlled trial of valproate in acutely manic bipolar patients, Pope et al. (1991) found that the

12 patients whose symptoms responded to valproate did not differ with respect to frequency of rapid cycling from the 5 valproate-treated patients who showed no response (McElroy et al. 1991). Also, antimanic response to valproate was not correlated with the degree of depression during mania. Similarly, in a double-blind, placebo-controlled trial conducted by Bowden et al. (1994), valproate was as effective in patients with rapid-cycling mania (defined in this study as four manic episodes within the past year) as in those with non-rapid-cycling mania.

Evidence suggesting that secondary or complicated mania responds well to valproate is similarly mixed. In an open study of 56 valproate-treated patients with mania, response was associated with the presence of nonparoxysmal abnormalities on electroencephalogram but not with neurological soft signs or abnormalities on computed axial tomography scans of brain (McElroy et al. 1988b). Nevertheless, there was a trend for responders to have histories of closed head trauma antedating the onset of their affective symptoms (Pope et al. 1988). Furthermore, case reports described successful valproate treatment of organic brain syndromes with affective features (Kahn et al. 1988) and mental retardation in patients with bipolar disorder or symptoms (Kastner et al. 1993; Sovner 1989). The diagnosis of schizoaffective disorder, bipolar type, has been associated with a less favorable valproate response than has the diagnosis of bipolar disorder (McElroy et al. 1992b; Tohen et al. 1994).

Side Effects and Toxicology

Valproate is generally well tolerated and has a low incidence of adverse effects and a favorable side-effect profile compared with other antiepileptics, lithium, and antipsychotics (Anonymous 1988; Beghi et al. 1986; Dreifuss 1989; Smith and Bleck 1991). For instance, valproate is less likely to cause cognitive impairment than are other antiepileptics (Beghi et al. 1986;

Vining 1987) and has been associated with a lower incidence of side effects than has lithium in bipolar patients (Vencovsky et al. 1983). In a double-blind, placebo-controlled trial of valproate versus lithium, Bowden et al. (1994) found the rate of premature termination for intolerance to be 11% in the lithium-treated group, whereas it was 6% for valproate and 3% for placebo. Like carbamazepine, valproate rarely causes renal side effects or EPS. Unlike carbamazepine, it rarely causes thyroid, cardiac, dermatological, or allergic effects. However, the drug is associated with both benign and potentially fatal side effects (for thorough reviews, see Beghi et al. 1986; Pellock and Willmore 1991; Rimmer and Richens 1985; Smith and Bleck 1991). Common dose-related side effects are gastrointestinal distress (e.g., anorexia, nausea, dyspepsia, indigestion, vomiting, and diarrhea), benign elevations in hepatic transaminase, and neurological symptoms (most commonly, tremor and sedation). Gastrointestinal complaints, benign hepatic transaminase elevations, and sedation are more likely to occur at the initiation of treatment and usually subside with dose reduction and/or over time.

Of significance is that gastrointestinal complaints are more frequent with valproic acid and sodium valproate than with the enteric-coated divalproex sodium formulation (Wilder et al. 1983). However, gastrointestinal complaints that persist despite dose reduction may be relieved by using divalproex sprinkle capsules or by the addition of a histamine-2 receptor antagonist (e.g., famotidine or cimetidine) (Stoll et al. 1991). Tremor can be managed with dose reduction or treatment with β-blockers. Coagulopathies, impaired platelet function, and transient thrombocytopenia (which are reversible with drug discontinuation) occur less frequently. Fairly frequent side effects that are often bothersome to patients include hair loss (which is usually transient), increased appetite, and weight gain. Hair loss may be minimized by cotreatment with a multivitamin containing zinc and selenium (Hurd et al. 1984).

Rare, idiosyncratic adverse effects that are not dose related but could be fatal include irreversible hepatic failure, acute hemorrhagic pancreatitis, and (extremely rarely) agranulocytosis. The risk of pancreatitis may be greater in mentally retarded adults treated with valproate (Buzan et al. 1995). Clear-cut risk factors for the development of valproate-associated irreversible hepatic failure have been identified in patients with epilepsy and include 1) young age (especially 2 years or younger), 2) administration of valproate in conjunction with other antiepileptics, and 3) presence of other medical or neurological abnormalities in addition to epilepsy. Since these factors were identified, the rate of valproate-associated fatal hepatic toxicity has decreased despite increased use of the drug. Thus, the overall rate of fatal hepatic toxicity decreased from 1 in 10,000 between 1978 and 1984 to 1 in 49,000 in 1985 and 1986. Furthermore, no hepatic fatalities have been reported in patients older than 10 years receiving valproate as antiepileptic monotherapy (Dreifuss et al. 1989).

Other serious side effects of valproate include teratogenicity (particularly neural tube defects with first-trimester exposure) and coma and death when taken in overdose. Offspring of mothers taking valproate have been reported to have an incidence of neural tube defects of 1%–1.5%. Minor dysmorphic syndromes have also been reported. Although the mechanism of valproate's teratogenicity is unknown, the formation of free radicals during the microsomal metabolism of valproate has been implicated. Valproate depletes selenium, a necessary component for the synthesis of glutathione peroxidase, which is an important free radical scavenger and antioxidant (Wilder 1992). Thus, multivitamins with trace metals (as well as folinic acid) have been recommended for women of childbearing potential who are taking valproate (and other antiepileptics) (Wilder 1992).

Regarding overdose, recovery from coma has occurred with serum valproate concentrations of greater than 2,000 µg/mL. In addition, serum valproate concentrations have been reduced by hemodialysis and hemoperfusion, and valproate-induced coma has been reversed with naloxone (Rimmer and Richens 1985). Because transient hepatic enzyme elevations, leukopenia, and thrombocytopenia are not predictive of life-threatening reactions (and thus, routine blood monitoring does not permit anticipation of hepatic failure or blood dyscrasias), it is generally not necessary to perform routine blood monitoring of hematological and hepatic function in epileptic patients receiving chronic antiepileptic medication (Pellock and Willmore 1991). Superior to routine laboratory screening is education of patients about the signs and symptoms of hepatic or hematological dysfunction and instructing them to report these symptoms if they occur, in conjunction with careful monitoring of the patient's clinical status.

Drug-Drug Interactions

Because valproate is highly protein bound and extensively metabolized by the liver, a number of potential drug-drug interactions may occur with other protein-bound or metabolized drugs (Fogel 1988; Levy et al. 1989; Rall and Schleifer 1985; Rimmer and Richens 1985). Thus, free fraction concentrations of valproate in serum can be increased and valproate toxicity precipitated by coadministration of other highly protein-bound drugs (e.g., aspirin) that can displace valproate from its protein-binding sites. Because valproate tends to inhibit drug oxidation—it is the only major antiepileptic that does not induce hepatic microsomal enzymes—serum concentrations of a number of metabolized drugs can be increased by the coadministration of valproate. Thus, valproate has been reported to increase serum concentrations of phenobarbital, phenytoin, and TCAs. Conversely, the metabolism of valproate can be increased, and valproate serum concentrations subsequently decreased, by coadministration of microsomal enzyme-inducing drugs such as carbamazepine;

drugs that inhibit metabolism may increase valproate concentrations in serum. Fluoxetine, for instance, has been reported to boost valproate concentrations (Sovner and Davis 1991).

Finally, neurological reactions may occur when valproate is administered with other neurotoxic drugs. For example, increased sedation and (extremely rarely) delirium have been reported when valproate is administered with antipsychotics (Costello and Suppes 1995). However, an initial report of the combination of valproate and clonazepam inducing absence status in three patients with absence epilepsy has not been replicated.

BENZODIAZEPINES

The benzodiazepines as a class are discussed in detail by Ballenger in Chapter 5 in this volume. Because these drugs have antiepileptic properties (i.e., diazepam in status epilepticus and clonazepam in absence epilepsy), their use in the treatment of bipolar disorder is briefly reviewed here.

In general, studies examining the efficacy of benzodiazepines in patients with bipolar disorder are inconsistent. Of four controlled studies evaluating clonazepam in the treatment of acute mania, clonazepam was found to be superior to placebo in one, superior to lithium in another, and comparable to haloperidol in a third (Chouinard 1987; Chouinard et al. 1983; Edwards et al. 1991). In the fourth study (Bradwejn et al. 1990), lorazepam was found to be superior to clonazepam, which had no significant antimanic effects.

All of these studies were confounded by small sample sizes, short durations of treatment, and difficulties in distinguishing putative specific antimanic effects from nonspecific sedative effects. Moreover, the first two studies were further confounded by the coadministration of neuroleptics. However, in a controlled study comparing lorazepam with haloperidol as adjuncts to lithium in the treatment of acute manic agitation, the two treatments appeared to be comparable (Lenox et al. 1992). This suggests that lorazepam (and perhaps other benzodiazepines) may be safe, effective alternatives to neuroleptics in the initial or early management of manic agitation until the effects of the primary mood-stabilizing agent become apparent.

Although there are no controlled studies of benzodiazepines in the treatment of bipolar depression, one open study reported the successful treatment of 21 (84%) of 25 depressed patients with open-label clonazepam (maximum daily doses of 1.5–6.0 mg) (Kishimoto et al. 1983). Of this group, 18 had major depression and 9 had bipolar depression, including 8 who had failed to respond to previous treatment with two or more antidepressants. However, treatment of panic disorder with various benzodiazepines has been associated with treatment-emergent depression (Tesar 1990).

Two studies have examined the prophylactic efficacy of benzodiazepines in patients with bipolar disorder. In the first, bipolar patients requiring combined maintenance treatment with lithium and haloperidol did equally well when their regimens were changed to lithium and clonazepam (Sachs et al. 1990). However, the second study (the only study to date attempting to assess the efficacy of clonazepam alone as a maintenance treatment) had to be prematurely terminated after the first five patients who were enrolled relapsed within the first 2–15 weeks of treatment (Aronson et al. 1989). Of note, the poor results observed in this study may have been due in part to the inclusion of lithium-refractory patients and to rapid tapering of antipsychotics before the initiation of clonazepam treatment (Chouinard 1989).

In summary, available studies have not yet definitively proven that benzodiazepines have specific antimanic, antidepressant, or long-term mood-stabilizing properties apart from their nonspecific sedative effects. However, benzodiazepines may be useful in the treatment of acute manic agitation either in place of or in conjunction with antipsychotics 1) until the effects of other primary mood-stabilizing agents become apparent and 2) in the short-term treatment of insomnia, anxiety, or catatonia associated with either mania or depression.

OTHER ANTIEPILEPTICS

Oxcarbazepine

Available in Europe but not yet available in the United States, oxcarbazepine (10,11-dihydro-10-oxo-carbamazepine), the 10-keto analogue of carbamazepine, has a chemical structure and antiepileptic profile similar to that of carbamazepine (Anonymous 1989; Dam and Jensen 1989). Oxcarbazepine has been shown to be as effective as carbamazepine in suppressing generalized tonic-clonic seizures and partial seizures, with and without secondary generalization. Preliminary reports also suggest that it may have antineuralgic effects.

Oxcarbazepine and carbamazepine, however, have significantly different pharmacokinetic profiles. Unlike carbamazepine, oxcarbazepine does not appear to induce the hepatic microsomal P450 enzyme system, and it is not metabolized to an epoxide with neurotoxic effects. Rather, oxcarbazepine is rapidly and extensively converted to the 10-hydroxy metabolite, an active metabolite responsible for most of the drug's antiepileptic effects. These differences suggest that oxcarbazepine may be an easier drug to administer, with fewer drug-drug interactions, and easier to tolerate with less neurotoxicity. Nevertheless, oxcarbazepine's most common side effects are tiredness, headache, dizziness, and ataxia. Also, it has been reported to cause allergic reactions and hyponatremia, although less frequently than does carbamazepine.

Four controlled studies assessing the efficacy of oxcarbazepine in the treatment of acute mania have shown that oxcarbazepine is superior to placebo and comparable to haloperidol and lithium after 14 days of treatment (Emrich

1990; Emrich et al. 1985; Müller and Stoll 1984). In these studies, the tolerability of oxcarbazepine was better than that of haloperidol and comparable to that of lithium. These results are limited, however, by the concomitant use of haloperidol (and in some cases lithium) in both treatment groups in the two largest studies (Emrich 1990). In addition, although the average oxcarbazepine dosage used in these studies was 1,400–2,400 mg/day, the optimal dosage range for the antimanic effects of oxcarbazepine has not yet been established.

Oxcarbazepine has not been tested in the treatment of acute major depression. However, two controlled studies have compared the prophylactic efficacy of oxcarbazepine with that of lithium in patients with bipolar disorder (Table 12–4). In the first study, Cabrera et al. (1986), using an oxcarbazepine dosage of only 900 mg/day, found significant decreases in the rates of recurrent manic and depressive episodes in both the oxcarbazepine- and the lithium-treated groups. In the second study, Wildgrube (1990) found a higher rate of relapse in patients maintained on oxcarbazepine than in those receiving lithium. However, the subjects in the oxcarbazepine-treated group were significantly older and more severely ill at the initiation of treatment than those in the group randomly assigned to lithium treatment. The small sample size in each study makes further interpretation of their data difficult, and larger studies are needed to establish the optimal dosage and therapeutic efficacy of oxcarbazepine as a maintenance agent for the treatment of bipolar disorder.

Phenytoin

Although there are no controlled studies of phenytoin in the treatment of bipolar disorder, open studies performed in the late 1940s and early 1950s indicated that phenytoin may be helpful in the treatment of psychiatric patients with acute mania or maniclike presentations (e.g., "excited psychoses") (Gutierrez-Esteinou and Cole 1988). For instance, in an open-label study of phenytoin in 60 state hospital psychiat-

ric patients, the best results were observed in the "excited" group, and improvement was shown in 73% of 16 patients with "excited schizophrenia" (*n* = 22) and 89% of 8 patients with mania (*n* = 9) (Kalinowsky and Putnam 1943). In a similar open-label trial of phenytoin in 73 psychotic patients, 11 of whom had manic-depressive illness, 5 of 9 patients in the manic phase and 1 of 2 in the depressive phase showed improvement (Kubanek and Rowell 1946). The authors concluded that phenytoin was useful in the treatment of "excited chronic psychoses." In yet another open-label study of 45 chronic patients with a wide range of diagnoses, 1 patient with mania and some patients with schizophrenia (only those with catatonia) showed improvement (Freyhan 1945). In short, although these studies are methodologically flawed and no controlled data yet indicate that phenytoin is effective in the treatment of mania, it may be considered as a treatment alternative for some patients resistant to lithium, carbamazepine, and valproate.

Lamotrigine

Lamotrigine, an anticonvulsant with established efficacy (mainly as adjunctive therapy) in partial seizures, is believed to act by inhibiting the stimulated presynaptic release of glutamate and may have antidepressant and/or mood-stabilizing effects. In a 6-month, open-label trial of 67 patients with treatment-refractory bipolar I and II disorders, lamotrigine was administered as monotherapy in 17 (25%) and as adjunctive therapy in 50 (75%) (Calabrese et al. 1995). Of 39 (58%) patients who presented in the depressed phase, 9 (23%) had moderate improvement in reduction of depressive symptoms and 18 (46%) showed marked improvement. Of 25 patients who presented in hypomanic, manic, or mixed states, 4 (16%) had moderate improvement in manic symptoms and 15 (60%) showed marked improvement. In a second open-label trial (Sporn and Sachs 1997), 16 patients with treatment-resistant bipolar I or II disorder re-

Table 12–4. Controlled studies of carbamazepine and oxcarbazepine as preventive therapy in patients with bipolar disorder

Study	N	Design	Concomitant medications	Duration (years)	Outcome
Okuma et al. 1981	12 CBZ; 10 P	CBZ v. P	Not specified, but permitted for breakthrough episodes	1	40% relapse on CBZ; 78% relapse on P
Placidi et al. 1986	20 CBZ; 16 L	CBZ v. L	TCAs, CPZ for breakthrough episodes	to 3	67% response rate for both groups
Watkins et al. 1987	19 CBZ; 18 L	CBZ v. L	Neuroleptics, antidepressants for breakthrough episodes	1.5	Mean time in remission: CBZ 16 months, L 9.4 months
Lusznat et al. 1988	20 CBZ; 21 L	CBZ v. L	Neuroleptics, antidepressants for breakthrough episodes	to 1	45% CBZ patients at 12 months, 25% L patients at 12 months, 25% CBZ rehospitalized, 50% L rehospitalized
Bellaire et al. 1988	46 CBZ; 52 L	CBZ v. L	ND	1	Mean reduction in number of episodes comparable: 1.8/year to 0.67/year CBZ, 1.7/year to 0.7/year L
Cabrera et al. 1986	4 OX; 6 L	OX v. L	Neuroleptics (1 OX, 2 L)	Up to 22	3/4 OX, 6/6 L had significant decrease in affective episodes
Wildgrube 1990	8 OX; 7 L	OX v. L	ND	Up to 33	6/8 OX, 3/7 L treatment failures

Note. CBZ = carbamazepine; OX = oxcarbazepine; ND = not described; TCAs = tricyclic antidepressants; CPZ = chlorpromazine; L = lithium.
Source. Reprinted from Keck PE Jr, McElroy SL, Nemeroff CB: "Anticonvulsants in the Treatment of Bipolar Disorder." *Journal of Neuropsychiatry and Clinical Neurosciences* 4:395–405, 1992. Used with permission.

ceived lamotrigine as adjunctive treatment for affective episodes. Eight (50%) of 16 patients were rated as responders, and lamotrigine appeared to exert antidepressant and mood-stabilizing effects in these patients.

Gabapentin

Gabapentin is a new anticonvulsant that is effective as adjunctive therapy in the treatment of partial seizures with and without secondary generalization. Four reports have described its effects in the treatment of psychiatric disorders (McElroy et al. 1997; Ryback and Ryback 1995; Short and Cooke 1995; Stanton et al. 1996). In one report (Stanton et al. 1996), gabapentin monotherapy appeared to ameliorate manic symptoms in patients with bipolar disorder. In a second report (Ryback and Ryback 1995), gabapentin produced improvement in behavioral dyscontrol in an adolescent with intermittent explosive disorder, organic mood disorder (secondary to closed head injury), and attention-deficit/hyperactivity disorder. Conversely, hypomanic symptoms were described in a patient with epilepsy when gabapentin was added to carbamazepine and lamotrigine (Short and Cooke 1995). Finally, McElroy et al. (1997) used open-label, adjunctive gabapentin to treat nine patients with bipolar I or II disorder who were experiencing hypomanic, manic, or mixed states inadequately responsive to mood stabilizers. Of the nine patients, seven had a moderate or marked reduction in manic symptoms by 1 month of gabapentin treatment. Another patient had moderate improvement after 3 months. Of these eight patients, six continued to have antimanic responses for follow-up periods ranging from 1 to 7 months. A double-blind, placebo-controlled study of gabapentin in patients with bipolar disorder was recently completed. No efficacy in the treatment of mania was demonstrated.

Barbiturate Antiepileptics

Barbiturate antiepileptics have not been well studied in the treatment of bipolar disorder. However, in an open study of primidone and/or mephobarbital in 27 patients with mood disorders refractory to lithium, carbamazepine, valproate, and phenytoin, 9 patients had sustained positive effects with primidone and 3 had positive effects with mephobarbital after failure of primidone treatment (Hayes 1993).

Acetazolamide

Inoue et al. (1984) in Japan reported that acetazolamide (a diuretic with antiepileptic properties) was effective in patients with atypical psychoses characterized by dreamy or confusional states and often associated with the premenstrual or puerperal period. Testing of this drug in bipolar patients—especially those

with associated confusion or perimenstrual or puerperal exacerbation of their symptoms— would therefore appear to be warranted.

CONCLUSION

Growing evidence indicates that a variety of antiepileptic drugs have beneficial effects in the treatment of bipolar disorder. To date, the antiepileptics best studied in the treatment of bipolar disorder are carbamazepine and valproate. These drugs have acute antimanic and long-term mood-stabilizing effects (and possibly acute antidepressant effects) in some bipolar patients, including those inadequately responsive to or intolerant of lithium. Other, less well-studied antiepileptic compounds, including oxcarbazepine and phenytoin, may also have mood-stabilizing effects. Although it is unclear whether benzodiazepines have specific mood-stabilizing effects, they are useful adjuncts to primary mood stabilizers in the treatment of acute manic agitation and catatonia.

It is important to remember that the antiepileptics may be synergistic with other mood-stabilizing agents—including one another—in the treatment of bipolar disorder that responds inadequately to monotherapy. Indeed, although viewed together as a class of drugs, the antiepileptics are in fact very different agents, possessing different chemical structures, pharmacological properties, pharmacokinetics, side effects, and efficacies in the treatment of epilepsy. Thus, even though carbamazepine and valproate may share similar predictors of response for bipolar disorder (e.g., dysphoric mania), different bipolar patients may respond to one agent but not to the other or may tolerate one agent better than the other, as is the case for patients with epilepsy. Clinicians therefore have a wide range of medications and combinations of medications to choose from when treating bipolar disorder. Furthermore, although the actions underlying the antiepileptic properties of these drugs may or may not be responsible for their mood-stabilizing effects, any future drugs with antiepileptic activity should be screened as putative antimanic, mood-stabilizing, or antidepressant agents.

REFERENCES

Albright PS, Burnham WM: Development of a new pharmacological seizure model: effects of anti-convulsants on cortical and amygdala-kindled seizures in the rat. Epilepsia 21: 681–689, 1980

American Psychiatric Association: Diagnostic and Statistical Manual of Mental Disorders, 3rd Edition. Washington, DC, American Psychiatric Association, 1980

Andrews DG, Schweitzer I, Marshall N: The comparative side effects of lithium, carbamazepine and combined lithium-carbamazepine in patients treated for affective disorders. Human Psychopharmacology 5:41–45, 1990

Anonymous: Sodium valproate. Lancet 2: 1229–1231, 1988

Anonymous: Oxcarbazepine. Lancet 2:196–198, 1989

Aronson TA, Skukla S, Hirschowitz J: Clonazepam treatment of five lithium-refractory patients with bipolar disorder. Am J Psychiatry 146: 77–80, 1989

Ballenger JC, Post RM: Therapeutic effects of carbamazepine in affective illness: a preliminary report. Communications in Psychopharmacology 2:159–175, 1978

Beghi E, DiMascio R, Sasanelli F, et al: Adverse reactions to antiepileptic drugs: a multicenter survey of clinical practice. Epilepsia 27:323–330, 1986

Bellaire W, Demish K, Stoll KD: Carbamazepine versus lithium in prophylaxis of recurrent affective disorders. Psychopharmacology (Berl) 96: 2875, 1988

Blom S: Tic douloureux treated with a new anticonvulsant: experiences with G 32883. Arch Neurol 2:357–366, 1963

Bourgeois BFD: Valproate: clinical use, in Antiepileptic Drugs, 3rd Edition. Edited by Levy RH, Dreifuss FE, Mattson RH, et al. New York, Raven, 1989, pp 633–642

Bowden CL, Brugger AM, Swann AC, et al: Efficacy of divalproex vs. lithium and placebo in the treatment of mania. JAMA 271:918–924, 1994

Bradwejn J, Shriqui C, Koszycki D, et al: Double-blind comparison of the effects of clonazepam and lorazepam in mania. J Clin Psychopharmacol 10:403–408, 1990

Brennan MJW, Sandyk R, Borsook D: Use of sodium valproate in the management of affective disorders: basic and clinical aspects, in Anticonvulsants in Affective Disorders. Edited by Emrich HM, Okuma T, Müller AA. Amsterdam, Excerpta Medica, 1984, pp 56–65

Brown D, Silverstone T, Cookson J: Carbamazepine compared to haloperidol in acute mania. International Journal of Clinical Psychopharmacology 48:89–93, 1987

Buzan RD, Firestone D, Thomas M, et al: Valproate-associated pancreatitis and cholecystitis in six mentally retarded adults. J Clin Psychiatry 56:529–532, 1995

Cabrera JF, Muhlbauer HD, Schley J, et al: Long-term randomized clinical trial of oxcarbazepine vs. lithium in bipolar and schizoaffective disorders: preliminary results. Pharmacopsychiatry 19:282–283, 1986

Calabrese JR, Delucchi GA: Spectrum of efficacy of valproate in 55 rapid-cycling manic depressives. Am J Psychiatry 147:431–434, 1990

Calabrese JR, Markovitz PJ, Kimmel SE, et al: Spectrum of efficacy of valproate in 78 rapid-cycling bipolar patients. J Clin Psychopharmacol 12: 53S–56S, 1992

Calabrese JR, Woyshville MJ, Kimmel SE, et al: Predictors of valproate response in bipolar rapid cycling. J Clin Psychopharmacol 13:280–283, 1993

Calabrese JR, Woyshville MJ, Bowden CL, et al: Spectrum of efficacy of lamotrigine in treatment-refractory manic depression. Second International Conference on Affective Disorders. Jerusalem, Israel, September 1995

Centers for Disease Control: Use of folic acid for prevention of spina bifida and other neural tube defects. JAMA 266:1190–1191, 1991

Chouinard G: Clonazepam in acute and maintenance treatment of bipolar affective disorder. J Clin Psychiatry 48:29S–36S, 1987

Chouinard G: Clonazepam in treatment of bipolar psychotic patients after discontinuation of neuroleptics (letter). Am J Psychiatry 146:1642, 1989

Chouinard G, Young SN, Annable L: Antimanic effect of clonazepam. Biol Psychiatry 18:451–486, 1983

Clothier J, Swann AC, Freeman T: Dysphoric mania. J Clin Psychopharmacol 12:13S–16S, 1992

Costello LE, Suppes T: A clinically significant interaction between clozapine and valproate. J Clin Psychopharmacol 15:139–140, 1995

Dalby MA: Antiepileptic and psychotropic effect of carbamazepine (Tegretol) in the treatment of psychomotor epilepsy. Epilepsia 12:325–334, 1971

Dam M, Jensen PK: Potential antiepileptic drugs: oxcarbazepine, in Antiepileptic Drugs, 3rd Edition. Edited by Levy RH, Dreifuss FE, Mattson RH, et al. New York, Raven, 1989, pp 913–924

Delcado-Escveta AV, Janz D: Consensus guidelines: preconception counseling management, and care of the pregnant woman with epilepsy. Neurology 42:149–160, 1992

Denicoff KD, Smith-Jackson EE, Disney ER, et al: Comparative prophylactic efficacy of lithium, carbamazepine, and the combination in bipolar disorder. J Clin Psychiatry 58:470–478, 1997

Desai NG, Gangadhar BN, Channabasavanna SM, et al: Carbamazepine hastens therapeutic action of lithium in mania, in Proceedings of the International Conference of New Directions in Affective Disorders, Jerusalem, Israel, September 1987

Dreifuss FE: Valproate toxicity, in Antiepileptic Drugs, 3rd Edition. Edited by Levy RH, Dreifuss FE, Mattson RH, et al. New York, Raven, 1989, pp 643–651

Dreifuss FE, Langer DH, Moline KA, et al: Valproic acid hepatic fatalities, II: U.S. experience since 1984. Neurology 39:201–207, 1989

Edwards R, Stephenson U, Flewett T: Clonazepam in acute mania: a double-blind trial. Aust N Z J Psychiatry 25:238–242, 1991

Emrich HM: Studies with oxcarbazepine (Trileptal) in acute mania. Int Clin Psychopharmacol 5: 83S–88S, 1990

Emrich HM, Wolf R: Valproate treatment of mania. Prog Neuropsychopharmacol Biol Psychiatry 16:691–701, 1992

Emrich HM, von Zerssen D, Kissling W, et al: On a possible role of GABA in mania: therapeutic efficacy of sodium valproate, in GABA and Benzodiazepine Receptors. Edited by Costa E, Dicharia G, Gessa GL. New York, Raven, 1981, pp 287–296

Emrich HM, Dose M, von Zerssen D: The use of sodium valproate, carbamazepine, and oxcarbazepine in patients with affective disorders. J Affect Disord 8:243–250, 1985

Fariello R, Smith MC: Valproate: mechanisms of action, in Antiepileptic Drugs, 3rd Edition. Edited by Levy RH, Dreifuss FE, Mattson RH, et al. New York, Raven, 1989, pp 567–575

Fogel BS: Combining anticonvulsants with conventional psychopharmacologic agents, in Use of Anticonvulsants in Psychiatry: Recent Advances. Edited by McElroy SL, Pope HG Jr. Clifton, NJ, Oxford Health Care, 1988, pp 77–94

Frankenburg FR, Tohen M, Cohen BM, et al: Long-term response to carbamazepine: a retrospective study. J Clin Psychopharmacol 8: 130–132, 1988

Freeman TW, Clothier JL, Pazzaglia P, et al: A double-blind comparison of valproate and lithium in the treatment of acute mania. Am J Psychiatry 149:108–111, 1992

Freyhan FA: Effectiveness of diphenylhydantoin in management of nonepileptic psychomotor excitement states. Arch Neurol Psychiatry 53: 370–374, 1945

Goodwin FK: Medical treatment of manic episodes, in Manic-Depressive Illness. Edited by Goodwin FK, Jamison KR. New York, Oxford University Press, 1990, pp 603–629

Gram L, Jensen PK: Carbamazepine toxicity, in Antiepileptic Drugs, 3rd Edition. Edited by Levy RH, Dreifuss FE, Mattson RH, et al. New York, Raven, 1989, pp 555–565

Grossi E, Sacchetti E, Vita A, et al: Carbamazepine vs. chlorpromazine in mania: a double-blind trial, in Anticonvulsants in Affective Disorders. Edited by Emrich HM, Okuma T, Müller AA. Amsterdam, Excerpta Medica, 1984, pp 177–187

Guscott R: Clinical experience with valproic acid in 22 patients with refractory bipolar mood disorder. Can J Psychiatry 37:590, 1992

Gutierrez-Esteinou R, Cole JO: Psychiatric effects of phenytoin and ethosuximide, in Use of Anticonvulsants in Psychiatry: Recent Advances. Edited by McElroy SL, Pope HG Jr. Clifton, NJ, Oxford Health Care, 1988, pp 59–76

Hayes SG: Long-term use of valproate in primary psychiatric disorders. J Clin Psychiatry 50: 35S–39S, 1989

Hayes SG: Barbiturate anticonvulsants in refractory affective disorders. Ann Clin Psychiatry 5: 35–44, 1993

Hernandez-Avila CA, Ortega-Soto HA, Jasso A, et al: Carbamazepine versus haloperidol for the treatment of acute manic episodes. Abstract presented at the 149th annual meeting of the American Psychiatric Association, New York, May 1996

Hurd RW, Van Rinsvelt HA, Wilder BJ, et al: Selenium, zinc, and copper changes with valproic acid: possible relation to drug side effects. Neurology 34:1394–1395, 1984

Inoue H, Hazama H, Hamazoe K, et al: Antipsychotic and prophylactic effects of acetazolamide (Diamox) on atypical psychosis. Folia Psychiatrica et Neurologica Japonica 38:425–436, 1984

Jacobsen FM: Low-dose valproate: a new treatment for cyclothymia, mild rapid-cycling disorders, and premenstrual syndrome. J Clin Psychiatry 54:229–234, 1993

Jones KL, Lacro RV, Johnson KA, et al: Pattern of malformations in the children of women treated with carbamazepine during pregnancy. N Engl J Med 320:186–188, 1989

Kahn D, Stevenson E, Douglas CJ: Effect of sodium valproate in three patients with organic brain syndromes. Am J Psychiatry 145:1010–1011, 1988

Kalinowsky LB, Putnam TJ: Attempts at treatment of schizophrenia and other non-epileptic psychoses with Dilantin. Archives of Neurology and Psychiatry 49:414–420, 1943

Kastner T, Finesmith R, Walsh K: Brief report: long-term administration of valproic acid in the treatment of affective symptoms in people with mental retardation. J Clin Psychopharmacol 13:448–451, 1993

Keck PE Jr, McElroy SL, Nemeroff CB: Anticonvulsants in the treatment of bipolar disorder. J Neuropsychiatry Clin Neurosci 4:395–405, 1992

Keck PE Jr, McElroy SL, Tugrul KC, et al: Valproate oral loading in the treatment of acute mania. J Clin Psychiatry 54:305–308, 1993

Ketter TA, Post RM: Clinical pharmacology and pharmacokinetics of carbamazepine, in Anticonvulsants in Mood Disorders. Edited by Joffe RT, Calabrese JR. New York, Marcel Dekker, 1994, pp 147–188

Ketter TA, Post RM, Worthington K: Principles of clinically important drug interactions with carbamazepine, part I. J Clin Psychopharmacol 11:198–203, 1991a

Ketter TA, Post RM, Worthington K: Principles of clinically important drug interactions with carbamazepine, part II. J Clin Psychopharmacol 11:306–313, 1991b

Kishimoto A, Ogura C, Hazama H, et al: Long-term prophylactic effects of carbamazepine in affective disorder. Br J Psychiatry 143:327–331, 1983

Klein E, Bental E, Lerer B, et al: Carbamazepine and haloperidol in excited psychoses. Arch Gen Psychiatry 41:165–170, 1984

Kramlinger KG, Post RM: The addition of lithium to carbamazepine: antidepressant efficacy in treatment-resistant depression. Arch Gen Psychiatry 46:794–800, 1989

Kubanek JL, Rowell RC: The use of Dilantin in the treatment of psychotic patients unresponsive to other treatments. Diseases of the Nervous System 7:47–50, 1946

Kupferberg AJ: Valproate: chemistry and methods of determination, in Antiepileptic Drugs, 3rd Edition. Edited by Levy RH, Dreifuss FE, Mattson RH, et al. New York, Raven, 1989, pp 577–582

Kutt H: Carbamazepine: chemistry and methods of determination, in Antiepileptic Drugs, 3rd Edition. Edited by Levy RH, Dreifuss FE, Mattson RH, et al. New York, Raven, 1989, pp 457–471

Lambert PA, Venaud G: Comparative study of valpromide versus lithium as prophylactic treatment in affective disorders. Nervure 17:1–9, 1994

Lambert PA, Cavaz G, Borselli S, et al: Action neuropsychotrope d'un nouvel anti-épileptique: le Dépamide. Ann Med Psychol (Paris) 1: 707–710, 1966

Lenox RH, Newhouse PA, Creelman WL, et al: Adjunctive treatment of manic agitation with lorazepam vs. haloperidol: a double-blind study. J Clin Psychiatry 53:47–52, 1992

Lenzi A, Lazzerini F, Grossi E, et al: Use of carbamazepine in acute psychosis: a controlled study. J Int Med Res 14:78–84, 1986

Lerer B, Moore N, Meyendorff E, et al: Carbamazepine versus lithium in mania: a double-blind study. J Clin Psychiatry 48:89–93, 1987

Leveil V, Nanquet R: A study of the action of valproic acid on the kindling effect. Epilepsia 18:229–234, 1977

Levy RH, Dreifuss FE, Mattson RH, et al (eds): Antiepileptic Drugs, 3rd Edition. New York, Raven, 1989

Loiseau P, Duche B: Carbamazepine: clinical use, in Antiepileptic Drugs, 3rd Edition. Edited by Levy RH, Dreifuss FE, Mattson RH, et al. New York, Raven, 1989, pp 533–554

Lusznat RM, Murphy DP, Nunn CMH: Carbamazepine vs. lithium in the treatment of prophylaxis of mania. Br J Psychiatry 153: 198–204, 1988

Macdonald RL: Carbamazepine: mechanisms of action, in Antiepileptic Drugs, 3rd Edition. Edited by Levy RH, Dreifuss FH, Mattson RH, et al. New York, Raven, 1989, pp 447–455

Mattson RH, Cramer JA, Damey PD, et al: Use of oral contraceptives by women with epilepsy. JAMA 256:238–240, 1986

Mattson RH, Cramer JA, Collins JF, et al: A comparison of valproate with carbamazepine for the treatment of complex partial seizures and secondarily generalized tonic-clonic seizures in adult. N Engl J Med 327:765–771, 1992

McElroy SL, Pope HG Jr (eds): Use of Anticonvulsants in Psychiatry: Recent Advances. Clifton, NJ, Oxford Health Care, 1988

McElroy SL, Keck PE Jr, Pope HG Jr, et al: Valproate in the treatment of rapid-cycling, bipolar disorder. J Clin Psychopharmacol 8: 275–279, 1988a

McElroy SL, Pope HG Jr, Keck PE Jr, et al: Treatment of psychiatric disorders with valproate: a series of 73 cases. Psychiatrie Psychobiologie 3: 81–85, 1988b

McElroy SL, Keck PE Jr, Pope HG Jr, et al: Correlates of antimanic response to valproate. Psychopharmacol Bull 27:127–133, 1991

McElroy SL, Keck PE Jr, Pope HG Jr, et al: Clinical and research implications of the diagnosis of dysphoric or mixed mania or hypomania. Am J Psychiatry 149:1633–1644, 1992a

McElroy SL, Keck PE Jr, Pope HG Jr, et al: Valproate in bipolar disorder: literature review and treatment guidelines. J Clin Psychopharmacol 12:42S–52S, 1992b

McElroy SL, Keck PE Jr, Stanton SP, et al: A randomized comparison of divalproex oral loading versus haloperidol in the initial treatment of acute psychotic mania. J Clin Psychiatry 57: 142–146, 1996

McElroy SL, Soutullo CA, Keck PE Jr, et al: A pilot trial of gabapentin in the treatment of bipolar disorder. Ann Clin Psychiatry 9:99–103, 1997

Möller MJ, Kissling W, Riehl T, et al: Double-blind evaluation of the antimanic properties of carbamazepine as a comedication to haloperidol. Prog Neuropsychopharmacol Biol Psychiatry 13:127–136, 1989

Morselli PL: Carbamazepine: absorption, distribution, and excretion, in Antiepileptic Drugs, 3rd Edition. Edited by Levy RH, Dreifuss FE, Mattson RH, et al. New York, Raven, 1989, pp 473–490

Müller AA, Stoll KD: Carbamazepine and oxcarbazepine in the treatment of manic syndromes: studies in Germany, in Anticonvulsants in Affective Disorders. Edited by Emrich HM, Okuma T, Müller AA. Amsterdam, Excerpta Medica, 1984, pp 134–147

Murphy DJ, Gannon MA, McGennis A: Carbamazepine in bipolar affective disorder. Lancet 2:1151–1152, 1989

Neumann J, Seidel K, Wunderlich BP: Comparative studies of the effect of carbamazepine and trimipramine in depression, in Anticonvulsants in Affective Disorders. Edited by Emrich HM, Okuma T, Müller AA. Amsterdam, Excerpta Medica, 1984, pp 160–166

Okuma T: Effects of carbamazepine and lithium on affective disorders. Neuropsychobiology 27: 138–145, 1993

Okuma T, Inanaga K, Otsuki S, et al: Comparison of the antimanic efficacy of carbamazepine and chlorpromazine. Psychopharmacology (Berl) 66:211–217, 1979

Okuma T, Inanaga K, Otsuki S, et al: A preliminary doubleblind study on the efficacy in prophylaxis of manic depressive illness. Psychopharmacology (Berl) 73:95–96, 1981

Okuma T, Yamashita I, Takahasi R, et al: Comparison of the antimanic efficacy of carbamazepine and lithium carbonate by double-blind controlled study. Pharmacopsychiatry 23:143–150, 1990

Pellock JM: Carbamazepine side effects in children and adults. Epilepsia 28:564S–570S, 1987

Pellock JM, Willmore LJ: A rational guide to routine blood monitoring in patients receiving antiepileptic drugs. Neurology 41:961–964, 1991

Penry JK, Dean JC: The scope and use of valproate in epilepsy. J Clin Psychiatry 40:17S–22S, 1989

Placidi GF, Lenzi A, Lazzerini F, et al: The comparative efficacy and safety of carbamazepine versus lithium: a randomized, double-blind 3 year trial in 83 patients. J Clin Psychiatry 47:490–494, 1986

Pope HG Jr, McElroy SL, Satlin A, et al: Head injury, bipolar disorder, and response to valproate. Compr Psychiatry 29:34–38, 1988

Pope HG Jr, McElroy SL, Keck PE Jr, et al: Valproate in the treatment of acute mania: a placebo-controlled study. Arch Gen Psychiatry 48:62–68, 1991

Post RM: Approaches to treatment-resistant bipolar affectively ill patients. Clin Neuropharmacol 11:93–104, 1988

Post RM: Non-lithium treatment for bipolar disorder. J Clin Psychiatry 51:9S–16S, 1990

Post RM, Ballenger JC, Uhde TW, et al: Efficacy of carbamazepine in manic-depressive illness: implications for underlying mechanisms, in Neurobiology of Mood Disorders. Edited by Post RM, Ballenger JC. Baltimore, MD, Williams & Wilkins, 1984a, pp 77–816

Post RM, Berettini W, Uhde TW, et al: Selective response to the anticonvulsant carbamazepine in manic depressive illness: a case study. J Clin Psychopharmacol 4:178–185, 1984b

Post RM, Uhde TW, Roy-Byrne PP, et al: Antidepressant effects of carbamazepine. Am J Psychiatry 143:29–34, 1985

Post RM, Uhde TW, Roy-Byrne PP, et al: Correlates of antimanic response to carbamazepine. Psychiatry Res 21:71–83, 1987

Post RM, Leverich GS, Rosoff AS, et al: Carbamazepine prophylaxis in refractory affective disorders: a focus on long-term follow-up. J Clin Psychopharmacol 10:318–327, 1990

Post RM, Altshuler LL, Ketter TA, et al: Antiepileptic drugs in affective illness: clinical and theoretical implications, in Advances in Neurology, Vol 55. Edited by Smith D, Treiman D, Trimble M. New York, Raven, 1991, pp 239–277

Post RM, Weiss SRB, Chuang DM: Mechanisms of action of anticonvulsants in affective disorders: comparison with lithium. J Clin Psychopharmacol 12:23S–35S, 1992

Prien RF, Gelenberg AJ: Alternatives to lithium for preventive treatment of bipolar disorder. Am J Psychiatry 146:840–848, 1989

Puzynski S, Klosiewicz L: Valproic acid amide as a prophylactic agent in affective and schizoaffective disorders. Psychopharmacol Bull 20: 151–159, 1984

Rall TW, Schleifer LS: Drugs effective in the therapy of the epilepsies, in The Pharmacological Basis of Therapeutics. Edited by Gilman AG, Goodman LS, Rall TW, et al. New York, Macmillan, 1985, pp 446–472

Rimmer E, Richens A: An update on sodium valproate. Pharmacotherapy 5:171–184, 1985

Rosa FWL: Spina bifida in infants of women treated with carbamazepine during pregnancy. N Engl J Med 324:674–677, 1991

Ryback R, Ryback L: Gabapentin for behavioral dyscontrol. Am J Psychiatry 152:1319, 1995

Sachs GS, Weilburg JB, Rosebaum JF: Clonazepam vs. neuroleptics as adjuncts to lithium maintenance. Psychopharmacol Bull 26:137–143, 1990

Seetharam MN, Pellock JM: Risk-benefit assessment of carbamazepine in children. Drug Saf 6:148–158, 1991

Short C, Cooke L: Hypomania induced by gabapentin. Br J Psychiatry 166:679–680, 1995

Simhandl CH, Denke E, Thau K: The comparative efficacy of carbamazepine low and high serum level and lithium carbonate in the prophylaxis of affective disorders. J Affect Disord 28:221–231, 1993

Small JG: Anticonvulsants in affective disorders. Psychopharmacol Bull 26:25–36, 1990

Small JG, Klapper MH, Milstein V, et al: Carbamazepine compared with lithium in the treatment of mania. Arch Gen Psychiatry 48: 915–921, 1991

Smith MC, Bleck TP: Convulsive disorders: toxicity of anticonvulsants. Clin Neuropharmacol 14: 97–115, 1991

Sovner R: The use of valproate in the treatment of mentally retarded persons with typical and atypical bipolar disorders. J Clin Psychiatry 50: 40S–43S, 1989

Sovner R, Davis JM: A potential drug interaction between fluoxetine and valproic acid. J Clin Psychopharmacol 11:389, 1991

Sporn J, Sachs G: The anticonvulsant lamotrigine in treatment-resistant manic-depressive illness. J Clin Psychopharmacol 17:185–189, 1997

Stanton SP, Keck PE Jr, McElroy SL: Treatment of acute mania with gabapentin (letter). Am J Psychiatry 154:287, 1996

Stoll AL, Vuckovic A, McElroy SL: Histamine 2-receptor antagonists for the treatment of valproate-induced gastrointestinal distress. Ann Clin Psychiatry 3:301–304, 1991

Stoll AL, Banov M, Kolbrener M, et al: Neurologic factors predict a favorable valproate response in bipolar and schizoaffective disorder. J Clin Psychopharmacol 14:311–313, 1994

Suppes T, McElroy SL, Gilbert J, et al: Clozapine in the treatment of dysphoric mania. Biol Psychiatry 32:270–280, 1992

Takezaki H, Hanaoka M: The use of carbamazepine (Tegretol) in the control of manic-depressive psychosis and other manic, depressive states. Clinical Psychiatry 13:173–182, 1971

Tesar GE: High potency benzodiazepines for short-term management of panic disorder: the U.S. experience. J Clin Psychiatry 51:4S–10S, 1990

Tohen M, Castillo J, Pope HG Jr, et al: Concomitant use of valproate and carbamazepine in bipolar and schizoaffective disorders. J Clin Psychopharmacol 14:67–70, 1994

Tohen M, Castillo J, Baldessarini RJ, et al: Blood dyscrasias with carbamazepine and valproate: a pharmacoepidemiological study of 2,228 patients at risk. Am J Psychiatry 152:413–418, 1995

Vencovsky E, Soucek K, Zatecká I: Comparison of side effects of lithium and dipropylacetamide (Depamide). Ceskoslovensk Psychiatrie 79: 223–227, 1983

Vining EPG: Cognitive dysfunction associated with antiepileptic drug therapy. Epilepsia 28: 18S–22S, 1987

Watkins SE, Callender K, Thomas DR, et al: The effect of carbamazepine and lithium on remission from affective illness. Br J Psychiatry 150: 180–182, 1987

Wilder BJ: Pharmacokinetics of valproate and carbamazepine. J Clin Psychopharmacol 12: 64S–68S, 1992

Wilder BJ, Karas BJ, Penry JK, et al: Gastrointestinal tolerance of divalproex sodium. Neurology 33:808–811, 1983

Wildgrube C: Case studies on prophylactic long-term effects of oxcarbazepine in recurrent affective disorders. Int Clin Psychopharmacol 5:89S–94S, 1990

Zona C, Tancredi V, Palma E, et al: Potassium currents in rat cortical neurons in culture are enhanced by the antiepileptic drug carbamazepine. Can J Physiol Pharmacol 68:545–547, 1990

Other Agents

THIRTEEN

Cognitive Enhancers

Deborah B. Marin, M.D., and
Kenneth L. Davis, M.D.

Identification of neurotransmitter deficits in the brains of patients with Alzheimer's disease (AD) has fostered the development of pharmacological strategies to alleviate these deficits (Davies and Maloney 1976). Consistent demonstration of central cholinergic depletion in patients with AD, in conjunction with the cholinergic system's involvement in learning, generated many studies that focused on cholinergic enhancement. Although the cholinergic approach has yielded some promising findings, the results to date have not revealed a consistently robust treatment for the cognitive disturbances seen in patients with AD (Chatellier and Lacomblez 1990; Davis et al. 1992; Farlow et al. 1992; Tariot et al. 1987a). It can be hypothesized that the variable results with the cholinergic replacement strategy in AD may be due in part to deficiencies in other neurotransmitters. If so, correction of deficits in multiple neurotransmitters would be expected to be more efficacious than a purely cholinergic approach.

An alternative to the palliative treatment of AD with neurotransmitter replacement strategies is the development of treatments that could slow the neurodegenerative process of AD and consequent cognitive decline. In this chapter, we review both strategies.

CHOLINERGIC AGENTS

Multiple lines of evidence support a critical role for cholinergic mechanisms in AD, including the following:

1. Centrally active anticholinergic agents produce cognitive deficits in humans (Drachman and Leavitt 1974; Dundee and Pandit 1972).
2. Cholinergic neurotransmission modulates memory and learning (Deutsch 1971).
3. Lesions of the central cholinergic system create learning and memory impairments that can be reversed with cholinomimetic administration (Bartus et al. 1987; Collerton 1986; Olton and Wenk 1987).
4. Postmortem studies of patients with AD document cholinergic cell loss in the septum and nucleus basalis of Meynert, decreased concentrations of choline acetyltransferase and acetylcholinesterase, and a correlation between these changes and degree of cognitive impairment (Davies and Maloney 1976; Perry et al. 1978).

Improvement of the overall functioning of the central cholinergic system could theoretically result from prevention of neuronal degeneration, increasing acetylcholine availability, and activation of postsynaptic cholinergic receptors. Of the several possible methods that could achieve these goals, three strategies have been clinically used: acetylcholine precursors, cholinesterase inhibitors, and postsynaptic agonists.

It has been reasoned that enhancing the availability of acetylcholine precursors could increase acetylcholine synthesis, thereby providing an increased pool of neurotransmitter for cholinergic transmission. Acetylcholine precursor treatments with choline or lecithin represented early attempts to enhance cholinergic transmission in AD. Little evidence supports the efficacy of the precursor loading approach (for review, see Bartus et al. 1985).

Cholinesterase Inhibitors

Physostigmine

History and discovery. The use of physostigmine and other cholinesterase inhibitors is based on the goal of enhancing cholinergic neurotransmission through inhibiting the breakdown of acetylcholine.

Structure. Physostigmine is a natural alkaloid that contains a tertiary amine.

Pharmacological profile. Physostigmine is a reversible anticholinesterase that effectively increases the concentration of acetylcholine at the sites of cholinergic transmission.

Pharmacokinetics and disposition. Physostigmine is absorbed in the gastrointestinal tract, subcutaneous tissue, and mucous membranes. It is hydrolyzed and inactivated within 2 hours, thus requiring multiple doses each day. Physostigmine readily crosses the blood-brain barrier.

Mechanism of action. Physostigmine enhances cholinergic transmission through its in-

creasing acetylcholine availability in the central nervous system (CNS).

Indications. Most studies in which physostigmine is administered parenterally have reported transient cognitive improvement in at least a subgroup of patients with AD (Mohs and Davis 1987). Oral administration of the compound has also been shown to have some efficacy. Some have speculated that long-term treatment with physostigmine may delay deterioration in patients with AD. Two studies with small patient samples suggest that long-term treatment with the medication may attenuate the course of cognitive decline (Beller et al. 1988; Jenike et al. 1990).

The limited efficacy of physostigmine may reflect the biological heterogeneity of patients and the pharmacological properties of the medication. There is significant interindividual variability in the gastrointestinal absorption, hepatic catabolism, hydrolysis, and CNS penetration of this compound (Whelpton and Hurst 1985). Blood levels required to achieve CNS concentrations necessary for cognitive enhancement may be associated with significant adverse effects, including gastrointestinal distress, hypotension, and bradycardia. Therefore, ineffective CNS penetration may have led to the lack of response in some patients tested with this drug. Novel drug delivery systems that overcome the blood-brain barrier problem have yet to be systematically tested.

Side effects. The side effects observed with physostigmine include depressed mood, anxiety, salivation, bradycardia, and gastrointestinal distress.

Drug-drug interactions. Physostigmine has been used primarily as a single agent for treating AD. As we describe later in this chapter, physostigmine has been shown to be safely administered in conjunction with selegiline (L-deprenyl).

Tetrahydroaminoacridine

History and discovery. Two pilot studies in patients with a diagnosis of AD suggested that 9-amino-1,2,3,4,-tetrahydroacridine (THA), administrated alone or in combination with lecithin, was associated with improvement in performances on psychometric tests and global assessments (Kaye et al. 1982; Summers et al. 1981). Summers et al. (1986) documented significant improvement in global status and psychometric performance in 16 subjects treated with THA. These earlier studies led to several multicenter trials to evaluate the efficacy of THA in patients with AD.

Structure. THA is an aminoacridine compound that is a reversible synthetic acetylcholinesterase inhibitor. It has an empirical formula of $C_{13}H_{14}N_2 \times HCl \times H_2O$.

Pharmacological profile. In vitro studies indicate that THA inhibits plasma and tissue acetylcholinesterase (Adem 1992). Unlike physostigmine, which interacts with the catalytic site of acetylcholinesterase, THA produces allosteric inhibition by binding to a hydrophobic region on the active surface of the enzyme (Adem 1992). THA has also been shown to interact with muscarinic and nicotinic receptors (Adem 1992). THA increases presynaptic acetylcholine release by blocking slow potassium channels and increases postsynaptic monoaminergic stimulation by interfering with the uptake of noradrenaline and serotonin (Drukarch et al. 1987, 1988). These latter characteristics of THA occur at concentrations higher than those required for acetylcholinesterase inhibition and therefore probably do not contribute to the drug's clinical effects.

Pharmacokinetics and disposition. THA is rapidly absorbed after oral administration; maximum concentrations in plasma are reached within 1–2 hours. THA is about 55% bound by plasma proteins and is metabolized by the cytochrome P450 system to multiple metabolites. After aromatic ring hydroxylation, the metabolites of THA undergo glucuronidation. The elimination half-life is 2–4 hours. THA is concentrated 10-fold in the brain, in part because of its high lipid solubility (Nielsen et al. 1989).

Mechanism of action. THA enhances cholinergic transmission through its increasing acetylcholine availability in the CNS.

Indications. Several double-blind, placebo-controlled studies have assessed the therapeutic efficacy of THA in larger patient samples. THA and lecithin administration produced minimal cognitive improvement in a study of 67 subjects (Chatellier and Lacomblez 1990). Statistically significant improvement was shown in Mini-Mental State Exam scores (Folstein et al. 1975) in another investigation of 39 patients (Gauthier et al. 1990). In a 6-week crossover trial, using an enriched-population design with 215 patients, Davis et al. (1992) found that the THA-treated group had significantly less decline in cognitive function than did the placebo-treated group, as assessed by the cognitive subscale of the Alzheimer's Disease Assessment Scale (ADAS-cog; Rosen et al. 1984). A 12-week parallel-group design study of 273 patients reported a significant dose-related improvement in cognition with THA treatment (Farlow et al. 1992). A double-blind, crossover study of 89 subjects showed that THA was superior to placebo in its effect on Mini-Mental State Exam scores (Sahakian and Coull 1993). A 30-week, double-blind, placebo-controlled, parallel-group trial with 653 patients showed the efficacy of THA when compared with placebo, and significant dose-response trends favored higher doses of the compound (Knapp et al. 1994).

In reviewing THA's efficacy, the different doses used across studies must be considered. Efficacy does seem to be dose dependent, and many of the early studies used low doses of the medication.

Side effects and toxicology. Side effects most often associated with THA include nausea, abdominal distress, tachycardia, and liver toxicity. Despite earlier reports of significant hepatic toxicity, THA is relatively safe (Summers et al. 1989). Hepatic toxicity is dose dependent and reversible.

Drug-drug interactions. Because THA undergoes extensive hepatic metabolism by the P450 system, drug-drug interactions may occur when this agent is given concurrently with others that undergo extensive metabolism through cytochrome P450. Coadministration of THA with theophylline has been shown to double theophylline's elimination half-life and plasma concentration.

Velnacrine

History and discovery. Velnacrine (HP 029) is a cholinesterase inhibitor for the treatment of AD. Animal studies determined that velnacrine significantly enhances long-term potentiation (considered an electrophysiological model for memory formation within the hippocampus) (Tanaka et al. 1989). The drug reverses scopolamine- or lesion-induced memory impairment in rodents (Fielding et al. 1989). Velnacrine has been shown to ameliorate the decline in short-term memory associated with aging in nonhuman primates (Jackson et al. 1995).

Structure. Velnacrine maleate is the maleate salt of an alcohol derivative of THA (Puri et al. 1990).

Pharmacological profile. Velnacrine inhibits both true cholinesterase and pseudocholinesterase and does not cause release of acetylcholine or act as a muscarinic agonist.

Pharmacokinetics and disposition. Velnacrine is well absorbed after oral administration. Mean peak plasma levels are attained 0.75–1.2 hours after dosing. The mean half-life range is 1.6–2.0 hours. Most of the drug is conjugated before excretion (Puri et al. 1990).

Indications. Patients with AD show marked intersubject variability in drug tolerance within the therapeutic dose range of velnacrine (Cutler et al. 1990). Double-blind, placebo-controlled studies have reported modest clinical improvement in patients with AD (Antuono 1995; Clipp and Moore 1995; Murphy et al. 1991; Zemlan et al. 1996). A 6-week dose-ranging study revealed that subjects who received velnacrine scored significantly better than subjects who received placebo on the ADAS-cog (Zemlan et al. 1996). A 24-week dose-ranging study that included 301 patients with AD found that the cognitive scores of the placebo-treated group deteriorated significantly more than those of the active medication group, and the results were dose dependent (Antuono 1995).

Side effects and toxicology. Side effects of velnacrine include dizziness, diarrhea, and headache. Reversible liver toxicity is observed in a dose-dependent manner with this compound (Murphy et al. 1991).

Drug-drug interactions. No specific drug-drug interactions have been observed with velnacrine, which is still undergoing clinical evaluation.

Donepezil

History and discovery. Donepezil (E2020) is a cholinesterase inhibitor that has been developed for the treatment of AD and is approved for this indication by the U.S. Food and Drug Administration.

Structure. The chemical structure for donepezil is (R,S)-1-benzyl-4[(5,6-dimethoxy-1-indanon)-2-yl]methylpiperidine hydrochloride (Ohnishi et al. 1993).

Pharmacological profile. Donepezil inhibits acetylcholinesterase in a mixed competitive-noncompetitive manner (Galli et al. 1994). Donepezil produces dose-dependent increases in extracellular acetylcholine concentration in the brain (Kawashima et al. 1994).

Pharmacokinetics and disposition. Donepezil is well absorbed after oral administration. In elderly subjects, the mean time to maximum peak plasma concentration is 5.2 ± 2.8 hours, and the mean half-life is 103.8 ± 40.6 hours (Mihara et al. 1993; Ohnishi et al. 1993). The time to maximum plasma concentration and the half-life both increase with age (Ohnishi et al. 1993). The inhibitor dissociation constant for donepezil is lower than that for THA (Nochi et al. 1995). Donepezil is mainly metabolized by the liver (Ohnishi et al. 1993).

Indications. A 12-week double-blind, placebo-controlled study with 161 patients demonstrated cognitive improvement on the ADAS-cog in individuals treated with 5 mg/day of donepezil.

Side effects and toxicology. In healthy elderly subjects, single oral dosing of the compound was tolerated (Ohnishi et al. 1993). Donepezil is not associated with liver toxicity in subjects with AD (S. L. Rogers et al. 1996).

Drug-drug interactions. No specific drug-drug interactions have been observed with donepezil.

Galanthamine

History and discovery. Galanthamine has been used clinically since the early 1960s in the treatment of paresis, paralysis, and myasthenia gravis (Mihailova et al. 1989). It has also been shown to reverse spatial memory deficits in hypocholinergic mice (Sweeney et al. 1988).

Structure. Galanthamine is a tertiary amine of the phenthrene group.

Pharmacological profile. Galanthamine is a potent inhibitor of acetylcholinesterase. In vivo, maximal inhibition of acetylcholinesterase is approached 30 minutes after oral administration (Thomsen et al. 1990).

Pharmacokinetics and disposition. Galanthamine is rapidly absorbed after oral administration. Cerebral concentrations that are three times higher than its plasma level are observed after its administration. Galanthamine's half-life of 7 hours is longer than that of THA or physostigmine (Thomsen et al. 1990). Metabolites include epigalanthamine and galanthaminone (Mihailova et al. 1989).

Indications. Eighteen patients with possible AD who received galanthamine for up to 6 months showed no statistically significant improvement on neuropsychological measures (Dal-Bianco et al. 1991).

Side effects and toxicology. Administration of galanthamine has been associated with agitation, sleeplessness, and irritability (Thomsen et al. 1990).

Summary

Several methodological issues must be considered in interpreting studies of cholinesterase inhibitors. Intersubject variability in bioavailability and inadequate dosing could attenuate response patterns. Crossover designs may include carryover effects that detract from a drug's effect in comparison with placebo. Repeated assessments lead to learning effects that can erroneously inflate a patient's response to medication and can produce carryover effects on discontinuation of the drug. Finally, another problem is the shifting baseline resulting from the progression of the severity of AD. The longer the study, the more this becomes a factor that needs to be addressed. Overall, double-blind, placebo-controlled studies suggest some therapeutic efficacy with these agents. These findings suggest that anticholinesterase therapy is likely to benefit a subgroup of patients with AD.

Cholinergic Agonists

The use of muscarinic agonists for cognitive enhancement is supported by their beneficial effects on memory and learning in hypo-cholinergic animals (Haroutunian et al. 1985).

Significant advances have been made in identifying muscarinic receptor subtypes. Research using molecular biology techniques has identified the presence of five muscarinic receptor subtypes, m1 through m5 (Ashkenazi et al. 1989; Birdsall et al. 1989; Bonner 1989; Bonner et al. 1987; Fukada et al. 1989). Studies with pharmacological antagonists have identified three classes of muscarinic receptors, M1, M2, and M3. The m1–m5 and M1–M3 systems overlap. Activation of the m1, m3, and m5 receptors causes cellular excitation, whereas activation of the m2 and m4 subtypes produces inhibitory effects (Ashkenazi et al. 1989; Bonner 1989).

Although muscarinic receptors play a significant role in memory, evidence suggests involvement of the nicotinic system in AD. The nicotinic receptors can be divided into super-high-, high-, and low-affinity subtypes (Nordberg et al. 1992). Brains of patients with AD show decrements in the high-affinity nicotinic sites (Nordberg et al. 1992). In animal studies, the nicotinic antagonist mecamylamine produces a dose-dependent impairment of memory comparable to that observed with scopolamine. The nicotinic and muscarinic systems appear to modulate performance jointly in learning and memory (Riekkinen et al. 1990).

Bethanechol

Bethanechol is a synthetic β-methyl analogue of acetylcholine. The agonist effects of bethanechol on M1 and M2 cholinergic receptors are believed to enhance cholinergic neuro-transmission. Studies in patients with AD have reported modest improvement with this agent (Harbaugh et al. 1989; Penn et al. 1988; Read et al. 1990).

Bethanechol must be administered by an intracerebroventricular route because it does not cross the blood-brain barrier. This route of administration has substantial risks, including perioperative complications, pneumocephalus,

seizures, and chronic subdural hematoma (Gauthier et al. 1986; Penn et al. 1988). Thus, bethanechol is not a viable option for cholinergic enhancement in patients with AD.

Arecoline

Arecoline is a natural alkaloid that has both muscarinic and nicotinic agonist properties. Its cholinergic agonist properties are thought to be responsible for its enhancement of cholinergic transmission. Arecoline has been shown to improve learning in healthy volunteer subjects (Sitaram et al. 1978). Modest improvement in picture recognition, verbal memory, and visuospatial construction after arecoline infusion has been observed in patients with AD (Christie et al. 1981; Raffaele et al. 1991; Tariot et al. 1988a).

Oxotremorine

Oxotremorine is a synthetic cholinergic agonist with a half-life of several hours. Oxotremorine administered to patients with AD produced no cognitive-enhancing effects and significant side effects, including panic and depression (Davis et al. 1987).

ENA 713

History and discovery. ENA 713 is an acetylcholinesterase inhibitor that was developed for the treatment of AD. ENA 713 has been shown to ameliorate learning deficits in basal forebrain–lesioned rats (Niigawa et al. 1995).

Structure. ENA 713 is a carbamate-type acetylcholinesterase inhibitor. The structure is (+)(s)-N-Ethyl-3-[l-dimethylaminoethyl]-N-methylphenyl-carbonate hydrogentartate.

Pharmacological profile. ENA 713 is a pseudo irreversible acetylcholinesterase inhibitor. This characteristic causes it to provide prolonged inhibition of acetylcholinesterase after the drug has been cleared from the plasma. ENA 713 shows selectivity for brain acetylcholinesterase, particularly in the hippocampus and cortex. A single 3-mg dose of ENA 713 produces 30%–40% inhibition of central acetylcholinesterase, with minimal inhibition of peripheral acetyl- or butylcholinesterase (Anand and Gharabawi 1996). Inhibition of acetylcholinesterase activity occurs within 30 minutes of administration. Phase 1 and 2 trials suggest that the therapeutic dose is 6–12 mg/day.

Pharmacokinetics and disposition. ENA 713 is rapidly absorbed, reaching peak plasma levels within 30 minutes, and lasting up to 6 hours (Niigawa et al. 1995).

Indications. A 13-week placebo-controlled study with 402 patients reported that 3 mg of ENA 713 twice a day improved cognition. Another double-blind, placebo-controlled study of 8 weeks' duration with 114 patients with AD found that 6–12 mg/day of ENA 713 improved cognitive function. Long-term studies of ENA 713 are in progress (Anand and Gharabawi 1996).

Side effects and toxicology. ENA 713 does not alter liver function, does not produce cardiac toxicity, and does not affect blood pressure. Side effects are cholinergic, with gastrointestinal symptoms being the most common adverse effects.

Drug-drug interactions. ENA 713 has no significant interactions with other drugs.

Nicotine

The reduction in nicotinic receptors in the brains of subjects with AD suggests the potential usefulness of strategies to provide additional stimulation of the remaining nicotinic receptors to enhance cognition in patients with AD (Sugaya et al. 1990). Nicotine administration has been shown both to improve the attentional component and to facilitate retention of the memory process (Warburton and Wesnes 1984). Intramuscular nicotine administration to primates improved performance on a delayed matching-to-sample task (Buccafusco and Jack-

son 1991). Intravenous nicotine administration to six patients with AD improved performance in recall (Newhouse et al. 1988). It is unfortunate that the anxiety and depressive symptoms associated with nicotine administration represent toxic effects that lessen the clinical utility of this compound.

Summary

None of the cholinergic agonist approaches tested to date has yielded the clinical benefit initially anticipated. Yet it may very well be that the potential benefits of postsynaptic enhancement have not been adequately tested. The diverse physiological effects of muscarinic and nicotinic activation limit the clinical usefulness of the agents currently used.

Development of therapies that are directed specifically at the receptors involved in cognition will enhance therapeutic efficacy and avoid undesirable side effects. Future directions in cholinergic enhancement may include manipulation of specific subtypes of both the muscarinic and the nicotinic receptors.

OTHER NEUROTRANSMITTER SYSTEMS

The heterogeneous nature of the neurochemical deficits in AD may significantly contribute to variable response patterns observed with anticholinesterases. Studies in animals also indicate the involvement of multiple neurotransmitter systems in learning and memory. For example, noradrenergic brain lesions negate cholinomimetic enhancement of memory. Clonidine administration restores the efficacy of cholinomimetic treatment in animals with combined noradrenergic and cholinergic lesions (Haroutunian et al. 1990). Postmortem studies show major neurotransmitter losses of the noradrenergic, corticotropin-releasing factor (CRF), and somatostatinergic systems in patients with AD. These findings suggest that anticholinesterase administration (in conjunction with an agent that augments another neurotransmitter system found to be deficient in AD) may be a more appropriate strategy for some patients.

Selegiline

History and Discovery

Selegiline has been used for the treatment of depression and Parkinson's disease. Use of selegiline for cognitive enhancement in AD is based on the following:

- The monoaminergic system is involved in cognitive behaviors and AD.
- Selegiline's antioxidant effect, through its inhibition of monoamine oxidase B, may prevent cell death.
- Selegiline interferes with the increased activity of monoamine oxidase B that is observed in patients with AD (Oreland and Gottfries 1986).

Structure

Selegiline [(−)-(R)-N,α-dimethyl-N-2-propynylphenthylamine hydrochloride] is a levorotatory acetylenic derivative of phenethylamine.

Pharmacological Profile

Selegiline is an irreversible monoamine oxidase inhibitor that selectively inhibits monoamine oxidase B at low doses.

Pharmacokinetics and Disposition

Selegiline is absorbed readily after oral administration. Three metabolites—N-desmethyldeprenyl (mean half-life 2 hours), amphetamine (mean half-life 18 hours), and methamphetamine (mean half-life 21 hours)—are found in serum and urine.

Indications

The results of four double-blind, placebo-controlled trials with small patient samples suggest that subchronic treatment with selegiline at 10 mg/day improves performance on attention, memory, and learning tasks (Agnoli et al. 1990; Mangoni et al. 1991; Piccinin et al. 1990; Tariot et al. 1987a, 1987b). Higher doses of selegiline were not as efficacious and were associated with more side effects (Tariot et al. 1987b). The beneficial effects of selegiline do not appear to result from its antidepressant action, because the monoamine oxidase A inhibitor tranylcypromine does not improve cognitive performance (Tariot et al. 1988b). The results for selegiline need to be replicated with larger patient samples and longer treatment trials to determine whether this agent will have clinically significant effects on cognition in patients with AD.

Side Effects and Toxicology

At low doses (10 mg/day), selegiline administration is not associated with tyramine sensitivity. Selegiline is well tolerated at low doses. Side effects include nausea, dizziness, abdominal discomfort, and dry mouth.

Drug-Drug Interactions

Selegiline administration to patients taking levodopa may lead to an exacerbation of levodopa-associated side effects. These effects may be reduced by lowering the dose of levodopa.

Combined Treatment Approaches

Animal and postmortem human studies suggest that a treatment approach using cholinergic-noradrenergic combinations may be more efficacious than cholinomimetic or monoaminergic agents alone. A pilot study with clonidine and physostigmine treatment in nine patients confirmed the safety of combining these agents in patients with AD (Davidson et al. 1989). One study noted that the combination of selegiline and a cholinesterase inhibitor was superior to administration of a cholinesterase alone, whereas two other investigations did not demonstrate significant cognitive improvement with the combination of a cholinesterase inhibitor and selegiline (Marin et al. 1995; Schneider et al. 1993; Sunderland et al. 1992). Inadequate physostigmine levels achieved in the latter trial may have led to spuriously poor results. Future studies are needed to determine the potential efficacy of combination treatments.

NEW APPROACHES

The approaches described here generally offer palliative treatment to augment the functioning of deficient neurotransmitter systems in patients with AD. Advances in the understanding of the biology of AD permit the development of strategies that may alter its underlying pathophysiology.

Glutamatergic Agents

Glutamatergic agents have not been systematically used for the treatment of AD. However, in this section, we review the rationale for and provide examples of potential glutamatergic agents for the treatment of AD.

History and Discovery

Glutamate is the major excitatory neurotransmitter of pyramidal neurons (Fonnum 1984). The postsynaptic effects of glutamate are mediated via several different receptor subtypes. These receptors can be classified according to their prototypic agonists (i.e., N-methyl-D-aspartate [NMDA], quisqualate, and kainate) (Foster and Fagg 1987).

Different receptor subtypes of the glutamatergic system have been implicated in memory processing. NMDA receptor blockade with aminophosphonopentanoic acid in the CA_1 region of the hippocampus prevents long-term potentiation (Collingridge and Bliss 1987). Binding of aminophosphonopentanoic acid to NMDA receptors disrupts spatial learning in a manner similar to that observed with hippocampal lesions (Morris et al. 1986). Antagonist binding to quisqualate and kainate receptors interferes with passive avoidance training in rodents (Danysz et al. 1988). Extensive loss of NMDA sites has been detected in the brains of

patients with AD (Greenamyre et al. 1985). Increased kainate receptor binding has been observed in postmortem studies (Geddes et al. 1985). Glutamate can induce neurotoxicity (Rothman and Olney 1987). The excitatory and neurotoxic effects of glutamate can occur through both NMDA and non-NMDA receptors (Greenamyre and Young 1989). NMDA and non-NMDA antagonists protect against injury caused by ischemia (Greenamyre and Young 1989; Rothman and Olney 1987). Thus, glutamate's wide CNS distribution and its neurotoxic properties implicate it as a potential contributor to the pathogenesis of several CNS neurodegenerative disorders.

Given that glutamate can enhance learning as well as produce neurotoxicity, determination of the optimal glutamatergic strategy must take into consideration the complex functions of glutamate and the various glutamatergic receptors. Both NMDA and non-NMDA sites could be potential targets for therapeutic approaches.

Glycine Site Inhibitors

Antagonism of the glycine modulatory site of the NMDA receptor could decrease neurotoxicity mediated by glutamate. 1-Hydroxy-3-amino-2-pyrrolidone (HA-966) and L-aminocyclobutane appear to inhibit NMDA-specific binding and to block NMDA responses (Hood et al. 1989; Watson et al. 1989). The glycine antagonists kynurenic acid and 7-chlorokynurenic acid do not interfere with passive avoidance in mice. These findings indicate that antagonism at the glycine site may interfere with glutamate's neurotoxicity without causing cognitive impairment (Chiamulera et al. 1991), a finding whose relevance to altering the course of AD depends on glutamate's involvement in cell death in patients with AD.

Non-NMDA Antagonists

Non-NMDA antagonism may provide a potential therapeutic strategy to decrease glutamatergic functioning and neurotoxicity. Antagonists of the non-NMDA receptors include

2,3-dihydroxy-6-nitro-7-sulfamoyl-benzo(F) quinoxaline (NBQX), 6,7-dinitroquinoxaline-2,3-dione (DNQX), and 6-cyano-7-nitro-quioxaline-2,3-dione (CNQX) (Honore et al. 1988; Sheardon et al. 1990). These agents have been shown to protect against the effects of ischemia by blocking non-NMDA sites (Sheardon et al. 1990). Clinical trials are necessary to determine whether these agents can interfere with cell death and alter the course of AD.

Partial Agonists

Given the complex sequelae of glutamatergic activation, a partial agonist approach is optimal. The glycine agonist milacemide enhances learning in normal and amnestic rodents (Handelmann et al. 1989). One clinical trial of this drug, however, did not enhance cognition and was accompanied by significant liver toxicity (Pomara et al. 1991). The partial glycine agonist D-cycloserine has also been shown to reverse memory impairments caused by scopolamine in healthy subjects (Jones et al. 1992). A 2-week, placebo-controlled, crossover study with 12 patients with AD did not find that D-cycloserine improved cognition when compared with placebo (Randolph et al. 1994). As with other glutamatergic-modulating agents, further clinical studies are necessary to test their potential efficacy.

Summary

Modulation of the glutamatergic system may provide several therapeutic strategies to enhance cognition and diminish the neuronal toxicity observed in patients with AD. No large-scale clinical trials yet conducted with glutamatergic modulators have found these agents to prevent neuronal damage, enhance memory, and have acceptable side-effect profiles.

Antiinflammatory Agents

History and Discovery

As with glutamatergic strategies, antiinflammatory agents have not been widely tested in the treatment of AD. However, basic science and epidemiological findings suggest the utility of these agents for AD treatment.

Several lines of evidence indicate the involvement of the immune system and inflammation in AD. Histochemical studies document the presence of several markers of inflammation in the brains of subjects with AD (Bauer et al. 1991; McGeer et al. 1989b; Styren et al. 1990). Furthermore, the immune response in the CNS has been shown to colocalize with senile plaques, suggesting a role for an immune response in the pathophysiology of AD (McGeer et al. 1989a).

Increased numbers of reactive glia and microglia (believed to be related to macrophages) have been observed in several postmortem studies of brains of AD subjects (Styren et al. 1990). Activated T lymphocytes, a hallmark of the cell-mediated response observed in chronic inflammatory states, have also been observed in postmortem studies of subjects with AD (McGeer et al. 1989b; J. Rogers et al. 1988). Complement proteins (including the membrane attack components) associated with the classical pathway have also been identified in senile plaques and tangles (McGeer et al. 1989a). The implications of the presence of complement proteins is that host cells can be inadvertently attacked and destroyed by these molecules.

Elevated concentrations of interleukins, agents that signal cell proliferation and the production of mediators of the inflammatory response, have also been noted in patients with AD. Specifically, concentrations of tumor necrosis factor, interleukin-1 (IL-1), and interleukin-6 (IL-6) have been elevated in patients with AD (Altstiel and Sperber 1991; Bauer et al. 1991; Fillit et al. 1991). The role of cytokines in amyloidogenesis is supported by their ability to stimulate amyloid precursor protein synthesis (Goldgaber et al. 1989). Acute-phase proteins—inflammatory response molecules that are induced by interleukins—have also been elevated in AD (Heinrich et al. 1990). C-reactive protein, α_2-macro-globulin, and α_1-antichymotrypsin concentrations are increased in patients with AD compared with age-matched control subjects (Abraham et al. 1988; Bauer et al. 1991; Matsubara et al. 1990; Rozmuller et al. 1990). Increased α_1-antichymotrypsin concentrations are particularly intriguing because the α_1-antichymotrypsin molecule is a component of senile plaques (Bauer et al. 1991). α_1-Antichymotrypsin may contribute to abnormal processing of amyloid precursor protein, leading to β-amyloid deposition (Bauer et al. 1991). It has been suggested that the immune system response in AD originates in the CNS.

The question that needs to be answered is what CNS events cause cytokine production. Whether local brain injury, an immunological process, or an autoimmune phenomenon induces the acute-phase response is unknown. Nonetheless, a definite immune response in AD could lead to cell death and enhance β-amyloid deposition. These data suggest that antiinflammatory therapy may slow progression of the illness. Evidence suggests that chronic exposure to antiinflammatory agents is protective against the development of AD. The prevalence of AD among patients at rheumatoid arthritis clinics—a population likely to have received chronic antiinflammatory therapy—was significantly less than that observed in the general population older than 64 years (McGeer et al. 1992b). Elderly patients with leprosy who had been treated with the antiinflammatory agent dapsone had significantly lower rates of dementia than did drug-free patients (McGeer et al. 1992a). A 6-month double-blind trial with the nonsteroidal antiinflammatory agent indomethacin documented that the conditions of patients with AD who received active drug declined significantly less than did those of patients who received placebo (J. Rogers et al. 1988). Future studies with antiinflammatory agents in patients with AD are necessary to determine the usefulness of antiinflammatory strategies.

CONCLUSION

Several strategies for cognitive enhancement have been attempted in patients with AD. An adequate acetylcholinesterase inhibitor has not yet been tested with all the necessary parameters. Combined neurotransmitter therapies have also not been adequately tested to determine the level of efficacy that could be achieved with this approach. Strategies to delay the progression of AD are now being explored and may provide the most effective means to treat the cognitive deterioration observed in patients who have AD.

REFERENCES

Abraham CR, Selkoe DJ, Potter H: Immunohistochemical identification of the serine protease inhibitor alpha-1 antichymotrypsin in the brain amyloid deposits of Alzheimer's disease. Cell 52:487–501, 1988

Adem A: Putative mechanisms of action of tacrine in Alzheimer's disease. Acta Neurol Scand 139: 69–74, 1992

Agnoli A, Martucci N, Fabbrini G, et al: Monoamine oxidase and dementia: treatment with an inhibitor of MAO-B activity. Dementia 1: 109–114, 1990

Altstiel LD, Sperber K: Cytokines in Alzheimer's disease. Prog Neuropsychopharmacol Biol Psychiatry 15:481–495, 1991

Anand R, Gharabawi G: Efficacy and safety results of the early phase studies with exelon (ENA 713) in Alzheimer's disease: an overview. J Drug Dev Clin Pract 8:109–116, 1996

Antuono PG: Effectiveness and safety of velnacrine for the treatment of Alzheimer's disease: a double-blind, placebo-controlled study. Mentane Study Group. Arch Intern Med 155:1766–1772, 1995

Ashkenazi A, Peralta EG, Winslow JW, et al: Functional diversity of muscarinic receptor subtypes in cellular signal transduction and growth. Trends Pharmacol Sci Suppl 10:16–22, 1989

Bartus RT, Dean RL, Pontecorvo MJ, et al: The cholinergic hypothesis: a historical overview, current perspective and future directions. Ann N Y Acad Sci 444:332–358, 1985

Bartus RT, Dean RL, Flicker C: Cholinergic psychopharmacology: an integration of human and animal research on memory, in Psychopharmacology: The Third Generation of Progress. Edited by Meltzer HY. New York, Raven, 1987, pp 219–232

Bauer J, Strauss S, Schreiter-Gasser U, et al: Interleukin-6 and alpha-2-macroglobulin indicate an acute phase response in the Alzheimer's disease cortices. FEBS Lett 285:111–114, 1991

Beller SA, Overall JE, Rhoades HM, et al: Long term outpatient treatment of senile dementia with oral physostigmine. J Clin Psychiatry 49:400–404, 1988

Birdsall N, Buckley N, Doods H: Nomenclature for muscarinic receptor subtypes recommended by symposium. Trends Pharmacol Sci Suppl 10:7–9, 1989

Bonner TI: New subtypes of muscarinic acetylcholine receptors. Trends Pharmacol Sci Suppl 10:11–15, 1989

Bonner TI, Buckley A, Young AC, et al: Identification of a family of muscarinic acetylcholine receptor genes. Science 237:527–532, 1987

Buccafusco JJ, Jackson W: Beneficial effects of nicotine administered prior to a delayed matching-to-sample task in young and aged monkeys. Neurobiol Aging 12:233–238, 1991

Chatellier G, Lacomblez L: Tacrine (tetrahydroaminoacridine; THA) and lecithin in senile dementia of the Alzheimer's type: a multi-center trial. BMJ 300:495–499, 1990

Chiamulera C, Costa S, Reggiani A: Effect of NMDA and strychnine-insensitive glycine site antagonist on NMDA-mediated convulsions and learning. Psychopharmacology 102:551–552, 1991

Christie JE, Shering A, Ferguson J, et al: Physostigmine and arecoline: effects of intravenous infusions in Alzheimer's presenile dementia. Br J Psychiatry 138:46–50, 1981

Clipp EC, Moore MJ: Caregiver time use: an outcome measure in clinical trial research on Alzheimer's disease. Clin Pharmacol Ther 58:228–236, 1995

Collerton D: Cholinergic function and intellectual decline in Alzheimer's disease. Neuroscience 19:1–28, 1986

Collingridge GL, Bliss TVP: NNMA receptors—their role in long-term potentiation. Trends Neurosci 10:288–293, 1987

Cutler NR, Murphy MF, Nash RJ, et al: Clinical safety, tolerance and plasma levels of the oral anticholinesterase 1,2,3,4-tetrahydro-9-aminoacradin-*I*-olmaleate (HP 029) in Alzheimer's disease: preliminary findings. J Clin Pharmacol 39:556–561, 1990

Dal-Bianco P, Maly J, Wober C, et al: Galanthamine treatment in Alzheimer's disease. J Neural Transm Suppl 33:59–63, 1991

Danysz W, Wroblewski JT, Costa E: Learning impairment in rats by *N*-methyl-D-aspartate receptor antagonist. Neuropharmacology 27:653–656, 1988

Davidson M, Bierer LM, Kaminsky R, et al: Combined administration of physostigmine and clonidine to patients with dementia of the Alzheimer type: a pilot safety study. Alzheimer Dis Assoc Disord 1:1–4, 1989

Davies P, Maloney AJ: Selective loss of central cholinergic neurons in Alzheimer's disease. Lancet 2:1403–1405, 1976

Davis KL, Hollander E, Davidson M, et al: Induction of depression with oxotremorine in Alzheimer's disease patients. Am J Psychiatry 144:468–471, 1987

Davis KL, Thal LJ, Gamzu ER, et al: A double-blind, placebo-controlled multicenter study of tacrine in Alzheimer's disease. N Engl J Med 327:1253–1259, 1992

Deutsch JA: The cholinergic synapse and the site of memory. Science 174:788–794, 1971

Drachman DA, Leavitt J: Human memory and the cholinergic system. Arch Neurol 30:113–121, 1974

Drukarch B, Kits S, Van der Meer EG, et al: 9-Amino-1,2,3,4-tetrahydroacridine (THA), an alleged drug for the treatment of Alzheimer's disease, inhibits acetylcholinesterase activity and slows outward K^+ current. Eur J Pharmacol 141:153–157, 1987

Drukarch B, Leysen JE, Stoof JC: Further analysis of the neuropharmacological profile of 9-amino-1,2,3,4-tetrahydroacridine (THA), an alleged drug for the treatment of Alzheimer's disease. Life Sci 42:1011–1017, 1988

Dundee JW, Pandit SK: Anterograde amnesic effects of pethidine, hyoscine, and diazepam in adults. Br J Pharmacol 44:140–144, 1972

Farlow M, Gracon SI, Hershey LA, et al: A controlled trial of tacrine in Alzheimer's disease. JAMA 268:2523–2529, 1992

Fielding S, Cornfeldt ML, Szewczak MR, et al: HP-029, a new drug for the treatment of Alzheimer's disease: its pharmacological profile. Paper presented at the 4th World Conference on Clinical Pharmacology and Therapeutics, West Berlin, Germany, July 28–30, 1989

Fillit H, Ding W, Buee L, et al: Elevated circulating tumor necrosis factor levels in Alzheimer's disease. Neurosci Lett 129:318–320, 1991

Folstein MF, Folstein SE, McHugh PR: Mini-Mental State: a practical method for grading the cognitive state of patients for the clinician. J Psychiatr Res 12:189–198, 1975

Fonnum F: Glutamate: a neurotransmitter in mammalian brain. J Neurochem 42:1–11, 1984

Foster AC, Fagg GE: Taking apart the NMDA receptor. Nature 329:395–396, 1987

Fukada K, Kubo T, Maeda A, et al: Selective effector coupling of muscarinic acetylcholine receptor subtypes. Trends Pharmacol Sci Suppl 10:4–10, 1989

Galli A, Nori F, Benini L, et al: Acetylcholinesterase protection and the anti-diisopropylfluorophosphate efficacy of E2020. Eur J Pharmacol 270:189–193, 1994

Gauthier S, Leblanc R, Quirion R, et al: Transmitter-replacement therapy in Alzheimer's disease using intracerebroventricular infusions of receptor agonists. Can J Neurol Sci 13:394–402, 1986

Gauthier S, Bouchard R, Lamontagne A, et al: Tetrahydroaminoacridine-lecithin combination treatment in patients with intermediate-stage Alzheimer's disease. N Engl J Med 322:1272–1276, 1990

Geddes JW, Monaghan DT, Cotman CW, et al: Plasticity of hippocampal circuitry in Alzheimer's disease. Science 230:1179–1181, 1985

Goldgaber D, Harris H, Hal T, et al: Interleukin-1 regulates synthesis of amyloid beta protein precursor mRNA in human endothelial cells. Proc Natl Acad Sci U S A 86:7606–7610, 1989

Greenamyre JT, Young AB: Excitatory amino acids and Alzheimer's disease. Neurobiol Aging 10:593–602, 1989

Greenamyre JT, Penney JB, Young AB: Alterations in L-glutamate binding in Alzheimer's and Huntington's diseases. Science 227:1496–1498, 1985

Handelmann GE, Nevins ME, Mueller LL, et al: Milacemide, a glycine prodrug, enhances performance of learning tasks in normal and amnestic rodents. Pharmacol Biochem Behav 34:823–838, 1989

Harbaugh RE, Reeder TM, Senter HJ, et al: Intracerebroventricular bethanechol chloride administration in Alzheimer's disease: results of a collaborative double-blind study. J Neurosurg 71:481–486, 1989

Haroutunian V, Kanof PD, Davis KL: Pharmacological alleviation of cholinergic lesion induced memory deficits in rats. Life Sci 37:945–952, 1985

Haroutunian V, Kanof PD, Tsuboyama G, et al: Restoration of cholinomimetic activity by clonidine in cholinergic plus adrenergic lesioned rats. Brain Res 507:261–266, 1990

Heinrich PC, Castell JV, Andus T: Interleukin-6 and the acute phase response. Biochem J 265:621–636, 1990

Honore T, Davies SN, Drejer J, et al: Quinoxalinediones: potent competitive non-NMDA glutamate receptor antagonist. Science 241:701–703, 1988

Hood WF, Sun ET, Cornpton RP, et al: 1-Aminocyclo-butane-1-carboxylate (ACBC): a specific antagonist of the N-methyl-D-aspartate receptor coupled glycine receptor. Eur J Pharmacol 161:281–282, 1989

Jackson WJ, Buccafusco JJ, Terry AV, et al: Velnacrine maleate improves delayed matching performance by aged monkeys. Psychopharmacology 119:391–398, 1995

Jenike MA, Albert MS, Baer L: Oral physostigmine as treatment for Alzheimer's disease: a long-term outpatient trial. Alzheimer Dis Assoc Disord 4:226–231, 1990

Jones RW, Wesnes KA, Kirby J: Effects of NMDA modulation in scopolamine dementia. Ann N Y Acad Sci 64:241–244, 1992

Kawashima K, Sato A, Yoshizawa M, Fjii T, et al: Effects of the centrally acting cholinesterase inhibitors tetrahydroaminoacrine and E2020 on the basal concentration of extracellular acetylcholine in the hippocampus of freely moving rats. Naunyn Schmiedebergs Arch Pharmacol 350:523–528, 1994

Kaye WH, Sitaram H, Weingartner H, et al: Modest facilitation of memory in dementia with combined lecithin and anticholinesterase treatment. Biol Psychiatry 17:275–280, 1982

Knapp MJ, Knopman DS, Solomon PR, et al: A 30-week randomized controlled trial of high-dose tacrine in patients with Alzheimer's disease. The Tacrine Study Group. JAMA 271:985–991, 1994

Mangoni A, Grassi MP, Frattola L, et al: Effects of a MAO-B inhibitor in the treatment of Alzheimer disease. Eur Neurol 31:100–107, 1991

Marin DB, Bierer LB, Ryan TM, et al: Physostigmine and deprenyl combination therapy for Alzheimer's disease. Psychiatry Res 58:181–189,1995

Matsubara E, Hirai S, Amari M, et al: Alpha-1 antichymotrypsin as a possible biochemical marker for Alzheimer-type dementia. Ann Neurol 28:561–567, 1990

McGeer PL, Akiyama H, Itagaki S, et al: Activation of the classical complement pathway in brain tissue of Alzheimer patients. Neurosci Lett 107:341–346, 1989a

McGeer PL, Akiyama H, Itagaki S, et al: Immune system response in Alzheimer's disease. Can J Neurol Sci 16:516–527, 1989b

McGeer PL, Harada N, Kimura H, et al: Prevalence of dementia amongst elderly Japanese with leprosy: apparent effect of chronic drug therapy. Dementia 3:146–149, 1992a

McGeer PL, McGeer EG, Rogers J, et al: Does antiinflammatory treatment protect against Alzheimer's disease? in Alzheimer's Disease: New Treatment Strategies. Edited by Khachaturian ZS, Blass JP. New York, Marcel Dekker, 1992b, pp 165–171

Mihailova D, Yamboliev I, Zhivkova Z, et al: Pharmacokinetics of galanthamine hydrobromide after single subcutaneous and oral dosage in humans. Pharmacology 39:50–58, 1989

Mihara M, Ohnishi A, Tomono Y, et al: Pharmacokinetics of E2020, a new compound for Alzheimer's disease, in healthy male volunteers. Int J Clin Pharmacol Ther Toxicol 31:223–229, 1993

Mohs RC, Davis KL: The experimental pharmacology of Alzheimer's disease and related dementias, in Psychopharmacology: The Third Generation of Progress. Edited by Meltzer HY. New York, Raven, 1987, pp 921–928

Morris RGM, Anderson E, Lynch GS, et al: Selective impairment of learning and blockade of long-term potentiation by an N-methyl-D-aspartate receptor antagonist, AP5. Nature 319:774–776, 1986

Murphy MF, Hardiman ST, Nash RJ, et al: Evaluation of HP 029 (velnacrine maleate) in Alzheimer's disease. Ann N Y Acad Sci 640:253–262, 1991

Newhouse PA, Sunderland T, Tariot PN, et al: Intravenous nicotine in Alzheimer's disease: a pilot study. Psychopharmacology (Berl) 95:171–175, 1988

Nielsen JA, Mena JEE, Williams IH, et al: Correlation of brain levels of 9-amino-1,2,3,4-tetrahydro-aminoacridine (THA) with neurochemical and behavioral changes. Eur J Pharmacol 173:53–64, 1989

Niigawa H, Tanimukai S, Takeda M, et al: Effects of SDZ ENA 713, novel acetylcholinesterase inhibitor, on learning of rats with basal forebrain lesions. Prog Neuropsychopharmacol Biol Psychiatry 19:171–186, 1995

Nochi S, Asakawa N, Sato T: Kinetic study on the inhibition of acetycholinesterase by 1-benzyl-4-[(5,6-dimethoxy-1-indanon)-2-yl]methylpiperidine hydrocholoride (E2020). Biol Pharm Bull 18:1145–1147, 1995

Nordberg A, Alafuzoff I, Winblad B: Nicotinic and muscarinic subtypes in the human brain: changes with aging and dementia. J Neurosci Res 31:103–111, 1992

Ohnishi A, Mihara M, Kamakura H, et al: Comparison of pharmacokinetics of E2020, a new compound for Alzheimer's disease, in healthy young and elderly subjects. J Clin Pharmacol 33:1086–1091, 1993

Olton DS, Wenk GL: Dementia: animal models of the cognitive impairments produced by degeneration of the basal forebrain cholinergic system, in Psychopharmacology: The Third Generation of Progress. Edited by Meltzer HY. New York, Raven, 1987, pp 941–953

Oreland L, Gottfries CG: Brain and monoamine oxidase in aging and in dementia of Alzheimer's type. Prog Neuropsychopharmacol Biol Psychiatry 10:533–540, 1986

Penn RD, Martin EM, Wilson RS, et al: Intraventricular bethanechol infusion in Alzheimer's disease: results of double-blind and escalating dose trials. Neurology 38:219–222, 1988

Perry EK, Tomlinson BE, Blessed G, et al: Correlation of cholinergic abnormalities with senile plaques and mental test scores in senile dementia. BMJ 2:1457–1459, 1978

Piccinin FL, Finali G, Piccirilli M: Neuropsychological effects of L-deprenyl in Alzheimer's type dementia. Clin Neuropharmacol 13:147–163, 1990

Pomara N, Mendels J, Lewitt PA, et al: Multicenter trial of milacemide in the treatment of Alzheimer's disease. Biol Psychiatry 29 (suppl):718, 1991

Puri SK, Hsu R, Ho I: Multiple dose pharmacokinetics, safety, and tolerance of velnacrine maleate in healthy elderly subjects: a potential therapeutic agent for Alzheimer's disease. J Clin Pharmacol 30:948–955, 1990

Raffaele KC, Berardi A, Morris P, et al: Effects of acute infusion of the muscarinic cholinergic agonist arecoline on verbal and visuo-spatial function in dementia of the Alzheimer type. Prog Neuropsychopharmacol Biol Psychiatry 15:643–648, 1991

Randolph C, Roberts JW, Tierney MC, et al: D-Cycloserine treatment of Alzheimer's disease. Alzheimer Dis Assoc Disord 8:198–205, 1994

Read SL, Frazee J, Shapira J, et al: Intracerebroventricular bethanechol for Alzheimer's disease: variable dose-related responses. Arch Neurol 47:1025–1030, 1990

Riekkinen P Jr, Sirvio J, Aaltonen M, et al: Effects of concurrent manipulations of nicotinic and muscarinic receptors on spatial and passive avoidance learning. Pharmacol Biochem Behav 54:405–410, 1990

Rogers J, Luber-Narod J, Styren SD, et al: Expression of immune-system-associated antigens by cells of the human central nervous system: relationship to the pathology of Alzheimer's disease. Neurobiol Aging 9:339–349, 1988

Rogers SL, Friedhoff LT, and the Donepezil Study Group: The efficacy and safety of donepezil in patients with Alzheimer's disease: results of a US multicentre, randomized, double blind, placebo controlled trial. Dementia 7:293–303, 1996

Rosen WG, Mohs RC, Davis K: A new rating scale for Alzheimer's disease. Am J Psychiatry 141:1356–1364, 1984

Rothman SM, Olney JW: Excitoxicity and the NMDA receptor. Trends Neurosci 7:299–302, 1987

Rozmuller JM, Stam FC, Eikelenboom P: Acute phase proteins are present in amorphous plaques in the cerebral but not in the cerebellar cortex of patients with Alzheimer's disease. Neurosci Lett 109:75–78, 1990

Sahakian BJ, Coull JT: Tetrahydroaminoacridine (THA) in Alzheimer's disease: an assessment of attentional and mnemonic function using CANTAB. Acta Neurol Scand Suppl 149:29–35, 1993

Schneider LS, Olin JT, Pawluczyk S: A double-blind crossover pilot study of L-deprenyl (selegiline) combined with cholinesterase inhibitors in Alzheimer's disease. Am J Psychiatry 150:321–323, 1993

Sheardon MJ, Nielsoen EO, Hansen AJ, et al: 2,3-Dihydroxy-6-nitro-7-sulfamoyl-benzo (F)quinoxaline: a neuroprotectant for cerebral ischemia. Science 247:571–574, 1990

Sitaram N, Weingartner H, Gillin JC: Human serial learning: enhancement with arecoline and impairment with scopolamine correlated with performance on placebo. Science 201:274–276, 1978

Styren SD, Civin WH, Rogers J: Molecular cellular and pathologic characterization of HLA-DR immunoreactivity in normal elderly and Alzheimer's disease brain. Exp Neurol 110:93–104, 1990

Sugaya K, Giacobini E, Chiappinelli VA: Nicotinic acetylcholine receptor subtypes in human frontal cortex: changes in Alzheimer's disease. J Neurosci Res 27:349–359, 1990

Summers WK, Viesselman JO, Marsh GM, et al: Use of THA in treatment of Alzheimer-like dementia: pilot study in twelve patients. Biol Psychiatry 16:145–153, 1981

Summers WK, Majovski LV, Marsh GM, et al: Oral tetrahydroaminoacridine in long-term treatment of senile dementia of the Alzheimer type. N Engl J Med 315:1241–1245, 1986

Summers WK, Koehler AL, Marsh GM, et al: Long-term hepatoxicity of tacrine. Lancet 1:729, 1989

Sunderland T, Molchan S, Lawlor B, et al: A strategy of "combination chemotherapy" in Alzheimer's disease: rationale and preliminary results with physostigmine plus deprenyl. Int Psychogeriatr 4 (suppl 2):291–309, 1992

Sweeney JE, Hohmann CF, Moran TM, et al: A long-acting cholinesterase inhibitor reverses spatial memory deficits in mice. Pharmacol Biochem Behav 31:141–147, 1988

Tanaka Y, Sakurai M, Hayashi S: Effect of scopolamine and HP 029, a cholinesterase inhibitor, on long term potentiation in hippocampal slices of the guinea pig. Neurosci Lett 98:179–183, 1989

Tariot PN, Cohen RM, Sunderland T, et al: L-Deprenyl in Alzheimer's disease. Arch Gen Psychiatry 44:427–433, 1987a

Tariot PN, Sunderland T, Weingartner H, et al: Cognitive effects of L-deprenyl in Alzheimer's disease. Psychopharmacology (Berl) 91:489–495, 1987b

Tariot PN, Cohen RM, Welkowitz JA, et al: Multiple-dose arecoline infusions in Alzheimer's disease. Arch Gen Psychiatry 45:901–905, 1988a

Tariot PN, Sunderland T, Cohen RM, et al: Tranylcypromine compared with L-deprenyl in Alzheimer's disease. J Clin Psychopharmacol 8:23–27, 1988b

Thomsen T, Bickel U, Fischer JP, et al: Stereoselectivity of cholinesterase inhibition by galanthamine and tolerance in humans. Eur J Clin Pharmacol 39:603–605, 1990

Warburton DM, Wesnes K: Drugs as research tools in psychology: cholinergic drugs and information processing. Neuropsychobiology 11:121–132, 1984

Watson GB, Bolanowski MA, Baganoff MP, et al: Glycine antagonist action of 1-aminocyclobutane-1-carboxylate (ACBC) in Xenopus oocytes injected with rat brain mRNA. Eur J Pharmacol 167:291–294, 1989

Whelpton R, Hurst P: Bioavailability of oral physostigmine (letter). N Engl J Med 313:1293–1294, 1985

Zemlan FP, Keys M, Richter RW, et al: Double blind, placebo controlled study of velnacrine in Alzheimer's disease. Life Sci 586:1823–1832, 1996

FOURTEEN

Sedative-Hypnotics

Seiji Nishino, M.D., Ph.D.,
Emmanuel Mignot, M.D., Ph.D., and
William C. Dement, M.D., Ph.D.

In this chapter, we examine some of the pharmacological properties of barbiturates, benzodiazepines, and other sedative-hypnotic compounds. Sedative drugs moderate excitement, decrease activity, and induce calmness, whereas hypnotic drugs produce drowsiness and facilitate the onset and maintenance of a state that resembles normal sleep in its electroencephalographical characteristics. Although these agents are central nervous system (CNS) depressants, they usually produce therapeutic effects at far lower doses than those that cause generalized depression of the CNS and coma.

Some sedative-hypnotic drugs retain other therapeutic uses as muscle relaxants (especially benzodiazepines), antiepileptic agents, or preanesthetic medications. Benzodiazepines are used widely as antianxiety drugs, and their effect on anxiety is believed to be truly distinct from their effect on sleepiness.

Sedative-hypnotics are important drugs to the neuroscientist. These substances modulate basic behaviors such as arousal and response to stress. Understanding their mode of action could thus help to elucidate neurochemical and neurophysiological control of these behaviors.

BENZODIAZEPINES

History

Benzodiazepines were first synthesized in the 1930s but were not systematically evaluated until 20 years later. The introduction in the early 1950s of chlorpromazine and meprobamate, which had sedative effects in animals, led to the decade of increasingly sophisticated in vivo pharmacological screening methods that were used to identify the sedative properties of benzodiazepines. Since the introduction of chlordiazepoxide, which was synthesized by Sternbach in 1957, into clinical medicine, more than 3,000 benzodiazepines have been synthesized. About 40 are in clinical use.

Several drugs chemically unrelated to the benzodiazepines have been shown to have sedative-hypnotic effects with a benzodiazepine-like profile, and it has been determined that these drugs act via the benzodiazepine receptor.

Most of the benzodiazepines on the market were selected for their high anxiolytic potential relative to CNS depression. Nevertheless, all benzodiazepines have sedative-hypnotic properties to various degrees, and some compounds that facilitate sleep have been used as hypnotics.

Mainly because of their remarkably low capacity to produce fatal CNS depression, benzodiazepines have displaced barbiturates as sedative-hypnotic agents.

Structure-Activity Relations

The term *benzodiazepine* refers to the portion of the structure composed of benzene rings (A) fused to a seven-membered diazepine ring (Figure 14–1). However, most of the older benzodiazepines contain a 5-aryl substituent (ring C) and a 1,4-diazepine ring, and the term has come to mean 1,4-benzodiazepines.

A substituent (most often chloride) at position 7 is essential for biological activity. A carbonyl at position 2 enhances activity and is generally present. Most of the newest products also substitute the 2 position, as with flurazepam. These general features are important for the metabolic fate of the compounds. Because the 7 and 2 positions of the molecule are resistant to all major degradative pathways, many of the metabolites retain substantial pharmacological activity.

Pharmacological Profile

The benzodiazepines share with the barbiturates anticonvulsant and sedative-hypnotic effects. In addition, they have the remarkable ability to reduce anxiety and aggression (Cook and Sepinwall 1975). Several lines of evidence indicate that benzodiazepines are powerful potentiators of γ-aminobutyric acid (GABA). Al-

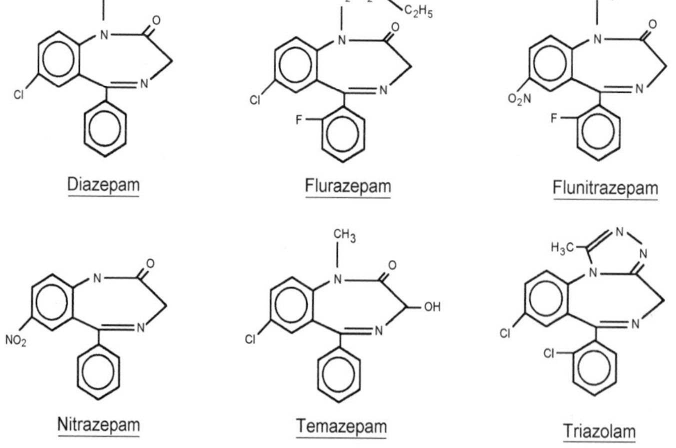

Figure 14–1.   Chemical structures for some commonly used benzodiazepines.

though this hypothesis is generally accepted, other neurotransmitters may also be involved in these actions.

Schmidt and colleagues in 1967 first reported that diazepam could potentiate the inhibitory effects of GABA on the spinal cord in cats. Later, it was shown that the effect of diazepam could be abolished if the endogenous content of GABA was depleted. This finding established that diazepam (and related benzodiazepines) did not act directly through GABA but modulated inhibitory transmission through GABA in some other way. It was subsequently reported that benzodiazepines bind specifically to neural elements in the mammalian brain with high affinity and that an excellent correlation exists between drug affinities for these specific binding sites and in vivo pharmacological potencies (Möhler and Okada 1977; Squires and Braestrup 1977). The binding of a benzodiazepine to this receptor site is enhanced in the presence of GABA or a GABA agonist, thereby suggesting that a functional (but independent) relationship exists between the GABA receptor and the benzodiazepine receptor (Tallman et al. 1978).

Barbiturates (and to some extent alcohol) also seem to produce anxiolytic and sedative effects at least partly by facilitating GABAergic transmission (see the section "Barbiturates"). This common action for chemically unrelated compounds can be explained by their ability to stimulate specific sites on the $GABA_A$ receptor complex.

The benzodiazepines bind with high affinity to the benzodiazepine receptor so that the action of GABA on its receptor is allosterically enhanced. Thus, GABA can produce stronger postsynaptic inhibition in the presence of a benzodiazepine.

The inhibitory effect of GABA is mediated by chloride ion channels. When the $GABA_A$ receptor is occupied by GABA or GABA agonists, such as muscimol, the chloride channels open, and chloride ions diffuse into the cell. One of the binding sites on the chloride ion channel is acti-

vated by barbiturates. Barbiturates appear to increase the duration of the open state of the chloride channel, whereas benzodiazepines increase the frequency of channel openings with little effect on duration (Enna and Möhler 1987; Richter and Holman 1982). Note that selective $GABA_A$ agonists, such as muscimol, have no sedative or anxiolytic properties; thus, the whole $GABA_A$ receptor complex (GABA/BZ-Cl⁻ channel) must be involved to show sedative-hypnotic properties.

Thus, it may be concluded that ω benzodiazepine agonists act as sedative-hypnotics by activating a specific benzodiazepine receptor that facilitates inhibitory GABAergic transmission. Other sedative-hypnotics, such as barbiturates and alcohol, also facilitate GABAergic transmission by acting on sites associated more directly with the chloride channel (Figure 14–2). Therefore, ω benzodiazepine agonists are assumed to potentiate only the ongoing, physiologically initiated action of GABA (at $GABA_A$ receptors), whereas barbiturates can cause inhibition at all GABAergic synapses regardless of whether these synapses are physiologically active. This fundamental difference between the allosteric effects of benzodiazepines within the $GABA_A$ receptor complex and the conducive effects of barbiturates on the chloride ion channel may explain why low doses of barbiturates have a pharmacological profile similar to that of benzodiazepines, whereas high doses of barbiturates cause a profound and sometimes fatal suppression of brain synaptic transmission.

In the mammalian CNS, two subtypes of ω receptors have been recognized. Benzodiazepine ω1 (or BZ1) receptors are sensitive to β-carbolines, imidazopyridines (e.g., zolpidem), and triazolopyridazines. Benzodiazepine ω2 (or BZ2) receptors have low affinity for these ligands and relatively high affinity for benzodiazepines. Benzodiazepine ω1 sites are enriched in the cerebellum, while ω2 sites are mostly present in the spinal cord, and both receptor subtypes are found in the cerebral cortex

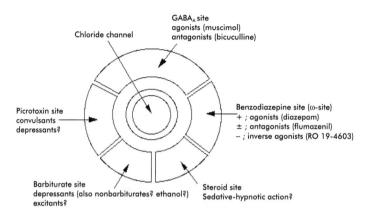

Figure 14–2. Diagrammatic representation of the complex macromolecular components of the γ-aminobutyric acid (GABA)–ergic receptor, chloride ionophores, and benzodiazepine binding sites. *Source.* Adapted from Olsen et al. 1991.

and hippocampus. Benzodiazepine $\omega 1$ and $\omega 2$ receptor subtypes are also located peripherally in adrenal chromaffin cells. Another subtype, $\omega 3$, was identified and commonly labeled the *peripheral benzodiazepine receptor subtype* because of its distribution on glial cell membranes in nonnervous tissues, such as adrenal, testis, liver, and kidney. It was later detected in the CNS, especially on the mitochondrial membrane and not in association with $GABA_A$ receptors. The $\omega 3$ subtype has high affinity for benzodiazepines and isoquinoline carboxamides. The functional role of this receptor is not known but may be involved in the sedative-hypnotic effects of some neuroactive steroids (pregnenolone, dehydroepiandrosterone, allopregnanolone, tetrahydrodeoxycorticosterone) (Edgar et al. 1997; Friess et al. 1996). These compounds are indeed metabolized through the mitochondrial benzodiazepine receptor and may also act directly on the $GABA_A/BZ\text{-}Cl^-$ to express their sedative-hypnotic effects (Rupprecht et al. 1996).

Ligand-gated ion channels mediate fast synaptic neurotransmission in the CNS. These ion channels include the molecularly related nicotinic acetylcholine receptors, glycine receptors, the serotonin-3 receptor (5-hydroxytryptamine-3, $5\text{-}HT_3$), and $GABA_A$ receptors. The structural feature common to all these receptors

is a four-membrane-spanning domain. Four or five subunits with this structure are assembled around a central channel pore, the gating of which is controlled by the respective neurotransmitters.

Regarding the structure of the $GABA_A$ receptor, molecular cloning studies have reported that many unrelated genes (α_{1-6}, β_{1-3}, γ_{1-3}, δ, and ρ) exist and contain a truly astonishing variety of $GABA_A$ receptor subtypes (Lüddens and Wisden 1991). The functional significance of these multiple subtypes is not entirely clear at present and must be studied further to better understand how the site of drug action affects various physiological functions (e.g., sleep, anxiety, muscle relation) and possibly the pathology of some psychiatric and sleep disorders.

Nonbenzodiazepine hypnotics (acting on the benzodiazepine receptor). Until about 1980, it was widely accepted that the benzodiazepine structure was a prerequisite for the anxiolytic profile and for recognition of and binding to the benzodiazepine receptor. However, more recently, two chemically unrelated drugs—the imidazopyridine zolpidem and the cyclopyrrolone zopiclone—have been shown to be useful sedative-hypnotics with benzodiazepine-like profiles (Figure 14–3). Other

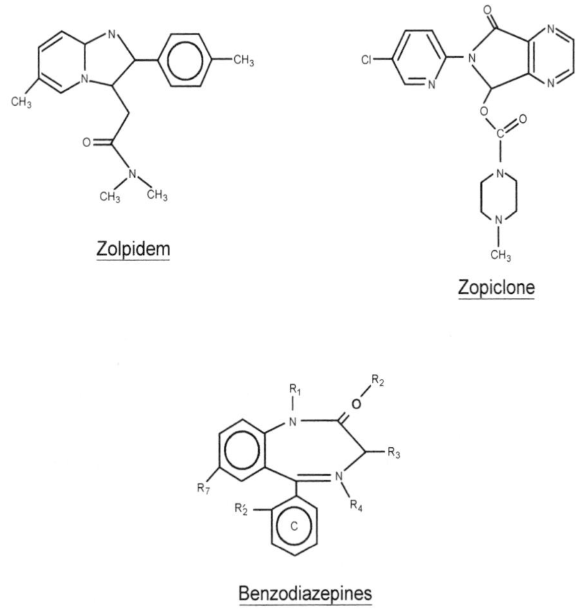

Figure 14–3. Two nonbenzodiazepine hypnotics—zolpidem (an imidazopyridine) and zoplicone (a cyclopyrrolone)—have been shown to be useful sedative-hypnotics with benzodiazepine-like profiles.

chemical classes of drugs that are structurally dissimilar to the benzodiazepines (e.g., triazolopyridazines) but act through the benzodiazepine receptor have also been developed and have anxiolytic activity in humans.

Nonbenzodiazepine hypnotics have a pharmacological profile slightly different from that of classic benzodiazepines. Zolpidem, for example, binds selectively to ω1 (BZ1) and has sedative-hypnotic properties when compared with other properties such as anxiolytic activity or muscle relaxation. Zolpidem and zopiclone have short half-lives—3 hours and 6 hours, respectively. These drugs were originally thought to not appreciably affect the rapid eye movement (REM) sleep pattern, whereas the quality of slow-wave sleep (SWS) may be slightly increased (Jovanovic and Dreyfus 1983; Shlarf 1992). Rebound effects (insomnia, anxiety), which are commonly seen following withdrawal of short-acting benzodiazepines, are minimal. These compounds also induce little respiratory depression and have less abuse potential than do

clinical benzodiazepine hypnotics. However, much longer clinical trials are needed to show whether the imidazopyridines or cyclopyrrolones have any significant advantages over the short to medium half-life benzodiazepines in the treatment of insomnia.

Natural ligands for benzodiazepine receptor in the brain. The presence of benzodiazepine receptors in the brain suggests that natural ligands modulate GABAergic transmission through these sites. Small amounts of benzodiazepines, such as diazepam and desmethyldiazepam, can be detected in human and animal tissues. This finding was confirmed with human brain tissue samples stored since the 1940s before the first synthesis of benzodiazepines (Sangameswaran et al. 1986). These benzodiazepines most likely originate from plants, such as wheat, corn, potatoes, or rice, and the levels detected are too low to be pharmacologically active (i.e., diazepam, <1 ng/g; desmethyldiazepam, 0.5 ng/g).

Other endogenous benzodiazepine-like substances with neuromodulatory effects probably exist in mammals. Endogenous ligands named *diazepam-binding inhibitors* or *endozepines* that bind to the benzodiazepine site on the GABA$_A$-ergic receptor complex have been identified and are being isolated by using biochemical purification protocols (Costa and Guidotti 1991; Marquardt et al. 1986; Rothstein et al. 1992). Their intrinsic action, like that of diazepam, is to potentiate GABA$_A$-receptor-mediated neurotransmission by acting as positive allosteric modulators of this receptor. Endozepines are present in the brain at pharmacologically active concentrations and may play a role both physiologically (e.g., regulation of memory, sleep, and learning) and pathologically (e.g., in panic attacks or hepatic encephalopathy) (Mullen et al. 1990; Nutt et al. 1990). Finally, endozepines have been involved in the neurological condition *idiopathic recurring stupor*, which is characterized by recurrent episodes of stupor or coma in the absence of any known toxic, metabolic, or structural brain damage. In this condition, the concentrations of endoz-

epines are greatly increased in the plasma of affected individuals, and stupor can be interrupted by flumazenil injections, a benzodiazepine antagonist. Thus, further knowledge of the roles of endozepines in physiological and pathological processes should be forthcoming once these endogenous ligands have been isolated and characterized (Rothstein et al. 1992).

Pharmacokinetics and Disposition

Benzodiazepines are generally absorbed rapidly and completely. Plasma binding is high (i.e., about 98% for diazepam). Benzodiazepines are very lipophilic (except for oxazepam), and penetration into the brain is rapid. For rapid onset of action, diazepam is available as an emulsion, which is administered intravenously for rapid control of epilepsy; midazolam is a water-soluble benzodiazepine suitable for intravenous injection.

The major metabolic pathways for the 1,4-benzodiazepines are shown in Figure 14–4. Medazepam is metabolized to diazepam, which is *N*-desmethylated to desmethyldiazepam.

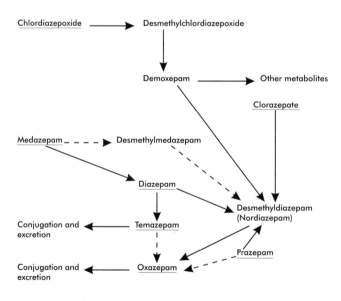

Figure 14–4. Metabolic pathways for the principal 1,4-benzodiazepines (solid and broken arrows denote major and minor pathways, respectively; commercially available drugs are underscored). Flurazepam, flunitrazepam, nitrazepam, and triazolam have separate metabolic pathways.

Chlordiazepoxide is also partly converted to desmethyldiazepam. Clorazepate is transformed to desmethyldiazepam.

Desmethyldiazepam is a critically important metabolite for biological activity because of its long half-life of more than 72 hours. Because diazepam's half-life is about 36 hours, the concentration of its desmethyl derivative soon exceeds that of diazepam during chronic administration. Desmethyldiazepam undergoes oxidation to oxazepam, which (like its 3-hydroxy analogue temazepam) is rapidly conjugated with glucuronic acid and excreted.

Among the various benzodiazepines, triazolam has a particularly short half-life (<4 hours), and flurazepam and nitrazepam both have long half-lives (Table 14–1). A major active metabolite of flurazepam, *N*-desalkylfluraze-

pam, has a very long half-life of about 100 hours.

Because benzodiazepines are often prescribed for long periods, their long-term pharmacokinetics are important. Diazepam and desmethyldiazepam reach plateau levels after a few weeks. Diazepam concentrations may then decline somewhat without much change in the concentration of the desmethyl metabolite.

Although benzodiazepines can stimulate liver metabolism in some animals, induction is of little clinical significance in humans.

Effects on Stages of Sleep

The hypnotic effects of benzodiazepines have been suggested to result from the modulatory effects of the GABAergic system on the raphe and locus coeruleus monoaminergic projec-

Table 14–1. **Pharmacokinetic properties of most commonly used hypnotic compounds acting on the benzodiazepine receptors (in the United States)**

Hypnotic compounds	Usual dose (mg)	T_{max}/Half-life (hours)	Active compound in blood (half-life)
Flurazepam (Dalmane)	15–30	0.5–1.0/48–150	Flurazepam, *N*-hydroxyethyl-flurazepam (1–4), *N*-desalkyl-flurazepam (46–120)
Quazepam (Doral)	7.5–15	2/20–40	Quazepam, oxoquazepam (20–40), *N*-desalkyl-2-oxoquazepam (*N*-desalkyl-flurazepam) (48–120)
Estazolam (ProSom)	1–2	1.6–1.9/13–35	Estazolam
Temazepam (Restoril)	15–30	1.5/8–20	Temazepam
Triazolam (Halcion)	0.125–0.25	1.3/2–6	Triazolam
Nonbenzodiazepines			
Zolpidem (Ambien)	5–10	0.8/1.5–2.4	Zolpidem
Zopiclone	3.75–7.5	1.1/3.5–6.5	Zopiclone, Zopiclone-*N*-oxide (3.5–6.0)

Note. T_{max} is the time required to reach the maximal plasma concentration. Half-life is the time required by the body to metabolize or inactivate half the amount of a substrate taken. The half-life of flurazepam is short, about 2.3 hours (0.5–3.0 hours). The half-life of flurazepam listed here includes that for *N*-desalkyl-flurazepam.

tions, but this hypothesis only partially explains their action. Magnocellular regions of the basal forebrain are now recognized as important sites for sleep-wake regulation and are likely to be involved (Szymusiak 1995). Neurons that are selectively active during SWS have been described in this structure, and GABAergic-cholinergic interactions at this level are believed to be involved in the initiation of sleep.

Another important site of action for benzodiazepines might be the suprachiasmatic nucleus (SCN). In SCN-lesioned animals, benzodiazepine treatment does not induce sleep (Edgar et al. 1993), but the hypnotic effect is restored if the SCN-lesioned animal is sleep deprived before drug administration. Benzodiazepines thus may facilitate the release of a sleep debt accumulated during wakefulness rather than produce de novo sleep (Mignot et al. 1992).

The effects of benzodiazepines on sleep architectures are well known (Table 14–2). Most benzodiazepines decrease sleep latency, especially when first used, and diminish the number of awakenings. All benzodiazepines increase time spent in Stage 2 sleep. Benzodiazepines also affect the quality of the SWS pattern. Thus, Stages 3 and 4 sleep are suppressed and remain

so during the period of drug administration. The decrease in Stage 4 sleep is accompanied by a reduction in nightmares.

Most benzodiazepines increase REM latency. The time spent in REM sleep is usually shortened; however, the reduction in percentage of REM sleep is minimal because the number of cycles of REM sleep usually increases late in the sleep time. Despite the shortening of SWS and REM sleep, the net effect of administration of benzodiazepines is usually an increase in total sleep time, so that the individual feels that the quality of sleep has improved. Furthermore, the hypnotic effect is greatest in subjects with the shortest baseline total sleep time.

If the benzodiazepine is discontinued after 3–4 weeks of nightly use, a considerable rebound in the amount and density of REM sleep and SWS may occur. However, this is not a consistent finding.

Because long-acting benzodiazepine hypnotics impair daytime performance and increase the risk of falls in geriatric patients, several shorter-acting compounds have been introduced and are the preferred choice for elderly patients (see section on the management of insomnia in the elderly in "General Consider-

Table 14–2. Comparative properties of benzodiazepines and barbiturates on sleep parameters

	Benzodiazepines	Barbiturates
Total sleep time	↑ tolerance with short-acting agents	↑ rapid tolerance
Stage 2 %	↑	↑
Slow-wave sleep (Stages 3 and 4) %	↓	↓ (slight)
REM latency	↑	↑
REM %	↓ (slight)	↓
Withdrawal	Rebound insomnia with short-acting agents Carryover effectiveness with long-acting agents REM rebound (slight)	Rebound decrease in Stage 2 and total sleep time REM rebound

Note. REM = rapid eye movement sleep.

ations in the Pharmacological Treatment of Insomnia" later in this chapter) (Figure 14–5). However, it has since been found that short-acting benzodiazepines induce rebound insomnia (a worsening of sleep difficulty beyond baseline levels on discontinuation of a hypnotic) (Kales et al. 1979), rebound anxiety, anterograde amnesia, and even paradoxical rage. Many other factors, such as the subtype of insomnia being treated and the dosage and duration of treatment, are also important to explain the occurrence of these specific side effects that may also be observed with other benzodiazepines. Nevertheless, enthusiasm for the shorter-acting compounds has been tempered.

Indications

Benzodiazepines are the drug treatment of choice in the management of anxiety, insomnia, and stress-related conditions. Although none of the currently available compounds has any significant advantage over the others, some drugs can be selected to match the patient's symptom patterns to the pharmacokinetics of the various drugs. If a patient has a persistent high level of anxiety, one of the precursors of desmethyl-diazepam such as diazepam or clorazepate is most appropriate. Patients with fluctuating anxiety may prefer to take shorter-acting compounds, such as oxazepam or lorazepam, when stressful circumstances occur or are expected.

An ideal hypnotic should induce sleep rapidly without producing sedation the next day. Both flurazepam and nitrazepam are inappropriately long-acting as hypnotics unless a persistent anxiolytic effect is desired the next day (see Figure 14–5). Even in such situations, diazepam given as one dose at night may be preferable. Oxazepam penetrates too slowly for a dependable hypnotic effect (slow onset of action). Both lorazepam and temazepam are appropriate treatments for insomnia, but the dosages available are quite high (Table 14–1). Triazolam is the shortest-acting hypnotic available. When very small doses of benzodiazepines (which were assumed to have no significant hypnotic action) are administered to patients with insomnia, sleep quality often improves greatly, and usually it is not necessary to use a benzodiazepine at a hypnotic dose as a first-choice treatment.

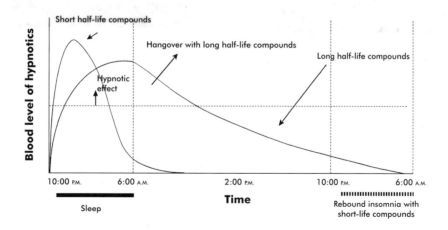

Figure 14–5. Duration of action of hypnotics and hangover and rebound insomnia. Hypnotics with long half-lives may impair daytime performance the day after drug administration, whereas short-acting compounds may induce rebound insomnia on discontinuation.

Benzodiazepines can increase the frequency of apnea and exacerbate oxygen desaturation in healthy subjects and in subjects with chronic bronchitis (Geddes et al. 1976). Although many reports suggest that benzodiazepines are safe in patients with obstructive sleep apnea, other authors disagree, and it seems wise to avoid hypnotics in patients with severe sleep apnea. One of the only other contraindications is myasthenia gravis, a condition in which muscle relaxation with benzodiazepines can exacerbate muscle atonia.

Benzodiazepines have many indications other than sleep induction and anxiolysis, such as epilepsy (see Keck and McElroy, Chapter 12, in this volume). Lorazepam and diazepam can be used for relaxation procedures, preoperative medication, and sedation during minor operations and investigations, often causing retrograde amnesia, a side effect that is sometimes desirable in this indication. Benzodiazepines have been used to manage alcohol withdrawal because cross-tolerance usually exists with alcohol, but large doses are often needed to suppress the withdrawal syndrome. Finally, benzodiazepines, especially clonazepam, are indicated in the treatment of many sleep disorders in adults and infants (see Reite, Chapter 30, in this volume).

Side Effects and Toxicology

When a benzodiazepine is taken at high doses, tiredness, drowsiness, and profound feelings of detachment are common but can be minimized by a careful dose adjustment. Headache, dizziness, ataxia, confusion, and disorientation are less common except in the elderly. A marked potentiation of the depressant effect of alcohol occurs. Other less common side effects include weight gain, skin rash, menstrual irregularities, impairment of sexual function, and, very rarely, agranulocytosis.

Because the safety of benzodiazepines in early pregnancy is not established, they should be avoided unless absolutely necessary. Diazepam is secreted in breast milk and may make the baby sleepy, unresponsive, and slow to feed.

Overdosage. The benzodiazepines are extremely widely prescribed, so it is not surprising that they are used in many suicide attempts. For adults, overdoses of benzodiazepines reportedly are not fatal unless alcohol or other psychotropic drugs are taken simultaneously. Typically, the patient falls asleep but is arousable and wakes after 24–48 hours. Treatment is supportive. A stomach pump is usually more punitive than therapeutic, and dialysis is usually useless because of high plasma binding.

Tolerance and dependence. Dependence, both psychological and physical, occurs with benzodiazepines as with other sedative-hypnotics. Abrupt discontinuation results in withdrawal phenomena such as anxiety, agitation, restlessness, and tension, which are usually delayed for several days because of the long half-life of the major metabolite, desmethyldiazepam. Even with the normal dosage, some patients have withdrawal effects. The fact that some patients gradually increase the dose suggests tolerance, but increases in dose are sometimes related to particularly stressful crises.

Psychological dependence is also common, based on the high incidence of repeat prescriptions, but it is mild, and the drug-seeking behavior is much less persistent than with barbiturates.

BARBITURATES

History

Barbital, one of the derivatives of barbituric acid, was introduced in 1903 and soon became extremely popular in clinical medicine because of its sleep-inducing and anxiolytic effects (Maynert 1965). In 1912, phenobarbital was introduced. In addition to its use as a sedative-hypnotic, phenobarbital has become one of the most important pharmacological treatments for epilepsy. Since then, more than 2,500 barbiturate analogues have been synthesized, of which about 50 have been made commercially available and only 20 of which are still on the market.

The success of barbiturates as sedative-hypnotics was largely overshadowed by the discovery of benzodiazepines in the late 1960s. With pharmacological properties very similar to those of barbiturates, these compounds have a much safer pharmacological profile. Thus, benzodiazepines have replaced barbiturates in many indications, especially for psychiatric conditions in which suicide is a possibility.

Pharmacological Profile

The main effects of barbiturates are sedation, sleep induction, and anesthesia. Some of the barbiturates, such as phenobarbital, also have selective anticonvulsant properties. The mechanisms of action of barbiturates are complex and still not fully understood. Nonanesthetic doses of barbiturates preferentially suppress polysynaptic responses. Pertinent to their sedative-hypnotic effects is the fact that the mesencephalic reticular activating system is extremely sensitive to these drugs (Killam 1962). The synaptic site of inhibition is either postsynaptic (e.g., at the level of cortical and cerebellar pyramidal cells and in the cuneate nucleus, substantia nigra, and thalamic relay neurons) or presynaptic (e.g., in the spinal cord). This inhibition occurs only at synapses where physiological inhibition is GABAergic and not glycinergic or monoaminergic. Thus, barbiturates, like benzodiazepines, potentiate GABA-mediated inhibitory processes in the brain. However, it remains unclear whether all of the effects of barbiturates are entirely mediated by GABAergic mechanisms.

Barbiturates do not displace benzodiazepines from their binding sites; instead, barbiturates enhance benzodiazepine binding by increasing the affinity of the receptor for benzodiazepines (Leeb-Lumberg et al. 1980). They also enhance the binding of GABA and its agonists to specific binding sites (Asano and Ogasawara 1981). These effects are almost completely dependent on the presence of chloride or other anions that are known to permeate the chloride channels associated with the GABA receptor complex, and they are competitively antagonized by picrotoxin (a convulsant) (Olsen et al. 1978). Taken together, these observations suggest that the macromolecular complex composed of $GABA_A$-ergic receptors, chloride ionophores, and binding sites for benzodiazepines (ω-site) is an important site of action for depressant barbiturates (see Figure 14–2).

Effects on stages of sleep. Barbiturates decrease sleep latency; however, they slightly increase fast electroencephalogram (EEG) activity during sleep. Barbiturates decrease body movement during sleep. Stage 2 sleep increases, whereas Stages 3 and 4 SWS generally decrease, except in some patients with anxiety and in patients who are addicted to barbiturates. REM sleep latency is prolonged, and both the total time spent in REM sleep and the number of REM cycles are diminished. With repeated nighttime administration, drug tolerance to the effects on sleep occurs in a few days. Discontinuation of barbiturates may lead to insomnia and disrupted sleep patterns (with a decrease in Stage 2 sleep) and increases in REM sleep (Kay et al. 1976).

Pharmacokinetics and Disposition

For hypnotic use, barbiturates are usually administered orally. Barbiturates are rapidly absorbed in the stomach, and their absorption decreases when the stomach is full. Because the sodium salts are rapidly dissolved, they are more rapidly absorbed than free acids.

Barbiturates are metabolized mainly in the liver, generally producing inactive polar metabolites that are rapidly excreted in the urine (Rall 1990). Changes in liver function can markedly alter the rate at which these compounds are inactivated. Chronic administration leads to pharmacokinetic tolerance even when low or infrequent doses of barbiturates are used (see the section "Drug-Drug Interactions" later in this chapter).

The rate of penetration of barbiturates into the CNS varies according to their lipophilicity. In general, liposolubility decreases latency to onset of action and duration of action. Thiopental, for example, enters the CNS rapidly and is used to rapidly induce anesthesia; barbitone crosses into the brain so slowly that it is inappropriate as a hypnotic drug.

Indications

Although clinical trials have shown that the barbiturates have sedative and hypnotic properties, they generally compare poorly with benzodiazepines. The patient feels "drugged" the next day, and there is always the risk of fatal overdose because of the depressant effect on respiration. Barbiturates suppress respiration, and the therapeutic dose of barbiturates may cause fatal respiratory depression in patients with sleep apnea. Patients with sleep apnea should therefore avoid taking barbiturates. Because of these risks, many clinicians have stopped using barbiturates as hypnotics and sedatives and prescribe them only as anticonvulsants.

The drugs are contraindicated in patients with porphyria because barbiturates enhance porphyrin synthesis. Liver function should be checked before and during drug administration. Liver dysfunction can significantly prolong the sedative effects of these drugs and may lead to fatal overdose.

Side Effects and Toxicology

In treating many patients who are prescribed barbiturates, it is difficult to control symptoms without producing oversedation. Patients typically oscillate between anxiety and torpor. Mental performance is often impaired, and patients should not drive or operate dangerous machinery.

Patients whose conditions have been stabilized for years with barbiturates must be considered drug dependent. Withdrawal leads to anxiety, agitation, trembling, and, frequently, convulsions. Substitution of a benzodiazepine that can be withdrawn more easily later is often successful.

Hypersensitive reactions (especially of the skin) may occur, and instances of megaloblastic anemia have been reported. An overdose of barbiturates leads to fatal respiratory and cardiovascular depression. Suicide attempts frequently involve overdoses of barbiturates, either taken alone or taken in combination with alcohol or other psychotropic drugs, particularly tricyclic antidepressants. Unfortunately, these suicide attempts are often successful. Severe poisoning results at 10 times the hypnotic dose, and twice that amount may be fatal.

Tolerance and dependence.   Tolerance to barbiturates occurs rapidly and is a result of both pharmacokinetic factors (e.g., liver-enzyme induction) and pharmacodynamic factors (e.g., neuronal adaptation to chronic drug administration). Cross-tolerance develops to alcohol, gas anesthetics, and other sedatives, including benzodiazepines.

Psychological dependence (i.e., drug-seeking behavior) is common. Patients typically visit several physicians to obtain more barbiturates. Intoxication may occur, as evidenced by impaired mental functioning, emotional instability, and neurological signs. Abrupt discontinuation after high dosage is likely to induce convulsions and delirium. After normal dosage, withdrawal phenomena include anxiety, insomnia, restlessness, agitation, tremor, muscle twitching, nausea and vomiting, orthostatic hypotension, and weight loss.

Drug-Drug Interactions

Barbiturates used with other CNS depressants can cause severe depression. Ethanol is the drug most frequently used, and interactions with antihistaminic compounds are also common.

Barbiturates may increase the activity of hepatic microsomal enzymes two- to threefold.

Clinically, this change is particularly important for patients who are also receiving metabolic competitors such as warfarin or digitoxin, for which careful control of plasma concentrations is vital (Rall 1990).

ALCOHOL-TYPE HYPNOTICS AND GAMMA-HYDROXYBUTYRATE

The alcohol type of hypnotics include the chloral derivatives, of which chloral hydrate, clomethiazole, and ethchlorvynol are still used occasionally in the elderly. Chloral hydrate is metabolized to another active sedative-hypnotic—trichloroethanol. These drugs have short half-lives (about 4–6 hours) and decrease sleep latency and number of awakenings; SWS is slightly depressed, but overall REM sleep time is largely unaffected. Chloral hydrate and its metabolite have an unpleasant taste and frequently cause epigastric distress and nausea. Undesirable side effects include light-headedness, ataxia, and nightmares. The chronic use of these drugs can lead to tolerance and occasionally to physical dependence. As with barbiturates, overdosage can lead to respiratory and cardiovascular depression, and therapeutic use of these drugs has largely been superseded by benzodiazepines.

γ-Hydroxybutyrate is a hypnotic agent that has been used mostly in the treatment of insomnia in narcoleptic patients (Scrima et al. 1990). Although the compound is structurally related to GABA, its mode of action involves specific non-GABAergic binding sites and a potent inhibitory effect on dopaminergic transmission (Vayer et al. 1987). The compound promotes SWS and REM sleep (Lapierre et al. 1990), but its effects on sleep architecture are short lasting, and repeated administration is usually necessary during the night. It is rarely used in other indications and is frequently abused by athletes because of its SWS-promoting effects, with resulting increases in growth hormone secretion (Chin et al. 1992). γ-Hydroxybutyrate is also commonly abused because of its euphoric effects (Chin et al. 1992).

ANTIHISTAMINES

Antihistamines, such as promethazine, diphenhydramine, and doxylamine, are sometimes prescribed as sleep inducers. They decrease sleep latency but do not increase total sleep time (Reite et al. 1997). These compounds are especially useful for patients who cannot sleep well because of acute allergic reactions or itching. Sedative antihistamines may also be prescribed in people who tend to abuse psychoactive drugs, because sedative antihistamines have not been shown to have abuse potential.

MELATONIN

Melatonin is a neurohormone produced by the pineal gland during the dark phase of the day-night cycle. In animals, melatonin has been implicated in the circadian regulation of sleep and in the seasonal control of reproduction. Studies suggest that melatonin administration may have some therapeutic effects in various disturbances of circadian rhythmicity such as jet lag (Arendt et al. 1987), shift work (Folkard et al. 1993), non-24-hour sleep-wake cycle in blind subjects (Arendt et al. 1988), and delayed sleep phase insomnia (Dahlitz et al. 1991), an effect associated with few side effects (e.g., headaches or nausea). High doses of melatonin (3–100 mg), which increase serum melatonin levels far beyond the normal nocturnal range, have been suggested to produce hypnotic effects in humans, especially in the elderly (Haimov et al. 1995). Lower, more physiological doses of melatonin (e.g., 0.3 mg) might also be active, but the data available to date are less convincing.

In humans, the production of melatonin during the dark period declines with age; this effect parallels declines in sleep quantity and quality (Van Coevorden et al. 1991). In one report, older patients with insomnia had a lower secretion of 6-sulphatoxymelatonin (the main melatonin metabolite) than did younger people or older subjects without insomnia (Haimov et al. 1994). These results suggest that deficiency in nocturnal melatonin secretion might contribute to disrupted sleep in the elderly; thus, in this population, insomnia is a particularly attractive indication for melatonin.

One of the difficulties in establishing therapeutic efficacy of melatonin is its short half-life (20–30 minutes). Bedtime melatonin administration reduces sleep latency but has few objective effects on sleep architecture. It is also unclear whether the hypnotic effect of a physiological or pharmacological dose is a direct effect on sleep or an indirect effect on circadian timing that subsequently gates the release of sleep or both. Finally, very few double-blind, placebo-controlled studies have been done, and most current reports are confounded by strong placebo effects in the context of a melatonin fad. Melatonin might be an effective hypnotic in some indications, but better controlled studies are needed to establish efficacy in specific indications. The purity of the products sold in health food stores is also a problem, and the long-term effects of melatonin administration in humans are unknown.

GENERAL CONSIDERATIONS IN THE PHARMACOLOGICAL TREATMENT OF INSOMNIA

Insomnia is a subjective complaint of insufficient, inadequate, or nonrestrictive sleep (see Buysse and Reynolds 1990). Disturbances in daytime functioning, such as fatigue, mood disturbances, and impaired performance, result from inadequate sleep. Insomnia is a common symptom. In 1983, a survey indicated that 35% of the general population reported having trouble sleeping in the past year, and 17% considered their problem serious (Mellinger et al. 1985). In the same survey, 7.1% of the popula-

tion had used a hypnotic in the past year (Mellinger et al. 1985).

Insomnia is a symptom that must be explored clinically before treatment is initiated. Sleep disturbances often indicate a larger psychiatric problem, such as depression. As mentioned above, a complaint of insomnia is also common with old age, especially in an institutional setting. In other cases, environmental factors (e.g., noise) and associated sleep disorders (periodic leg movements, sleep apneas, parasomnias) may be involved.

A useful initial approach to the patient with insomnia is to consider the duration of the complaint. Insomnia can occur as a transient (1–2 days), short-term (more than a few days to a few months), or chronic disturbance (several months or even years). The duration of insomnia not only suggests its cause (see Table 14–3) but also provides some guidance on how to use hypnotics.

Transient insomnias are typically caused by an environmental acute stressor or jet lag and shift work. In this indication, pharmacotherapy with benzodiazepine hypnotics or other hypnotics has no risks because dependence on the treatment is unlikely to develop if the therapy lasts less than a week to 10 days.

Short-term (a few days to a few months) insomnias are particularly important to recognize because they may evolve into chronic, psychophysiological insomnia if not or inadequately treated. Typically, patients develop insomnia during a stressful period of their lives (e.g., work or personal difficulties). The condition frequently worsens if untreated, and the patient worries excessively about his or her sleep, which evolves toward a behaviorally learned, chronic insomnia that does not resolve once the stressful period is over. In this indication, the use of benzodiazepine hypnotics on a daily basis is also dangerous because it may lead to tolerance and dependence. Reassurance regarding the favorable resolution of the stressful event is important, and the patient should be instructed to use hypnotic medications intermittently (e.g.,

Table 14–3. **Nosological classification of insomnia (International Classification of Sleep Disorders Diagnostic Criteria)**

Category	% of patients with corresponding diagnosis[a]	Description
Psychophysiological	15	Transient or persistent insomnia that develops as a result of psychological factors, physiological tension/arousal, and negative conditioning
Idiopathic insomnia	<5	Insomnia and daytime dysfunction, which begin in childhood and continue into adulthood
Associated with sleep-induced respiratory impairment	5–10	Frequent respiratory pauses or hypoxia (e.g., sleep apnea, alveolar hypoventilation) that lead to brief arousals during the night
Associated with periodic leg movements and restless legs	12	Repetitive, stereotyped jerking leg movements or unpleasant dysesthesias in legs on falling asleep, which frequently interrupt sleep
Associated with psychiatric disorders	35	Insomnia associated with behavioral symptoms and underlying biological disturbances of psychiatric disorders (including affective, anxiety, psychotic, and personality disorders)
Associated with neurological disorders	~5	Insomnia associated with neurological disorders, such as cerebral degenerative disorders, dementia, and parkinsonism
Associated with other medical disorders	~5	Insomnia associated with other medical disorders, such as nocturnal cardiac ischemia, chronic obstructive pulmonary disease, and sleep-related asthma; sleep is expected to improve when the underlying condition is treated
Associated with chronic drugs and alcohol use	12	Insomnia associated with use of, tolerance to, or withdrawal from CNS-active agents, including stimulants, sedative-hypnotics, and alcohol
Sleep state misperception	5–10	Subjective insomnia complaint that is not substantiated by polysomnography
Transient sleep-wake disorders[b]	NA	Rapid time-zone change (jet lag) or schedule or work shift change results in symptoms of insomnia during new, desired sleep hours, and sleepiness during new, desired wake hours
Persistent sleep-wake disorders[b]	NA	A frequently changing sleep-wake schedule, delayed or advanced sleep phase syndrome, non-24-hour sleep-wake pattern, or irregular sleep-wake pattern results in symptoms of insomnia during desired sleep hours and sleepiness during desired wake hours

Note. CNS = central nervous system; NA = not available.
[a]Estimated from approximately 2,000 patients with a diagnosed disorder of initiating and maintaining sleep by 20 centers; contributed by the Association of Sleep Disorders Centers National Case Series (Coleman 1983).
[b]These diagnoses are classified as disorders of the circadian rhythm sleep disorders in the *International Classification of Sleep Disorders* diagnostic criteria (American Sleep Disorders Association 1990).
Source. Adapted from Buysse and Reynolds 1990.

every few days, as needed) to avoid the development of tolerance. An education in sleep hygiene (not taking naps even when very tired, having regular wake-up times, avoiding caffeine and alcohol) is also important to reduce the possibility of evolution into a chronic problem.

Chronic insomnia first should be evaluated with a sleep log for a 2-week period. Most commonly, some degree of sleep state misperception is present, and patients with insomnia greatly exaggerate the complaint (i.e., they sleep more than they claim and take less time to fall asleep than they report). In most cases, insomnia has developed as the result of psychological factors and negative conditioning, as mentioned above. In rare cases, insomnia began in childhood and has persisted in adulthood (idiopathic insomnia). In chronic insomnia, improved sleep hygiene and various behavioral techniques that aim to reduce negative conditioning (stimulus control therapy), sleep restriction, and phototherapy are often helpful on a long-term basis, but these methods are only successful if the patient is motivated and if specialized clinical supervision is available. The most appropriate use of drugs is in patients in whom sleep disturbance is clearly causing some daytime dysfunction. If the clinician decides to use pharmacotherapy, it is always helpful to start with the lowest dose of hypnotic possible (hypnotic medications are frequently overdosed) to reduce the risk of tolerance and dependence and to try to avoid daily use.

Insomnia can also be classified on the basis of individual clinical features—that is, as sleep initiation, sleep maintenance, or termination (early-morning awakening). In this context, the most important pharmacological properties to consider when selecting a hypnotic for treatment are how quickly it acts and how long the effects last (see Table 14–1 for commonly used compounds). The rate of absorption is the most critical factor determining onset of action. T_{max} (time required to reach the maximal plasma concentration) is the pharmacological parameter that best predicts onset of action. After absorp-

tion, hypnotics are distributed to various organs; distribution and drug elimination influence the duration of action. The elimination half-life (see Table 14–1) usually provides a good first estimate of the duration of action for drugs that have comparable absorption and distribution profiles. Hypnotics with long durations of action are helpful for patients who have difficulty both initiating and maintaining sleep. One advantage of these long-acting compounds is that rebound insomnia is often delayed and milder if the drug has to be withdrawn (see Figure 14–5). Patients who have difficulty initiating sleep might prefer short-acting compounds; however, for these compounds, it may be necessary, paradoxically, to switch to longer-acting hypnotics before withdrawal of all hypnotic treatment.

The importance of determining whether insomnia is the symptom of an underlying neuropsychiatric condition must be emphasized (see Table 14–3). For depression, trazodone (25–50 mg), amitriptyline (10 mg), trimipramine (25–50 mg), or doxepin (25–50 mg) can be used as hypnotics or in combination with other hypnotics. Most schizophrenic patients also have persistent insomnia (initiation and maintenance of sleep), and phenothiazines, such as chlorpromazine, thioridazine, and levomepromazine, are effective therapies. When psychotic symptoms are associated with insomnia, butyrophenones, such as haloperidol, also can be used. For insomnia associated with anxiety disorders, hypnotics supplemented with anxiolytics can be used, and this treatment may prevent rebound insomnia and its related anxiety.

Sleep disturbances are very frequent complaints in old age, and treatment must be initiated carefully in this population (see also Salzman et al., Chapter 28, in this volume). About 12% of the United States population is older than 60 years, and this population receives 35%–40% of all sedative-hypnotic prescriptions (Gottlieb 1990).

Before starting pharmacological therapy, all possible causes of insomnia should be examined (i.e., psychophysiological, associated with drugs and alcohol, disturbance of the sleep-wake cycle, associated with periodic leg movements, sleep apnea, or other physical or psychiatric conditions). Before selecting a specific hypnotic, the clinician should consider the pharmacological properties, side-effect profiles, patients' medical health and histories, and patients' histories of sedative-hypnotic use. The special case of melatonin has been discussed earlier in this chapter. Hypnotics or their active metabolites often accumulate during chronic use in elderly patients, and this accumulation may cause cognition problems, disorientation, confusion, and, occasionally, falls. Hypnotics with short or intermediate half-lives are thus recommended, and the lowest dose possible should be used. Compounds with a short half-life, such as triazolam or zolpidem, may be effective for problems with sleep initiation and sleep fragmentation. Zolpidem has little muscle relaxant effect and may be preferable. Compounds with an intermediate hypnotic profile, such as estazolam and temazepam, are also reported to be effective in elderly patients. Hypnotics with intermediate half-lives may alter less daytime performance and memory and are less likely to induce rebound insomnia after withdrawal compared with regular hypnotics.

CONCLUSION

The mechanism of action of most currently available hypnotics (barbiturates, alcohol, benzodiazepines, zolpidem, and zopiclone) involves a modulatory effect of GABAergic activity. These compounds stimulate GABAergic transmission by acting on the GABA$_A$/BZ-Cl$^-$ macromolecular complex, known to contain multiple modulatory binding sites and many receptor subtypes. This recently discovered molecular diversity suggests that new GABAergic hypnotic compounds with better side-effect profiles will be developed in the future.

Other non-GABAergic hypnotics, including mostly sedative antidepressants, antihista-

mines, and melatonin, are viable strategies in the treatment of insomnia. Their prescription, as for other regular benzodiazepine-like hypnotic compounds, should be guided by the knowledge that insomnia is a heterogeneous condition that should be explored clinically before any pharmacological treatment is initiated.

REFERENCES

American Sleep Disorders Association: The International Classification of Sleep Disorders: Diagnostic and Coding Manual. Rochester, MN, American Sleep Disorders Association, 1990

Arendt J, Aldhous M, Marks V, et al: Some effects of jet-lag and their alleviation by melatonin. Ergonomics 30:1379–1393, 1987

Arendt J, Aldhous M, Wright J: Synchronisation of a disturbed sleep-wake cycle in a blind man by melatonin treatment. Lancet 1:772–773, 1988

Asano T, Ogasawara N: Chloride-dependent stimulation of GABA and benzodiazepine receptor binding by pentobarbital. Brain Res 225: 212–216, 1981

Buysse DJ, Reynolds III CF: Insomnia, in Handbook of Sleep Disorders. Edited by Thorpy MJ. New York, Marcel Dekker, 1990, pp 375–433

Chin M, Kreutzer RA, Dyer JL: Acute poisoning from γ-hydroxybutyrate in California. West J Med 156:380–384, 1992

Coleman RM: Diagnosis, treatment, and follow-up of about 8,000 sleep/wake disorder patients, in Sleep/Wake Disorders; National History, Epidemiology, and Long Term Evolution. Edited by Guilleminault C, Lugaresi E. New York, Raven, 1983, pp 29–35

Cook L, Sepinwall J: Behavioral analysis of the effects and mechanisms of action of benzodiazepines. Adv Biochem Psychopharmacol 14:1–28, 1975

Costa E, Guidotti A: Diazepam binding inhibitor (DBI): a peptide with multiple biological actions. Life Sci 49:325–344, 1991

Dahlitz M, Alvarez B, Vignan J, et al: Delayed sleep phase syndrome response to melatonin. Lancet 337:1121–1124, 1991

Edgar DM, Dement WC, Fuller CA: Effect of SCN-lesions on sleep in squirrel monkeys: evidence for opponent processes in sleep-wake regulation. J Neurosci 13:1065–1079, 1993

Edgar DM, Seidel WF, Gee KW, et al: CCD-3693: an orally bioavailable analog of the endogenous neuroactive steroid, pregnanolone, demonstrates potent sedative hypnotic action in the rat. J Pharmacol Exp Ther 282:420–429, 1997

Enna SJ, Möhler H: γ-Aminobutyric acid (GABA) receptors and their association with benzodiazepine recognition sites, in Psychopharmacology: The Third Generation of Progress. Edited by Meltzer HY. New York, Raven, 1987, pp 265–272

Folkard S, Arendt J, Clark M: Can melatonin improve shift workers' tolerance of the night shift? Some preliminary findings. Chronobiol Int 10:315–320, 1993

Friess E, Lance M, Holster F: The effects of 'neuroactive' steroids upon sleep in human and rats (abstract). J Sleep Res 5:S69, 1996

Geddes DM, Rudorf M, Saunders KB: Effect of nitrazepam and flurazepam on the ventilatory response to carbon dioxide. Thorax 31:548–551, 1976

Gottlieb GL: Sleep disorders and their management: special considerations in the elderly. Am J Med 88:29S–33S, 1990

Haimov I, Laudon M, Zisapel N, et al: Sleep disorders and melatonin rhythms in elderly people. BMJ 309:167, 1994

Haimov I, Lavie P, Lauden M, et al: Melatonin treatment of sleep onset insomnia in the elderly. Sleep 18:598–603, 1995

Jovanovic UJ, Dreyfus JF: Polygraphical sleep recording in insomniac patients under zopiclone or nitrazepam. Pharmacology 27 (suppl 2): 136–145, 1983

Kales A, Shlarf MB, Kales JD, et al: Rebound insomnia: a potential hazard following withdrawal of certain benzodiazepines. JAMA 241:1691–1695, 1979

Kay DC, Blackburn AB, Buckingham JA, et al: Human pharmacology of sleep, in Pharmacology of Sleep. Edited by Williams RL, Karakan I. New York, Wiley, 1976, pp 83–210

Killam K: Drug action on the brainstem reticular formation. Pharmacol Rev 14:175–224, 1962

Lapierre O, Montplaisir J, Lamarre M, et al: The effect of gamma-hydroxybutyrate on nocturnal and diurnal sleep of normal subjects: further consideration on REM sleep-triggering mechanisms. Sleep 13:24–30, 1990

Leeb-Lumberg F, Snowman A, Olsen RW: Barbiturate receptor sites are coupled to benzodiazepine receptors. Proc Natl Acad Sci U S A 77: 7467–7472, 1980

Lüddens H, Wisden W: Function and pharmacology of multiple GABA_A receptor subunit. Trends Pharmacol Sci 12:49–51, 1991

Marquardt H, Todaro GJ, Shoyab M: Complete amino acid sequences of bovine and human endozepines: homology with rat diazepam binding inhibitor. J Biol Chem 261:9727–9731, 1986

Maynert EW: Sedative and hypnotics, II: barbiturates, in Drill's Pharmacology in Medicine. Edited by DiPalma IR. New York, McGraw-Hill, 1965, pp 188–209

Mellinger GD, Balter MB, Uhlenhuth EH: Insomnia and its treatment: prevalence and correlates. Arch Gen Psychiatry 42:225–232, 1985

Mignot E, Edgar DM, Miller JD, et al: Strategies for the development of new treatments in sleep disorders medicine, in Target Receptors for Anxiolytics and Hypnotics: From Molecular Pharmacology to Therapeutics. Edited by Mendelewicz J, Racagni G, Karger AG. Basel, Karger, 1992, pp 129–150

Möhler H, Okada T: Benzodiazepine receptor: demonstration in the central nervous system. Science 198:849–851, 1977

Mullen KD, Szauter KM, Kaminsky-Russ K: "Endogenous" benzodiazepine activity in physiological fluids of patients with hepatic encephalopathy. Lancet 336:81–83, 1990

Nutt DJ, Glue P, Lawson C, et al: Flumazenil provocation of panic attacks. Arch Gen Psychiatry 47:917–925, 1990

Olsen RW, Tick MK, Miller T: Dihydropicotoxine binding to crayfish muscle sites possibly related to γ-aminobutyric acid receptor-ionophores. Mol Pharmacol 14:381–390, 1978

Olsen RW, Bureau MH, Endo S, et al: The GABA_A receptor family in the mammalian brain. Neurochem Res 16:317–325, 1991

Rall TR: Hypnotics and sedatives; ethanol, in The Pharmacological Basis of Therapeutics, 8th Edition. Edited by Gilman AG, Rall TW, Niles AS, et al. New York, Pergamon, 1990, pp 345–382

Reite M, Ruddy J, Nagel K: Concise Guide to Evaluation and Management of Sleep Disorders, 2nd Edition. Washington, DC, American Psychiatric Press, 1997

Richter JA, Holman JR Jr: Barbiturates: their in vivo effects and potential biochemical mechanisms. Prog Neurobiol 18:275–319, 1982

Rothstein JD, Guidotti A, Tinuper P, et al: Endogenous benzodiazepine receptor ligands in idiopathic recurring stupor. Lancet 340:1002–1004, 1992

Rupprecht R, Hauser CAE, Trapp T, et al: Neurosteroids: molecular mechanisms of action and psychopharmacological significance. J Steroid Biochem Mol Biol 56:163–168, 1996

Sangameswaran L, Fales HM, Friedrich P, et al: Purification of a benzodiazepine from bovine brain and detection of benzodiazepine like immunoreactivity in human brain. Proc Natl Acad Sci U S A 83:9236–9240, 1986

Schmidt RF, Vogel ME, Zimmermann M: Effect of diazepam on presynaptic inhibition and other spinal reflexes. Naunyn Schmiedebergs Arch Pharmacol 258:69–82, 1967

Scrima L, Hartman PG, Johnson FH, et al: The effects of gamma-hydroxybutyrate on the sleep of narcolepsy patients: a double-blind study. Sleep 13:479–490, 1990

Shlarf MB: Pharmacology of classic and novel hypnotic drugs, in Target Receptors for Anxiolytics and Hypnotics: From Molecular Pharmacology to Therapeutics. Edited by Mendelwicz J, Racagni G. Basel, Karger, 1992, pp 109–116

Squires RF, Braestrup C: Benzodiazepine receptors in rat brain. Nature 266:732–734, 1977

Szymusiak R: Magnocellular nuclei of the basal forebrain: substrates of sleep and arousal regulation. Sleep 18:478–500, 1995

Tallman JF, Thomas JW, Gallager DW: GABAergic modulation of benzodiazepine binding site sensitivity. Nature 274:383–385, 1978

Van Coevorden A, Mockel J, Laurent E, et al: Neuroendocrine rhythms and sleep in aging men. Am J Physiol 260:651–661, 1991

Vayer P, Mandel P, Maitre M: Gamma-hydroxybutyrate, a possible neurotransmitter. Life Sci 41:1547–1557, 1987

FIFTEEN

Stimulants in Psychiatry

Jan Fawcett, M.D., and
Katie A. Busch, M.D.

The marked and varied effects of amphetamine, despite its relatively simple structure and its potential for abuse and dependence, have made it a topic of interest and controversy since it was first synthesized in 1887.

Today, the major areas of medical use of stimulants are the treatment of narcolepsy, for which amphetamine or methylphenidate (MPH) is used to relieve the symptoms of sleepiness and involuntary sleeping without affecting the etiology of the illness, and in the treatment of attention-deficit/hyperactivity disorder (ADHD) in children, which continues to generate scientific, medical, and public controversy. Stimulants are also of possible value in treating adult attention-deficit disorder or residual ADHD, and they are still used in the treatment of obesity despite significant medical and scientific doubts as to their long-term benefits in maintaining weight loss and concerns about abuse and dependence. Other proposed uses of stimulants include the treatment of affective disorders and certain organic brain disorders and their use in cancer patients receiving high doses of opiates for pain. These uses are discussed later in this chapter.

Dextroamphetamine (DAMPH) and MPH are the two most commonly used stimulants in psychiatry and medicine. They have both similarities and differences in effect. In this chapter, we focus on these two compounds as primary examples of stimulant medications. We consider their mechanisms of action and the current evidence concerning their therapeutic and adverse effects and the hazards associated with their use. Other weaker but clinically used stimulants, such as phentermine and pemoline, will be discussed in their clinical contexts.

HISTORY AND DISCOVERY

Amphetamines were used by both sides in World War II. It has been contended that Japan had large supplies of amphetamines that were placed on the open market after the war, leading to an epidemic of amphetamine abuse and cases of amphetamine psychosis, first in Japan in the 1950s and then in the United States in the 1960s (Fischman 1987). In 1958, the piperazine derivative of amphetamine, MPH, was first introduced to treat hyperactivity in children (Anders and Ciaranello 1977).

Narcolepsy was probably the first disorder for which amphetamine was used clinically

(Prinzmetal and Bloomberg 1935). Amphetamine revolutionized therapy for this condition and, although its use was not curative, it was noted that "the drug may enable the patient to become symptom free" (Connell 1968, p. 235). The effective dose ranged as high as 30–50 mg, taken in divided doses two or three times daily.

It was later found that amphetamine itself may have beneficial effects, particularly in the milder epileptic states, and it has been used as the sole method of medication for epilepsy, with varying results. Connell pointed out that in 1968, it was more common for amphetamine to be used in combination with other anticonvulsant drugs than by itself. This is in accordance with the observations of Hoffman and Lefkowitz (1993), who noted that amphetamine "can obtund the maximal electroshock seizure discharge" (p. 211).

Amphetamines were also widely used in the treatment of drug addiction and alcoholism to offset sleepiness and lethargy. This continued until the recognition of the dangers of amphetamine dependence and abuse of amphetamines, "together with the vicious cycle of amphetamine to counteract effect of sedatives, followed by sedatives to counteract the use of amphetamines (e.g., insomnia)" (Connell 1968, p. 235). This realization led to the discontinuation of amphetamine use in the treatment of these conditions.

Connell mentioned that Bradley and Bowen (1941) had reported the use of amphetamines to modify antisocial behavior in children. He summarized clinical observations of the effects of amphetamine as showing that "when children are withdrawn or lethargic, the amphetamines tended to make them more alert, more accessible to persons and the environment" (Connell 1968, p. 236).

The "paradoxical" effect of amphetamine noted in psychopathic adults was also seen in aggressive, noisy children; children who were hyperactive tended to move more quietly, to be calmer, and to quarrel less when taking amphetamines. These observations appear to precede those of the effect of amphetamine and MPH in hyperkinetic children with a diagnosis of what is now called ADHD.

The next historical use of amphetamines, and perhaps one of its most common uses, was in the treatment of obesity. Connell (1968) commented that there was "an increasing body of opinion suggesting that the contribution of amphetamines to the long-term treatment of obesity is small or nonexistent and does not justify their use now that the dangers of dependency and abuse are so much better known" (p. 236).

The epidemic of amphetamine abuse peaked in the United States in the 1960s and 1970s and was in decline by 1978, when the cocaine epidemic was well under way (Foltin and Fischman 1991). In 1970, amphetamine and its derivatives were scheduled under the Controlled Substances Act.

From the perspective of the history of stimulants, the indications for their use have considerably narrowed over the years. The reasons for this probably include the realization of the risks of abuse and dependence on these agents, that newer and more effective agents have been shown to work in treating some of these conditions, and that the stimulants have simply been shown to be ineffective and have thus fallen into disuse. At the same time, an interest in the clinical use of stimulants in psychiatry remains, as evidenced by case reports of positive treatment responses in patients with particular types of affective disorders and some other psychiatric conditions. These areas of possible effectiveness for the stimulants are reviewed in the "Indications" section of this chapter.

STRUCTURE-ACTIVITY RELATIONS

Phenylisopropylamine (amphetamine) is a relatively simple structure and forms the template for a wide variety of pharmacologically active substances. Although amphetamine is a central nervous system (CNS) stimulant, minor modifications of it result in agents that can produce a broad spectrum of effects, including decongestant, anorectic, antidepressant (bupropion and the monoamine oxidase inhibitor [MAOI] tranylcypromine), and hallucinogenic (Glennon 1987). As noted by Glennon (1987), although health professionals and the lay public may assume that all amphetamine derivatives could possess amphetamine-like characteristics, this is not necessarily the case. Although amphetamine itself has (most notably) CNS stimulant, anorectic, and vasoconstrictor properties, a review of its structure-activity relations shows that its major properties (plus psychomimetic, MAO inhibition, and neurotransmitter uptake effects) can be enhanced by structural modification at the expense of other effects.

With respect to the behavioral properties of the simple phenylisopropylamines, two general groups, the CNS stimulant and the hallucinogenic properties, can be considered. The phenylisopropylamine molecule can be arbitrarily divided into three structural components: 1) the aromatic nucleus, 2) the terminal amine, and 3) the isopropyl side chain. In general, substitution on the aromatic nucleus of amphetamine results in agents that are less potent or inactive as CNS stimulants (Glennon 1987). The substitution of two or more methoxy groups plus ethyl, methyl, or bromine groups on the aromatic nucleus creates hallucinogens of various potencies.

Several popular hallucinogens of abuse result from the substitution of methylenedioxy substitutions on two carbons of the aromatic ring. This results in 2,3-methylenedioxyamphetamine (MDA) or 3,4-MDA, known as the "love drug," which has behavioral properties distinct from those of either amphetamine or other typical hallucinogens. The end monomethyl analogue of 3,4-MDA, N-methyl-3,4-methylenedioxymethamphetamine (MDMA) or "XTC" ("Ecstasy"), is perhaps one of the best-known contemporary stimulant hallucinogens of abuse (Glennon 1987). These compounds have often been called "designer drugs" because their structure-activity relations have been used to design new derivatives of a

known agent, the resulting drugs not yet being covered under the Controlled Substances Act of 1970.

Methamphetamine may have stronger CNS stimulant properties than does amphetamine. The d-isomer of amphetamine has been generally found to have far more potent CNS stimulant effects than does the l-isomer. In contrast, the l-isomers of the hallucinogenic phenylisopropylamines have more potent hallucinogenic effects (Glennon 1987). Removal of an α-methyl group of amphetamine leads to the formation of phenylethylamine, which has little CNS-stimulating effect because of its rapid breakdown by MAO-B. The removal of an α-methyl group of a hallucinogenic phenylisopropylamine usually results in retention of activity but a decrease in potency. In contrast, 3,4-MDA is unique because it seems to have both stimulant and hallucinogenic effects and may produce effects that are distinct from these properties. However, it is also unique in that it possesses a methylenedioxy group on the aromatic ring in the 3,4 position. The addition of a methyl group to the terminal chain to produce MDMA appears to increase the potency of its CNS stimulant effects while somewhat decreasing its hallucinogenic activity (Glennon 1987).

There have been contradictory reports in the literature about the relative effects of d- and l-isomers of amphetamine on mood activation and neurohormone responses and effects that are presumed to result from increases in norepinephrine and dopamine systems. Smith and Davis (1977) showed in control subjects that DAMPH was more efficacious than MPH, which was more efficacious than l-amphetamine, in increasing euphoric and activating moods; this result presumably reflects the potency of dopamine actions. In contrast, Janowsky and Davis (1976) found that MPH had 1.5 times the ability of DAMPH to increase activation of psychosis in schizophrenic patients. In both studies, DAMPH was about twice as effective as l-amphetamine. The drugs were given orally in the former study and intravenously in the latter, which could explain the difference.

Studies of the effects of the *d*- and *l*-isomers on growth hormone, adrenocorticotropic hormone, cortisol, and prolactin secretion have varied in both animals and humans and are therefore inconclusive. Older reports (Arnold et al. 1972, 1976) suggested that levoamphetamine or *d,l*-amphetamine might have clinical superiority in the treatment of hyperkinetic children. This claim, together with the short half-life of DAMPH, has led to the marketing of a preparation containing four salts of levo- and DAMPH (DAMPH saccharate, amphetamine aspartate, DAMPH sulfate, and amphetamine sulfate). Studies comparing this formulation (Adderall) with MPH have not yet been published but will be useful in estimating any clinical advantages of this combination. Available formulations are listed in Table 22–3 in Chapter 22, this volume).

The *d*-threo enantiomer of MPH is believed to be responsible for the therapeutic activity (Patrick et al. 1981).

PHARMACOLOGICAL PROFILE

Amphetamine produces stimulating effects on the CNS such as arousal, wakefulness, euphoria, lessening of fatigue, and increased energy and self-confidence. Another central action is the inhibition of appetite. In humans, both cocaine and amphetamine produce behaviors characterized by repetitious arrangement of objects. Such behaviors may be analogous to stereotyped behaviors induced by amphetamines in animals (Patrick et al. 1981).

Amphetamine is a weak base; one theory for its mechanism of action is its dissipation of the pH gradient intracellularly (see next section, "Mechanism of Action").

Because of the basic nature of amphetamine and its excretion pattern, both hydration and the use of ammonium chloride, 500 mg every 3–4 hours, to acidify the urine accelerate its excretion and possibly shorten the duration of the amphetamine reaction. Urine pH should be kept below 5 (Tinklenburg and Berger 1977). The major metabolite of MPH is ritalinic acid, which is inactive. Thin-layer chromatographic analysis of human plasma collected 2 hours after administration of labeled MPH indicates that more than 75% of the total radioactivity is ritalinic acid, whereas compounds appearing to be parahydroxyritalinic acid and 6-oxoritalinic acid make up approximately 1%–2% of the activity, respectively (Patrick et al. 1987).

Clinical concentrations of MPH in blood are 2–20 ng/mL, which is below that of most psychotherapeutic agents. Such a minute amount requires sensitive analytical methodology for therapeutic drug monitoring, often requiring gas chromatography–mass spectrometry methods. Like amphetamine, MPH accumulates in highly perfused tissues and accumulates rapidly in the brain within 1–5 minutes after intravenous administration. Although typical doses of amphetamine result in significantly higher plasma concentrations than do typical doses of MPH, it appears that the pharmacological actions of MPH in humans can be attributed solely to the parent compound (Patrick et al. 1987).

MECHANISM OF ACTION

The two prototypic stimulants amphetamine and MPH, although they have some similar net effects, also have differences in structure-activity relations and mechanisms of action. As noted by Seiden et al. (1993), "both the releasing and uptake-inhibiting actions of [amphetamine] are mediated by the catecholamine uptake transporter" (p. 640). In 1959, Axelrod et al. demonstrated that epinephrine could be rapidly and selectively taken up by the heart, spleen, and glandular organs, each of which has sympathetic innervation. It was subsequently discovered that norepinephrine-containing neurons could bind or take up norepinephrine against a concentration gradient; later, it was found that the uptake transporter could release catecholamines (CAs) as well as reclaim them back into the nerve terminals.

Further investigation found that amphetamine apparently inhibits the uptake and release of dopamine or norepinephrine or both. The catecholamine transporter normally moves dopamine from the outside to the inside of the cell. However, in the presence of some drugs, such as amphetamine, the direction of transport appears to be reversed, and dopamine is moved from the inside to the outside of the cell through a mechanism called *exchange diffusion*, which occurs at low doses (1–5 mg/kg) of amphetamine. Moderate to high doses of amphetamine (>5 mg/kg) cause the release of dopamine through exchange diffusion across the cell membrane, passive diffusion of amphetamine into the cell, and an interaction between amphetamine and the vesicle membrane transporter. A passive diffusion of amphetamine into the storage vesicle, causing alkalization of the vesicle, results in the release of dopamine from the vesicles as well, which is then subject to release by the cell membrane. These mechanisms, as well as a blocking of reuptake of dopamine by amphetamine, all lead to an increase in synaptic norepinephrine and dopamine. Other antidepressant medications acting on catecholamines, including both dopamine and norepinephrine, tend to exert their action by simply blocking the reuptake mechanism.

MPH appears to release dopamine stored in the vesicles alone, whereas amphetamine releases dopamine from newly synthesized pools and increases dopamine diffusion from the vesicles into the cell. This mechanism appears to distinguish amphetamine from antidepressant medication in terms of its rapidity of onset of effect and from MPH in terms of its potency. Further support for these differentiations includes the findings that blocking catecholamine synthesis by α-methyl-p-tyrosine interferes with dopamine release by both amphetamine and MPH, whereas reserpine, which releases dopamine from storage sites in vesicles, interferes

significantly only with MPH effects and does not totally inhibit amphetamine effects. This again differentiates the two dopamine storage pools—1) vesicular storage, which is dependent on an inward proton pump and the maintenance of low intravesicular pH, and 2) cytoplasmic storage, which has neither of these requirements (Seiden et al. 1993).

The structure of amphetamine is similar to that of both norepinephrine and dopamine. Part of the mechanism related to the vesicular action of amphetamine is that it is a weak base and causes alkalinization of the storage vesicles. Amphetamine also induces the release of [^{3}H]serotonin from chromaffin granules from the adrenal medulla (Sulzer and Rayport 1990). Although amphetamine competitively inhibits MAO in vitro, it appears to be a weak MAOI in moderate doses in vivo. Evidence suggests that amphetamine in high doses may act as a competitive inhibitor for MAO-A (Mantle et al. 1976; Miller et al. 1980). This effect seems to be less significant physiologically than the catecholamine-releasing effects of the drugs.

Brown et al. (1978) showed that, although amphetamine given in doses of 20 mg to control subjects causes stimulation of both growth hormone and cortisol, MPH in the same dose causes stimulation of only growth hormone. The elation caused by MPH was found to be correlated with elevation of growth hormone. This led Brown et al. (1978) to suggest that the elation response may be related to the dopamine effects of both stimulants, whereas the cortisol response may be related to the norepinephrine effects of amphetamine alone. The norepinephrine effects of amphetamine may explain its higher incidence of increased pulse and hypertension.

In studies with human subjects, Nurnberger et al. (1984) showed that DAMPH-induced excitation is due to stimulation of the CNS by dopamine, whereas cardiovascular effects, increased blood pressure, and increased norepinephrine levels in serum result from noradrenergic effects that can be blocked by propranolol. Kuczenski and Segal (1997) compared the potency of MPH with amphetamine in the rat brain, showing "considerably lower" levels of dopamine and norepinephrine release and no effect on serotonin release with MPH, in contrast to amphetamine.

Nicola et al. (1996) used specific dopamine, subtype 1 (D_1), and D_2 receptor blockers in mice and found that "dopamine and amphetamine [by increasing endogenous extracellular dopamine levels] reduce excitatory synaptic transmission in the nucleus accumbens by activating presynaptic dopamine receptors with D_1-like properties" (p. 1602). Sloviter et al. (1978) first noticed the similarity between the effects of high doses of DAMPH in rats and the behavioral syndrome caused by intense activation of the serotonin receptor. Those researchers pursued studies showing that responsiveness of the amphetamine syndrome could be blocked by either serotonin synthesis inhibition or receptor blockade. This finding suggests that amphetamine acts indirectly through the serotonin system by activating serotonin receptors, possibly through the displacement of endogenous serotonin.

Data published by Colado et al. (1997) provide evidence that the hallucinogenic stimulant MDMA ("Ecstasy") produces serotonergic neurotoxicity by the formation of free radicals, whereas fenfluramine produces similar effects by some other unidentified mechanism.

INDICATIONS

The *Physicians' Desk Reference* (PDR; 2001) lists two indications approved by the U.S. Food and Drug Administration for DAMPH: 1) narcolepsy and 2) ADHD. The indications listed for MPH are 1) attention-deficit disorders in children and 2) narcolepsy. Other therapeutic uses of stimulant medications are controversial, principally because they have become drugs of abuse when sold illicitly or prescribed irresponsibly. As a result, amphetamine is a Schedule II

and MPH a Schedule III substance under the Controlled Substances Act of 1970. Moreover, certain states (e.g., Wisconsin) have passed even more restrictive legislation limiting the use of stimulants to specific indications. Stimulants are prohibited in some European countries.

Are stimulants ineffective in relation to their risks and thus without a place in psychiatric practice? Or has concern over the abuse potential of these drugs in certain vulnerable populations led to a suppression of their use in cases in which they could be medically useful (and even possibly lifesaving), as in severe, treatment-refractory depression?

Since 1987, there have been at least three published reviews of the use of psychostimulants and several reviews preliminary to case reports. Of the major reviews, Chiarello and Cole (1987) dealt with the use of stimulants in general psychiatry, Satel and Nelson (1989) focused on the use of psychostimulants in the treatment of affective disorders, and Ayd and Zohar (1987) emphasized the role of stimulants in treatment-resistant affective disorders. Based on these reviews, the efficacy of DAMPH alone in treating patients with affective disorders is controversial. This is based on the fact that no double-blind studies have been done since 1962. Many of the studies that have been reported have shown high rates of response to placebo that were not exceeded by DAMPH response rates and were done on a short-term basis. Chiarello and Cole (1987) pointed out that the studies were not adequate to conclude whether DAMPH did in fact have therapeutic effects for some patients, and data may have been analyzed in such a way that the authors missed positive effects. However, Satel and Nelson (1989) observed that studies of imipramine (IMI) compared with placebo carried out at approximately the same time, presumably with similar methodology and interpretation, showed that IMI was superior to placebo in 15 of 24 studies. This was a more robust outcome than could be drawn from the three or four double-blind, placebo-controlled studies in which DAMPH was used in doses ranging from 10 to 30 mg/day.

MPH was studied in four reported double-blind trials in the late 1960s and early 1970s, in doses of up to 30–40 mg/day, showing modest responses in comparison to placebo. Clinical effects were evident in some patients. Pemoline was also studied in double-blind, placebo-controlled trials in the mid- to late 1970s and was shown to have modest effects when given as a sole treatment. The studies of these three major stimulants and critical reviews of these studies seem to echo the conclusion that, although some effects might be noted in some patients, the evidence as to whether these responses will persist over time is mixed. No good evidence would establish stimulants as a responsible first-line treatment in patients with depressive illness when the benefits of these drugs in placebo-controlled studies are compared with those of other available antidepressant medications.

Open studies have a significant disadvantage compared with placebo-controlled studies in that they do not account for placebo response. (These studies also tend to be published more often if they are positive than if they turn out to have negative results.) On the other hand, open studies tend to have more flexible dose ranges and may provide useful information about the type of clinical responses seen and in what type of patients they are seen, because they may not treat groups of more highly selected patients.

Five open studies of amphetamine, benzedrine, or DAMPH have been completed and have involved 185 subjects, ranging from hospitalized patients with retardation or agitation to those with neurotic depressions. According to various criteria, improvement was seen in 30%–76% of the subjects. In two open studies of MPH used to treat various types of depressive disorders at doses of 30–60 mg/day, improvement was reported in 76%–82% of subjects.

In addition, a number of uncontrolled studies and case reports have been reported in which stimulants, most frequently MPH, have been used for the treatment of depression in various types of medically ill patients. Between 1956 and 1991, studies of 159 medically ill patients were reported and showed positive responses in 68%–98% of patients (Kraus and Burch 1992). One study in adult patients with cancer showed a response in 23 of 30 patients (77%), whereas another similar study showed response in 14 of 17 patients (82%) (Fernandez et al. 1987). From 1988 to 1992, four studies (Angrist et al. 1992; Fernandez et al. 1988a, 1988b; Holmes et al. 1989) presented 38 case reports of patients with human immunodeficiency virus (HIV)-related neuropsychiatric symptoms, including depression; 86% (33) of the subjects showed some improvement, and 65% (25) showed moderate to marked improvement.

Two studies (Johnson et al. 1992; Lazarus et al. 1992) described case reports of response to MPH in poststroke patients with depression. One showed that 70% of subjects improved, and the other showed that 80% improved with doses ranging from 5 mg twice daily to total doses of 40 mg/day. In a subsequent study, Lazarus et al. (1994) showed a more rapid onset of response with MPH compared with nortriptyline therapy. The average response time for MPH responders was 2.4 days compared with 27 days for the nortriptyline group. Gwirtsman et al. (1994) reported the results of a study in which MPH was given in one or two doses of 5–15 mg in addition to tricyclic antidepressants (TCAs). Improvement was seen at 1 week in 30% of the patients and at 2 weeks in 63% of the patients starting the trial, suggesting that the combination produced an accelerated response. A report by Fernandez et al. (1995) found that MPH in a dosage of 30 mg/day produced a response and an onset of response that were equivalent to those produced by desipramine (DMI) given at 150 mg/day in depressed acquired immunodeficiency syndrome (AIDS) patients. In an open trial of DAMPH at a median dose of 10 mg/day, Wagner et al. (1997) found a rapid onset of improvement of depression and low energy in 18 of 19 AIDS patients. Olin and Masand (1996) reported a chart review of 59 cancer patients treated for depression with either DAMPH or MPH over 5 years at Massachusetts General Hospital. Those authors noted some improvement in 83% of patients, substantial improvement in 73%, and no differences in efficacy between stimulants or across diagnostic categories for depression.

A review of open series and case reports of medically ill patients with various diagnoses showed that stimulants had two important advantages. The first advantage was the rapidity of response; most authors agreed that a response was evident within 2–3 days—much earlier than the average time for other antidepressants. The second advantage often cited was the dearth of side effects compared with other antidepressant medications, especially in medically ill patients. (The question of side effects and hazards is reviewed in the "Side Effects and Toxicology" section later in this chapter.)

Stimulants as Potentiators for Antidepressant Medications

The literature has supported the use of stimulants as augmenters of antidepressant medications in treatment-resistant patients. In 1971, Wharton et al. published a paper that had been read at the annual meeting of the American Psychiatric Association in 1969. The researchers reported on seven patients with recurrent refractory psychotic depressive illness, five of whom had had repeated courses of electroconvulsive therapy. Five of the patients recovered within 2 weeks of receiving IMI at 150 mg/day and MPH 10 mg twice daily (Wharton et al. 1971). The other two patients recovered more gradually without requiring electroconvulsive therapy. Wharton et al. (1971) documented a rise in serum IMI levels after the addition of MPH, and they hypothesized that this rapid increase in blood levels might be related to the enhanced response. Five of the patients who could be followed up maintained their response for 2–3 years. Subsequently, in a letter to the *American Journal of Psychiatry*,

Flemenbaum (1971) reported on "six to ten" patients (p. 239) treated with MPH-IMI combinations and noted a rapid onset of effect and correction of hypotension associated with TCA medication. However, Flemenbaum did note three cases of young patients with labile hypertension who had hypertensive episodes associated with the MPH-IMI combination.

Cooper and Simpson (1973) reported another case, that of a 61-year-old patient with a 19-year history of depressive disorder. The patient had not benefited from various treatment modalities and sustained a partial response with 300 mg/day of IMI but still required hospitalization; however, marked improvement occurred with the addition of a maximum dose of 40 mg of MPH. Cooper and Simpson reported an almost 20-fold increase in IMI levels and a 50% increase in DMI levels. In this case, within 2 weeks after MPH was withdrawn, plasma IMI and DMI levels had returned to baseline values, and the patient apparently relapsed. The authors presented this as a confirmation of the observation by Perel et al. (1969) that IMI metabolism was inhibited by MPH.

Drimmer et al. (1983) presented the case of a patient with a diagnosis of bipolar depression with hypomania who had had a depressive episode and was not helped by up to 350 mg/day of amoxapine. The patient was then treated with DMI at a dosage of 200 mg/day and sustained marked improvement in mood and agitation within 3 days of the addition of MPH at a dose of 10 mg twice daily (Drimmer et al. 1983). The patient experienced a relapse after MPH was gradually withdrawn and again responded to its reinstatement at a dosage of up to 40 mg/day. No significant increases in DMI levels were noted in this patient. The authors believed that the rapidity of response when MPH was added to DMI, as well as the lack of DMI increase, argued against the hypothesis that a mechanism of enhancement of TCA levels was responsible for the potentiating effect of MPH. Rather, they argued that the dopaminergic effects of MPH were more likely to be the basis for its potentiating effects on IMI and DMI treatment.

Myers and Stewart (1989) further commented on the rapidity of onset of a DMI-MPH combination in the case of a 69-year-old male patient admitted for the treatment of transitional cell carcinoma of the bladder. The patient had developed suicidal ideation and was threatening to jump out of his fourth-floor hospital window. However, within 2 days of administration of this combination, he was no longer suicidal and was able to enjoy watching television. He relapsed within 4 days of discontinuation of MPH but then responded to 400 mg/day of DMI (Myers and Stewart 1989).

Although the mechanism of action of the combination of IMI or DMI plus MPH is unclear, the available case reports suggest that it may be an effective combination for patients with treatment-resistant depression. This combination has the advantage of rapid response and relatively few hazards, except for the possibility of elevated blood pressure in patients with histories of labile hypertension.

Metz and Shader (1991) reported four cases of patients refractory to TCAs, three of whom either had partial responses to fluoxetine or relapsed on fluoxetine under stress but improved when 9.375–18.750 mg/day of pemoline was added. These responses were monitored and observed to last for 9–23 months. The addition of either DAMPH or pemoline to fluoxetine is suggested by these case reports as a way of treating partial responses in patients taking fluoxetine or in those who have relapsed in treatment. Although the use of stimulants with other antidepressants has not been documented in a double-blind study (which is not surprising, considering the expense of double-blind, placebo-controlled studies, the lack of commercial interest in these older stimulants, and the relatively small percentage of patients treated with antidepressants who require stimulant potentiation), published case reports suggest the efficacy and probable safety of this combination in patients with depression that has been resistant to successful treatment with existing antidepressant agents.

MAOIs are currently used mainly to treat depression that has proven refractory to other antidepressant medications, some cases of "atypical depression," and severe panic or anxiety disorders that are unresponsive to other pharmacological therapies. Because of their potential for interactions with dietary substances and other medications, as well as their frequent side effects, MAOIs are usually not used until after treatment with other medications has failed. However, clinicians who treat depressive illnesses that are resistant to conventional pharmacological treatment still encounter patients who not only require MAOIs but also may have failed to respond to these agents and to electroconvulsive therapy. In patients with highly resistant depression, the stakes become higher in many cases because hopelessness induced by the depressive illness is augmented by the reality of a lack of response and a further increased risk of suicide.

Feighner et al. (1985) reported on the use of a combination of MAOI, TCA, and stimulant therapy for treatment-resistant depression. The researchers cited 16 subjects, 13 of whom improved when various MAOIs were potentiated by either DAMPH or MPH. Fawcett et al. (1991) presented 32 cases of patients who were refractory to long series of trials with TCAs, selective serotonin reuptake inhibitors (SSRIs) (in some cases), and (in 14 cases) electroconvulsive therapy without a response to treatment. Seventy-eight percent of these patients responded with the addition of either pemoline or DAMPH to one to four different MAOIs in their maximum tolerated doses. DAMPH was given in dosages of 10–40 mg four times daily and pemoline in dosages of 18.75–37.50 mg three times daily to patients receiving maximum tolerated doses of 40–120 mg of MAOIs. The patients' ages ranged from 20 to the early 80s (Fawcett et al. 1991). Neither of these two reports of stimulant potentiation of MAOIs reported any serious side effects except for the possible switching of several patients into hypomania or mania in the series conducted by

Fawcett et al. (1991). Both studies reviewed older literature in which three cases of death had ensued after the administration of MAOIs potentiated with DAMPH (Dally 1962; Krisko et al. 1969; Lloyd and Walker 1965; Mason 1962; Smilkstein et al. 1987; Stockley 1973; Zeck 1961). Two of these three cases involved elevated blood pressure, hyperpyrexia, seizures, and death; one case did not show elevation of blood pressure but did show hyperpyrexia, seizures, and death. These cases were reported in the literature in the early to late 1960s.

Although the use of stimulants with MAOIs is contraindicated in PDR, in addition to the observations of Feighner et al. (1985), in some patients with high-risk depression for whom all other treatments have failed, the use of stimulants to potentiate MAOIs has proved helpful and even lifesaving.

The decision to prescribe stimulants should be based on a clinical history of treatment-resistant or treatment-refractory illness. This is true of other uses of stimulants in treating depression (such as their use in treating medically ill stroke patients, elderly patients, or treatment-resistant patients), as well as the use of stimulants to potentiate MAOIs in patients with highly treatment-resistant depressive illness. The patient's medical status and his or her capacity for careful compliance with the prescribed regimen should be evaluated. In making these clinical decisions, careful judgment should be used in evaluating the risks and benefits and determining what is best for an individual patient.

The use of stimulants may not be necessary in the average patient; however, we believe that although the continual emergence of new antidepressant medications may increase patients' chances of treatment response, a significant percentage of patients, because of idiosyncratic differences or medical conditions, do not respond at all to these medications or cannot tolerate their effects. These patients may find themselves in severe states of impairment or even at risk for death by suicide. These patients may benefit from the use of stimulants alone or in combination to potentiate other available antidepressant medications. The clinical literature on the possible usefulness of stimulants must be available to psychiatrists, as well as to those who legislate the use of these substances. The latter group may be motivated more by their concern for potential danger and may not be fully aware of the potential benefits of psychostimulants to patients who may not otherwise recover and regain control of their lives.

Summary of the Use of Stimulants in Depression

Although double-blind studies performed in the 1960s did not produce data strongly supporting the efficacy of stimulants in treating a broad range of depressed patients, it is important to recognize that the designs of these studies were highly flawed. Placebo response rates were extremely high, making it difficult for stimulants to show a higher rate of effectiveness. Although these studies do not offer support for the efficacy of stimulants used alone in the treatment of depression, they certainly do not convincingly rule out the possibility that stimulants may be effective for some patients.

Open studies point in a slightly different direction, emphasizing the value of stimulants in treating patients with severe medical illnesses, poststroke patients, elderly patients, patients with severe heart disease, and AIDS patients, all of whom had concurrent depression and increased risks associated with side effects to antidepressant medications. Three reports support a possible role for stimulants in the treatment of patients recovering from moderate brain injury; 88 subjects were involved in these studies (Hornstein et al. 1996; Mooney and Haas 1993; Plenger et al. 1996). Low to moderate doses of MPH and DAMPH reduced depression and apathy and improved cognitive functions. One study of 38 patients also showed a reduction in anger and temper outbursts compared with patients given placebo, whereas an open study of MPH (0.3 mg/kg twice a day) in 12 patients with chronic closed head injury found no benefit (Speech et al. 1993). The effectiveness of MPH in the treatment of negative symptoms in dementia has been reported (Galynker et al. 1997).

A case report noted improvement of prominent apathy secondary to multiple subcortical infarcts, and single photon emission computed tomography and reaction time showed selective improvement of frontal system function. Wroblewski et al. (1992) reported a trend toward a lesser incidence of seizures in 30 patients with active seizure disorders taking MPH. Their results provide some reassurance that giving MPH to brain-injured patients is not likely to increase the risk of seizure.

In general, these case reports were positive, showing a high rate of improvement in patients with a relatively low rate of side effects and a rapid response time of 2–3 days. It has been noted that case reports are generally published when they are positive; thus, the efficacy of stimulants in these patients may be overestimated.

The use of stimulants to potentiate other antidepressant medications in patients with either treatment-resistant depression or partial response has been raised in several studies—including their use with MAOIs, despite the PDR's warnings against this practice. The use of stimulants to predict TCA response showed some theoretical interest, but the movement to more widespread use of SSRIs diminishes the significance and value of this early research.

Some studies have reviewed the hypothesis that dopamine hypofunction may play a significant role in depressive illness. D'haenen and Bossuyt (1994) reported an increase in D_2 receptor density in depressed patients. These studies, viewed in the context of antidepressant effects reported with the use of the dopamine agonists bromocriptine, piribedil, and pergolide, further strengthen the hypothesis that the dopamine system is an important mechanism in at least some depressed patients (Bouckoms and Mangini 1993; Post et al. 1978; Theohar et al. 1981). The therapeutic use of stimulants in selected patients appears to have a growing theoretical and empirical basis, particularly in view of the limited dopaminergic effects of most standard antidepressant medications.

Other Uses of Stimulants in Psychiatry and Medicine

ADHD in children has been a continually accepted indication for the use of psychostimulants. This use has not been without some social controversy concerning the use of drugs in children and the possibilities of adverse side effects. Possible effects include growth retardation, which has not been substantiated, and possible negative cognitive effects that seem to result from overdose in some children, as well as overuse or inappropriate use as the result of poor clinical diagnosis.

Barkley (1977) reviewed 15 studies of the use of amphetamines in children with ADHD, involving a total of 915 patients. The studies had various designs, including the use of hospital staff, teachers, clinicians, and parents as judges of response. The studies reviewed showed that, on average, symptoms improved in 74% of subjects and were unchanged or worsened in 26%. Fourteen of these reports were studies of MPH that involved a total of 866 patients and used clinicians, parents, and teachers as judges of outcome. These studies showed that, on average, symptoms improved in 77% of subjects and were unchanged or worsened in 23%. Pemoline was used in two studies of 105 subjects. In these studies, clinicians and teachers judged outcome, and symptoms improved in 73% of subjects and were unchanged or worsened in 27%. In another eight studies, 417 children had a mean improvement rate of 39% compared with a mean rate of unchanged or worsening symptoms of 61%.

Barkley (1977) concluded in this review that most children taking psychostimulant medications are judged as improved, whereas a small percentage are not. The author also concluded that follow-up studies find the long-term psychosocial adjustment of these children to be essentially unaffected by stimulant treatment. Barkley then noted that the search needed to consider specific variables for measures of improvement rather than just general improvement, as many studies up until that time had tended to do.

More recently, Schachar and Tannock (1993) looked for evidence of a sustained effect of stimulant treatment in children with ADHD. Eighteen studies were identified with a duration of at least 3 months. Seventeen were studies of MPH, and one was a study of DAMPH; none involved pemoline or slow-release stimulants. Eleven of these studies were randomized, controlled trials, whereas seven used quasi-experimental designs without randomization. The results of the randomized, controlled trials showed the psychostimulants to provide a greater benefit than did the nonrandomized trials. This finding suggested to the researchers that the "efficacy of extended treatment may have been underestimated because more seriously disturbed children were assigned to medication treatment than to control treatments in nonrandomized trials" (p. 81). Reviewing 11 randomized, controlled studies that collectively involved 271 children medicated for an average of 6 months, the authors found that "results of 8 out of the 11 randomized controlled trials indicate clear beneficial effects of prolonged treatment with MPH on the core behavioral features of ADHD, that is, poor sustained attention, impulsiveness, and excessive motor activity" (p. 89).

Of the three studies that failed to find extended stimulant treatment to be efficacious, one was discounted because of an attrition rate of more than 50%. The results of a second study indicated that prolonged MPH treatment did reduce the severity of poor symptoms, but the improvements were comparable in magnitude to those obtained with IMI.

It was also shown that the beneficial effects of treatment dissipate rapidly when treatment is terminated. Stimulant treatment did not appear to reduce symptoms to a level considered to be

in the range of normal behavior. It was concluded that few children made sufficient progress to become symptom free at the end of the trial. In addition, although short-term treatment had a significant effect on social and academic symptoms, extended treatment produced a far less clear result. Schachar and Tannock (1993) further concluded that future studies of extended treatment must address questions about the development of drug tolerance, as well as concerns about long-term adverse effects, such as abnormal movement and dysphoria.

The modest effectiveness of MPH indicated by these studies suggests a need to combine medication with educational interventions and psychological therapies. Satterfield et al. (1987) showed indirect evidence for the superior effectiveness of combining intensive multimodal therapy and MPH over medication alone. However, no direct evidence exists in longer-term studies to support this contention (Satterfield et al. 1981, 1987; Schachar and Tannock 1993).

Psychostimulants have been shown to be helpful in treating the core symptoms of ADHD in children, both acutely and over at least a 6-month period. It is also clear that the effect of psychostimulants is toward improvement and not total suppression of symptoms—the symptoms return when medications are discontinued. There is still concern about the long-term effects of these medications and of ADHD itself in terms of delinquency and other conduct disturbances.

Klein and Wender (1995) reviewed the use of MPH in children with ADHD, concluding that "at appropriately high doses of MPH, a large proportion of children are not only better, many are well. In addition to having the cardinal features of their disorder eliminated, appropriately medicated children experience improvement in other important functional domains, such as in social interactions with parents, teachers, and peers, in academic performance, and in self-esteem" (p. 429). Spencer et al. (1996b) found "155 studies of 5,778 children, adolescents, and adults documenting the efficacy of stimulants in an estimated 70% of subjects" (p. 409). They further found that "the literature clearly documents that stimulants not only improve abnormal behaviors of ADHD, but also self-esteem, cognition, and social and family function" (p. 409). The recent major 14-month multicenter study of MPH reported that the drug was superior to behavior therapy in children with ADHD (MTA Cooperative Group 1999). This study included 579 children.

Wender et al. (1985) described the use of stimulants in adults with similar problems of attention, concentration, and focus, terming this syndrome *adult attention deficit disorder.* Their study involved patients meeting the Utah criteria for residual ADHD, which included a history of core symptoms of childhood ADHD having been reported by a parent using the Conners Teacher Rating Scale (Sprague et al. 1974). Wender et al. (1985) found that, although pemoline was not more effective than placebo, MPH reduced core symptoms. This reduction occurred (sometimes dramatically) in 57% of subjects taking MPH and in 11% taking placebo.

Spencer et al. (1995) replicated the results of Wender et al. (1985) in a randomized, 7-week, placebo-controlled, crossover study of 23 adults with ADHD, using standardized instruments for the diagnosis of ADHD and separate assessments of ADHD. With a "robust" dose of MPH (1.0 mg/kg/day), Spencer et al. (1995) found "a marked therapeutic response for methylphenidate treatment of ADHD symptoms that exceeded the placebo response (78% vs 4%, $P < 0.0001$)" (p. 434).

Of particular interest is a report by Castellanos et al. (1996) based on the measurement of homovanillic acid levels in cerebrospinal fluid. In this study, 45 boys met DSM-III (American Psychiatric Association 1980) criteria for ADHD before beginning double-blind trials of MPH, DAMPH, or placebo. This study replicated the results of a prior study that found a significant correlation between homovanillic acid levels in cerebrospinal fluid and ratings of hy-

peractivity in subjects taking placebo. It also showed that, after baseline symptom severity was controlled for, higher homovanillic acid levels in cerebrospinal fluid predicted better response, whereas lower homovanillic acid levels were associated with worsening on some measures.

Spencer et al. (1996a) described another interesting finding in a study of 124 children and adolescents who were compared with 109 control subjects. Using appropriate correction by age and parental height, the authors found small but significant height differences that were evident in early- but not in late-adolescent children with ADHD. The height differences were unrelated to the use of psychotropic medications. The investigators concluded that "ADHD may be associated with temporary deficits in growth in height in mid-adolescence that may normalize by late adolescence. This effect appears to be mediated by ADHD and not its treatment" (p. 1460).

Stimulants have long been accepted as valuable in treating narcolepsy, which is often treated by psychiatrists as well as by neurologists and general physicians. The chronic use of stimulants in many cases reduces episodes of daytime sleepiness, which can cause impairment and danger, especially if the sleepiness occurs while the patient is driving. Stimulants do not reverse the cataplexy that some narcoleptic patients experience, but either TCAs or SSRIs in combination with stimulants may be helpful for this condition.

Although several studies have suggested that stimulants may improve negative symptoms in schizophrenic patients, others have shown that stimulants may worsen positive symptoms of schizophrenia, such as delusions and hallucinations (Lieberman et al. 1990). There is also evidence that schizophrenic patients have high rates of comorbid substance abuse, perhaps as a consequence of the blunted affectivity associated with negative symptoms of the disease.

In one report, Insel et al. (1983) reported positive effects of DAMPH given to patients with obsessive-compulsive disorder. The experience of these authors suggests that these patients also had lower levels of anxiety when DAMPH was used.

Khantzian et al. (1984) presented three cases of cocaine abuse in which patients were treated with MPH, all three of whom demonstrated improvement. This experience led to the hypothesis that cocaine abuse may be associated with the presence of dysthymic disorder or chronic depression without the full neurovegetative symptomatology of major depression. It was further hypothesized that the "normalizing effect of MPH with the pilot cases makes a compelling argument for more extensive clinical study to test the possibility that a minimal brain dysfunction syndrome or attention deficit disorder or a variant contributes to cocaine dependence" (pp. 110–111). This hypothesis was also based on the fact that the patients did not develop tolerance to MPH. It was also mentioned that the authors had treated four other subjects who had abused cocaine and who did not have symptoms of attention-deficit disorder. Khantzian et al. (1984) observed dose escalations without prolonged facilitation of cocaine abstinence. Hence, initial observations indicated that only a subpopulation of abusers respond favorably to MPH treatment of cocaine abuse. This had led to a proposal a while back for further study of the use of MPH in cocaine abusers with symptoms of ADHD (H. D. Kleber, personal communication, May 1993).

SIDE EFFECTS AND TOXICOLOGY

The effects of amphetamine include the alpha and beta actions that are common to indirectly acting sympathomimetic drugs. Amphetamine given orally raises both systolic and diastolic blood pressure. Heart rate is often reflexively slowed, and, with large doses, cardiac arrhythmias may occur. Cardiac output is not enhanced by therapeutic doses, and cerebral blood flow is little changed (Hoffman and Lefkowitz 1993).

Smooth muscles respond to amphetamine in general as they do to other sympathomimetic drugs. There is a contractile effect on the urinary bladder sphincter, an effect that has been used in treating enuresis and incontinence. Pain and difficulty in micturition can therefore occur. Amphetamine may cause relaxation of the intestine and may delay the movement of intestinal contents, but the opposite effect may also be seen. The response of the human uterus varies, but usually an increase in tone occurs. Contraindications for amphetamine include advanced arteriosclerosis, symptomatic cardiovascular disease, moderate to severe hypertension, hyperthyroidism, as well as a history of drug abuse (PDR 2001).

Side effects noted with therapeutic doses of amphetamine also include mild gastrointestinal disturbance, anorexia, dry mouth, tachycardia, cardiac arrhythmias, insomnia, and restlessness (Meyler 1966). Headache, palpitations, dizziness, vasomotor disturbances, agitation, confusion, dysphoria, apprehension, and delirium have also been also mentioned. Other side effects that have been documented include flushing, pallor, a swaying sensation, excessive sweating, and muscular pains. Tiredness and sleepiness, as well as lethargy and listlessness, together with a mild depression of mood, may occur when the effect wears off.

The unsupervised use of amphetamine or the abuse of this substance involves taking doses in excess of therapeutic doses to experience the psychological effects of the drug, such as euphoria. This excess use also leads to a tendency to loquaciousness and diminution of inhibitions. Tolerance is progressive in some individuals, and drug dependence may occur.

The effects of large doses of amphetamine include marked euphoria and overcheerfulness, restlessness, rapid and slurred speech, and tension, anxiety, and irritability. Other effects may include excessively dry mouth, producing a tendency to rub the tongue along the inside of the lower lip; tachycardia and cardiac arrhythmias; brisk reflexes, dilation of the pupils, and occasionally, a sluggish response to light; fine tremor of the limbs; and weight loss. Amphetamine psychosis, which has been described in detail elsewhere (Connell 1968), presents as a paranoid psychosis in a setting of clear consciousness. A rare confusional state may occur for a short time, but this is usually short lived. After withdrawal in a patient who has taken large quantities of amphetamine, excessive tiredness and sleepiness may be noted. More important, however, the patient may experience severe depression with suicidal ideation and the danger of suicide attempts.

Although most studies of stimulants in general psychiatry have emphasized the lack of side effects or adverse events associated with their use, some reports have suggested caution and careful monitoring in prescribing stimulant medications for psychiatric patients. Several reports have suggested the possibility of hypertension as a side effect, particularly in patients with hypertension illness or labile hypertension. There have been an increasing number of reports of cerebral hemorrhage and cerebral angiitis with the use of intravenous stimulants or the ingestion of large amounts. However, it appears that in these cases, either self-administered overdoses were being taken by individuals who were abusing drugs or the medications were not being given under medical supervision (Bergstrom and Keller 1992; Brust 1992; Carson et al. 1987; Citron et al. 1970; Harrington et al. 1983; Imanse and Vanneste 1990; Kalant and Kalant 1975; Lazarus et al. 1992; Ragland et al. 1993; C. L. Rumbaugh et al. 1971; D. L. Rumbaugh 1971; Trugman 1988). In addition, increasing reports of cardiomyopathy and myocardial infarction have been noted in patients who had abused stimulants intravenously and, less commonly, in those taking high oral doses (Call et al. 1982; O'Neill et al. 1983; Packe et al. 1990).

The increasingly widespread use of the stimulant phentermine in combination with the serotonin-releasing drug fenfluramine as an anorexigenic combination ("Phen-Fen") has fo-cused increasing attention on the hazards of this combination. McCann et al. (1997), reporting on the increased incidence of primary pulmonary hypertension arising in populations using this combination, stated that "whether concomitant use of other drugs that share certain pharmacological actions with fenfluramine (e.g., phentermine, selective serotonin reuptake inhibitors, and tricyclic antidepressants) influence the risk of developing PPH has not been determined" (p. 670). However, Connolly et al. (1997), reporting on 24 cases of valvular heart disease associated with phentermine-fenfluramine, stated that pulmonary hypertension has been associated with phentermine alone, based on a study by Heuer (1978), and further pointed out that phentermine interferes with the pulmonary clearance of serotonin (Morita and Mehendale 1983).

Graham and Green (1997) reported on another 28 cases of valvular disease associated with the use of the phentermine-fenfluramine combination. The mean duration of treatment was 10 months (range 2–36 months) when symptoms first developed. The average dose of phentermine was 30 mg (range 15–60 mg), and the average dose of fenfluramine was 60 mg (range 10–120 mg). A dose of phentermine of more than 30 mg/day was significantly ($P = 0.02$) associated with multivalvular disease. The possible valvular effects have led to the withdrawal of fenfluramine from the U.S. market.

Recently, attention has been drawn to the possible association of liver toxicity with the use of pemoline (PDR 1998). Thirteen cases of acute hepatic failure have been reported since pemoline was first marketed in 1973. The rate of reported cases (which could be an underestimate) is 4–17 times that expected in the general population. Of the 13 cases reported since May 1996, 11 resulted in death or transplantation, usually within 4 weeks of the onset of signs or symptoms of liver failure. The earliest onset of hepatic abnormalities occurred within 6 months after initiation of treatment. This resulted in a labeling warning that pemoline should not be "ordinarily considered as first line drug therapy for ADHD" (Pemoline—Abbott Laboratories package insert).

Sterling et al. (1996) presented a case of pemoline-induced autoimmune hepatitis in a 46-year-old woman receiving the drug for the management of multiple sclerosis. That the hepatitis was autoimmune in nature was based on elevations of antinuclear antibodies, antithyroid antibodies, and immunoglobulins A and M. These features disappeared after normalization of the patient's liver enzymes and remained absent for 6 months after prednisone therapy.

Berkovitch et al. (1995) reported a case of fatal fulminant failure after transplantation failure and, calculating the relative risk, found a significant association suggesting causation. However, Shevell and Schreiber (1997), in a descriptive meta-analysis of the literature, concluded that current assumptions about the risk of acute hepatic failure posed by pemoline use alone are overestimates; those authors recommend monitoring of hepatic function during pemoline therapy.

Risk of Abuse or Addiction

The epidemic of amphetamine abuse during the 1960s gave rise to the subsequent abuse of stimulants both orally and intravenously, as well as to the development of "designer drugs" with both stimulant and hallucinogenic potency. These phenomena have underscored the risks of stimulant abuse and dependence and have focused attention on the availability and possible misuse of psychostimulant drugs.

Findings of high rates of coexisting abuse of alcohol, cocaine, opiates, and (in some cases) stimulants in patients with Axis I disorders were reported in the Epidemiologic Catchment Area study sampled in 1980–1984 by Regier et al. (1990). That survey found the prevalence of amphetamine abuse or dependence within the 6 months preceding the survey (6-month prevalence) to be 0.2%, whereas the prevalence of

abuse or dependence at any time during the respondents' lifetime (lifetime prevalence) was 1.7%. Sixty-six percent of patients who had amphetamine abuse or dependence had a comorbid mental disorder; 33% had a comorbid affective disorder and 33% a comorbid anxiety disorder.

Blumberg et al. (1971) reported the findings of a chromatographic examination of urine samples in 332 young psychiatric patients: 24.1% had at least one positive test for amphetamines. Robinson and Wolkind (1970) reported that 16 of 54 (29.6%) patients in a psychiatric hospital had evidence of nonprescribed amphetamines in their urine.

These studies (although they are from a period when stimulant abuse was close to its peak, in the late 1960s) demonstrated the high rate of abuse of stimulant medications among psychiatric patients. On the other hand, we are aware of few, if any, reports of stimulant abuse among patients who have no histories of drug or alcohol abuse and whose use of psychostimulants for the treatment of psychiatric disorders such as major depression is medically supervised.

The classifications of stimulants as Class II or III narcotic substances requiring regulation (and in some cases, triplicate prescription) are based on the recognition of the addictive potential of these stimulants. The concern about addictive potential is also reflected in some state laws contraindicating the use of stimulants for any treatment indication, such as depression or other psychiatric indications, other than those specifically spelled out in that state's laws. However, reports of the use of stimulants in clinical practice have described very few incidents of diagnosed patients increasing the dose, becoming dependent, or abusing stimulant medications. Metz and Shader (1991) described the case of a patient with a history of stimulant abuse who abused MPH. Several authors and reviewers of the literature on stimulants have stated that there simply are no studies showing that patients being treated for depression or other specific psychiatric syndromes are prone to abuse or to become addicted to stimulants.

It is increasingly recognized that co-morbidity exists between affective disorders, personality disorders, and even addictive disorders such as alcoholism. Clinical discretion in the treatment of patients with comorbid addictive disorders with stimulants is certainly always indicated. It has yet to be confirmed, however, that patients with depression or other specific medical or psychiatric indications for the use of stimulants are at any higher risk for abuse of or addiction to these agents than are patients without these conditions. It therefore seems that concerns about the abuse or addictive potential of stimulants need not automatically be interpreted as constituting a risk for patients who might benefit from their use under the care of a skilled psychiatrist. This question needs to be examined in terms of the risks and benefits related to the clinical state of each patient. It should be recognized that in a significant percentage of patients, their severe, debilitating, and even life-threatening depressive illnesses do not respond to available antidepressant medications. In the discussion that follows, we consider some theoretical reasons that stimulants may add an ingredient of response in these patients when other medications fail.

A report from the Drug Abuse Warning Network (DAWN) (Carabillo 1978) presented a collection of episodic reports obtained from hospital emergency rooms, medical examiners, and crisis intervention centers in the continental United States. These reports documented incidents conforming to the definition of *drug abuse*, or the nonmedical use of a substance for psychic effects, dependence, or self-destruction. *Drug abuse* was further defined as the use of prescription drugs in a manner inconsistent with accepted medical practice. DAWN surveys of incidents from July 1, 1973, through September 30, 1976, showed a marked difference in the reporting of abuse of various stimulants in the anorectic class. Amphetamine, methamphetamine, and phenmetrazine were ranked highest, whereas phentermine was in the middle ranges, and mazindol and chlorphentermine were ranked at the bottom of the list.

The relation of cumulative DAWN incidents of anorectic drug abuse to dosage units prescribed for these drugs was tabulated for the period from July 1, 1973, to December 30, 1975. Amphetamine and methamphetamine were still ranked highest, by rate as well as by mention, whereas phentermine and chlorphentermine were in the middle range, and diethylpropion, fenfluramine, mazindol, and benzphetamine were at the low end. A comparison of DAWN-reported incidents and total prescriptions for various anorexiants from July 1973 to December 1975 again showed reports involving amphetamine preparations to be five times those involving phenmetrazine, which was five times those of diethylpropion, phentermine, benzphetamine, and mazindol. Some of the anorexiants, such as diethylpropion, may be less often abused because of patterns of metabolic conversion of limited capacity to form the primary metabolites seen with modest doses. It is considered unlikely, in view of this, that the rapid incremental effects seen with increasing doses of DAMPH would be obtainable with diethylpropion, according to this report. More recent DAWN (1994) emergency room reports found that 1.9% reported amphetamine, 3.4% reported methedrine, 0.1% reported unspecified stimulants, and 0.2% reported MPH use, suggesting a similar liability among stimulants to that reported in more detail in 1973.

When tested for self-administration and "liking," amphetamine and cocaine score at the top of all such measures. Phenmetrazine and diethylpropion are also chosen above placebo 60%–80% of the time, and 40%–60% of subjects exclusively choose active drug. Phenyl-propanolamine and mazindol were chosen at placebo levels despite their identification as stimulants by subjects discriminating between them and placebo. Caffeine, despite its widespread consumption in caffeinated beverages, resulted in experimentally low doses being chosen above placebo levels by about half of the subjects tested. High doses of caffeine (i.e., the equivalent of more than three cups of coffee) were avoided by most of the subjects tested (Foltin and Fischman 1991).

It can therefore be readily seen that stimulant drugs do present hazards of abuse and dependence. However, patients with specific psychiatric disorders, such as major depression and adult attention hyperactivity disorder, may have a decreased risk of abuse, particularly in medically supervised environments.

DRUG-DRUG INTERACTIONS

Burrell et al. (1969) reported that MPH may interfere with the metabolism of drugs such as IMI. Their findings were supported by Cooper and Simpson (1973), as well as by an original report by Wharton et al. (1971). This might indicate that the mechanism for this effect on DMI metabolism may be the inhibition of cytochrome P450 enzyme systems, suggesting a possible increase of other drugs metabolized by various subfamilies of this system. A second possible drug interaction is the use of stimulants with other potential stimulant drugs taken for other purposes, such as phenylpropanolamine used as a decongestant and other over-the-counter medicines that might produce significant hypertension. Cerebral hemorrhage has been reported in a few cases of patients taking phenylpropanolamine alone, and its combination with psychostimulants might prove hazardous for some patients via this mechanism.

Although we have reported on the use of stimulants with MAOIs and found no apparent interactions (Fawcett et al. 1991), any such use should be carefully monitored for the possibility of hypertensive reactions or hyperpyrexia. Three or four cases of severe interactions producing hypertension, hyperpyrexia, convulsions, and death have been reported. The use of psychostimulants in significant doses may overwhelm the effect of antihypertensive medications and produce clinically significant hypertension in some individuals.

CONCLUSION

Psychostimulants are potent substances that should be used only after careful clinical diagnosis (both psychiatric and medical). This use should be followed with great clinical care in selected patients. The informed and careful use of these substances may produce benefits for individuals with significant psychiatric disorders who are not responsive to currently available treatment. Stimulants should be prescribed by skilled clinicians who are familiar with their potential clinical (e.g., behavior, nervousness, mania) and medical (e.g., tachycardia, elevated blood pressure, sweats) side effects, toxic effects, and drug-drug interactions.

REFERENCES

American Psychiatric Association: Diagnostic and Statistical Manual of Mental Disorders, 3rd Edition. Washington, DC, American Psychiatric Association, 1980

Anders TF, Ciaranello RD: Pharmacologic treatment of minimal brain dysfunction syndrome, in Psychopharmacology: From Theory to Practice. Edited by Barchas JD, Berger PA, Ciaranello RD, et al. New York, Oxford University Press, 1977, pp 425–435

Angrist B, D'Hollosy M, Sanfilipo M, et al: Central nervous system stimulants as symptomatic treatments for AIDS-related neuropsychiatric impairment. J Clin Psychopharmacol 12:268–272, 1992

Arnold LE, Wender PH, McCloskey K, et al: Levoamphetamine and dextroamphetamine: comparative efficacy in the hyperkinetic syndrome. Arch Gen Psychiatry 27:816–822, 1972

Arnold LE, Huestis RD, Smeltzer DJ, et al: Levoamphetamine vs dextroamphetamine in minimal brain dysfunction. Arch Gen Psychiatry 33:292–301, 1976

Axelrod J, Weil-Malherbe H, Tomchick R: The physiological disposition of ^{3}H-epinephrine and its metabolite metanephrine. J Pharmacol Exp Ther 127:251–256, 1959

Ayd FJ, Zohar J: Psychostimulant (amphetamine or methylphenidate) therapy for chronic and treatment-resistant depression, in Treating Resistant Depression. Edited by Zohar J, Belmaker RH. New York, PMA Publishing, 1987, pp 343–355

Barkley RA: A review of stimulant drug research with hyperactive children. J Child Psychol Psychiatry 18:137–165, 1977

Bergstrom DL, Keller C: Drug-induced myocardial ischemia and acute myocardial infarction. Critical Care Nursing Clinics of North America 4 (2):273–278, 1992

Berkovitch M, Pope E, Phillips J, et al: Pemoline-associated fulminant liver failure: testing the evidence for causation. Clin Pharmacol Ther 57:696–698, 1995

Blumberg AG, Cohen M, Heaton AM, et al: Covert drug abuse among voluntary hospitalized psychiatric patients. JAMA 217:1659–1661, 1971

Bouckoms A, Mangini L: Pergolide: an antidepressant adjuvant for mood disorders? Psychopharmacol Bull 29:207–211, 1993

Bradley C, Bowen M: Amphetamine (benzedrine) therapy of children's behavior disorders. Am J Orthopsychiatry 11:92–103, 1941

Brown WA, Corriveau DP, Ebert MH: Acute psychologic and neuroendocrine effects of dextro-amphetamine and methylphenidate. Psychopharmacology (Berl) 58:189–195, 1978

Brust JCM: Stroke and substance abuse, in Stroke: Pathophysiology, Diagnosis, and Management, 2nd Edition. Edited by Barnett HJM, Mohr JP, Stein BM, et al. New York, Churchill Livingstone, 1992, pp 875–893

Burrell JM, Black M, Wharton RN, et al: Inhibition of imipramine metabolism by methylphenidate (abstract). Federation Proceedings 28:418, 1969

Call TD, Hartneck J, Dickinson WA, et al: Acute cardiomyopathy secondary to intravenous amphetamine abuse. Ann Intern Med 97:559–560, 1982

Carabillo EA: U.S.A. Drug Abuse Warning Network, in Central Mechanisms of Anorectic Drugs. Edited by Garattini S, Samanin R. New York, Raven, 1978, pp 461–471

Carson P, Oldroyd K, Phadke K: Myocardial infarction due to amphetamine. BMJ 294:1525–1526, 1987

Castellanos FX, Elia J, Kruesi MJ, et al: Cerebrospinal fluid homovanillic acid predicts behavioral response to stimulants in 45 boys with attention deficit/hyperactivity disorder. Neuropsychopharmacology 14:125–137, 1996

Chiarello RJ, Cole JO: The use of psychostimulants in general psychiatry. Arch Gen Psychiatry 44:286–295, 1987

Citron BP, Halpert M, McCarron M, et al: Necrotizing angiitis associated with drug abuse. N Engl J Med 283:1003–1011, 1970

Colado MI, O'Shea E, Granados R, et al: In vivo evidence for free radical involvement in the degeneration of rat brain 5-HT following administration of MDMA ("Ecstasy") and *p*-chloramphetamine but not the degeneration following fenfluramine. Br J Pharmacol 121:889–900, 1997

Connell PH: The use and abuse of amphetamines. Practitioner 200:234–243, 1968

Connolly HM, Crary JL, McGoon MD, et al: Valvular heart disease associated with fenfluramine-phentermine. N Engl J Med 337:581–588, 1997

Cooper TB, Simpson GM: Concomitant imipramine and methylphenidate administration: a case report. Am J Psychiatry 130:6, 1973

Dally PJ: Fatal reaction associated with tranylcypromine and methylamphetamine. Lancet 1:1235–1236, 1962

D'haenen HA, Bossuyt A: Dopamine D$_2$ receptor density in depression measured with single photon emission computed tomography. Biol Psychiatry 35:128–132, 1994

Drimmer EJ, Gitlin MJ, Gwirtsman HE: Desipramine and methylphenidate combination treatment for depression: case report. Am J Psychiatry 140:241–242, 1983

Drug Abuse Warning Network: Annual E.R. Department Data (DAWN Series No 14–17). U.S. Department of Health and Human Services, 1994

Fawcett J, Kravitz HM, Zajecka JM, et al: CNS stimulant potentiation of monoamine oxidase inhibitors in treatment-refractory depression. J Clin Psychopharmacol 11:127–132, 1991

Feighner JP, Herbstein J, Damlouji N: Combined MAOI, TCA and direct stimulant therapy of treatment resistant depression. J Clin Psychiatry 46:206–209, 1985

Fernandez F, Adams F, Holmes VF, et al: Methylphenidate for depressive disorders in cancer patients. Psychosomatics 28:455–459, 1987

Fernandez F, Adams F, Levy JK, et al: Cognitive impairment due to AIDS-related complex and its response to psychostimulants. Psychosomatics 29:38–46, 1988a

Fernandez F, Levy JK, Galizzi H: Response of HIV-related depression to psychostimulants: case reports. Hospital and Community Psychiatry 39:628–631, 1988b

Fernandez F, Levy JK, Samley HR, et al: Effects of methylphenidate in HIV-related depression: a comparative trial with desipramine. Int J Psychiatry Med 25:53–67, 1995

Fischman MW: Cocaine and the amphetamines, in Psychopharmacology: The Third Generation of Progress. Edited by Meltzer HY. New York, Raven, 1987, pp 1543–1553

Flemenbaum A: Methylphenidate: a catalyst for the tricyclic antidepressants? Am J Psychiatry 128:239, 1971

Foltin RW, Fischman MW: Assessment of abuse liability of stimulant drugs in humans: a methodological survey. Drug Alcohol Depend 28:3–48, 1991

Galynker I, Ieronimo C, Miner C, et al: Methylphenidate treatment of negative symptoms in patients with dementia. J Neuropsychiatry Clin Neurosci 9:231–239, 1997

Glennon RA: Psychoactive phenylisopropylamines, in Psychopharmacology: The Third Generation of Progress. Edited by Meltzer HY. New York, Raven, 1987, pp 1627–1634

Graham DJ, Green L: Further cases of valvular heart disease associated with fenfluramine-phentermine (letter). N Engl J Med 337:635, 1997

Gwirtsman HE, Szuba MP, Toren L, et al: The antidepressant response to tricyclics in major depressives is accelerated with adjunctive use of methylphenidate. Psychopharmacol Bull 39:157–164, 1994

Harrington H, Heller HA, Dawson D, et al: Intracerebral hemorrhage and oral amphetamine. Arch Neurol 40:503–507, 1983

Heuer L: Pulmonary hypertension. Cher Prax 23:497, 1978

Hoffman BB, Lefkowitz RJ: Catecholamines and sympathomimetic drugs, in The Pharmacological Basis of Therapeutics, 8th Edition. Edited by Gilman AG, Goodman LS, Rall TW, et al. New York, Macmillan, 1993, pp 187–220

Holmes VF, Fernandez F, Levy JK: Psychostimulant response in AIDS-related complex patients. J Clin Psychiatry 50:5–8, 1989

Hornstein A, Lennihan L, Seliger G, et al: Amphetamine in recovery from brain injury. Brain Inj 10:145–148, 1996

Imanse J, Vanneste J: Intraventricular hemorrhage following amphetamine abuse. Neurology 40:1318–1319, 1990

Insel TR, Hamilton JA, Guttmacher LB, et al: d-Amphetamine in obsessive-compulsive disorder. Psychopharmacology (Berl) 80:231–235, 1983

Janowsky D, Davis JM: Methylphenidate, dextroamphetamine, and levoamphetamine. Arch Gen Psychiatry 33:304–308, 1976

Johnson ML, Roberts MD, Rossa R, et al: Methylphenidate in stroke patients with depression. Am J Phys Med Rehabil 71:239–241, 1992

Kalant H, Kalant OJ: Death in amphetamine users: causes and rates. Canadian Medical Association Journal 112:299–304, 1975

Khantzian EJ, Gawin F, Kleber HD, et al: Methylphenidate (Ritalin®) treatment of cocaine dependence—a preliminary report. J Subst Abuse Treat 1:107–112, 1984

Klein RG, Wender P: The role of methylphenidate in psychiatry. Arch Gen Psychiatry 52:429–433, 1995

Kraus MF, Burch EA: Methylphenidate hydrochloride as an antidepressant: controversy, case studies and review. South Med J 85:985–991, 1992

Krisko I, Lewis E, Johnston JE: Severe hyperpyrexia due to tranylcypromine-amphetamine toxicity. Ann Intern Med 70:559–564, 1969

Kuczenski R, Segal D: Effects of methylphenidate on extracellular dopamine, serotonin and norepinephrine: comparison with amphetamine. J Neurochem 68:2032–2037, 1997

Lazarus LW, Winemiller DR, Lingam VR, et al: Efficacy and side effects of methylphenidate for post-stroke depression. J Clin Psychiatry 53:447–449, 1992

Lazarus L, Moberg P, Langsley PR, et al: Methylphenidate and nortriptyline in the treatment of poststroke depression. Arch Phys Med Rehabil 75:403–406, 1994

Lieberman JA, Kinon BJ, Loebel AD: Dopaminergic mechanisms in idiopathic and drug-induced psychoses. Schizophr Bull 16:97–110, 1990

Lloyd JTA, Walker DRH: Death after combined dexamphetamine and phenelzine. BMJ 2:168–169, 1965

Mantle TJ, Tipton KF, Garrett NJ: Inhibition of monoamine oxidase by amphetamine and related compounds. Biochem Pharmacol 25:2073–2077, 1976

Mason A: Fatal reaction associated with tranylcypromine and methylamphetamine. Lancet 1:1073, 1962

McCann UD, Seiden LS, Rubin LJ, et al: Brain serotonin neurotoxicity and primary pulmonary hypertension from fenfluramine and dexfenfluramine. JAMA 278:666–672, 1997

Metz A, Shader RI: Combination of fluoxetine with pemoline in the treatment of major depressive disorder. Int Clin Psychopharmacol 6:93–96, 1991

Meyler L: The Side Effects of Drugs. Amsterdam, Excerpta Medica Foundation, 1966

Miller HH, Shore PA, Clarke DE: In vivo monoamine oxidase inhibition by *d*-amphetamine. Biochem Pharmacol 29:1347–1354, 1980

Mooney GF, Haas LF: Effect of methylphenidate on brain injury-related anger. Arch Phys Med Rehabil 74:153–160, 1993

Morita T, Mehendale HM: Effects of chlorphentermine and phentermine on the pulmonary disposition of 5-hydroxytryptamine in the rat in vivo. American Review of Respiratory Disease 127:747–750, 1983

The MTA Cooperative Group: A 14-month randomized clinical trial of treatment strategies for attention-deficit/hyperactivity disorder. Arch Gen Psychiatry 56:1073–1086, 1999

Myers WC, Stewart JT: Use of methylphenidate. Hospital and Community Psychiatry 40:754, 1989

Nicola SM, Kombian SB, Malenka RC: Psychostimulants depress excitatory synaptic transmission in the nucleus accumbens via presynaptic D1-like dopamine receptors. J Neurosci 26:1591–1604, 1996

Nurnberger JI, Simmons-Alling S, Kessler L, et al: Separate mechanisms for behavioral, cardiovascular, and hormonal responses to dextroamphetamine in man. Psychopharmacology (Berl) 84:200–204, 1984

Olin J, Masand P: Psychostimulants for depression in hospitalized cancer patients. Psychosomatics 37:57–62, 1996

O'Neill ME, Arnolda LF, Coles DM, et al: Acute amphetamine cardiomyopathy in a drug addict. Clin Cardiol 6:189–191, 1983

Packe GE, Garton MJ, Jennings K: Acute myocardial infarction caused by intravenous amphetamine abuse. British Heart Journal 64:23–24, 1990

Patrick KS, Kilts CD, Breese GR: Synthesis and pharmacology of hydroxylated metabolites of methylphenidate. J Med Chem 24:1237–1240, 1981

Patrick KS, Mueller RA, Gualtieri CT, et al: Pharmacokinetics and actions of methylphenidate, in Psychopharmacology: The Third Generation of Progress. Edited by Meltzer H. New York, Raven, 1987, pp 1387–1395

Perel JM, Black N, Wharton RN, et al: Inhibition of imipramine metabolism by methylphenidate (abstract). Federation Proceedings 28:418, 1969

Physicians' Desk Reference, 55th Edition. Montvale, NJ, Medical Economics, 2001

Plenger PM, Dixon CE, Castillo RM, et al: Subacute methylphenidate treatment for moderate to moderately severe traumatic brain injury: a preliminary double-blind placebo-controlled study. Arch Phys Med Rehabil 77:536–540, 1996

Post RM, Gerner RH, Carman JS: Effects of a dopamine agonist piribedil in depressed patients. Arch Gen Psychiatry 35:609–615, 1978

Prinzmetal M, Bloomberg W: The use of benzedrine for the treatment of narcolepsy. JAMA 105:2051–2054, 1935

Ragland AS, Ismail Y, Arsura EL: Myocardial infarction after amphetamine use. Am Heart J 125:247–249, 1993

Regier DA, Farmer ME, Rae DS, et al: Comorbidity of mental disorders with alcohol and other drug abuse: results from the Epidemiologic Catchment Area (ECA) study. JAMA 264:2511–2518, 1990

Robinson AE, Wolkind SN: Amphetamine abuse amongst psychiatric inpatients: the use of gas chromatography. Br J Psychiatry 116:643–644, 1970

Rumbaugh CL, Bergeron RT, Fang HCH, et al: Cerebral angiographic changes in the drug abuse patient. Radiology 101:335–344, 1971

Rumbaugh DL, Bergeron RT, Scanlan RL, et al: Cerebral vascular changes secondary to amphetamine abuse in the experimental animal. Radiology 101:345–351, 1971

Satel SL, Nelson JC: Stimulants in the treatment of depression: a critical overview. J Clin Psychiatry 59:241–249, 1989

Satterfield JH, Satterfield BT, Cantwell DP: Three multi-modal treatment of 100 hyperactive boys. Behavioral Pediatrics 98:650–655, 1981

Satterfield JH, Satterfield BT, Shell AM: Therapeutic interventions to prevent delinquency in hyperactive boys. J Am Acad Child Adolesc Psychiatry 26:56–64, 1987

Schachar R, Tannock R: Childhood hyperactivity and psychostimulants: a review of extended treatment studies. J Child Adolesc Psychopharmacol 3:81–97, 1993

Seiden LS, Sabol KE, Ricaurte GA: Amphetamine: effects on catecholamine systems and behavior. Annu Rev Pharmacol Toxicol 32:639–677, 1993

Shevell M, Schreiber R: Pemoline-associated hepatic failure: a critical analysis of the literature. Pediatr Neurol 16(1):14–16, 1997

Sloviter E, Drust EG, Connor JD: Evidence that serotonin mediates some behavioral effects of amphetamine. J Pharmacol Exp Ther 6:348–352, 1978

Smilkstein MJ, Smolinske SC, Rumack BH: A case of MAO inhibitor/MDMA interaction: agony after ecstasy. Clinical Toxicology 25:149–152, 1987

Smith RC, Davis JM: Comparative effects of d-amphetamine/amphetamine and methylphenidate on mood in man. Psychopharmacology (Berl) 53:1–12, 1977

Speech TH, Rao SM, Osmon DC, et al: A double-blind controlled study of methylphenidate treatment in closed head injury. Brain Inj 7:333–338, 1993

Spencer T, Wilens T, Biederman J, et al: A double-blind, crossover comparison of methylphenidate and placebo in adults with childhood-onset attention-deficit hyperactivity disorder. Arch Gen Psychiatry 52:434–443, 1995

Spencer T, Biederman J, Harding M, et al: Growth deficits in ADHD children revisited: evidence for disorder-associated growth delays? J Am Acad Child Adolesc Psychiatry 35:1460–1469, 1996a

Spencer T, Biederman J, Wilens T, et al: Pharmacotherapy of attention-deficit hyperactivity disorder across the life cycle. J Am Acad Child Adolesc Psychiatry 35:409–432, 1996b

Sprague RL, Cohen M, Werry JS: Normative data on the Conners Teacher's Rating Scale and Abbreviated Scale (technical report). Urbana-Champaign, University of Illinois Children's Research Center, 1974

Sterling MJ, Kane M, Grace ND: Pemoline-induced autoimmune hepatitis. Am J Gastroenterol 91:2233–2234, 1996

Stockley IH: Drug interactions: monoamine oxidase inhibitors, I: interactions with sympathomimetic amines. The Pharmaceutical Journal 210:590–594, 1973

Sulzer D, Rayport S: Amphetamine and other psychostimulants reduce pH gradients in midbrain dopaminergic neurons and chromaffin granules: a mechanism of action. Neuron 5:797–808, 1990

Theohar C, Fischer-Cornelssen K, Akesson H, et al: Bromocriptine as antidepressant: double-blind comparative study with imipramine in psychogenic and endogenous depression. Current Therapeutic Research 30:830–842, 1981

Tinklenburg JR, Berger PA: Treatment of abusers of non-addictive drugs, in Psychopharmacology: From Theory to Practice. Edited by Barchas JD, Berger PA, Ciaranello RD, et al. New York, Oxford University Press, 1977, pp 386–403

Trugman JM: Cerebral arteritis and oral methylphenidate. Lancet 1:584–585, 1988

Wagner GH, Rabkin JG, Rabkin R: Dextro-amphetamine as a treatment for depression and low energy in AIDS patients: a pilot study. J Psychosom Res 42:407–411, 1997

Wender PH, Reimherr FW, Wood D, et al: A controlled study of methylphenidate in the treatment of attention deficit disorder, residual type, in adults. Am J Psychiatry 142:547–552, 1985

Wharton RN, Perel JM, Dayton PG, et al: A potential clinical use for methylphenidate with tricyclic antidepressants. Am J Psychiatry 127:1619–1625, 1971

Wroblewski BA, Leary JM, Phelan AM, et al: Methylphenidate and seizure frequency in brain injured patients with seizure disorders. J Clin Psychiatry 53:86–89, 1992

Zeck P: The dangers of some antidepressant drugs. Med J Aust 2:607–608, 1961

SIXTEEN

Electroconvulsive Therapy

Gary S. Figiel, M.D.,
William M. McDonald, M.D.,
W. Vaughn McCall, M.D., and
Charles Zorumpski, M.D.

The clinical practice of electro-convulsive therapy (ECT) developed from the work of Ladhaus von Meduna (1985) on the therapeutic benefits of camphor monobromide–induced convulsions in patients with schizophrenia. Following his lead, in 1938 Cerletti and Bini reported that convulsions could be safely induced in humans by an electrical stimulus (Cerletti 1940). Since that time, ECT has been found to be consistently effective in the treatment of depression, mania, and schizophrenia (Abrams 1992).

In this chapter, we review the use of ECT in the treatment of psychiatric disorders, most notably depression but also including mania, schizophrenia, and Parkinson's disease. The mechanism of action of ECT is discussed within the context of its anticonvulsant and amnestic effects and in relation to the supplemental use of rapid-rate transcranial magnetic stimulation (rTMS). Finally, we provide an overview of the literature on the potential side effects and com-plications of ECT and discuss recommendations for its use in clinical practice.

USE OF ECT

The use of ECT declined from the 1960s to the 1980s, but since then its use has steadily increased. ECT is most commonly administered to patients with depression, followed by those with schizophrenia and mania. Probably because of the increased incidence of depression in women, they are more likely to receive ECT than are men. Middle and upper socioeconomic groups are more frequently administered ECT. Consistent with this finding, ECT is much more commonly used in private hospitals than in public facilities. No doubt reflecting the safe and effective way that ECT can now be administered, recent studies have shown a significant increase in the number of elderly patients receiving ECT. Unfortunately, there may still be a significant lack of access to ECT in many metropolitan areas. It is hoped that ongoing education of physicians and the public will ensure the availability of ECT to all who might benefit from it (Sackeim et al. 1995).

EFFICACY OF ECT

Major Depression

ECT is most commonly used for the treatment of depression. An American Psychiatric Association (APA) Task Force reported that ECT is an effective treatment in up to 80% of patients with either unipolar or bipolar major depression (American Psychiatric Association 1990). ECT should no longer be considered a treatment of last resort but may be considered as a treatment of first choice when a rapid clinical response is essential in severely ill patients, when a history of a positive response to ECT or of medication refractoriness or intolerance is present, and, finally, when patients and family request ECT over other treatment options.

ECT Compared With Antidepressants and Predictors of Response

Although ECT has commonly been reported to be more effective when compared with antidepressants, the literature from which this conclusion is drawn has major methodological flaws. In most studies, subtherapeutic doses of antidepressants were used. Nonetheless, ECT has been found to be equal to or superior to all pharmacological agents with which it has been compared.

Clinical predictors of response to ECT remain elusive. Potential positive predictors of response include increasing age and the presence of psychotic and catatonic symptoms. Several studies have reported that patients with longer current episodes of depression are less likely to respond to ECT. Surprisingly, the presence of the endogenous or melancholic subtypes of depression has not been able to predict a positive response to ECT.

Prudic et al. (1996) reported that patients in whom one or more tricyclic antidepressant trials had failed before ECT responded less favorably to ECT than did patients in whom adequate antidepressant trials had not failed before ECT. Additional work from the same group suggests that these findings may not pertain to newer second-generation antidepressants (Prudic et al. 1996; Sackeim et al. 1995).

A large number of preexisting structural abnormalities observed on brain magnetic resonance imaging (MRI) scans appear in many elderly depressed patients referred for ECT. Preliminary observations suggest that these preexisting structural brain changes may predispose some elderly depressed patients to a less favorable response from ECT and to an increased risk for developing ECT-induced interictal delirium (Hickie et al. 1995). Clearly, these research areas are of tremendous potential clinical significance and require further study.

Stimulus Dosing in Electroconvulsive Therapy for Treatment of Depression

Questions about the proper management of the electrical stimulus have been central to the science and practice of ECT since the inception of the treatment. Issues in stimulus dosing have included 1) whether the stimulus should be subconvulsive or convulsive; 2) what is the optimal stimulus waveform; 3) if a convulsive stimulus is desired, to what degree the stimulus intensity should be in excess of the convulsive threshold; and 4) which physiological parameters provide useful feedback to continuously refine stimulus dosing throughout the ECT course.

Convulsive, subconvulsive, and sham stimulation.   The use of nonconvulsive electrical stimulation to treat psychological problems preceded the introduction of ECT by decades. Most of the treatments involved administering static electricity to parts of the body not limited to the head (Grover 1924). This practice faded from American psychiatry as it became clear that subconvulsive stimulation was associated with a *poorer* outcome than conventional psychotherapy in psychoneurotic patients (Hargrove et al. 1953).

The elements of *modified* ECT (including muscle relaxation and general anesthesia) were described early in the history of ECT. The wide-scale adoption of these modifications raised new questions as to whether the seizure was central to the antidepressant efficacy of ECT or whether anesthesia alone would be just as effective. The Northwick Park trial (Crow et al. 1982) and the Leicestershire trial (Brandon et al. 1984) are examples of two "sham" ECT studies in which anesthesia alone was compared with real ECT. It was convincingly demonstrated that real ECT was more effective, especially for the most severe forms of depression (Brandon et al. 1984; Crow et al. 1982).

Thus, the effectiveness of ECT was clearly linked to the production of a seizure. Neither anesthesia alone without the electrical stimulus nor the use of subconvulsive stimuli appears to have real merit in the treatment of depression.

Stimulus waveform.   Given that a convulsive stimulus is necessary for the antidepressant effects of ECT, a nearly infinite number of variations were available for formulating the stimulus waveform. The earliest ECT devices delivered a sinusoidal stimulus, probably because that was the standard waveform for domestic use. Other waveforms available on early ECT devices included the "chopped" sine wave, the unidirectional pulse square wave, and the alternating brief pulse square wave. Although some investigators had a suspicion that sine wave stimuli may have produced slightly better antidepressant effects than did brief pulse stimuli, these suspicions were overwhelmed by convincing data that sine wave ECT produced more memory side effects than brief pulse ECT, irrespective of the placement of the stimulating electrode (Weiner et al. 1986). The more severe memory side effects produced by sinusoidal stimuli may be explained by the slower rise time for each sine

wave cycle as compared with the brief pulse cycle. Consequent to its slower rise time, much of the sine wave stimulus is subconvulsive and thus presumably adds nothing to the therapeutic effect of ECT, adding only to its side effects. The abrupt rise in the brief pulse waveform allows for the entire stimulus to be above the convulsive threshold (suprathreshold). Because much of the sine wave stimulus is "wasted" in the subconvulsive range, it would be predicted that brief pulse stimuli would be more efficient, requiring a stimulus of smaller magnitude to produce a seizure.

These expectations were borne out in the studies of Weiner (1980), which showed that brief pulse stimuli could provoke a seizure with only one-third of the energy required with sine wave stimuli. Brief pulse ECT devices now dominate the American scene, virtually replacing the sine wave devices for the reasons described above (Farah and McCall 1993).

Magnitude of the stimulus dose.   The consensus regarding the need for convulsive (as opposed to subconvulsive) stimuli and brief pulse waveforms would seem to make stimulus dosing in ECT a straightforward process, except for the question of how much the stimulus should exceed the convulsive threshold. For years, ECT practitioners were satisfied that the answer to this question was found in the work of Ottosson (1962), who compared routine ECT with ECT modified by pretreatment with intravenous lidocaine. He found that seizures induced by lidocaine-modified ECT were shorter than those induced by routine ECT. Thus, a direct relation was found between seizure duration and antidepressant effect. From this work it was widely accepted that stimulus doses producing seizures longer than 25–30 seconds had an antidepressant effect (American Psychiatric Association 1978).

This clinical wisdom was shattered with the groundbreaking work of Sackeim in the late 1980s. Sackeim et al. (1993) showed that if the magnitude of the electrical stimulus was just barely above the convulsive threshold, then ECT was ineffective with right-unilateral-stimulating electrode placement, despite the production of electrographic seizures typically in excess of 25 seconds. In contrast, bilateral ECT was fully effective with stimuli minimally above or 2.5 times above the seizure threshold, but excess memory side effects accrued only at the higher stimulus dose (Sackeim et al. 1993). These dose-response relationships are true to the extent that the stimulus exceeded the convulsive threshold for a given patient, and they are not related to the absolute magnitude of the stimulus dose. This situation is analogous to the pharmacological treatment of depression with tricyclic antidepressants: serum blood levels are more important than the absolute oral dose in determining both efficacy and side effects.

These findings led to the following conclusions: 1) with right-unilateral electrode placement, the stimulus should be substantially (≥2.5 times) above the convulsive threshold to ensure the efficacy of ECT, and 2) with bilateral electrode placement, the stimulus should not be excessively above the convulsive threshold to avoid undue memory side effects. The convulsive threshold varies by a factor of at least 40-fold in large patient samples, thus making the mean threshold for a group of patients useless for individual cases (Sackeim et al. 1991). It is clear that the convulsive threshold is related to age, sex, race, choice of stimulating electrode placement, and, perhaps, cranial dimensions (Colenda and McCall 1996; McCall et al. 1993; Sackeim et al. 1991). Still, these factors predict only a small amount of the variance in the convulsive threshold. Statistical models to predict the convulsive threshold fare poorly, especially in patients with high thresholds (Colenda and McCall 1996).

The bulk of the evidence thus suggests that it is important to determine the dose of the stimulus as a proportion of the convulsive threshold and that the convulsive threshold of each patient should be known, preferably by measuring convulsive threshold early in the ECT course. The most accurate means of measuring the convulsive threshold for a given patient is empirical observation: giving intentionally subconvulsive stimuli at the first treatment and, in the same session, following with successively larger stimuli until a seizure is produced. This stimulus "titration" technique defines the convulsive threshold for each patient.

Refinement of stimulus dosing during electroconvulsive therapy. The report of Sackeim et al. (1993) that threshold right-unilateral ECT produced seizures of ≥25 seconds without antidepressant efficacy cast into doubt the clinical wisdom that the stimulus dose was therapeutic if the electrographic seizure lasted 25 seconds. Investigators have scrambled to find a physiological marker of treatment adequacy to replace seizure duration. The most promising candidate is seizure morphology. Ottosson (1962) reported that lidocaine changed the shape of ECT seizures and affected duration, although the first finding is largely overlooked. Lidocaine-modified seizures, in addition to being less efficacious than standard ECT seizures, were characterized by loss of spike activity and poor postictal suppression (Ottosson 1962).

This finding is now extended by evidence that seizure morphology indeed varies with ECT techniques of different efficacies. In general, greater seizure intensity is apparent as ECT techniques progress from lower (right-unilateral, low stimulus intensity) to higher (bilateral, high stimulus intensity) efficacy (Krystal et al. 1993). Electrode placement and stimulus intensity have independent and additive effects on seizure morphology. Seizures of greater intensity are characterized by higher peak ictal amplitudes, greater stereotypy of the ictal discharge, greater symmetry and coherence between the left and right cerebral hemispheres, and more profound postictal suppression. Preliminary evidence suggests that greater seizure intensity is predictive of greater likelihood of response and/or faster response (McCall and Farah 1994; Nobler et al. 1993).

Recommendations for stimulus dosing.
Our recommendations for stimulus dosing are
made with the following two caveats: 1) recommendations can be made only in regard to major
depression; it is unknown whether dosing strategies for other diagnoses should be the same or
different; and 2) dosing recommendations can
be made only in the context of the chosen electrode placement and the patient's clinical condition. It is clear that a supraconvulsive stimulus is
necessary to obtain ECT's antidepressant effect. It is likely that any supraconvulsive stimulus
will have antidepressant efficacy with bilateral
electrode placement, but a stimulus at least 2.5
times the convulsive threshold is required for
right-unilateral ECT in most patients. Those
patients with the most serious complications of
major depression (i.e., active suicidal behavior in
the hospital, catatonia, or food refusal) merit an
approach most likely to yield quick antidepressant results. In such circumstances, bilateral
ECT with a relatively high, fixed dose could be
justified; stimulus dose titration would not be
required because concern about cognitive side
effects becomes a purely secondary issue, based
on the severity of the patient's clinical status.
However, whether fixed, high-dose right-unilateral ECT could provide an equally fast and
effective response needs to be examined.

Mania

Early anecdotal reports suggested that ECT was
beneficial in the treatment of mania. Since 1970,
several retrospective studies have consistently
confirmed these earlier observations (Mukherjee et al. 1994). Small et al. (1988) conducted
a major prospective controlled trial in which the
efficacy of ECT was compared with that of lithium in the treatment of mania. The results of
this study showed that patients who received
ECT improved more during the first 8 weeks of
treatment than did patients who received lithium. After 8 weeks of treatment, ECT and lithium were comparable in efficacy. In addition,
the authors observed that patients who had

mixed symptoms of depression and mania responded particularly well to ECT.

Controversy persists over whether unilateral ECT is as effective as bilateral ECT in the
treatment of mania. Unfortunately, in most
studies of ECT in which unilateral ECT was
found not to be as effective as bilateral ECT in
the treatment of mania, either the amount of
electrical charge used or the percentage by
which the electrical stimulus exceeded the seizure threshold was not reported.

Schizophrenia

Fink and Sackeim (1996) provided an excellent
review on the use of ECT in the treatment of
schizophrenia. The authors cautiously noted
that most studies examining the efficacy of
ECT in treating schizophrenia do not meet
present standards for scientific methodology.
Nonetheless, the authors concluded that ECT
is a highly effective treatment for psychosis and
that ECT should be considered particularly in
patients with first episodes of schizophrenia, especially when they have symptoms of agitation,
increased psychomotor activity, delirium, or
delusions. The authors also concluded that
ECT was effective in treating schizophrenia
when catatonia or positive symptoms of psychosis were present. They speculated that by using
ECT early in the course of schizophrenia, the
progressive, debilitating effects of the illness
may be avoided.

Of interest is that the literature to date
suggests that ECT combined with neuroleptics is probably more effective than ECT or
neuroleptics alone in treating schizophrenia.
In general, the conclusions of the authors are
consistent with the recommendations of the
APA Task Force report, which stated that
"ECT is an effective treatment for schizophrenia in the following clinical conditions:
1) patients with catatonia; or 2) when affective
symptoms are present; or 3) when there is a
history of a previous favorable response to
ECT" (American Psychiatric Association

1990, p. 8). Clearly, there is a need for further research in this area.

Parkinson's Disease

For the past two decades, ECT has been reported to be effective in the treatment of patients with Parkinson's disease (Rasmussen and Abrams 1991). These reports have included patients with and without psychiatric illnesses. Favorable predictors of response include advanced age, severe disability ("on-off" syndromes), and painful dyskinesias. Reduction in symptoms of Parkinson's disease tends to occur during the first several sessions of ECT. However, the effects from ECT are not permanent and usually last from several days to several months, although prolonged improvement has been reported in a few patients. Although maintenance ECT studies in patients with Parkinson's disease are lacking, our clinical experience has suggested that the therapeutic benefits of ECT in these patients can be sustained with maintenance ECT. Unilateral ECT appears to be as effective as bilateral ECT in treating Parkinson's disease. However, because of the increased risk for ECT-induced interictal delirium in patients with Parkinson's disease, careful consideration must be given to the amount of electrical charge administered, the type of electrode placement used, and the frequency of treatments (Figiel et al. 1991).

Neuroleptic Malignant Syndrome

Although ECT has been reported to be effective in treating neuroleptic malignant syndrome, some cardiac complications have been reported in patients with neuroleptic malignant syndrome treated with ECT. Until more clinical studies are completed, however, we agree with the APA Task Force's recommendations that ECT should be reserved for patients with neuroleptic malignant syndrome who are refractory to or intolerant of standard medical treatments (American Psychiatric Association 1990).

CONTRAINDICATIONS TO ECT

Although there are no absolute contraindications to ECT, several clinical conditions may increase the risk of complications from ECT:

- Recent myocardial infarction
- Any illness that increases intracranial pressure
- Medical conditions that may disrupt the blood-brain barrier (e.g., multiple sclerosis, recent cerebrovascular accident)
- Aneurysm
- Bleeding disorders

When treating high-risk patients with ECT, clinicians must understand the effects of ECT on cerebral and cardiac physiology and combine this information with data from the extant ECT literature to help develop individual risk-benefit ratios.

PRETREATMENT MEDICAL EVALUATION FOR ECT

All patients should be given a thorough medical and neuropsychiatric evaluation before beginning ECT. Particular emphasis should be placed on diseases affecting the central nervous system (CNS) and the cardiovascular system. The pre-ECT evaluation should include a physical examination, a mental status examination, a medical history, and a review of systems. The patient's mental status should be evaluated before ECT is begun and monitored closely before the administration of all ECT sessions.

Along with the physical examination, some basic laboratory tests (blood count and electrolytes) and an electrocardiogram should be done in all patients before ECT. Clinicians should obtain a chest X ray in patients with a history of cardiac or pulmonary disease. Finally, spine films should be considered in patients with a history of back pain, positive findings on physical examination, or medical conditions that may affect the skeletal system.

Information obtained from the patient's neuropsychiatric history must include the following:

- History of prior ECT and any complications
- History of dementia
- History of any other neurological illnesses
- Any symptoms or signs on neurological examination suggestive of increased intracranial pressure
- Any other medical conditions that may affect the CNS

On the basis of the examination, some patients may need a brain imaging scan before ECT. Whether all patients referred for ECT should routinely receive brain scans needs to be reevaluated.

From a cardiac standpoint, the clinician must determine the patient's cardiovascular risk factors and whether the patient has angina. The patient's exercise tolerance should also be estimated. On the basis of this information, the clinician can decide whether a cardiology consult is needed before ECT. One of the best means to reduce the incidence of ECT-induced cardiac complications is to ensure that the patient has received optimum medical management before undergoing ECT.

In general, patients are given their cardiac (except lidocaine), pulmonary (except theophylline), and glaucoma (except anticholinesterases) medications 1–2 hours before a treatment. Theophylline has been associated with status epilepticus during ECT. As a result, we recommend discontinuing theophylline during ECT if clinically feasible. If not, blood levels of theophylline should be closely monitored and patients maintained on the lowest clinically effective dose. Patients with glaucoma who are receiving echothiophate should be switched to another medication because echothiophate can adversely interact with succinylcholine. In dia-

betic patients, hypoglycemic medications are usually withheld on the morning of treatment to minimize the risk of hypoglycemia. In general, patients with epilepsy should continue taking their anticonvulsants during ECT. If difficulty arises in eliciting seizures, a decrease in dose of the anticonvulsant can be considered.

The APA Task Force on ECT recommends that, in general, all psychotropic medications should be discontinued before ECT (American Psychiatric Association 1990). When neuroleptics are necessary to control agitation or psychotic symptoms, a high-potency neuroleptic is probably preferable to minimize any hypotension that may develop during ECT. There is no convincing evidence that antidepressants administered during ECT either augment the antidepressant properties of ECT or increase the speed of response.

Concerns have been raised over whether monoamine oxidase inhibitors can be used safely with anesthesia. At Emory University, we require a 48-hour washout of monoamine oxidase inhibitors before ECT. Lithium is also usually discontinued at least 48 hours before ECT because of a potentially increased risk of delirium during ECT.

Benzodiazepines can interfere with the induction of a seizure during ECT, thereby resulting in a decreased efficacy from the treatments. As a result, benzodiazepines should be reduced to the lowest possible dose or stopped before ECT. Patients taking benzodiazepines should be on a stable dose for 24–48 hours before ECT to reduce the risk of prolonged seizures or status epilepticus during ECT. Finally, informed consent should be obtained from all patients before ECT. Patients deemed to be incompetent may require the appointment of a legal guardian for consent (Sackeim et al. 1995).

TREATMENT TECHNIQUE

ECT sessions are usually scheduled for the morning. The patient's bladder and rectum should be emptied before treatment. Patients should have nothing to eat or drink for at least 6–8 hours before receiving a treatment. The ECT treatment team consists of a psychiatrist, an anesthesiologist (or nurse anesthetist), and a nursing team specially trained in ECT. The ECT treatment area should have resuscitative equipment available in case a medical emergency arises.

The standard anesthetic agent used is methohexital, a short-acting barbiturate. Methohexital is given in a dose of approximately 1 mg/kg. Immediately after the onset of methohexital's effect, a muscle relaxant is administered intravenously. Succinylcholine, in doses of 0.75–1.50 mg/kg, is a widely used depolarizing blocking agent. In patients with musculoskeletal disease, a nondepolarizing agent can be considered. Anticholinergic agents, such as atropine or glycopyrrolate, have often been used to prevent ECT-induced bradycardia and to minimize airway secretions. An anticholinergic agent should always be used if a β-blocker is used to control the ECT-induced rise in blood pressure and heart rate. Atropine (0.4–1.0 mg) or glycopyrrolate (0.2–0.4 mg) can be given either intramuscularly 30 minutes before the treatment or intravenously at the time of the treatment. At Emory University, we prefer to administer atropine intravenously at the time of the treatment because of its potent vagolytic effects.

Caffeine sodium benzoate (usual dose = 120–140 mg) may be administered intravenously during ECT to maintain adequate seizure duration. Caffeine appears to lengthen seizure duration during ECT without lowering the seizure threshold. At present, it is not known whether caffeine either augments ECT's antidepressant effects or increases the speed of response during a course of ECT. Thus, it seems the use of caffeine during ECT should be reserved for patients who are having short seizures during ECT and who do not require or cannot tolerate higher stimulus doses.

The patient is oxygenated by positive-pressure ventilation from the onset of anesthesia un-

til spontaneous respiration is resumed. In addition, the patient is monitored with a pulse oximeter and should likewise have blood pressure and heart rate continuously monitored. Before the electrical stimulus is administered, a rubber bite block is inserted into the patient's mouth.

In bilateral ECT, electrodes are placed frontotemporally, with the center of each electrode approximately 1 inch (2.54 cm) above the center of an imaginary line whose endpoints are the tragus of the ear and the external canthus of the eye.

With unilateral ECT, d'Elia electrode placement is believed to be the safest and most effective (Weiner and Coffey 1986). In this technique, one electrode is placed over the nondominant frontotemporal area, and the other electrode is placed high on the nondominant centroparietal scalp, just lateral to the midline vertex. Weiner and Coffey (1986) elegantly described in depth the potential clinical benefits from the d'Elia electrode placement when using unilateral ECT.

Typically, a seizure lasting 30–90 seconds occurs during treatment. The seizure is monitored by electroencephalography. Seizures lasting longer than 3 minutes should be terminated. This can easily be done by administering a second dose of methohexital. The motor manifestations of the seizure can be monitored by inflating a blood pressure cuff on the right ankle before the muscle relaxant is administered. By placing the blood pressure cuff on the right ankle, it is possible to monitor a generalized seizure when nondominant (right) unilateral ECT is used because the isolated limb is contralateral to the stimulated hemisphere. Patients are usually alert and oriented 20–45 minutes after receiving a treatment.

CARDIAC COMPLICATIONS IN PATIENTS RECEIVING ECT

ECT often produces transient systemic hypertension and abrupt transitions in cardiac rate, which can result in myocardial ischemia or arrhythmias. The increased incidence of cardiac complications among elderly patients is probably associated with the increased rate of preexisting cardiac illnesses such as hypertension, coronary artery disease, and arrhythmias. On the basis of these observations, several authors have recommended the use of prophylactic cardiac medications to dampen cardiovascular responses during ECT in elderly patients with cardiovascular disease.

Research has now documented that labetalol (a short-acting drug with both α- and β-blocking activity), nifedipine (a calcium channel–blocking agent with vasodilating effects), and several other cardiac medications can be safely used to attenuate the cardiac response during ECT (Cattan et al. 1990; Figiel et al. 1993, 1994; Zielinski et al. 1993).

Using noncardiac-modified ECT, Cattan et al. (1990) retrospectively found that 23% (17) of 81 patients older than 65 who were receiving ECT had cardiac complications. The rate of cardiac complications was significantly higher among the 39 patients older than 80 (14 patients, or 36%) than among the 42 patients ages 65–80 (5 patients, or 12%).

Zielinski et al. (1993) prospectively examined the type and incidence of ECT-induced cardiac complications in 40 elderly patients with preexisting cardiac disease who received noncardiac-modified ECT. They observed that, of these 40 patients, 8 (20%) experienced major cardiac complications during ECT, and 14 (35%) had minor cardiac complications during ECT (mainly transient reversible arrhythmias). Not surprisingly, the authors found a higher incidence of ECT-induced cardiac complications in patients with preexisting cardiac disease. No deaths occurred, and 38 of the 40 cardiac patients were able to complete their course of ECT.

Two prospective studies using cardiac-modified ECT (Figiel et al. 1993, 1994) were completed at Emory University. Neither study used a control group. The cardiac protocol for these two studies was identical. At the first treatment, the dose of labetalol was determined on the basis of the patient's age and cardiac status. In general, a starting dose of 10 mg was used. Whenever the maximum heart rate during ECT exceeded 100 beats/minute, the dose of labetalol was increased by 5 mg at subsequent treatments (the maximum dose of labetalol administered at any one treatment was 20 mg). In addition, whenever a patient experienced two successive recordings of systolic blood pressures exceeding 210 mm Hg, 10 mg of nifedipine in addition was given sublingually before induction with anesthesia at all subsequent treatments.

A total of 38 elderly patients (mean age 70 years) participated in the first study (Figiel et al. 1993). Preexisting cardiac disease was common in these patients (26 patients, or 68%). We used the same criteria for cardiac complications as those used by Cattan et al. (1990) and Zielinski et al. (1993), and we observed no cardiac complications at any ECT treatment of these 38 patients (Figiel et al. 1993).

In addition, we completed a second prospective, cardiac-modified ECT study in which we used the identical cardiac protocol described above (labetalol and nifedipine). A total of 57 consecutive elderly patients (mean age 75 years) participated in this study. Of these patients, 44 (77%) had preexisting cardiac disease. Only 2 patients (4%) developed minor ECT-induced cardiac complications. Two patients developed brief episodes of orthostatic hypotension in the recovery room. Neither of these patients had any clinical symptoms, and both were treated by 15 additional minutes of bed rest and intravenous fluids (Figiel et al. 1994).

Early anecdotal reports suggested that β-blockers might not be safe for use during ECT without the concomitant use of anticholinergic medications. On the basis of these earlier observations, we strongly urge that adequate doses of an anticholinergic medication (intravenous atropine, 0.4–0.8 mg, or glycopyrrolate, 0.2 mg) be used to prevent bradycardias whenever β-blockers are used during ECT. To help prevent ECT-induced hypotension, we additionally strongly recommend that all patients be adequately hydrated before undergoing ECT and that psychotropic medications be discontinued whenever possible. Given these caveats, however, the results of the two cardiac-modified ECT studies (Figiel et al. 1993, 1994) suggest that labetalol and nifedipine can be used safely in elderly patients during ECT.

Although ECT in general is safe and effective for elderly patients, significant ECT-induced cardiac complications are not uncommon. Recently, nicardipine (a short-acting calcium channel blocker that can be given intravenously) has been substituted for nifedepine, and esmolol (a short-acting pure beta blocker) has been used to supplement or replace labetalol in patients with significant tachycardia. It seems reasonable to suggest that, by attenuating the cardiovascular response during ECT, one might expect a decrease in the incidence of cardiac complications during ECT in the elderly. This belief is supported by the two cardiac-modified ECT studies described earlier (Figiel et al. 1993, 1994). In the absence of contraindications to the use of β-adrenergic–blocking agents, and after appropriate consultation with an anesthesiologist and a cardiologist, we and others recommend consideration of cardiac-modified ECT in elderly patients referred for ECT, particularly those who have preexisting cardiac disease.

FREQUENCY AND NUMBER OF TREATMENTS

We agree with the APA Task Force's recommendations that an ECT course should be completed when a plateau in response occurs (American Psychiatric Association 1990). There are no convincing data to support that additional treatments beyond this point reduce the rate of relapse after ECT (Barton et al. 1973). In addition, these recommendations also imply that, rather than giving a predetermined number of ECT sessions, the patient's clinical status during the course of ECT should dictate the number of treatments given.

The elegant work of Lerer et al. (1995) has shown that ECT administered twice weekly is no less effective than treatments administered three times a week. One advantage of a more frequent treatment schedule is a faster rate of response. On the other hand, a disadvantage is the potential development of more cognitive side effects from ECT. Given these observations, we believe that the frequency of ECT treatments should be tailored to the individual patient's needs. For example, a patient with a severe, life-threatening illness will benefit from a faster rate of response and should be given more frequent treatments. In patients for whom the risk of cognitive side effects from ECT is a concern (i.e., those with Alzheimer's disease, Parkinson's disease, or severe frontal lobe and caudate hyperintensities on brain MRI scan, as well as those receiving outpatient ECT), a less frequent ECT treatment schedule is certainly a reasonable choice.

COGNITIVE SIDE EFFECTS OF ECT

The greatest area of concern with ECT has to do with the potential development of adverse cerebral and cognitive changes. The technique by which ECT is administered determines the incidence and severity of cognitive side effects that may develop during a course of ECT.

The degree of amnesia incurred during a course of ECT is greater with bilateral ECT than with unilateral ECT. In the area of ECT-induced memory loss, one of the most important findings in recent years has been the mild effects on memory when right-unilateral ECT is administered with a brief pulse stimulation. Many patients who receive bilateral ECT treatments do not complain of significant memory problems. However, some patients receiving bilateral ECT may report memory deficits lasting for as long as 6 months to several years after receiving ECT.

It has been clearly shown that a sine wave stimulus produces greater amnestic effects than does a brief and ultrabrief stimulus pulse. In addition, Sackeim et al. (1991, 1993) reported that, within a specific waveform, the magnitude by which an electrical dose exceeds the seizure threshold (rather than the absolute electrical dose) may be related to the severity of cognitive defects that develop during ECT. Finally, Lerer et al. (1995) consistently reported that twice-weekly treatments produced less cognitive impairment than did treatments administered three times a week.

Interictal ECT-induced delirium is not an uncommon side effect in the elderly (Figiel and Coffey 1990). Interictal ECT-induced delirium is defined as a delirium meeting DSM-IV criteria (American Psychiatric Association 1994) that develops during a course of ECT and persists on days when the patient does not receive a treatment. This side effect is primarily observed in the elderly receiving ECT and increases in incidence with advancing age. ECT-induced interictal delirium is associated with prolonged hospitalizations and an increased risk of falls. Among the elderly, additional risk factors for interictal delirium are 1) Parkinson's disease, 2) Alzheimer's disease, 3) one or more cardiovascular risk factors, and 4) preexisting structural changes in the caudate nucleus observed on brain scans.

As a rule, an ECT-induced interictal delirium is a short-lived, reversible side effect if identified early. Once it has been identified, treatments should be held until the delirium resolves. Subsequent treatments should be administered less frequently at a lower electrical charge.

Does Electroconvulsive Therapy Cause Brain Damage?

Human autopsy studies of patients who have received ECT have shown no convincing evidence of irreversible brain damage when ECT is administered with current techniques. These findings are supported by a brain MRI study in which no significant structural brain changes were found immediately or 6 months after the completion of ECT. The reader is referred to excellent review articles on these areas of research (Devanand et al. 1994; Weiner 1984).

Effects of Electroconvulsive Therapy on Cerebral Physiology

Immediately after an ECT treatment, the electroencephalogram shows generalized slowing. This slowing tends to increase and persist longer after successive treatments. After a course of ECT is completed, slow-wave activity gradually decreases, and the electroencephalogram reverts to baseline activity within 3 months (Weiner et al. 1986). Rarely, electroencephalogram abnormalities may persist for more than 3 months. Prior electroencephalogram abnormalities may increase the risk for developing prolonged abnormalities after ECT, but the clinical significance of these abnormalities is unknown.

Electrically induced seizures in animals and humans have been shown to produce transient increases in permeability of the blood-brain barrier (Laursen et al. 1991). These findings are consistent with a brain MRI study in which increased T-1 relaxation times were observed after ECT (Scott et al. 1990). Laursen et al. (1991) reported that the ECT-induced increase in blood-brain barrier permeability is associated with an increased stimulus intensity and an increased number of ECT treatments. In addition, Bolwig et al. (1977) were able to decrease changes in blood-brain barrier permeability during ECT by blocking ECT-induced hypertensive response with high-spinal anesthesia. Because a disturbed blood-brain barrier may predispose some patients toward ECT-induced neurological complications, work is needed to examine the ways by which ECT-induced changes in blood-brain barrier permeability can be minimized, such as by attenuating the ECT-induced cardiovascular response or by reducing the amount of the stimulus charge.

The combination of increased CO_2 production, decreased pH, and systemic hypertension leads to a doubling of cerebral blood flow during ECT (Broderston et al. 1973; Posner et al. 1969). The transiently increased cerebral blood flow results in a sharp rise in both intracranial and intraocular pressure (Maltbie et al. 1980). Methods that limit the accumulation of CO_2, such as forced hyperventilation, or that attenuate the increase in blood pressure tend to decrease the rise in intracranial pressure associated with ECT.

PROPHYLACTIC SOMATIC TREATMENT OF PATIENTS WITH ACUTE RESPONSE TO ECT

The debate over appropriate prophylactic treatment for patients with an acute response to ECT has focused on the clinical decision to continue either antidepressant therapy or maintenance ECT. Confusion in this area persists because of the lack of controlled studies comparing the efficacy of antidepressants with that of maintenance ECT.

Two studies (Aronson et al. 1987; Spiker et al. 1985) evaluated adult patients after an acute course of ECT for psychotic depression and found a relapse rate of 68% (*n* = 53 patients) at 1 year. Spiker et al. (1985) found a 1-year relapse rate of 50% in patients with delusional depression who initially responded to an acute course of ECT. Aronson et al. (1987) followed up patients with delusional depression who responded to either medication or ECT and found that 80% of the medication-responsive group and 95% of the ECT-responsive patients relapsed in the first year after hospitalization. These studies did not compare the adequacy of either the initial (pre-ECT) or the continuation medication trial.

Sackeim et al. (1990) followed up 58 patients for 1 year after ECT and found a differential relapse rate of 64% in those with major depression (with and without psychotic features) in whom an adequate pre-ECT medication trial had failed. In contrast, the relapse rate in patients who did not receive an adequate pre-ECT antidepressant trial was only 32%. Other clinical and demographic factors were not significant in predicting relapse. Significantly, the adequacy of the post-ECT maintenance medication was not correlated with relapse. However, as in the studies cited above, the maintenance medications post-ECT were not standardized, and the evaluation of the pre-ECT medication trial was retrospective. The conclusion of this study is intuitively appealing: Patients whose symptoms do not respond to antidepressant medication before ECT are those most likely to relapse during maintenance medication. As is true of depressed patients with psychotic features, the relapse rates of almost two-thirds of patients in 1 year remain alarmingly high.

The elderly are particularly prone to increased disability from depression and form a substantial proportion of patients in an acute ECT program. Data from naturalistic studies confirm that the relapse rates for elderly patients treated with ECT are also quite high. These rates have varied from 67% in 6 months (Karlinsky and Shulman 1984) to 75% in 1 year (Murphy 1983). The elderly may therefore be at increased risk for relapse after acute ECT.

Continuation/Maintenance Electroconvulsive Therapy in Major Depression

The high relapse rates of depressed patients receiving antidepressants after ECT have led clinicians to use alternative therapies, such as continuation/maintenance ECT, in patients who are at high risk for recurrence of their mood disorder. *Continuation ECT* is defined as ECT that continues for up to 6 months after the acute ECT course. Continuation ECT is differentiated from *maintenance ECT*, which is defined as ECT that continues for more than 6 months after the index course. In this chapter, the term *prophylactic ECT* is used to refer to any ECT treatments given as continuation or mainte-nance. Many of the studies reviewed here do not differentiate patients receiving continuation ECT from those receiving maintenance ECT, although treatment indications, side effects, and outcomes may be different for these two types of prophylactic ECT.

APA clinical guidelines (American Psychiat-ric Association 1990) for candidates for prophy-lactic ECT include patients who have recurring affective episodes that are responsive to ECT and/or who are resistant or intolerant to, or noncompliant with, antidepressant medica-tions. Prophylactic ECT strategies are increas-ingly being used to treat major depression and bipolar disorder in patients thought to be at high risk for relapse. In a 1985 survey of private hos-pitals, 64% of the hospitals that provided ECT also provided prophylactic ECT (Levy and Albrecht 1985). Kramer (1987) found a similar use pattern, with 59% of respondents using con-tinuation/maintenance ECT primarily for re-current depression.

Most of the studies examining maintenance ECT are case reports (Thienhaus et al. 1990). The more recent reports follow a naturalistic design with relatively few subjects but generally describe a marked decrease in the number of hospitalizations, hospital days, and depressive symptoms; increased functional status; and sta-ble cognitive functioning for the period of con-tinuation ECT (Clarke et al. 1989; Decina et al. 1987; Loo et al. 1991; Thienhaus et al. 1990; Thornton et al. 1990). These positive results have been extended primarily to elderly popula-tions (Jaffe et al. 1989; Loo et al. 1991; Thienhaus et al. 1990).

In a prospective study, Clarke et al. (1989) used continuation ECT in 27 patients who re-ceived an acute course of ECT because of a his-tory of medication intolerance or resistance. The rate of rehospitalization was six times lower (8%) in patients who completed a 5-month course of continuation ECT than in patients who did not complete the protocol (47%). There are few other prospective studies, and no controlled trials, of continuation/maintenance ECT. Guidelines for the use of prophylactic ECT therefore remain vague primarily because of the paucity of data on which to base these guidelines. Monroe (1991) has delineated the contradiction of the increasing use of continua-tion/maintenance ECT and the lack of research defining the parameters of administering the treatments and potential side effects and contra-indications. At the time of Monroe's review, the available studies of continuation/maintenance ECT included only 325 patients with depres-sion (including 85 with bipolar disorder and 121 with psychotic depression).

TREATMENT RECOMMENDATIONS

1. Patients who have failed previous trials of medication and are therefore relatively medication resistant. A significant mi-nority of patients with major depression are rel-atively medication resistant despite adequate medication trials. Sackeim et al. (1990) found that the most important factor in relapse after an acute course of ECT is whether the patient re-ceived an adequate pretreatment medication trial. In patients who had undergone an ade-quate pretreatment medication trial, the relapse rate after ECT was found to be twofold higher (64% vs. 32%) (Sackeim et al. 1990). Shapira et al. (1995) also found that patients who had re-ceived an adequate pretreatment pharmaco-therapy trial relapsed at a significantly higher rate when they received lithium maintenance therapy. Interestingly, Grunhaus et al. (1990) re-ported a relapse rate of only 17% in patients in whom a previous medication trial had failed and who received up to 12 weeks of maintenance ECT.

Patients in whom an adequate medication trial has failed before ECT should be informed of the risk of relapse and given the option of con-tinuation ECT for 6 months, followed by main-tenance medication. The clinical decision of whether to continue ECT beyond 6 months should be made on an individual basis, weighing the risks (primarily cognitive effects vs. the risk of suicide or recurrent psychosis) and benefits (long-term effects of a period of mood stability).

2. Patients who are severely ill. Some researchers have found that the 1-year relapse rate in patients with psychotic depression treated with medication alone may be as high as 95% (Aronson et al. 1987; Spiker et al. 1985). Petrides et al. (1994) retrospectively examined the records of patients with delusional depression treated with prophylactic ECT and found the relapse rate at 1 year to be only 42%. They compared their findings with those from the study by Aronson et al. (1987). Both patient groups were drawn from the same institution, although prophylactic ECT was not available at the time that Aronson et al. (1987) reported relapse rates of 95% in patients with delusional depression who were taking antidepressants. Vanelle et al. (1994) prospectively administered maintenance ECT (defined as ECT for more than 6 months after the index course), often with concomitant antipsychotic medication, approximately once a month for 1 year to a group of patients with psychotic depression and found full or partial remission in 80% of patients. Grunhaus et al. (1990) also found an excellent clinical response in patients with psychotic depression who were administered prophylactic ECT. Prophylactic ECT may therefore be a viable option in patients with delusional depression and should be discussed with these patients and their families.

3. Patients who cannot tolerate the side effects of antidepressant medication, because of either concomitant medical illness or a personal sensitivity to antidepressant side effects, or who are noncompliant with their medication trial. Most of the patients who cannot tolerate the side effects of antidepressant medication, because of either concomitant medical illness or a personal sensitivity to antidepressant side effects, can be tried on maintenance medication after a successful course of

ECT. Many patients who are acutely ill may be extremely sensitive to the side effects of medications but may tolerate the same medication once they have responded to acute treatment. Conditions associated with depression, such as malnutrition and dehydration, may worsen the orthostatic hypotension from tricyclic antidepressants. In a patient with agitated depression, minimal activation from the selective serotonin reuptake inhibitors may be experienced as extreme agitation. Once the depressive episode has remitted, patients can usually tolerate an additional medication trial. Patients who are noncompliant with their antidepressant medication should be evaluated on an individual basis, and, after discussions with the patient and the family, the risks and benefits of prophylactic ECT should be weighed against an additional medication trial.

PROCEDURAL GUIDELINES FOR CONTINUATION ECT

Treatment Parameters

At Emory University, the electrode placement and dose parameters used in the index course are maintained during maintenance ECT. Retrospective reviews have not found stimulus placement to affect outcome (Petrides et al. 1994), although no systematic studies have compared unilateral and bilateral placement in prophylactic ECT.

Treatment Intervals, Frequency, and Duration

There are few guidelines on what frequency of continuation ECT is optimal to maintain mood stability. The intervals between courses of prophylactic continuation ECT in the studies reviewed vary from 3–5 weeks (Loo et al. 1991) to 4–8 weeks (Thienhaus et al. 1990). Other clinicians argue that treatments should be gradually tapered from once a week to once a month, depending on clinical response (Aronson et al. 1987; Clarke et al. 1989; Matzen et al. 1988).

Kramer (1987) surveyed 51 clinicians in 24 states and found the frequency and duration of maintenance ECT to vary from two treatments per week extending to once every 3–4 weeks over 30 months, to one treatment every 6 months over 60 months, to as long as 48 years. In Kramer's survey, clinicians described continuing ECT until the patient was asymptomatic for a predetermined period ranging from 1 month to 2 years.

Grunhaus et al. (1990) assessed individual patients' clinical histories and assigned them to either abbreviated maintenance ECT (i.e., once or twice a week for 4–12 weeks) or full maintenance ECT (i.e., gradually tapering ECT to once a month over 3 months and continuing once a month for 6 months). Abbreviated maintenance was used when symptoms were unresponsive to medication after the index episode and lasted more than 12 months or when the patient relapsed after a successful course of ECT or had difficulties tolerating continuation pharmacotherapy. Full maintenance was used in patients who relapsed after a successful course of ECT despite adequate pharmacotherapy. Among 10 patients, these authors found an excellent response in 6 (5 of 6 receiving abbreviated maintenance; 1 of 4 receiving full maintenance), particularly in those with delusional depression.

In a prospective study, Vanelle et al. (1994) administered maintenance ECT with an average frequency of once every 3.5–3.9 weeks for 1 year and found that 64% of patients needed shorter intervals to prevent a recurrence of their depressive disorders. The patients who required a shorter interval were older and had a longer duration of illness. Vanelle et al. (1994) posited that the older patients may have had a shorter time to relapse, a suggestion that is consistent with data showing that older patients tend to have accelerated mood cycles (Zis et al. 1980).

Recommendations for Treatment

The greatest risk of relapse after ECT is within the first few months after acute treatment (Clarke et al. 1989; Sackeim et al. 1990; Shapira et al. 1995). During this crucial period, many patients and their families describe a recurrence of symptoms of depression when treatment intervals are extended by even a few days. This pattern of response has resulted in the development of a continuation ECT protocol at Emory University in which treatment intervals between continuation ECT are extended in increments—from once a week for the first four treatments, to every 10 days for the next three treatments, then every 2 weeks for the final 4 months. During the 6 months of continuation ECT, treatments are not extended beyond every 2 weeks, because a high relapse rate is seen during the 6 months when continuation ECT treatments are extended beyond every 2 weeks. If a patient becomes symptomatic, the treatment interval is again shortened for additional treatments until the patient is clinically stable. The patient is then returned to the longest ECT treatment interval during which he or she remained healthy. Patients are encouraged to continue in ECT for at least 6 months. In the final month of continuation ECT, treatment with an antidepressant is initiated. However, which antidepressant drug can be safely and effectively used during continuation ECT requires further study. Patients who relapse quickly after discontinuation of continuation ECT should be considered for maintenance ECT.

Informed Consent

Individual hospital policies and state laws dictate the procedure for obtaining informed consent. Patients in outpatient ECT usually are subject to the same guidelines as are applicable to the ambulatory surgery service in the treating hospital. In general, the same policies governing consent for the index ECT course apply to the prophylactic course of ECT. The consent procedures have been reviewed extensively elsewhere (Abrams 1992; American Psychiatric Association 1978, 1990; Greenberg et al. 1993). A new consent should be obtained before each course of prophylactic ECT, when a patient changes from inpatient and outpatient status, and at least every 6 months. The patient's primary physician should also document at the beginning of each ECT course (i.e., at the time of the consent) the justification for the prophylactic ECT.

Cognitive Complications

There are few data on the cognitive changes of patients receiving repeated ECT over a period of months to years. Most reports have focused on acute ECT and have shown either transient changes in memory or no neuroanatomical changes on MRI (Coffey et al. 1988). Most of the available reports in which prophylactic ECT has been used describe only minor subjective complaints, and few studies report objective neuropsychological testing. Grunhaus et al. (1990) reported that the patients in their study experienced minor memory difficulties (recent recall and names) that returned to normal within 6–8 months. Patients in a study by Vanelle et al. (1994) (mean age 70 ± 13 years) described either no subjective memory problems ($n = 8$) or minor subjective cognitive complaints ($n = 14$). Petrides et al. (1994) noted only minor subjective memory problems in 30 patients (mean age 52 ± 15 years) receiving an average of seven continuation ECT treatments over 2 months. Thienhaus et al. (1990) found stable cognitive function (as measured on the Mini-Mental State Exam [Folstein et al. 1975]) in six elderly patients (mean age 71 ± 5 years) over 1–5 years of prophylactic ECT.

Summary

Prophylactic ECT is an effective and cost-efficient alternative to medication in a selected subgroup of patients with recurrent depression, particularly in elderly patients and those with a history of medication resistance and delusional depression. Patients in these subgroups may benefit from a period of mood stabilization with continuation ECT that is followed by maintenance medication. There is, however, a paucity

of prospective research on prophylactic ECT, despite the increasing use of this treatment in clinical practice. Future research should focus on identification of selected subpopulations who may benefit from prophylactic medication compared with ECT, standardization of the techniques for administering the treatments, potential cardiac and cognitive side effects of repeated treatments, and cost-effectiveness of prophylactic ECT.

MECHANISMS OF ACTION

More than 100 theories have been proposed to explain the therapeutic effects of ECT. These range from hypotheses about psychological and psychodynamic processes to neurotransmitter changes, neuroendocrine effects, and alterations in second-messenger systems and gene expression (Sackeim 1994). On the basis of current information, it seems that certain theories about ECT can be discarded. For example, there is little evidence that anesthetics or muscle relaxants produce sustained clinical benefits in CNS disorders. Similarly, there is no convincing evidence that ECT produces structural brain damage or that the memory-impairing effects of ECT are necessary for clinical improvement (Devanand et al. 1994; Weiner 1984). The latter is particularly important because memory loss has been a popular lay theory. Current ECT practice, which includes the use of vigorous oxygenation, brief electrical pulses, titrated electrical dosing, and unilateral electrode placement, is largely directed toward diminishing memory impairment to the greatest extent possible. Other psychological explanations for the effects of ECT are equally implausible.

Most serious efforts to understand the mechanisms of ECT's effects have centered on changes in CNS neurotransmitter systems and/or biochemical processes. For useful reviews of the biochemical effects of electrically induced seizures, the reader is referred to excellent papers by Nutt and Glue (1993) and

Fochtmann (1994). The problem in identifying these mechanisms lies in the fact that ECT affects many CNS systems, and it is difficult to have confidence in mechanisms of action in illnesses that are poorly defined at a neurochemical level. Furthermore, much of the neurochemical information about ECT comes from studies of electroconvulsive shock (ECS) in animals, in which the assumption is made that the effects of repeated seizures in presumably normal animals are relevant to actions in patients with psychiatric disorders (Lerer et al. 1984).

A strategy for examining the mechanism of action of ECT is to examine the effects of ECT on CNS processes for which there is more detailed basic science information. The assumption here is that the effects of ECT on those CNS systems that are involved in the better-understood disorders have a higher likelihood of being related to clinical effects. Although none of these strategies is entirely satisfactory, in this chapter, we concentrate on the latter approach and discuss specific examples in which ECT mechanisms may be closer to being understood.

Anticonvulsant Effects

The anticonvulsant effects of ECT include increases in seizure threshold and decreases in seizure duration (Sackeim et al. 1991). There is now considerable information about the cellular correlates of seizures (McNamara 1994), and it is of interest to determine whether these insights are relevant to the anticonvulsant effects of ECT. Given the role of γ-aminobutyric acid (GABA) as the major fast inhibitory transmitter in the CNS and as a target for several antiepileptic drugs (e.g., barbiturates, benzodiazepines, loreclezole) (Macdonald and Olsen 1994), it seems reasonable to expect changes in this transmitter system over a course of ECT. Indeed, data from studies in animals have demonstrated increases in the threshold for convulsant drugs that act via $GABA_A$ receptors (bicuculline and pentylenetetrazol) after ECS

(Nutt et al. 1981; Plaznik et al. 1989). Furthermore, GABA levels have been shown to increase in certain CNS regions after ECS (Green et al. 1982), suggesting an increase in tonic inhibition in these regions after several seizures. At the receptor level, there is evidence for increases in the $GABA_B$ receptors that mediate pre- and postsynaptic inhibition in the CNS (Lloyd et al. 1985).

An intriguing finding in rodents is that repeated seizures cause the release of an anticonvulsant substance into cerebrospinal fluid. Anticonvulsant activity can be transferred to naive animals by intracerebroventricular injections of cerebrospinal fluid from animals who have experienced seizures (Tortella and Long 1985, 1988). Tortella et al. (1989) provided evidence that the anticonvulsant is an endogenous opioid and that treatment with naloxone, a broad-spectrum opiate receptor antagonist, blocks the anticonvulsant effects of ECS in animals. There is also evidence for upregulation of specific δ opiate binding sites (e.g., sites for D-alanine-D-leucine enkephalin [DADLE]) after repeated seizures (Hitzemann et al. 1987). Whether similar changes occur in humans remains speculative.

Amnestic Effects

There is evidence that muscarinic cholinergic receptors contribute to some forms of memory, and in humans, antimuscarinic agents are associated with memory impairment (Krueger et al. 1992). In animals, the effects of ECS on central muscarinic systems have been variable (Fochtmann 1994). However, some studies suggest that ECT diminishes muscarinic binding in the cortex and hippocampus. There is also evidence for diminished behavioral responses to muscarinic agonists, decreases in brain choline acetyltransferase, and decreases in brain acetylcholine levels (Nutt and Glue 1993). Taken together, these findings suggest that alterations in CNS muscarinic systems may contribute to memory impairment.

Investigators believe that long-term potentiation is a synaptic mechanism that may be involved in memory processing and that disruption of this process could contribute to anterograde amnesia. The term *long-term potentiation* typically refers to a persistent enhancement of glutamate-mediated excitatory synaptic transmission that follows repeated synaptic use. ECS and generalized seizures disrupt the formation of long-term potentiation in animals and also produce memory impairment (Anwyl et al. 1987; Stewart and Reid 1993). Several ECS-induced changes, including effects on muscarinic and adrenergic neurotransmission, could contribute to the inhibition of long-term potentiation. Furthermore, the enhanced inhibition that may contribute to the anticonvulsant effects of ECT could also play a role because these inhibitory systems can modulate efficacy at excitatory synapses (Kuba and Kumamoto 1990).

Parkinson's Disease

ECT can be helpful in treating the motor symptoms of Parkinson's disease independent of its effects on affective symptoms. The effectiveness of antimuscarinic drugs in treating parkinsonian symptoms suggests that the effects of ECT on central muscarinic systems may be relevant (Fochtmann 1988). However, ECT also alters central dopaminergic systems that are more fundamentally involved in Parkinson's disease (Fochtmann 1994). Acutely, ECS increases dopamine levels in the frontal cortex and striatum and has variable effects on basal dopamine levels. Furthermore, dopamine autoreceptor sensitivity is diminished after ECS, an effect that would tend to augment dopamine release. There is also evidence that dopamine, subtype 1 (D_1), receptor agonists cause increased stimulation of adenylate cyclase after ECS. However, D_1 dopamine receptor binding is increased in the substantia nigra (Fochtmann et al. 1989), but not in the striatum (Nowak and Zak 1989), after ECS.

Phencyclidine-Induced Psychosis

Some evidence indicates that ECT can be an effective treatment in patients with phencyclidine-induced psychosis, producing benefit with a small number of treatments (Dinwiddie et al. 1988). It appears that a major effect of phencyclidine in the CNS occurs via open channel block of N-methyl-D-aspartate (NMDA)–type glutamate receptors. Of importance is the observation that phencyclidine-induced block shows voltage dependence and the block is long-lived, the ion channel closing around the phencyclidine molecule (MacDonald et al. 1991). Relief of NMDA channel block requires that NMDA ion channels open at depolarized membrane potentials (Huettner and Bean 1988). Thus, neuronal membrane depolarization and receptor agonist exposure are required for phencyclidine to exit the channel. Although it is not certain that blocking of NMDA ion channels is critical for phencyclidine psychosis, it is interesting that ECT-induced seizures would be expected to relieve phencyclidine block. That is, during a seizure, neurons depolarize (caused by synaptic excitation and action potential firing) and glutamate is released at synapses. These events would work in conjunction to rapidly relieve phencyclidine-induced block and could provide a rationale for the effectiveness of ECT.

Major Psychiatric Disorders

Much of the above discussion of ECT mechanisms has been highly speculative. Until more information about the cellular and synaptic pathophysiology of psychiatric disorders is available, it seems unlikely that the beneficial effects of ECT will be well understood. Certainly many of the effects outlined above could contribute, including effects on central dopaminergic and cholinergic systems. Furthermore, the usefulness of anticonvulsants as mood stabilizers makes it possible that the anticonvulsant effects of ECT could be important in the management of affective disorders. This latter hypothesis is attractive in that it could explain ECT's therapeutic effects in both mania and depression (Sackeim 1994). However, data directly indicating a therapeutic requirement for the anticonvulsant effects of ECT are lacking.

Because of the efficacy of psychotropic medications, there has been considerable interest in determining how the effects of ECT compare with known drug effects. Particular emphasis has been placed on examining the effects on biogenic amines. Of interest is that certain antidepressants cause β_1-adrenergic receptor subsensitivity, and similar effects occur with ECT (Nutt and Glue 1993). ECT has multiple other effects on the adrenergic system, including increases in norepinephrine turnover and α_1-adrenergic receptor sensitivity and possibly decreases in presynaptic α_2-adrenergic receptors. ECT also appears to enhance the function of the serotonergic transmitter system, producing increased behavioral sensitivity to serotonin receptor agonists and possibly increases in 5-hydroxytryptamine, subtype 2, receptor binding in the cerebral cortex (Fochtmann 1994; Nutt and Glue 1993; Sackeim 1994). The latter effect differs from changes induced by chronic antidepressant drug treatment.

RAPID-RATE TRANSCRANIAL MAGNETIC STIMULATION

Often asked is the question "What new treatment will eventually replace ECT?" Since its initial use, numerous other treatments have come and gone in psychiatry, but the use of ECT has persisted. Most recently, rTMS has yielded exciting preliminary results in the treatment of depression. However, given the highly safe and effective manner in which ECT can now be administered, the question asked should no longer be whether rTMS will replace ECT, but how rTMS can complement ECT in the treatment of psychiatric disorders (Pascual-Leone et al. 1996).

rTMS allows magnetic stimuli to stimulate the cerebral cortex noninvasively (Pascual-Leone et al. 1996). Lesion and imaging studies suggest that left prefrontal lobe dysfunction is pathophysiologically linked to depression. On the basis of these observations, several groups have begun to examine whether rTMS administered to the left prefrontal lobe may be of benefit in treating some patients with depression. In a randomized, placebo-controlled study, rTMS was found to be effective in treating 11 of 17 patients with psychotic depression (Pascual-Leone et al. 1996). The authors found that rTMS was most effective when applied over the left frontal lobe anterior to the motor cortex. However, the therapeutic benefits of rTMS were transient, lasting less than 1 month. Potential benefits of rTMS include the absence of anesthesia and absent or minimal cardiac and cognitive side effects. Potential side effects from rTMS are headaches and a small risk for developing a seizure during treatment.

The fact that rTMS uses subconvulsive stimuli challenges the long-held belief that a generalized seizure is required for ECT to be effective. We hope that continued study of the mechanism of action of rTMS will further the understanding of ECT and in turn allow clinicians to better understand the pathophysiology of depression and to provide the safest and most effective care to patients.

CONCLUSION

Nearly 60 years have passed since ECT was first used in the treatment of psychiatric disorders. The lack of rigorous scientific studies during the early use of ECT in part allowed controversy to develop over the use of ECT. Despite this ongoing controversy, ECT continues to be an extremely important tool in the treatment of several psychiatric disorders. This no doubt reflects the highly safe and effective manner in which ECT can now be administered. It is hoped that adequate research funding will be available in the future to further advance the study of ECT and to ensure that ECT will be adequately available to all patients who might benefit from it.

REFERENCES

Abrams R: Electroconvulsive Therapy, 2nd Edition. New York, Oxford University Press, 1992, pp 3–9

American Psychiatric Association: Report of the Task Force on Electroconvulsive Therapy of the American Psychiatric Association. Washington, DC, American Psychiatric Association, 1978

American Psychiatric Association: The Practice of Electroconvulsive Therapy: Recommendations for Practice, Training, and Privileging. Task Force Report on ECT. Washington, DC, American Psychiatric Association, 1990

American Psychiatric Association: Diagnostic and Statistical Manual of Mental Disorders, 4th Edition. Washington, DC, American Psychiatric Association, 1994

Anwyl R, Walshe J, Rowan M: Electroconvulsive treatment reduces long-term potentiation in rat hippocampus. Brain Res 435:377–379, 1987

Aronson TA, Shukla S, Hoff A: Continuation therapy after ECT for delusional depression: a naturalistic study of prophylactic treatments and relapse. Convulsive Therapy 3:241–259, 1987

Barton JL, Mehta S, Snaith RP: The prophylactic value of extra ECT in depressive illness. Acta Psychiatr Scand 49:386–392, 1973

Bolwig TG, Hertz MM, Westergaard E: Acute hypertension causing blood-brain barrier breakdown during epileptic seizures. Acta Neurol Scand 56:335–342, 1977

Brandon S, Cowley P, McDonald C, et al: Electroconvulsive therapy: results in depressive illness from the Leicestershire trial. BMJ 288:22–25, 1984

Broderston P, Paulson OB, Bolwig TG, et al: Cerebral hyperemia in electrically induced epileptic seizures. Arch Neurol 28:334–338, 1973

Cattan RA, Barry PP, Mead G, et al: Electroconvulsive therapy in octogenarians. J Am Geriatr Soc 38:753–758, 1990

Cerletti U: L'elettroshock. Rivista Sperimentale Freniatria 64:209–310, 1940

Clarke TB, Coffey CE, Hoffman GW, et al: Continuation therapy for depression using outpatient electroconvulsive therapy. Convulsive Therapy 5:330–337, 1989

Coffey CE, Figiel GS, Djang WT, et al: Effects of ECT on brain structure: a pilot prospective magnetic resonance imaging study. Am J Psychiatry 145:701–706, 1988

Colenda CC, McCall WV: A statistical model predicting the seizure threshold for right unilateral electroconvulsive therapy in 106 patients. Convulsive Therapy 12:3–12, 1996

Crow TJ, Deakin JFW, Johnstone EC, et al: Mechanism of action of ECT: relevance of clinical evidence. Paper presented at the 13th Congress of the Collegium Internationale Neuro-Psychologicum, Jerusalem, Israel, June 1982

Decina P, Guthrie EB, Sackheim HA, et al: Continuation ECT in the management of relapses of major affective episodes. Acta Psychiatr Scand 75:559–562, 1987

Devanand DP, Dwork AJ, Hutchinson ER, et al: Does ECT alter brain structure? Am J Psychiatry 151:957–970, 1994

Dinwiddie SH, Drevets WC, Smith DR: Treatment of phencyclidine-associated psychosis with ECT. Convulsive Therapy 4:230–235, 1988

Farah A, McCall WV: Electroconvulsive therapy stimulus dosing: a survey of contemporary practices. Convulsive Therapy 9:90–94, 1993

Figiel GS, Coffey CE: Brain magnetic resonance imaging findings in ECT-induced delirium. J Neuropsychiatry Clin Neurosci 2:53–58, 1990

Figiel GS, Hassen M, Krishnan KRR, et al: ECT induced delirium in depressed patients with Parkinson's disease. J Neuropsychiatry Clin Neurosci 3:405–411, 1991

Figiel GS, DeLeo B, Zorumski CF, et al: Combined use of labetalol and nifedipine in controlling the cardiovascular response from ECT. J Geriatr Psychiatry Neurol 6:20–24, 1993

Figiel GS, McDonald L, LaPlante R: Cardiac modified ECT in the elderly (letter). Am J Psychiatry 151:790–791, 1994

Fink M, Sackeim HA: Convulsive therapy in schizophrenia? Schizophr Bull 22:27–39, 1996

Fochtmann LJ: A mechanism for the efficacy of ECT in Parkinson's disease. Convulsive Therapy 4:321–327, 1988

Fochtmann LJ: Animal studies of electroconvulsive therapy: foundations for future research. Psychopharm Bull 30:321–444, 1994

Fochtmann LJ, Cruciani R, Aiso M, et al: Chronic electroconvulsive shock increases D1 receptor binding in rat substantia nigra. Eur J Pharmacol 167:305–306, 1989

Folstein MF, Folstein SE, McHugh PR: Mini-Mental State: a practical method for grading the cognitive state of patients for the clinician. J Psychiatr Res 12:189–198, 1975

Green AR, Sant K, Bowdler JM, et al: Further evidence for a relationship between changes in GABA concentration in rat brain and enhanced monoamine mediated behavioral responses following repeated electroconvulsive shock. Neuropharmacology 21:981–984, 1982

Greenberg PE, Stiglin LE, Finkelstein SN, et al: Depression: a neglected major illness. J Clin Psychiatry 54:419–424, 1993

Grover BB: Handbook of Electrotherapy. Philadelphia, PA, Davis, 1924

Grunhaus L, Pande AC, Hasket RF: Full and abbreviated courses of maintenance electroconvulsive therapy. Convulsive Therapy 6:130–138, 1990

Hargrove EA, Bennett AE, Ford FR: The value of subconvulsive electrostimulation in the treatment of some emotional disorders. Am J Psychiatry 8:612–616, 1953

Hickie I, Scott E, Mitchell P, et al: Subcortical hyperintensities on magnetic resonance imaging: clinical correlates and prognostic significance in patients with severe depression. Biol Psychiatry 37:151–160, 1995

Hitzemann RJ, Hitzemann BA, Blatt S, et al: Repeated electroconvulsive shock: effect on sodium dependency and regional distribution of opioid binding sites. Mol Pharmacol 31:562–566, 1987

Huettner JE, Bean BP: Block of N-methyl-D-aspartate-activated current by the anticonvulsant MK-801: selective binding to open channels. Proc Natl Acad Sci U S A 85:1307–1311, 1988

Jaffe R, Dubin WR, Roemer R, et al: Continuation and maintenance ECT—efficacy and safety. Paper presented at the 142nd annual meeting of the American Psychiatric Association, San Francisco, CA, May 1989

Karlinsky H, Shulman KI: The clinical use of electroconvulsive therapy in old age. J Am Geriatr Soc 32:183–186, 1984

Kramer BA: Maintenance ECT: a survey of practice. Convuls Ther 3:260–268, 1987

Krueger RB, Sackeim HA, Gamzu ER: Pharmacological treatment of the cognitive side effects of ECT: a review. Psychopharm Bull 28:409–424, 1992

Krystal AD, Wiener RD, McCall WV, et al: The effects of ECT stimulus dose and electrode placement on the ictal electroencephalogram: an intraindividual cross-over study. Biol Psychiatry 24:759–767, 1993

Kuba K, Kumamoto E: Long-term potentiation in vertebrate synapses: a variety of cascades with common subprocesses. Prog Neurobiol 34:197–269, 1990

Laursen H, Gjerris A, Bolwig TG, et al: Cerebral edema and vascular permeability to serum proteins following electroconvulsive shock in rats. Convulsive Therapy 7:237–244, 1991

Lerer B, Weiner RD, Belmaker RH (eds): ECT: Basic Mechanisms. Washington, DC, American Psychiatric Association, 1984

Lerer B, Shapira B, Calev A, et al: Antidepressant and cognitive effects of twice- versus three-times weekly ECT. Am J Psychiatry 152:564–570, 1995

Levy SD, Albrecht E: Electroconvulsive therapy: a survey of use in the private psychiatric hospital. J Clin Psychiatry 46:125–127, 1985

Lloyd KG, Thuret F, Pilc A: Upregulation of gamma-aminobutyric acid (GABA)$_B$ binding sites in rat frontal cortex: a common action of repeated administration of different classes of antidepressants and electroshock. J Pharmacol Exp Ther 235:191–199, 1985

Loo H, Galinowski A, de Carvalho W, et al: The clonidine test in posttraumatic stress disorder. Am J Psychiatry 148:810, 1991

Macdonald RL, Olsen RW: GABA$_A$ receptor channels. Annu Rev Neurosci 17:569–602, 1994

MacDonald JF, Bartlett MC, Mody I, et al: Actions of ketamine, phencyclidine and MK-801 on NMDA receptor currents in cultured mouse hippocampal neurons. J Physiol (Lond) 432:483–508, 1991

Maltbie AA, Wingfield MS, Volow MR, et al: Electroconvulsive therapy in the presence of brain tumor. J Nerv Ment Dis 168:400–405, 1980

Matzen TA, Martin RL, Watt TJ, et al: The use of maintenance electroconvulsive therapy for relapsing depression. Jefferson Journal of Psychiatry 6:52–58, 1988

McCall WV, Farah BA: Greater ictal EEG regularity during RUL ECT is associated with greater treatment efficiency (abstract). Convulsive Therapy 11:69, 1994

McCall WV, Shelp FE, Weiner RD, et al: Convulsive threshold differences in right unilateral and bilateral ECT. Biol Psychiatry 24:759–767, 1993

McNamara JO: Cellular and molecular basis of epilepsy. J Neurosci 14:3413–3425, 1994

Meduna L: Autobiography, part 1. Convulsive Therapy 1:43–57, 1985

Monroe RRJ: Maintenance electroconvulsive therapy. Psychiatr Clin North Am 14:947–960, 1991

Mukherjee S, Sackeim HA, Schnur DB: Electroconvulsive therapy of acute mania episodes: a review of 50 years' experience. Am J Psychiatry 151:169–176, 1994

Murphy E: The prognosis of depression in old age. Br J Psychiatry 142:111–119, 1983

Nobler MS, Sackeim HA, Solomou M, et al: EEG manifestations during ECT: effects of electrode placement and stimulus intensity. Biol Psychiatry 34:321–330, 1993

Nowak G, Zak J: Repeated electroconvulsive shock (ECS) enhances striatal D1 dopamine receptor turnover in rats. Eur J Pharmacol 167:307–308, 1989

Nutt DJ, Glue P: The neurobiology of ECT: animal studies, in The Clinical Science of Electroconvulsive Therapy. Edited by Coffey CE. Washington, DC, American Psychiatric Association, 1993, pp 213–234

Nutt DJ, Cowen PJ, Green AR: Studies of the postictal rise in seizure threshold. Eur J Pharmacol 71:287–295, 1981

Ottosson JO: Seizure characteristics and therapeutic efficiency in electroconvulsive therapy: an analysis of the antidepressant efficiency of grand mal and lidocaine-modified seizures. J Nerv Ment Dis 135:239–251, 1962

Pascual-Leone A, Rubio B, Pallardo F, et al: Rapid-rate transcranial magnetic stimulation of left dorsolateral prefrontal cortex in drug-resistant depression. Lancet 348:233–237, 1996

Petrides G, Dhossche D, Fink M, et al: Continuation ECT: relapse prevention in affective disorders. Convulsive Therapy 10:189–194, 1994

Plaznik A, Kostowski W, Stefanski R: The influence of antidepressive treatment on GABA related mechanisms in the rat hippocampus: behavioral studies. Pharmacol Biochem Behav 33:749–753, 1989

Posner JB, Plum F, Van Poznak A: Cerebral metabolism during electrically induced seizures in man. Arch Neurol 28:388–395, 1969

Prudic J, Haskett RF, Mulsant B, et al: Resistance to antidepressant medications and short-term clinical response to ECT. Am J Psychiatry 153:985–992, 1996

Rasmussen K, Abrams R: Treatment of Parkinson's disease with electroconvulsive therapy. Psychiatr Clin North Am 14:925–934, 1991

Sackeim HA: Central issues regarding the mechanism of action of electroconvulsive therapy: directions for future research. Psychopharm Bull 30:281–308, 1994

Sackeim HA, Prudic J, Devanand DP, et al: The impact of medication resistance and continuation pharmacotherapy on relapse following response to electroconvulsive therapy in major depression. J Clin Psychopharmacol 10:96–104, 1990

Sackeim HA, Devanand DP, Prudic J: Stimulus intensity, seizure threshold and seizure duration: impact on the efficacy and safety of electroconvulsive therapy. Psychiatr Clin North Am 14:803–843, 1991

Sackeim HA, Prudic J, Devanand DP, et al: Effects of stimulus intensity and electrode placement on the efficacy and cognitive effects of electroconvulsive therapy. N Engl J Med 328:839–846, 1993

Sackeim HA, Devanand DP, Nobler MS: Electroconvulsive therapy, in Psychopharmacology: The Fourth Generation of Progress. Edited by Bloom FE, Kupfer DJ. New York, Raven, 1995, pp 1123–1141

Scott AIF, Douglass RHB, Whitfield A, et al: Time course of cerebral magnetic resonance changes after electroconvulsive therapy. Br J Psychiatry 156:551–553, 1990

Shapira B, Gorfine M, Lerer B: A prospective study of lithium continuation therapy in depressed patients who have responded to electroconvulsive therapy. Convulsive Therapy 11:80–85, 1995

Small JG, Klapper MH, Kellams JJ, et al: Electroconvulsive therapy compared with lithium in the management of manic states. Arch Gen Psychiatry 45:727–732, 1988

Spiker DG, Stein J, Rich CL: Delusional depression and electroconvulsive therapy: one year later. Convulsive Therapy 1:167–172, 1985

Stewart C, Reid I: Electroconvulsive stimulation and synaptic plasticity in the rat. Brain Res 620:139–141, 1993

Thienhaus OJ, Margletta S, Bennet JA: A study of the clinical efficacy of maintenance ECT. J Clin Psychiatry 51:141–144, 1990

Thornton JE, Mulsant BH, Dealy R, et al: A retrospective study of maintenance electroconvulsive therapy in a university-based psychiatric practice. Convulsive Therapy 6:121–129, 1990

Tortella FC, Long JB: Endogenous anticonvulsant substance in rat cerebrospinal fluid after a generalized seizure. Science 228:1106–1108, 1985

Tortella FC, Long JB: Characterization of opioid peptide-like anticonvulsant activity in rat cerebrospinal fluid. Brain Res 456:139–146, 1988

Tortella FC, Long JB, Hong J-S, et al: Modulation of endogenous opioid systems by electroconvulsive shock. Convulsive Therapy 5:261–273, 1989

Vanelle JM, Loo H, Galinowski A, et al: Maintenance ECT in intractable manic-depressive disorders. Convulsive Therapy 10:195–205, 1994

Weiner RD: ECT and seizure threshold: effects of stimulus wave form and electrode placement. Biol Psychiatry 15:225–241, 1980

Weiner RD: Does electroconvulsive therapy cause brain damage? Behav Brain Sci 7:1–53, 1984

Weiner RD, Coffey CE: Minimizing therapeutic differences between bilateral and unilateral nondominant ECT. Convulsive Therapy 2:261–265, 1986

Weiner RD, Rogers HJ, Davidson SR, et al: Effects of electroconvulsive therapy upon brain electrical activity. Ann N Y Acad Sci 462:270–281, 1986

Zielinski RJ, Roose SP, Devanand DP, et al: Cardiovascular complications of ECT in depressed patients with cardiac disease. Am J Psychiatry 150:904–909, 1993

Zis AP, Grof P, Webster M, et al: Prediction of relapse in recurrent affective disorder. Psychopharmacol Bull 16:47–49, 1980

SECTION II

Psychopharmacological Treatment

Donald F. Klein, M.D., Section Editor

SEVENTEEN

Treatment of Depression

Dennis S. Charney, M.D.,
Robert M. Berman, M.D., and
Helen L. Miller, M.D.

The effectiveness of the pharmacological treatment of depression compares very favorably with the pharmacological treatment of chronic medical disorders, such as hypertension and diabetes. The spectrum of available antidepressant medications permits the clinician to select a specific antidepressant drug based on depressive subtype and coexisting medical conditions. For patients who do not respond to the initial antidepressant drug prescribed, a range of options exists for subsequent drug treatment approaches. In this chapter, we review the clinical strategies involved in the drug treatment of depressed patients.

HISTORICAL BACKGROUND

The most dramatic and fundamental discoveries in the pharmacotherapy of psychiatric disorders took place in the two decades after World War II. In the early 1950s, several investigators noted that iproniazid, initially used to treat tuberculosis, caused an elevation of mood in some patients (Crane 1956). In the United States, Kline and colleagues started to use iproniazid in depressed patients. Kline's original impetus to try iproniazid for treatment of depression was further supported by the effects (e.g., hyperalertness and hyperactivity) of that drug on laboratory animals. The clinical efficacy of iproniazid in the treatment of depression was quickly established (Kline 1970; Loomer et al. 1957, 1958). Consequently, additional irreversible monoamine oxidase inhibitors (MAOIs) were synthesized, found to be effective for depression, and approved for general use. After about 5 years of widespread use, the highly effective MAOIs became increasingly less popular in the treatment of depression because of their side-effect profile. Over the past decade, reversible selective MAOIs were introduced in Europe and South America, and these medications have a favorable side-effect profile with reduced tyramine sensitivity. The future availability of those compounds in the United States may enhance psychiatrists' interest in this class of antidepressant drugs.

At approximately the same time that iproniazid was reported to be an antidepressant, Roland Kuhn (1958) was testing the tricyclic compound G 2022355 (imipramine) in the treatment of psychiatric patients in Switzerland. Kuhn observed that imipramine, although lacking antipsychotic properties, improved depressed mood in some schizophrenic patients. Subsequently, imipramine was documented as an effective antidepressant (Kuhn 1970a, 1970b, 1989). The mechanism of action underlying imipramine's antidepressant properties was not initially known. Subsequently, it was determined that the ability of imipramine to inhibit the reuptake of norepinephrine and serotonin (5-HT) was related to its antidepressant activity (Carlsson et al. 1968; Glowinski and Axelrod 1964). This discovery facilitated the development of other tricyclic antidepressants (TCAs) that inhibited monoamine reuptake, with variable potency.

A search began in the 1970s for drugs that would selectively enhance the function of one of the monoamine systems rather than all three. A specific and potent dopamine reuptake inhibitor, nomifensine, was synthesized and used with success in the treatment of depression; however, hematological side effects (i.e., hemolytic anemia) precluded its wide use.

The search also led to the development of compounds with primary actions on serotonin. Fluoxetine was the first available selective serotonin reuptake inhibitor (SSRI) to be marketed for the treatment of depression (Beasley et al. 1991, 1992). Subsequently, other SSRIs— sertraline (Amin et al. 1989), paroxetine (Rickels et al. 1992), fluvoxamine (Wilde et al. 1993), and citalopram (Montgomery and Djarv 1996)—have been developed and are useful for treating major depression. Further preclinical understanding has led to the strategy of developing agents that specifically target multiple monoamine receptors or reuptake sites. Examples of this generation of antidepressant agents include venlafaxine (an SSRI and noradrenergic reuptake inhibitor), nefazodone (a specific 5-HT$_2$ antagonist and weak SSRI), and mirtazapine (a 5-HT$_2$, 5-HT$_3$, and α_2-adrenergic antagonist).

PHARMACOTHERAPY FOR THE ACUTE DEPRESSIVE EPISODE

Early recognition and treatment of depressive illness may have important implications for treatment responsiveness. The shorter the episode of depression prior to initiating treatment, the higher the chances of recovery are and the lower the impairment in social and vocational adjustment will be (Keller et al. 1982a, 1982b; Lavori et al. 1984).

Medical Evaluation

The initial evaluation of patients presenting with depressive symptoms should include a careful medical history, a physical examination, and appropriate laboratory testing. Clinicians must consider the possible existence of physical illnesses that may present as depression or have depression as an associated symptom. Medical conditions that should be considered when evaluating depressed patients are listed in Table 17–1. In some cases, treatment of the underlying medical condition is sufficient to eliminate depressive symptoms. However, in many cases, depressive symptoms will persist, necessitating the use of antidepressant drugs. Drug-induced depression will occasionally be encountered. The drug classes listed in Table 17–2 have been associated with depressive symptoms. The patient's medication should be reviewed and drugs that are less centrally active substituted when possible.

Another rationale for a comprehensive medical assessment is that the identification of specific medical disorders will influence the choice of antidepressant drugs. The blockade of neurotransmitter receptors by antidepressant drugs is related to numerous side effects of antidepressant drugs and drug-drug interactions. Table 17–3 summarizes the relationship between specific receptors and antidepressant-induced side effects. The antidepressants with the highest and lowest affinity for these receptors are listed (Richelson 1991; Richelson and

Table 17–1. Medical conditions associated with depressive symptoms

Cardiovascular disease
  Cardiomyopathy
  Cerebral ischemia
  Congestive heart failure
  Myocardial infarction
Neurological disorders
  Alzheimer's disease
  Multiple sclerosis
  Parkinson's disease
  Head trauma
  Narcolepsy
  Brain tumors
  Wilson's disease
Cancer
  Pancreatic cancer
  Lung cancer
Endocrine disorders
  Hypothyroidism
  Hyperthyroidism
  Cushing's disease
  Addison's disease
  Hyperparathyroidism
  Hypoparathyroidism
  Hypoglycemia
  Pheochromocytoma
  Carcinoid
  Ovarian failure
  Testicular failure
Infectious diseases
  Syphilis
  Mononucleosis
  Hepatitis
  Acquired immunodeficiency syndrome
  Tuberculosis
  Influenza
  Encephalitis
  Lyme disease
Nutritional deficiencies
  Folate
  Vitamin B_{12}
  Pyridoxine (B_6)
  Riboflavin (B_2)
  Thiamine (B_1)
  Iron

Nelson 1984). Antidepressant drug recommendations based on coexisting specific medical disorders are reviewed in Table 17–4 (Richelson 1989).

In addition, stimulants may be considered a treatment alternative in some medically ill populations. Although placebo-controlled trials offer little support for the antidepressant efficacy of stimulants in major depression, multiple studies support their usefulness in medically ill geriatric populations with depressive symptoms characterized by apathy (Satel and Nelson 1989).

Cardiovascular disease. The SSRIs (fluoxetine, sertraline, paroxetine) and bupropion are preferred in patients with heart conduction disease, orthostatic hypotension, ventricular arrhythmias, and/or ischemic heart disease. These drugs have little or no effect on heart rate, heart rhythm, or blood pressure. Although the SSRIs have not been systematically evaluated in patients with cardiovascular disease, they do not

Table 17–2. Classes of drugs associated with depressive symptoms

Drugs of abuse
  Phencyclidine
  Marijuana
  Amphetamines
  Cocaine
  Opiates
  Sedative-hypnotics
  Alcohol
Antihypertensive drugs
  Reserpine
  Propranolol
  Methyldopa
  Guanethidine
  Clonidine
Gastrointestinal drugs
  Cimetidine
Cytotoxic agents
Corticosteroids
Oral contraceptives

Table 17–3. Relationship between blockade of neurotransmitter receptors and antidepressant-induced side effects

Receptor subtype	Side effects	Receptor affinity[a]	
		High	**Low**
Histamine-1 receptor	Sedation	Doxepin ++++	Venlafaxine 0
	Weight gain	Trimipramine ++++	Nefazodone ±
	Hypotension	Amitriptyline +++	Bupropion ±
	Potentiation of CNS depressants	Maprotiline +++	Trazodone +
		Mirtazapine +++	Desipramine +
			Nortriptyline +
Muscarinic receptors	Dry mouth	Amitriptyline +++	Bupropion 0
	Blurred vision	Clomipramine +++	Trazodone 0
	Urinary retention	Protriptyline +++	Nefazodone 0
	Constipation		Venlafaxine 0
	Memory dysfunction		Mirtazapine 0
	Tachycardia		SSRIs ±
			Nortriptyline +
			Desipramine +
			SSRIs +
α₁ Receptors	Postural hypotension	Doxepin ++++	Venlafaxine 0
	Reflex tachycardia	Trimipramine ++++	Bupropion 0
	Potentiation of antihypertensive effects of prazosin	Trazodone ++++	Mirtazapine +
		Nefazodone +++	SSRIs +
		Amoxapine +++	
α₂ Receptors	Blockade of antihypertensive effects of clonidine, α-methyldopa, guanfacine	Mirtazapine +++	Bupropion 0
		Trimipramine ++	Venlafaxine 0

	Amitriptyline	++	SSRIs	+
	Trazodone	++	Nefazodone	+
Serotonin-2 receptors				
Ejaculatory dysfunction	Amoxapine	++++	Bupropion	0
Hypotension	Nefazodone	+++	Venlafaxine	0
Alleviation of migraine headaches	Trazodone	+++	SSRIs	±
	Doxepin	++	Desipramine	±
	Amitriptyline	++		

Note. 0 = no affinity; ± = negligible affinity; + = weak affinity; ++ = moderate affinity; +++ = high affinity; ++++ = very high affinity; CNS = central nervous system; SSRIs = selective serotonin reuptake inhibitors.

[a]Drugs with higher receptor affinity are associated with a greater frequency of receptor-mediated side effects.

Source. Adapted from Cusack et al. 1994; Richelson 1991.

prolong either the P-R or the QRS intervals or cause orthostatic hypotension as TCAs do. No serious cardiovascular side effects have been reported with SSRIs, except for several cases of severe sinus node slowing (Buff et al. 1991; Ellison et al. 1990; Feder 1991; Glassman et al. 1993).

One investigation of bupropion in depressed patients with severe heart disease (Roose et al. 1991) found it to be free of effects on heart conduction and contractility. Neither SSRIs nor bupropion has yet been carefully investigated in patients with arrhythmias and heart failure (Glassman and Preud'homme 1993).

TCAs have been used safely in patients with preexisting cardiac disease for many years, but these drugs generally should be avoided as first-choice antidepressants in these patients. The effects of TCAs to slow intraventricular conduction, as reflected in the increased QRS, P-R, and Q-T_c intervals on the electrocardiogram, may pose a risk to patients with prolonged conduction times or heart block and patients taking quinidine or other type 1 antiarrhythmics. The orthostatic hypotension and rebound tachycardia produced by TCAs are risks in patients with congestive heart failure, particularly those with left ventricular impairment, and in patients taking drugs such as diuretics or vasodilators (Glassman and Preud'homme 1993).

In the past, it had been suggested that certain preexisting arrhythmias would benefit from TCA treatment because, at therapeutic plasma concentrations, TCAs suppress arrhythmias, and their cardiac effects are similar to those of class I antiarrhythmic drugs (Glassman and Bigger 1981; Glassman et al. 1987; Rawling and Fozzard 1979; Weld and Bigger 1980). However, several multicenter studies reported that class I antiarrhythmic drugs are associated with increased mortality when administered to patients with ventricular arrhythmias postmyocardial infarction (Cardiac Arrhythmia Suppression Trial Investigators 1989; Cardiac Arrhythmia Suppression Trial II Investigators 1992; Horowitz et al. 1987; Morganroth and

Table 17–4.   **Antidepressant drugs of choice for depressed patients with comorbid medical disorders**

Comorbid disorder	Drugs of choice
Cardiovascular	
Congestive heart failure or ischemic heart disease	For each of these conditions, SSRIs (fluoxetine, sertraline, or paroxetine) or bupropion is preferred.
Conduction disturbance	Of the tricyclic antidepressants, nortriptyline or desipramine is best.
Tachycardia	
Orthostatic hypotension	
Neurological	
Seizure disorder	Desipramine, MAOIs, venlafaxine, SSRIs, mirtazapine (avoid bupropion, clomipramine, maprotiline)
Organic brain syndrome	SSRIs, bupropion, trazodone
Migraine headaches	Amitriptyline, trazodone, amoxapine, doxepin
Parkinson's disease	Amitriptyline, doxepin, SSRIs (avoid amoxapine)
Chronic pain	SSRIs, amitriptyline, doxepin
Stroke	SSRIs
Gastrointestinal	
Peptic ulcer disease	Doxepin, trimipramine
Chronic diarrhea	Doxepin, trimipramine, amitriptyline
Chronic constipation	SSRIs, bupropion, trazodone, nefazodone
Sexual	
Erectile failure	Bupropion, nefazodone, trazodone
Anorgasmia	Bupropion, desipramine, nefazodone, trazodone
Ophthalmological	
Angle-closure glaucoma	SSRIs, bupropion, trazodone, nefazodone

Note.   SSRIs = selective serotonin reuptake inhibitors; MAOIs = monoamine oxidase inhibitors.
Source.   Adapted from Richelson 1989.

Goin 1991; Pratt et al. 1990). Studies have also documented that these antiarrhythmic drugs may have a mortality risk when used in patients with atrial fibrillation (Coplen et al. 1990; Falk 1989; Selzer and Wray 1964). Class I antiarrhythmic drugs are sodium channel blockers. TCAs have class I antiarrhythmic properties. Thus, Glassman and colleagues (1993) suggested that TCAs may have mortality risks similar to those of antiarrhythmics when used in depressed patients with a recent myocardial infarction and, perhaps, in a wider range of cardiac disease. Investigators have hypothesized that the risk of using class I antiarrhythmics increases proportionately with the severity of ischemic heart disease (Bigger 1990; Echt et al. 1991).

Venlafaxine has been associated with sustained elevated blood pressure in a dose-dependent manner, with approximately 13% of patients taking doses greater than 300 mg/day experiencing clinically significant elevations (Feighner 1995). In approximately one-third of patients, blood pressure will eventually diminish, as evidenced during 1-year follow-up studies (Feighner 1995). The risk of hypertension appears reduced with the extended release formulation, which is used at lower total daily doses. Still, concurrent administration of antihypertensive medications may be warranted in some cases (Feighner 1995). Both trazodone and nefazodone have been associated with hypotension (Robinson et al. 1996). Further studies are needed to assess the safety of these medications in patients with underlying conduction abnormalities and ischemic heart disease.

Neurological disease. Desipramine, MAOIs, SSRIs, and trazodone are preferred for depressed patients with seizure disorders or for patients at risk for seizures based on predisposing factors such as head trauma, multiple central nervous system (CNS) medications, and substance abuse. These drugs lower the seizure threshold less than other antidepressant drugs do, with a 1.0%–1.5% incidence of seizures during the first 2 years of treatment (see Rosenstein et al. 1993). Mirtazapine has also been associated with a low incidence of seizures (R. Davis and Wilde 1995). Three antidepressant drugs—maprotiline, clomipramine, and bupropion—should be particularly avoided in these patients at risk for seizures (Jick et al. 1983; Settle 1992; Trimble 1978). Maprotiline causes an increased incidence of seizures with rapid dose escalation and higher doses (Dessain et al. 1987). Clomipramine has been reported to have a high seizure risk (Peck et al. 1983; Trimble 1978). Bupropion should be avoided in patients at risk for seizure disorders because in doses higher than 300 mg/day, it has an observed seizure rate approximately twice that observed with most other antidepressants (Davidson 1989; Johnston et al. 1991). Use of the extended release formulation appears to lower the risk.

Depression is a common sequela of stroke, occurring in an estimated 30% of patients. SSRIs may be safer than TCAs in treatment of these patients because of their lower incidence of cardiovascular side effects and lack of anticholinergic properties.

Confusion in patients with organic brain syndromes can be exacerbated by anticholinergic effects of antidepressant drugs. Therefore, drugs such as SSRIs, trazodone, maprotiline, amoxapine, bupropion, and venlafaxine are indicated in those patients. These agents should also be used in patients with other conditions, such as neurogenic bladder and prostate disease, that may worsen as a result of cholinergic receptor blockade.

Evidence indicates that migraine headaches may be effectively treated with serotonin receptor antagonists, particularly the 5-HT_{1D} receptor antagonist sumatriptan (Humphrey 1992). Therefore, antidepressant drugs such as amoxapine and trazodone, with high affinity for serotonin receptors, may be useful for depressed patients with migraines.

Depression occurs in approximately 50% of patients with Parkinson's disease. Reduced serotonin function is evident in parkinsonian patients with depression (Mayeux et al. 1984). SSRIs may be particularly helpful in these patients. The anticholinergic effects of antidepressants such as amitriptyline and doxepin reduce the motor deficits of Parkinson's disease. Amoxapine should be avoided because of its dopamine receptor–blocking actions.

Cancer. About 25% of patients with cancer report clinically significant depressive symptoms. Selection of antidepressant drugs should be based on cancer-related somatic problems. Patients experiencing significant weight loss and reduced appetite may benefit from TCAs that increase appetite and produce weight gain. On the other hand, the anticholinergic effects of TCAs may be contraindicated in cancer patients recovering from abdominal surgery or stomatitis. SSRIs, bupropion, nefazodone, or mirtazapine should be used in these patients.

Allergic disease. Antidepressant drugs such as doxepin, trimipramine, amitriptyline, and maprotiline, which have strong antihistamine properties, are indicated for depressed patients with severe allergic disorders such as dermatological allergies and idiopathic pruritus.

Gastrointestinal disease. Depressed patients with peptic ulcer disease may particularly benefit from trimipramine and doxepin because of their strong anticholinergic and histamine-2

(H$_2$) antagonist properties. Drugs with potent anticholinergic effects should be avoided in treatment of depressed patients with chronic constipation. Conversely, these drugs may be useful for depressed patients with chronic diarrhea.

Sexual dysfunction. TCAs, SSRIs, and MAOIs have been reported to reduce erectile function and, therefore, should be avoided in patients with erectile impotence (Segraves 1992). In contrast, bupropion does not produce erectile dysfunction and when used in patients with a history of TCA-induced erectile failure, normal function is restored (Gardner and Johnston 1985). Trazodone, nefazodone, and mirtazapine may also prove useful in this depressed population.

Inability to ejaculate, greatly delayed ejaculation, and anorgasmia have been reported with use of TCAs, MAOIs, and SSRIs (Segraves 1992). Bupropion is not associated with these side effects and is the drug of choice for patients prone to the development of these symptoms (Gardner and Johnston 1985).

Ophthalmic disease. Antidepressant drugs with little or no anticholinergic effects should be used in depressed patients with angle-closure glaucoma.

Psychiatric Evaluation

The initial psychiatric evaluation of the depressed patient should focus on determining whether other psychiatric disorders coexist with the depression and identifying depressive disorder subtype. The existence of comorbid psychiatric disorders will influence the choice of antidepressant. For example, SSRIs are the drug of choice for patients with comorbid depression and obsessive-compulsive disorder (OCD) (Goodman et al. 1990). Furthermore, preliminary evidence suggests that the SSRIs may be indicated for patients with posttraumatic stress disorder (PTSD) (Nagy et al. 1993) and for

obese patients (Marcus et al. 1990). MAOIs may be the most effective agent for depressed patients with panic disorder (Sheehan et al. 1983a); however, SSRIs may be a preferable first-line agent in this population. Evidence (discussed in greater detail later in this chapter; see section, "Depressive Subtypes and Antidepressant Response") indicates that specific depressive subtypes (i.e., atypical depression, delusional depression, bipolar depression) respond preferentially to specific antidepressant agents.

FACTORS INFLUENCING THE ANTIDEPRESSANT DRUG OF CHOICE

Symptomatic Predictors of Antidepressant Response

Most studies indicate that depressed patients with melancholia respond better to TCAs than do patients with nonmelancholic depression (Paykel 1972; Raskin and Crook 1976; Simpson et al. 1976). Of the individual symptoms, psychomotor retardation, loss of interest, and anhedonia are the best prognostic indicators of antidepressant response (Downing and Rickels 1973; Hollister and Overall 1965; Overall et al. 1966; Paykel 1972; Raskin and Crook 1976; Simpson et al. 1976). In contrast, sleep and appetite disturbances are not predictive of antidepressant response (for review, see Joyce and Paykel 1989).

Regarding specific antidepressant choice, multiple studies suggest that SSRIs and TCAs are equivalently effective in various depressed populations, including severely depressed inpatient and outpatient melancholic samples (e.g., Feighner et al. 1993; Moller et al. 1993; Stuppaeck et al. 1994). Furthermore, many melancholic patients who are refractory to TCAs have subsequently responded to SSRIs (e.g., Amsterdam et al. 1994). Nevertheless, in the subgroup of melancholic depressed inpatients, treatment efficacy has been best established for the TCAs, which may prove more efficacious than the SSRIs (Danish University Antidepressant Study Group 1990; Roose et al. 1994). Further studies are needed to confirm this latter conclusion. Venlafaxine has been reported to be more effective in inpatients with melancholia than fluoxetine or placebo (Clerk et al. 1994; Guelfi et al. 1995).

In patients with nonmelancholic depression, TCAs are superior to placebo (Quitkin et al. 1989). Consistent evidence maintains that depressed patients with an associated personality disorder or narcissistic, hypochondriacal, or histrionic personality traits respond less well to TCAs than do subjects without personality disorders (Bielski and Friedel 1976; Hirschfeld et al. 1986; Paykel 1979; Pfohl et al. 1984; Shawcross and Tyrer 1985). MAOIs or SSRIs may be helpful for these patients.

Neurobiological Predictors of Antidepressant Response

Numerous research studies have attempted to identify neurobiological predictors of antidepressant response (Joyce and Paykel 1989). The results of these investigations have generally been disappointing. The hypothesis suggesting the existence of norepinephrine- and serotonin-deficient depressive subtypes has not been confirmed (Berman et al. 1996). Furthermore, characterization of the depression by levels of the norepinephrine metabolite 3-methoxy-4-hydroxyphenylglycol (MHPG) or the serotonin metabolite 5-hydroxyindoleacetic acid (5-HIAA) has not been of practical use in the selection of antidepressant drugs. Preliminary data suggest that low cerebrospinal fluid (CSF) 5-HIAA relates to therapeutic responses to zimeldine (Aberg-Wistedt et al. 1981), clomipramine (van Praag 1977), imipramine (Goodwin et al. 1973), and nortriptyline (Asberg et al. 1973).

The ratio of serum tryptophan (the amino acid precursor of serotonin) to large neutral amino acids has been found to have modest value (25% of the variance) in predicting clinical response to amitriptyline, clomipramine, and paroxetine (Møller et al. 1983, 1990). The ratio

of tyrosine (the amino acid precursor of norepinephrine and dopamine) to large neutral amino acids may relate to nortriptyline (Møller et al. 1985) and maprotiline (Møller et al. 1986) responses.

A series of investigations have examined whether the effect of single doses of a stimulant drug (e.g., amphetamine, methylphenidate) on mood is predictive of antidepressant response. Mood elevation after stimulant administration has been found to be associated with a therapeutic response to imipramine (P. Brown and Brawley 1983; Sabelli et al. 1983; van Kammen and Murphy 1978) and desipramine (Ettigi et al. 1983; Sabelli et al. 1983; Spar and La Rue 1985). An absent or dysphoric mood response after stimulant administration has been proposed to predict therapeutic responses to amitriptyline (P. Brown and Brawley 1983; Sabelli et al. 1983; Spar and La Rue 1985) and nortriptyline (Sabelli et al. 1983). Similar to the studies involving urinary MHPG and amino acid ratios, the high variability in the findings limits therapeutic application.

Blunted suppression of cortisol after dexamethasone administration (Carroll 1982) usually normalizes during successful antidepressant treatment (Greden et al. 1983; Holsboer et al. 1982), and failure to normalize is associated with poor outcome and early relapse (Greden et al. 1983; Targum 1984). However, the lack of cortisol suppression by dexamethasone is not associated with a greater likelihood of responding to antidepressant treatment in general (W. A. Brown and Shuey 1980; Greden et al. 1983) or to specific antidepressant drugs (W. A. Brown and Qualls 1981; Gitlin and Gerner 1986; Greden et al. 1981). It has been suggested, however, that this neuroendocrine dysfunction is associated with lack of response to placebo or psychotherapy and the need for antidepressant drugs or electroconvulsive therapy (ECT) (Peselow et al. 1986; Rush 1983).

Preliminary data indicate that a reduced rapid eye movement (REM) latency is associated with a poor placebo response (Coble et al.

1979) and a positive response to TCAs (Coble et al. 1979; Hochli et al. 1986; Kupfer et al. 1976, 1980; Svendsen and Christensen 1981).

DEPRESSIVE SUBTYPES AND ANTIDEPRESSANT RESPONSE

The treatments of choice for depressive subtypes are considered in the following sections (Table 17–5).

Unipolar Major Depression

An extensive review of overall efficacy of antidepressant drug treatment in uncomplicated unipolar major depression indicates that approximately 65% of patients treated with antidepressants improve compared with 30% given placebos (J. M. Davis 1985). To date, one antidepressant drug does not stand out as having better efficacy than others. Therefore, the initial choice of an antidepressant drug for a patient with unipolar major depression, with or without melancholia, depends on the associated medical conditions and the drug-induced side effects. Purchase price may be a factor to consider when selecting an antidepressant, because the generic TCAs are much less expensive than the SSRIs and bupropion.

The discovery of the TCAs represented a

Table 17–5.   **Treatments of choice for depressive subtypes**

Major depression
  All antidepressants have equal efficacy.
  Choice of antidepressant is based on side effects, comorbid medical conditions, family
    history of drug treatment response, and previous response to antidepressants.
Atypical depression
  Monoamine oxidase inhibitors (MAOIs) have superior efficacy to tricyclic antidepressants
    (TCAs).
  Selective serotonin reuptake inhibitors (SSRIs) need further study. Superior to placebo
    but not imipramine.
Delusional depression
  Antidepressant alone usually is ineffective.
  Antidepressant and antipsychotic combination is effective in many patients.
  Electroconvulsive therapy is probably the most effective treatment.
Bipolar depression
  All antidepressants may produce mania or hypomania (bupropion may be least likely).
  MAOIs may be more effective than TCAs.
  Lithium may be more effective than in unipolar depression.
  Lithium-MAOI and lithium-carbamazepine combinations may be effective for patients
    with refractory conditions.
Dysthymic disorder
  Antidepressant efficacy may be reduced compared with major depression.
  MAOIs may be more effective than TCAs.
  SSRIs appear effective.
Geriatric depression
  Drug of choice is based largely on side-effect profile.
  Low or absent anticholinergic properties—desipramine, nortriptyline, SSRIs, bupropion.
  Reduced cardiovascular adverse effects—desipramine, nortriptyline, SSRIs, bupropion.
  Generally use lower doses. ECT is often beneficial.
Comorbid psychiatric disorders
  Panic disorder—bupropion and trazodone are not effective.
  Obsessive-compulsive disorder—SSRIs are the drugs of choice.
  Eating disorders—SSRIs may be the drugs of choice.

major breakthrough in clinical psychiatry. The efficacy of this class of antidepressants for moderate and severe depression is unquestioned. Although the use of these medications as a first-choice agent is appropriate in many cases, these compounds are being used less often because of the availability of newer antidepressant drugs with less adverse side-effect profiles and less lethality with overdose.

The availability of the SSRIs has provided another therapeutic option for the clinician. In fact, fluoxetine is the most widely used antidepressant in the United States. SSRIs are appropriate first-choice antidepressant drugs because of their broad spectrum of efficacy, favorable side-effect profile, and lack of lethality with overdose. The SSRIs are effective in psychiatric disorders that frequently occur in combination with depression, such as OCD and PTSD, conditions for which TCAs (except clomipramine) are generally ineffective. Note that the SSRIs have adverse side effects, such as headache, tremor, nausea, diarrhea, insomnia, agitation, and nervousness, that may need to be attended to. Sexual dysfunction (particularly anorgasmia in men and women) and ejaculatory disturbances are more common with these drugs than with TCAs. In addition, paroxetine, sertraline, and fluoxetine inhibit cytochrome P450 (CYP) enzymes, thereby reducing the metabolism of drugs such as warfarin, phenytoin, and digoxin, which are metabolized by this system (Bergstrom et al. 1992; Crewe et al. 1992). Nefazodone, SSRIs, and TCAs may significantly inhibit metabolism of terfenadine and astemizole. Because the parent compounds of these antihistamines may cause fatal arrhythmias, these agents should not be prescribed with the aforementioned antidepressants (Nemeroff et al. 1996; Riesenman 1995).

Bupropion is an antidepressant with different neurochemical properties from those of other available antidepressant drugs. It has weak effects on noradrenergic and serotonin reuptake; its dopamine-enhancing actions are sufficiently weak to make this an unlikely mechanism of action. Bupropion is comparable in efficacy to the TCAs (Feighner et al. 1986; Ferguson et al. 1994) and the SSRIs (Feighner et al. 1991) for major depression. Anecdotal evidence indicates that bupropion may be useful in patients with bipolar disorder, particularly for maintenance prophylaxis (Haykal and Akiskal 1990; Shopsin 1983; Wright et al. 1985). Bupropion is generally well tolerated and has fewer side effects than do the TCAs. It does not cause sedation, weight gain, sexual dysfunction, or anticholinergic effects and has minimal cardiovascular toxicity and low lethality with overdose. A therapeutic disadvantage is that bupropion is not effective for treatment of panic disorder and OCD (Sheehan et al. 1983b).

MAOIs (e.g., tranylcypromine, phenelzine, isocarboxazid) are extremely effective antidepressant agents. As described later in this chapter, they may be superior to other antidepressants in the treatment of atypical depression (Liebowitz et al. 1988). In addition, they are effective for treatment of panic disorder (Sheehan et al. 1983b), PTSD (Kosten et al. 1991), social phobia (Liebowitz et al. 1986), and bulimia (Walsh et al. 1984). The factor limiting the use of MAOIs is their side-effect profile. The available MAOIs are irreversible inhibitors of the enzyme monoamine oxidase. Patients must avoid foods containing tyramine because the inability of peripheral monoamine oxidase to metabolize tyramine may lead to hypertension and (rarely) cerebral hemorrhage or death (Cooper 1989). Other MAOI side effects include weight gain, orthostatic hypotension, delayed ejaculation, insomnia, and the spectrum of anticholinergic signs and symptoms.

A relatively new development is the introduction of short-acting reversible inhibitors such as moclobemide, which is currently not available in the United States. These drugs are less vulnerable to the tyramine reaction and often have fewer side effects compared with the MAOIs. Several preliminary treatment trials indicate that these drugs may have a therapeutic spectrum of action similar to that of reversible

MAOIs (Lecrubier and Guelfi 1990).

Nefazodone and trazodone are antidepressants that are distinguished biochemically from the TCAs, SSRIs, and MAOIs. They have moderate serotonin reuptake inhibition properties but are also postsynaptic serotonin receptor antagonists. Their principal metabolite—*m*-chlorophenylpiperazine (m-CPP)—is a nonselective serotonin receptor agonist. Controlled trials indicate that nefazodone and trazodone are similar in efficacy to other antidepressants. However, they may not be particularly useful for treating panic disorder (Charney et al. 1986), and there is no evidence that they are effective for treating OCD. Their side-effect profiles are notable for a lack of anticholinergic effects and low lethality with overdose. Their principal adverse effects are sedation, light-headedness, confusion, orthostatic hypotension, nausea, and (in rare cases with trazodone) priapism.

Mirtazapine is the newest addition to the pharmaceutical armamentarium for the treatment of depression in the United States. This medication has a novel pharmacological profile and is distinguished by its potent antagonist activity at the α_2-adrenergic, 5-HT$_2$, and 5-HT$_3$ receptors. Additionally, significant histaminergic antagonism may contribute to mirtazapine's potential side effects of drowsiness, dry mouth, and constipation. In multiple efficacy studies, mirtazapine was shown to be effective in treating moderate to severe major depression, with responsiveness similar to that of TCAs (R. Davis and Wilde 1995). Notably, preliminary experience with this drug worldwide suggests that it has a high therapeutic index, and no known deaths due to overdose have been cited to date. Further studies are needed to investigate the role of mirtazapine in patients with medical complications and those refractory to treatment.

Atypical Depression

The current general consensus is that a nonmelancholic atypical depressive syndrome exists that responds preferentially to MAOIs (Liebo-

witz et al. 1988; Quitkin et al. 1990, 1991). This syndrome generally meets criteria for unipolar depression, bipolar depression, or dysthymic disorder, but excessive mood reactivity (i.e., complete, transient remission from depressed mood in response to positive environmental factors) and two or more of the associated features of overeating, oversleeping, extreme fatigue, and chronic oversensitivity to rejection are also present (Liebowitz et al. 1988; F. Quitkin, personal communication, June 1993). In comparison to TCAs, MAOIs have superior efficacy for the symptoms associated with atypical depression, as well as for borderline and labile personality and self-rated interpersonal sensitivity (Liebowitz et al. 1988).

In considering the initial antidepressant drug trial in atypical depression, the clinician must balance the greater response to MAOIs (i.e., phenelzine) against their greater side-effect risk. MAOIs are appropriate as first-line treatment in this disorder. However, since recent reports indicate that SSRIs are effective in this subtype (McGrath et al. 2000), these drugs may be tested first.

Delusional Depression

Considerable data from descriptive, neurobiological, and treatment response investigations suggest that delusional depression is a distinct subtype of depressive illness (for review, see Joyce and Paykel 1989). The evidence is convincing that patients with delusional depression have a poorer response to TCAs than do patients with nondelusional depression. The recommended pharmacological treatment for delusional depression is a combination of antidepressant and antipsychotic drugs (Charney and Nelson 1981; Nelson and Bowers 1978; Spiker et al. 1985). The antipsychotic dose is generally less than that required to treat the psychotic symptoms associated with schizophrenia. The antipsychotic drug will elevate antidepressant blood levels, necessitating lower antidepressant drug doses and, when appropriate, monitoring blood levels. No evidence suggests that specific antidepressant or antipsychotic drugs are more effective in delusional depression. In patients with a medication-refractory delusional depression, ECT is a treatment alternative.

Bipolar Depression

The concept that bipolar and unipolar affective disorders are distinct entities is based on family studies, a variety of biological studies, clinical characteristics, course of illness, and treatment response (for review, see Joyce and Paykel 1989). During treatment of a patient's depressed phase of bipolar disorder, the clinician must avoid eliciting a manic episode. Most studies indicate that essentially all antidepressant drugs can induce mania in bipolar patients (Bunney 1977; Prien et al. 1973). Preliminary evidence suggests that bupropion and the SSRIs may potentially confer a reduced likelihood of a manic switch (Peet 1994; Stoll et al. 1994).

Some evidence indicates that bipolar depressed patients are more likely to have an antidepressant response to lithium than are unipolar depressed patients (Baron et al. 1975; Goodwin et al. 1972; Mendels et al. 1979; Noyes et al. 1974). Anecdotal reports propose that bipolar depression (especially when characterized by anergia, psychomotor retardation, and hypersomnia) may be more responsive to phenelzine, lithium, and tranylcypromine (Himmelhoch et al. 1972) than to TCAs. Of concern, a growing literature has suggested that antidepressant medications in bipolar depressed subjects may lead to cycle acceleration, with such acceleration potentially associated with greater treatment resistance (see Post and Weiss 1995). In some bipolar depressed patients refractory to standard treatment, carbamazepine alone or carbamazepine plus lithium is effective (Post 1991).

Dysthymic Disorder

Dysthymia was first recognized as a disorder in 1980, with the publication of DSM-III (American Psychiatric Association 1980). Dysthymic disorder is generally conceptualized as an illness with an insidious onset that begins at an early age. Dysthymic disorder and major depression may be diagnosed simultaneously in some subjects. The coexistence of dysthymic disorder with a major depressive episode is referred to as *double depression* (Keller et al. 1983). This background is important when reviewing the dysthymia literature, because it has not been as well characterized as other affective disorders, and the biology and treatment of dysthymic disorder are not well understood.

Dysthymic disorder appears to respond to a variety of antidepressant agents, including TCAs, MAOIs, and SSRIs (Bakish et al. 1994; Howland 1991; Marin et al. 1994; Rosenthal et al. 1992; Thase et al. 1996). Data suggest that MAOIs may be superior to TCAs in the treatment of this disorder, but this issue is unresolved.

Some theoretical issues cloud research into treatment of dysthymic disorder, particularly the degree to which it is distinct from major depression as opposed to a varying expression of the same illness. For example, although the concept of a double depression is a useful one, it is not clear that a person with both dysthymic disorder and major depression in fact has two illnesses as opposed to a single illness varying in severity over time (Garvey et al. 1989).

The risks of nontreatment should be emphasized. Studies have found that most subjects with dysthymic disorder go on to develop major depression. Patients with double depression who recover from an episode of major depression but continue to have dysthymic symptoms are at greater risk for relapse into major depression. The risk of relapse increases the longer the episode of dysthymia continues (Keller et al. 1992).

Geriatric Depression

Depression in the geriatric population (older than 65 years) constitutes a major public health problem and is often underdiagnosed and undertreated (National Institutes of Health Consensus Development Panel 1992). This underdiagnosis is partially a result of the insidious nature of depression in elderly people. In contrast to a young adult's presentation, depressed mood in an elderly person may be less prominent than other depressive symptoms such as changes in appetite and sleep, loss of interest, anergia, and social withdrawal; these changes may appear to be caused by aging and attendant medical problems.

Although relatively few controlled studies of antidepressant efficacy have been conducted in depressed patients older than 60, most antidepressants are believed to be equally efficacious for geriatric depression as for nongeriatric depression (for review, see Salzman 1993). Very little is known about antidepressant efficacy in very old depressed patients (those older than 85).

The risk of adverse drug side effects is increased in elderly people for several reasons. Elderly patients are more likely to have concomitant medical disorders, to be more sensitive to drug side effects, and to take other medications, which increases drug-drug interactions. In addition, drugs are excreted more slowly and metabolized less efficiently in elderly people compared with younger people. Therefore, lower antidepressant doses may be warranted in the elderly, and treatment nonresponse or unexpected side effects should prompt therapeutic drug level monitoring. Antidepressant medications should be initiated at low doses and increased very gradually (Neshkes and Jarvik 1987).

The efficacy studies of TCAs favor nortriptyline and desipramine because they are less likely than other TCAs to produce orthostatic hypotension (which can lead to falls and fractures) and because they have fewer adverse anticholinergic, cardiovascular, and sedative effects. Monitoring plasma levels of nortriptyline and desipramine and electrocardiograms will facilitate effective and safe use (Reynolds et al. 1992; Salzman 1993).

SSRIs may be particularly useful for elderly patients. The low incidence of cardiovascular side effects and lack of anticholinergic properties offer advantages over most other antidepressant classes (Altamura et al. 1989; Cohn et al. 1990; Dunner et al. 1992). As with the TCAs, the SSRIs should be initiated at low doses (fluoxetine, 5 mg; sertraline, 12.5 mg; paroxetine, 10 mg) and increased slowly as needed. The reduced inhibition of cytochrome P450 of citalopram and sertraline compared with fluoxetine and paroxetine suggests that their use is favored over other SSRIs in treating elderly patients taking concomitant medications.

Bupropion has been shown to be as efficacious for elderly patients as are other antidepressant drugs (Branconnier et al. 1983; Kane et al. 1983). Like the SSRIs, it does not produce anticholinergic side effects or orthostatic hypotension. The activating effects of bupropion may be a disadvantage for some individuals. As more experience is gained with bupropion in treating elderly patients, it may emerge as one of the drugs of choice for this population.

The sedative properties and lack of anticholinergic effects of nefazodone, trazodone, and mirtazapine may offer advantages to elderly depressed patients who are agitated. However, nefazodone and trazodone may cause orthostatic hypotension, which limits their usefulness in treating elderly patients.

Although the MAOIs (especially phenelzine) are not widely prescribed for elderly patients, these drugs are effective and safe for the treatment of geriatric depression. In low doses, psychomotor stimulants may diminish depressed mood, loss of interest, and anergia in some elderly individuals.

ECT is extremely effective in the treatment of depression in elderly patients. When the depression is very severe or is accompanied by delusions, ECT is the treatment of choice. A limitation of the use of ECT is that relapse after effective ECT is common, and usually alternative maintenance treatment is needed (Sackeim et al. 1990). Another disadvantage of ECT for elderly patients is transient post-ECT confusion. Use of unilateral treatments with a brief-pulse current to reduce confusion after the procedure may be helpful (Kramer 1987).

DURATION OF TREATMENT

Many patients with depressive illness are prone to relapse if antidepressant treatment is not continued. Data indicate that 50% or more of patients experiencing an episode of depression will eventually have a recurrence (Angst 1990; Lee and Murray 1988). The continuation of TCAs for 6 months after resolution of depressive symptoms reduces the relapse rate by more than 50% compared with placebo (Prien and Kupfer 1986). These data have led to the recommendation that pharmacological treatment for a first episode of depression should continue for 6 months after a patient's symptoms have responded to an antidepressant medication. Patients with recurrent major depression require longer-term antidepressant drug maintenance.

Unfortunately, long-term clinical trials designed to develop guidelines for chronic antidepressant drug use are limited. Most of the available data are based on studies of 1-year antidepressant drug maintenance. TCAs, MAOIs, and SSRIs have all been shown to reduce relapse rates by more than 50% during this period compared with placebo (Doogan and Caillard 1992; Eric 1991; Georgotas et al. 1989; Montgomery et al. 1988, 1991). In addition, patients maintained on a full dosage of imipramine for 3 years had a 20% relapse rate compared with an 80% relapse rate on placebo (Frank et al. 1990). Only one controlled study has evaluated the efficacy of an antidepressant beyond 3 years. An extension of the original 3-year maintenance study of imipramine to 5 years found that imipramine continued to have a clinically significant prophylactic effect (Kupfer et al. 1992).

These studies strongly support the continued efficacy of full-dose antidepressant therapy in preventing relapse over a period of several years. The clinical implications of this work are

that patients who have recovered from an initial depressive episode or prior depressive episodes spaced far apart (i.e., greater than 5 years) should receive maintenance antidepressant therapy for 6 months to 1 year. However, patients with prior depressive episodes that occurred less than 3 years apart should probably be given full-dose maintenance antidepressant therapy for at least 3, and probably up to 5, years. Patients with frequent recurrent depressive episodes may require lifetime treatment with antidepressants.

Maintenance antidepressant therapy should be discontinued with a slow taper. Involvement of a significant other, friend, or close family member to help the patient monitor for the return of symptoms and, if necessary, alert the treating clinician is also helpful.

THERAPEUTIC MONITORING OF ANTIDEPRESSANT BLOOD LEVELS

Therapeutic plasma levels have been established only for imipramine, desipramine, and nortriptyline (American Psychiatric Association Task Force Report 1985). However, information is available on other antidepressants for which blood levels may be useful in the treatment of refractory patients or elderly depressed patients to determine whether drug dosage is adequate (for review, see Preskorn 1989; Preskorn and Fast 1991).

For some antidepressants, therapeutic drug monitoring enables the clinician to maximize therapeutic dosage. Most studies have reported an association between plasma levels of nortriptyline, imipramine, and desipramine and clinical efficacy (Glassman et al. 1977; Nelson et al. 1982; Risch et al. 1979). The available evidence suggests that a curvilinear relationship may exist between nortriptyline plasma levels and antidepressant efficacy, with maximal therapeutic efficacy achieved with levels of 50–175 ng/mL. Thus, if the nortriptyline plasma level is less than 50 ng/mL or greater than 175 ng/mL, a dose change may be warranted. Evidence supports a linear relationship between plasma levels of imipramine plus desipramine (to which imipramine is metabolized) and clinical response. A similar relationship has been identified between desipramine plasma levels and therapeutic efficacy. Therefore, increasing drug doses to raise serum levels of imipramine and desipramine above a threshold value may convert nonresponders to responders.

Most investigations support a more limited role for the plasma levels of antidepressants other than nortriptyline, imipramine, or desipramine. In these cases, a plasma level determination might be useful when abnormal metabolism or poor compliance is suspected.

Monitoring of antidepressant drug levels may also help the clinician avoid drug toxicity. For some antidepressant drugs, a relationship exists between plasma concentration and toxicity. Data indicate that the effects of TCAs on cardiac function (i.e., delayed intraventricular conduction and rhythm disturbances) and on brain neuronal activity (i.e., seizures, delirium) are concentration dependent (Preskorn 1989). The same may be true for other antidepressants such as bupropion that show a dose-dependent increase in drug-induced seizures (Preskorn 1991). The SSRIs may not require therapeutic drug monitoring, because relationships to clinical response or adverse effects have not been identified.

Therapeutic antidepressant drug monitoring may assist in the evaluation of drug-drug interactions. Many pharmacological agents, which are commonly coadministered with antidepressants, may alter steady-state antidepressant drug levels. For example, drugs that stimulate the hepatic microsomal enzyme system (e.g., anticonvulsants, barbiturates, chronic alcohol use, glutethimide, chloral hydrate, nicotine, oral contraceptives) will lower drug levels of most antidepressant drugs. On the other hand, TCA levels are increased by neuroleptics and stimulants that inhibit hepatic metabolism. Coadministration of fluoxetine and TCAs in-

creases TCA blood levels as a result of hepatic metabolism inhibition via CYP2D6 (Bergstrom et al. 1992). Sertraline and citalopram may have less inhibitory effects on CYP2D6 than do other SSRIs (Crewe et al. 1992; Preskorn et al. 1994). Inhibition of CYP2D6 will also increase levels of anticonvulsants, neuroleptics, certain antiarrhythmic drugs, and β-adrenergic–blocking drugs. Dosages of these drugs may need to be adjusted in patients receiving SSRIs.

ANTIDEPRESSANT DRUGS AND SUICIDE

Antidepressant drugs are extremely effective in both acute treatment of depression and prevention of recurrence. However, whether antidepressant drugs can reduce the incidence of suicide in depressed patients has not been established. Some data suggest that SSRIs may be more effective than standard antidepressants in decreasing suicidal ideation, but these data are preliminary and inconsistent. This issue has been a great concern for clinicians and patients because of the suggestion that the SSRI fluoxetine may precipitate or exacerbate suicidal ideation or behavior (Beasley et al. 1991; Mann and Kapur 1991; Power and Cowen 1992; Teicher et al. 1990).

Several reviews have examined the data relevant to the question of whether antidepressant pharmacotherapy is associated with the emergence of suicidal ideation and behavior. These studies indicate that although suicidal ideation may emerge rarely during antidepressant treatment of depressed patients, these responses occur with essentially all types of antidepressant drugs, and a causal relationship to antidepressant drugs has not been established. Furthermore, the emergence or intensification of suicidal ideation and behavior with antidepressant drugs is not limited to patients with primary depression. Patients with a history of impulsive-aggressive behavior appear to be particularly prone to these effects (Mann and Kapur

1991; Power and Cowen 1992).

Suicidal ideation or behavior may be more frequent in patients who are nonresponsive, have unrecognized akathisia, and have attempted suicide previously. Patients should be informed of this rare adverse reaction and must be instructed to immediately contact their clinician should these symptoms occur (Mann and Kapur 1991).

APPROACHES TO TREATMENT OF REFRACTORY DEPRESSION

Despite the well-documented effectiveness of antidepressant drugs, a significant proportion—approximately 10%–30%—of the depressed patient population does not respond adequately to treatment. Based on the relatively high prevalence of depression, a substantial number of patients are not adequately responding to treatment (Nierenberg et al. 1991).

For the purposes of this discussion, we have used a definition that has a lower threshold than that generally used in clinical practice. *Refractory depression* is defined as an episode of major depression, not secondary to a medical or drug-induced condition, that fails to respond (or to maintain a response) to an adequate trial of an antidepressant drug of established efficacy. An *adequate trial* is defined as 6 weeks of treatment with the antidepressant at a dosage considered therapeutic.

Once it has been established that a patient is resistant to an antidepressant, several options are available to the treating clinician: maximizing the trial of that same antidepressant, changing to a different antidepressant, or selecting a drug combination or nonpharmacological treatment, such as ECT (Table 17–6).

Maximizing the Antidepressant Drug Trial

When a patient does not respond to an antidepressant, a clinician may maximize the response

Table 17–6. Therapeutic options for treatment-refractory depressed patients

Treatment	Efficacy	Replicability
Lithium augmentation of antidepressants	+++	+++
Electroconvulsive therapy	+++	+++
Thyroid (T$_3$) augmentation of antidepressants	++–+++	++
Stimulant augmentation of antidepressants	+–++	++
TCA and MAOI combination	+	++
Estrogen	0–+	++
Desipramine and fluoxetine combination	++–+++	+
High-dose MAOI	++	+
Repetitive transcranial magnetic stimulation	++	+
Antiglucocorticoid therapy	+–++	+
Pindolol augmentation of SSRI	0–+++	+

Note. Efficacy was rated as follows: 0 = ineffective; + = slightly effective; ++ = moderately effective; +++ = very effective. Replication refers to the extent to which the efficacy of the treatment has been investigated; it was rated as follows: + = open studies and/or only one controlled study conducted; ++ = several controlled studies conducted but further investigation indicated for complete evaluation; +++ = highly replicated and consistent degree of efficacy reported. T$_3$ = triiodothyronine; TCA = tricyclic antidepressant; MAOI = monoamine oxidase inhibitor; SSRIs = selective serotonin reuptake inhibitor.

to that same antidepressant by increasing its dose and/or the duration of the trial. Measuring the plasma levels of certain antidepressants may help determine whether a dosage adjustment is needed.

Use of higher than conventional doses of other antidepressant medications may be considered in cases of highly refractory depression; however, dosages should be increased very slowly, with frequent monitoring for side effects, including serial electrocardiogram monitoring if indicated.

Changing Treatment Strategies

Medication substitution. When a patient does not respond to an adequate antidepressant trial, the clinician often decides to change to a different antidepressant. The choice of the next antidepressant should involve those considerations ordinarily included in the initial selection of an antidepressant, such as side-effect profile, past antidepressant trial responses, family history of antidepressant responses, course of illness, premorbid personality, and depressive subtype.

Another method that has been advocated in selecting another antidepressant is consideration of its neuropharmacological properties. For example, if the patient's depression did not respond to an adequate trial with fluoxetine (a potent blocker of serotonin reuptake), then a trial with desipramine (a potent blocker of norepinephrine reuptake) is indicated. This rationale has become a basis for a common clinical practice, but its validity has not been confirmed in systematic clinical trials (Nolen et al. 1988). Some evidence suggests that two SSRIs— fluoxetine (Beasley et al. 1990) and fluvoxamine (Delgado et al. 1988)—may be effective in some patients in whom treatment with TCAs was unsuccessful.

Treatment with MAOIs may be useful for depressed patients whose condition has not responded to TCAs such as imipramine. In a double-blind crossover trial, phenelzine was reported to be effective in approximately two-thirds of patients whose symptoms had not responded to imipramine (McGrath et al. 1993). These chronically depressed, nonmelancholic, mood-reactive patients had many symptoms characteristic of atypical depression. In another double-blind crossover study, 75% of a group of anergic bipolar depressed patients had been refractory to treatment with imipramine, but many patients had therapeutic responses to tranylcypromine (Thase et al. 1992). Thus, these results suggest that many depressed patients characterized by anergia, psychomotor retardation, and symptoms of atypical depression will have therapeutic responses to MAOIs despite previous treatment resistance to TCAs.

Electroconvulsive therapy. As discussed earlier in this chapter, most investigations suggest that ECT has efficacy equal or superior to that of TCAs or MAOIs in the treatment of severe depression. A possible exception is that ECT is not effective for treating atypical depression. The results from several centers indicate that ECT is often effective in cases of depression unresponsive to TCAs (Avery and Winokur 1977; Devanand et al. 1991). For example, in the British Cooperative Study, ECT resulted in a 50% response rate in those patients whose conditions did not improve with imipramine (Clinical Psychiatry Committee of the British Medical Research Council 1965). In a study of 153 endogenously depressed patients who were imipramine nonresponders, 120 (78%) responded to ECT (Avery and Lubrano 1979).

ECT is particularly indicated in patients with psychotic depression. In one study, co-administration of an antipsychotic and a TCA in a delusionally depressed sample resulted in a total drug response rate of 70% compared with 22% for a single agent (Charney and Nelson 1981). Nevertheless, seven of the eight who had inadequate responses to the antipsychotic-TCA treatment responded to ECT. For most patients with psychotic depression, ECT or the antipsychotic-TCA combination is the treatment of choice.

Selecting an Antidepressant Drug Combination

TCAs and MAOIs. The rationale for combining a TCA with an MAOI was based on the monoamine deficiency hypothesis of depression. The combined ability of TCAs to inhibit presynaptic reuptake of biogenic amines and MAOIs to reduce metabolic breakdown of biogenic amines theoretically results in increased neurotransmitters in the synapse.

Most initial reports of combined TCA-MAOI therapy in the treatment of refractory depression were encouraging. However, most of these studies used open designs with no placebo control or comparison treatment groups (Pande et al. 1991; Razani et al. 1983; Schmauss et al. 1988; White and Simpson 1981). To date, no controlled study has confirmed an advantage in efficacy when a TCA is combined with an MAOI compared with either agent given alone. Despite early alarm about adverse side effects associated with this combination, the relative safety of this approach has been substantiated, provided low to moderate doses of an MAOI are added to an ongoing trial of a moderate dose of a TCA (Pande et al. 1991). An occasional patient may benefit from this treatment approach (Tyrer and Murphy 1990).

Desipramine or bupropion with fluoxetine. Several uncontrolled studies have found that when desipramine and fluoxetine are used in combination, they have a synergistic effect. In several cases when desipramine was added to fluoxetine, patients rapidly improved. These patients had been unresponsive to desipramine or fluoxetine alone (Eisen 1989). A case series of 30 treatment-refractory depressed patients reported an 87% response rate to combination treatment (Weilburg et al. 1989). Bupropion has also been reported in open-label trials to augment SSRI response (Spier 1998). Double-blind, placebo-controlled studies are needed to document the efficacy of such treatment combinations.

Augmentation Strategies

Antidepressants and stimulants. The combination of a TCA and methylphenidate is usu-ally mentioned as a treatment approach to refractory depression. However, to our knowledge, no studies of its efficacy have used a comparison treatment group. In the most frequently cited report, seven treatment-refractory patients with psychotic depression were given 20-mg doses of methylphenidate in addition to an imipramine regimen. Five of the seven patients had rapid and robust improvements (Wharton et al. 1971). However, the clinical improvement may have been the result of methylphenidate-induced increases in imipramine plasma levels. In a single case report, robust and rapid resolution of a patient's intractable depression occurred when methylphenidate was added to ongoing desipramine treatment. No concomitant change in plasma desipramine level occurred (Drimmer et al. 1983). In more recent case series of SSRI-refractory depressed patients, methylphenidate (10–40 mg/day) (Stoll et al. 1996) and pemoline (9.875–37.5 mg/day) (Metz and Shader 1991) augmentation resulted in marked reduction in depressive symptoms.

A report on clinical experience with a combination of either pemoline or dextroamphetamine and an MAOI in 32 depressed patients who were severely refractory to treatment indicated that the combination was safe and effective (Fawcett et al. 1991). Six patients became manic ($n = 1$) or hypomanic ($n = 5$). This treatment approach may be a viable option for severely ill patients.

Lithium augmentation of antidepressant action. DeMontigny et al. (1981, 1983) hypothesized that lithium's ability to increase presynaptic transmission of serotonin would potentiate TCA-induced postsynaptic serotonergic supersensitivity, resulting in enhanced efficacy of transmission in the brain serotonergic system. Although other mechanisms for lithium's effectiveness are possible, the discovery of this treatment approach represents the potential effect that a hypothesis generated from basic neuroscience research may have on the development and implementation of new treatment strategies.

Very strong data from more than 20 investigations support the effectiveness of adding lithium carbonate to ongoing antidepressant treatment in treatment-refractory depressed patients (Austin et al. 1991; Charney et al. 1991; Kramlinger and Post 1989). Whether starting an antidepressant and lithium concomitantly is equally efficacious in treating refractory depression has not been determined. Similarly, it is not known whether the lithium-antidepressant combination is necessary for preventing relapse and, if not, which agent should be used alone for prophylaxis. Preliminary observations indicate that the effectiveness of lithium augmentation is sustained and reduces the relapse rate—particularly in patients who had an acute, marked response to lithium augmentation (Nierenberg et al. 1990).

The earliest reports of lithium augmentation found that in patients whose symptoms did not respond to standard treatment with antidepressants, depressive symptomatology decreased dramatically within 48–72 hours after lithium was added (DeMontigny et al. 1981). Subsequent controlled investigations reported a more variable response to lithium. Only a fraction of patients whose condition responds to lithium augmentation will have dramatic responses within a week of adding lithium. More commonly, the response is gradual, with a response latency of up to 3 weeks.

The overall response rate of patients with treatment-refractory depression is approximately 50%, with patients with nonpsychotic melancholic depression or bipolar depression most likely to respond. However, many patients with nonmelancholic depression or delusional depression also respond to lithium augmentation. Lithium appears to be effective when added to all classes of antidepressant drugs, including carbamazepine. No evidence supports any superiority of one antidepressant type when lithium is added.

A controlled fixed-dose lithium investigation was conducted to determine proper lithium dose. This study and clinical experience suggest that lithium should be used in the typical fashion, titrating doses to a lithium level of 0.5–0.8 mEq/L (Stein and Bernadt 1993).

Lithium and monoamine oxidase inhibitors.   Shortly after lithium carbonate was introduced in the United States for the treatment of bipolar disorders, two reports (Himmelhoch et al. 1972; Zall 1971) on using lithium and an MAOI together were published. The rationale seemed related less to biological theory and more to a growing awareness that lithium alone was not always effective in the acute treatment of bipolar depression. In these open, uncontrolled trials, an MAOI was added to ongoing lithium administration in 24 lithium-resistant subjects. Most had already failed to respond to TCAs alone. Nineteen of 24 had substantial improvement after the MAOI was added. In a more recent investigation, 11 of 12 well-defined refractory unipolar depressed patients who had not responded to other lithium-antidepressant combinations were successfully treated when tranylcypromine was added to lithium (Price et al. 1985). Further investigation should help clarify whether the sequence in which an MAOI and lithium are combined affects efficacy (Nelson and Byck 1982).

Thyroid hormones and antidepressant drugs.   In 1963, Prange reported a case of hyperthyroidism in which imipramine seemed to induce a toxic reaction. Based on this clinical observation and the preclinical evidence that thyroid hormone enhances adrenergic receptor sensitivity, Prange reasoned that modest amounts of triiodothyronine (T_3) might accelerate imipramine's antidepressant activity without producing toxicity. In a placebo-controlled study of 20 depressed (but not treatment-refractory) patients, a more rapid onset of antidepressant action was observed in the imipramine-T_3 group compared with the imipramine-placebo group (Prange et al. 1969). Several other studies also found that a T_3-TCA combination provided a more rapid relief of symptoms than a TCA alone. The general trend in these studies was for women to respond better than men.

These favorable reports of T_3's effect on the rate of TCA response stimulated investigation into the efficacy of the T_3-TCA combination in refractory depression. Open studies (Banki 1975; Earle 1969; Ogura et al. 1974; Schwartz et al. 1984; Tsutsui et al. 1979) showed that when T_3 was added to TCAs in treatment-refractory depressed patients, about two-thirds of the cases had a favorable outcome. The significance of any conclusion drawn from these studies is weakened by several methodological flaws, including the absence of standardized diagnostic and treatment response rating criteria and a nonblind design. The results of controlled studies are less consistent. Two studies reported antidepressant effects of T_3 augmentation (Goodwin et al. 1982; Joffe and Singer 1991), whereas two other investigations did not (Gitlin et al. 1987; Thase et al. 1989). However, a placebo-controlled comparison of lithium and T_3 augmentation of TCAs in treatment-refractory patients with unipolar depression found that both of these agents were equal in efficacy and superior to placebo (Joffe et al. 1993). The effectiveness of thyroid hormone augmentation is not related to varying degrees of subclinical hypothyroidism in depressed patients.

Estrogen.   In the 1930s, several reports were published on the use of estrogen for depression occurring around the time of menopause. The rationale for the use of estrogen for treatment was that symptoms (including depression) occurring during menopause were the result of declining hormone levels. The findings of these studies were inconsistent, ranging from conclusions that estrogen had no proven value to assertions that it was a specific treatment for involutional melancholia. A more recent investigation failed to demonstrate an antidepressant effect of estrogen in perimenopausal patients (Coope 1981). However, a double-blind, pla-

cebo-controlled study used much higher doses of conjugated estrogen (Premarin at doses of up to 25 mg/day) in pre- and postmenopausal treatment-refractory depressed patients. Depression ratings significantly improved, but no complete remission occurred in the estrogen-treated patients (Klaiber et al. 1979). No significant association of estrogen response with menopausal status was found. The authors speculated that estrogen might exert an antidepressant action by augmenting central noradrenergic activity. However, preclinical studies indicated that the effect of estrogen on brain serotonin function may mediate some of its actions (Fischette et al. 1984).

Few reports of combined antidepressant-estrogen treatment have been published. In studies comparing imipramine plus estrogen with imipramine alone, the combination showed no clear advantage (Oppenheim 1984; Prange 1972; Shapira et al. 1985). Several case reports suggested possible beneficial effects of adding contraceptives to antidepressants for treatment of refractory depression (Sherwin 1991).

At present, insufficient data exist to support an estrogen trial early in the course of treatment for patients with treatment-refractory depression. In addition, the side effects of long-term estrogen administration to pre- and postmenopausal depressed women have not been definitively determined.

PROMISING APPROACHES

The depression treatment literature is rich with a variety of other pharmacological and nonpharmacological approaches. However, their efficacy in refractory depression has not been studied sufficiently to warrant detailed inclusion in this chapter. Pharmacological approaches of interest include the use of S-adenosylmethionine (Rosenbaum et al. 1990). Examples of innovative nonpharmacological approaches for depressed patients with hypothesized biological rhythm disturbances include sleep deprivation and bright-light treatment (Levitt et al. 1991).

Another developing antidepressant strategy directly targets the hypothalamic-pituitary-adrenal (HPA) axis. Abnormalities of the HPA axis were among the first and most consistently identified findings in depressed subjects. Such findings include elevated CSF corticotropin-releasing hormone (CRH) levels, elevated cortisol levels, and diminished sensitivity to dexamethasone suppression. In preclinical and clinical studies, chronic antidepressant treatment normalized these findings. Therefore, agents that directly reduce the hypercortisolemia in depressed subjects were tested for antidepressant activity (Murphy and Wolkowitz 1993).

In two open-trial studies (Murphy et al. 1991; Wolkowitz et al. 1993), refractory depressed patients consistently showed clinical improvement during administration of a regimen of steroid suppressant therapy, including aminoglutethimide, metyrapone, and ketoconazole. In the first study (Murphy et al. 1991), 6 of 10 initial study subjects who completed the trial had either a full ($n = 4$) or a partial ($n = 2$) remission. In the second study (Wolkowitz et al. 1993), 7 of 10 initial study subjects who completed the trial had an average 30% decrease in Hamilton Rating Scale for Depression scores. A preliminary placebo-controlled study of 20 medication-free depressed subjects reported no differences between ketoconazole- and placebo-treated patients; however, the subgroup of patients with high baseline cortisol levels did respond significantly better to ketoconazole than to placebo (Wolkowitz et al. 1996). Because of potential serious side effects, such as hepatotoxicity and hypoadrenalism, an antiglucocorticoid strategy should not be used in the general population until further placebo-controlled studies validate its effectiveness.

A novel strategy in the treatment of major depression is the concomitant use of a serotonin autoreceptor antagonist with an SSRI to enhance serotonergic function. In preliminary, open-label studies, pindolol, a serotonin antagonist and β-adrenergic blocker, has strongly augmented SSRIs in resistant depression and rapidly accelerated treatment response (Artigas et al. 1994; Blier and Bergeron 1995). To date, placebo-controlled studies of this strategy have reported mixed results. Results from our group with fluoxetine have not been favorable (Berman et al. 1996); however, other researchers have found that a fluoxetine-pindolol combination hastens response in a subgroup of patients who are predominantly treatment-naive with nonchronic depressions (Isaac et al. 1996). Further evaluation of this pharmacological approach is necessary.

A novel nonpharmacological approach to the treatment of depression involves the application of repetitive transcranial trains of magnetic stimulation (rTMS) over the left prefrontal cortex, an area consistently implicated in the pathophysiology of major depression. rTMS likely depolarizes cortical neurons in a generalized region; therefore, it bears some similarity to ECT. However, rTMS confers only a modest risk of seizure. rTMS was first applied to nondepressed subjects and had effects on mood (Bickford et al. 1987). In one study of five highly refractory depressed subjects, two patients had robust improvement after rTMS treatment, with 17-item Hamilton Rating Scale for Depression scores decreasing from 23 to 3 and 20 to 12 (George et al. 1995). Both patients had failed to respond to 10 or more previous antidepressant trials. Further work is under way to elaborate these findings. Controlled, blinded trials are needed to establish further the effectiveness of this potential treatment.

THE FUTURE OF PHARMACOLOGICAL TREATMENT OF DEPRESSIVE ILLNESS

Clinicians now have an impressive drug armamentarium from which to treat depressive illness. Severe depressive illness in most patients will have good therapeutic responses to antidepressant drugs, with an acceptable degree of adverse side effects. Furthermore, various effective drug treatment approaches have been developed for most patients whose symptoms do not respond to the initial antidepressant drug used.

However, important deficits persist in knowledge relevant to the pharmacological treatment of depression. Descriptive and biological markers capable of identifying subtypes of depressive illness characterized by therapeutic responses to specific antidepressants are lacking. The mechanisms of action of antidepressant drugs have not been established. This limits the discovery of new, more effective, rapid-acting antidepressant drugs.

The future development of antidepressant drugs likely will move beyond drugs with therapeutic properties related to monoamine reuptake or metabolism inhibition because of recent data suggesting that these systems may not be primary in the pathophysiology of depression (Berman et al. 1996). Further understanding of the effects of antidepressant drug action at sites distal to receptor recognition sites may provide new approaches for developing new classes of antidepressant drugs.

REFERENCES

Aberg-Wistedt A, Jostell KG, Ross SB, et al: Effects of zimeldine and desipramine on serotonin and noradrenaline uptake mechanisms in relation to plasma concentrations and to therapeutic effects during treatment of depression. Psychopharmacology (Berl) 74:297–305, 1981

Altamura AC, DeNovelis F, Guercetti G, et al: Fluoxetine compared with amitriptyline in elderly depression: a controlled clinical trial. Int J Clin Pharmacol Res 9:391–396, 1989

American Psychiatric Association: Diagnostic and Statistical Manual of Mental Disorders, 3rd Edition. Washington, DC, American Psychiatric Association, 1980

American Psychiatric Association Task Force Report: Tricyclic antidepressants: blood level measurements and clinical outcome. Am J Psychiatry 142:155–182, 1985

Amin M, Lehmann H, Mirmiran J: A double-blind, placebo-controlled dose-finding study with sertraline. Psychopharmacol Bull 25:164–167, 1989

Amsterdam J, Maislin G, Potter L: Fluoxetine efficacy in treatment resistant depression. Prog Neuropsychopharmacol Biol Psychiatry 18: 243–261, 1994

Angst J: Natural history and epidemiology of depression, in Results of Community Studies in Prediction and Treatment of Recurrent Depression. Edited by Cobb J, Goeting N. Southampton, England, Duphar Medical Relations, 1990, pp 121–154

Artigas F, Perez V, Alvarez E: Pindolol induces a rapid improvement of depressed patients treated with serotonin reuptake inhibitors. Arch Gen Psychiatry 51:248–251, 1994

Asberg M, Bertilsson L, Tuck D, et al: Indoleamine metabolites in cerebrospinal fluid of depressed patients before and during treatment with nortriptyline. Clin Pharmacol Ther 14:277–286, 1973

Austin MP, Souza FG, Goodwin GM: Lithium augmentation in antidepressant-resistant patients: a quantitative analysis. Br J Psychiatry 159: 510–514, 1991

Avery D, Lubrano A: Depression treated with imipramine and ECT: the DeCardis study reconsidered. Am J Psychiatry 136:559–562, 1979

Avery D, Winokur G: The efficacy of electroconvulsive therapy and antidepressants in depression. Biol Psychiatry 12:507–524, 1977

Bakish D, Ravindran A, Hooper C, et al: Psychopharmacological treatment response of patients with a DSM-III diagnosis of dysthymic disorder. Psychopharmacol Bull 30:53–59, 1994

Banki CM: Triiodothyronine in the treatment of depression. Orv Hetil 116:2543–2546, 1975

Baron M, Gershon ES, Rudy V, et al: Lithium carbonate response in depression: prediction by unipolar/bipolar illness, average-evoked response, catechol-O-methyltransferase, and family history. Arch Gen Psychiatry 32:1107–1111, 1975

Beasley CM Jr, Sayler ME, Cunningham GE, et al: Fluoxetine in tricyclic refractory major depressive disorder. J Affect Disord 20:193–200, 1990

Beasley CM Jr, Dornseif BE, Bosomworth JC, et al: Fluoxetine and suicide: a meta-analysis of controlled trials of treatment for depression. BMJ 303:685–692, 1991

Beasley CM, Masica DN, Potvin JH: Fluoxetine: a review of receptor and functional effects and their clinical implications. Psychopharmacology (Berl) 107:1–10, 1992

Bergstrom RF, Peyton AL, Lemberger L: Quantification and mechanism of the fluoxetine and tricyclic antidepressant interaction. Clin Pharmacol Ther 51:239–248, 1992

Berman RM, Krystal JH, Charney DS: Mechanism of action of antidepressants: monoamine hypotheses and beyond, in Biology of Schizophrenia and Affective Disease. Edited by Watson SJ. Washington, DC, American Psychiatric Press, 1996, pp 295–368

Bickford RG, Guidie N, Fortesque P, et al: Magnetic stimulation of human peripheral nerve and brain: response enhancement by magneto-electrical technique. Neurosurgery 20:110–116, 1987

Bielski RJ, Friedel RO: Prediction of tricyclic antidepressant response: a critical review. Arch Gen Psychiatry 33:1479–1489, 1976

Bigger JT Jr: Implications of the Cardiac Arrhythmia Suppression Trial for antiarrhythmic drug treatment. Am J Cardiol 65:3D–10D, 1990

Blier P, Bergeron R: Effectiveness of pindolol with selected antidepressant drugs in the treatment of major depression. J Clin Psychopharmacol 15:217–222, 1995

Branconnier RJ, Cole JO, Ghazvinian S, et al: Clinical pharmacology of bupropion and imipramine in elderly depressives. J Clin Psychiatry 44 (5, sec 2):130–133, 1983

Brown P, Brawley P: Dexamethasone suppression test and mood response to methylphenidate in primary depression. Am J Psychiatry 140:990–993, 1983

Brown WA, Qualls CB: Pituitary-adrenal disinhibition in depression: marker of a subtype with characteristic clinical features and response to treatment. Psychiatry Res 4:115–128, 1981

Brown WA, Shuey I: Response to dexamethasone and subtype of depression. Arch Gen Psychiatry 37:747–751, 1980

Buff DD, Brenner R, Kirtane SS, et al: Dysrhythmia associated with fluoxetine treatment in an elderly patient with cardiac disease. J Clin Psychiatry 52:174–176, 1991

Bunney WE: The switch process in manic-depressive psychosis. Ann Intern Med 87:319–335, 1977

Cardiac Arrhythmia Suppression Trial (CAST) Investigators: Preliminary report: effect of encainide and flecainide on mortality in a randomized trial of arrhythmia suppression after myocardial infarction. N Engl J Med 321:406–412, 1989

Cardiac Arrhythmia Suppression Trial II Investigators: Effect of the antiarrhythmic agent moricizine on survival after myocardial infarction. N Engl J Med 327:227–233, 1992

Carlsson A, Fuxe K, Ungerstedt U: The effect of imipramine on central 5-hydroxytryptamine neurons. J Pharm Pharmacol 20:150–151, 1968

Carroll BJ: The dexamethasone suppression test for melancholia. Br J Psychiatry 140:292–304, 1982

Charney DS, Nelson JC: Delusional and non-delusional unipolar depression: further evidence for distinct subtypes. Am J Psychiatry 138:328–333, 1981

Charney DS, Woods SW, Goodman WK, et al: Drug treatment of panic disorder: the comparative efficacy of imipramine, alprazolam and trazodone. J Clin Psychiatry 47:580–585, 1986

Charney DS, Delgado PL, Southwick SM, et al: Current hypotheses of the mechanism of antidepressant treatments: implications for the treatment of refractory depression, in Advances in Neuropsychiatry and Psychopharmacology, Vol 2: Refractory Depression. Edited by Amsterdam JD. New York, Raven, 1991, pp 23–40

Clerk GE, Ruimy P, Verdeau-Pailles J, et al: A double-blind comparison of venlafaxine and fluoxetine in patients hospitalized for major depression and melancholia. Int Clin Psychopharmacol 9:139–143, 1994

Clinical Psychiatry Committee of the British Medical Research Council: Clinical trial of the treatment of depressive illness. BMJ 1:881–886, 1965

Coble PA, Kupfer DJ, Spiker DG, et al: EEG sleep in primary depression: a longitudinal placebo study. J Affect Disord 1:131–138, 1979

Cohn CK, Shrivastava R, Mendels J, et al: Double-blind, multicenter comparison of sertraline and amitriptyline in elderly depressed patients. J Clin Psychiatry 51 (12, suppl B):28–33, 1990

Coope J: Is estrogen therapy effective in the treatment of menopausal depression? Journal of the Royal College of General Practitioners 31: 134–140, 1981

Cooper AJ: Tyramine and irreversible monoamine oxidase inhibitors in clinical practice. Br J Psychiatry 155 (suppl 6):38–45, 1989

Coplen SE, Antman EM, Berlin JA, et al: Efficacy and safety of quinidine therapy for maintenance of sinus rhythm after cardioversion: a meta-analysis of randomized control trials. Circulation 82:1106–1116, 1990

Crane GE: The psychiatric side-effects of iproniazid. Am J Psychiatry 112:494–501, 1956

Crewe HK, Lennard MS, Tucker GT, et al: The effect of selective serotonin re-uptake inhibitors on cytochrome P4502D6 (CYP2D6) activity in human liver microsomes. Br J Pharmacol 34: 262–265, 1992

Cusack B, Nelson A, Richelson E: Binding of antidepressants to human brain receptors: focus on newer generation of compounds. Psychopharmacology 114:559–565, 1994

Danish University Antidepressant Study Group: Paroxetine: a selective serotonin reuptake inhibitor showing better tolerance, but weaker antidepressant effect than clomipramine in a controlled multicenter study. J Affect Disord 18: 289–299, 1990

Davidson J: Seizures and bupropion: a review. J Clin Psychiatry 50:256–261, 1989

Davis JM: Antidepressant drugs, in Comprehensive Textbook of Psychiatry, Vol 4, 4th Edition. Edited by Kaplan HI, Saddock BJ. Baltimore, MD, Williams & Wilkins, 1985, pp 765–794

Davis R, Wilde MI: Mirtazapine: a review of its pharmacology and therapeutic potential in the management of major depression. CNS Drugs 5:389–402, 1995

Delgado PL, Price LH, Charney DS, et al: Efficacy of fluvoxamine in treatment-refractory depression. J Affect Disord 15:55–60, 1988

DeMontigny CF, Grunberg AF, Deschenes JP: Lithium induces rapid relief of depression in tricyclic antidepressant drug non-responders. Br J Psychiatry 138:252–256, 1981

DeMontigny CF, Ceurnoyer G, Morissette R, et al: Lithium carbonate addition in tricyclic antidepressant-resistant unipolar depression. Arch Gen Psychiatry 40:1327–1334, 1983

Dessain EC, Schatzberg AF, Woods BT, et al: Maprotiline treatment in depression. Arch Gen Psychiatry 43:86–90, 1987

Devanand DP, Sacheim HA, Prudic J: Electroconvulsive therapy in the treatment-resistant patient. Psychiatr Clin North Am 14:905–923, 1991

Doogan DP, Caillard V: Sertraline in the prevention of depression. Br J Psychiatry 160:217–222, 1992

Downing RW, Rickels K: Predictors of response to amitriptyline and placebo in three outpatient treatment settings. J Nerv Ment Dis 156: 109–129, 1973

Drimmer EJ, Gitlin MJ, Gwirtouran HE: Desipramine and methylphenidate combination treatment of depression: case report. Am J Psychiatry 140:241–242, 1983

Dunner DL, Cohn JB, Walshe TI, et al: Two combined, multicenter double-blind studies of paroxetine and doxepin in geriatric patients with major depression. J Clin Psychiatry 53 (2 suppl):57–60, 1992

Earle BV: Thyroid hormone and tricyclic antidepressants in resistant depressions. Am J Psychiatry 126:1667–1669, 1969

Echt DS, Liebson PR, Mitchell LB, et al: Mortality and morbidity in patients receiving encainide, flecainide, or placebo: the Cardiac Arrhythmia Suppression Trial. N Engl J Med 324:781–788, 1991

Eisen A: Fluoxetine and desipramine: a strategy for augmenting antidepressant response. Pharmacopsychiatry 22:272–273, 1989

Ellison JM, Milofsky JE, Ely E: Fluoxetine-induced bradycardia and syncope in two patients. J Clin Psychiatry 51:385–386, 1990

Eric L: A prospective, double-blind, comparative, multicentre study of paroxetine and placebo in preventing recurrent major depressive episodes. Biol Psychiatry 29 (suppl 11):254S–255S, 1991

Ettigi PG, Hayes PE, Narasimhacharr N, et al: d-Amphetamine response and dexamethasone suppression test as predictors of treatment outcome in unipolar depression. Biol Psychiatry 18:499–504, 1983

Falk RH: Flecainide-induced ventricular tachycardia and fibrillation in patients treated for atrial fibrillation. Ann Intern Med 111:107–111, 1989

Fawcett J, Kravitz HM, Sajecka JM, et al: CNS stimulant potentiation of monoamine oxidase inhibitors in treatment-refractory depression. J Clin Psychopharmacol 11:127–132, 1991

Feder R: Bradycardia and syncope induced by fluoxetine (letter). J Clin Psychiatry 52:139, 1991

Feighner J: Cardiovascular safety in depressed patients: focus on venlafaxine. J Clin Psychiatry 56(12):574–579, 1995

Feighner J, Hendrickson G, Miller L, et al: Double-blind comparison of doxepin vs bupropion in outpatients with major depressive disorder. J Clin Psychopharmacol 6:27–32, 1986

Feighner J, Gardner E, Johnson J, et al: Double-blind comparison of bupropion and fluoxetine in depressed outpatients. J Clin Psychiatry 52:329–355, 1991

Feighner J, Cohn J, Fabre L, et al: A study comparing paroxetine, placebo and imipramine in depressed patients. J Affect Disord 28:71–79, 1993

Ferguson J, Cunningham L, Merideth C, et al: Bupropion in tricyclic antidepressant nonresponders with unipolar major depressive disorder. Ann Clin Psychiatry 6:153–160, 1994

Fischette CT, Biegon A, McEwen B: Sex steroid modulation of the serotonin behavioral syndrome. Life Sci 35:1197–1206, 1984

Frank E, Kupfer DJ, Perel JM, et al: Three-year outcomes for maintenance therapies in recurrent depression. Arch Gen Psychiatry 47:1093–1099, 1990

Gardner EA, Johnston JA: Bupropion: an antidepressant without sexual pathophysiological action. J Clin Psychopharmacol 5:24–29, 1985

Garvey MJ, Cook BL, Tollefson GD, et al: Antidepressant response in chronic major depression. Compr Psychiatry 30:214–217, 1989

George MS, Wassermann EM, Williams WA, et al: Daily repetitive transcranial magnetic stimulation (rTMS) improves mood in depression. NeuroReport 6:1853–1856, 1995

Georgotas A, McCue RE, Cooper TB: A placebo controlled comparison of nortriptyline and phenelzine in maintenance therapy of elderly depressed patients. Arch Gen Psychiatry 46:783–786, 1989

Gitlin MJ, Gerner RH: The dexamethasone suppression test and response to somatic treatment: a review. J Clin Psychiatry 47:16–21, 1986

Gitlin MJ, Weiner H, Fairbanks L: Failure of T_3 to potentiate tricyclic antidepressant response. J Affect Disord 13:267–272, 1987

Glassman AH, Bigger JT Jr: Cardiovascular effects of therapeutic doses of tricyclic antidepressants: a review. Arch Gen Psychiatry 38:815–820, 1981

Glassman AH, Preud'homme XA: Review of the cardiovascular effects of heterocyclic antidepressants. J Clin Psychiatry 54 (2, suppl):16–22, 1993

Glassman AH, Perel JM, Shostak M, et al: Clinical implications of imipramine plasma levels for depressive illness. Arch Gen Psychiatry 34:197–204, 1977

Glassman AH, Roose SP, Giardina EGV, et al: Cardiovascular effects of tricyclic antidepressants, in Psychopharmacology: The Third Generation of Progress. Edited by Meltzer HY. New York, Raven, 1987, pp 1437–1442

Glassman AH, Roose SP, Bigger JT Jr: The safety of tricyclic antidepressants in cardiac patients: risk-benefit reconsidered. JAMA 269:2673–2675, 1993

Glowinski J, Axelrod J: Inhibition of uptake of tritiated-noradrenaline in the intact rat brain by imipramine and structurally related compounds. Nature 204:1318–1319, 1964

Goodman WK, Price LH, Delgado PL, et al: Specificity of serotonin reuptake inhibitors in the treatment of obsessive-compulsive disorder: comparison of fluvoxamine and desipramine. Arch Gen Psychiatry 47:577–585, 1990

Goodwin FK, Murphy DL, Dunner DL, et al: Lithium response in unipolar versus bipolar depression. Am J Psychiatry 129:44–47, 1972

Goodwin FK, Post RM, Murphy DL: CSF amine metabolites and therapies of depression. Scientific Proceedings in Summary Form: The One Hundred Twenty-Sixth Annual Meeting of the American Psychiatric Association, Honolulu, HI, May 7–11, 1973, pp 24–25

Goodwin FK, Prange AJ, Post RM, et al: Potentiation of antidepressant effects by L-tri-iodothyronine in tricyclic nonresponders. Am J Psychiatry 139:34–38, 1982

Greden JF, Kronfol Z, Gardner R, et al: Dexamethasone suppression test and selection of antidepressant medications. J Affect Disord 3:389–396, 1981

Greden JF, Gardner R, King D: Dexamethasone suppression tests in anti-depressant treatment of melancholia: the process of normalization and test-retest reproducibility. Arch Gen Psychiatry 40:493–500, 1983

Guelfi JD, White C, Hackett D, et al: Effectiveness of venlafaxine in patients hospitalized for major depression and melancholia. J Clin Psychiatry 56:450–458, 1995

Haykal RF, Akiskal HS: Bupropion as a promising approach to rapidly cycling bipolar II patients. J Clin Psychiatry 51:450–455, 1990

Himmelhoch JM, Detre T, Kupfer DJ, et al: Treatment of previously intractable depressions with tranylcypromine and lithium. J Nerv Ment Dis 155:216–220, 1972

Hirschfeld RMA, Klerman GL, Andreasen NC, et al: Psycho-social predictors of chronicity in depressed patients. Br J Psychiatry 148:648–654, 1986

Hochli D, Riemann D, Zulley J, et al: Initial REM sleep suppression by clomipramine: a prognostic tool for treatment response in patients with a major depressive disorder. Biol Psychiatry 21:1217–1220, 1986

Hollister LE, Overall JE: Reflections on the specificity of action of antidepressants. Psychosomatics 6:361–365, 1965

Holsboer F, Liebl R, Hofschuster E: Repeated dexamethasone suppression test during depressive illness: normalization of test result compared with clinical improvement. J Affect Disord 4:93–101, 1982

Horowitz LN, Zipes DP, Bigger JT Jr, et al: Proarrhythmia, arrhythmogenesis or aggravation of arrhythmia—a status report. Am J Cardiol 59:54E–56E, 1987

Howland RH: Pharmacotherapy of dysthymia: a review. J Clin Psychopharmacol 11(2):83–92, 1991

Humphrey P: 5-Hydroxytryptamine receptors and drug discovery, in Serotonin Receptor Subtypes: Pharmacological Significance and Clinical Implications (International Academic and Biomedical Drug Research, Vol 1). Edited by Langer SZ, Brunello N, Racagni G, et al. Basel, Switzerland, Karger, 1992, pp 129–139

Isaac MT, Tome MB, Hart R: Serotonergic autoreceptor blockade in the reduction of antidepressant latency: a controlled trial. Program and Abstracts on New Research in Summary Form: the 149th Annual Meeting of the American Psychiatric Association, New York City, May 4–9, 1996, p 154

Jick H, Dinan BJ, Hunter JR, et al: Tricyclic antidepressants and convulsions. J Clin Psychopharmacol 3:182–185, 1983

Joffe RT, Singer W: Thyroid hormone potentiation of antidepressants, in Advances in Neuropsychiatry and Psychopharmacology, Vol 2: Refractory Depression. Edited by Amsterdam JD. New York, Raven, 1991, pp 185–190

Joffe RT, Singer W, Levitt AJ, et al: A placebo-controlled comparison of lithium and triiodothyronine augmentation of tricyclic antidepressants in unipolar refractory depression. Arch Gen Psychiatry 50:387–393, 1993

Johnston JA, Lineberry CG, Ascher JA, et al: A 102-center prospective study of seizure in association with bupropion. J Clin Psychiatry 52:450–456, 1991

Joyce PR, Paykel ES: Predictors of drug response in depression. Arch Gen Psychiatry 46:89–99, 1989

Kane JM, Cole K, Sarantakos S, et al: Safety and efficacy of bupropion in elderly patients: preliminary observations. J Clin Psychiatry 44 (5, sec 2):134–136, 1983

Keller MB, Shapiro RW, Lavori PW, et al: Recovery in major depressive disorder: analysis with the life table and regression models. Arch Gen Psychiatry 39:905–910, 1982a

Keller MB, Shapiro RW, Lavori PW, et al: Relapse in major depressive disorder: analysis with the life table. Arch Gen Psychiatry 39:911–915, 1982b

Keller MB, Lavori PW, Endicott J, et al: "Double depression": two year follow-up. Am J Psychiatry 140:289–294, 1983

Keller MB, Lavori PW, Mueller TI, et al: Time to recovery, chronicity, and levels of psychopathology in major depression: a 5-year prospective follow-up of 431 subjects. Arch Gen Psychiatry 49:809–816, 1992

Klaiber EL, Bouerman DM, Vogel W, et al: Estrogen therapy for severe persistent depression in women. Arch Gen Psychiatry 36:550–554, 1979

Kline NS: Monoamine oxidase inhibitors: an unfinished picaresque tale, in Discoveries in Biological Psychiatry. Edited by Ayd FJ, Blackwell B. Philadelphia, PA, JB Lippincott, 1970, pp 194–204

Kosten TR, Frank JB, Dan E, et al: Pharmacotherapy for posttraumatic stress disorder using phenelzine or imipramine. J Nerv Ment Dis 179:366–370, 1991

Kramer BA: Electroconvulsive therapy use in geriatric depression. J Nerv Ment Dis 175:233–235, 1987

Kramlinger KG, Post RM: The addition of lithium to carbamazepine: antidepressant efficacy in treatment-resistant depression. Arch Gen Psychiatry 46:794–800, 1989

Kuhn R: The treatment of depressive states with G22355 (imipramine) hydrochloride. Am J Psychiatry 115:459–464, 1958

Kuhn R: Foreword, in Tofranil® (Imipramine). Berne, Switzerland, Verlag Stamplfi, 1970a, pp vi–vii

Kuhn R: The imipramine story, in Discoveries in Biological Psychiatry. Edited by Ayd FJ, Blackwell B. Philadelphia, PA, JB Lippincott, 1970b, pp 205–217

Kuhn R: The discovery of modern antidepressants. Psychiatric Journal of the University of Ottawa 14:249–252, 1989

Kupfer DJ, Foster FG, Reich L, et al: EEG sleep changes as predictors in depression. Am J Psychiatry 133:622–626, 1976

Kupfer DJ, Spiker DG, Coble PA, et al: Depression, EEG sleep, and clinical response. Compr Psychiatry 21:212–220, 1980

Kupfer DJ, Frank E, Perel JM, et al: Five-year outcome for maintenance therapies in recurrent depression. Arch Gen Psychiatry 49:769–773, 1992

Lavori PW, Keller MB, Klerman GL: Relapse in affective disorders: a reanalysis of the literature using life table methods. J Psychiatr Res 18:13–21, 1984

Lecrubier Y, Guelfi JD: Efficacy of reversible inhibitors of monoamine oxidase-A in various forms of depression. Acta Psychiatr Scand Suppl 360:18–23, 1990

Lee AS, Murray AM: The long term outcome of Maudsley depressives. Br J Psychiatry 153:741–751, 1988

Levitt AJ, Joffe RT, Kennedy SH: Bright light augmentation in antidepressant nonresponders. J Clin Psychiatry 52:336–337, 1991

Liebowitz MR, Fyer AJ, Gorman JM, et al: Phenelzine in social phobia. J Clin Psychopharmacol 6:93–98, 1986

Liebowitz MR, Quitkin FM, Stewart JW, et al: Antidepressant specificity in atypical depression. Arch Gen Psychiatry 45:129–137, 1988

Loomer HP, Saunders JC, Kline NS: Iproniazid, an amine oxidase inhibitor, as an example of a psychic energizer. Congressional Record, 1957, pp 1382–1390

Loomer HP, Saunders JC, Kline NS: A clinical and pharmaco-dynamic evaluation of iproniazid as a psychic energizer (Psychiatric Research Report No 8). Washington, DC, American Psychiatric Association, 1958, pp 129–141

Mann JJ, Kapur S: The emergence of suicidal ideation and behavior during antidepressant pharmacotherapy. Arch Gen Psychiatry 48:1027–1033, 1991

Marcus MD, Wing RR, Ewing L, et al: A double blind, placebo-controlled trial of fluoxetine plus behavior modification in the treatment of obese binge-eaters and non-binge eaters. Am J Psychiatry 147:876–881, 1990

Marin D, Kocsis J, Frances A, et al: Desipramine for the treatment of "pure" dysthymia versus double depression. Am J Psychiatry 151:1079–1080, 1994

Mayeux R, Stern Y, Cote L, et al: Altered serotonin metabolism in depressed patients with Parkinson's disease. Neurology 34:642–646, 1984

McGrath PJ, Stewart JW, Nunes EV, et al: A double-blind crossover trial of imipramine and phenelzine for outpatients with treatment-refractory depression. Am J Psychiatry 150:118–123, 1993

McGrath P, Stewart JW, Janal MN, et al: A placebo-controlled study of fluoxetine versus imipramine in the acute treatment of atypical depression. Am J Psychiatry 157:344–350, 2000

Mendels J, Ramsey TA, Dyson WL, et al: Lithium as an antidepressant. Arch Gen Psychiatry 36:845–846, 1979

Metz A, Shader RI: Combination of fluoxetine and pemoline in the treatment of major depressive disorder. Int Clin Psychopharmacol 6:93–96, 1991

Moller H, Berzewski H, Eckmann F, et al: Double-blind multicenter study of paroxetine and amitriptyline in depressed inpatients. Pharmacopsychiatry 26:75–78, 1993

Møller SE, Honore P, Larsen OB: Tryptophan and tyrosine ratios to neutral amino acids in endogenous depression: relation to antidepressant response to amitriptyline and lithium/L-tryptophan. J Affect Disord 5:67–79, 1983

Møller SE, Odum K, Kirk L, et al: Plasma tyrosine/neutral amino acid ratio correlated with clinical response to nortriptyline in endogenously depressed patients. J Affect Disord 9:223–229, 1985

Møller SE, de Beurs P, Timmerman L, et al: Plasma tryptophan and tyrosine ratios to competing amino acids in relation to antidepressant response to citalopram and maprotiline. Psychopharmacology (Berl) 88:96–110, 1986

Møller SE, Bech P, Bjerrum H, et al: Plasma ratio tryptophan/neutral amino acids in relation to clinical response to paroxetine and clomipramine in patients with major depression. J Affect Disord 18:59–66, 1990

Montgomery S, Djarv L: The antidepressant efficacy of citalopram. Int Clin Psychopharmacol 11S:29–33, 1996

Montgomery SA, Dufour H, Brion S, et al: The prophylactic efficacy of fluoxetine in unipolar depression. Br J Psychiatry 153 (suppl 3):69–76, 1988

Montgomery SA, Doogan DP, Burnside R: The influence of different relapse criteria on the assessment of long-term efficacy of sertraline. Int Clin Psychopharmacol 6 (suppl 2):37–46, 1991

Morganroth J, Goin JE: Quinidine-related mortality in the short-to-medium-term treatment of ventricular arrhythmias: a meta-analysis. Circulation 84:1977–1983, 1991

Murphy BEP, Wolkowitz OM: The pathophysiologic significance of hyperadrenocorticism: antiglucocorticoid strategies. Psychiatric Annals 23:682–690, 1993

Murphy BE, Dhar V, Ghadirian AM, et al: Response to steroid suppression in major depression resistant to antidepressant therapy. J Clin Psychopharmacol 11:121–126, 1991

Nagy LM, Morgan CA III, Southwick SM, et al: Open prospective trial of fluoxetine for posttraumatic stress disorder. J Clin Psychopharmacol 13:107–113, 1993

National Institutes of Health Consensus Development Panel on Depression in Late Life: Diagnosis and treatment of depression in late life (NIH consensus conference). JAMA 268:1018–1024, 1992

Nelson JC, Bowers MB: Delusional unipolar depression: description and drug response. Arch Gen Psychiatry 35:1321–1328, 1978

Nelson JC, Byck R: Rapid response to lithium in phenelzine non-responders. Br J Psychiatry 141:85–86, 1982

Nelson JC, Jatlow P, Quinlan DM, et al: Desipramine plasma concentration and antidepressant response. Arch Gen Psychiatry 39:1419–1422, 1982

Nemeroff CB, DeVane CL, Pollock BG: Newer antidepressants and the cytochrome P450 system. Am J Psychiatry 153:311–320, 1996

Neshkes RE, Jarvik LF: Affective disorders in the elderly. Annu Rev Med 38:445–456, 1987

Nierenberg AA, Price LH, Charney DS: After lithium augmentation: a retrospective follow-up of patients with antidepressant-refractory depression. J Affect Disord 18:167–175, 1990

Nierenberg AA, Keck PE Jr, Samson J, et al: Methodological considerations for the study of treatment-resistant depression, in Advances in Neuropsychiatry and Psychopharmacology, Vol 2: Refractory Depression. Edited by Amsterdam JD. New York, Raven, 1991, pp 1–12

Nolen WA, van de Putte JJ, Dijken WA, et al: Treatment strategy in depression, I: non-tricyclic and selective reuptake inhibitors in resistant depression: a double-blind partial crossover study on the effects of oxaprotiline and fluvoxamine. Acta Psychiatr Scand 78:668–675, 1988

Noyes R, Dempsey GM, Blum A, et al: Lithium treatment of depression. Compr Psychiatry 15:187–193, 1974

Ogura C, Okuma T, Uchida Y, et al: Combined thyroid (triiodothyronine)-tricyclic antidepressant treatment in depressive states. Folia Psychiatrica et Neurologica Japonica 28:179–186, 1974

Oppenheim G: Rapid mood cycling with estrogen: implications for therapy. J Clin Psychiatry 45:34–35, 1984

Overall JE, Hollister LE, Johnson M, et al: Nosology of depression and differential response to drugs. JAMA 195:946–948, 1966

Pande AC, Calarco MM, Grunhaus LJ: Combined MAOI-TCA treatment in refractory depression, in Advances in Neuropsychiatry and Psychopharmacology, Vol 2: Refractory Depression. Edited by Amsterdam JD. New York, Raven, 1991, pp 115–122

Paykel ES: Depressive typologies and response to amitriptyline. Br J Psychiatry 120:147–156, 1972

Paykel ES: Predictors of treatment response, in Psychopharmacology of Affective Disorders. Edited by Paykel ES, Coppen A. Oxford, England, Oxford University Press, 1979, pp 193–220

Peck AW, Stern WC, Watkinson C: Incidence of seizures during treatment with tricyclic antidepressant drugs and bupropion. J Clin Psychiatry 44 (5, sec 2):197–201, 1983

Peet M: Induction of mania with selective serotonin re-uptake inhibitors and tricyclic antidepressants. Br J Psychiatry 164:549–550, 1994

Peselow ED, Loutin A, Wolkin A, et al: The dexamethasone suppression test and response to placebo. J Clin Psychopharmacol 6:286–291, 1986

Pfohl B, Stangl D, Zimmerman M: The implications of DSM-III personality disorders for patients with major depression. J Affect Disord 7:309–318, 1984

Post RM: Anticonvulsants as adjuncts or alternatives to lithium in refractory bipolar illness, in Advances in Neuropsychiatry and Psychopharmacology, Vol 2: Refractory Depression. Edited by Amsterdam JD. New York, Raven, 1991, pp 155–165

Post R, Weiss S: The neurobiology of treatment-resistant mood disorders, in Psychopharmacology: The Fourth Generation of Progress. Edited by Bloom F, Kupfer D. New York, Raven, 1995, pp 1605–1611

Power AC, Cowen PJ: Fluoxetine and suicidal behaviour: some clinical and theoretical aspects of a controversy. Br J Psychiatry 161:735–741, 1992

Prange AJ: Paroxysmal auricular tachycardia apparently resulting from combined thyroid-imipramine treatment. Am J Psychiatry 119:994–995, 1963

Prange AJ: Estrogen may well affect response to antidepressant. JAMA 219:143–144, 1972

Prange AJ, Wilson IC, Rabon AM, et al: Enhancement of imipramine antidepressant activity by thyroid hormone. Am J Psychiatry 126:457–469, 1969

Pratt GM, Brater DC, Harrell FE Jr, et al: Clinical and regulatory implications of the Cardiac Arrhythmia Suppression Trial. Am J Cardiol 65:103–105, 1990

Preskorn SH: Tricyclic antidepressants: the whys and hows of therapeutic drug monitoring. J Clin Psychiatry 50 (7, suppl):34–42, 1989

Preskorn SH: Should bupropion dosage be adjusted based upon therapeutic drug monitoring? Psychopharmacol Bull 27:637–643, 1991

Preskorn SH, Fast GA: Therapeutic drug monitoring for antidepressants: efficacy, safety, and cost effectiveness. J Clin Psychiatry 52 (6, suppl):23–33, 1991

Preskorn SH, Alderman J, Chung M, et al: Pharmacokinetics of desipramine coadministered with sertraline or fluoxetine. J Clin Psychopharmacol 14:90–98, 1994

Price LH, Gharney DS, Heninger GR: Efficacy of lithium-tranylcypromine treatment in refractory depression. Am J Psychiatry 142:619–623, 1985

Prien RF, Kupfer DJ: Continuation drug therapy for major depressive episodes: how long should it be maintained? Am J Psychiatry 143:18–23, 1986

Prien RF, Klett J, Caffey EM: Lithium carbonate and imipramine in prevention of affective episodes. Arch Gen Psychiatry 29:420–425, 1973

Quitkin FM, McGrath P, Liebowitz MR, et al: Monoamine oxidase inhibitors in bipolar endogenous depressives. J Clin Psychopharmacol 1:70–74, 1989

Quitkin FM, McGrath PJ, Stewart JW, et al: Atypical depression, panic attacks, and response to imipramine and phenelzine. Arch Gen Psychiatry 47:935–941, 1990

Quitkin FM, Harrison W, Stewart JW, et al: Response to phenelzine and imipramine in placebo nonresponders with atypical depression. Arch Gen Psychiatry 48:319–323, 1991

Raskin A, Crook TA: The endogenous-neurotic distinction as a predictor of response to antidepressant drugs. Psychol Med 6:59–70, 1976

Rawling DA, Fozzard HA: Effects of imipramine on cellular electrophysiological properties of cardiac Purkinje fibers. J Pharmacol Exp Ther 209:371–375, 1979

Razani J, White KL, White J, et al: The safety and efficacy of combined amitriptyline and tranylcypromine antidepressant treatment: a controlled trial. Arch Gen Psychiatry 40:657–661, 1983

Reynolds CF III, Frank E, Perel JM, et al: Combined pharmacotherapy and psychotherapy in the acute and continuation treatment of elderly patients with recurrent major depression: a preliminary report. Am J Psychiatry 149:1687–1692, 1992

Richelson E: Antidepressants: pharmacology and clinical use, in Treatments of Psychiatric Disorders: A Task Force Report of the American Psychiatric Association. Washington, DC, American Psychiatric Association, 1989, pp 1773–1786

Richelson E: Side effects of old and new generation antidepressants: a pharmacologic framework. J Clin Psychiatry 9:13–19, 1991

Richelson E, Nelson A: Antagonism by antidepressants of neurotransmitter receptors of normal human brain in vitro. J Pharmacol Exp Ther 230:94–102, 1984

Rickels K, Amsterdam J, Clary C, et al: The efficacy and safety of paroxetine compared with placebo in outpatients with major depression. J Clin Psychiatry 53 (suppl):30–32, 1992

Riesenman C: Antidepressant drug interactions and the cytochrome P450 system: a critical appraisal. Pharmacotherapy 15 (6, pt 2):84S–99S, 1995

Risch SC, Huey LY, Janowsky DS: Plasma levels of tricyclic antidepressants and clinical efficacy: review of the literature—parts I and II. J Clin Psychiatry 40:4–16, 58–69, 1979

Robinson DS, Roberts DL, Smith JM, et al: The safety profile of nefazodone. J Clin Psychiatry 57 (suppl 2):31–38, 1996

Roose SP, Palack GW, Glassman AH, et al: Cardiovascular effects of bupropion in depressed patients with heart disease. Am J Psychiatry 148:512–516, 1991

Roose SP, Glassman AH, Attia E, et al: Comparative efficacy of selective serotonin reuptake inhibitors and tricyclics in the treatment of melancholia. Am J Psychiatry 151:1735–1739, 1994

Rosenbaum JF, Fava M, Falk WE, et al: The antidepressant potential of oral *S*-adenosyl-L-methionine. Acta Psychiatr Scand 81:432–436, 1990

Rosenstein D, Nelson J, Jacobs S: Seizures associated with antidepressants: a review. J Clin Psychiatry 54:289–299, 1993

Rosenthal J, Hemlock C, Hellerstein DJ, et al: A preliminary study of serotonergic antidepressants in treatment of dysthymia. Prog Neuropsychopharmacol Biol Psychiatry 16:933–941, 1992

Rush AJ: Cognitive therapy of depression: rationale, techniques and efficacy. Psychiatr Clin North Am 6:105–127, 1983

Sabelli HC, Fawcett J, Javaid JJ, et al: The methylphenidate test for differentiating desipramine responsive from nortriptyline responsive depression. Am J Psychiatry 140:212–214, 1983

Sackeim HA, Prudic J, Devanand DP, et al: The impact of medication resistance and continuation pharmacotherapy on relapse following response to electroconvulsive therapy in major depression. J Clin Psychopharmacol 10:96–104, 1990

Salzman C: Pharmacologic treatment of depression in the elderly. J Clin Psychiatry 54 (2, suppl):23–28, 1993

Satel S, Nelson J: Stimulants in the treatment of depression: a critical overview. J Clin Psychiatry 50:241–249, 1989

Schmauss M, Kapfhammer HP, Meyer P, et al: Combined MAO-inhibitor and tri-(tetra) cyclic antidepressant treatment in therapy resistant depression. Prog Neuropsychopharmacol Biol Psychiatry 12:523–532, 1988

Schwartz G, Halaris A, Baxter L: Normal thyroid function in desipramine nonresponders compared to responders by the addition of L-tri-iodothyronine. Am J Psychiatry 141: 1614–1616, 1984

Segraves RT: Sexual dysfunction complicating the treatment of depression. J Clin Psychiatry 10: 75–83, 1992

Selzer A, Wray HW: Quinidine syncope: paroxysmal ventricular fibrillations occurring during treatment of chronic atrial arrhythmias. Circulation 30:17–26, 1964

Settle EC Jr: Antidepressant side effects: issues and options. J Clin Psychiatry 10:48–61, 1992

Shapira B, Oppenheim G, Zohar J, et al: Lack of efficacy of estrogen supplementation to imipramine in resistant female depressives. Biol Psychiatry 20:576–579, 1985

Shawcross CR, Tyrer P: Influence of personality on response to monoamine oxidase inhibitors and tricyclic antidepressants. J Psychiatr Res 19:557–562, 1985

Sheehan DV, Ballenger J, Jacobsen G: Treatment of endogenous anxiety with phobic, hysterical and hypochondriacal symptoms. Arch Gen Psychiatry 40:125–138, 1983a

Sheehan DV, Davidson J, Manschreck T, et al: Lack of efficacy of a new antidepressant (bupropion) in the treatment of panic disorder with phobias. J Clin Pharmacol 3:28–31, 1983b

Sherwin BB: Estrogen and refractory depression, in Advances in Neuropsychiatry and Psychopharmacology, Vol 2: Refractory Depression. Edited by Amsterdam JD. New York, Raven, 1991, pp 209–218

Shopsin B: Bupropion's prophylactic efficacy in bipolar affective illness. J Clin Psychiatry 44 (5, sec 2):163–169, 1983

Simpson GM, Lee HL, Cuche Z, et al: Two doses of imipramine in hospitalized endogenous and neurotic depressions. Arch Gen Psychiatry 33: 1093–1102, 1976

Spar JA, La Rue A: Acute response to methylphenidate as a predictor of outcome of treatment with TCAs in the elderly. J Clin Psychiatry 46:466–469, 1985

Spier SA: Use of bupropion with SRI's and venlafaxine. Depress Anxiety 7:73–75, 1998

Spiker DG, Weiss JC, Dealy RS, et al: The pharmacological treatment of delusional depression. Am J Psychiatry 142:430–436, 1985

Stein G, Bernadt M: Lithium augmentation therapy in tricyclic-resistant depression: a controlled trial using lithium in low and normal doses. Br J Psychiatry 162:634–640, 1993

Stoll AL, Mayer PV, Kolbrener M, et al: Antidepressant-associated mania: a controlled comparison with spontaneous mania. Am J Psychiatry 151: 1642–1645, 1994

Stoll AL, Srinavasan SP, Diamond L, et al: Methylphenidate augmentation of serotonin selective reuptake inhibitors: a case series. J Clin Psychiatry 75:73–76, 1996

Stuppaeck C, Geretsegger C, Whitworth A, et al: A multicenter double-blind trial of paroxetine versus amitriptyline in depressed inpatients. J Clin Psychopharmacol 14:241– 246, 1994

Svendsen K, Christensen PDG: Duration of REM sleep latency as predictor of effect of antidepressant therapy. Acta Psychiatr Scand 64:238–243, 1981

Targum SD: Persistent neuroendocrine dysregulation in major depressive disorder: a marker for early relapse. Biol Psychiatry 19: 305–318, 1984

Teicher MH, Glod C, Cole JO: Emergence of intense suicidal preoccupation during fluoxetine treatment. Am J Psychiatry 147:207–210, 1990

Thase ME, Kupfer DJ, Jarret DB: Treatment of imipramine-resistant recurrent depression, I: an open clinical trial of adjunctive L-triiodothyronine. J Clin Psychiatry 50:385–388, 1989

Thase ME, Mallinger AD, McKnight D, et al: Treatment of imipramine-resistant recurrent depression, IV: a double-blind crossover study of tranylcypromine for anergic bipolar depression. Am J Psychiatry 149:195–198, 1992

Thase ME, Fava M, Halbreich U, et al: A placebo-controlled, randomized clinical trial comparing sertraline and imipramine for the treatment of dysthymia. Arch Gen Psychiatry 53: 777–784, 1996

Trimble MR: Nonmonoamine oxidase inhibitor antidepressants and epilepsy: a review. Epilepsia 19:241–250, 1978

Tsutsui S, Yamazaki Y, Namba T, et al: Combined therapy of T$_3$ and antidepressants in depression. J Int Med Res 7:138–146, 1979

Tyrer P, Murphy S: Efficacy of combined antidepressant therapy in resistant neurotic disorder. Br J Psychiatry 156:115–118, 1990

van Kammen DP, Murphy DL: Prediction of imipramine antidepressant response by a one day *d*-amphetamine trial. Am J Psychiatry 135:1179–1184, 1978

van Praag HM: New evidence of serotonin deficient depressions. Neuropsychobiology 3:56–63, 1977

Walsh BT, Stewart JW, Roose SP, et al: Treatment of bulimia with phenelzine: a double-blind, placebo-controlled study. Arch Gen Psychiatry 41:1105–1109, 1984

Weilburg JB, Rosenbaum JF, Biederman J, et al: Fluoxetine added to non-MAOI antidepressants converts nonresponders to responders: a preliminary report. J Clin Psychiatry 50:447–449, 1989

Weld FM, Bigger JT Jr: Electrophysiological effects of imipramine on ovine cardiac Purkinje and ventricular muscle fibers. Circ Res 46:167–175, 1980

Wharton RN, Perel JM, Dayton PG, et al: A potential clinical use for methylphenidate (Ritalin) with tricyclic antidepressants. Am J Psychiatry 127:1619–1625, 1971

White K, Simpson G: Combined MAOI-tricyclic antidepressant treatment: a reevaluation. J Clin Psychopharmacol 1:264–282, 1981

Wilde M, Plosker G, Benfield P: Fluvoxamine: an updated review of its pharmacology, and therapeutic use in depressive illness. Drugs 46:895–924, 1993

Wolkowitz OM, Reus VI, Manfredi F, et al: Ketoconazole administration in hypercortisolemic depression. Am J Psychiatry 150:810–812, 1993

Wolkowitz OM, Reus VI, Vinogradov S, et al: Antiglucocorticoids in depression and schizophrenia. Program and Abstracts on New Research in Summary Form: the 149th Annual Meeting of the American Psychiatric Association, New York City, May 4–9, 1996, p 152

Wright D, Galloway L, Kim J, et al: Bupropion in the long-term treatment of cyclic mood disorders: mood stabilizing effects. J Clin Psychiatry 46:22–25, 1985

Zall H: Lithium carbonate and isocarboxazid: an effective drug approach in severe depressions. Am J Psychiatry 127:136–139, 1971

EIGHTEEN

Treatment of Bipolar Disorder

Charles L. Bowden, M.D.

RATIONALE FOR TREATMENT

Many of the treatments for bipolar disorder have established efficacy and provide not only symptomatic control but also improved social and vocational functioning. The subsyndromal variations of bipolar disorder—based on both symptom constellation and illness course—have major differences in prognosis and require different treatment strategies.

SYMPTOMATIC AND ILLNESS COURSE FEATURES AFFECTING PHARMACOTHERAPY

The recommendations here are intended for both bipolar I and II groups, with the caveat that experimental data from bipolar II patients are limited. A major difference between mania and hypomania affecting treatment is that hypomania is much more likely to escape detection by the psychiatrist and to be rationalized as healthy function by the patient. Both factors thus increase the possibility of incorrect diagnosis and of poor compliance with treatment.

The criteria for diagnosis of depression in bipolar disorder require the presence of a major depressive episode. This is in part based on evidence that the symptom profile and severity of the depression in bipolar disorder are relatively similar to those of major depression (Katz et al. 1982). However, the frequency of certain symptoms differs in bipolar patients compared with unipolar patients. Hypersomnia and psychomotor retardation are more common in bipolar depression, and anxiety and agitation are less common (Beigel and Murphy 1971; Katz et al. 1982). As many as 25% of bipolar patients may have three or four depressive episodes before their first manic episode (Angst et al. 1978). If the clinician does not recognize a bipolar pattern, then prolonged treatment of the patient with antidepressants, with the attendant risks of precipitating manic episodes and increasing cycle frequency, may result. Attention to several factors during assessment may reduce such erroneous diagnostic classification. The more frequent and the greater the number of depressive episodes, the greater the likelihood of bipolar disorder (Goodwin and Jamison 1990). A high frequency of either bipolar depression or major depression in a patient's relatives is positively associated with the likelihood that the patient's mood disorder is bipolar.

Approximately one-half of all manic patients will have psychotic symptoms. Patients with psychotic features have responded less well to lithium than patients without psychosis in some, but not all, studies (Goodwin and Jamison

1990). Psychotic symptomatology was reduced more in divalproex-treated than in lithium-treated patients in a large, well-designed study (Bowden et al. 1994). Schizoaffective patients refractory to standard antimanic therapies have been reported to respond well to clozapine (Suppes et al. 1992).

Bipolar disorder is strongly associated with several other disorders: migraine, obsessive-compulsive disorder (OCD), panic disorder, and attention-deficit/hyperactivity disorder (ADHD). Although some of this association may be a function of overlapping criteria (e.g., ADHD), much appears to indicate some shared etiopathology. The presence of these comorbid conditions does have treatment implications. Valproate is beneficial for migraine (for which it is approved by the U.S. Food and Drug Administration [FDA] for prophylaxis) and possibly for panic attacks and OCD (Deltito 1994; Herridge and Pope 1985; Lum et al. 1990; Primeau et al. 1990). Valproate also appears to be effective in mania comorbid with substance abuse, but this finding is only based on an open study (Brady et al. 1995). Therefore, the presence of such additional problems in a patient with bipolar disorder would predispose to initiation of treatment with valproate.

Mixed or depressive manic patients respond less well to both acute and chronic treatment with lithium than do patients with pure or elated mania (Bowden 1995; Keller et al. 1986; Swann et al. 1997). Additional features that may aid in identifying patients with mixed mania include older age at first onset of illness, fewer episodes per unit of time, a positive dexamethasone suppression test, and no family history of mood disorder.

Patients with a greater frequency of episodes have quite low response rates to lithium during both acute and prophylactic treatment (Dunner and Fieve 1974; Kukopulos et al. 1983). *Rapid cycling* is defined as four or more episodes of any combination of depression and mania during a 12-month period. A smaller group of patients has much more frequent cycles, even within a

day (Frye et al. 1996; Kramlinger and Post 1995). Drug-induced precipitation of mania in these patients appears to presage more frequent cycling (Altshuler et al. 1995; Keller et al. 1992).

Patients with concurrent substance abuse (including alcoholism) respond less well to lithium than do patients without substance abuse but may respond well to valproate (Brady et al. 1995). The substance abuse must be eliminated through direct intervention. Concurrent attention to the bipolar illness is warranted. Some substance abuse appears to be an effort either to extend manic symptoms or to alleviate dysphoric symptoms of the disorder, and it may resolve with alleviation of the manic or depressive episode. Because approximately one-half of both bipolar I and II patients have concurrent substance abuse, close attention to this problem during evaluation or at times of breakthrough episodes is important (Regier et al. 1988).

A wide range of medical disorders results in disturbance of mood, either concurrently or as sequelae of the medical disorder. Most late-onset bipolar disorders are in this category. When possible, treatment should concurrently be aimed at the primary disorder. Patients with secondary bipolar disorders tend to have mixed symptomatology and more manic than depressed episodes. Lithium is relatively ineffective in treatment of these conditions. Uncontrolled studies suggest more favorable responses with carbamazepine or valproate (D. Kahn et al. 1988; Tohen et al. 1990).

PHARMACOTHERAPIES

General Principles of Drug Treatment

Charting of mood has a special role in bipolar disorder management. Because of the fluctuating mood states and varying symptom presentations requiring changing medication regimens, as well as the nearly uniform long-term treatment required, it can be difficult to glean drug treatment–clinical response relationships from the traditional medical record with progress notes. Charting offers a graphically succinct means of capturing several domains of treatment and response on one sheet.

Benzodiazepines often relieve insomnia and related agitation and restlessness. Their adjunctive use is particularly important early in treatment, before the mood stabilizer becomes effective, and as needed to normalize sleep during maintenance treatment. Although standard doses of any benzodiazepine may be helpful, two drugs warrant special consideration. Lorazepam has the advantage of parenteral administration to the patient unable or unwilling to take oral medication. Clonazepam has a long duration of action, thus reducing the need for frequent dosing and producing consistent sedation both at night and (if needed) during the day. Additionally, clonazepam (one of a small number of drugs that is metabolized by nitrogen reduction) is not pharmacokinetically altered by enzyme inducers such as carbamazepine. Sedating antidepressants such as trazodone, which are often used for sleep induction in major depression, should generally be avoided in bipolar disorder because of the risk of cycle acceleration.

Many patients with bipolar disorder are exquisitely sensitive to chemical agents that may destabilize mood (Goodwin and Jamison 1990). The clinician should inquire about such medication or substance use and, when warranted, couple this with toxicological screening. Although antidepressants are the most important group in this regard, some patients are destabilized by a panoply of substances, such as mild quantities of alcohol, topical steroids, medications for glaucoma, or mild use of stimulants.

Most patients with bipolar disorder receive a combination of drugs rather than monotherapy as maintenance treatment. Although some of this polypharmacy is attributable to failure to discontinue a medication that is no longer needed, most authorities believe that combined drug therapy is needed to achieve the best possible clinical response in a substantial number of patients.

The two types of combined drug therapy are 1) concurrent use of two or more mood-stabilizing drugs and 2) use of a mood-stabilizing agent plus one or more adjunctive drugs. Reports have been published on the effectiveness and good tolerance of all such combinations of the first type (Kramlinger and Post 1989). More caution should be exercised in combining valproate and carbamazepine. Carbamazepine may increase the percentage of a potentially hepatotoxic valproate metabolite (Ketter et al. 1992). The adjunctive drugs used in the second type of combined drug therapy are generally limited to benzodiazepines, antipsychotics, and/or antidepressants.

If improvement occurs after addition of the second drug, the clinician should consider gradually tapering the dosage of the first drug because no other procedure ensures that the improvement is associated with the two drugs in combination rather than the second drug alone. Combined drug therapy warrants closer monitoring for adverse effects and greater utilization of plasma concentration monitoring to ensure that drug concentrations have not strayed outside the ranges generally deemed safe and effective.

Acute Mania and Hypomania

Lithium, valproate, and carbamazepine have relatively well-established efficacy in acute mania. Lithium and the divalproex form of valproate are approved by the FDA for this indication. Lithium is most likely to be effective in patients with elated manic symptomatology but not mixed manic features. Response rates in these patients may be as high as 90%. Lithium is much less effective in patients with mixed mania (Bowden 1995; Himmelhoch et al. 1991; Prien et al. 1988; Secunda et al. 1985) or rapid cycling (Dunner and Fieve 1974; Kukopulos et al. 1983). More severely ill and psychotically manic patients may also respond less well to lithium than do acutely ill manic patients. Lithium is generally poorly tolerated in elderly patients, in whom cognitive and gastrointestinal adverse effects are especially prominent (Shulman et al. 1987).

One randomized, placebo-controlled study of lithium in acute mania has been conducted. Forty-nine percent of the patients had a moderate or better response within 3 weeks of vigorous lithium treatment without any use of neuroleptics. This represents a highly and clinically significant difference over placebo. Thirty-one percent of patients' conditions were actually worse at last assessment. Dropout rates and adverse events were somewhat higher in patients treated with lithium than in those treated with valproate (Bowden et al. 1994).

The time to initial (albeit not full) response is generally 7–14 days for those patients who are treated successfully with lithium. However, initial improvement may not occur sooner than the third or fourth week for some patients. Because the behavior of the acutely manic patient is often disruptive and dangerous, adjunctive medications are often required during this lag period. Lithium plasma concentrations required for acutely manic patients are often somewhat higher than those needed for maintenance therapy, and maintenance dosage should be decreased to compensate for reduced renal clearance after recovery from a manic episode (Goodwin and Zis 1979). Although a loading-dose strategy does not appear to be effective for lithium, the dosage should be increased as rapidly as tolerated until either the patient responds or a plasma level of 1.2–1.4 mEq/L is reached. Although lithium has many serious adverse effects, most will not be problematic during treatment of acute episodes. Common side effects with acute treatment are gastrointestinal irritation, tremor, metallic taste, and cognitive dulling.

In a double-blind, parallel-group study in hospitalized acutely manic patients, divalproex and lithium were equally effective, and both were significantly better than placebo (Bowden et al. 1994). Significant improvement with valproate was present from the fifth day of treatment. Dropout rates, particularly for reasons of adverse effects, were lower in valproate-treated than in lithium-treated subjects. The symptoms that had the earliest and most robust response to valproate were largely those constituting the primary manic syndrome: elevated mood, reduced need for sleep, and excessive activity. Those symptom areas (e.g., accelerated speech, poor judgment) that are elevated in mania but not specific thereto were less responsive to either drug.

The quality and scope of double-blind, placebo-controlled studies of valproate effectiveness in acute mania are better than those for lithium. Two placebo-controlled studies have reported highly clinically significant clinical superiority of divalproex over placebo (Bowden et al. 1994; Pope et al. 1991). The divalproex form has better gastrointestinal tolerability than valproic acid (Wilder et al. 1983). Divalproex is as effective in acute treatment of patients with mixed mania as in those with pure mania and those with rapid cycling (Bowden et al. 1994; Calabrese and Delucchi 1990).

Divalproex can be administered in a loading dose of 20–30 mg/kg, which results in a partial response within 1–3 days (Keck et al. 1993). The adverse effects of divalproex most likely to occur during acute treatment include gastrointestinal irritation, tremor, sedation, and cognitive dulling. A serum level between 45 and 110 µg/mL provides a relatively wide range for therapeutically effective yet well tolerated treatment (Bowden et al. 1996).

The one placebo-controlled study of carbamazepine was a crossover design with 19 patients that did not allow comparison of relative efficacy. Nevertheless, more than a dozen controlled studies indicate that carbamazepine is effective in acute mania (Post et al. 1988). Comparisons with lithium indicate lesser efficacy for carbamazepine. Of the two parallel-group comparisons with lithium, one found a lower response rate with carbamazepine than with lithium (Lerer et al. 1987). The other, composed of a relatively treatment-refractory sample, reported only a 33% response rate for both drugs (Small et al. 1991). Comparisons with neuroleptics have shown equivalent response rates, whereas lithium was generally superior to neuroleptics in controlled trials (Goodwin and Jamison 1990). Carbamazepine was more effective in treatment of patients with mixed mania than in those with pure mania. It is less effective in rapid-cycling than in non-rapid-cycling patients (Denicoff et al. 1994; Okuma et al. 1990).

Carbamazepine requires cautious initial administration. A starting dose of 200 mg twice a day with a gradual increase to levels greater than 4 µg/mL will often prevent or reduce sedation, cognitive dulling, diplopia, gastrointestinal irritability, and psychomotor slowing, which otherwise are relatively common early adverse effects. Carbamazepine causes induction of the 3A4 isoform of the P450 family of oxidative enzymes. This induction is generally clinically identifiable at about the fourth to eighth week of treatment. This complicates management, requiring relatively frequent plasma level measurement and dosage increases to return to the range at which initial response occurred. Similarly, other medications metabolized through 3A4 will likely require an increased dosage. In the case of several of these drugs (oral contraceptives, bupropion, alprazolam, nefazodone), concurrent use is inadvisable because of the marked lowering of plasma levels (Ketter et al. 1995). Rashes, which lead to discontinuation in 10%–15% of patients, can include severe hemorrhagic responses (e.g., Stevens-Johnson syndrome). Regular monitoring of white blood cell and platelet count is important, although the relatively common 20%–30% reduction in granulocyte count and platelet count warrants more frequent monitoring rather than discontinuation of the medication.

Dosage should be increased as tolerated until a response occurs or a carbamazepine concentration of 12 µg/mL is achieved. Despite the lack of strong plasma level–response guidelines, plasma concentration monitoring every 2–3 months is still warranted. This ensures that the concentration is not moving upward or downward despite a stable dosage, serves as a check on compliance, and establishes that the patient is within the concentration range at which a positive initial response occurred.

Acute Depression

Direct experimental data about drug efficacy in bipolar depression are inadequate. Only two double-blind, randomized, parallel-group, placebo-controlled studies of bipolar patients have been published (Calabrese et al. 1999; Cohn et al. 1989). Consequently, recommendations for treatment of bipolar depression are based largely on data that are either outdated, derived from research on a different disease (i.e., major depression), or both. The response rate of bipolar and unipolar depression to tricyclic antidepressants (TCAs) appears to be similar (Koslow et al. 1983). Bipolar depression specifically characterized by anergia is more responsive to monoamine oxidase inhibitors (MAOIs) than to TCAs (Himmelhoch et al. 1991). Initial dosages and patterns of dosage escalation and dosage ranges do not differ from those for major depression. With the exception of the risks of mood destabilization (expressed as either hypomania, rapid cycling, or both), the side-effect profile does not differ.

Because selective serotonin reuptake inhibitors (SSRIs) have a favorable side-effect profile, they are promising agents for bipolar depression. Positive results have been reported with fluoxetine and paroxetine. Fluoxetine was superior to placebo and nonsignificantly better than imipramine in one placebo-controlled study (Cohn et al. 1989). The patients treated with fluoxetine had fewer side effects than those treated with imipramine. Bupropion has also been reported to be more effective than a TCA with a lower rate of induction of mania in a randomized, blinded small open study (Shopsin 1983).

Results of a consensus survey of experts favored bupropion and SSRIs as initial treatment for bipolar depressive episodes (Frances et al. 1996). Given the greater likelihood of cognitive impairment, autonomic overstimulation, hypotension, sedation, and weight gain, as well as the potential lethality in suicide attempts, associated with all TCAs, their use should generally be limited to secondary choices or to patients who have benefited from and tolerated them well in previous depressive episodes. Among the SSRIs, the long half-life of fluoxetine is a potential disadvantage, because plasma levels would not decline by 50% for approximately 1 month after discontinuing the drug if the patient developed hypomania.

If the patient is unresponsive, is intolerant, or has a medical contraindication to these agents, electroconvulsive therapy (ECT) may be implemented. ECT has been reported to be superior to TCAs in bipolar depression, although the studies have substantial methodological limitations (Goodwin and Jamison 1990). A recent randomized trial suggested that lamotrigine, an approved antiepileptic drug, may be effective in bipolar depressive episodes (Calabrese et al. 1999).

Several studies—only one of which was prospective and controlled—indicated that all of the above classes of antidepressants can either precipitate manic or (more often) hypomanic episodes or destabilize the course of illness, which results in a rapid-cycling course (Frye et al. 1996; Prien et al. 1984; Wehr and Goodwin 1987). The frequency of development of drug-induced mania is not established, although studies suggest that it may occur in approximately 30% of patients with bipolar disorder (Frye et al. 1996). The few studies that have not reported this adverse effect have tended to exclude the very subjects who would be at risk for mood destabilization (Kupfer et al. 1988; Lewis and Winokur 1982). Furthermore, concurrent lithium does not consistently prevent the development of manic episodes (Quitkin et al. 1981). Based on this increasingly strong evidence for mood disturbance from antidepressants, the recommendation for use of antidepressants in

bipolar disorder has changed to that of limiting them to administration during depressive episodes.

Maintenance Treatment

Bipolar disorder is in nearly all instances recurrent and chronic, with no tendency for the patient to mature out of the disease. Single episodes of mania are rare. Furthermore, the risks of not treating prophylactically include the disease's suicide rate of approximately 15%, the strong likelihood of recurrent episodes, and the serious social and vocational morbidity associated with the illness.

Early maintenance-phase studies of lithium's superiority over placebo were substantially more conclusive for maintenance treatment than for acute treatment, with early studies showing an approximate 2:1 superiority of lithium over placebo (Baastrup et al. 1970; Davis 1976). Lithium discontinuation is followed by a high rate of relapse, with most new episodes being of manic rather than depressed type (Suppes et al. 1992).

Studies indicate that a substantial number of patients have inadequate long-term responses to lithium therapy. A naturalistic follow-up of outpatients with bipolar disorder found that the outcome was no better for patients given lithium maintenance therapy than for those taking no medication (Goldberg et al. 1995; Harrow et al. 1990). Even among patients with an initial successful response to lithium for 2 years, only about half continued to have an unequivocally good response in subsequent years (Maj et al. 1989).

Part of the poor response over time may be related to inadequate dosing. Gelenberg and colleagues (1989) found that relapse rates were higher among patients with plasma levels maintained at 0.4–0.6 mEq/L than among patients with plasma levels maintained at 0.8–1.0 mEq/L. The difference in relapse rates was only for manic episodes—suggesting, as do most studies, that lithium's prophylactic benefits are largely for new manic or hypomanic episodes. Additionally, the differences held only for patients with one or two prior episodes and thus cannot be generalized to patients with frequent episodes (Gelenberg et al. 1989).

The dosage of lithium needed to maintain a desired serum level is generally somewhat lower during maintenance treatment than during an acute manic episode (Vahip et al. 1995). Lithium's side effects are much more problematic during maintenance therapy than during acute therapy. Additional problems unlikely to occur during acute treatment include weight gain, acne, hypothyroidism, polydipsia, and polyuria. The group of side effects most likely to cause poor compliance or discontinuation of lithium are those that affect the central nervous system. These include impaired cognition, impaired short-term memory, poor coordination, muscular weakness, and lethargy (Jamison et al. 1979). Thyroid function should be assessed approximately every 6 months because of the high frequency of hypothyroidism during lithium treatment and the potential for hypothyroidism to then compromise the patient's clinical response (Citrome 1995).

The combination of a relatively low percentage of patients with good long-term outcomes, the frequency and functional severity of side effects, and lithium's very narrow therapeutic index has stimulated studies of alternative mood stabilizers.

A randomized, open comparison of valproate and lithium for an 18-month period reported good efficacy for both drugs, with somewhat more favorable results among valproate-treated patients (Lambert and Venaud 1992). In a randomized, double-blind study of bipolar I patients treated for 1 year with divalproex, lithium, or placebo, divalproex was somewhat more effective than lithium in duration of time in maintenance treatment. In fewer divalproex-treated than placebo-treated patients, treatment was prematurely terminated for mania or depression. Patients whose acute mania was treated with divalproex and who received divalproex during the maintenance phase also had better outcomes than those who received lithium or placebo. Divalproex was somewhat better tolerated than lithium (Bowden et al. 2000).

Valproate's dosage and plasma levels appear to be the same for maintenance treatment as those used for acute treatment. As with lithium, additional side effects must be considered. Transient hair loss may occur after several weeks of therapy. Selenium and zinc may provide some protection against hair loss. Increased appetite and weight gain may occur, in what is probably a dose-dependent response. Although cognitive dulling may occur, it appears to be dose related and generally manageable by adjustment of timing of valproate dosage or reduction of dosage.

Carbamazepine has been inadequately studied in maintenance-phase treatment. Lusznat and colleagues (1988) found no significant differences between lithium and carbamazepine among patients treated for up to a year, although a larger percentage of carbamazepine-treated patients relapsed during treatment. Small and colleagues (1991) reported a trend favoring lithium over carbamazepine in the long-term maintenance-phase treatment of initially hospitalized, treatment-refractory manic patients. Carbamazepine was inferior to lithium in a random assignment study without concomitant medication (Lerer et al. 1987). Another small study found that carbamazepine was superior to placebo; however, nearly all patients received supplemental neuroleptics (Goncalves and Stoll 1985). This and the Lerer study suggest (albeit without much data) that antipsychotic medication may be needed when carbamazepine is used.

Dosing approaches for carbamazepine require some modification during months 2–6 of treatment. Sometime during this period, most patients undergo hepatic enzyme induction, thus requiring a consequent increase in carbamazepine dose to restore the plasma level that was initially effective. In addition to the acute-phase side effects, several additional side effects require monitoring during maintenance-phase treatment. Hematological and hepatic function should be monitored. Hyponatremia may be clinically significant, particularly in older patients. Carbamazepine lowers not only its own levels but also those of all oxidatively metabolized drugs (Jann et al. 1985; E. M. Kahn et al. 1990). Careful inquiry as to continued efficacy of such other drugs and use of drug-level monitoring (when available) will ward off most problems of this type.

Selection of a Mood Stabilizer

As a result of randomized studies comparing divalproex and lithium, the rationale for selection of a primary mood-stabilizing agent has changed. Lithium appears to be most useful for patients with elated manic episodes and for patients who have shown good responses and tolerability during previous episodes (Bowden et al. 1994). Divalproex appears to be more effective than lithium for patients with mixed mania, rapid cycling, concurrent substance abuse, and secondary mania (Bowden and Rhodes 1997). Divalproex is generally better tolerated than lithium, especially regarding cognition, and poses fewer serious risks. These advantages are particularly clinically important in adolescents and elderly persons with bipolar disorder (Papatheodorou et al. 1995; Tohen et al. 1990). Overall, these studies suggest a broader spectrum of efficacy for divalproex than for lithium. However, lithium may be highly effective in the subset of patients for whom it provides benefit.

CONCLUSION

Early studies are assessing the effectiveness of olanzapine, risperidone, lamotrigine, topiramate, and gabapentin for various aspects of bipolar disorder. Recognition of the complex presentations of bipolar disorder, the spectrum of conditions with elements of bipolar symptomatology, and its episodic course and the excitement engendered by evidence of the effectiveness of a new treatment—divalproex—have stimulated interest in the disorder. Important studies of symptomatology, illness course, and potential new treatments are in progress and are likely to affect patient care even beyond the information summarized in this chapter. Close attention to this developing information will substantially improve the quality of care psychiatrists can provide for patients with this disease.

REFERENCES

Altshuler LL, Post RM, Leverich GS, et al: Antidepressant-induced mania and cycle acceleration: a controversy revisited. Am J Psychiatry 152: 1130–1138, 1995

Angst J, Felder W, Stassen HH: The course of affective disorders, I: change of diagnosis of monopolar, unipolar, and bipolar illness. Archiv für Psychiatrie Nervenkrankheiten 226:57–64, 1978

Baastrup PC, Poulsen JC, Schou M, et al: Prophylactic lithium: double-blind discontinuation in manic-depressive and recurrent-depressive disorders. Lancet 2:326–330, 1970

Beigel A, Murphy DL: Assessing clinical characteristics of the manic state. Am J Psychiatry 128: 688–694, 1971

Bowden CL: Predictors of response to divalproex and lithium. J Clin Psychiatry 56:25–30, 1995

Bowden CL, Rhodes LJ: Treatment of acute mania, in Current Psychiatric Therapy, 2nd Edition. Edited by Dunner DL. Philadelphia, PA, WB Saunders, 1997, pp 253–261

Bowden CL, Brugger AM, Swann AC, et al: Efficacy of divalproex vs lithium and placebo in the treatment of mania. JAMA 271:918–924, 1994

Bowden CL, Janicak PG, Orsulak P, et al: Relation of serum valproate concentration to response in mania. Am J Psychiatry 153:765–770, 1996

Bowden CL, Calabrese JR, McElroy SL, et al: A randomized, placebo-controlled 12-month trial of divalproex and lithium in treatment of patients with bipolar I disorder. Divalproex Maintenance Study Group. Arch Gen Psychiatry 57:481–489, 2000

Brady KT, Sonne S, Anton R, et al: Valproate in the treatment of acute bipolar affective episodes complicated by substance abuse: a pilot study. J Clin Psychiatry 56:118–121, 1995

Calabrese JR, Delucchi GA: Spectrum of efficacy of valproate in 55 patients with rapid-cycling bipolar disorder. Am J Psychiatry 147:431–434, 1990

Calabrese JR, Bowden CL, Sachs GS, et al: A double-blind placebo-controlled study of lamotrigine monotherapy in outpatients with bipolar I depression. J Clin Psychiatry 60:79–88, 1999

Citrome L: The use of lithium, carbamazepine, and valproic acid in a state operated psychiatric hospital. Journal of Pharmacy Technology 11: 55–59, 1995

Cohn JB, Collins G, Ashbrook E, et al: A comparison of fluoxetine, imipramine, and placebo in patients with bipolar depressive disorder. Int Clin Psychopharmacol 4:313–322, 1989

Davis JM: Overview: maintenance therapy in psychiatry, II: affective disorders. Am J Psychiatry 133:1–13, 1976

Deltito JA: Valproate treatment for the difficult-to-treat patient with OCD (letter). J Clin Psychiatry 55:500, 1994

Denicoff KD, Blake KD, Smith-Jackson EE, et al: Morbidity in treated bipolar disorder: a one-year prospective study using daily life chart ratings. Depression 2:95–104, 1994

Dunner DL, Fieve RR: Clinical factors in lithium carbonate prophylaxis failure. Arch Gen Psychiatry 30:229–233, 1974

Frances A, Docherty JP, Kahn DA: The expert consensus guideline series: treatment of bipolar disorder. J Clin Psychiatry 57:3–88, 1996

Frye MA, Altshuler LL, Szuba MP, et al: The relationship between antimanic agent for treatment of classic or dysphoric mania and length of hospital stay. J Clin Psychiatry 57:17–21, 1996

Gelenberg AJ, Kane JM, Keller MB, et al: Comparison of standard and low serum levels of lithium for maintenance treatment of bipolar disorder. N Engl J Med 321:1489–1493, 1989

Goldberg JF, Harrow M, Grossman LS: Course and outcome in bipolar affective disorder. Am J Psychiatry 152:379–384, 1995

Goncalves N, Stoll KD: Carbam pin bei manischen syndromen. EINE kontrollierte doppel blind studie [Carbamazepine in manic syndromes: a controlled double-blind study]. Nervenerzt 56:43–47, 1985

Goodwin FK, Jamison KR: Manic-Depressive Illness. New York, Oxford University Press, 1990

Goodwin FK, Zis AP: Lithium in the treatment of mania: comparisons with neuroleptics. Arch Gen Psychiatry 36:840–844, 1979

Harrow M, Goldberg JF, Grossman LS, et al: Outcome in manic disorders: a naturalistic follow-up study. Arch Gen Psychiatry 47:665–671, 1990

Herridge PL, Pope HG Jr: Treatment of bulimia and rapid-cycling bipolar disorder with sodium valproate: a case report. J Clin Psychopharmacol 5:229–230, 1985

Himmelhoch JM, Thase MF, Mallinger AG, et al: Tranylcypromine versus imipramine in anergic bipolar depression. Am J Psychiatry 148: 910–916, 1991

Jamison KR, Gerner RH, Goodwin FK: Patient and physician attitudes toward lithium: relationship to compliance. Arch Gen Psychiatry 36:866–869, 1979

Jann MW, Ereshefsky L, Saklad SR, et al: Effects of carbamazepine on plasma haloperidol levels. J Clin Psychopharmacol 5:106–109, 1985

Kahn D, Stevenson E, Douglas CJ: Effect of sodium valproate in three patients with organic brain syndromes. Am J Psychiatry 145:101–111, 1988

Kahn EM, Schulz SC, Perel JM, et al: Change in haloperidol level due to carbamazepine—a complicating factor in combined medication for schizophrenia. J Clin Psychopharmacol 10: 54–57, 1990

Katz MM, Robins E, Croughan J, et al: Behavioral measurement and drug response characteristics of unipolar and bipolar depression. Psychol Med 12:25–36, 1982

Keck PE Jr, McElroy SL, Tugrul KC, et al: Valproate oral loading in the treatment of acute mania. J Clin Psychiatry 54:305–308, 1993

Keller MB, Lavori PW, Coryell W, et al: Differential outcome of pure manic, mixed/cycling, and pure depressive episodes in patients with bipolar illness. JAMA 255:3138–3142, 1986

Keller MB, Lavori PW, Kane JM, et al: Subsyndromal symptoms in bipolar disorder: a comparison of standard and low serum levels of lithium. Arch Gen Psychiatry 49:371–376, 1992

Ketter TA, Pazzaglia P, Post RM: Synergy of carbamazepine and valproic acid in affective illness: case report and review of literature. J Clin Psychopharmacol 12:276–282, 1992

Ketter TA, Jenkins JB, Schroeder DH, et al: Carbamazepine but not valproate induces bupropion metabolism. J Clin Psychopharmacol 15:327–330, 1995

Koslow SH, Maas JW, Bowden CL, et al: CSF and urinary biogenic amines and metabolites in depression and mania: a controlled, univariate analysis. Arch Gen Psychiatry 40:999–1010, 1983

Kramlinger KG, Post RM: The addition of lithium carbonate to carbamazepine: antidepressant efficacy in treatment-resistant depression. Arch Gen Psychiatry 46:794–800, 1989

Kramlinger KG, Post RM: Ultra-rapid and ultradian cycling in bipolar affective illness. Br J Psychiatry 167:95/31.1– 95/31.10, 1995

Kukopulos A, Caliari B, Tundo A, et al: Rapid cyclers, temperament, and antidepressants. Compr Psychiatry 24:249–258, 1983

Kupfer DJ, Carpenter LL, Frank E: Possible role of antidepressants in precipitating mania and hypomania in recurrent depression. Am J Psychiatry 145:804–808, 1988

Lambert PA, Venaud G: Comparative study of valpromide versus lithium as prophylactic treatment in affective disorders. Nervure Journal de Psychiatrie 7:1–9, 1992

Lerer B, Moore N, Meyendorff E, et al: Carbamazepine versus lithium in mania: a double-blind study. J Clin Psychiatry 48:89–93, 1987

Lewis JL, Winokur G: The induction of mania: a natural history study with controls. Arch Gen Psychiatry 39:303–306, 1982

Lum M, Fontaine R, Elie R, et al: Divalproex sodium's antipanic effect in panic disorder: a placebo-controlled study. Biol Psychiatry 27:164A–165A, 1990

Lusznat R, Murphy DP, Nunn CMH: Carbamazepine vs lithium in the treatment and prophylaxis of mania. Br J Psychiatry 153:198–204, 1988

Maj M, Priozzi R, Kemali D: Long-term outcome of lithium prophylaxis in patients initially classified as complete responders. Psychopharmacology 98:535–538, 1989

Okuma T, Yamashita I, Takahashi R, et al: Comparison of the antimanic efficacy of carbamazepine and lithium carbonate by double-blind controlled study. Pharmacopsychiatry 23:143–150, 1990

Papatheodorou G, Kutcher SP, Katic M, et al: The efficacy and safety of divalproex sodium in the treatment of acute mania in adolescents and young adults. J Clin Psychopharmacol 15:110–116, 1995

Pope HG Jr, McElroy SL, Keck PE Jr, et al: Valproate in the treatment of acute mania: a placebo-controlled study. Arch Gen Psychiatry 48:62–68, 1991

Post RM, Roy-Byrne PP, Uhde TW: Graphic representation of the life course of illness in patients with affective disorder. Am J Psychiatry 145:844–848, 1988

Prien RF, Kupfer DJ, Mansky PA, et al: Drug therapy in the prevention of recurrences in unipolar and bipolar affective disorders: report of the NIMH Collaborative Study Group comparing lithium carbonate, imipramine, and a lithium carbonate-imipramine combination. Arch Gen Psychiatry 41:1096–1104, 1984

Prien RF, Himmelhoch JM, Kupfer DJ: Treatment of mixed mania. J Affect Disord 15:9–15, 1988

Primeau F, Fontaine R, Beauclair L: Valproic acid and panic disorder. Can J Psychiatry 35:248–250, 1990

Quitkin FM, Kane J, Rifkin A, et al: Prophylactic lithium carbonate with and without imipramine for bipolar I patients: a double-blind study. Arch Gen Psychiatry 38:902–907, 1981

Regier DA, Boyd JH, Burke JDJ, et al: One-month prevalence of mental disorders in the United States: based on five Epidemiological Catchment Area sites. Arch Gen Psychiatry 45:977–986, 1988

Secunda S, Katz MM, Swann A, et al: Mania: diagnosis, state measurement and prediction of treatment response. J Affect Disord 8:113–121, 1985

Shopsin B: Bupropion's prophylactic efficacy in bipolar affective illness. J Clin Psychiatry 44:163–169, 1983

Shulman KI, Mackenzie S, Hardy B: The clinical use of lithium carbonate in old age: a review. Prog Neuropsychopharmacol Biol Psychiatry 11:159–164, 1987

Small JG, Klapper MH, Milstein V, et al: Carbamazepine compared with lithium in the treatment of mania. Arch Gen Psychiatry 48: 915–921, 1991

Suppes T, McElroy SL, Gilbert J, et al: Clozapine in the treatment of dysphoric mania. Biol Psychiatry 32:270–280, 1992

Swann AC, Bowden CL, Morris D, et al: Depression during mania: treatment response to lithium or divalproex. Arch Gen Psychiatry 54: 37–42, 1997

Tohen M, Watemaux CM, Tsuang MT, et al: Four-year follow-up of twenty-four first-episode manic patients. J Affect Disord 19: 76–86, 1990

Vahip S, Ozkan B, Ayan A, et al: Elevation of plasma lithium at the end of mania and some biochemical correlates. Abstract presented at the Second International Conference on New Directions in Affective Disorders, Jerusalem, Israel, 1995, p 31

Wehr TA, Goodwin FK: Can antidepressants cause mania and worsen the course of affective illness? Am J Psychiatry 144:1403–1411, 1987

Wilder BJ, Karas BJ, Penry JK, et al: Gastrointestinal tolerance of divalproex sodium. Neurology 33:808–811, 1983

NINETEEN

Treatment of Schizophrenia

Herbert Y. Meltzer, M.D., and
S. Hossein Fatemi, M.D., Ph.D.

The treatment of schizophrenia is based on the skillful integration of pharmacotherapy and psychosocial interventions. Never before has there been as broad an array of drugs to treat the full range of deficits that are variably present in this illness, including positive, negative, and disorganization symptoms; depressive symptoms; and cognitive disturbances. These developments in pharmacological treatments are taking place in the context of significant changes in how treatment is provided to persons with schizophrenia; these changes are, in large part, the result of deinstitutionalization of even the most seriously and persistently ill schizophrenic patients and the increasingly prominent role of managed care in deciding who will provide treatment, what treatments will be available, and for how long. The purpose of this chapter is to provide an integrative approach to the treatment of schizophrenia. Extensive discussion of specific antipsychotic drugs is found elsewhere in this volume (see Marder, Chapter 8; Owens and Risch, Chapter 9; and Stanilla and Simpson, Chapter 10, in this volume).

HISTORICAL BACKGROUND

Dementia praecox and schizophrenia were recognized by Emil Kraepelin and Eugen Bleuler approximately 100 and 90 years ago, respectively. The disorder that these concepts represent has, to the best of our knowledge, been present throughout human history. Before the introduction of pharmacotherapy in the 1950s, in the great majority of cases, schizophrenia led to lifelong psychosis with very poor outcome.

Opiates and sedatives, as well as insulin coma therapy, were used in the first half of the twentieth century without producing specific improvement in psychopathology or changing the course of illness. The first effective somatic treatment was electroconvulsive therapy

Preparation of this manuscript was supported by a Center Grant from the National Institute of Mental Health (MH-48481) and grants from the Esel, Lattner, and Lauerate Foundations, and Ms. Debra Schuller.

The excellent secretarial support of Ms. Diantha McLeod and Ms. Dina Kauffman is greatly appreciated.

(ECT), which remains in limited use.

The discovery and testing of chlorpromazine, a tricyclic phenothiazine compound, in 1954 by Laborit, Delay, and Deniker in France was the beginning of the modern era of the pharmacotherapy of schizophrenia. Their careful, pioneering studies were the first reliable demonstration of pharmacological treatment of psychosis, which ranks as among the most important discoveries in all of medicine.

Elucidation of the role of receptor blockade in the action of chlorpromazine led to the discovery of many other phenothiazines with antipsychotic efficacy (e.g., fluphenazine, perphenazine, and thioridazine), as well as other classes of agents that included effective antipsychotic drugs (e.g., haloperidol, sulpiride, molindone, pimozide, and thiothixene). It was noted that all these agents produce extrapyramidal side effects (EPS)—that is, dystonic reactions, muscle rigidity, tremor, loss of associated movements, and akathisia (an intense restlessness that leads to repetitive limb movements and pacing [Adler et al. 1989]). After months to years of neuroleptic treatment, abnormal involuntary movement of the tongue, lips, face, and limbs, known as *tardive dyskinesia*, or permanent dystonias, referred to as *tardive dystonia*, developed in some, but not all, patients.

Antipsychotic drugs that are potent dopamine receptor antagonists are referred to as the *typical* or *conventional* neuroleptics because at usual clinical doses they produce the neurological side effects noted above. It is now established that the antipsychotic efficacy of these agents is the result of blockade of D_2 dopamine receptors in the mesolimbic system of the brain, whereas their EPS are the result of blockade of the same group of receptors in the basal ganglia (K. L. Davis et al. 1991). These two processes appear to be inextricably linked. However, as noted later in this chapter, there is controversy as to whether lower doses of these agents, which do not produce EPS, might be clinically effective by producing sufficient blockade of dopaminergic transmission in the mesolimbic system

and sparing that in the basal ganglia (McEvoy et al. 1991).

The search for medications that have antipsychotic properties but that do not produce as many or as severe EPS as the conventional neuroleptic drugs led to the discovery, in 1959, of clozapine, a dibenzodiazepine, which produces virtually no EPS in humans, even though other members of the same chemical class, loxapine and amoxapine, produce significant EPS at clinically effective doses (Meltzer 1996, 1997). Clozapine was introduced into clinical practice in 1969 but was withdrawn because of its ability to produce agranulocytosis (Meltzer 1997). It was reintroduced in 1989 after it was found to be more effective than the first generation of antipsychotic drugs in many patients with treatment-resistant schizophrenia (Kane et al. 1988). It had also been observed that clozapine did not produce tardive dyskinesia or tardive dystonia but, in fact, actively suppressed the symptoms of both conditions in many, but not all, patients; this finding disproved the strongly held belief that any antipsychotic drug that could alleviate the symptoms of tardive movement disorders would also produce them (Kane and Marder 1993).

Unlike the typical neuroleptic drugs mentioned earlier, clozapine is not a potent antagonist of the D_2 receptor in vivo or in vitro (Fatemi et al. 1996). As is discussed below, clozapine has a complex pharmacology (Fatemi et al. 1996).

The hypothesis that clozapine's novel effects derive from potent antagonism of the serotonin (5-HT) 5-HT_{2A} receptor (Meltzer et al. 1989), coupled with the earlier finding of weak blockade of the D_2 receptor, led to the development of a group of drugs with similar properties (e.g., risperidone, olanzapine, quetiapine, and ziprasidone). However, as noted below, these drugs differ from clozapine in many other pharmacological properties (Schotte et al. 1996). It is still uncertain as to whether the potent 5-HT_{2A}/weak D_2 antagonism hypothesis is correct. These drugs, which are sometimes referred to as *serotonin-dopamine antagonists*, are currently being assessed for their superiority to the typical neuroleptic drugs and their advantages and disadvantages relative to clozapine. They are frequently referred to as *atypical* antipsychotic drugs because of the dissociation between antipsychotic activity and EPS (Meltzer 1995b).

TREATMENT OBJECTIVES

Psychopathology

Schizophrenia is usually first recognized during late adolescence or early adulthood with the appearance of positive symptoms (i.e., delusions, hallucinations, thought disturbance, and bizarre behavior) (Carpenter 1987). The onset of these symptoms may be gradual or abrupt. It is now recognized that there are antecedents to psychosis in childhood and early adolescence (e.g., disturbances in motor behavior, attention, interpersonal relationships in some patients with schizophrenia) (Baum and Walker 1995; Murray et al. 1992). So-called negative symptoms (i.e., lack of spontaneity, decreased motivation, flat affect, anhedonia, and anergia) may precede or follow the development of psychosis (Kibel et al. 1993; Liddle 1987; Murray et al. 1992). A third syndrome, disorganization (i.e., incoherence, inappropriate affect, loose associations, and poverty of thought content), has also been recognized as an independent domain of psychopathology (Liddle 1987; Liddle and Barnes 1990; Meltzer and Zureick 1989).

Patients will show varying levels of each of these three syndromes. DSM-IV (American Psychiatric Association 1994) criteria for schizophrenia require that delusions, hallucinations, disorganized speech, or disorganized behavior be present at least 1 month before the diagnosis can be made. Negative symptoms, along with at least one of the four positive or disorganization symptoms described above, can satisfy Criterion A in the DSM-IV diagnostic criteria.

When patients first present for treatment, they usually manifest one or more of the positive or disorganization symptoms mentioned above. These symptoms may be severe and of acute onset, in which case they are usually quite disturbing to the patient or family. However, they may be of gradual onset and may not be disturbing to the patient or family for a variety of reasons. In this case, the symptoms may have been present for some time and may not have received medical attention because they were not manifested in such a way as to be noticeable or because those in close contact with the individual did not recognize the need for medical attention. There is some evidence that prolonged psychosis prior to antipsychotic drug treatment may be associated with worse long-term outcome (Wyatt 1991; Wyatt et al. 1997).

The treatment of schizophrenia traditionally has focused—and, unfortunately, in many places still focuses—mainly on the treatment of positive symptoms. The primary reasons for this emphasis are that positive symptoms are relatively easy to detect and that the typical neuroleptic drugs have the ability to ameliorate these symptoms in the large majority of patients. Since the seminal paper of Crow (1980), the treatment of negative symptoms has been appreciated as an important, if elusive, target of antipsychotic drug treatment.

Carpenter (1987, 1994) has promoted the desirability of distinguishing between *primary negative symptoms*—negative symptoms that are enduring and unrelated to positive symptoms, EPS resulting from treatment with antipsychotic drugs, depression, or other types of psychopathology—and *secondary negative symptoms*—symptoms that result from one or more of the factors above and presumably would remit if that factor(s) was effectively treated. Although having obvious face validity, this distinction is not easy to make in clinical practice and from the patient's perspective is of little significance. However, to the extent that making such a distinction can lead to increased awareness of those components of the illness that are supposedly causing the secondary negative symptoms (i.e., positive symptoms, EPS, and depression), it is of some importance. Primary negative symptoms should be the target of therapeutic intervention in their own right.

Cognitive Impairment

Patients with schizophrenia have widespread, multifaceted impairments in neurocognitive measures such as executive function, attention, and working memory. Cognitive impairment in schizophrenia is an early feature of the illness (Saykin et al. 1991). Indeed, some aspects of this deficit may precede the development of psychotic symptoms. For most patients, once the deficit is established at the end of the first episode, the extent of impairment changes only marginally over time, although clearly there are significant numbers of patients in whom the impairment is progressive and reaches the proportions characteristic of severe dementia (Goldberg et al. 1993). It is important to treat the cognitive disturbance as well as the symptoms of schizophrenia and to assess the role of such disturbance on work and social function (Cassens et al. 1990; Green 1996).

The range of cognitive tests applied to patients with schizophrenia is enormous. The frequency and extent of abnormalities vary with the test. It has been estimated that about 40% of patients with schizophrenia have impaired neurocognition (Braff et al. 1991; Goldberg et al. 1988). The major deficits are in executive function (abstraction/flexibility), attention, verbal learning and memory, spatial and verbal working memory, semantic memory, and psychomotor performance (Braff et al. 1991; Saykin et al. 1991). These abnormalities in cognition are believed to be the result of abnormalities in the frontal and temporal lobes and in the connectivity between these regions (Weinberger 1987).

Mood Disturbance

In addition to positive, negative, and disorganization symptoms and cognitive dysfunction, patients with schizophrenia have affective disturbances. Flat affect and inappropriate affect are components of negative symptoms and disorganization, respectively, but patients with schizophrenia may have varying degrees of depressive and hypomanic or manic symptoms as well. When these mood symptoms are a prominent part of the clinical picture and precede the core schizophrenic symptoms, patients are appropriately diagnosed as having *schizoaffective disorder, depressed or bipolar type.* The mood symptoms accompanying schizophrenia or schizoaffective disorder must be the target of therapy as well.

The importance of detecting and treating depressive symptoms in schizophrenia has been discussed by Siris et al. (1981). Approximately half of patients with schizophrenia will experience a significant depressive episode during the course of their illness. When this episode follows an acute exacerbation of positive symptoms, it is called a *postpsychotic depression.* Between 9% and 13% of patients with schizophrenia commit suicide, and as many as 50% make suicide attempts with varying severity of intent (Roy 1982). These attempts may reflect the despair patients with schizophrenia experience because of the disabling effects of their illness and the lack of efficacy of treatments offered to them.

Social and Work Function and Quality of Life

The positive, negative, disorganization, and affective symptoms experienced by patients with schizophrenia, together with the cognitive disturbance, lead to great *disability in social and work function.* This is particularly true in developed countries, where a high level of cognitive function may be needed for most jobs. Only about 20% of patients with schizophrenia are employed.

Another concept of importance in evaluating the adequacy of treatment in schizophrenia is *quality of life* (Awad 1992). Quality of life, which refers to the individual's subjective sense of well-being, has been surprisingly neglected in discussions of schizophrenia, in part because of the impairment in insight in many patients with schizophrenia and the limited goals that clinicians have established for themselves with regard to patients with this illness. There is no generally accepted definition of quality of life. The concept can entail the subjective assessment of both medical and nonmedical aspects of life. Nonmedical aspects include social status, economic well-being, and fulfillment of personal aspirations.

An individual's assessment of the quality of his or her life is affected by many factors, including premorbid level of functioning and degree of awareness of the severity of impairment in cognition, with subsequent demoralization and depression. In addition, the side effects of medication (e.g., EPS, weight gain, impaired sexual function not due to loss of libido) and the disfiguring aspects of tardive dyskinesia can lead to poor quality of life.

Substance Abuse

A large and growing proportion of patients with schizophrenia have substance abuse and dependence problems involving alcohol, stimulants (including cocaine), and even psychotomimetic agents such as phencyclidine (Buckley et al. 1994; Mueser et al. 1990). Although estimates vary widely, it can be safely concluded that between 25% and 50% of schizophrenia patients abuse alcohol or illicit drugs at some point in their illness. These agents may produce in some patients a transient sense of well-being that results from the temporary relief of depression or anhedonia. However, in the long run, use of these substances greatly diminishes quality of life because of the role of these substances in increasing psychotic symptomatology, impairing cognitive function, or producing medical problems such as liver failure. Substance abuse in schizophrenia is closely associated with, and often causally related to, medication noncompliance (Mueser et al. 1990; Weiden et al. 1991).

Summary

It is of essential importance in the treatment of schizophrenia to recognize that the major psychopathological dimensions of the schizophrenia syndrome (e.g., positive, negative, disorganization, and depressive symptoms) may be independent of one another and of cognitive dysfunction (Meltzer 1992). The severity of impairment in these domains is often very disparate. The Type I, Type II model of schizophrenia proposed by Crow (1980) suggested that positive symptoms and negative symptoms were independent and that the former, but not the latter, respond to typical neuroleptic drugs. We have found that negative symptoms and cognition are more relevant to quality of life than are positive symptoms.

TREATMENT OF THE ACUTE PHASE OF PSYCHOSIS

Stages of the Illness

Acute Psychosis

The acute phase of schizophrenia is currently organized, for purposes of treatment, into three phases, although, as we shall argue, it may be important to consider a fourth phase.

1. *Period of markedly increased positive symptoms* (referred to as *acute exacerbations*). Control of positive symptoms and preparing the patient for long-term treatment are the essential components of treatment during this phase of the illness.
2. *Phase of symptom remission following an acute exacerbation.* There is evidence that during this period patients will relapse within days to months if neuroleptic treatment is stopped (Gilbert et al. 1995). The goals of treatment during this phase are suppression of symptoms, prevention of relapse, and rehabilitation of the work and social function of the patient.
3. *Residual phase.* In this period, which only

some patients enter, the propensity for an acute exacerbation to recur when neuroleptic drugs are stopped is greatly diminished. During this period, patients may not require neuroleptics to remain nonpsychotic. They may still have negative symptoms and cognitive dysfunction, however. In rare cases, individuals show no major symptoms. The major goal of this period of treatment is to focus on reintegration and socialization.

Prodromal Phase

A fourth phase of schizophrenia emerging as a target for treatment, the *prodromal* phase, is actually the first phase of the illness, occurring before the onset of psychosis (McGorry et al. 1995). There is now evidence that incipient features of schizophrenia are present during this period, which may even begin at birth but for clinical purposes is usually considered to be the period several months to several years before the psychosis emerges (Baum and Walker 1995; Murray et al. 1992). During this period, patients exhibit some of the symptoms of schizotypal patients—for example, magical thinking, mildly bizarre behavior, increased problems with attention and concentration, decreased school or work performance, increased irritability or withdrawal, ritualistic or socially unacceptable behaviors, loss of or failure to develop appropriate interest in sexual activity.

It is of great importance to determine 1) whether pharmacological and psychosocial interventions at this stage of the illness might be effective and 2) whether the benefits of treatment at this phase would outweigh the risks of the interventions, considering that a proportion of those individuals who would receive treatment would not be destined to develop schizophrenia even though they are manifesting schizotypal symptoms and have decreased social and intellectual function. Clearly, as biological tests to identify individuals with vulnerability to develop schizophrenia are developed, treat-

ments for this phase of the evolution of schizophrenia will be of the greatest importance. It is conceivable that effective interventions in the prodromal phase will prevent the development of acute episodes and thus obviate treatment in that period as well as maintenance treatment.

Acute Phase of Psychosis

Periods of acute psychosis may occur during the first episode or any time thereafter, even when patients are compliant with previously effective dosages of medication. Acute psychosis may occur during periods of increased stress from the environment but can also occur without apparent exogenous events contributing. It is not uncommon for patients to experience as many as 20 to 30 acute episodes of psychosis; such recurrence may be the result of noncompliance, failure to prescribe clozapine, if needed, for patients with neuroleptic-, risperidone-, or olanzapine-resistant schizophrenia, or the poor organization of mental health services for patients who would otherwise be compliant. There is concern that each episode of psychosis or prolonged periods of psychosis without treatment may have long-term adverse consequences (Wyatt 1991).

First-Episode Schizophrenia

The patient with first-episode schizophrenia may present with florid psychotic symptoms that have been present for as long as several years or as brief as a few days. The duration of psychosis prior to presentation depends on the severity and type of symptoms, the extent to which the patient can hide them from detection, the sensitivity of the observers in the environment, and the availability of treatments, among other factors. The first challenge with such patients is to establish the diagnosis and to rule out any other psychiatric or medical, especially neurological, conditions that may be present. Schizophrenia may be difficult to differentiate from mania during the first episode. Characteristic manic symptoms may be absent or less prominent than delusions and hallucinations, which may be paranoid rather than grandiose in some manic patients. It is, therefore, sometimes prudent to defer the diagnosis of schizophrenia until definitive information about the character and course of the illness is available.

The initial decision to be made in the treatment of a patient with first-episode schizophrenia is whether hospitalization is required. Assuming that managed care does not preclude hospitalization because of failure to meet narrow criteria (e.g., danger to self or others), it is necessary to evaluate a number of factors to decide whether to hospitalize the patient. An intensive evaluation is necessary to rule out organic factors that may be producing the psychosis. It may not be possible to do this evaluation conveniently or safely on an outpatient basis. However, if symptoms are relatively mild and an evaluation of the family and environment suggests the availability of considerable support and the absence of stressors, it may be possible to conduct such an evaluation on an outpatient basis. However, first-episode patients who are initially treated as outpatients often fail to continue treatment because the clinician, in the limited time available, cannot establish a relationship with the patient in the initial interview. Hospitalization is strongly recommended for patients who are in severely stressful situations, whether these occur at home, school, or work. Removing the patient from these stressful situations, sometimes even without administering antipsychotic medication, can lead to a rapid remission (Young and Meltzer 1980).

It may be necessary to seek civil commitment for some patients. The clinician should avoid taking this step, if possible, by attempting to obtain a voluntary admission. This process may take additional time and, thus, can be difficult to carry out in a managed care environment in which time of contact with new patients is restricted—to as little as 45 minutes in some instances. In some jurisdictions, civil commitment requires prolonged hospitalization even if there is no clinical need for it after a relatively brief period of time.

The duration of hospitalization for first-episode patients should be kept relatively short, since there is no evidence that prolonged hospitalization achieves any greater benefit than brief hospitalizations. In a managed care environment, the duration of the first hospitalization may be only a few days. If this is the case, it is of great importance that the clinician establish a relationship with the patient that will lead to continuing contact after discharge and a good chance of compliance with treatment. Contact with the family during the hospitalization by the clinician is critical to ensuring continuing contact with the patient and compliance.

During the first episode, whether evaluation is on an outpatient or inpatient basis, it is essential to establish the history of the illness, the family history of mental illness, the use of illicit drugs or alcohol, the presence of other medical conditions that may be directly associated with psychosis, or the use of medications that may produce psychosis. Generally, it is useful to obtain a brain imaging study to examine for structural abnormalities. A computed tomography (CT) or magnetic resonance imaging (MRI) examination will reveal any organic abnormalities that may be contributing to the clinical picture.

Psychopharmacological Treatment of the Acute Phase

The initial treatment of an acute psychosis requires consideration of drug, dosage, and route of administration. Oral medication may be acceptable and sufficient for many patients. One of the atypical agents may be preferred because of their low risk of EPS. Patients who present in the emergency room with severe agitation or threatening harm to themselves or others require being isolated in a safe room. They may also require restraining of their limbs. The latter should be done with great care for the psychological well-being of the patient, but physical safety for patient and staff is the preeminent consideration. Patients who are this severely ill will ordinarily require parenteral medication.

The most commonly used medication for this purpose at present is haloperidol, with chlorpromazine as a second choice. Haloperidol, 5 mg intramuscularly, is effective in calming many patients within 30 minutes. If the response is insufficient, the injection may be repeated at intervals of 1 hour after vital signs are checked. There is no clear evidence of a safe upper limit in such a situation. Parenteral administration of a benzodiazepine such as lorazepam may also be a useful augmentation of the neuroleptic. Monitoring vital signs is crucial during this period. In the most severe cases, emergency ECT may be needed.

Conventional neuroleptics and the atypical antipsychotics are effective in treating an acute exacerbation of schizophrenia (Arvanitis et al. 1997; Beasley et al. 1996; Chouinard et al. 1993; J. M. Davis et al. 1989) and effect remission of psychosis in about 75% of patients within days to months. About 10% of first-episode patients fail to respond to typical neuroleptics and may have to be treated with an atypical antipsychotic or clozapine.

Time Course of Response in an Acute Episode

It may be expected that some decrease in agitation, anxiety, and sleeplessness will occur shortly after the initiation of antipsychotic treatment. Some patients show a rapid decrease in positive symptoms, but more often it is several days before any appreciable decrease is noted. Most patients show a near maximal response by 6 weeks of treatment. If a satisfactory remission of positive symptoms is not achieved with a typical neuroleptic by 6 weeks, assuming that the dose is adequate, a switch to an atypical antipsychotic drug is indicated.

Choice of Antipsychotic for Acute Treatment

The choice of which oral medication to use during acute exacerbations depends on a number of factors. There is no convincing evidence for any advantages in efficacy among the conventional antipsychotic drugs (Baldessarini et al. 1988; Kane and Marder 1993). This has been attributed to the fact that the efficacy of these agents is based solely on their ability to block D_2 receptors in mesolimbic areas of the brain, including the nucleus accumbens, the stria terminalis, and the olfactory tubercle (K. L. Davis et al. 1991). These agents differ in affinities for other receptors, including α_1- and α_2-adrenergic receptors, muscarinic receptors, and H_1 histamine receptors (Richelson and Nelson 1984). This suggests that the antipsychotic efficacy of these agents has little to do with actions at these receptors.

The differences in pharmacology among the conventional antipsychotic drugs are relevant to their side-effect profiles, which provide some basis for choosing among them. It is likely that the potent anticholinergic effects of thioridazine are the basis for its low EPS profile. However, there is no evidence that thioridazine is any *less* likely to produce tardive dyskinesia than any of the other conventional neuroleptic drugs. The antimuscarinic property of the conventional antipsychotic drugs may also contribute to memory impairment and urinary retention. H_1 receptors in brain have an important role in arousal and the regulation of appetite. Loxapine, *cis*-thiothixene, and chlorpromazine are conventional neuroleptics that have higher affinities for the H_1 receptor than does the classic antihistamine diphenhydramine. Haloperidol and molindone have low affinities for these receptors and thus might be chosen when it is of particular importance to minimize sedation and appetite stimulation. Neuroleptic drugs, with the exception of molindone, cause significant blockade of the α_1 receptor at clinically effective doses, which leads to varying degrees of postural hypotension, nasal congestion, dizziness, and tachycardia. The most potent of these neuroleptics in this regard are chlorpromazine, thioridazine, and haloperidol. The least potent α_1 antagonists are loxapine and molindone. The blockade of α_2 receptors by conventional neuroleptics is relatively weak and is not related to any particular side effect.

Extrapyramidal Side Effects

The side effects associated with D_2 receptor blockade are more or less unavoidable with the conventional neuroleptic drugs. Low-potency agents such as chlorpromazine and thioridazine have the least EPS, whereas high-potency agents such as fluphenazine and haloperidol have the most. Parkinsonian side effects (e.g., dystonic reactions, including opisthotonos) may be manifest from the first dose. These side effects are usually treated by intravenous administration of diphenhydramine or intramuscular administration of trihexyphenidyl. More frequent are symptoms that occur after several days to weeks of treatment, such as muscle rigidity, loss of associated movement, masked facies, and drooling. These parkinsonian side effects are usually treated by lowering the dose and/or administering an oral antiparkinsonian agent (e.g., trihexyphenidyl or benztropine mesylate, which are potent anticholinergic agents, or amantadine, a dopaminomimetic agent). Increases in serum prolactin levels are present with all the conventional neuroleptic drugs (Meltzer and Fang 1976). The increases are greater in females than in males and sometimes produce galactorrhea, a condition that may be treated with pergolide mesylate or bromocriptine, both of which are direct-acting dopamine agonists.

Dosage of Neuroleptics

The dosages of conventional antipsychotic agents and galenic forms are given in Table 19–1. In general, the lowest dosages of the dosage ranges listed in Table 19–1 should be used. Fixed-dose studies reviewed by Marder (see Chapter 8 in this volume) suggest that low doses of haloperidol, and presumably the other conventional drugs as well, are as effective as higher dosages in the treatment of acute psychosis. Increasing the dose of these agents when patients fail to respond rapidly is not recommended. The addition of a benzodiazepine may produce a further calming effect prior to the onset of efficacy of lower doses of neuroleptic drugs. Some pa-

tients may require higher doses of neuroleptic drugs to respond adequately, but it is likely that such patients may actually be neuroleptic resistant, as described below, and should be treated with clozapine or perhaps another atypical antipsychotic drug.

Atypical Antipsychotic Drugs

Although clozapine was the first atypical antipsychotic drug discovered, it is not recommended at this time as a first-line treatment for patients with schizophrenia because of the increased risk of agranulocytosis. But the side-effect burden of the newer atypical agents such as risperidone, olanzapine, quetiapine, and ziprasidone is such that they may be considered as first-line agents. The clinical pharmacology of these drugs is discussed elsewhere in this volume (see Chapters 8–10). Remarks here will be confined to an overview of their role in the treatment of schizophrenia based on current knowledge.

The atypical drugs share an ability to produce fewer EPS than the conventional neuroleptics, though dose considerations are critical. As previously mentioned, many patients with schizophrenia will respond to low doses of typical neuroleptic drugs that produce few or no EPS. The problem is that many clinicians prescribe higher doses than are needed. It should be noted that there is no evidence that any of the newer atypical antipsychotic drugs produce agranulocytosis at the same level that clozapine does, so weekly monitoring of white blood cell (WBC) counts is not needed.

Risperidone. Risperidone, a benzisoxazole compound, was the first novel atypical antipsychotic drug introduced after clozapine. It has been very rapidly adopted because of its low incidence of EPS and because its efficacy is as good as—and possibly superior to—that of conventional antipsychotics (Chouinard et al. 1993; Marder and Meibach 1994; Peuskens 1995). Like clozapine, risperidone is more potent as a 5-HT_{2A} antagonist than as a D_2 antagonist.

Table 19–1. Antipsychotic drugs available in the United States, dosage ranges, and dosage forms

Drug	Dosage range (mg)	Parenteral dosage (mg)	Galenic form(s)
Conventional			
Butyrophenone			
Haloperidol (Haldol)	5–30	5–10	Oral, liquid, injection
Haloperidol decanoate (Haldol-D)		25–100 q 1–4 weeks	
Dibenzoxazepine			
Loxapine succinate (Loxitane)	40–100	25	Oral, liquid, injection
Diphenylbutylpiperidine			
Pimozide (Orap)	2–6		Oral
Indole			
Molindone hydrochloride (Moban)	50–225		Oral, liquid
Phenothiazines			
Acetophenazine maleate (Tindal)	40–120	—	Oral
Chlorpromazine hydrochloride (Thorazine)	200–800	25–50	Oral, liquid, injection, suppository
Fluphenazine hydrochloride (Prolixin)	2–60	1.25–2.5	Oral, liquid, injection
Fluphenazine decanoate (Prolixin-D)		12.5–50 q 1–4 weeks	
Fluphenazine enanthate (Prolixin-E)		12.5–50 q 1–4 weeks	
Mesoridazine besylate (Serentil)	75–300	25	Oral, liquid, injection
Perphenazine (Trilafon)	8–32	5–10	Oral, liquid, injection
Thioridazine hydrochloride (Mellaril)	150–800		Oral, liquid
Trifluoperazine hydrochloride (Stelazine)	5–20	1–2	Oral, liquid, injection
Thioxanthenes			
Thiothixene hydrochloride (Navane)	5–30	2–4	Oral, liquid, injection
Atypical			
Benzisothiazolyl			
Ziprasidone (Zeldox)	40–160	10	Oral, liquid, injection
Benzisoxazole			
Risperidone (Risperdal)	2–8		Oral, liquid
Dibenzothiazepine			
Quetiapine fumarate (Seroquel)	150–750	—	Oral
Dibenzodiazepine			
Clozapine (Clozaril)	100–900	—	Oral
Thienobenzodiazepine			
Olanzapine (Zyprexa)	7.5–30	—	Oral

The studies mentioned above, and reviewed by Owens and Risch in this volume (see Chapter 9), clearly indicate that risperidone is at least as effective as haloperidol for treating acute exacerbations and may be more effective for treating negative symptoms. These advantages of risperidone over haloperidol in terms of EPS and negative symptoms have proven to be important for fostering compliance and preventing relapse. Risperidone has been found to produce improvement in working memory in a recent clinical trial (Green et al. 1997). These benefits are important for justifying the additional expense of this medication.

Clinical experience indicates that risperidone is sometimes effective in patients who fail to respond adequately to typical neuroleptic drugs, but the rate of positive response with this drug is not as high as that for clozapine. Indeed, in patients who are stable on clozapine, the attempt to switch to risperidone leads to a high rate of relapse. This should not be taken as an indication that risperidone is always ineffective in patients who do not respond adequately to typical neuroleptic drugs.

Risperidone, at the lower end of its dosage range (1–4 mg), has been shown to be comparable to olanzapine, ziprasidone, and quetiapine in EPS liability. If higher doses are used, however, risperidone may produce more EPS than do these agents. Risperidone at a mean dose of 6.1 mg/day produced more EPS and required benztropine more frequently than did clozapine (Daniel et al. 1996). Trials of 4–6 weeks at the lower doses (1–6 mg/day) are indicated to optimize the response to risperidone in relation to EPS. There is no evidence at present to conclude that the risk of tardive dyskinesia is less with risperidone than with conventional neuroleptic drugs.

Risperidone produces less weight gain than clozapine (Daniel et al. 1996). Risperidone is associated with increases in serum prolactin levels that are comparable to those with typical neuroleptic drugs (Umbricht and Kane 1995). Risperidone has been found to induce activation

(e.g., hypomanic symptoms) in some patients. Depot and skin patch formulations of risperidone are in development and should prove useful for patients who are unwilling or unable to take oral medication consistently.

Olanzapine. Olanzapine, at doses of 10–15 mg/day, has been shown to be effective for the treatment of acute psychotic episodes in both first-episode and chronic schizophrenia patients (Beasley et al. 1996; Tollefson et al. 1997b). Once-a-day administration makes olanzapine convenient to use and appears not to produce significant EPS at recommended (10–15 mg/day) or even slightly higher doses (Beasley et al. 1996; Tollefson et al. 1997b). Thus, olanzapine may be better tolerated than risperidone in some patients who are very prone to develop EPS when higher doses are needed.

A significant number of patients appear to require as much as 20 mg/day of olanzapine. As with risperidone, there is evidence that olanzapine is superior to haloperidol in the treatment of both negative and positive symptoms. A path analysis found evidence that olanzapine has a beneficial effect on primary negative symptoms (Tollefson and Sanger 1997). There is some evidence that olanzapine may be efficacious in treatment-resistant patients.

Findings from a study by Tollefson et al. (1997a) suggest that olanzapine, compared with haloperidol, may be associated with lower risk for producing tardive dyskinesia. Treatment-emergent tardive dyskinesia in 707 olanzapine-treated patients over a median period of exposure of 237 days (range 42–964) was 7.0% compared with a rate of 16.2% in 197 patients treated with haloperidol for a median of 203 days. Analysis of Abnormal Involuntary Movement Scale (AIMS) data showed the same results.

The major side effects of olanzapine appear to be significant weight gain and sedation. Olanzapine does not produce increases in serum prolactin levels at clinically effective doses.

Thus, some female patients may find olanzapine more acceptable than risperidone if they are sensitive to elevated prolactin levels. There is some evidence that compliance with olanzapine is superior to that with typical neuroleptic drugs. Preliminary data suggest that olanzapine has beneficial effects on some cognitive functions (H. Y. Meltzer and S. M. McGurk, unpublished observations). Like risperidone, olanzapine has been found to produce in some patients activation that may be hypomanic in nature. Skin patch and depot formulations of olanzapine are in development.

Quetiapine.　　Quetiapine, another serotonin-dopamine receptor antagonist, was approved by the Food and Drug Administration (FDA) in 1998. It has preclinical effects in animal models of EPS that are very similar to those of clozapine. Quetiapine was shown to be superior to placebo and equivalent to chlorpromazine in early clinical trials in hospitalized schizophrenic patients (Goldstein and Arvanitis 1995; Small et al. 1997). There was no evidence that quetiapine was more effective than haloperidol in the treatment of positive or negative symptoms during a 6-week trial (Arvanitis et al. 1997).

Twice-a-day administration is necessary for quetiapine (Casey 1996). The effective dosage range appears to be between 200 and 750 mg/day, with an optimal dosage of perhaps 300 mg/day (Arvanitis et al. 1997).

Quetiapine produces no increase in serum prolactin levels and has significant advantages in terms of EPS, appearing to be no more likely than placebo to produce EPS (Arvanitis et al. 1997; Casey 1996). As with olanzapine, the major side effects of quetiapine are weight gain, postural hypotension, and sedation. Quetiapine produces some increases in liver enzymes, but these do not appear to be clinically significant. Another possible side effect of quetiapine is cataract development; thus, ophthalmologic examination should be performed early in treatment and every 6 months thereafter.

Ziprasidone.　　Ziprasidone, the last of the serotonin-dopamine antagonists to be discussed here, has just received FDA approval but is associated with Q-T$_c$ prolongation (Seeger et al. 1995). In addition to its antagonism of 5-HT$_{2A}$, 5-HT$_{2C}$, and D$_2$ receptors, ziprasidone is a potent 5-HT$_{1A}$ agonist—a feature that may have advantages for treating anxiety and depression in schizophrenia (Seeger et al. 1995). Early clinical trials indicate that ziprasidone is effective in treating positive, negative, and mood symptoms in patients with acute exacerbations. It is also effective in delaying relapse in patients with chronic schizophrenia.

Ziprasidone has a favorable profile with regard to elevations of serum prolactin and EPS or akathisia. It appears to produce less weight gain than the other atypical antipsychotic drugs, though studies involving direct comparisons are needed to firmly establish this. It is not yet known whether ziprasidone is effective in treating patients with neuroleptic-resistant schizophrenia or in diminishing the risk of developing tardive dyskinesia.

Clozapine.　　Because of its ability to produce agranulocytosis, clozapine is not considered to be a first-line treatment (Marder and Van Putten 1988). However, it is highly effective in neuroleptic-responsive patients as well. Clozapine will be discussed in detail later in this chapter in the context of neuroleptic resistance.

There is some evidence that clozapine is superior to typical neuroleptic drugs in patients with non-treatment-resistant schizophrenia (see Meltzer and Ranjan 1996 for review), particularly in terms of cognitive measures (Lee et al. 1994). There is no evidence to date as to its superiority to other atypical neuroleptic drugs in non-treatment-resistant schizophrenia patients. However, until there is evidence to the contrary, it is reasonable to assume that clozapine has the least risk of producing EPS or tardive movement disorders of any of the atypical antipsychotic drugs.

It is not recommended at this point that

clozapine be used for first-episode schizophrenia. However, clinicians should be alert to the possibility that if adequate trials of typical or other atypical antipsychotic drugs produce only control of positive symptoms, unsatisfactory outcome in other important dimensions (e.g., negative symptoms, cognition, mood, and suicidality) provides the basis for a clozapine trial.

Choice of an Atypical Antipsychotic Drug

For the clinician, choosing between the new, atypical antipsychotic drugs and the conventional neuroleptic agents represents a challenge. The benefits of the newer agents that have been demonstrated in controlled clinical trials are impressive. However, it is still necessary to show that these benefits can be achieved in routine clinical practice, where patients cannot be carefully selected and where polypharmacy may interfere with the actions of these agents.

The apparent advantages of risperidone and olanzapine over haloperidol in treating negative symptoms would appear to favor these two agents over quetiapine and ziprasidone. It must be emphasized, however, that the studies on which this suggestion is based did not directly compare these agents.

It is also necessary to understand the magnitude of the advantages of atypical agents over conventional neuroleptic drugs in making the decision as to which drug to choose. Large-scale clinical trials can show statistically significant differences that may not be very significant clinically.

Finally, the importance of significant advantages with regard to effects on cognitive function must be emphasized. As previously mentioned, risperidone, olanzapine, and clozapine have been shown in most, but not all, studies to have positive effects on certain aspects of cognitive function. Data for the effects of quetiapine and ziprasidone on cognition are needed. More data on the cognitive effects of all the atypical antipsychotic drugs, along with follow-up data to indicate whether these effects translate into

clinically significant differences (e.g., in the ability to work), are needed.

MAINTENANCE TREATMENT

Conventional neuroleptic drugs are still the most widely used treatment following the end of an acute episode, despite the evidence that the atypical antipsychotic drugs have considerable advantages for many patients. The choice between these classes of drugs is discussed later in this section. There is strong evidence that without continuous treatment with an effective antipsychotic agent, nearly all schizophrenic patients will relapse within a 12- to 24-month period. The rate of relapse is approximately 3.5% per month, so within 2 years of the acute episode nearly all schizophrenic patients will have relapsed. However, the rate of development of tardive dyskinesia is 4%–5% per year (Glazer et al. 1993; Kane et al. 1984), so those patients who continue to take conventional neuroleptic drugs indefinitely do so at some significant risk. For many patients, however, only mild forms of tardive dyskinesia develop, and these symptoms may be suppressed by the antipsychotic agent.

A number of studies have sought to define the most appropriate minimum dosage for effective maintenance treatment in schizophrenia (Hogarty et al. 1988; Kane et al. 1985; Marder et al. 1984, 1987). Markedly lower doses than those used to treat acute episodes may be effective. For most patients, doses in the moderate range are indicated for maintenance treatment (e.g., 5–15 mg/day of haloperidol or 12.5–25 mg of fluphenazine decanoate every 2 weeks) (Levinson et al. 1990; Rifkin et al. 1990; Van Putten et al. 1990). Hogarty et al. (1988) found that social adjustment was superior in patients receiving lower doses of neuroleptics for maintenance treatment. Higher doses provide little added protection and increase the risk or severity of EPS. Should moderate doses not prove satisfactory, the choice of the clinician is to raise the dose, with probable worsening of EPS, or to switch to an atypical antipsychotic drug. The latter may be the more satisfactory choice in most patients.

Depot neuroleptic drugs are used in many clinics to ensure adequate delivery of medication. Visiting nurses or case managers help ensure that patients receive injections at scheduled times. Either fluphenazine decanoate at doses of 12.5–25 mg every 2 weeks or haloperidol decanoate at doses of 50–100 mg every 2–4 weeks is of great value in ensuring compliance. Unfortunately, there are as yet no long-acting preparations of the novel antipsychotic drugs.

The importance of striving for compliance with treatment in schizophrenic patients cannot be overstated. Relapse rates due to noncompliance of as high as 50% within a year after discharge from hospital for an acute episode have been reported (Weiden et al. 1991). Factors associated with poor compliance include persistent psychotic symptoms, poor insight with denial of illness, dissatisfaction with care providers, persistent EPS, and poor social support. Case management and family education may decrease noncompliance. However, use of depot neuroleptics or more effective oral medications with low EPS potential is probably the most important element in a compliance program.

Management of Side Effects of Neuroleptics

Side effects of treatment with conventional neuroleptics are common (Ayd 1961; Casey 1991; Chakos et al. 1992) and are the chief reason for poor compliance with treatment (Van Putten 1974; Weiden et al. 1991). For sake of convenience, they may be divided into neurological (Table 19–2) and nonneurological adverse effects (Table 19–3).

Neurological Side Effects

The main neurological side effects of neuroleptics are EPS (acute dystonic reactions, parkinsonism, akathisia), tardive dyskinesia and other tardive movement disorders, neuroleptic malignant syndrome (NMS), and seizures (Table 19–2). Ayd (1961) reported on the incidence of side effects in more than 3,000 patients evaluated for as many as 6 years and noted that 38% of patients showed EPS: 2% had dystonia, 15% parkinsonism, and 21% akathisia. In a prospective study of 70 "first-episode" schizophrenic patients (Chakos et al. 1992), 38% of patients showed no EPS, whereas 38% had one form of EPS, 21% two forms, and 3% all three forms. Parkinsonism was observed in 34% of patients, acute dystonia in 36%, and akathisia in 18%. Acute EPS were associated with both higher baseline psychopathology and better treatment outcome.

Acute dystonic reactions.   Acute dystonic reactions typically occur within the first 4 days of neuroleptic treatment and are more common in young male patients who are receiving high-potency neuroleptics (Casey 1991). These reactions are characterized by sustained, involuntary muscular spasms, most often involving the facial, head, or neck muscles; examples include spasm of masticatory muscles (trismus), spasm of the orbicularis oculi (blepharospasm), oculogyric crises (fixed upward gazing of the eyes), torticollis, dysarthria, and dysphagia. Such spasms are painful and very distressing and may go undetected or be misinterpreted by staff.

Treatment of acute dystonia includes one or more parenteral injections of an anticholinergic (e.g., benztropine mesylate 2 mg intramuscularly) or antihistamine (e.g., diphenhydramine 50 mg intravenously) drug. Oral anticholinergic drugs are generally administered thereafter. If there is a recurrence, then the neuroleptic dosage should be reduced or a switch should be made to an atypical agent. Prophylactic use of anticholinergics to avoid the development of EPS is not indicated because of the risk of anticholinergic toxicity and the possible increase in the risk for tardive dyskinesia (Boodhood and Sadler 1991).

Table 19–2. **Neurological side effects of conventional neuroleptic drugs**

Side effect	Characteristics	Prevalence	Risk factors	Management
Acute dystonia	Oculogyric crises; dysarthria; acute neck and truncal spasms	2%–90%	Young males; high-potency neuroleptics	Reduce dosage or switch to a different drug class; administer anticholinergic or antihistamine (benztropine mesylate 2 mg im/po or diphenhydramine 50 mg iv)
Parkinsonism	Tremor; cogwheel rigidity; bradykinesia	2%–90%	Dose related	Reduce dosage; administer anticholinergic
Akathisia	Subjective and objective motor restlessness	35%	Dose related; low serum iron status?	Reduce dosage or switch to another drug class; administer benzodiazepine (diazepam 2 mg three times a day), β-blocker (propranolol 10–40 mg twice a day)
Tardive dyskinesia	Involuntary choreic or athetoid movements, orofacial and peripheral	5%–50%	Female gender; age; brain disease; concomitant antiparkinsonian treatments?; history of EPS; affective symptoms; diabetes	Reduce or discontinue neuroleptic; administer vitamin E 400–1,200 mg, switch to clozapine
Neuroleptic malignant syndrome	Pyrexia; muscle rigidity; autonomic instability; clouding of consciousness; elevated CK	0.1%–1%	High, rapid neuroleptic dosing; agitation; organic brain impairment	Rule out other medical conditions; discontinue neuroleptic; use supportive measures; administer dopamine agonist (bromocriptine 15–30 mg); administer muscle relaxant (dantrolene 100–400 mg)
Seizures	Grand mal; myoclonic	0.1%	Dosage; epileptogenic tendency; organic brain impairment	Reduce dosage; administer concomitant anticonvulsant drug (valproate 400–1,000 mg)

Note. im = intramuscular; po = oral; EPS = extrapyramidal side effects; CK = creatine kinase.

Table 19–3. Nonneurological side effects of conventional neuroleptic drugs

Side effect	Characteristics	Prevalence	Management
Sedation	Tolerance developing over time	~70%	Reduce dosage; switch to nonsedating drug; add L-dopa or methylphenidate
Weight gain		15%–20%	Use practical measures; monitor for diabetes
Hypotension	Antiadrenergic effect	10%–30%	Reduce dosage; switch to a different drug class
Anticholinergic effects	Cognitive impairment; blurred vision; dry mouth; constipation; sexual dysfunction	~60%	Reduce dosage; switch to a low anticholinergic drug
Hormonal	Elevated prolactin; reduced testosterone	Variable	Treat breast abscess if one develops; reduce dosage; add bromocriptine; switch to olanzapine or quetiapine
Marrow toxicity	Agranulocytosis	<0.1%	Obtain hematologist consult; discontinue neuroleptic
Jaundice	Cholestatic	<0.1%	Investigate for other causes; switch to another drug
Retinitis pigmentosa		Low	Avoid high doses of thioridazine

Parkinsonism. Parkinsonism, which is similar to idiopathic Parkinson's disease, consists of tremor, rigidity, and bradykinesia and appears to be a direct (i.e., dose-related) consequence of dopamine receptor blockade in the nigrostriatal pathway (Casey 1991). These symptoms generally emerge after a few days of neuroleptic treatment and are more common in older patients. More than 60% of patients may show one or more of the features of parkinsonism.

Early detection of parkinsonism is important because it is readily treated with the addition of an anticholinergic drug or a dopaminomimetic drug (e.g., amantadine 100 mg twice a day). With patients who manifest parkinsonism at low doses of neuroleptics, a switch should be made to an atypical agent, because these patients may be at increased risk for tardive dyskinesia (Barnes 1990).

Akathisia. Akathisia is a syndrome of subjective and objective motor restlessness associated with neuroleptic treatment. Patients experience anxiety, inner restlessness, inability to stand still, and constant pacing (Adler et al. 1989). It may be very distressing for the patient and is a chief cause of neuroleptic noncompliance (Van Putten 1974; Weiden et al. 1991). Akathisia is often overlooked or misinterpreted as anxiety or worsening of psychosis.

Anticholinergic drugs are of limited use in the treatment of akathisia, but the addition of a β-blocker (e.g., propranolol 20 mg twice a day) or a benzodiazepine (e.g., diazepam 2 mg three times a day) may be more effective (Adler et al. 1989). Reducing neuroleptic dosage and switching to an atypical antipsychotic are the other alternatives for the management of akathisia.

Tardive dyskinesia and other tardive movement disorders. Tardive dyskinesia and tardive dystonia are serious, potentially irreversible side effects of long-term neuroleptic treatment that are characterized by the late appearance of choreiform or athetoid movements of body regions, particularly in the orofacial and truncal regions (Barnes 1990; Casey 1991). Although neuroleptic dosage and duration of treatment have been implicated as risk factors, their association with tardive dyskinesia is inconsistent (Barnes 1990). Old age, female gender, affective disorders, and evidence of organic brain impairment are risk factors for tardive dyskinesia. Diabetes has also been established as a risk factor (Woerner et al. 1993). Acute EPS have been associated specifically with vulnerability to tardive dyskinesia (Barnes 1990).

Current management strategies for tardive dyskinesia reflect its proposed pathophysiology. First, the risk of tardive dyskinesia may be minimized through use of the lowest effective dose of neuroleptic for the shortest duration of time, clinical circumstances permitting. Discontinuation of neuroleptics alone results in a 50% improvement in tardive dyskinesia by 3 months in more than a third of patients, with further improvement over time (Glazer et al. 1990). Second, reduction in neuroleptic dose may alleviate symptoms of tardive dyskinesia, although often these symptoms initially worsen as part of a withdrawal dyskinesia. Third, several classes of agents have been tried for the treatment of tardive dyskinesia. Dopaminergic and dopamine-depleting agents and vitamin E have been tried in the treatment of tardive dyskinesia, but the results are at best inconsistent (Feltner and Hertzman 1993).

At present, clozapine is the best treatment option for moderate to severe, persistent tardive dyskinesia (Lieberman et al. 1991; Meltzer and Luchins 1984). For patients with severe tardive dyskinesia or dystonia, switching to clozapine is usually desirable.

Neuroleptic malignant syndrome. NMS is an uncommon (incidence < 0.9%), potentially fatal complication of neuroleptic treatment. It is characterized by the development of fever, rigidity, autonomic instability, altered consciousness, and elevated creatine kinase (CK) activity

(Meltzer 1973) and raised WBC count in the absence of any other medical condition that might explain these symptoms (Kellam 1990; Rosebush and Stewart 1989). Rapid increases in dosage of neuroleptic drugs, parenteral administration, agitation, and diagnosis of affective disorder are all risk factors for the development of NMS (Kellam 1990). NMS may develop after removal of antiparkinsonian agents.

When NMS is suspected, the patient must have a thorough physical examination and organic and septic workup to rule out other causes. If no other causes are evident, then immediate cessation of neuroleptics (and lithium, if present) and provision of full supportive measures are recommended. A dopamine agonist (e.g., bromocriptine 30 mg/day) and a muscle relaxant (e.g., dantrolene 400 mg/day) should be given as adjunctive therapy. ECT may also be given to manage acute psychotic symptoms during NMS (Hermesh et al. 1987). The risk of recurrence on reexposure to neuroleptics—approximately 30% of patients have a recurrence of NMS—may be minimized by delaying rechallenge by 2 weeks post NMS and by using an antipsychotic of an alternative class (Rosebush and Stewart 1989). Switching to a low-EPS atypical antipsychotic is recommended.

Seizures. Standard neuroleptic drugs lower the seizure threshold. A history of epilepsy or organic brain impairment is a risk factor for the development of seizures in persons taking neuroleptics. However, seizures occur uncommonly during treatment and are more likely to arise during neuroleptic withdrawal, particularly when complicated by withdrawal from benzodiazepines or other agents.

Nonneurological Side Effects

Nonneurological adverse effects of standard antipsychotic medication (Table 19–3) are, in general, of lesser morbidity but may be distressing for patients and may limit the choice and ultimate dosage of neuroleptic.

Most patients experience some sedative effects while taking neuroleptics. Sedation is more commonly associated with low-potency agents that possess prominent antiadrenergic and antimuscarinic effects (e.g., mesoridazine) than with other, higher-potency agents. Tolerance usually develops, although if sedation persists, then divided doses and adjustment of time when doses are taken, neuroleptic dose reduction, *or* substitution is a worthwhile management strategy.

Weight gain is a particular problem with clozapine and olanzapine, and, apparently, with this weight gain, there is an increased risk for diabetes. Increases of 5%–10% of base weight are often noted. Dietary counseling and exercise programs are desirable. Weight gain with other atypical and typical antipsychotics is less frequent and less extensive.

Hypotension is a frequent cardiovascular side effect attributable to an α_1 antiadrenergic effect and more commonly seen with low-potency agents. Tachycardia may also be observed, as may nonspecific T-wave changes on the electrocardiogram (ECG), which result from atropine-like effects on the myocardium.

Common anticholinergic adverse effects include blurred vision, precipitation of glaucoma, dry mouth, reduced gastrointestinal tract motility, urinary hesitancy, and impotence. Anticholinergic toxicity, ranging from subtle memory impairment to delirium, may result from concomitant use of anticholinergic drugs; the elderly are particularly prone to this problem. These adverse effects may be avoided by careful clinical observation and judicious management of neuroleptic dosage and any concomitant medications.

Hyperprolactinemia, the chief endocrine side effect of standard neuroleptics, is a direct consequence of blockade of pituitary dopamine receptors (Meltzer and Fang 1976). Hyperprolactinemia accounts for amenorrhea in female patients and for galactorrhea, which may rarely result in a breast abscess.

Leukocytosis, eosinophilia, or leukopenia may occur with treatment with standard neuro-leptics, especially phenothiazines. Agranulocytosis, however, occurs in only 1 of 2,000 patients receiving standard neuroleptics. Because WBC counts are typically not monitored with these drugs, a proportion of these cases are fatal, so the mortality rate may be comparable to that with clozapine. Leukopenia (WBC $\leq$ 3,000/mm^3) may forewarn the clinician of impending agranulocytosis, and neuroleptic medication should be withdrawn.

Neuroleptics uncommonly induce hepatitis with a cholestatic pattern that generally is self-limiting and resolves with brief cessation of treatment.

Dermatological reactions, hypersensitivity urticaria, photosensitivity, or slate-gray hyperpigmentation occurs in fewer than 5% of patients receiving standard neuroleptics. These effects are managed conservatively, with dermatological consultation as necessary. Retinitis pigmentosa has been described in patients receiving doses of thioridazine above 800 mg/day, so low doses of thioridazine are advocated in long-term maintenance therapy.

It is important to recognize that adverse effects can also occur from interactions with other drugs (Goff and Baldessarini 1993). Such effects may result from alterations in the metabolism of neuroleptics (e.g., carbamazepine induces the hepatic microsomal system that metabolizes haloperidol, with the result that plasma levels are lowered) or additive toxic effects (e.g., combined anticholinergic effects with concomitant use of tricyclic antidepressant medications). Almost all antidepressants will raise antipsychotic blood levels as a result of metabolic interactions. Although such an effect amounts to increasing the dose of neuroleptics, antidepressants increase vulnerability to psychosis. Lithium may induce neurotoxic reactions when combined with neuroleptics. Patients need to be alerted in advance to these potential adverse effects. Commonly prescribed drugs that interact with antipsychotics include alcohol, anticonvulsants, anxiolytics, antidepressants, antihypertensives, cimetidine, disulfiram, and lithium.

Discontinuation of Neuroleptic Treatment

Because of the high probability of relapse, indefinite maintenance treatment with an antipsychotic is prudent. A targeted, or intermittent, maintenance strategy has been used to reduce relapse in stable patients. This strategy relies heavily on the patient's and relatives' ability to recognize prodromal symptoms of relapse: anxiety, irritability, sleep disturbance, perceptual aberrations, oddity of behavior, and paranoid ideas of reference. Intensive psychosocial and educative support are also necessary. Studies have indicated that patients on targeted strategies not only fare significantly worse in terms of relapse (both higher rates and greater severity) but also show only modest reductions in overall side effects when compared with patients who are continued on conventional maintenance treatment.

Augmentation of Neuroleptic Drugs

Various augmenting agents have been used to enhance conventional or atypical antipsychotic drug response and to treat other, specific associated symptoms (Table 19–4). In general, these drugs, when added to neuroleptics or atypical antipsychotics, have at best only marginal effects on both positive and negative symptoms (Christison et al. 1991; Meltzer 1992). Anticonvulsants and lithium may produce clinically significant improvement in aggression.

Some preliminary findings have shown encouraging benefits in treating persistent positive and negative symptoms with selective serotonin reuptake inhibitors (SSRIs) (Goff et al. 1991; Silver and Nassar 1992).

Benzodiazepines have also been shown to be helpful in ameliorating persistent psychotic symptoms in some patients (Meltzer 1992; Wolkowitz and Pickar 1991). However, these effects are, at best, modest and must be weighed against the adverse effects of these agents and also the potential for rebound psychotic and anxiety symptoms, which are particularly associated with the withdrawal of high-potency triazolobenzodiazepines such as alprazolam.

When negative symptoms predominate, the use of L-dopa, bromocriptine, or methylphenidate to accentuate dopaminergic activity may be of benefit, although this strategy may be associated with a risk of precipitating a relapse of positive symptoms.

Anticonvulsant drugs, such as valproate and carbamazepine, appear to be ineffective as a primary treatment for schizophrenia (Carpenter and Strauss 1991), but they may be of use in persistently psychotic patients who manifest impulsive or violent behavior (Meltzer 1992). Patients who have electroencephalogram (EEG) abnormalities or episodic dyscontrol behaviors may also derive benefit from adjunctive anticonvulsant therapy.

Finally, the role of ECT in the treatment of the persistently psychotic patient has come under renewed scrutiny (Sajatovic and Meltzer 1993). Maintenance ECT may be of value in the management of treatment-refractory schizophrenia and can result in reduction in positive symptoms and rates of rehospitalization

Table 19–4. Neuroleptic augmentation strategies in treatment-refractory schizophrenia

Symptom(s)	Adjunctive treatment
Persistent positive symptoms	Lithium, anticonvulsants, electroconvulsive therapy
Persistent negative symptoms	L-Dopa, bromocriptine, benzodiazepine
Depressive symptoms	Antidepressants, lithium
Hypomania	Lithium
Anxiety	Benzodiazepine
Aggression	Anticonvulsants, lithium

(Sajatovic and Meltzer 1993). However, ECT needs to be given at least monthly.

PHARMACOTHERAPY OF ANTIPSYCHOTIC DRUG–RESISTANT SCHIZOPHRENIA

Clozapine

Clozapine, a dibenzodiazepine chemically related to loxapine, was first identified as a promising antipsychotic that produces few or no EPS (for review, see Baldessarini and Frankenburg 1991). At least six controlled studies demonstrated that clozapine had superior efficacy compared with typical antipsychotic drugs for the treatment of neuroleptic-responsive schizophrenia (e.g., Ekblöm and Haggström 1974; Fischer-Cornelssen and Ferner 1976; Gerlach et al. 1974). However, in 1975, eight patients treated with clozapine died from agranulocytosis in southwestern Finland (Amsler et al. 1977). All of these cases of agranulocytosis occurred within the first 4 months of treatment. The overall incidence of agranulocytosis is thought to be 1%.

Clozapine was withdrawn from general use in Europe and from further clinical trials in the United States. However, clinical experience with clozapine over the next decade suggested that clozapine not only caused lower EPS but also was devoid of risk for tardive dyskinesia (Casey 1989). Moreover, additional clinical evidence for its superiority in efficacy was obtained, although not from controlled studies (Juul Povlsen et al. 1985; Kuha and Miettinen 1986; Lindström 1988).

These studies led to the first controlled trial of clozapine in treatment-resistant schizophrenia, which was conducted by one of the present authors (H. Y. M.) and colleagues (Kane et al. 1988). In a double-blind trial of 6 weeks' duration, clozapine and chlorpromazine were compared in nearly 300 hospitalized patients with treatment-resistant schizophrenia. Treatment

resistance was defined as the failure to respond to at least three separate trials of neuroleptics, from at least two different chemical classes, over a 5-year period at dosages equivalent to 1,000 mg/day of chlorpromazine or greater for a period of 6 weeks.

As a result of this study, clozapine was approved for use in neuroleptic-responsive and -resistant schizophrenic patients by the FDA in 1989. By the end of 1996, it had been administered to approximately 175,000 patients in the United States, with about 90,000 having remained in treatment for at least 6 months. Numerous other countries also approved clozapine as a result of this study.

Subsequent experience has also indicated that the response to clozapine may either be very rapid (≤6 weeks) in about 30% of patients (Stern et al. 1994) or delayed (6 weeks to 6 months) in another 30% (Lieberman et al. 1994; Meltzer 1995a).

Efficacy

Effect on psychopathology.   Clozapine has been found to be significantly superior to typical neuroleptics in reducing the total score on the Brief Psychiatric Rating Scale (BPRS) Positive Symptoms subscale as well as the scores on individual items that constitute this subscale (i.e., Conceptual Disorganization, Hallucinatory Behavior, Suspiciousness, and Unusual Thought Content) (Claghorn et al. 1987; Kane et al. 1988; Pickar et al. 1992).

Effect on negative symptoms.   Kane et al. (1988), in their controlled trial of clozapine in treatment-resistant schizophrenia, found clozapine to be clearly more effective than chlorpromazine in reducing scores on the BPRS Negative Symptoms subscale (i.e., Emotional Withdrawal, Blunted Affect, Psychomotor-Retardation, and Disorientation). Clozapine has been reported to decrease significantly scores on the BPRS Withdrawal/Retardation subscale (Meltzer 1989a).

Clozapine is also effective in ameliorating the negative symptoms in patients who do not have notable positive symptoms (Meltzer and Zureick 1989). Pickar et al. (1992) found significantly more improvement in scores on the BPRS Negative Symptoms subscale, but not in those on the Scale for the Assessment of Negative Symptoms (SANS), in clozapine-treated patients compared with fluphenazine-treated patients.

Clozapine has been reported to produce a significant decrease in ratings on the Schedule for Affective Disorders and Schizophrenia–C (SADS-C) Disorganization factor, which includes loose association, poverty of thought content, incoherence, and inappropriate affect (Meltzer 1992). The effect of clozapine on the Disorganization cluster of the SADS-C was superior to its effect on both the Positive and Negative subscales of that same schedule.

Clozapine is effective in improving some of these deficits in patients with treatment-resistant schizophrenia. Hagger et al. (1993) studied cognitive function and psychopathology in 36 patients with treatment-resistant schizophrenia before initiation of clozapine and at 6 weeks and 6 months of clozapine treatment. Compared with 26 healthy control subjects, the schizophrenic patients were noted to have deficits in measures of memory, executive function, and attention. With clozapine treatment, significant improvement occurred in retrieval from reference memory at 6 weeks and 6 months and in some measures of executive function (Wechsler Intelligence Scale for Children—Revised Maze Test), attention (Wechsler Adult Intelligence Scale—Revised Digit Symbol subtest), and recall memory (Verbal List Learning Test) at 6 months.

Effect on mood symptoms.   Clozapine has been reported to be effective in decreasing both manic and depressive symptoms in patients with treatment-resistant schizoaffective disorder (McElroy et al. 1991; Naber and Hippius 1990; Naber et al. 1989, 1992; Owen et al. 1993; Wood

and Rubinstein 1990). Overall, clozapine was found to be more effective in schizoaffective patients than in schizophrenic patients.

In a prospective study, clozapine markedly reduced suicidality, especially low- and high-probability suicide attempts, in patients with treatment-resistant schizophrenia and schizoaffective disorder (Meltzer and Okayli 1995). This decrease in suicidality was associated with improvement in depression and hopelessness, as measured by the Hamilton Rating Scale for Depression (Hamilton 1960). These findings could be the basis for reevaluation of the risk-benefit assessment of clozapine. Thus, the overall morbidity and mortality for treatment-resistant schizophrenia could be less with clozapine than with typical neuroleptic drugs because of decreased suicidality. Suicide has been reported to occur in 9%–13% of schizophrenic patients, whereas the risk of agranulocytosis from clozapine is less than 1%, and the mortality is approximately 0.01% (Alvir et al. 1993).

Dosage and Administration

The recommended starting dosage of clozapine is 12.5–25 mg/day to test for possible hypotension. The dosage of clozapine may be increased by 25 mg every other day until it reaches 100 mg/day. This can be done on an outpatient basis if the patient is able to adhere to the prescribed schedule or if there are family members or case managers who can assist the patient. The total dose can then be increased by 50 mg every other day until a dosage of 300–450 mg/day is reached. Twice-a-day dosage is recommended, because the half-life of clozapine is 16 hours (Choc et al. 1987; Jann et al. 1993). The dosage need not exceed 450–600 mg/day in most adults age 60 years or younger in the initial phase of treatment. However, if response at 600 mg/day is unsatisfactory, the dosage should be further increased up to a maximum of 900 mg/day. The dosage of clozapine required in the elderly is usually 200–300 mg/day but may be as low as 5–100 mg/day (Kronig et al. 1995). No data are available as to whether lower dosages of clozapine are needed for maintenance treatment. Clozapine is effective in adolescent patients with schizophrenia (Birmaher et al. 1992). The dosage may have to be reduced because of sedation and hypersalivation.

To date, no fixed-dose studies have been done to determine the optimal dosage in treatment-resistant schizophrenia. In the United States, dosages of 400–600 mg/day (mean dosage 444 mg/day) are most common, whereas in Europe, dosages in the range of 200–500 mg/day or lower (mean dosage 284 mg/day) are most often used (Fleischhacker et al. 1994; Naber et al. 1989). The reasons for this discrepancy are unknown at this time but could be related to more common use of concomitant neuroleptic drugs in Europe.

In general, clozapine is best given as monotherapy from the start. If this is not clinically feasible, then the medication regimen should be simplified as much as possible so that the patient is receiving a single neuroleptic such as haloperidol (in oral form only). Patients should be withdrawn from typical neuroleptic drugs as the dosage of clozapine is increased to 450 mg/day. Benzodiazepines should be avoided because of the risk (based mainly on case reports) of respiratory depression with concomitant use of clozapine and benzodiazepines during the initial phases of treatment. The duration of a trial with clozapine before it is considered to be ineffective may be as long as 6 months (Lieberman et al. 1994; Meltzer 1989b, 1995a; Safferman et al. 1991).

Clozapine and Extrapyramidal Symptoms

Clozapine produces remarkably few EPS (Lieberman et al. 1991, 1994) and can suppress tardive dyskinesia or dystonia (Chengappa et al. 1994; Lieberman et al. 1994). The rate of suppression may be slow, with some patients showing no change until after 6 months of treatment. The rate of akathisia in clozapine-treated patients is also low (Chengappa et al. 1994; Claghorn et al. 1987). These features give clozapine very significant advantages over typical neuroleptics and possibly other atypical antipsychotic agents as well.

Side Effects

The side effects of clozapine have been reviewed by Safferman et al. (1991). Important side effects of clozapine and their management are highlighted in Table 19–5. The most serious of these is agranulocytosis, which is reported to occur in slightly fewer than 1% of patients receiving clozapine (Alvir et al. 1993). Since early 1998 the weekly blood testing requirement has become every other week after the initial 6 months of treatment with clozapine. The peak risk period for developing agranulocytosis is in the first 18 weeks of treatment; as yet, there are no useful predictors as to which patients are likely to develop this side effect. Age and female gender may be risk factors for the development of clozapine-related agranulocytosis (Alvir et al. 1993). For patients who show an abrupt or marked fall in WBC count or whose WBC count falls to between 3,500/mm^3 and 3,000/mm^3 inclusive, the WBC count should be checked twice a week. If the WBC count falls below 3,000/mm^3 but is not less than 2,000/mm^3, clozapine should be stopped and the WBC count monitored daily. A WBC count of less than 2,000/mm^3 or an absolute neutrophil count of less than 1,000/mm^3 is an indication for immediate cessation of clozapine. When the WBC count falls below 1,500/mm^3 or the absolute neutrophil count reaches 500/mm^3, clozapine therapy should *never* be resumed.

Agranulocytosis is an indication for hospitalization and the institution of reverse isolation. A full infectious disease workup is mandatory, and often the prophylactic use of antibiotics is advisable. The use of one of the known granulocyte-stimulating factors will help to restore normal bone marrow production (Gerson and Meltzer 1992; Lieberman and Alvir 1992).

Major motor seizures occur at a rate of approximately 3% at 300 mg/day and 6% at 600 mg/day of clozapine (Sajatovic and Meltzer 1993). Myoclonus occurs less frequently. Neither major motor seizures nor myoclonus is a

Table 19–5. Side effects of clozapine

Side effect	Incidence	Action
Agranulocytosis	0.8%	Monitor WBC weekly for the first 6 months, then every other week; if WBC < 2,000/mm^3: stop clozapine; hospitalize; treat infection aggressively; never give clozapine again
Seizures	3%, dose related	Decrease dose of clozapine; add phenytoin or valproate
Tachycardia	>25%	Treat if heart rate is >140 bpm or patient is symptomatic; add low dose of β-blocker
Hypertension	9%	Monitor; add β-blocker if BP high or hypertension persistent
Hypotension	9%	Monitor; encourage fluid intake; alter dosage regimen
Dizziness	20%	Tolerance often develops; monitor; alter dosage regimen
Sedation	40%, dose related	Give maximum dosage at night; reduce total daily dose; add methylphenidate 20–40 mg/day
Weight gain	Variable, >3%	Reduce diet; prescribe exercise
Hypersalivation	31%	Benztropine mesylate or clonidine may help
Constipation	14%	Prescribe laxative, if required
Nausea	5%	Use supportive measures

Note. WBC = white blood cell; bpm = beats per minute; BP = blood pressure.

cause for discontinuation of clozapine; rather, they should be treated either by reduction in the dosage of clozapine or by addition of an anticonvulsant agent. Valproic acid is usually effective but may increase clozapine levels. Carbamazepine should be avoided because of the risk of agranulocytosis, but when necessary for seizure control, carbamazepine and clozapine can be given.

The other main side effects of clozapine are cardiovascular effects, sedation, weight gain, and hypersalivation. The chief cardiovascular effects are orthostatic hypotension, tachycardia, and ECG changes. Other than tachycardia, which is persistent, these effects are seen early in treatment, are short lived, and seldom result in discontinuation of clozapine. Sedation is a less serious but common and distressing side effect. It is generally observed early in treatment, and

tolerance develops over time. Another common side effect of clozapine is weight gain, with reported rates varying from 1% to 85% (average 38%); the weight gain associated with clozapine is greater than that associated with haloperidol (Hummer et al. 1995). Simple strategies, including dietary advice, exercise, and weight monitoring, are usually effective. Most of the gain occurs in the first 4 months. Hypersalivation, another common side effect of clozapine, generally occurs at night, again often in the initial phases of treatment (Ben-Aryeh et al. 1996). If the hypersalivation becomes troublesome or persistent, the addition of benztropine mesylate or clonidine (an α_1 receptor agonist) will usually relieve this side effect. Constipation and nausea are also side effects of clozapine. Some patients cannot tolerate clozapine or refuse to try it.

Availability

Numerous fiscal and political constraints influence the availability of clozapine for patients with treatment-refractory schizophrenia. When these constraints preclude a trial of clozapine, the use of the more traditional neuroleptic augmentation strategies is advisable. Some of the most commonly used augmenting agents, and their relative indications, are listed in Table 19–4. Recently the FDA approved a generic form of clozapine, which does not require registration and may be less costly.

Relationship Between Clinical Efficacy and Plasma Concentrations

The half-life of clozapine after twice-a-day dosing at steady state is about 16 hours (range 6–33). Thus, a steady state is achieved after about 1 week of twice-a-day administration at a constant dosage (Choc et al. 1987). Current evidence suggests that of the major metabolites of clozapine, norclozapine may be partially active, and clozapine-N-oxide may be pharmacologically inactive, but this issue needs further elucidation.

There is some evidence that plasma levels of clozapine may be a useful guide to optimally efficacious dosage. It appears that dosages that achieve plasma levels higher than 350–370 ng/mL are maximally effective in treatment-resistant schizophrenia (Hasegawa et al. 1993; Lieberman et al. 1994; Perry et al. 1991). There is no evidence of a therapeutic window. Some patients do respond at lower plasma levels. Clozapine plasma levels are most commonly measured by high-pressure liquid chromatography (Lovdahl et al. 1991).

Plasma levels of clozapine should be obtained in patients who have inadequate response. Also, it may be useful to check clozapine levels once the dosage exceeds 600 mg/day, because the incidence of seizures increases significantly at dosages higher than 600 mg/day, and because high plasma concentrations of clozapine are associated with seizures (Simpson

and Cooper 1978). Finally, it may be possible, in selected cases, to exceed the recommended limit of 900 mg/day if there is poor response, if plasma levels are lower than 370 ng/mL, and there are no serious or troublesome side effects.

Factors that have been found to affect plasma levels of clozapine include gender, smoking, and certain drugs. Phenytoin has been reported to lower the clozapine concentration (Miller 1991). Valproate and fluvoxamine increase plasma levels of clozapine by decreasing its metabolism.

Partial Response to Clozapine

Partial response to clozapine may be approached in a variety of ways. Clinical experience indicates that addition of a low dose of a high-potency neuroleptic drug to clozapine has been found to be helpful in ameliorating positive symptoms in some partial responders. Concomitant ECT may also be useful in some of these patients, but maintenance ECT may be needed to sustain the benefits (Sajatovic and Meltzer 1993).

Antidepressants and mood stabilizers have also been used as adjuncts in treating depressive or manic symptoms among schizoaffective patients. SSRIs, including fluoxetine, sertraline, fluvoxamine, and paroxetine, are the antidepressants of choice (Cassady and Thacker 1992). It may be prudent not to initiate clozapine and lithium simultaneously given a few reports of increased neurotoxicity (Blake et al. 1992; Pope et al. 1991); but once a stable dosage of clozapine has been attained, lithium can safely be added in most cases. Valproic acid may also be used. Carbamazepine is absolutely contraindicated because of increased risk of agranulocytosis.

For persistent anxiety symptoms, benzodiazepines or buspirone may be added. A few earlier reports of cardiorespiratory collapse with concomitant use of benzodiazepines caused great concern; however, subsequent clinical experience has shown that this combination is safe in most medically healthy patients. Again, benzodiazepines should be added preferably only after a stable dose of clozapine has been achieved.

Recommendations for Pharmacological Treatment of Resistant Schizophrenia

After determining that a patient has not had a satisfactory response to typical neuroleptic drugs, despite adequate dosage and duration of treatment, and that compliance has been adequate, the choice of pharmacotherapy is between initiating treatment with clozapine immediately or trying one or more of the novel antipsychotic drugs first.

At present, clinical experience with risperidone and olanzapine indicates that some proportion of patients with neuroleptic-resistant schizophrenia will respond to adequate doses of these agents, but the appropriate dosage range and duration of a trial are not known.

What is known is that clozapine will be more effective than standard neuroleptics in a high proportion of such patients (i.e., at least 60%) (Lieberman et al. 1994; Meltzer and Ranjan 1996) but that there is somewhat increased risk and more difficult administration attached.

Patients and their families should be given, when possible, sufficient information about the potential benefits and risks of all pharmacological treatment options and encouraged to make an informed choice. Because clozapine is the drug for which there is the best evidence for efficacy and tolerability in treatment-resistant schizophrenia patients, a decision to go directly to clozapine should be supported. However, some patients or mental health providers will wish to try olanzapine, quetiapine, or risperidone before clozapine in order to avoid the need for biweekly blood drawing and the risk of agranulocytosis. This, too, is a reasonable approach. Should there be an unsatisfactory response to either of these agents, it would appear prudent to proceed directly to clozapine without the need for a trial of the other agent—or of

ziprasidone once it has been approved for use, in the absence of any empirical evidence that it is effective in cases of neuroleptic-resistant schizophrenia.

CONCLUSION

Significant advances have been made in defining appropriate treatment strategies for patients with schizophrenia (Meltzer and Ranjan 1995). A broad view of treatment objectives that includes much more than positive symptom control is essential. Neuroleptic drugs are still widely used for acute and maintenance treatment of schizophrenia, but atypical antipsychotic drugs are rapidly displacing them. Olanzapine, risperidone, quetiapine, and ziprasidone may qualify as first-line drugs because of fewer side effects and superior efficacy compared with standard neuroleptics. As a group, the atypical antipsychotic agents have advantages in terms of EPS, negative symptoms, and compliance. Clozapine is the treatment of choice in schizophrenic patients who fail to respond to other antipsychotic drugs and has demonstrated efficacy in a wide range of outcome measures. The efficacy of alternative treatments for patients with neuroleptic-resistant schizophrenia, including neuroleptic augmentation strategies or adjunctive ECT, is now less clear, and these treatments are probably best reserved for patients who either refuse or cannot tolerate clozapine treatment. The advent of clozapine and other new antipsychotics offers encouragement and optimism for the treatment of persons with schizophrenia and provides a neurobiological framework on which to explore the pathophysiology of schizophrenia.

REFERENCES

Adler LA, Angrist B, Reiter S, et al: Neuroleptic-induced akathisia: a review. Psychopharmacology (Berl) 97:1–11, 1989

Alvir JMJ, Lieberman JA, Safferman AZ, et al: Clozapine-induced agranulocytosis: incidence and risk factors in the United States. N Engl J Med 329:162–167, 1993

American Psychiatric Association: Diagnostic and Statistical Manual of Mental Disorders, 4th Edition. Washington, DC, American Psychiatric Association, 1994

Amsler HA, Teerenhovi L, Barth E, et al: Agranulocytosis in patients treated with clozapine: a study of the Finnish epidemic. Acta Psychiatr Scand 56:241–248, 1977

Arvanitis LA, Miller BG, Seroquel Trial 13 Study Group: Multiple fixed doses of "Seroquel" (quetiapine) in patients with acute exacerbation of schizophrenia: a comparison with haloperidol and placebo. Biol Psychiatry 42:233–246, 1997

Awad G: Quality of life of schizophrenic patients on medications and implications for new drug trials. Hospital and Community Psychiatry 43:262–265, 1992

Ayd FJ: A summary of drug-induced extrapyramidal reactions. JAMA 175:1054–1060, 1961

Baldessarini RJ, Frankenburg FF: Clozapine: a novel antipsychotic agent. N Engl J Med 324:746–754, 1991

Baldessarini RJ, Cohen BM, Teicher MH: Significance of neuroleptic dose and plasma level in the pharmacological treatment of psychoses. Arch Gen Psychiatry 45:79–91, 1988

Barnes TRE: Movement disorder associated with antipsychotic drugs: the tardive syndromes. International Review of Psychiatry 2:355–366, 1990

Baum KM, Walker EF: Childhood behavioral precursors of adult symptom dimensions in schizophrenia. Schizophr Res 16:111–120, 1995

Beasley CM, Tollefson G, Tran P, et al: Olanzapine versus placebo and haloperidol: acute phase results of the North American double-blind olanzapine trial. Neuropsychopharmacology 14:111–123, 1996

Ben-Aryeh H, Jungerman T, Szargel R, et al: Salivary flow-rate and composition in schizophrenic patients on clozapine: subjective reports and laboratory data. Biol Psychiatry 39:946–949, 1996

Birmaher B, Baker R, Kapur S, et al: Clozapine for the treatment of adolescents with schizophrenia. J Am Acad Child Adolesc Psychiatry 31:160–164, 1992

Blake LM, Marks RC, Luchins DJ: Reversible neuroleptic symptoms with clozapine. J Clin Psychopharmacol 12:297–299, 1992

Boodhood JA, Sadler WM: Anticholinergic antiparkinsonian drugs in psychiatry. Br J Hosp Med 46:167–169, 1991

Braff DL, Heaton R, Kuck J, et al: The generalized pattern of neuropsychological deficits in outpatients with chronic schizophrenia with heterogeneous Wisconsin Card Sorting Test results. Arch Gen Psychiatry 48:891–898, 1991

Buckley P, Way L, Meltzer HY: Substance abuse among patients with treatment-resistant schizophrenia: characteristics and implications for clozapine therapy. Am J Psychiatry 151:154–159, 1994

Carpenter WT Jr: The phenomenology and course of schizophrenia: treatment implications, in Psychopharmacology: A Third Generation of Progress. Edited by Meltzer HY. New York, Raven, 1987, pp 1121–1128

Carpenter WT Jr: The deficit syndrome. Am J Psychiatry 151:327–329, 1994

Carpenter WT Jr, Strauss JS: The prediction of outcome in schizophrenia, IV: eleven-year follow up of the Washington IPSS Cohort. J Nerv Ment Dis 179:517–525, 1991

Casey DE: Clozapine: neuroleptic-induced EPS and tardive dyskinesia. Psychopharmacology (Berl) 99 (suppl):S47–S53, 1989

Casey DE: Neuroleptic drug-induced extrapyramidal syndromes and tardive dyskinesia. Schizophr Res 4:109–120, 1991

Casey DE: 'Seroquel' (quetiapine): preclinical and clinical findings of a new atypical antipsychotic. Expert Opinion on Investigational Drugs 5:939–957, 1996

Cassady SL, Thacker GK: Addition of fluoxetine to clozapine (letter). Am J Psychiatry 149:1274, 1992

Cassens G, Inglis ALK, Appelbaum PS, et al: Neuroleptics: effects on neuropsychological function in chronic schizophrenic patients. Schizophr Bull 16:477–499, 1990

Chakos MH, Mayerhoff DI, Loebel AD, et al: Incidence and correlates of acute extrapyramidal symptoms in first episode of schizophrenia. Psychopharmacol Bull 28:81–86, 1992

Chengappa KN, Shelton M, Baker R, et al: The prevalence of akathisia in patients receiving stable doses of clozapine. J Clin Psychiatry 55:142–145, 1994

Choc MG, Lehr RG, Hsuan F, et al: Multiple-dose pharmacokinetics of clozapine in patients. Pharm Res 4:402–405, 1987

Chouinard G, Jones B, Remington G, et al: A Canadian multicenter placebo-controlled study of fixed doses of risperidone and haloperidol in the treatment of chronic schizophrenic patients. J Clin Psychopharmacol 13:25–40, 1993

Christison GW, Kirch DJ, Wyatt RJ: When symptoms persist: choosing among alternative somatic treatments for schizophrenia. Schizophr Bull 17:217–245, 1991

Claghorn J, Honigfeld G, Abuzzahab FS, et al: The risks and benefits of clozapine versus chlorpromazine. J Clin Psychopharmacol 7:377–384, 1987

Crow TJ: Schizophrenia: more than one molecular process. BMJ 280:66–68, 1980

Daniel DG, Goldberg TE, Weinberger DR, et al: Different side-effect profiles of risperidone and clozapine in 20 outpatients with schizophrenia or schizoaffective disorder: a pilot study. Am J Psychiatry 153:417–419, 1996

Davis JM, Barter JT, Kane JM: Antipsychotic drugs, in Comprehensive Textbook of Psychiatry/V, 5th Edition. Edited by Kaplan HI, Sadock BJ. Baltimore, MD, Williams & Wilkins, 1989, pp 1591–1626

Davis KL, Kahn RS, Ko G, et al: Dopamine in schizophrenia: a review and reconceptualization. Am J Psychiatry 148:1474–1486, 1991

Ekblöm B, Haggström JE: Clozapine (Leponex) compared with chlorpromazine: a double-blind evaluation of pharmacological and clinical properties. Current Therapeutic Research 16:945–957, 1974

Fatemi SH, Meltzer HY, Roth BL: Atypical antipsychotic drugs: clinical and preclinical studies, in Handbook of Experimental Pharmacology, Vol 120: Antipsychotics. Edited by Csernansky JG. Heidelberg, Springer-Verlag, 1996, pp 77–116

Feltner DE, Hertzman M: Progress in the treatment of tardive dyskinesia: theory and practice. Hospital and Community Psychiatry 44:25–34, 1993

Fischer-Cornelssen KA, Ferner VJ: An example of European multicenter trials: multispectral analysis of clozapine. Psychopharmacol Bull 2:34–39, 1976

Fleischhacker WW, Hummer M, Kurz M, et al: Clozapine dose in the United States and Europe: implications for therapeutic and adverse effects. J Clin Psychiatry 55 (no 9, suppl B):78–81, 1994

Gerlach I, Koppelhus P, Helweg E, et al: Clozapine and haloperidol in a single-blind cross-over trial: therapeutic and biochemical aspects in the treatment of schizophrenia. Acta Psychiatr Scand 50:410–424, 1974

Gerson SL, Meltzer HY: Mechanisms of clozapine-induced agranulocytosis. Drug Saf 7:17–25, 1992

Gilbert PL, Harris MJ, McAdams LA, et al: Neuroleptic withdrawal in schizophrenic patients: a review of the literature. Arch Gen Psychiatry 52:173–188, 1995

Glazer WM, Morgenstein H, Schooler N, et al: Predictors of improvement in tardive dyskinesia following discontinuation of neuroleptic medication. Br J Psychiatry 157:585–592, 1990

Glazer WM, Morgenstein H, Doucette JT: Predicting the long-term risk of tardive dyskinesia in outpatients maintained on neuroleptic medication. J Clin Psychiatry 54:133–139, 1993

Goff DC, Baldessarini RJ: Drug interactions with antipsychotic agents. J Clin Psychopharmacol 13:57–65, 1993

Goff DC, Midha KK, Brotman AW, et al: An open trial of buspirone added to neuroleptics in schizophrenic patients. J Clin Psychopharmacol 11:193–197, 1991

Goldberg TE, Calls JR, Weinberger DR, et al: Performance of schizophrenic patients on putative neuropsychological tests of frontal lobe function. Int J Neurosci 42:51–58, 1988

Goldberg TE, Greenberg RD, Griffin SJ, et al: The effect of clozapine on cognition and psychiatric symptoms in patients with schizophrenia. Br J Psychiatry 162:43–48, 1993

Goldstein JF, Arvanitis LA: ICI204,636 (Seroquel); a dibenzthiazepine atypical antipsychotic: review of preclinical pharmacology and highlights of phase II clinical trial. CNS Drug Review 1:50–73, 1995

Green MF: What are the functional consequences of neurocognitive deficits in schizophrenia? Am J Psychiatry 153:321–330, 1996

Green MF, Marshall BD Jr, Wirshing WC, et al: Does risperidone improve verbal working memory in treatment-resistant schizophrenia? Am J Psychiatry 154:799–804, 1997

Hagger C, Buckley P, Kenny JT, et al: Improvement in cognitive functions and psychiatric symptoms in treatment-refractory schizophrenic patients receiving clozapine. Biol Psychiatry 34:702–712, 1993

Hamilton M: A rating scale for depression. J Neurol Neurosurg Psychiatry 23:56–62, 1960

Hasegawa M, Gutierrez-Esteinou R, Way L, et al: Relationship between clinical efficacy and clozapine plasma concentrations in schizophrenia: effect of smoking. J Clin Psychopharmacol 13:383–390, 1993

Hermesh H, Aizenburg D, Weizman A: A successful electroconvulsive treatment of neuroleptic malignant syndrome. Acta Psychiatr Scand 75: 237–239, 1987

Hogarty GE, Anderson CM, Reiss DJ, et al: Family psychoeducation, social skills training, and maintenance chemotherapy in the aftercare treatment of schizophrenia, II: two-year effects of a controlled study on relapse and adjustment. Arch Gen Psychiatry 48:340–347, 1988

Hummer M, Kemmler G, Kurz M, et al: Weight gain induced by clozapine. Eur Neuropsychopharmacol 5:437–440, 1995

Jann MW, Grimstey SR, Gray EC, et al: Pharmacokinetics and pharmaco-dynamics of clozapine. Clin Pharmacokinet 24:161–176, 1993

Juul Povlsen U, Noring V, Fog R, et al: Tolerability and therapeutic effect of clozapine: a retrospective investigation of 216 patients treated with clozapine for up to 12 years. Acta Psychiatr Scand 71:176–185, 1985

Kane J, Marder SR: Psychopharmacologic treatment of schizophrenia. Schizophr Bull 19: 287–302, 1993

Kane JM, Woener M, Weinhold P, et al: Incidence of tardive dyskinesia: five-year data from a prospective study. Psychopharmacol Bull 20:39–40, 1984

Kane JM, Rifkin A, Woerner M, et al: High-dose versus low-dose strategies in the treatment of schizophrenia. Psychopharmacol Bull 21: 533–537, 1985

Kane J, Honigfeld G, Singer J, et al [Clozaril Collaborative Study Group]: Clozapine for the treatment-resistant schizophrenic: a double-blind comparison with chlorpromazine. Arch Gen Psychiatry 45:789–796, 1988

Kellam AMP: The (frequently) neuroleptic malignant syndrome. Br J Psychiatry 157:169–173, 1990

Kibel DA, Laffont I, Liddle PF: The composition of the negative syndrome of chronic schizophrenia. Br J Psychiatry 162:744–750, 1993

Kronig M, Munne R, Szymanski S, et al: Plasma clozapine levels and clinical response for treatment refractory schizophrenic patients. Am J Psychiatry 152:179–182, 1995

Kuha S, Miettinen E: Long-term effect of clozapine in schizophrenia: a retrospective study of 108 chronic schizophrenics treated with clozapine for up to 7 years. Nordisk Psykiatrisk Tidsskrift 40:225–230, 1986

Lee MA, Thompson P, Meltzer HY: Effects of clozapine on cognitive function in schizophrenia. J Clin Psychiatry 55 (no 9, suppl B):82–87, 1994

Levinson DF, Simpson GM, Single H, et al: Fluphenazine dose, clinical response and extrapyramidal symptoms during acute treatment. Arch Gen Psychiatry 47:761–768, 1990

Liddle PF: The symptoms of chronic schizophrenia: a reexamination of the positive-negative dichotomy. Br J Psychiatry 151:145–15l, 1987

Liddle PF, Barnes TR: Syndromes of chronic schizophrenia. Br J Psychiatry 157:558–561, 1990

Lieberman JA, Alvir JMJ: A report of clozapine-induced agranulocytosis in the United States: incidence and risk factors. Drug Saf 7 (suppl):1–2, 1992

Lieberman JA, Saltz BL, Johns CA, et al: The effects of clozapine on tardive dyskinesia. Br J Psychiatry 158:503–510, 1991

Lieberman J, Safferman A, Pollack S, et al: Clinical effects of clozapine in chronic schizophrenia: response to treatment and predictors of outcome. Am J Psychiatry 151:1744–1752, 1994

Lindström LH: The effect of long-term treatment with clozapine in schizophrenia: a retrospective study in 96 patients treated with clozapine for up to 13 years. Acta Psychiatr Scand 77: 524–529, 1988

Lovdahl MJ, Perry PJ, Miller DD: The assay of clozapine and N-desmethylclozapine in human plasma by high-performance liquid chromatography. Ther Drug Monit 13:69–72, 1991

Marder SR, Meibach RC: Risperidone in the treatment of schizophrenia. Am J Psychiatry 151: 825–835, 1994

Marder SR, Van Putten T: Who should receive clozapine? Arch Gen Psychiatry 45:865–867, 1988

Marder SR, Van Putten T, Mentz J, et al: Costs and benefits of two doses of fluphenazine. Arch Gen Psychiatry 41:1025–1029, 1984

Marder SR, Van Putten T, Mintz J, et al: Low- and conventional-dose maintenance therapy with fluphenazine decanoate: two-year outcome. Arch Gen Psychiatry 44:518–521, 1987

McElroy SL, Dessain EC, Pope HG Jr, et al: Clozapine in the treatment of psychotic mood disorders, schizoaffective disorder, and schizophrenia. J Clin Psychiatry 52:411–414, 1991

McEvoy JP, Hogarty GE, Steingard S: Optimal dose of neuroleptic in acute schizophrenia: a controlled study of neuroleptic threshold and higher haloperidol dose. Arch Gen Psychiatry 48:739–745, 1991

McGorry PD, McFarlane C, Patton GC, et al: The prevalence of prodromal features of schizophrenia in adolescence: a preliminary survey. Acta Psychiatr Scand 92:241–249, 1995

Meltzer HY: Rigidity, hyperpyrexia and coma following fluphenazine enanthate. Psychopharmacologia 29:337–346, 1973

Meltzer HY: Clinical studies on the mechanism of action of clozapine: the dopamine-serotonin hypothesis of schizophrenia. Psychopharmacology (Berl) 99 (suppl):S18–S27, 1989a

Meltzer HY: Duration of a clozapine trial in neuroleptic-resistant schizophrenia (letter). Arch Gen Psychiatry 46:672, 1989b

Meltzer HY: Dimensions of outcome with clozapine. Br J Psychiatry 160:46–53, 1992

Meltzer HY: Clozapine: is another view valid? Am J Psychiatry 152:821–825, 1995a

Meltzer HY: The concept of atypical antipsychotics, in Advances in the Neurobiology of Schizophrenia, Vol 1. Edited by den Boer JA, Westenberg HGM, van Praag HM. London, Wiley, 1995b, pp 265–273

Meltzer HY: A career in biological psychiatry, in The Psychopharmacologists: Interviews by David Healy. London, Chapman & Hall, 1996, pp 509–538

Meltzer HY: The clozapine story, in The Handbook of Psychopharmacology Trials. Edited by Hertzman M, Feltner DE. New York, New York University Press, 1997, pp 137–156

Meltzer HY, Fang VS: Effect of neuroleptics on serum prolactin in schizophrenic patients. Arch Gen Psychiatry 33:279–286, 1976

Meltzer HY, Luchins DJ: Effect of clozapine in severe tardive dyskinesia: a case report. J Clin Psychopharmacol 4:286– 287, 1984

Meltzer HY, Okayli G: The reduction of suicidality during clozapine treatment in neuroleptic-resistant schizophrenia: impact on risk-benefit assessment. Am J Psychiatry 152:183–190, 1995

Meltzer HY, Ranjan R: Recent advances in the pharmacotherapy of schizophrenia. Acta Psychiatr Scand Suppl 384:95–101, 1995

Meltzer HY, Ranjan R: Efficacy of novel antipsychotic drugs in treatment-refractory schizophrenia, in Handbook of Experimental Pharmacology, Vol 120: Antipsychotics. Edited by Csernansky JG. Heidelberg, Springer-Verlag, 1996, pp 333–358

Meltzer HY, Zureick JL: Negative symptoms in schizophrenia. A target for new drug development, in Clinical Pharmacology in Psychiatry, Vol 1. Edited by Dahl SG, Gram LF. Berlin, Springer, 1989, pp 68–77

Meltzer HY, Matsubara S, Lee JC: Classification of typical and atypical antipsychotic drugs on the basis of dopamine D-1, D-2 and serotonin$_2$ pKi values. J Pharmacol Exp Ther 251:238–246, 1989

Miller DD: Effect of phenytoin on plasma clozapine concentrations in two patients. J Clin Psychiatry 52:23–25, 1991

Mueser KT, Yarnold PR, Levinson DF, et al: Prevalence of substance abuse in schizophrenia: demographic and clinical correlates. Schizophr Bull 16:31–53, 1990

Murray RM, O'Callaghan E, Castle DJ, et al: A neurodevelopmental approach to the classification of schizophrenia. Schizophr Bull 18: 319–331, 1992

Naber D, Hippius H: The European experience with use of clozapine. Hospital and Community Psychiatry 41:886–890, 1990

Naber D, Leppig M, Grohman R, et al: Efficacy and adverse effects of clozapine in the treatment of schizophrenia and tardive dyskinesia—a retrospective study of 387 patients. Psychopharmacology (Berl) 99 (suppl):S73–S76, 1989

Naber D, Holzbach R, Perro C, et al: Clinical management of clozapine patients in relation to efficacy and side-effects. Br J Psychiatry 160:54–59, 1992

Owen RR, Gutierrez-Esteinou R, Hsiao J, et al: Effects of clozapine and fluphenazine treatment on responses to m-chlorophenylpiperazine infusions in schizophrenia. Arch Gen Psychiatry 50:636–644, 1993

Perry PJ, Miller DD, Arndt SV, et al: Clozapine and norclozapine plasma concentrations and clinical response of treatment-refractory schizophrenic patients. Am J Psychiatry 148:231–235, 1991

Peuskens J: Risperidone in the treatment of patients with chronic schizophrenia: a multi-national multi-centre, double-blind parallel-group study versus haloperidol. Br J Psychiatry 166:712–726, 1995

Pickar D, Owen RR, Litman RE, et al: Clinical and biological response to clozapine in patients with schizophrenia. Arch Gen Psychiatry 49:345–353, 1992

Pope HG Jr, McElroy SL, Keck PE, et al: Valproate in the treatment of acute mania. Arch Gen Psychiatry 44:113–118, 1991

Richelson E, Nelson A: Antagonism by neuroleptics of neurotransmitter receptors of normal human brain in vitro. Eur J Pharmacol 103:197–204, 1984

Rifkin A, Karajgi B, Doddi S, et al: Dose and blood levels of haloperidol in treatment of mania. Psychopharmacol Bull 76:144–146, 1990

Rosebush PI, Stewart TD: A prospective analysis of 24 episodes of neuroleptic malignant syndrome. Am J Psychiatry 146:717–725, 1989

Roy A: Suicide in chronic schizophrenia. Br J Psychiatry 141:171–177, 1982

Safferman A, Lieberman J, Kane J, et al: Update on the clinical efficacy and side effects of clozapine. Schizophr Bull 17:247–261, 1991

Sajatovic M, Meltzer HY: The effect of short-term electroconvulsive treatment plus neuroleptic in treatment-resistant schizophrenia and schizoaffective disorder. Convulsive Therapy 9:167–175, 1993

Saykin AJ, Gur RC, Gur RJ, et al: Neuropsychological function in schizophrenia: selective impairment in learning and memory. Arch Gen Psychiatry 48:618–624, 1991

Schotte A, Janssen PFM, Gommeren W, et al: Risperidone compared with new and reference antipsychotic drugs: in vitro and in vivo receptor binding. Psychopharmacology (Berl) 124: 57–73, 1996

Seeger TF, Seymour PA, Schmidt AW, et al: Ziprasidone (CP-88,059): a new antipsychotic with combined dopamine and serotonin receptor antagonist activity. J Pharmacol Exp Ther 275:101–113, 1995

Silver H, Nassar A: Fluvoxamine improves negative symptoms in treated chronic schizophrenia: an add-on double-blind, placebo-controlled study. Biol Psychiatry 31:698–704, 1992

Simpson GM, Cooper TA: Clozapine plasma levels and convulsions. Am J Psychiatry 135:99–100, 1978

Siris SG, Harmon GK, Endicott J: Postpsychotic depressive symptoms in hospitalized schizophrenic patients. Arch Gen Psychiatry 38: 1122–1123, 1981

Small JG, Hirsch SR, Arvanitis LA, et al [Seroquel Study Group]: Quetiapine in patients with schizophrenia: a high- and low-dose double-blind comparison with placebo. Arch Gen Psychiatry 54:549–557, 1997

Stern R, Kahn R, Davidson M, et al: Early response to clozapine in schizophrenia. Am J Psychiatry 151:1817–1818, 1994

Tollefson GD, Sanger TM: Negative symptoms: a path analytic approach to a double-blind, placebo- and haloperidol-controlled clinical trial with olanzapine. Am J Psychiatry 154:466–474, 1997

Tollefson GD, Beasley CM, Tamura RN, et al: Blind, controlled long-term study of the comparative incidence of treatment-emergent tardive dyskinesia with olanzapine or haloperidol. Am J Psychiatry 154:1248–1259, 1997a

Tollefson GD, Beasley CM, Tran PV, et al: Olanzapine versus haloperidol in the treatment of schizophrenia and schizoaffective and schizophreniform disorders: results of an international collaborative trial. Am J Psychiatry 154:457–465, 1997b

Umbricht D, Kane JM: Risperidone: efficacy and safety. Schizophr Bull 21:593–604, 1995

Van Putten T: Why do schizophrenic patients refuse to take their drugs? Arch Gen Psychiatry 31:67–72, 1974

Van Putten T, Marder SR, Mintz J: A controlled dose comparison of haloperidol in newly admitted schizophrenic patients. Arch Gen Psychiatry 47:754–758, 1990

Weiden PJ, Dixon L, Frances A, et al: Neuroleptic noncompliance in schizophrenia, in Schizophrenia Research. Edited by Tamminga CA, Schulz SC. New York, Raven, 1991, pp 285–296

Weinberger DR: Implications of normal brain development for the pathogenesis of schizophrenia. Arch Gen Psychiatry 44:660–669, 1987

Woerner MG, Saltz BL, Kane JM, et al: Diabetes and the development of tardive dyskinesia. Am J Psychiatry 150:966–968, 1993

Wolkowitz OM, Pickar D: Benzodiazepines in the treatment of schizophrenia: a review and reappraisal. Am J Psychiatry 148:714–726, 1991

Wood MJ, Rubinstein M: An atypical responder to clozapine. Am J Psychiatry 147:369, 1990

Wyatt RJ: Neuroleptics and the natural course of schizophrenia. Schizophr Bull 17:325–351, 1991

Wyatt RJ, Green MF, Tuma AH: Long-term morbidity associated with delayed treatment of first admission schizophrenic patients: a re-analysis of the Camarillo State Hospital data. Psychol Med 27:261–268, 1997

Young MA, Meltzer HY: The relationship of demographic, clinical and outcome variables to neuroleptic treatment requirements. Schizophr Bull 6:88–101, 1980

TWENTY

Treatment of Anxiety Disorders

C. Barr Taylor, M.D.

The psychopharmacological treatment of panic and other anxiety disorders has changed dramatically in the past 10 years. The changes in treatment were initiated by the publication of DSM-III (American Psychiatric Association 1980), which allowed for uniform diagnoses, by the epidemiological evidence of the high prevalence of these disorders, by the development of new pharmacological and cognitive therapies, and by a general increase in research in this area. Even 10 years ago, benzodiazepines were the customary psychopharmacological treatment in the United States for most anxiety disorders. Now a variety of agents has been shown to be effective. The psychological treatment of anxiety disorders also has expanded and has been better integrated into the pharmacological treatment (Taylor and Arnow 1988).

PANIC DISORDER

Panic disorder (with and without agoraphobia) is the most common anxiety disorder, occurring in 2%–6% of the population (Myers et al. 1984). The target symptoms of panic disorder include panic attacks, anticipatory and generalized anxiety, avoidance (agoraphobia), and, to varying degrees, worry, somatic symptoms, and even obsessions. Panic disorder is a long-term disorder, with frequent relapses, changes in symptomatology, and comorbidity. Of the latter, depression and alcohol use and abuse are particularly relevant in considering which psychopharmacological agents to use.

Short-Term, Acute Treatment

The short-term goals of psychopharmacological treatment are symptom relief and initiation of psychoeducational or psychological therapies. In many patients, the target symptoms are alleviated and work, family, and social functioning improve within 8 weeks of treatment with combinations of psychological and pharmacological therapies.

Antidepressants

Antidepressants should be considered the first line of treatment for patients with panic disorder, especially if depression is present. Of all the antidepressants, imipramine has been used the longest and has been most extensively investigated. However, research has substantiated the

431

benefit of serotonin reuptake inhibitors (SRIs). Based on their effectiveness and favorable side-effect profile, they should now be considered the first drug of choice (Coplan et al. 1996).

Serotonin reuptake inhibitors. The SRIs, including fluoxetine, paroxetine, fluvoxamine, and clomipramine, have proven to be effective antipanic agents at least in the short term (Den Boer and Westenberg 1990; Modigh et al. 1992; Oehrberg et al. 1995; Pecknold et al. 1995).

Patients with panic disorder sometimes have a reaction, characterized by feelings of restlessness, sweating, flushing, or even increased anxiety, to SRIs at the usual starting dose. This reaction is similar to that with other antidepressants and may even be more common with SRIs, especially clomipramine, than with other psychopharmacological treatments. To avoid or minimize this "jitteriness reaction," many clinicians begin with one-quarter to one-half the usual SRI dose, increasing the medication as tolerated and needed. Low doses of benzodiazepines can also be used on an as-needed basis to counteract this syndrome temporarily.

Sexual dysfunction is a common side effect of SRIs. Sexual dysfunction can involve loss of interest in sex and/or alteration in physiological arousal, including difficulty with orgasm and ejaculation (Gitlin 1994).

Because SRIs (and other antidepressants) can precipitate manic episodes, a careful history of hypomanic episodes should be obtained and/or a positive family history of bipolarity should be documented and other medications considered as appropriate. Some patients report dizziness, paresthesias, tremor, anxiety, nausea, and other symptoms when SRIs are abruptly discontinued. This so-called serotonin withdrawal syndrome usually occurs after 2 days and resolves within 3 weeks (Price et al. 1996; Zajecka et al. 1997). The syndrome appears to be minimized if SRIs are discontinued over a few weeks.

Tricyclics. The benefits of imipramine for reducing the frequency of panic attacks were first noted by D. F. Klein and Fink in 1962. Since then, several studies have substantiated its benefits. The largest study involved 1,168 patients in 14 countries and compared imipramine, alprazolam, and placebo (Cross-National Collaborative Panic Study 1992). At the end of the study, the effects of the two active drugs were similar to each other, and both drugs were superior to placebo for most outcome measures.

Imipramine should be started at doses of 25–50 mg and increased gradually. Most patients achieve a therapeutic benefit at 150–250 mg, although the dose can be increased to 300 mg. Mavissakalian and Perel (1995) found a positive dose-response relationship between imipramine and clinical improvement. Different dose ranges had different clinical effects. For phobias, the best total drug plasma level was in the range of 110–140 ng/mL; higher levels had a detrimental effect. For panic, the probability of response increased quickly with greater plasma levels and then tapered off, with no improvement at levels beyond 140 ng/mL. About 25% of patients with panic disorder who begin taking imipramine experience the "jitteriness syndrome" mentioned above. In patients who find these symptoms intolerable, imipramine can be reduced to very low doses (10 mg) and increased gradually.

Desipramine would theoretically work as well as imipramine because it is the main metabolite of imipramine. However, imipramine may be more serotonergic than desipramine, which may give imipramine greater efficacy, assuming that the serotonin system is important in panic disorder. Clomipramine has been shown to be effective for panic in European studies (Amin et al. 1977). Amitriptyline and nortriptyline may also be effective, but fewer studies are available, and the studies are less well designed (Ballenger 1986).

Monoamine oxidase inhibitors. Monoamine oxidase inhibitors (MAOIs) are also effective antipanic and antiphobic agents. Of the three available MAOIs, phenelzine has been studied most extensively and has been shown to be as efficacious as imipramine. Isocarboxazid and tranylcypromine are probably also effective. Recently, so-called reversible and selective MAOIs have been developed. In theory, they should be effective for panic disorder, and at least one study has found this to be the case (Bakish et al. 1993). They appear to be as effective as traditional MAOIs. In comparison with irreversible and nonselective MAOIs, such drugs have reduced tyramine-potentiating effects.

Other antidepressants.　Trazodone has been shown to be less effective than imipramine or alprazolam (Charney et al. 1986). Nefazodone, which is chemically related to trazodone, has been shown to reduce anxiety in depressed patients, but little information is available on its effect in patients with panic disorder (Fawcett et al. 1995). Some of the newer antidepressants may prove to be of benefit. Case reports suggest, for instance, that venlafaxine, a drug that inhibits the neuronal reuptake of both serotonin and norepinephrine and has been shown to be an effective antidepressant, may help to reduce panic attacks (Geracioti 1995).

Benzodiazepines

The benzodiazepines are effective for reducing panic attacks, phobic behavior, and anticipatory anxiety. Of the many benzodiazepines, alprazolam has been studied most extensively. The results of two large cross-national trials have been reported (Ballenger et al. 1988; Cross-National Collaborative Panic Study 1992). In the first large multicenter trial, 526 patients were randomized to receive either alprazolam or placebo. Of these, 86% of the alprazolam subjects completed the trial compared with only 50% of the placebo subjects. At the primary comparison point (week 4 of the study), 82% of the subjects receiving alprazolam were considered moderately improved or better compared with 42% of the placebo group. At that point, 50% of the alprazolam group compared with 28% of the

placebo group had no panic attacks. For those subjects who completed the trial, no significant difference in total number of panic attacks or in disability ratings was found between subjects taking alprazolam and those taking placebo, although the former were much less fearful and avoidant than the latter.

Different benzodiazepines are probably equally effective at comparable doses. For example, diazepam is about one-tenth as effective as alprazolam, and, if given at doses of 20–60 mg, diazepam appears to be as effective as alprazolam (Dunner et al. 1986). However, at those doses, diazepam causes relatively more sedation than alprazolam, and this side effect may limit its usefulness. Clonazepam has also been shown to be effective. It is as potent as alprazolam and has the advantage of a longer half-life (Tesar et al. 1991). Lorazepam (mean daily dose of 7 mg) was as effective as alprazolam in one study (Schweizer et al. 1990).

The choice of a benzodiazepine depends on potency, half-life, and evidence of effectiveness from clinical studies. Although effective, alprazolam has the disadvantage of a short half-life. Thus, frequent dosing may be necessary (as often as six times a day in rare cases), and some patients complain of breakthrough anxiety, either in the morning or between doses. A sustained-release form of alprazolam appears to avoid this problem (Carter et al. 1995). Alprazolam should be initiated at 0.25–0.50 mg three times a day. Doses should be increased every 4–6 days as needed and tolerated. Clonazepam should be initiated at 0.5 tablet per day and increased every 3–5 days to therapeutic goals. Some investigators recommend that the medication be increased until the patient is symptom free. However, one study found no relationship between dose and outcome. In a study of alprazolam, 13 of 14 patients with a serum level between 15 and 77 ng/mL, achieved with doses between 1 and 6 mg/day, reached zero panic attacks at the end of the study (Wincor et al. 1991). A study of 2 or 6 mg of alprazolam compared with placebo found only a few statistically significant differences between the two groups, and both doses were better than placebo (Lydiard et al. 1992). Furthermore, higher doses require longer withdrawal.

Benzodiazepines should be used cautiously in the elderly. Among the short-half-life drugs, high-potency compounds (e.g., lorazepam, alprazolam) may be more toxic than low-potency compounds (e.g., oxazepam) in the elderly.

Benzodiazepines often produce sedation, increase the effects of alcohol, can produce dyscoordination, and are associated with dependence and withdrawal (Busto et al. 1986). Benzodiazepine withdrawal occurs even after only 4–8 weeks of use. Moreover, studies suggest that withdrawal-like phenomena can be precipitated by benzodiazepine receptor antagonists after as brief as 1 day of benzodiazepine administration (Spealman 1986).

After benzodiazepines have been used for a few weeks or more, a careful plan of discontinuation is needed. The withdrawal syndrome can be severe enough to cause epileptic seizures, confusion, and psychotic symptoms (Noyes et al. 1986; Owen and Tyrer 1983; Taylor and Arnow 1988). For most patients, withdrawal symptoms are more diffuse, including anxiety, insomnia, panic, tremor, muscle twitching, perceptual disturbances, and depersonalization (Busto et al. 1986; Owen and Tyrer 1983; Taylor and Arnow 1988). Profound insomnia is a sign that the symptoms are related more to withdrawal than to return of anxiety, because this symptom is rare with anxiety. Possibly because of these side effects, many patients are reluctant to stop taking the benzodiazepines.

Pecknold et al. (1988) found no rebound and only 7% of patients with clinically significant withdrawal symptoms when a slow, flexible taper was used. Benzodiazepine doses should be reduced more slowly at the end of the taper (Rickels et al. 1990). During withdrawal from alprazolam, it may be easier to switch patients to clonazepam, because clonazepam can be given in fewer doses (Patterson 1990). Cognitive-behavior therapy (Bruce et al. 1995) and

carbamazepine (E. Klein et al. 1994) may help facilitate withdrawal.

Previous drug or alcohol abuse is a risk factor for dependence and increased use of benzodiazepines (Haskell et al. 1986; Lennane 1986). Such a history is not an absolute contraindication to benzodiazepine use, but these drugs should be used with particular caution in this population. When the clinician is considering benzodiazepine use for chronically anxious patients, he or she should document the patient's diagnosis and status, carefully monitor medications, and apply other forms of therapy concurrently.

Other Medications

Buspirone, which may have antianxiety properties, does not appear to be effective for panic disorder (Sheehan et al. 1990). Neuroleptics are generally not useful because of their acute and long-term toxicity, and they may even exacerbate panic symptoms. However, atypical neuroleptics, such as clozapine, may prove to be effective anxiolytics in psychotic disorders because of their serotonin (5-HT) antagonistic properties. Anticonvulsants, such as carbamazepine and valproic acid, have been reported to be effective in case reports (Keck et al. 1993).

Concomitant Psychoeducation and Psychotherapy

Psychoeducation should be used in combination with medication. Other psychotherapeutic approaches may also be of benefit and perhaps even enhance the outcome. Cognitive-behavior approaches have been shown to reduce panic attacks and avoidance significantly and have been the most extensively evaluated interventions (Brown and Barlow 1995; Taylor and Arnow 1988; Welkowitz et al. 1991; Zinbarg et al. 1992). Other psychological therapies also have shown benefit (Ost 1988; Shear et al. 1994). Most cognitive therapy interventions require at least 12–18 hours of treatment spaced over 3–6 months with follow-up sessions to deal with relapse, although more rapid and less costly interventions may prove equally effective (Lidren et al. 1994; Newman et al. 1997; Swinson et al. 1995).

Long-Term Treatment

Panic disorder is a chronic, long-term condition, and the length of pharmacological treatment remains controversial. Most of the studies reported in the previous section have focused on only short-term outcomes. Current clinical practice generally involves a trial of 3–6 months of an effective medication. More controversial is continued therapy for an additional 6–12 months or longer. We do know that relapse rates are very high after medication is discontinued. Depending on the medication, concomitant psychological treatment, the length of follow-up, and the criteria, relapse rates of between 20% and 80% have been reported (Ballenger 1992). With medication alone, probably fewer than half of patients remain well after medication has been discontinued for 6 months or longer. Ballenger (1992) asserted that the medications shown to be effective have few adverse physical effects; therefore, the length of treatment should only be based on questions of effectiveness.

The evidence that patients with depression, another long-term condition, have better outcomes with maintenance medication should also be considered (Kupfer et al. 1992). In light of the controversies surrounding long-term medication use, and because the medication may no longer be necessary, it is good practice to routinely discontinue the medication after 6 months to a year, especially if patients are taking benzodiazepines. Patients should remain off of the medication for at least a month before being restarted on it to give adequate time for adjustment after discontinuation.

Clinicians usually reinstate the medication previously used if it was successful or prescribe a new medication if it might have an advantage over the medication previously used.

Refractory Cases

Most panic disorders can be treated successfully with one medication, often the first one tried. However, some patients may require combinations of medications. The combinations that have been reported to be successful tend to be similar to those reported for depression, such as the use of a tricyclic and an SRI (Coplan et al. 1996; Tiffon et al. 1994). If such combined therapy fails, then addition of a benzodiazepine or some of the other agents mentioned earlier in this chapter can be considered.

GENERALIZED ANXIETY DISORDER

Generalized anxiety disorder (GAD), like panic disorder, is common, occurring in at least 2%–3% of the population (Weissman et al. 1978). The main features of GAD are chronic cognitive, behavioral, and physiological symptoms of hyperarousal and anxiety. GAD commonly occurs with other anxiety disorders and depression, and the latter should always be considered when symptoms of GAD are present. When depression or panic disorder is present, it should be treated first.

Benzodiazepines have been the mainstay of treatment for patients with GAD (Thompson 1996). Benzodiazepines are effective in the short run for reducing symptoms of GAD. Different types of benzodiazepines at equivalent doses are equally effective for generalized anxiety, and the agent used should be chosen on the basis of potency, half-life, and side effects.

The issues discussed earlier in this chapter regarding the use of benzodiazepines for panic disorder apply to GAD. In 1980, after reviewing studies on benzodiazepine effects, the British Medical Association concluded that the effects of such drugs do not persist beyond 3–4 months. However, other experts have argued that benzodiazepines are effective for much longer. For instance, Haskell et al. (1986) studied 194 patients with a history of diazepam use. The patients taking long-term diazepam were as symptomatic as patients presenting for anxiety treatment. Yet, 158 of the 194 had tried to discontinue diazepam at some time, and, of these, 142 reported the reemergence of anxiety symptoms. However, the patients believed that they were deriving benefit from treatment.

The problems with benzodiazepines have prompted an intensive search for alternative agents effective in reducing symptoms of GAD. Buspirone, an azapirone derivative and a 5-HT$_{1A}$ partial agonist, has been shown to be as effective as benzodiazepines and significantly better than placebo in controlled clinical trials (Goldberg and Finnerty 1979; Napoliello 1986; Rickels et al. 1982; Wheatley 1982) at doses of 20–40 mg. In these trials, improvement continued from pretreatment through the fourth week of treatment and paralleled but was somewhat slower than that of the benzodiazepines (Rickels et al. 1990).

Buspirone produces less drowsiness, psychomotor impairment, and alcohol potentiation and has less potential for addiction or abuse compared with the benzodiazepines. Buspirone seems to be most helpful in anxious patients who do not demand immediate relief of symptoms, including patients who have taken benzodiazepines (Rickels 1990). A meta-analysis of GAD treatment studies found that diazepam had a somewhat greater effect than buspirone (Cox et al. 1992). Some investigators add buspirone to reduce rebound symptoms during discontinuation from benzodiazepines (Udelman and Udelman 1990). Buspirone will not block the potential serious withdrawal effects of benzodiazepines and should not be used instead of a gradual benzodiazepine withdrawal.

An important and perhaps overlooked finding is that imipramine may have anxiolytic effects (Hoehn-Saric et al. 1988; Kahn et al. 1986; McLeod et al. 1990). Imipramine had a significant effect on reducing anticipatory anxiety in the cross-national alprazolam and imipramine trial, but the effect was only significantly different by the eighth week of treatment. Doses lower than those used for panic disorder are of-

ten effective in GAD. Treatment may not be effective until patients have been taking medication for a month or longer.

Serotonin reuptake blockers may prove to have significant antianxiety effects. Clomipramine has been shown to be effective in at least one uncontrolled study (Wingerson et al. 1992).

Venlafaxine (Effexor XR) has been approved for generalized anxiety disorder. Published studies have reported efficacy both in acute studies (Davidson et al. 1999; Rickels et al. 2000) and in 6-month continuation trials (Gelenberg et al. 2000).

Partial benzodiazepine agonists (e.g., bretazenil and abecarnil) were exciting new potential anxiolytics a few years ago (Ballenger et al. 1992; Haefely et al. 1992) with low risk of dependence, but studies have failed to demonstrate efficacy.

The cognitive-behavioral treatment of GAD has been less well evaluated than that of panic disorder. A combination of relaxation and related techniques aimed at decreasing hyperarousal—cognitive-behavior therapy, skills training and coping, and alteration in lifestyle factors as appropriate—is often beneficial (Borkovec and Costello 1993; Miller et al. 1995; Taylor 1978; Taylor and Arnow 1988), but long-term controlled studies are lacking. Traditional psychodynamic therapies are often effective in alleviating symptoms of chronic anxiety.

SOCIAL PHOBIA

Social phobia is a common, disabling, and often unrecognized anxiety disorder, occurring in about 1%–2% of the population (Myers et al. 1984). Although social phobia shares many features of panic disorder and often occurs with it, it has separate phenomenological features. For instance, the five most common fears of people with social phobia are 1) public speaking, 2) eating in public, 3) writing in public, 4) using public lavatories, and 5) being stared at or being the center of attention, whereas the most common fears of people with panic disorder are 1) driving or traveling, 2) going to stores, 3) being in crowds, 4) eating in restaurants, and 5) using elevators (Uhde et al. 1991). People with social phobia do not have spontaneous panic attacks and do not panic when they are alone or asleep. They also have low rates of dyspnea. Fear of negative evaluation is the critical cognitive feature of social phobia. Many people with social phobia also have avoidant personality disorder, characterized by chronic patterns of shyness and avoidance. Patients with avoidant personality disorder appear very similar to patients with generalized social phobia (Hofmann et al. 1995). Social phobia is often quite disabling and results in extreme anxiety, avoidance, work and social impairment, depression, and substance abuse (Liebowitz et al. 1985).

The pharmacological treatment of social phobia had lagged behind that of other anxiety disorders. However, studies have found that fluoxetine, sertraline, fluvoxamine, and paroxetine can be effective treatments of social phobia (Marshall and Schneier 1996). Paroxetine was the first SSRI approved for social phobia. Multiple acute studies have demonstrated that paroxetine is both superior to placebo and highly effective in the disorder (e.g., Baldwin et al. 1999; Stein et al. 1998). In addition, fluvoxamine has also been reported to be highly effective (Stein et al. 1999).

High-potency benzodiazepines, particularly alprazolam and clonazepam, have been reported to reduce symptoms of social phobia (Davidson et al. 1991; Lydiard et al. 1988; Reiter et al. 1990). Gabapentin also appears to be effective in the disorder (Pande et al. 1999).

Liebowitz et al. (1988) decided to use MAOIs to treat social phobia after observing that MAOIs are useful in a variety of phobias and reduce excessive interpersonal sensitivity in patients with atypical depression. In a sample of 74 patients, phenelzine was superior to both atenolol and placebo, with no significant differences between the latter two agents (Liebowitz et al. 1992).

Reversible MAOIs, a class of medications that is selective for isoenyzme A of monoamine oxidase and that binds reversibly so that it has less risk for hypertensive crises than the standard MAOIs, may also be effective for social phobia. For instance, Versiani et al. (1992) found that moclobemide, an experimental reversible MAOI, was nearly as effective as phenelzine and superior to placebo. A U.S. multicenter trial did not find moclobemide to differ from placebo (Noyes et al. 1997). However, other studies point to modest effects (International Multicenter Clinical Trial Group on Moclobemide 1997). Development of this compound has been halted in the United States.

β-Blockers also have been used to treat social phobia, with mixed results. For performance anxiety, β-blockers have been shown to benefit activities such as pistol shooting, bowling, stringed instrument playing, and public speaking (Liebowitz et al. 1991). Doses of 10–40 mg of propranolol taken about 1 hour before such performances can reduce symptoms of sympathetic activity, such as sweating and tremor, that may serve as cues for anxiety and fear. The early β-blocker studies focused on performance anxiety, and this subgroup of persons with social phobia may respond differently than individuals with generalized social fears. A small controlled trial found that propranolol and placebo had no effect in patients receiving behavioral treatment (Falloon et al. 1981).

Uncontrolled trials also found that buspirone, in doses up to 60 mg/day, had some benefits in patients with social phobia (Liebowitz et al. 1991). Buspirone had no effect on exposure therapy in a controlled clinical trial (Clark and Agras 1991).

As with panic disorder, cognitive-behavior therapy is an appropriate adjunctive treatment to psychopharmacology in social phobia. A major line of basic research in behavior therapy has been devoted to one type of social phobia—that of speech phobia. This research has led to a number of treatment approaches, including systematic desensitization, social skills training, imaginal flooding, applied relaxation training, graduated exposure, anxiety management, and a variety of cognitive-restructuring procedures (i.e., self-instructional training, rational-emotive therapy, and cognitive-behavior group therapy) (Liebowitz et al. 1985).

In one study, cognitive-behavior treatment programs were compared with phenelzine, alprazolam, or placebo administered to patients with social phobia (Gelernter et al. 1991). All patients improved in all groups. Patients treated with phenelzine plus self-exposure had greater improvement than other groups did on a measure of trait anxiety. Comparative studies are needed before the relative benefits of psychopharmacological and psychological treatments alone and in combination are known.

OBSESSIVE-COMPULSIVE DISORDER

Obsessive-compulsive disorder (OCD) is much more common than formerly thought, with a 6-month point prevalence of 1%–2% and a lifetime prevalence of 2%–3% (Myers et al. 1984; Robins et al. 1984). Five medications—clomipramine, fluoxetine, fluvoxamine, paroxetine, and sertraline—have proven effective in reducing OCD symptoms (Jefferson and Greist 1996). Nevertheless, many patients continue to experience symptoms.

Given apparent comparable efficacy, either clomipramine or an SRI should be considered the drug of first choice for OCD, after taking into account the relatively different side effects of clomipramine (a tricyclic) compared with the SRIs (Goodman et al. 1992). At the end of one large trial, obsessive and compulsive symptoms in patients given clomipramine had decreased by 35%–42% on the Yale-Brown Obsessive-Compulsive Scale, the standard instrument for measuring improvement, compared with 2%–5% in placebo groups (Clomipramine Collaborative Study Group 1991). Significant improvement was generally not seen until after about 6 weeks of clomipramine treatment with doses up to 300 mg.

Research on the effectiveness and use of SRIs for OCD has shown that many patients' symptoms decline in 2–3 weeks, but clinical response may be delayed considerably (4 weeks in the fluoxetine and 6 weeks in the fluvoxamine multicenter trials); thus, a trial of 10–12 weeks is recommended before concluding lack of efficacy (Jefferson and Greist 1996). In the early studies, relatively high doses of SRIs were used. However, it is not clear if patients would have responded to lower doses if given more time. A preliminary fixed-dose study comparing 10 weeks of single daily doses of 20, 40, or 60 mg of fluoxetine with placebo did not find a clear-cut advantage of the 40- or 60-mg doses over the 20-mg dose (Wheadon 1991). Jefferson and Greist (1996) recommended that an OCD drug trial should not be considered complete until a patient has been treated with a minimum daily dose of the following (assuming tolerability): clomipramine 250 mg, fluoxetine 60 mg, fluvoxamine 300 mg, paroxetine 60 mg, and sertraline 200 mg.

If patients' symptoms do not respond to clomipramine or an SRI at adequate doses and time, then another SRI (or clomipramine) should be tried. If a partial response occurs, initiation of combined treatment may be appropriate. At this point in the history of OCD, combined treatments are largely based on case reports and single-case design rather than rigorous studies. Currently recommended strategies are to add agents such as buspirone, lithium, or fenfluramine, which may modify serotonergic function, to ongoing SRI or clomipramine therapy.

Buspirone has also been studied in treatment-resistant OCD patients. The results have been mixed; some studies show a benefit and others do not (Goodman et al. 1992). Buspirone added to the SSRI regimen for OCD patients has been reported to be effective in open trials but not in controlled studies (Schatzberg et al. 1997).

Before the advent of SRIs, neuroleptics were used to treat OCD, often with little effect. However, in carefully selected patients, neuroleptics may be of use, particularly if the patient has tics (such as Tourette's disorder), delusions, or schizotypal personality disorder (Goodman et al. 1992). Clozapine seemed to help one patient with very severe OCD refractory to extensive medication trials, electroconvulsive therapy, and capsulotomy. However, several studies have reported that obsessive-compulsive symptoms appeared to worsen during the course of treatment of schizophrenia with clozapine or risperidone (Jefferson and Greist 1996).

Clonazepam has been used to treat OCD to some effect (Hewlett et al. 1990). Trazodone has been shown to potentiate fluoxetine in patients with depression (Nierenberg et al. 1992) and may be useful as an adjunct to fluoxetine, but it does not seem to be effective by itself (Pigott et al. 1992).

The length of psychopharmacological treatment for OCD is unknown. OCD is a chronic illness, and patients are likely to require medication indefinitely. Relapse after discontinuation of medications is likely (Pato et al. 1988).

Behavioral treatments may provide a better long-term result than psychopharmacological ones. Of 40 patients who had been treated 6 years earlier with exposure therapy for 3 or 6 weeks and with clomipramine or placebo for 36 weeks, 47% remained much improved (O'Sullivan et al. 1991). The few patients who were taking tricyclics at follow-up assessment were no more improved than those who were not taking medications or were taking other drugs, and the patients given clomipramine during treatment were no more improved at follow-up than their placebo-taking counterparts. The study suggests that psychopharmacological treatment may enhance psychological therapies. However, one study found no benefit of adding imipramine to exposure therapy (Foa et al. 1992).

POSTTRAUMATIC STRESS DISORDER

Posttraumatic stress disorder (PTSD) has a lifetime prevalence of at least 1% (Helzer et al. 1987). The psychopharmacological treatment of PTSD is in its early stages and is reviewed only briefly here.

Most of the psychopharmacology trials for PTSD have focused on veterans. Some evidence suggests that United States veterans and civilians with PTSD are different populations and may have different responses to medications. For instance, in a study of fluoxetine, veterans' conditions improved less than did those of patients in a trauma clinic (van der Kolk et al. 1994).

Open trials of various tricyclic antidepressants have reported some benefit for some PTSD symptoms (Burstein 1984; Falcon et al. 1985; Kauffman et al. 1987). MAOIs have also been shown to be effective in open trials (Davidson et al. 1987; Hogben and Cornfield 1981; Shen and Park 1983). An 8-week, double-blind, randomized comparison of imipramine (average dose 240 mg/day), phenelzine (average dose 71 mg/day), and placebo was conducted with 34 veterans (Frank et al. 1988). Patients in both active-drug groups improved, especially for the symptoms of nightmares, flashbacks, and intrusive recollections, but no change was observed for symptoms of avoidance. Overall, the patients who received phenelzine had greater (but not significantly so) improvement than the patients who received imipramine.

Inhibitors of adrenergic activity, such as propranolol and clonidine, have also been used with some success; however, these medications seem to have been more effective in combination with tricyclics (Kinzie and Leung 1989).

Many other medications have been tried in the treatment of PTSD. On the assumption that kindling plays an important pathophysiological role in PTSD, agents that reduce kindling (e.g., carbamazepine, lithium, and valproate) have been tried. Carbamazepine reduced aggressive outbursts and anger in veterans with PTSD

(Lipper et al. 1986; Wolf et al. 1988). Lithium, which affects multiple neurotransmitter systems, has been effective in open-label studies of relatively few patients (Bunney and Garland-Bunney 1987; Kitchner and Greenstein 1985). In an open clinical trial, 10 of 16 Vietnam War veterans taking valproate had significantly improved conditions (Fesler 1991). Benzodiazepines may reduce some symptoms but have been associated with an increase in anger (Feldman 1987). No reports have been published on the use of SRIs.

After reviewing the psychopharmacological studies of PTSD, Silver et al. (1990) concluded that the positive symptoms of PTSD (e.g., reexperiencing of the event and increased arousal) often respond to medication, whereas negative symptoms (e.g., avoidance and withdrawal) respond poorly. Over time, the field has moved more to using SSRIs as first-line agents (Marshall et al. 1996), and sertraline has now received FDA approval. It appears to be more effective in women than in men.

β-Blockers can be considered for treatment of persistent symptoms of autonomic arousal in patients who have no medical contraindications. Medications that have been shown to have antiaggressive properties can be used in patients with extreme anger or irritability.

Psychological interventions should be used in combination with psychopharmacology. However, as with psychopharmacology, few controlled trials are available to guide practice in this area.

REFERENCES

American Psychiatric Association: Diagnostic and Statistical Manual of Mental Disorders, 3rd Edition. Washington, DC, American Psychiatric Association, 1980

Amin MM, Ban TA, Pecknold JC, et al: Clomipramine (Anafranil) and behaviour therapy in obsessive-compulsive and phobic disorders. J Int Med Res 5 (suppl 5):33–37, 1977

Bakish D, Saxena BM, Bown R, et al: Reversible monoamine oxidase-A inhibitors in panic disorder. Clin Neuropharmacol 16 (suppl 2):S77–S82, 1993

Ballenger JC: Pharmacotherapy of the panic disorders. J Clin Psychiatry 47 (suppl 6):27–32, 1986

Ballenger JC: Medication discontinuation in panic disorder. J Clin Psychiatry 53 (suppl 3):26–31, 1992

Ballenger JC, Burrows G, DuPont R, et al: Alprazolam in panic disorder and agoraphobia: results from a multicenter trial, I: efficacy in short-term treatment. Arch Gen Psychiatry 45:413–422, 1988

Ballenger JC, McDonald S, Noyes R Jr, et al: The first double-blind, placebo-controlled trial of a partial benzodiazepine agonist, abecarnil (ZK 112-119), in generalized anxiety disorder. Adv Biochem Psychopharmacol 47:431–437, 1992

Borkovec TD, Costello E: Efficacy of applied relaxation and cognitive behavioral therapy in the treatment of generalized anxiety disorder. J Consult Clin Psychol 61:611–619, 1993

Brown TA, Barlow DH: Long-term outcome in cognitive-behavioral treatment of panic disorder: clinical predictors and alternative strategies for assessment. J Consult Clin Psychol 63:754–765, 1995

Bruce TJ, Spiegel DA, Gregg SF, et al: Predictors of alprazolam discontinuation with and without cognitive behavior therapy in panic disorder. Am J Psychiatry 152:1156–1160, 1995

Bunney WE Jr, Garland-Bunney GL: Mechanisms of action of lithium in affective illness: basic and clinical implications, in Psychopharmacology: The Third Generation of Progress. Edited by Meltzer HY. New York, Raven, 1987, pp 533–565

Burstein A: Treatment of post-traumatic stress disorder with imipramine. Psychosomatics 25:681–687, 1984

Busto U, Sellers EM, Naranjo CA, et al: Withdrawal reaction after long-term therapeutic use of benzodiazepines. N Engl J Med 315:854–859, 1986

Carter CS, Fawcett J, Hertzman M, et al: Adinazolam-SR in panic disorder with agoraphobia: relationship of daily dose to efficacy. J Clin Psychiatry 56:202–210, 1995

Charney DS, Woods SW, Goodman WK, et al: Drug treatment of panic disorder: the comparative efficacy of imipramine, alprazolam, and trazodone. J Clin Psychiatry 47:580–586, 1986

Clark DB, Agras WS: The assessment and treatment of performance anxiety in musicians. Am J Psychiatry 148:598–605, 1991

Clomipramine Collaborative Study Group: Clomipramine in the treatment of patients with obsessive-compulsive disorder. Arch Gen Psychiatry 48:730–738, 1991

Coplan JD, Pine DS, Papp LA, et al: An algorithm-oriented treatment approach for panic disorder. Psychiatric Annals 26:192–201, 1996

Cox BJ, Swinson RP, Lee PS: Meta-analysis of anxiety disorder treatment studies (letter). J Clin Psychopharmacol 12:300–301, 1992

Cross-National Collaborative Panic Study, Second Phase Investigators: Drug treatment of panic disorder: comparative efficacy of alprazolam, imipramine, and placebo. Br J Psychiatry 160:191–202, 1992

Davidson J, Walker JI, Kilts C: A pilot study of phenelzine in the treatment of post-traumatic stress disorder. Br J Psychiatry 150:252–255, 1987

Davidson JRT, Ford SM, Smith RD, et al: Long-term treatment of social phobia with clonazepam. J Clin Psychiatry 52 (suppl 11):16–20, 1991

Davidson JR, Dupont RL, Hedges D, et al: Efficacy, safety, and tolerability of venlafaxine extended release and buspirone in outpatients with generalized anxiety disorder. J Clin Psychiatry 60:528–535, 1999

Den Boer JA, Westenberg HG: Serotonin function in panic disorder: a double blind placebo controlled study with fluvoxamine and ritanserin. Psychopharmacology 102:85–94, 1990

Dunner DL, Ishiki D, Avery DH, et al: Effect of alprazolam and diazepam on anxiety and panic attacks in panic disorder: a controlled study. J Clin Psychiatry 47:458–460, 1986

Falcon S, Ryan C, Chamberlain K, et al: Tricyclics: possible treatment for posttraumatic stress disorder. J Clin Psychiatry 46:385–388, 1985

Falloon IR, Lloyd GG, Harpin RE: The treatment of social phobia: real-life rehearsal with non-professional therapists. J Nerv Ment Dis 169:180–184, 1981

Fawcett J, Marcus RN, Anton SF, et al: Response of anxiety and agitation symptoms during nefazodone treatment of major depression. J Clin Psychiatry 56 (suppl 6):37–42, 1995

Feldman TB: Alprazolam in the treatment of posttraumatic stress disorder (letter). J Clin Psychiatry 48:216–217, 1987

Fesler FA: Valproate in combat-related posttraumatic stress disorder. J Clin Psychiatry 52:361–364, 1991

Foa EB, Kozak MJ, Steketee GS, et al: Treatment of depressive and obsessive-compulsive symptoms in OCD by imipramine and behavioral therapy. Br J Clin Psychol 31:279–292, 1992

Frank JB, Kosten TR, Giller EL Jr, et al: A randomized clinical trial of phenelzine and imipramine for posttraumatic stress disorder. Am J Psychiatry 145:1289–1291, 1988

Gelenberg AJ, Lydiard RB, Rudolph RL, et al: Efficacy of venlafaxine extended-release capsules in nondepressed outpatients with generalized anxiety: a 6-month randomized controlled trial. JAMA 283:3082–3088, 2000

Gelernter CS, Uhde TW, Cimbolic P, et al: Cognitive-behavioral and pharmacological treatments for social phobia: a controlled study. Arch Gen Psychiatry 48:938–945, 1991

Geracioti TD Jr: Venlafaxine treatment of panic disorder: a case series. J Clin Psychiatry 56:408–410, 1995

Gitlin MJ: Psychotropic medications and their effects on sexual function: diagnosis, biology, and treatment approaches. J Clin Psychiatry 55:406–413, 1994

Goldberg HL, Finnerty RJ: The comparative efficacy of buspirone and diazepam in the treatment of anxiety. Am J Psychiatry 136:1184–1187, 1979

Goodman WK, McDougle CJ, Price LH: Pharmacotherapy of obsessive compulsive disorder. J Clin Psychiatry 53 (suppl 4):29–37, 1992

Haefely W, Facklam M, Schoch P, et al: Partial agonists of benzodiazepine receptors for the treatment of epilepsy, sleep, and anxiety disorders, in GABAergic Synaptic Transmission. Edited by Biggio G, Concas A, Costa E. New York, Raven, 1992, pp 379–394

Haskell D, Cole JO, Schniebolk S, et al: A survey of diazepam patients. Psychopharmacol Bull 22:434–438, 1986

Helzer JE, Robins LN, McEvoy L: Post-traumatic stress disorder in the general population: findings of the Epidemiological Catchment Area Survey. N Engl J Med 317:1630–1634, 1987

Hewlett WA, Vinogradov S, Agras WS: Clonazepam treatment of obsessions and compulsions. J Clin Psychiatry 51:158–161, 1990

Hoehn-Saric R, McLeod DR, Zimmerli WD: Differential effects of alprazolam and imipramine in generalized anxiety disorder: somatic versus psychiatric symptoms. J Clin Psychiatry 49:293–301, 1988

Hofmann SG, Newman ME, Becker E, et al: Social phobia with and without avoidant personality disorder: preliminary behavior therapy outcome findings. J Anxiety Disord 9:1–13, 1995

Hogben GL, Cornfield RB: Treatment of traumatic war neurosis with phenelzine. Arch Gen Psychiatry 38:440–445, 1981

International Multicenter Clinical Trial Group on Moclobemide in Social Phobia: Moclobemide in social phobia—a double-blind, placebo-controlled clinical study. Eur Arch Psychiatry Clin Neurosci 247:71–80, 1997

Jefferson JW, Greist JH: The pharmacotherapy of obsessive-compulsive disorder. Psychiatric Annals 26:202–209, 1996

Kahn RJ, McNair DM, Lipman RS, et al: Imipramine and chlordiazepoxide in depression and anxiety disorders, II: efficacy in anxious outpatients. Arch Gen Psychiatry 43:79–95 , 1986

Kauffman CD, Reist C, Djenderedijan A, et al: Biological markers of affective disorders and posttraumatic stress disorder: a pilot study with desipramine. J Clin Psychiatry 48:366–367, 1987

Keck PE Jr, McElroy SL, Tugrul KC, et al: Antiepileptic drugs for the treatment of panic disorder. Neuropsychobiology 27:150–153, 1993

Kinzie JD, Leung P: Clonidine in Cambodian patients with posttraumatic stress disorder. J Nerv Ment Dis 177:546–550, 1989

Kitchner I, Greenstein R: Low dose lithium carbonate in the treatment of posttraumatic stress disorder: brief communication. Mil Med 150:378–381, 1985

Klein DF, Fink M: Psychiatric reaction patterns to imipramine. Am J Psychiatry 119:4324–4338, 1962

Klein E, Colin V, Stolk J, et al: Alprazolam withdrawal in patients with panic disorder and generalized anxiety disorder: vulnerability and effect of carbamazepine. Am J Psychiatry 151:1760–1766, 1994

Kupfer DJ, Frank E, Perel JM, et al: Five-year outcome for maintenance therapies in recurrent depression. Arch Gen Psychiatry 49:769–773, 1992

Lennane KJ: Treatment of benzodiazepine dependence. Med J Aust 144:594–597, 1986

Lidren DM, Watkins PL, Gould RA, et al: A comparison of bibliotherapy and group therapy in the treatment of panic disorder. J Consult Clin Psychol 62:865–869, 1994

Liebowitz MR, Gorman JM, Fyer AJ, et al: Social phobia: review of a neglected anxiety disorder. Arch Gen Psychiatry 42:729–736, 1985

Liebowitz MR, Gorman JM, Fyer AJ, et al: Pharmacotherapy of social phobia: an interim report of a placebo-controlled comparisons of phenelzine and atenolol. J Clin Psychiatry 49:252–257, 1988

Liebowitz MR, Schneier FR, Hollander E, et al: Treatment of social phobia with drugs other than benzodiazepines. J Clin Psychiatry 52 (suppl 11):10–15, 1991

Liebowitz MR, Schneier F, Campeas R, et al: Phenelzine vs. atenolol in social phobia: a placebo-controlled comparison. Arch Gen Psychiatry 49:290–300, 1992

Lipper S, Davidson JR, Grady TA, et al: Preliminary study of carbamazepine in post-traumatic stress disorder. Psychosomatics 27:849–854, 1986

Lydiard RB, Laraia MT, Howell EF, et al: Alprazolam in the treatment of social phobia. J Clin Psychiatry 49:17–19, 1988

Lydiard RB, Lesser IM, Ballenger JC, et al: A fixed-dose study of alprazolam 2 mg, alprazolam 6 mg, and placebo in panic disorder. J Clin Psychopharmacol 12:96–103, 1992

Marshall RD, Schneier FR: An algorithm for the pharmacotherapy for social phobia. Psychiatric Annals 26:210–216, 1996

Marshall RD, Stein DJ, Liebowitz MR, et al: A pharmacotherapy algorithm in the treatment of posttraumatic stress disorder. Psychiatric Annals 26:217–226, 1996

Mavissakalian MR, Perel JM: Imipramine treatment of panic disorder with agoraphobia: dose ranging and plasma level-response relationships. Am J Psychiatry 152:673–682, 1995

McLeod DR, Hoehn-Saric R, Zimmerli WD, et al: Treatment effects of alprazolam and imipramine: physiological versus subjective changes in patients with generalized anxiety disorder. Biol Psychiatry 28:849–861, 1990

Miller JJ, Fletcher K, Kabat-Zinn J: Three-year follow-up and clinical implications of a mindfulness meditation-based stress reduction intervention in the treatment of anxiety disorders. Gen Hosp Psychiatry 17:192–200, 1995

Modigh K, Westberg P, Erickson E: Superiority of clomipramine over imipramine in the treatment of panic disorder: a placebo-controlled trial. J Clin Psychopharmacol 12:251–261, 1992

Myers JK, Weissman MM, Tischler GL, et al: Six-month prevalence of psychiatric disorders in three communities: 1980–1982. Arch Gen Psychiatry 41:959–967, 1984

Napoliello MJ: An interim multicentre report on 7,677 anxious geriatric out-patients treated with buspirone. British Journal of Clinical Practice 40:71–73, 1986

Newman MG, Kenardy J, Herman S, et al: Comparison of palmtop-computer-assisted brief cognitive-behavioral treatment to cognitive-behavioral treatment for panic disorder. J Consult Clin Psychol 65:178–183, 1997

Nierenberg AA, Cole JO, Glass L: Possible trazodone potentiation of fluoxetine: a case series. J Clin Psychiatry 53:83–85, 1992

Noyes R Jr, Perry PJ, Crowe R, et al: Seizures following the withdrawal of alprazolam. J Nerv Ment Dis 174:50–52, 1986

Noyes R, Moroz G, Davidson JRT, et al: Moclobemide in social phobia: a controlled dose-response trial. J Clin Psychopharmacol 17:247–254, 1997

Oehrberg S, Christiansen PE, Behnke K, et al: Paroxetine in the treatment of panic disorder: a randomised, double-blind, placebo-controlled study. Br J Psychiatry 167:374–379, 1995

Ost LG: Applied relaxation vs progressive relaxation in the treatment of panic disorder. Behav Res Ther 26:13–22, 1988

O'Sullivan G, Noshirvani H, Marks I, et al: Six-year follow-up after exposure and clomipramine therapy for obsessive compulsive disorder. J Clin Psychiatry 52:150–155, 1991

Owen RT, Tyrer P: Benzodiazepine dependence: a review of the evidence. Drugs 25:385–398, 1983

Pande AC, Davidson JRT, Jefferson JW, et al: Treatment of social phobia with gabapentin: a placebo-controlled study. J Clin Psychopharmacol 19:341–348, 1999

Pato MT, Zohar-Kadouch R, Zohar J, et al: Return of symptoms after discontinuation of clomipramine in patients with obsessive-compulsive disorder. Am J Psychiatry 145:1521–1525, 1988

Patterson JF: Withdrawal from alprazolam dependency using clonazepam: clinical observations. J Clin Psychiatry 51 (suppl):47–49, 1990

Pecknold JC, Swinson RP, Krich K, et al: Alprazolam in panic disorder and agoraphobia: results from a multicenter trial, III: discontinuation effects. Arch Gen Psychiatry 45:429–436, 1988

Pecknold JC, Luthe L, Iny L, et al: Fluoxetine in panic disorder: pharmacologic and tritiated platelet imipramine and paroxetine binding study. J Psychiatry Neurosci 20:193–198, 1995

Pigott TA, L'Heureux F, Rubenstein CS, et al: A double-blind, placebo controlled study of trazodone in patients with obsessive-compulsive disorder. J Clin Psychopharmacol 12:156–162, 1992

Price JS, Waller PC, Wood SM, et al: A comparison of the post-marketing safety of four selective serotonin re-uptake inhibitors including the investigation of symptoms occurring on withdrawal. Br J Clin Pharmacol 42:757–763, 1996

Reiter SR, Pollack MH, Rosenbaum JF, et al: Clonazepam for the treatment of social phobia. J Clin Psychiatry 51:470–472, 1990

Rickels K: Buspirone in clinical practice. J Clin Psychiatry 51 (suppl):51–54, 1990

Rickels K, Weisman K, Norstad N, et al: Buspirone and diazepam in anxiety: a controlled study. J Clin Psychiatry 43:81–86, 1982

Rickels K, Schweizer E, Case WG, et al: Long-term therapeutic use of benzodiazepines, I: effects of abrupt discontinuation. Arch Gen Psychiatry 47:899–907, 1990

Rickels K, Pollack MH, Sheehan DV, et al: Efficacy of extended-release venlafaxine in nondepressed outpatients with generalized anxiety disorder. Am J Psychiatry 157:968–974, 2000

Robins LN, Helzer JE, Weissman MM, et al: Lifetime prevalence of specific psychiatric disorders in three sites. Arch Gen Psychiatry 412:958–967, 1984

Schatzberg AF, Cole JO, DeBattista C: Manual of Clinical Psychopharmacology, 3rd Edition. Washington, DC, American Psychiatric Press, 1997, p 258

Schweizer E, Pohl R, Balon R, et al: Lorazepam vs. alprazolam in the treatment of panic disorder. Pharmacopsychiatry 23:90–93, 1990

Shear MK, Pilkonis PA, Cloitre M, et al: Cognitive behavioral treatment compared with nonprescriptive treatment of panic disorder. Arch Gen Psychiatry 51:395–401, 1994

Sheehan DV, Raj AB, Sheehan KH, et al: Is buspirone effective for panic disorder? J Clin Psychopharmacol 10:3–11, 1990

Shen WW, Park S: The use of monoamine oxidase inhibitors in the treatment of traumatic war neurosis: case report. Mil Med 148:430–431, 1983

Silver JM, Sandberg DP, Hales RE: New approaches in the pharmacotherapy of post-traumatic stress disorder. J Clin Psychiatry 51 (suppl 10):33–38, 1990

Spealman RD: Disruption of schedule-controlled behavior by Ro 15-1788 one day after acute treatment with benzodiazepines. Psychopharmacology 88:398–400, 1986

Swinson RP, Fergus KD, Cox BJ, et al: Efficacy of telephone-administered behavioral therapy for panic disorder with agoraphobia. Behav Res Ther 33:465–469, 1995

Taylor CB: Relaxation training and related techniques, in Behavior Modification: Principles and Clinical Applications. Edited by Agras WS. Boston, MA, Little, Brown, 1978, pp 134–162

Taylor CB, Arnow B: The Nature and Treatment of Anxiety Disorders. New York, Free Press, 1988

Tesar GE, Rosenbaum JF, Pollack MH, et al: Double-blind, placebo-controlled comparison of clonazepam and alprazolam for panic disorder. J Clin Psychiatry 52:69–76, 1991

Thompson PM: Generalized anxiety disorder treatment algorithm. Psychiatric Annals 26:227–232, 1996

Tiffon L, Coplan JD, Papp LA, et al: Augmentation strategies with tricyclic or fluoxetine treatment in seven partially responsive panic disorder patients. J Clin Psychiatry 55:66–69, 1994

Udelman HD, Udelman DL: Concurrent use of buspirone in anxious patients during withdrawal from alprazolam therapy. J Clin Psychiatry 51 (suppl):46–50, 1990

Uhde TW, Tancer ME, Black B, et al: Phenomenology and neurobiology of social phobia: comparison with panic disorder. J Clin Psychiatry 52 (suppl 11):31–40, 1991

van der Kolk BA, Dreyfuss D, Michaels M, et al: Fluoxetine in posttraumatic stress disorder. J Clin Psychiatry 55:517–522, 1994

Versiani M, Nardi AE, Mundim FD, et al: Pharmacotherapy of social phobia: a controlled study with moclobemide and phenelzine. Br J Psychiatry 161:353–360, 1992

Weissman MM, Myers JK, Harding PS: Psychiatric disorders in a U.S. urban community. Am J Psychiatry 135:459–462, 1978

Welkowitz LA, Papp LA, Cloitre M, et al: Cognitive-behavior therapy for panic disorder delivered by psychopharmacologically oriented clinicians. J Nerv Ment Dis 179:473–477, 1991

Wheadon DE: Placebo controlled multi-center trial of fluoxetine in OCD. Paper presented at the 5th World Congress of Biological Psychiatry, Florence, Italy, June 12, 1991

Wheatley D: Buspirone: multicenter efficacy study. J Clin Psychiatry 43:92–94, 1982

Wincor MZ, Munjack DJ, Palmer R: Alprazolam levels and response in panic disorder: preliminary results. J Clin Psychopharmacol 11:48–51, 1991

Wingerson D, Nguyen C, Roy-Byrne PP: Clomipramine treatment for generalized anxiety disorder (letter). J Clin Psychopharmacol 12:214–215, 1992

Wolf ME, Alavi A, Mosnaim AD: Posttraumatic stress disorder in Vietnam veterans: clinical and EEG findings; possible therapeutic effects of carbamazepine. Biol Psychiatry 23:642–644, 1988

Zajecka J, Tracy KA, Mitchell S: Discontinuation symptoms after treatment with serotonin reuptake inhibitors: a literature review. J Clin Psychiatry 58:291–297, 1997

Zinbarg RT, Barlow DH, Brown JA, et al: Cognitive-behavioral approaches to the nature and treatment of anxiety disorders. Annu Rev Psychol 43:235–267, 1992

TWENTY-ONE

Treatment of Noncognitive Symptoms in Alzheimer's Disease and Other Dementias

Murray A. Raskind, M.D., and
Elaine R. Peskind, M.D.

Alzheimer's disease (AD) afflicts at least 4 million people in the United States (St. George-Hyslop 2000). The primary symptoms of AD are acquired impairment of memory and other intellectual functions. Noncognitive problems also are highly prevalent in AD and in other late-life disorders causing dementia (Ballard et al. 1995; Wragg and Jeste 1989) and are the most common precipitants of institutional placement (O'Donnell et al. 1992). The most troublesome are psychotic and disruptive agitated behaviors, such as physical and verbal aggression, uncooperativeness with activities necessary for personal hygiene and safety, wandering, delusions and hallucinations, and motoric hyperactivity.

In this chapter, we review the psychopharmacological management of these behaviors in AD and other disorders causing dementia. We also review the management of depression complicating dementia.

PREVALENCE OF PSYCHOTROPIC DRUG USE IN DISORDERS CAUSING DEMENTIA

Most patients with AD who manifest disruptive behaviors are given psychotropic medication as a part of their treatment regimens (Salzman 1987). Rovner and colleagues (1986) documented noncognitive behavioral problems in the majority of patients (*n* = 38) from a random sample of 50 residents of a proprietary nursing home. Among the 40% (*n* = 20) of patients with five or more behavioral problems, the most frequently reported were disruptiveness, restlessness, noisiness, and aggressive behaviors.

Beers et al. (1988) reviewed psychotropic medication use in intermediate-care-facility residents in Massachusetts and found that 50% of all elderly residents were receiving a psychotropic medication, 26% were receiving antipsychotic medication, and 28% were receiving sedative-hypnotics (primarily benzodiaze-pines and sedating antihistamines).

Buck (1988) examined the administration of psychotropic medications to Medicaid recipi-ents residing continuously in nursing homes in Illinois. Of these residents, 60% received at least one psychotropic medication during the year. Avorn and colleagues (1989) surveyed a random sample of 55 nursing homes in Massachusetts and found that more than 50% of the residents were taking at least one psychoactive medi-cation.

PSYCHOPHARMACOLOGICAL MANAGEMENT OF DISRUPTIVE AGITATED BEHAVIORS

Antipsychotic Drugs

General clinical issues.   The rationale for the use of antipsychotic drugs is partially based on phenomenological similarities of some dis-ruptive behaviors in patients with dementia to signs and symptoms of schizophrenia in nonelderly patients. For example, delusions and hallucinations are common in AD (Cummings et al. 1987; Wragg and Jeste 1989). It should be emphasized that psychotic behaviors in AD are often qualitatively different from those that complicate schizophrenia.

In AD and in other disorders causing de-mentia, the most common delusions are rela-tively unelaborated paranoid beliefs, such as that money or property has been stolen. System-atized complex delusions with bizarre content and grandiose delusions are uncommon. Often, the delusions accompanying AD appear to be related to underlying memory deficits. Al-though these beliefs meet formal criteria for delusions, they are in some ways unlike the delu-sions of schizophrenia for which the anti-psychotic drugs have proved so effective. These phenomenological differences may explain why antipsychotic drugs are less effective in AD than in schizophrenia (Schneider et al. 1990).

Nonpsychotic disruptive behaviors, such as motor restlessness, aggressive verbal and physi-cal outbursts, persistent pacing, and unco-operativeness, also may occur in the absence of delusions and/or hallucinations. Patients with AD who have disruptive agitated behaviors but no discernible psychosis often have been in-cluded in antipsychotic drug outcome trials. Inclusion of such agitated but not psychotic patients with AD in treatment trials of anti-psychotic drugs may have contributed to the rel-atively small magnitude of reported anti-psychotic efficacy in patients with AD (see the next subsection).

Because the adverse effects of antipsychotic drugs, particularly extrapyramidal effects, can be very troubling for elderly patients with de-mentia (Devanand et al. 1989), the clinician should carefully weigh risks and benefits before prescribing antipsychotic drugs for delusions and hallucinations that are not bothersome ei-ther to the patient or to caregivers. In these in-stances, the potential adverse effects of anti-psychotic medications, such as extrapyramidal rigidity and excessive sedation, may complicate management more than they improve the pa-tient's quality of life. On the other hand, several studies have reported that psychotic symptoms in AD are associated with more rapid cognitive deterioration (Drevets and Rubin 1989; Jeste et al. 1992; Lopez et al. 1991; Y. Stern et al. 1987). Long-term studies are needed to clarify whether pharmacological control of psychotic symp-toms would modify disease progression.

Outcome trials.   Relatively few placebo-controlled studies have provided interpretable data. Furthermore, many of the studies com-pleted before publication of DSM-III (Ameri-can Psychiatric Association 1980) used some-what confusing diagnostic nomenclature and occasionally used the term *psychotic* to connote severe dementia rather than the presence of de-lusions and/or hallucinations.

In one of these early studies, chlor-promazine was compared with placebo in a double-blind crossover design (Seager 1955). Global ratings of disturbed behaviors favored chlorpromazine over placebo, but sedation and falls were more common in the chlorpromazine group. Acetophenazine was superior to placebo for assaultiveness, nocturnal wandering, irritability, hyperexcitability, and abnormal fear (L. D. Hamilton and Bennett 1962a). Excessive sedation was a major adverse effect of acetophenazine. Significant differences favoring haloperidol compared with placebo were noted in ratings of hallucinations, restlessness, and uncooperativeness (Sugerman et al. 1964). In the haloperidol group, a substantial number of subjects developed unsteady gait and/or pseudoparkinsonian signs. In this study, the patients who were most severely agitated prior to randomization had the best response to haloperidol.

Other studies completed before DSM-III was published did not report an advantage for antipsychotic medications compared with placebo. A common feature of these studies was the absence of target signs and symptoms (e.g., hallucinations, delusions, severe agitation, and severe hyperactivity) that responded better to antipsychotic medication than to placebo in the three studies described above. Trifluoperazine was compared with placebo in patients with the target symptoms of apathy, withdrawal, and cognitive and behavioral deterioration (e.g., incontinence, loss of ambulation, and severe disorientation) (L. D. Hamilton and Bennett 1962b). Trifluoperazine was no more effective than placebo in this study and induced troublesome sedation and parkinsonian signs.

Thiothixene was compared with placebo in a study of patients with dementia in whom the target symptoms were primarily cognitive deficits (Rada and Kellner 1976). Global improvement was noted equally in the thiothixene and placebo groups. The placebo response in this study has also been found in more recent placebo-controlled trials of antipsychotic medications (see later in this section).

Several studies have been conducted since the publication of DSM-III and DSM-III-R (American Psychiatric Association 1987). Patients with chronic schizophrenia beginning in early life were excluded from the samples. In addition, these studies required that either psychotic symptoms (i.e., delusions and hallucinations) or disruptive nonpsychotic behaviors be present as target symptoms.

Two studies have been carried out in very elderly typical community nursing home patients (mean age > 80 years). Barnes et al. (1982) randomized 60 patients (mean age 83 years) whose symptoms met criteria for either AD or multi-infarct dementia and who had psychotic or nonpsychotic disruptive behaviors to receive either thioridazine, loxapine, or placebo. Ratings of excitement and uncooperativeness on the Brief Psychiatric Rating Scale (Overall and Gorham 1962) had significantly greater improvement with either active drug than with placebo. However, suspiciousness and hostility decreased both with active drug and with placebo. Global improvement was greater for active drug than for placebo, but only one-third of the patients taking active medication were rated as either moderately or markedly improved. Finkel et al. (1995) randomized 33 nursing home residents (mean age 85 years) with agitated behavior to thiothixene or placebo. Behavioral improvement as quantified by the Cohen-Mansfield Agitation Inventory (Cohen-Mansfield 1986) significantly favored thiothixene, but the magnitude of difference between active drug and placebo was modest. Psychotic signs and symptoms per se were not identified or quantified in this study. These two studies suggest real but limited efficacy for antipsychotic drugs in typical nursing home populations of behaviorally disturbed and very old patients with dementia.

In a younger (mean age 73 years) state psychiatric hospital sample of behaviorally disturbed patients with AD and multi-infarct dementia, haloperidol or loxapine was significantly more effective than placebo for suspiciousness, hallucinatory behavior, excitement, hostility, and uncooperativeness (Petrie et al.

1982). Thirty-two percent of loxapine patients and 35% of haloperidol patients were moderately or markedly improved compared with 9% of placebo patients.

Devanand and colleagues (1998) completed a random assignment, parallel-group, double-blind, placebo-controlled study in which "standard"-dose haloperidol (2–3 mg/day), low-dose haloperidol (0.5–0.75 mg/day), and placebo were compared in a 6-week trial with a subsequent crossover phase. Haloperidol at 2–3 mg/day showed moderate efficacy and was significantly superior to low-dose haloperidol and placebo, which did not differ from each other in measures of both efficacy and side effects. These findings suggest that doses of haloperidol below 1 mg/day are often subtherapeutic.

There is now considerable experience in using atypical antipsychotic agents in the treatment of noncognitive symptoms of Alzheimer's disease. The available data suggest efficacy of risperidone, quetiapine, and olanzapine.

The Lewy body variant of AD presents clinically with extrapyramidal rigidity, fluctuating cognitive impairment, and an increased incidence of psychotic symptoms as compared with typical AD (Byrne et al. 1991). In addition to the diffuse neuritic plaques characteristic of AD, this variant shows subcortical, limbic, and neocortical Lewy bodies (Perry et al. 1990) at postmortem examination. Patients with the Lewy body variant of AD appear particularly susceptible to extrapyramidal adverse effects of typical antipsychotic drugs (McKeith et al. 1992). Anecdotal reports suggest that the atypical antipsychotic drug risperidone potentially may reduce psychotic symptoms with fewer parkinsonian adverse effects than those of typical antipsychotics (e.g., haloperidol) in Lewy body variant AD (Allen et al. 1995; Lee et al. 1994).

The important question of long-term antipsychotic drug maintenance was addressed by an antipsychotic drug discontinuation study in patients with dementia whose disturbed behaviors appeared to decline with antipsychotic medication and who had then been given chronic antipsychotic maintenance therapy. Risse et al. (1987) substituted placebo for maintenance antipsychotic medication in nine male patients with dementia. At the end of the 6-week substitution period, two were rated as more agitated, two were unchanged, and five actually were rated as less agitated. These results suggest the need for further study of antipsychotic medication discontinuation trials in behaviorally stable patients with dementia who appear to have benefited from past antipsychotic treatment. Such discontinuation trials also are consistent with federal policies as stipulated in the Omnibus Budget Reconciliation Act (OBRA) of 1987 (Kelly 1989).

Drugs With Pharmacological Effects on Serotonin Systems

The loss of serotonergic neurons in the brain stem raphe nuclei and decreased concentrations of the serotonin metabolite 5-hydroxyindoleacetic acid (5-HIAA) in postmortem brain tissue and in cerebrospinal fluid (Blenow et al. 1991; Zweig et al. 1988) indicate a serotonergic deficiency in AD. The efficacy of serotonergic drugs, such as trazodone, buspirone, and selective serotonin uptake inhibitors (SSRIs), for treatment of disruptive agitated behaviors in AD is suggested by anecdotal reports (Colenda 1988; Pinner and Rich 1988; Sakauye et al. 1993; Simpson and Foster 1986; Tiller et al. 1988) and a few placebo-controlled studies.

In a double-blind, placebo-controlled crossover study, Lawlor et al. (1994) treated 10 patients with AD and behavioral complications (troublesome agitation, depression, psychosis, or anxiety) with trazodone (up to 150 mg/day), buspirone (30 mg/day), and placebo. Trazodone produced a small but significant behavioral improvement compared with placebo, whereas buspirone had no apparent effect. Levy (1994) used buspirone to treat 20 patients with AD and behavioral disturbances rated as at least moderately troublesome on the Behavioral Pathology in Alzheimer's Disease Rating Scale (BEHAVE-AD) (Reisberg et al. 1987; see also Reisberg et al. 1996) in a single-blind dose-escalation study. After a 2- to 4-week psychotropic drug washout period, subjects were given placebo for 1 week and then progressively increasing weekly doses (15, 30, 45, and 60 mg) of buspirone. At least one dose of buspirone was significantly more effective than placebo for global behavioral score, aggression, and anxiety.

Because trazodone and buspirone have relatively low toxicity, both drugs merit further investigation in parallel-group studies that encourage titration to relatively high dosage levels.

Lebert et al. (1994) conducted an open 8-week pilot study of fluoxetine (20 mg/day) in 10 patients with AD. Ratings of emotional lability, irritability, anxiety, and fear-panic were significantly improved following fluoxetine treatment. Surprisingly, the rating of "reduced mood" was unaffected by fluoxetine. Positive effects of the SSRI citalopram as compared with placebo on both anxiety and affective symptoms in patients with dementia also have been reported (Nyth and Gottfries 1990). The efficacy of citalopram in depression complicating AD is discussed later in this chapter (see section, "Depression Complicating AD and Other Disorders Causing Dementia").

Antimanic Drugs

The effectiveness of carbamazepine for the hyperactivity, aggressive behaviors, and temper outbursts seen in patients in the manic phase of bipolar disorder has prompted open trials of these drugs for treatment of disruptive agitated behaviors in patients with AD or other disorders causing dementia (Chambers et al. 1982; Gleason and Schneider 1990; Marin and Greenwald 1989). The most convincing data supporting carbamazepine efficacy were reported by Tariot et al. (1994). In a non-

randomized, placebo-controlled pilot study, they reported decreased agitation with minimal adverse effects in 25 nursing home patients with dementia.

The anticonvulsant and antimanic drug sodium valproate was evaluated in an open-label study of 4 patients who had AD complicated by disruptive agitated behaviors but who did not have clear psychotic signs or symptoms (Mellow et al. 1993). Substantial behavioral improvement was observed in 2 of the 4 patients, and no adverse effects were noted. Additional controlled studies are under way with valproate.

Benzodiazepines

The use of benzodiazepines in patients with dementia and disturbed behaviors was reviewed by R. G. Stern and colleagues (1991). Several placebo-controlled studies of benzodiazepines were completed in the 1960s and 1970s. Although specific subject diagnoses are difficult to determine, these studies probably included mostly patients with AD and other disorders causing dementia.

Sanders (1965) compared oxazepam with placebo in elderly (mean age 81) "emotionally disturbed" patients. Although oxazepam was superior to placebo after 6 weeks of treatment, no difference was found between the placebo-treated and oxazepam-treated patients at the end of the 8-week treatment period. Agitation and anxiety had the most favorable response to active treatment. These data suggest that tolerance to the benzodiazepine may have developed by the end of the treatment protocol.

Thioridazine and diazepam were compared in a non-placebo-controlled study of the control of behavioral symptoms associated with "senility" (Kirven and Montero 1973). Although both drugs were associated with symptomatic reduction, the trend was in favor of thioridazine. As with the Sanders (1965) study, the data suggested that tolerance may have developed to the benzodiazepine by the end of the treatment protocol. In both of these studies, psychotic symptoms, such as delusions and/or hallucinations, were not specifically rated.

In another study (Coccaro et al. 1990), the efficacy of an antipsychotic drug (haloperidol), a benzodiazepine (oxazepam), and a sedating antihistamine (diphenhydramine) were compared for the treatment of agitated behaviors in a group of elderly institutionalized patients, most of whom met criteria for AD. These behaviors decreased in all treatment groups over the 8-week period, but there was no differential response to the three psychotropic drugs. This study does not provide evidence favoring benzodiazepines for the treatment of behaviorally disturbed patients with dementia, given that oxazepam appeared to be even less effective than the other two drugs.

Cholinesterase Inhibitors

Cholinesterase inhibitor therapy was conceptualized as a specific therapy for the cognitive deficits presumably secondary to the presynaptic cholinergic lesion of AD (Whitehouse et al. 1982). Uncontrolled studies suggest possible efficacy of cholinesterase inhibitors for noncognitive symptoms, such as apathy, agitation, and delusions (Cummings and Kaufer 1996). In the 30-week pivotal study establishing the efficacy of tacrine for memory and other cognitive deficits of AD (Knapp et al. 1994), effects of tacrine on noncognitive symptoms as quantified by the noncognitive subscale of the Alzheimer's Disease Assessment Scale (Rosen et al. 1984) were evaluated in an exploratory analysis (Raskind et al. 1997). Subjects with AD randomized to receive tacrine (160 mg/day—the recommended target dose) more frequently showed improvement or stabilization of pacing, delusions, and poor cooperation than did subjects with AD randomized to receive placebo. These data suggest that the cholinergic deficiency of AD may contribute to at least some noncognitive behavioral disturbances in this disorder. Data on this issue will shortly be available for the two new cholinesterase inhibitors

now FDA approved for the treatment of Alzheimer's disease.

PRACTICAL MANAGEMENT OF DISRUPTIVE BEHAVIORS IN AD AND OTHER DISORDERS CAUSING DEMENTIA

Antipsychotic drugs should still be the first agents tried for the management of disruptive behaviors in dementia. Before antipsychotic medications are instituted, the clinician must evaluate the general medical condition of the patient to rule out a medical etiology for disruptive behaviors (e.g., pain, thyrotoxicosis) or an adverse effect of a nonpsychotropic medication (e.g., theophylline, L-dopa). Environmental and behavioral approaches also should be instituted when possible. For example, the pacing behavior of patients in the middle stages of AD is best treated by providing a secure environment in which patients can get up and walk around at any time of the day or night. Pacing not clearly attributable to delusions or hallucinations appears unresponsive to psychotropic medication, and akathisia from antipsychotic medications may exacerbate pacing. Collaboration with a clinical psychologist or other mental health professional knowledgeable in behavioral techniques can prove rewarding (Teri et al. 1992).

The choice of a particular antipsychotic drug should be based on the tolerability of the adverse effects of a given agent by the patient to whom it will be prescribed. Haloperidol and other high-potency drugs are more likely to produce parkinsonian signs and symptoms than are low-potency antipsychotic drugs such as thioridazine. However, thioridazine and other low-potency drugs are more likely to produce anticholinergic adverse effects (e.g., urinary retention, constipation, dry mouth, blurred vision, central anticholinergic delirium), orthostatic hypotension, and excess sedation than are high-potency antipsychotic drugs such as haloperidol. The newer atypical antipsychotic drugs have a low propensity to produce either extrapyramidal or anticholinergic adverse effects and therefore must be considered first-line agents instead of typical antipsychotics.

Antipsychotic drugs should be started at a low but constantly prescribed dose. The dose should be increased gradually, perhaps every week, if the desired therapeutic effect has not been achieved and adverse effects are either not present or well tolerated. Dividing the total dose into a two- or three-times-a-day regimen may avoid excessive peak plasma drug concentrations that could increase acute adverse effects. Divided dosing does, however, increase demands on caregivers and nursing personnel.

As should be apparent from this review of clinical outcome trials of psychotropic drugs other than antipsychotics for disruptive behaviors in AD and other disorders causing dementia, no well-established guidelines are available for selecting a psychotropic medication for patients in whom antipsychotic drugs are either ineffective or poorly tolerated. Buspirone has the advantage of a relatively benign adverse-effect profile. Trazodone may also be effective, but orthostatic hypotension or excessive sedation may complicate the use of trazodone in some patients. Violent behavior may respond to carbamazepine or valproate. These drugs are reasonably well tolerated, though sedation and ataxia may occur. Short-half-life benzodiazepines may be useful if subjective anxiety is prominent or can be reasonably inferred from the patient's behavioral problems. However, benzodiazepines have a high incidence of ataxia and excessive sedation and can impair cognitive function in elderly patients (Sunderland et al. 1989). Furthermore, tolerance to the therapeutic antianxiety or antiagitation effects of the benzodiazepines may occur. It also appears likely that cholinesterase inhibitors prescribed as cognitive enhancers will have positive effects on noncognitive behavioral problems in some patients with AD.

DEPRESSION COMPLICATING AD AND OTHER DISORDERS CAUSING DEMENTIA

Because depression per se can impair cognitive function (Cohen et al. 1982), the recognition and effective treatment of depression complicating a disorder causing dementia offer the potential for both improving mood and maximizing the patient's cognitive abilities. Studies have found a high prevalence of depressive signs and symptoms in AD (Reifler et al. 1986; Rovner et al. 1986) that are associated with added functional impairment (Pearson et al. 1989).

Although anecdotal reports suggest that antidepressant drugs are effective in the treatment of depression complicating AD and other disorders causing dementia (Jenike 1985), only a few placebo-controlled studies have been performed. Reifler and colleagues (1989) compared imipramine with placebo in a double-blind study of major depressive episode complicating AD. Patients were still living in the community but were in the middle stages of AD (Mini-Mental State Exam [Folstein et al. 1975] mean score = 17) and had depression of mild to moderate severity (Hamilton Rating Scale for Depression [M. Hamilton 1960] mean score = 19). Patients were given imipramine (mean dose 83 mg/day; mean plasma level of imipramine plus desmethylimipramine 116 ng/mL) or placebo for 8 weeks. Significant reduction in depressive signs and symptoms was documented in both the imipramine and the placebo groups, but the amount of improvement was indistinguishable between groups. AD outpatients with depressive symptoms respond positively to participation in an antidepressant treatment outcome trial. Whether a tricyclic antidepressant specifically ameliorates depressive symptomatology in doses well tolerated in patients with AD has yet to be confirmed.

Interpretation of the Reifler et al. (1989) study is complicated because the emergence of adverse effects limited the amount of imipramine prescribed. A higher dose of imipramine might have been even more effective than the substantial placebo group response.

Tricyclic antidepressants also have been evaluated in a placebo-controlled study of depression (both major depressive episode and dysthymia) complicating stroke (Lipsey et al. 1984). A substantial proportion of the subjects in this study likely had at least mild multi-infarct dementia. In this study (Lipsey et al. 1984), nortriptyline was more effective than placebo for depressive signs and symptoms. The SSRI citalopram was compared with placebo in a small group of patients with dementia (unspecified type) with depressive symptomatology (Nyth et al. 1992). Citalopram was modestly but significantly more effective than placebo and was well tolerated. Sertraline also has been reported to improve depressed affect in advanced AD (Volicer et al. 1994). Similar data are available for paroxetine and fluoxetine. Additional placebo-controlled studies of SSRIs for the treatment of depression complicating AD and other neurodegenerative disorders causing dementia are needed.

CONCLUSION

Further studies are necessary to provide rational guidelines for the psychopharmacological management of noncognitive behavioral problems complicating AD and other disorders causing dementia. Extrapolations from the large body of psychotherapeutic drug outcome studies in younger patients with diseases such as schizophrenia and depression starting in adolescence or middle age often are not relevant to elderly patients with dementia. Careful evaluations of newer antipsychotic agents with reduced extrapyramidal toxicity, such as risperidone, quetiapine, and olanzapine, may improve the applicability of the general class of antipsychotic drugs for behaviorally disturbed patients with dementia. Placebo-controlled outcome studies of drugs such as buspirone and trazodone can establish or refute the hints of efficacy derived from anecdotal reports. The antimanic drugs, particularly carbamazepine and sodium valproate, also deserve evaluations in well-designed clinical trials. The potential positive effects of "cognitive-acting" drugs such as the cholinesterase inhibitors tacrine and donepezil should not be discounted in future outcome trials. Careful attention to accurate phenomenological descriptions of specific types of behavioral problems may help to establish therapeutic specificity of a drug for a given behavioral problem.

REFERENCES

Allen RL, Walker Z, D'Ath PJ, et al: Risperidone for psychotic and behavioural symptoms in Lewy body dementia (letter). Lancet 346:185, 1995

American Psychiatric Association: Diagnostic and Statistical Manual of Mental Disorders, 3rd Edition. Washington, DC, American Psychiatric Association, 1980

American Psychiatric Association: Diagnostic and Statistical Manual of Mental Disorders, 3rd Edition, Revised. Washington, DC, American Psychiatric Association, 1987

Avorn J, Dreyer P, Connelly MA, et al: Use of psychoactive medication and the quality of care in rest homes. N Engl J Med 320:227–232, 1989

Ballard CG, Saad K, Patel A, et al: The prevalence and phenomenology of psychotic symptoms in dementia sufferers. Int J Geriatr Psychiatry 10:477–485, 1995

Barnes R, Veith R, Okimoto J, et al: Efficacy of antipsychotic medications in behaviorally disturbed dementia patients. Am J Psychiatry 139:1170–1174, 1982

Beers M, Avorn J, Soumerai SB, et al: Psychoactive medication use in intermediate-care facility residents. JAMA 260:3016–3020, 1988

Blenow KAJ, Wallin A, Gottfries CG, et al: Significance of decreased lumbar CSF levels of HVA and 5-HIAA in Alzheimer's disease. Neurobiol Aging 13:107–113, 1991

Buck JA: Psychotropic drug practice in nursing homes. J Am Geriatr Soc 36:409–418, 1988

Byrne EJ, Lennox GG, Godwin-Austen RB, et al: Dementia associated with cortical Lewy bodies: proposed clinical diagnostic criteria. Dementia 2:283–284, 1991

Chambers CA, Bain J, Rosbottom R, et al: Carbamazepine in senile dementia and overactivity—a placebo controlled double blind trial. IRCS Journal of Medical Science 10:505–506, 1982

Coccaro EF, Kramer E, Zemishlany Z, et al: Pharmacologic treatment of noncognitive behavioral disturbances in elderly demented patients. Am J Psychiatry 147:1640–1656, 1990

Cohen RM, Weingartner HW, Smallberg A, et al: Effort and cognition in depression. Arch Gen Psychiatry 39:593–597, 1982

Cohen-Mansfield J: Agitated behaviors in the elderly, II: preliminary results in the cognitively deteriorated. J Am Geriatr Soc 34:722–727, 1986

Colenda CC: Buspirone in treatment of agitated demented patient (letter). Lancet 1:1169, 1988

Cummings JL, Kaufer D: Neuropsychiatric aspects of Alzheimer's disease: the cholinergic hypothesis revisited. Neurology 47:876–883, 1996

Cummings JL, Miller B, Hill MA, et al: Neuropsychiatric aspects of multi-infarct dementia and dementia of the Alzheimer type. Arch Neurol 44:389–393, 1987

Devanand DP, Sackheim HA, Brown RP, et al: A pilot study of haloperidol treatment of psychosis and behavioral disturbance in Alzheimer's disease. Arch Neurol 46:854–857, 1989

Devanand DP, Marder K, Michaels KS, et al: A randomized, placebo-controlled dose-comparison trial of haloperidol for psychosis and disruptive behaviors in Alzheimer's disease. Am J Psychiatry 155:1512–1520, 1998

Drevets WC, Rubin E: Psychotic symptoms and the longitudinal course of senile dementia of the Alzheimer type. Biol Psychiatry 25:39–48, 1989

Finkel SI, Lyons JS, Anderson RL, et al: A randomized, placebo-controlled trial of thiothixene in agitated, demented nursing home patients. Int J Geriatr Psychiatry 10:129–136, 1995

Folstein MF, Folstein SE, McHugh PR: Mini-Mental State: a practical method for grading the cognitive state of patients for the clinician. J Psychiatr Res 12:189–198, 1975

Gleason RP, Schneider LS: Carbamazepine treatment of agitation in Alzheimer's outpatients refractory to neuroleptics. J Clin Psychiatry 51:115–118, 1990

Hamilton LD, Bennett JL: Acetophenazine for hyperactive geriatric patients. Geriatrics 17:596–601, 1962a

Hamilton LD, Bennett JL: The use of trifluoperazine in geriatric patients with chronic brain syndrome. J Am Geriatr Soc 10:140–147, 1962b

Hamilton M: A rating scale for depression. J Neurol Neurosurg Psychiatry 23:56–62, 1960

Jenike MA: MAO inhibitors as treatment for depressed patients with primary degenerative dementia (Alzheimer's disease). Am J Psychiatry 142:763–764, 1985

Jeste DV, Wragg RE, Salmon DP, et al: Cognitive deficits with Alzheimer's disease with and without delusions. Am J Psychiatry 149:184–189, 1992

Katzman R: The prevalence and malignancy of Alzheimer's disease: a major killer. Arch Neurol 33:217–218, 1976

Kelly M: The Omnibus Budget Reconciliation Act of 1987: a policy analysis. Nurs Clin North Am 24:791–794, 1989

Kirven LE, Montero EF: Comparison of thioridazine and diazepam in the control of nonpsychotic symptoms associated with senility: double-blind study. J Am Geriatr Soc 21:546–551, 1973

Knapp MJ, Knopman DS, Solomon PR, et al: A 30 week randomized controlled trial of high dose tacrine in patients with Alzheimer's disease. JAMA 271:985–991, 1994

Lawlor BA, Radcliffe J, Molchan SE, et al: A pilot placebo-controlled study of trazodone and buspirone in Alzheimer's disease. Int J Geriatr Psychiatry 9:55–59, 1994

Lebert F, Pasquier F, Petit H: Behavioural effects of fluoxetine in dementia of Alzheimer type (letter). International Journal of Geriatric Society 9:590–591, 1994

Lee H, Cooney JM, Lawlor BA: The use of risperidone, an atypical neuroleptic, in Lewy body disease. Int J Geriatr Psychiatry 9:415–417, 1994

Levy MA: A trial of buspirone for the control of disruptive behaviors in community-dwelling patients with dementia. Int J Geriatr Psychiatry 9:841–848, 1994

Lipsey JR, Pearlson GD, Robinson RG, et al: Nortriptyline treatment of post-stroke depression: a double blind study. Lancet 1:297–300, 1984

Lopez OL, Becker JT, Brenner RP, et al: Alzheimer's disease with delusions and hallucinations: neuropsychological and electroencephalographs correlates. Neurology 41:906–912, 1991

Marin DB, Greenwald BS: Carbamazepine for aggressive agitation in demented patients (letter). Am J Psychiatry 146:805, 1989

McKeith I, Fairbairn A, Perry R, et al: Neuroleptic sensitivity in patients with senile dementia of Lewy body type. BMJ 305:673–678, 1992

Mellow AM, Solano-Lopez C, Davis S: Sodium valproate in the treatment of behavioral disturbance in dementia. J Geriatr Psychiatry Neurol 6:28–32, 1993

Nyth AL, Gottfries CG: The clinical efficacy of citalopram in treatment of emotional disturbances in dementia disorders (a Nordic multicenter study). Br J Psychiatry 157:894–901, 1990

Nyth AL, Gottfries CG, Lyby K, et al: A controlled multicenter clinical study of citalopram and placebo in elderly depressed patients with and without concomitant dementia. Acta Psychiatr Scand 86:138–145, 1992

O'Donnell BF, Drachman DA, Barnes HJ, et al: Incontinence and troublesome behaviors predict institutionalization in dementia. J Geriatr Psychiatry Neurol 5:45–52, 1992

Overall JE, Gorham DR: The Brief Psychiatric Rating Scale. Psychol Rep 10:799–812, 1962

Pearson JL, Teri L, Reifler BV, et al: Functional status and cognitive impairment in Alzheimer's disease patients with and without depression. J Am Geriatr Soc 37:1117–1121, 1989

Perry RH, Irving D, Blessed G, et al: Senile dementia of Lewy body type: a clinically and neuropathologically distinct form of Lewy body dementia in the elderly. J Neurol Sci 95:119–139, 1990

Petrie WM, Ban TA, Berney S, et al: Loxapine in psychogeriatrics: a placebo- and standard-controlled clinical investigation. J Clin Psychopharmacol 2:122–126, 1982

Pinner E, Rich CL: Effects of trazodone on aggressive behavior in seven patients with organic mental disorders. Am J Psychiatry 145:1295–1296, 1988

Rada RT, Kellner R: Thiothixene in the treatment of geriatric patients with chronic organic brain syndrome. J Am Geriatr Soc 24:105–107, 1976

Raskind MA, Sadowsky CH, Sigmund WR, et al: Effect of tacrine on language, praxis and noncognitive behavioral problems in Alzheimer's disease. Arch Neurol 54:836–840, 1997

Reifler BV, Larson E, Teri L, et al: Dementia of Alzheimer's type and depression. J Am Geriatr Soc 34:855–859, 1986

Reifler BV, Teri L, Raskind M, et al: Double-blind trial of imipramine in Alzheimer's disease patients with and without depression. Am J Psychiatry 146:45–49, 1989

Reisberg B, Borenstein J, Salob SP, et al: Behavioural symptoms in Alzheimer's disease: phenomenology and treatment. J Clin Psychiatry 48 (5, suppl):9–15, 1987

Reisberg B, Auer SR, Monteiro IM: Behavioral Pathology in Alzheimer's Disease (BEHAVE-AD) rating scale. Int Psychogeriatr 8 (suppl 3): 301–308, 1996

Risse SC, Cubberly L, Lampe TH, et al: Acute effects of neuroleptic withdrawal in elderly dementia patients. Journal of Geriatric Drug Therapy 2:65–67, 1987

Rosen WG, Mohs RC, Davis KL: A new rating scale for Alzheimer's disease. Am J Psychiatry 141: 1356–1364, 1984

Rovner BW, Kafonek S, Filipp L, et al: Prevalence of mental illness in a community nursing home. Am J Psychiatry 143:1446–1449, 1986

Sakauye KM, Camp CJ, Ford PA: Effects of buspirone on agitation associated with dementia. Am J Geriatr Psychiatry 1:82–84, 1993

Salzman C: Treatment of the elderly agitated patient. J Clin Psychiatry 48 (5, suppl):19–22, 1987

Sanders JF: Evaluation of oxazepam and placebo in emotionally disturbed aged patients. Geriatrics 20:739–746, 1965

Schneider LS, Pollock VE, Lyness SA: A meta-analysis of controlled trials of neuroleptic treatment in dementia. J Am Geriatr Soc 38: 553–563, 1990

Seager CP: Chlorpromazine in treatment of elderly psychotic women. BMJ 1:882–885, 1955

Simpson DM, Foster D: Improvement in organically disturbed behavior with trazodone treatment. J Clin Psychiatry 47:191–193, 1986

Stern RG, Duffelmeyer ME, Zemishlani Z, et al: The use of benzodiazepines in the management of behavioral symptoms in dementia patients. Psychiatr Clin North Am 14:375–384, 1991

Stern Y, Mayeux R, Sano M, et al: Predictions of disease course in patients with probable Alzheimer's disease. Neurology 37:1649–1653, 1987

St. George-Hyslop P: Piecing together Alzheimer's. Sci Am 283:75–83, 2000

Sugerman AA, Williams BH, Adlerstein AM: Haloperidol in the psychiatric disorders of old age. Am J Psychiatry 120:1190–1192, 1964

Sunderland T, Weingartner T, Cohen RM, et al: Low-dose oral lorazepam administration in Alzheimer subjects and age-matched controls. Psychopharmacology (Berl) 99:129–133, 1989

Tariot PN, Erb R, Leibovici A, et al: Carbamazepine treatment of agitation in nursing home patients with dementia: a preliminary study. J Am Geriatr Soc 42:1160–1166, 1994

Teri L, Rabins P, Whitehouse P, et al: Management of behavior disturbance in Alzheimer disease: current knowledge and future directions. Alzheimer Dis Assoc Disord 6:77–88, 1992

Tiller JW, Dakis JA, Shaw JM: Short-term buspirone treatment in disinhibition with dementia (letter). Lancet 2:510, 1988

Volicer L, Rheaume Y, Cyr D: Treatment of depression in advanced Alzheimer's disease using sertraline. J Geriatr Psychiatry Neurol 7: 227–229, 1994

Whitehouse PJ, Price DL, Struble RG, et al: Alzheimer's disease and senile dementia: loss of neurons in the basal forebrain. Science 215: 1237–1239, 1982

Wragg RE, Jeste DV: Overview of depression and psychosis in Alzheimer's disease. Am J Psychiatry 146:577–587, 1989

Zweig RM, Ross CA, Hedreen J, et al: The neuropathology of aminergic nuclei in Alzheimer's disease. Ann Neurol 24:233–242, 1988

TWENTY-TWO

Treatment of Childhood and Adolescent Disorders

Mina K. Dulcan, M.D.,
Joel Bregman, M.D.,
Elizabeth B. Weller, M.D., and
Ronald Weller, M.D.

SPECIAL ISSUES IN THE PSYCHOPHARMACOLOGICAL TREATMENT OF CHILDREN AND ADOLESCENTS

In this chapter, we emphasize the ways in which the practice of psychopharmacology with children and adolescents differs from that with adults. Unless otherwise specified, *children* refers to individuals age 4 years through adolescence. Detailed discussions of specific drugs can be found in Section I of this textbook. For those disorders and their respective treatments that are similar in youths and adults, the reader should also refer to other chapters in this section. This chapter details the treatment of disorders that occur in both adults and children that are not covered in other chapters of this text, such as attention-deficit/hyperactivity disorder (ADHD), Tourette's disorder, mental retardation, and autistic disorder. Whenever possible, DSM-IV (American Psychiatric Association 1994) terminology is used.

A number of texts provide more extensive information on the use of medications in pediatric psychiatry (e.g., Findling and Blumer 1998; Greenhill and Osman 2000; Kutcher 1997; Riddle 1995a, 1995b; Werry and Aman 1999). The clinical aspects of the diagnosis and treatment of developmental psychopathology may be found in Dulcan and Martini (1999).

The clinical practice of pediatric psychopharmacology is impeded by the relative lack of controlled empirical trials. There are numerous examples of medications that appeared to be effective in anecdotal reports, case series, and open trials that were not shown to be more effective than placebo in double-blind studies.

Evaluation

The evaluation of a young person is complicated by the interaction of psychopathology with the child's environment and with developmental processes. An interview with at least one parent or adult caregiver is essential. Information from teachers is desirable in all cases, and indispensable in ADHD. Standardized symptom rating scales supplement the clinical interview regarding the primary diagnosis, possible comorbidity, and baseline levels of target symptoms (Achenbach 1991). A recent medical history and physical examination are necessary, with laboratory follow-up as indicated. A drug screen or pregnancy test may be required. Whenever a student's functioning in school is impaired, psychoeducational testing (including, at a minimum, intelligence quotient [IQ] and academic achievement tests) should be obtained. Additional testing for learning disabilities may be needed.

Treatment Planning

Psychiatric diagnosis, specific target symptoms, and the strengths and weaknesses of the patient, the family, the school, and the community all enter into the choice of intervention strategies. Parents and their child (as clinically and developmentally appropriate) are included in a discussion about the disorder and a review of treatment options, parent and child motivation, available resources, potential risks and benefits of each intervention, and the risks of no treatment. In clinical psychopharmacology, therapeutic contact to form and maintain a treatment alliance is essential. Other interventions may be primary or used together with medications as determined by target symptoms and data on efficacy for the specific diagnosis. These may include parent guidance or training in behavior modification; special assistance at school; and individual, family, and group psychotherapy. For the most seriously impaired children, hospitalization or day treatment may be needed.

Ethical Issues

The careful physician attempts to balance the risks of medication, the risks of the untreated disorder, and the expected benefits of medication relative to other treatments. It is usually prudent to delay the use of a new psychotropic drug in children and young adolescents until substantial clinical experience has been accumu-

lated for its use in adults.

Adults may misinterpret a youngster's response to the environment either as evidence for a need for medication or as improvement because of a medication. Adults may seek to use drugs instead of investigating the family or institutional dynamics that may be provoking and maintaining such behavior and/or implementing more time-consuming, difficult, and expensive therapeutic or behavioral management strategies. Perceived levels of a child's symptoms may be more closely related to the adult's tolerance of the behaviors than to objective data.

Consent for drug treatment of children is a complex issue (Popper 1987) that can be made even more difficult in clinical situations, such as when divorced parents are feuding over the child's treatment. Informed consent is best considered an ongoing process rather than a single event. The legal minimum age for giving informed consent varies from state to state, but "assent" to medication use is considered possible to obtain from a patient older than 7 years (Popper 1987). Formal consent forms (although often required by law or by institutional guidelines) are less useful than a discussion documented in the medical record that includes the topic, parties present, understanding of the disorder and prognosis, therapeutic options with risks and benefits, questions asked, subsequent consent, and the opportunity to ask further questions (Schouten and Duckworth 1993). Published information sheets for parents, youths, and teachers are now available to supplement discussion with the physician regarding specific medications (Dulcan 1999).

The Food and Drug Administration

Once a drug is approved for any indication, the U.S. Food and Drug Administration (FDA) regulates only the company's advertising of the drug, not the prescribing behavior of physicians. In addition, the "administration of an approved drug in a way that is not approved by the FDA is not research and does not call for special consent or review if it is given solely in the patient's interest" (American Academy of Pediatrics 1996, p. 144). Because pharmaceutical companies have had little incentive to undertake the time, expense, and perceived excessive potential liability associated with testing drugs in children, nearly all psychopharmacological agents and indications (and three-fourths of the drugs used in pediatrics as well [American Academy of Pediatrics 1996]) lack pediatric labeling and are "unapproved" or "off-label" for children. As a result, the FDA guidelines as published in the *Physicians' Desk Reference* (PDR) cannot be relied on for appropriate indications, age ranges, or doses for children. Although lack of approval for an age group or a disorder does not imply improper or illegal use, it is prudent to inform the family of these labeling issues, as well as of evidence in the literature for safe and effective use (Appler and McMann 1989). Recent FDA regulations recognizing additional methods (including data from existing nonindustry sponsored trials) to support pediatric labeling claims and the FDA's encouragement of drug manufacturers to establish safety and efficacy and to determine pharmacokinetics and appropriate doses in children may lead to more complete labeling information and to commercial sponsorship of more drug trials in children (Coté et al. 1996). A special section in the *Journal of the American Academy of Child and Adolescent Psychiatry* (May 1999) summarized existing data.

The Meaning of Medication

Emanative effects are the indirect and inadvertent cognitive and social (i.e., nonpharmacological) consequences of prescribing a drug. These can be positive or negative and may influence the child's self-esteem or attributions of the source of problems and their solution or the parent's or teacher's view of the child.

A placebo response may occur, especially in ADHD, Tourette's disorder, depression, overanxious disorder, and autistic disorder. This result is not surprising, given children's suggest-

ibility, the power of adult influence, the "magical thinking" that is normal in young children, and the natural waxing and waning of symptoms. In the clinical situation, the parent, teacher, or child may have such significant positive or negative expectancies about the drug that a single-blind, placebo-drug crossover trial is indicated. Examples of situations that may require such a trial include initiating stimulant medication for ADHD or determining whether a chronically administered drug is still required and effective, is no longer needed, is ineffective, or is even exacerbating the condition (Doherty et al. 1987; Fine and Jewesson 1989; McBride 1988; Ullmann and Sleator 1986; Varley and Trupin 1983).

Measurement of Outcome

The physician should specify target symptoms and obtain affective, behavioral, and physical baseline and posttreatment data. Side effects that are tolerable in adults may be unacceptable in the long-term treatment of children. Children's cognitive limitations in identifying and reporting physical symptoms or changes in mood require a skilled clinician to detect drug-induced changes. Therapeutic and side effects can be assessed by interviews and rating scales for patients, parents, and teachers. (For compendia of scales, see Aman 1999; Klein et al. 1994; Zametkin and Yamada 1999.) Other means of assessment include direct observation by the clinician, physical examination, and, where appropriate, laboratory or psychometric tests to evaluate attention or learning.

Compliance

Faithful adherence to a prescribed regimen requires the cooperation of one or both parents, the child, and often additional caregivers and school personnel. Pediatric medications may be incorrectly used because of parental factors such as lack of perceived need for drug, carelessness, inability to afford medication, misunderstanding of instructions, complex schedules of administration (Briant 1978), and family dynamics. Both developmental and psychopathological factors may impede the patient's cooperation (Firestone 1982). Media attention to alleged inappropriate use of medications (especially Ritalin and Prozac) has made some families and teachers highly resistant to pharmacotherapy. Small group teaching (Knight et al. 1990) or a medication manual (Bastiaens 1992; Bastiaens and Bastiaens 1993) may be useful in educating young patients about their medications and may improve adherence.

Some children cannot or will not swallow pills. Some drugs are available in elixir form or can be dissolved in juice. Problems with this method of administration may include unpleasant taste, incompatibility resulting in precipitation of the medication, and inaccurate dosing (J. L. Geller et al. 1992). If necessary, a behavior modification program may be implemented to shape pill-swallowing behavior (Pelco et al. 1987).

Developmental Toxicology

Developmental toxicology refers to the unique or especially severe side effects resulting from interaction between a drug and a patient's stage or process of physical, cognitive, or emotional development. Interference with a child's learning in school or development of social relationships within the family or with peers can have lasting effects. Behavioral toxicity (negative effects on mood, behavior, or learning) often develops before physical side effects are observed, especially in young children (Campbell et al. 1985).

Metabolism and Kinetics

Dosage may be determined empirically or by extrapolation from adult doses according to weight or age. Unfortunately, dosage studies in children are rare. Few data exist on the parameters that determine pharmacokinetics in chil-

dren (Briant 1978). Young children absorb some drugs more rapidly than adults, leading to higher peak levels (Jatlow 1987). Young children may require divided doses to minimize fluctuations in blood level (particularly for tricyclic antidepressants [TCAs]), although more frequent doses may reduce medication compliance. Age-related factors that may influence distribution include uptake by actively growing tissue and proportional size of organs and tissue masses. In children, drugs such as lithium (which are primarily distributed in body water) have a proportionally larger volume of distribution and, therefore, lower concentration (Jatlow 1987). By age 1 year, glomerular filtration rate and renal tubular mechanisms for secretion reach adult levels. Hepatic enzyme activity develops early, and rate of drug metabolism is related to liver size. Prepubertal children have relatively large livers and may require a larger dose per kilogram of body weight of drugs that are primarily metabolized by the liver (Briant 1978). Near the time of puberty, the rate of hepatic drug transformation often decreases abruptly toward adult levels, and more careful monitoring is required (Jatlow 1987). The pubertal increase in gonadal hormones may be contributory to this slower processing of drugs by the liver (Ryan et al. 1986). Proportion of fat (which serves as a reservoir for lipid-soluble compounds) increases during the first year of life, followed by a gradual loss until (in girls) the pubertal increase (Briant 1978). Children tend to have less protein binding of drugs, when compared with adults, leaving a greater proportion of the drug biologically active.

ATTENTION-DEFICIT/ HYPERACTIVITY DISORDER

Assessment for Treatment

We refer to ADHD in this section, although much of the research discussed here used diagnostic systems other than DSM-IV. DSM-IV delineates three subtypes: predominantly inattentive (roughly corresponding to attention-deficit disorder [ADD] without hyperactivity), predominantly hyperactive-impulsive (found mostly in preschool children), and combined (similar to ADD with hyperactivity). Parent interviews and standardized rating scales (Achenbach 1991; Barkley 1998) are the core of the assessment process. The interview with the child may not confirm or deny the diagnosis of ADHD, but it provides information about alternative or comorbid diagnoses and the child's own view of his or her problems. Some children and most adolescents with ADHD are able to pay attention and maintain behavioral control while in the office setting. Few have insight into their own difficulties or the willingness or ability to report them accurately. Information from the school, including reports of behavior, learning, and attendance, as well as grades and test scores, is essential. Psychoeducational testing is indicated to assess possible low IQ or specific developmental disorders (learning disabilities) that may be masquerading as ADHD or may coexist with ADHD. Achievement testing helps in educational planning. Sensory deficits (e.g., vision or hearing) and medical or social etiologies of poor attention must be ruled out.

Parent and teacher rating scales yield valuable information efficiently (Achenbach 1991; Barkley 1998). Comparison with normative groups by age and sex can help distinguish normal variants in levels of attention, activity, and impulse control from the disorder of ADHD. The broad-spectrum scales can also be used to screen for comorbidity. There are many choices (see Barkley 1998 and Klein et al. 1994 for reviews), but the most commonly used and best normed and validated are the Child Behavior Checklist (Achenbach 1991), the Teacher Report Form of the Child Behavior Checklist (Achenbach 1991; Edelbrock et al. 1984), and the Conners Parent and Teacher Rating Scales (Conners 1969; Goyette et al. 1978).

Selection of Treatment[1]

Although medication is the most powerful and best documented intervention for ADHD, the number and variety of symptoms and the limitations of medication efficacy may require multimodality treatment (MTA Cooperative Group 1999a, 1999b). Optimal clinical management includes regular appointments (every week or two during titration, and then at least monthly except in very mild cases) to assess medication efficacy, side effects, and need for other treatment for specific remaining target symptoms. Education of parents, including techniques of behavior management, is virtually always needed. Specific developmental disorders (learning disabilities) or lags in achievement because of inattention are frequent and may require tutoring or special class placement. Social skills deficits may respond to group therapy. Because raising a child with ADHD exacerbates family discord, family therapy may be essential if medication or behavior modification is to be effective.

Behavior modification addresses symptoms that medication does not, and some parents prefer it to medication treatment. However, most parents find that behavior management training is more difficult to sustain and more costly than pharmacotherapy, and the child's generalization of improvement to new situations is minimal. Targeted behavioral interventions are effective in the short term in improving behavior, social skills, and academic performance but are less useful in reducing inattention, hyperactivity, or impulsivity (Abikoff and Gittelman 1984). Time-limited interventions, whether pharmacological or psychosocial, have limited ability to produce long-lasting behavior change in children with ADHD. These youngsters often require both instruction to remedy deficits in social or academic skills and contingency management to induce them to use the skills (Pelham and Bender 1982).

---

[1] For more detail, see the American Academy of Child and Adolescent Psychiatry practice parameters (1997a).

For many youngsters with ADHD, neither stimulant medication nor behavior therapy alone is sufficient to normalize behavior and academic performance (DuPaul and Rapport 1993). There are nonresponders to each intervention. Neither observed social skills nor peer ratings of popularity typically normalize with stimulant treatment alone (Ullman and Sleator 1985; Whalen et al. 1989). Some short-term studies have found intensive behavior modification and methylphenidate to have additive effects in children who showed partial response to either intervention; in many cases, this approach yielded performance indistinguishable from that of normal peers (Gittelman et al. 1980; Pelham and Bender 1982; Pelham and Murphy 1986; Pelham et al. 1980, 1986). The combination of intensive classroom behavior therapy with a low dose of methylphenidate produces the same efficacy as a high dose of medication alone (Carlson et al. 1992). Practical implications are that the combination may be more expensive and less feasible than medication alone, but it may be especially useful for children who cannot tolerate a higher dose of medication. More generally, it has been very difficult to verify that psychosocial treatments have any additive effect to carefully monitored pharmacotherapy for the core symptoms of ADHD.

The decision to medicate is based on persistent ADHD symptoms that are not due to another treatable cause and that are sufficiently severe to cause functional impairment at school and usually at home and with peers. The child's parents must be willing to monitor medication and to attend appointments. Clinical attention is required to avoid possible lowering of the child's self-esteem and self-efficacy, stigmatization by peers, and dependence by parents and teachers on medication rather than making needed changes in the environment. Patients themselves, parents, and teachers can be instructed that medication enables the youngster to accomplish what he or she wishes to do; it does not "make" him or her do anything. Children and adolescents should be given full credit for im-

provement and helped to take an appropriate amount of responsibility for their difficulties. A useful analogy is the assistance provided by leg braces or eyeglasses.

Whether ADHD in an individual patient will respond to a specific medication is difficult to predict. Neurological soft signs, electroencephalogram (EEG), and neurochemical measures do not appear to be useful predictors of stimulant responsivity (Halperin et al. 1986; Zametkin et al. 1986). Reduced response to stimulants in children with ADHD who have comorbid anxiety is controversial (Tannock et al. 1995).

It has now been amply documented that ADHD symptoms often continue into adulthood, resulting in considerable impairment (Wender 1995). The same drugs used for children continue to be effective, although side-effect profiles may differ in degree.

Stimulants

In most circumstances, a stimulant drug is the first pharmacological choice for a patient with ADHD. Although drug abuse does not result from properly monitored prescribed stimulants, caution may be indicated in the presence of conduct disorder or preexisting chemical dependency. If the risk of drug abuse by the patient or the patient's peers or family is high, a nonstimulant drug may be preferable to methylphenidate or dextroamphetamine.

In preschool children, stimulant efficacy is more variable, and the rate of side effects is higher, especially sadness, irritability, clinginess, insomnia, and anorexia (Barkley 1988; N. J. Cohen et al. 1981; Conners 1975; Schleifer et al. 1975). Stimulants can, however, reduce oppositional and aggressive behavior and increase on-task behavior in preschoolers, especially when used with a contingency management program (Speltz et al. 1987). Stimulants should be used in this age group in more severe cases or in situations in which parent training and placement of the child in a highly structured, well-staffed preschool program have been unsuccessful or are not possible.

Stimulants are effective in the treatment of adolescents with cognitive and/or behavioral symptoms of ADHD (R. T. Brown and Sexson 1989; S. W. Evans and Pelham 1991; Klorman et al. 1990). Contrary to popular belief, youngsters who are positive responders as children do not require a change in drug at puberty. Adolescents whose conditions are newly diagnosed may be started on a stimulant.

Children with ADHD frequently have comorbid conduct disorder with verbal and physical aggression. Stimulants have been shown to decrease aggressive behavior in these patients (Hinshaw 1991). Anecdotal reports indicate that stimulants improve academic performance in some children who have attention deficits without hyperactivity (Famularo and Fenton 1987).

Bupropion

Bupropion may decrease hyperactivity and aggression and perhaps improve cognitive performance of children with ADHD and conduct disorder (Conners et al. 1996). One blind, controlled crossover study found that efficacy of bupropion was statistically equal to that of methylphenidate in decreasing behavioral and cognitive symptoms of ADHD (Barrickman et al. 1995).

α-Adrenergic Agonists

Despite limited empirical data, the antihypertensive agents clonidine and guanfacine are used as adjuncts to stimulant medication or as third-line alternative drugs (Connor et al. 1999). Clonidine is useful in modulating mood and activity level and improving cooperation and frustration tolerance in a subgroup of children with ADHD, especially those who are very highly aroused, hyperactive, impulsive, defiant, irritable, explosive, and labile (Hunt et al. 1990). Clonidine often improves ability to fall asleep, whether insomnia is a result of ADHD overarousal, oppositional refusal to go to bed, or stimulant effect or rebound (T. E. Brown and

Gammon 1992). Although clonidine has no direct effect on attention, it may be used alone in children with a family or personal history of tics or those who are nonresponders or negative responders to stimulants. It is most useful in combination with a stimulant when stimulant response is only partial or when stimulant dose is limited by side effects (Hunt et al. 1991). The addition of clonidine may allow a lower dose of stimulant medication (Hunt et al. 1991). Questions have been raised about the safety of the combination of clonidine and methylphenidate, however (see later subsection on clonidine and Wilens et al. 1999).

Guanfacine hydrochloride has a longer half-life and a more favorable side-effect profile than does clonidine. Preliminary animal and human data suggest positive cognitive effects. Guanfacine hydrochloride has been used for similar indications as those for clonidine—that is, for children who cannot tolerate clonidine's sedative effect or in whom clonidine has too short a duration of action, leading to rebound effects on tics, sleep, or behavior. Only data from open trials are available (Chappell et al. 1995; Horrigan and Barnhill 1995; Hunt et al. 1995).

Tricyclic Antidepressants

A TCA may be used to treat ADHD if stimulants exacerbate tics or Tourette's disorder (Riddle et al. 1988) or if the patient or a parent is at high risk for abusing or selling a stimulant. In addition, a TCA may be indicated if stimulants are ineffective or if side effects (especially dysphoria, weight loss, or severe rebound) are unacceptable. Their narrower margin of safety makes them a second or third choice, especially in prepubertal children. Although depressive symptoms in children with ADHD have not been found to differentially predict positive outcome of TCA treatment, a TCA may decrease depressive symptoms in youngsters with ADHD, and it avoids the risk of stimulant-induced dysphoria (Biederman et al. 1989a). The longer duration of action does not require a dose at school and minimizes rebound effects.

Drawbacks include the inconvenience and expense of electrocardiogram (ECG) monitoring, serious potential cardiac side effects (especially in prepubertal children), the danger of accidental or intentional overdose, and troublesome anticholinergic and sedating side effects. There have been case reports of sudden death in children taking desipramine (Riddle et al. 1993). (See section "Depressive Disorders" later in this chapter for a discussion.)

TCAs reduce symptoms of ADHD better than placebo does but not as well as stimulants do (Pliszka 1987). TCAs do not cause impairment on cognitive tests, but they yield minimal improvement on these measures, in comparison to stimulant effects (Biederman et al. 1989a; Donnelly et al. 1986; Rapport et al. 1993). At present, the TCAs used most often for ADHD are nortriptyline and imipramine, although desipramine is occasionally used (especially in older adolescents). Amitriptyline has an unacceptable level of anticholinergic and sedative side effects. (The use of TCAs in young patients is discussed later in this chapter in "Depressive Disorders.")

Selective Serotonin Reuptake Inhibitors (SSRIs)

Although there has been considerable clinical interest in the use of SSRIs in the treatment of ADHD, only anecdotal data are available. SSRIs do not appear to be efficacious for the core symptoms of ADHD but may be useful as adjuncts for secondary or comorbid mood and behavior symptoms (Gammon and Brown 1993).

Assessment of Response

Multiple outcome measures are essential. The direction and magnitude of effects in various domains (i.e., cognitive, behavioral, social) are typically inconsistent among children and even for a specific child. A particular dose of medication often produces improvement in some areas of functioning, but no change or worsening in oth-

ers, and stimulant dose-response curves vary in shape (Rapport et al. 1987). Data from parents and teachers on behavior and academic performance are essential prior to initiating stimulant medication and at regular intervals during treatment (Barkley et al. 1988). The Child Attention Problems (CAP; Barkley 1990) is a brief teacher rating scale derived from the Teacher Report Form of the Child Behavior Checklist (Achenbach 1991) that is convenient to use weekly to assess treatment outcome (see Table 22–1 and Table 22–2). It covers both overactivity/impulsivity and inattention symptoms. In the absence of any intervention, rating scale scores tend to decline from the first administration to the second and then rise with frequent repeated administration (Diamond and Deane 1988). The Conners Abbreviated Teacher Rating Scale (Goyette et al. 1978) can be used to measure drug response. It is not ideal as a diagnostic screen, however, because it overlooks children with attention deficits without hyperactivity (Ullmann et al. 1985) and is overinclusive of oppositional and aggressive children, even without ADHD. The IOWA Conners is a short form that was developed to separate inattention and overactivity ratings from oppositional defiance (Loney and Milich 1982; Pelham et al. 1989). It is useful in following treatment progress in children with comorbid ADHD and oppositional defiant disorder. Use of the Academic Performance Rating Scale (DuPaul et al. 1991) ensures that learning as well as behavior receives attention in the school setting. Systematic observations of behavior (Barkley et al. 1988) and measures of academic productivity and accuracy (Gadow and Swanson 1985; Pelham 1985) may also be useful in assessing a drug's effect.

Use of Stimulants

Stimulants include methylphenidate, dextroamphetamine, Adderall (a combination of four amphetamine salts), and magnesium pemoline.

Table 22–1. Child Attention Problems (CAP) Rating Scale

Child's name: _____   Child's age: _____

Today's date: _____   Child's sex: Male   [ ]

Filled out by: _____   Female [ ]

Below is a list of items that describes pupils. For each item that describes the pupil **now or within the past week,** check whether the item is **Not true, Somewhat or Sometimes true,** or **Very or Often true.** Please check all items as well as you can, even if some do not seem to apply to this pupil.

	Not true	Somewhat or Sometimes true	Very or Often true
1. Fails to finish things he/she starts	[ ]	[ ]	[ ]
2. Can't concentrate, can't pay attention for long	[ ]	[ ]	[ ]
3. Can't sit still, restless, or hyperactive	[ ]	[ ]	[ ]
4. Fidgets	[ ]	[ ]	[ ]
5. Daydreams or gets lost in his/her thoughts	[ ]	[ ]	[ ]
6. Impulsive or acts without thinking	[ ]	[ ]	[ ]
7. Difficulty following directions	[ ]	[ ]	[ ]
8. Talks out of turn	[ ]	[ ]	[ ]
9. Messy work	[ ]	[ ]	[ ]
10. Inattentive, easily distracted	[ ]	[ ]	[ ]
11. Talks too much	[ ]	[ ]	[ ]
12. Fails to carry out assigned tasks	[ ]	[ ]	[ ]

Please feel free to write any comments about the pupil's work or behavior in the last week.

Source.   Reprinted with permission of Craig Edelbrock, Ph.D.

Initiation of Treatment

The physician should explicitly debunk common myths about stimulant treatment. Stimulants do not have a paradoxical sedative action, do not lead to drug abuse, and often continue to be indicated and effective after puberty.

No predictors are available to help specify which stimulant will be best for a particular child. A substantial number of children respond to one stimulant but not to another (Elia et al. 1991). Therefore, if one stimulant is insufficiently effective, another should be tried before using another drug class. Methylphenidate is the most commonly used and best studied stimulant. Dextroamphetamine is less expensive and has a longer duration of action than methylphenidate. Disadvantages include negative attitudes of pharmacists toward dextroamphetamine, its exclusion from many formularies, and higher potential for abuse. Dextroamphetamine may have a mildly increased incidence of side effects such as appetite suppression and compulsive behaviors. The risk of pemoline-induced chemical hepatitis (Nehra et al. 1990), although

Table 22–2. Child Attention Problems (CAP) Rating Scale scoring

Each of the 12 items is scored 0, 1, or 2.

Total score = sum of the scores on all items

Subscores:

    Inattention: Sum of scores on items 1, 2, 5, 7, 9, 10, and 12

    Overactivity: Sum of scores on items 3, 4, 6, 8, and 11

Scores recommended as the upper limit of the normal range (93rd percentile):

	Boys	Girls
Inattention	9	7
Overactivity	6	5
Total score	15	11

Source. Reprinted with permission of Craig Edelbrock, Ph.D.

rare, and the higher incidence of involuntary movements limit the usefulness of pemoline.

Longer-acting stimulant preparations are appealing when the duration of action of the standard formulations is very short (2.5–3 hours), severe rebound occurs, or the administration of medication every 4 hours (or at school) is inconvenient, stigmatizing, or impossible. The most commonly used long-acting forms are Ritalin Sustained Release [SR], Dexedrine Spansule, and Adderall. Excessively high doses may result if a child chews a SR tablet or a spansule instead of swallowing it. A new form of long-acting methylphenidate appears to provide improved daytime coverage and is about to be released in the United States.

Stimulant medication should be initiated with a low dose and titrated every week or two, using half or whole pills, within the usual recommended range, according to response and side effects, using body weight as a rough guide (see Table 22–3). An alternative strategy is a systematic trial using a range of doses (Greenhill et al. 1996). Preschool children or patients with ADHD, predominantly inattentive type, may

be more sensitive to both therapeutic and side effects of stimulants; therefore, lower doses may be indicated. Starting with only a morning dose may be useful in assessing drug effect through comparing morning and afternoon school performance. The need for an after-school dose or medication on weekends is individually determined by considering target symptoms. A third dose after school improves behavior without increasing sleep problems (Kent et al. 1995).

Continuation, Maintenance, and Monitoring

The physician should work closely with parents on dose adjustments and obtain regular reports from teachers and annual academic testing. Children should not be responsible for their own medications because these youngsters are impulsive and forgetful at best, and most dislike the idea of taking medication, even when they can verbalize its positive effects and cannot identify any side effects. They will often avoid, "forget," or simply refuse to take a dose of medication. Pemoline requires obtaining liver enzyme measures at baseline and every 2 weeks thereafter. Parents should be instructed to notify the clinician promptly if the child develops vomiting or persistent abdominal distress, nausea, lethargy, or malaise.

Management of Side Effects

Patients should be monitored for changes in pulse, blood pressure, and weight and for the appearance of growth retardation, dysphoria, or tics. Most side effects are similar for all stimulants (see Table 22–4). Giving medication after meals minimizes anorexia. Insomnia may be caused by ADHD symptoms, oppositional refusal to go to bed, separation anxiety, or stimulant rebound or effect. Preexisting sleep problems are common in patients with ADHD. Stimulants may either worsen or improve irritable mood (Gadow 1992). Children with comorbid anxiety and African American male adolescents may be at risk for mildly elevated blood pressure while taking stimulants (R. T.

Table 22–3.   Clinical use of most commonly prescribed stimulant medications

	Methylphenidate	Dextroamphetamine	Adderall
How supplied (mg)	5, 10, 20 Sustained release: 20	5, 10 Elixir (5 mg/5 mL) Spansule: 5, 10, 15	5, 10, 20, 30
Usual starting dose (mg)	5–10 once or twice a day	2.5 or 5.0 once or twice a day	5–10 once or twice a day
Usual single dose range (mg/kg/dose)	0.3–0.7	0.15–0.5	0.15–0.5
Usual daily dose range (mg/day)	10–60	5–40	5–30
Maintenance number of doses per day	2–4	2–3	1–2
Behaviorally equivalent doses (mg)[a]	10 twice a day Sustained release: 20 mg every morning	5 twice a day Spansule: 10 mg every morning	5 twice a day

[a]Pelham et al. 1995, 1999.

Brown and Sexson 1989; Urman et al. 1995), but other cardiovascular side effects are exceedingly rare (Safer 1992).

The use of stimulants in patients with a personal or family history of tics has been controversial because of concern that new, persistent tics might be precipitated. Existing data suggest that tics may appear or worsen in some children who are at genetic risk. The physician must balance the impairment resulting from tics compared with that from ADHD symptoms, considering the efficacy and side-effect profile of alternative medications. With appropriate informed consent and careful clinical monitoring, stimulants may still be the medication of first choice.

Although stimulant-induced growth retardation has been a concern, any decrease in expected weight gain is small, despite statistical significance in studies. The effect on height is rarely clinically significant. The magnitude is dose related and appears to be greater with dextroamphetamine than with methylphenidate or pemoline (Greenhill 1981). Growth retardation can be minimized by using drug holidays. Tolerance to this effect has been reported. Medication-free summers (if clinically appropriate) may facilitate height or weight normalization (Klein et al. 1988). A study of young adults treated in childhood with methylphenidate showed no decrement in final height (Klein and Mannuzza 1988).

Rebound effects, increased excitability, activity, talkativeness, irritability, and insomnia, beginning 3–15 hours after a dose, may be seen daily or for up to several days after sudden withdrawal of high daily doses of stimulants. These effects may resemble a worsening of the original symptoms (Zahn et al. 1980). Management strategies include increased structure after school, a dose of medication in the afternoon that is smaller than the midday dose, the use of a long-acting formulation, and the addition of either clonidine or guanfacine.

There is no evidence that stimulants produce a decrease in the seizure threshold. In con-

Table 22–4. Side effects of stimulant medications

Common initial side effects (try dose reduction)
Anorexia
Weight loss
Irritability
Abdominal pain
Headaches
Emotional oversensitivity, crying easily
Less common side effects
Insomnia
Dysphoria (especially at higher doses)
Decreased social interest
Impaired cognitive test performance (especially at very high doses)
Less than expected weight gain
Rebound overactivity and irritability (as dose wears off)
Anxiety
Nervous habits (e.g., picking at skin, pulling hair)
Hypersensitivity, rash, conjunctivitis, or hives
Withdrawal effects
Insomnia
Rebound attention-deficit/hyperactivity disorder symptoms
Depression (rare)
Rare but potentially serious side effects
Motor tics
Exacerbation or precipitation of Tourette's disorder
Depression
Growth retardation (reversible when drug stopped)
Tachycardia
Hypertension
Psychosis with hallucinations
Stereotyped activities or compulsions
Side effects reported with pemoline only
Choreiform movements
Dyskinesias
Night terrors
Lip licking or biting
Chemical hepatitis (elevated serum glutamic-oxaloacetic transaminase and serum glutamic-pyruvic transaminase, jaundice, epigastric pain) (very rare) (Patterson 1984)

Source. Adapted from Dulcan MK, Popper CW: *Concise Guide to Child and Adolescent Psychiatry.* Washington, DC, American Psychiatric Press, 1991. Copyright 1991, American Psychiatric Press. Used with permission.

trast to popular lay belief, taking stimulants prescribed for ADHD does not result in addiction.

Discontinuation

If symptoms are not severe outside of the school setting, the young person should have an annual drug-free trial in the summer of at least 2 weeks but longer if possible. If school behavior and academic performance are stable, a carefully monitored trial off medication during the school year (but *not* at the beginning) will provide data on whether medication is still needed. The duration of medication treatment is individually determined by whether drug-responsive target symptoms are still present. Treatment may be required through adolescence and into adulthood.

Treatment Resistance

Stimulant tolerance is reported anecdotally, but noncompliance should be the first possibility considered when medication appears to have become ineffective. Decreased drug effect may also be due to a reaction to stress at home or school, attenuation of an initial positive placebo effect, or lower efficacy of a generic preparation. True tolerance may be more likely with the long-acting formulations (Birmaher et al. 1989). If tolerance occurs, another stimulant may be substituted.

If several stimulants in appropriate doses have been found to be ineffective for an individual child, several strategies are possible. More intensive psychosocial treatment may be indicated. An innovative strategy for difficult-to-manage cases is the combination of short-acting and longer-acting stimulant medications (Fitzpatrick et al. 1992). Bupropion is an alternative possibility. If a stimulant is partially effective, clonidine or guanfacine may be added. A TCA trial may be successful in stimulant nonresponders. Anecdotal data suggest the use of fluoxetine in combination with methylphenidate (Gammon and Brown 1993), but there is little evidence of efficacy for the core symptoms of ADHD.

Use of Bupropion

The clinical history should include a search for seizures and factors that predispose to seizures (e.g., head trauma, other central nervous system pathology, other drugs that lower the seizure threshold, or eating disorders). An EEG may be indicated prior to starting bupropion if an eating disorder or a seizure diathesis is possible. Bupropion is administered in two or three daily doses, beginning with a dose of 37.5 or 50 mg twice a day, with gradual titration over 2 weeks to a usual maximum of 250 mg/day (300–400 mg/day in adolescents). A single dose should not exceed 150 mg. Blood levels do not appear to be useful. Allergic reactions are relatively common, including rash, urticaria, and rare serum sickness. Other side effects include drowsiness, fatigue, nausea, anorexia, dizziness, and "spaciness" (Barrickman et al. 1995; Conners et al. 1996). Bupropion may exacerbate tics (T. Spencer et al. 1993). Side effects seen in adults may be expected, and seizures are possible at daily doses greater than 450 mg.

Use of Clonidine

Initiation of Treatment

The clinician should take reasonable precautions before starting clonidine, including a thorough cardiovascular history, a recent clinical cardiac examination, measurement of baseline blood pressure and pulse, and possibly an ECG. History of syncope and finding of bradycardia or heart block on baseline ECG are relative contraindications. Laboratory blood studies may include a complete blood count (CBC) with differential and fasting glucose (if personal or family history suggests diabetes). Clonidine is initiated at a low dose of 0.05 mg (one-half of the smallest manufactured tablet) at bedtime. This converts the side effect of initial sedation into a benefit. An alternative strategy is to begin with 0.025 mg four times a day.

Continuation, Maintenance, and Monitoring

The dose of clonidine is titrated gradually over several weeks to 0.15–0.30 mg/day (0.003–0.01 mg/kg/day) in three or four divided doses. Very young children (age 5–7 years) may require lower initial and maintenance doses. The transdermal form (skin patch) may improve compliance and reduce variability in blood levels. It lasts only 5 days in children (compared with 7 days in adults) (Hunt et al. 1990). Once the daily dose is determined using pills, an equivalent size patch may be substituted (0.1, 0.2, or 0.3 mg/day). The patch may be cut to adjust the dose. Note that patches do not adhere well in hot, humid climates.

Clonidine has a slow onset of therapeutic action, in part because of the gradual dose increase needed to minimize side effects, and perhaps due to the time required for receptor downregulation (Hunt et al. 1991). Significant clinical response is not seen for as long as a month, and maximal effect may be delayed for another several months.

Management of Side Effects

Clonidine's most troublesome side effect is sedation, but this effect tends to decrease after several weeks. Dry mouth, nausea, and photophobia have been reported, with hypotension and dizziness possible at high doses. The skin patch often causes local pruritic dermatitis and may cause a toxic reaction if chewed or swallowed. Depression may occur, most often in patients with a history of depressive symptoms in themselves or their families (Hunt et al. 1991). Glucose tolerance may decrease, especially in those at risk for diabetes.

Four deaths have been reported to the FDA of children who at one time had been taking both methylphenidate and clonidine, but the evidence linking the drugs to the deaths is tenuous, at best (Wilens et al. 1999). Pending further clarification, extra caution is advised when treating children with cardiac or cardiovascular disease or when combining clonidine with other medications. Erratic compliance with medication increases the risk of adverse cardiovascular events. Families should be cautioned repeatedly about this problem, and clonidine should not be prescribed if it cannot be administered reliably. The acute onset of dizziness, fatigue, light-headedness, sedation, syncope, or near-syncope, especially if it occurs during or after exercise, should prompt closer clinical monitoring and cardiology consultation (Cantwell et al. 1997).

Discontinuation

When clonidine is discontinued, it should be tapered rather than stopped suddenly to avoid a withdrawal syndrome consisting of increased motor restlessness, headache, agitation, and elevated blood pressure and pulse rate (Leckman et al. 1986).

Use of Guanfacine

The use of guanfacine is similar to that of clonidine. Compared with clonidine, guanfacine has fewer and less significant side effects (particularly sedation and hypotension) and a longer half-life. It is typically given in divided doses two or three times a day, starting with 0.5 mg (one-half of a 1-mg tablet) in the morning or at bedtime. The daily dose is increased by 0.5-mg increments every 3–4 days. The usual maximum dose is 3 mg/day. One mg of guanfacine is equivalent to 0.1 mg of clonidine. When switching between the two agents, one can be tapered down as the other is increased.

Use of Tricyclic Antidepressants

When treating ADHD, the clinician may start nortriptyline at 10 or 25 mg/day and may increase the dosage as tolerated until a clinical effect or a maximum of 4.5 mg/kg/day (usual dose 2 mg/kg/day), given in two divided doses, is reached. The serum level (50–150 ng/mL) may relate to therapeutic response (Wilens et al. 1993). Imipramine (or desipramine) is begun at 10 or 25 mg/day and increased weekly to a maxi-

mum dose of 5 mg/kg/day (divided into three doses per day in prepubertal children). Plasma levels do not predict efficacy. Some patients respond to a daily dose as low as 2 mg/kg. The use of TCAs in children and adolescents is discussed in the next section.

A note of caution is necessary: The combination of imipramine and methylphenidate has been associated with a syndrome of confusion, affective lability, marked aggression, and severe agitation that disappeared when the medications were stopped (Grob and Coyle 1986). The mechanism may be methylphenidate's interference with hepatic metabolism of imipramine, resulting in a longer half-life and elevated blood levels.

MOOD DISORDERS

Bipolar Disorders

Assessment for Treatment

Adolescents may develop a clinical picture similar to that in adults. Diagnosis in prepubertal children is controversial (Biederman et al. 1998). Clinical assessment should be done by interviewing the child and the parents together and then each individually. When assessing the child, it is important to ask age-specific questions that cover the DSM-IV criteria. Children with mania can be distinguished from children with ADHD by their higher total score and distinctive pattern of item endorsement on the clinician-completed Mania Rating Scale (MRS; Fristad et al. 1995). A careful history can often differentiate the child with mania from a child with hyperactivity or conduct disorder. In mania, a cyclic history is more common; in conduct disorder and ADHD, symptoms are more chronic. Obtaining a family psychiatric history may also be useful.

Medical conditions that may cause secondary mania, such as multiple sclerosis, seizure disorders, brain tumors, treatment with steroids, and drug abuse, must be ruled out. Similar to the workup for any child with a first episode of psychosis, the baseline workup for a youth with mania might include magnetic resonance imaging (MRI) or computed tomography (CT) scan. The medical evaluation should include routine blood studies, including CBC with differential, electrolytes, thyroid function tests, blood urea nitrogen (BUN), creatinine, and creatinine clearance.

Selection of Treatment

For the most part, the physician must extrapolate from data on the successful psychopharmacological treatment of adults with bipolar disorder.

Lithium carbonate is the drug most commonly used to stabilize mood in children (Weller et al. 1986). Although mania in children and adolescents that is treated with lithium may become easier to manage, the dramatic positive response to lithium observed in adults with mania is uncommon. Youngsters with mania who have preadolescent onset of psychopathology have a poorer response to lithium than those with adolescent-onset mania without prepubertal psychopathology (Strober et al. 1988). In a study in which researchers used lithium to treat aggressive behavior in children and adolescents, positive responders had mood symptoms, a family history of mood disorders, and/or lithium-responsive relatives (Youngerman and Canino 1978).

Because the degree of symptom abatement with lithium is often disappointing, other medications such as carbamazepine and valproic acid have been tried, although no double-blind, placebo-controlled studies have been done in children and adolescents with bipolar disorder. Some clinicians advocate using valproate even before a trial of lithium and/or carbamazepine. Practice is based on anecdotal clinical experience (West et al. 1994) and extrapolation from the treatment of adults. The clinician should obtain consent from parents or guardians and assent from the patient before starting mood-stabilizing medication in a child or adolescent.

The clinician should make clear to the responsible adult that data substantiating the efficacy of treating children and adolescents with mania or hypomania with these agents are limited. (The use of carbamazepine is discussed in the section, "Aggression," later in this chapter.)

Assessment of Response

Treatment of bipolar disorder in youths is best done by experienced clinicians who can assess response. The MRS can be used to assess response because total scores decrease with successful treatment. The Beigel-Murphy (Beigel et al. 1971) scale can also be used with adolescents.

Use of Lithium

Initiation of treatment. In children, traditional practice is to start lithium at 300 mg/day for several weeks and slowly increase the dose to 900 mg/day. If the clinician uses a weight-based dosage guide for prepubertal children, therapeutic levels can be safely attained in a much shorter time (Weller et al. 1986). The higher glomerular filtration rate in children, compared with adults, usually requires a higher mg/kg dose before puberty. Published nomograms can be used to calculate dosages based on blood levels after single test doses (Alessi et al. 1994; B. Geller and Fetner 1989; Malone et al. 1995b). Lithium's half-life could permit once-a-day dosing in adolescents, although children have more rapid lithium clearance than do adults, and multiple divided doses may be necessary to maintain therapeutic levels. In addition, some patients have gastrointestinal distress when they take the entire day's dose at bedtime. Lithium is therefore usually given two or three times a day with meals. Divided doses have the disadvantage of potentially decreasing adherence to the prescribed regimen, however. Some clinicians use slow-release lithium to sustain the therapeutic effect throughout the day while avoiding multiple doses. No systematic studies in children have compared the efficacy and side effects of different dosing schedules.

In general, the blood level should not exceed 1.4 mEq/L. Peak serum levels will occur within 1–2 hours after ingestion. Steady-state serum levels are achieved after 5 days. Blood should be drawn for a serum level 8–12 hours after the patient ingested the last evening dose and before the first morning dose. For children, an 8:00 A.M. sampling time is most commonly used. Some clinicians suggest that lithium may be maintained at higher blood levels in preschool-aged children. There are, however, no published data supporting the safety and efficacy of this practice.

Continuation, maintenance, and monitoring. A child or adolescent being treated with lithium carbonate should have a psychiatric visit at least once a month to ensure that the lithium is tolerated well and to monitor compliance. Although in the acute manic phase, serum levels up to 1.4 mEq/L are tolerated well, clinical experience suggests that maintenance levels can be lower (i.e., 0.6–1.2 mEq/L). Although it is theoretically possible to substitute saliva levels of lithium for serum levels (Weller et al. 1987), this approach has not yet become common in clinical practice. BUN, creatinine, and creatinine clearance should be periodically measured because lithium may cause alterations in kidney function. Lithium may produce goiter and/or hypothyroidism; therefore, a thyroid-stimulating hormone (TSH) test should be obtained every 4–6 months.

Management of side effects. Lithium is well tolerated by most children and adolescents, although children younger than 7 years are more prone to side effects, especially with higher lithium doses and serum levels (Hagino et al. 1995). The most common side effects in children (i.e., tremor, weight gain, development or exacerbation of enuresis, polyuria, polydipsia, and polyphagia; Weller et al. 1986) rarely require discontinuation of lithium. Acne may be induced or aggravated, especially in adolescents. Lithium carbonate is deposited in bones, but it is

not known whether this has any significant effect on a growing child whose epiphyseal plate is not closed. Lithium has not been reported to interfere with the growth of children. The effect of lithium on cognitive functioning in children has not been studied in detail. Hypokalemia is a very rare side effect that can be managed by dietary supplementation (e.g., two bananas, two large carrots, two cups of skim milk, half of a honeydew melon, or an avocado daily). Such supplementation may be preferable to giving potassium tablets, which can further irritate the gastrointestinal tract and which have a taste that most children dislike.

When a child is taking lithium carbonate, the patient and the family should be taught to be especially cautious when the patient develops an illness with fever, vomiting, or diarrhea; uses rigorous dieting to lose weight; or takes diuretics or nonsteroidal antiinflammatory agents. Any of these situations should immediately be brought to the psychiatrist's attention. Lithium should be discontinued while a patient has fever, vomiting, or diarrhea. Vigorous exercise in hot weather can also lead to lithium toxicity, and parents should be cautioned to be sure the patient drinks enough water. Nonsteroidal antiinflammatory agents (other than aspirin), which are often taken by adolescent girls to relieve menstrual distress, can increase lithium levels and even lead to lithium intoxication. Wide swings in salt intake can produce erratic lithium levels, between ineffective and toxic.

Discontinuation. Gradual tapering off of medication is recommended. The patient should be followed up closely after discontinuing medication and should be checked for signs of relapse to mania or for symptoms of depression so that episodes can be treated early and hospitalization avoided. The kindling hypothesis and data on adult treatment resistance following intermittent treatment suggest special caution regarding discontinuation of mood stabilizers.

No studies address the issue of how long

lithium should be continued. A naturalistic study (Strober et al. 1990) found that adolescents who discontinued their lithium were three times more likely to relapse compared with those who continued the medication. Most relapses occurred within the first year after cessation of treatment. Once lithium is started, it seems advisable to continue for at least 6 months and preferably for a year. If studies of lithium termination in adults are applicable, an even longer duration of treatment might be considered.

Use of Valproate

Initiation of treatment. Baseline liver function tests are necessary before starting treatment with valproate because it can cause hepatotoxicity, although this effect is extremely rare in patients older than 10 years; the greatest risk is for patients younger than 3 years (Trimble 1990). Other initial laboratory studies include CBC with differential, creatinine, BUN, and TSH.

Valproic acid is available in tablets, capsules (Depakene), and an elixir of 250 mg/5 mL (16-ounce bottles). Depakote, an enteric-coated tablet combining sodium valproate and valproic acid (available in 125, 250, and 500 mg), is recommended to avoid gastrointestinal side effects. Valproic acid should be started at a dose of 250 mg/day (500 mg in adolescents) and increased by 250 mg every 4 days, not to exceed 60 mg/kg/day. The usual range for adolescent acute mania is 1,000–1,750 mg/day. Although valproic acid can be given in a single bedtime dose, it is usually administered in two divided daily doses. Plasma levels are minimally useful.

Continuation, maintenance, and monitoring. Liver function tests should be done periodically, although routine liver function studies may not detect idiosyncratic liver failure. Parents should be instructed to notify the clinician promptly if the child develops vomiting, easy bruising, or persistent abdominal distress, nausea, lethargy, or malaise.

Management of side effects. Side effects of valproate include nausea, vomiting, anorexia, lethargy, and abdominal pain, although these may be minimized by starting with a low dose and titrating up slowly. Hepatotoxicity is possible, but when valproate is discontinued, recovery of liver enzymes occurs within several weeks. A very rare complication of valproate treatment of children and adolescents is (potentially fatal) pancreatitis, which usually occurs within the first 12 months of treatment (Trimble 1990). However, most patients who experience this complication are taking multiple anticonvulsants. Neutropenia and thrombocytopenia as well as macrocytic anemia have been reported in valproate-treated patients. Little is known about the longer-term effects of the use of valproate during development, although data from its use to treat children with seizure disorders do not suggest unique problems, with the exception of mildly decreased bone mineral density (Sheth et al. 1995) and, in girls, polycystic ovaries and/or hyperandrogenism following chronic valproate use (Geller 1998).

Treatment resistance. If mania is resistant to treatment, several options can be considered. However, it should always be remembered that although such strategies have been used in adults (see Chapter 18), few, if any, studies of their efficacy or safety have been done in children and adolescents.

A possible strategy is the addition of an antipsychotic agent, most commonly haloperidol, although the newer atypical antipsychotics may have fewer side effects. Despite an isolated report of complications from the simultaneous use of haloperidol and lithium in adult patients, most patients tolerate this combination fairly well. Clinical experience suggests that the use of haloperidol or an atypical neuroleptic should be considered in treating mania in patients with psychosis who have obsessive or compulsive traits and frequent rumination or who have comorbid diagnoses (e.g., Tourette's disorder) that might respond to haloperidol.

Electroconvulsive therapy has rarely been used in treatment-resistant manic teenagers.

Depressive Disorders

In the past 20 years, recognition that mood disorders can present in children and adolescents has resulted in increased interest in diagnosing and treating depression in young patients. The successful pharmacological treatment of mood disorders in this age group awaits well-designed multicenter double-blind, placebo-controlled studies.

Assessment for Treatment

The clinician should conduct an assessment using DSM-IV criteria, including interviewing both the parents and the child and obtaining information from the child's school. It is important to remember that most children with mood disorders have a family history of such disorders. Parental depression may color the reporting of the child's psychopathology. However, the child and a parent may be simultaneously depressed. Reports from the teacher, who can observe the child objectively in comparison with other students, can be a very important part of the evaluation. Although teacher evaluations may be more difficult to obtain and may be less accurate for high school students, information from the school is still valuable. The most disturbed youths often come to the attention of the school counselor, the school nurse, or the principal because of poor attendance or declining academic performance.

Interview-based assessment measures include the Child Depression Rating Scale—Revised (CDRS-R; Poznanski et al. 1985), which is similar to the Hamilton Rating Scale for Depression (Hamilton 1967) and combines information from the clinician, child, parent, and teacher. Self-report is also important. In children, the Children's Depression Inventory (CDI; Kovacs 1985) is frequently used, although it performs better as a screen than as a diagnostic instrument. It may underestimate the degree of

depression because children can determine the "normal" response and answer accordingly. In one study, the CDI did not differentiate children with depression from those with conduct disorder (Fristad et al. 1988). In adolescents, the Beck Depression Inventory (BDI; Beck et al. 1961) can be used.

Selection of Treatment

The clinician should not underestimate the importance of working with school personnel and parents by educating them about the illness. Also, individual and/or group therapies may address social deficits that cannot be remedied with medication alone.

Published algorithms exist based on clinical experience and extrapolation from data on adults (e.g., see Ambrosini et al. 1995; Hughes et al. 1999; Johnston and Fruehling 1994). Selection of the first drug may be influenced by the patient's target symptoms, comorbidity, risk of impulsive behavior, family history of disorder and drug response, and side-effect profile of the drugs. Remarkably few empirical data on children and adolescents are available to guide therapeutic choices (see Emslie et al. 1999 for a review).

SSRIs, including fluoxetine, sertraline, paroxetine, and venlafaxine, may be effective in the treatment of depression in children and adolescents. Long-term effects of these medications on growing children are not known. Their advantages over TCAs include the absence of cardiac side effects and relative safety in overdose. As with other antidepressants, hypomania or mania can be precipitated.

Several open-label studies report improvement in depressed children and adolescents (some of whom did not respond to TCAs) treated with fluoxetine. One rigorous double-blind, placebo-controlled trial in children and adolescents with depression found that fluoxetine yielded significantly greater improvement in depressive symptoms than did placebo (Emslie et al. 1997). Fluoxetine is started at 20 mg/day or less. Most patients do not need more than 40 mg/day. Fluoxetine is sometimes prescribed on an every-other-day basis because of the long half-life of the drug and its active metabolites. (The use of fluoxetine is discussed in the subsection, "Obsessive-Compulsive Disorder," later in this chapter.)

Open trials of sertraline in adolescents with a major depressive episode were promising in reducing symptoms of depression and anxiety. The most troublesome side effects were insomnia, feelings of tension and restlessness, drowsiness, anorexia, weight change, headaches, and nightmares (Ambrosini et al. 1999; McConville et al. 1996). An open trial of bupropion in adolescents with major depressive disorder was promising (Arredondo et al. 1993).

In open studies, 75% of child and adolescent patients whose depression was treated with TCAs responded positively. However, only one of the (relatively few) double-blind, placebo-controlled studies found an advantage of imipramine over placebo (Preskorn et al. 1987). In adolescents, no double-blind study shows the efficacy of TCAs over placebo. Existing studies, however, have small sample sizes, lack of data on how subtypes and predictors of response differ with development, and problems with limited duration of treatment and insufficiently sensitive measures of response (Conners 1992; Strober et al. 1992).

Assessment of Response

To fully assess response to medication, the clinician should obtain input from the child, parent, and school personnel. Depending on the patient's age, the CDI, the BDI, or the abbreviated CDRS-R can be used to assess changes in symptomatology (Overholser et al. 1995).

Medication Use

See Hughes et al. 1999 for a recent algorithm.

Use of Tricyclic Antidepressants

Initiation of treatment. Pharmacokinetics for TCAs are different in children than in ado-

lescents or adults. The smaller fat-to-muscle ratio in children leads to a decreased volume of distribution, and most children do not have the buffer of a relatively large volume of fat in which the drug can be stored. Children have larger livers relative to body size, leading to faster metabolism (Sallee et al. 1986), more rapid absorption, and lower protein binding than in adults (Winsberg et al. 1974); these factors all contribute to a shorter half-life in younger children. As a result, children probably need a higher weight-corrected dose of TCAs than do adults. Prepubertal children are prone to rapid dramatic swings in blood levels from toxic to ineffective and should be given divided doses to produce more stable levels (Ryan 1992). Plasma levels vary widely at a given fixed dose.

TCAs' quinidine-like effect slows cardiac conduction time and repolarization. Children and adolescents may develop mildly increased pulse and blood pressure and small, statistically significant, but usually clinically benign, ECG changes (intraventricular conduction defects; e.g., lengthened P-R interval that may progress to a first-degree atrioventricular heart block and occasional widening of the QRS complex), especially at doses equivalent to greater than 3 mg/kg/day of imipramine or desipramine (Bartels et al. 1991; Biederman et al. 1989b, 1993; Fletcher et al. 1993; Leonard et al. 1995; Schroeder et al. 1989; Winsberg et al. 1975). In one carefully monitored sample of nearly 200 children and adolescents, desipramine in doses up to 5 mg/kg/day produced increases in diastolic blood pressure, heart rate, and ECG conduction parameters that were statistically significant but not clinically meaningful or symptomatic (Biederman 1991). Prolongation of the Q-T$_c$ interval may be a sensitive indicator of cardiac effect (Wilens et al. 1996). The tendency of prepubertal children to have wider swings in blood levels may place them at higher risk for serious cardiac conduction changes. Approximately 5% of the population has a genetic defect in TCA metabolism, which causes these individuals to be "slow hydroxylators," increasing risk for toxicity.

Five cases (three prepubertal children, one 12-year-old girl, and one 14-year-old boy) have been reported of unexplained sudden death during desipramine treatment, and in three of these cases, death occurred following exercise (Popper and Zimnitzky 1995; Riddle et al. 1990/1991, 1993). A causal relationship between the medication and the deaths has not been established. The evidence appears to suggest that treatment with desipramine in usual doses is associated with only a slight added risk of sudden death beyond that occurring naturally (Biederman et al. 1995). Desipramine may represent a greater risk than other TCAs, however. Because of these concerns, clinical practice now favors nortriptyline or imipramine as the first choice among the tricyclics in the treatment of prepubertal children.

Before initiating treatment with a TCA, the clinician should perform a complete physical examination, including baseline vital signs. He or she should obtain a careful history for cardiac symptoms such as chest pain, dyspnea, actual or near syncope, palpitation, or tachycardia. Congenital hearing impairment may signal Jervell-DeLange syndrome, which is associated with cardiac abnormalities and increased risk of sudden death (Ambrosini et al. 1995). The clinician should examine the family history for possible contraindications to TCA use, such as arrhythmias (especially long–Q-T syndrome), unexplained fainting, conduction defects, cardiomyopathy, early cardiac disease, or sudden death (Liberthson 1996).

An ECG should be performed prior to initiating treatment. If abnormalities are seen in a routine ECG, an ECG with a rhythm strip should be obtained and interpreted by a pediatric cardiologist. If the history suggests head trauma or seizures, an EEG is indicated prior to starting treatment because TCAs lower the seizure threshold. Parents must be reminded to supervise closely the administration of medication and to keep pills in a safe place.

Treatment should be initiated with a small dose of the TCA and gradually increased. Some experts believe that plasma level monitoring may be helpful in determining optimum dose (if a laboratory that measures TCA levels reliably is available) (Preskorn et al. 1988), although this is controversial. TCAs have long half-lives; hence, once-a-day dosing is adequate for antidepressant effect. The short half-life of TCAs in prepubertal children can produce daily withdrawal symptoms if medication is given only once a day. If this occurs, or if comorbid ADHD is present, a thrice-daily regimen may be preferred. For imipramine, the daily dose should not exceed 5 mg/kg or 200 mg, whichever is smaller. Equivalent doses for other TCAs should be used. Most studies of TCAs in childhood depression have used imipramine and nortriptyline. Serial ECGs after each dose increase of 50–100 mg/day are recommended when the daily dose is above 2.5 mg/kg of imipramine or 1.0 mg/kg/day of nortriptyline (Wilens et al. 1996). Table 22–5 lists titration parameters for monitoring vital signs and ECG.

Table 22–5. Guidelines for the use of tricyclic antidepressants in children and adolescents

	Children	Adolescents
P-R interval (seconds)	0.2	0.2
QRS interval (seconds)	0.12 130% of baseline	0.12
Q-T$_c$ interval (seconds)	0.48	0.48
Resting heart rate (beats/minute)	110–130	110–120
Chronic blood pressure (mm Hg)	120/80	140/90

Note. **Electrocardiogram and vital sign limits to titration:** reduce dose or discontinue drug if reached.
Source. Wilens et al. 1996.

Continuation, maintenance, and monitoring. Once the symptoms respond to the antidepressant (after approximately 3–8 weeks), the medication should be continued for at least 4–6 months. Throughout this period, the clinician should continue to monitor side effects and response. Monitoring the medication with plasma levels is recommended by some to ensure compliance and avoid toxicity (Preskorn et al. 1988). Periodic ECGs should be obtained if the dose exceeds 3 mg/kg/day. Unexplained withdrawal symptoms may indicate that poor compliance is resulting in missed doses. Because of the predictability of TCA-induced ECG changes, a rhythm strip is useful in monitoring compliance.

Management of side effects. If ECG changes appear, alternatives include decreasing the dose or switching to another antidepressant. The most common side effects of TCAs are dry mouth, tremor, constipation, and tachycardia. Drowsiness and dizziness sometimes occur at initiation of treatment. However, with proper instruction in how to manage transient postural hypotension, most children tolerate this side effect and adjust to it. Dry mouth can usually be managed by instructing the patient to chew sugarless gum or wax or to sip water or diet drinks. These techniques will help keep the mouth moist while minimizing the risk of dental cavities and weight gain. In extreme cases that do not respond to these measures, a 1% solution of pilocarpine can be formulated by local pharmacists. If a TCA-induced tremor becomes intolerable, decreasing the dosage should be considered. Constipation is a common problem, for which a regular toileting schedule, a high-fiber diet, and increased liquids are helpful. Bedtime snacks of popcorn are fun for children and provide good roughage. In the occasional situation in which a stool softener is needed, Colace (200 mg at bedtime) can be used. Behavioral toxicity may be manifested by irritability, mania, agitation, anger, aggression, forgetfulness, or confusion. A drug blood level is often required to dif-

ferentiate central nervous system toxicity from exacerbation of the primary condition. The physician should be alert to the risk of intentional overdose or accidental poisoning, not only by the patient but also by other family members, especially young children. Switching to mania may occur, which would demand discontinuation of the TCA and addition of a mood stabilizer (B. Geller et al. 1993).

Discontinuation. After a child or adolescent has been asymptomatic for 4–6 months, stopping the medication should be considered. It is not advisable to stop the medication when the patient is confronting stressful life events. Some clinicians now maintain their young patients on TCAs chronically, especially when a patient has had multiple episodes of unipolar depression.

Sudden cessation of moderate or higher doses results in a flulike anticholinergic withdrawal syndrome with malaise, nausea, cramps, vomiting, headaches, and muscle pains. Other manifestations may include social withdrawal, hyperactivity, depression, agitation, and insomnia (Petti and Law 1981; Ryan 1990). TCAs should therefore be tapered off over a 2- to 3-week period, especially if the patient has been taking medication for a long time.

SCHIZOPHRENIA

Assessment for Treatment

Schizophrenia is often difficult to diagnose prior to adulthood, especially in prepubertal children. In addition to thorough medical, neurological, psychiatric, and developmental assessment, target symptoms for treatment should be identified. Before beginning medication, the clinician should ensure that a complete physical examination and baseline laboratory workup (including CBC with differential, liver profile, and urinalysis) have been done.

Selection of Treatment

The cornerstone of treatment is an intensive and comprehensive program that may include a highly structured environment, remediation of specific developmental deficits, social skills training, family psychoeducational treatment, and supportive reality-based individual psychotherapy. Special education placement or the assistance of a full-time aide in a mainstream classroom is commonly required. Day treatment, hospitalization, or long-term residential treatment may be needed. Medication is indicated if positive psychotic symptoms (e.g., delusions or hallucinations) cause significant impairment or interfere with other interventions. Disabling negative symptoms (e.g., apathy and social withdrawal) may also be indications for drug treatment, given the potential therapeutic effects of the newer neuroleptics.

A variety of neuroleptics appear to have modest efficacy in children and adolescents (Campbell et al. 1999). In general, however, schizophrenia in young patients is less responsive to pharmacotherapy than is that in adults, and substantial impairment continues, even if the more florid symptoms such as hallucinations, anxiety, and agitation abate (Campbell et al. 1985). Although no evidence suggests superior efficacy of one traditional neuroleptic over another, the lower-potency compounds (e.g., chlorpromazine and thioridazine) are best avoided because of sedation, cognitive dulling, and memory deficits that can interfere with learning in school and in treatment programs. Concerns regarding the development of tardive dyskinesia (TD) in long-term use of the typical neuroleptics and the prominence of negative symptoms in young schizophrenic patients suggest that clozapine may prove to be useful (Teicher and Glod 1990), although it is likely to be replaced by the even newer antipsychotic medications being developed. A double-blind trial found clozapine to be superior to haloperidol for both positive and negative symptoms in children and adolescents with early-onset schizophrenia (Kumra et al. 1996). Risperidone is rapidly becoming a preferred drug in adults and may be indicated for young schizophrenic patients as well, but only small case series reports have been published (Armenteros et al. 1997; Quintana and Keshavan 1995; Simeon et al. 1995). Negative as well as positive symptoms may improve. Although risperidone's side-effect profile is more benign than that of other neuroleptics, children appear to be more sensitive than adults to developing extrapyramidal symptoms on this drug (Mandoki 1995).

Assessment of Response

Full efficacy may require several months to appear (as long as 6–9 months for clozapine and risperidone). Parent and teacher reports are essential, in addition to self-reports from adolescents. Standardized clinician ratings such as the Positive and Negative Syndrome Scales derived from the Children's Psychiatric Rating Scale are sensitive to neuroleptic-induced improvement in children (E. K. Spencer et al. 1994).

Initiation of Treatment

TD has been documented in children and adolescents after as brief a period of treatment as 5 months (Herskowitz 1987), and it may appear even during periods of constant medication dose (see Wolf and Wagner 1993 for a review). Initiation of chronic neuroleptic treatment during the developmental period may yield a greater risk of TD than exposure that begins in adulthood. Before the clinician prescribes a neuroleptic and periodically thereafter, he or she should carefully examine each patient for abnormal movements by using a scale such as the Abnormal Involuntary Movement Scale (AIMS; Munetz and Benjamin 1988). Parents and patients (as they are able) should receive regular explanations of the risk of movement disorders.

Prior to clozapine treatment, an EEG is needed because of the increased frequency of seizures and EEG abnormalities in adolescents while taking this drug.

Antipsychotic drugs are highly lipophilic. Chlorpromazine has been reported to have a lower plasma concentration in children than in adults after the same weight-adjusted dose (Rivera-Calimlim et al. 1979). However, the magnitude of the difference exceeds that expected from the small proportional excess of adipose tissue in children compared with adults, probably because of children's increased efficiency of hepatic biotransformation (Jatlow 1987). Developmental changes in protein binding may be influential as well.

Doses must be titrated with careful attention to positive and negative effects. Age, weight, and severity of symptoms do not provide clear dose guidelines. The initial dose should be very low, with gradual increments, no more than once or twice a week. Loading doses or rapid titration does not accelerate clinical improvement but does increase side effects and decrease compliance. Children metabolize these drugs more rapidly than do adults but also require lower plasma levels for efficacy. Common doses for children are 0.25–6.0 mg of haloperidol or 10–200 mg of chlorpromazine, or the equivalent, per day. Older adolescents with schizophrenia may require doses of neuroleptics in the adult range. Young adolescents fall in between, and doses must be empirically determined. Even less is known about optimal doses of the atypical neuroleptics. Although a single daily dose (usually at bedtime) is generally preferred for maintenance, divided doses may be used during titration (especially in hospitalized patients) to minimize side effects and permit finer dose adjustments.

Continuation, Maintenance, and Monitoring

Efficacy and side effects must be monitored regularly. A standard protocol should be followed for clozapine (see Towbin et al. 1994 for recommendations). Neuroleptics should be maintained at the lowest effective dose. Although current practice with adults with schizophrenia is to maintain neuroleptic treatment indefinitely, for children the lack of clarity in diagnosis and the possibility of developmental toxicity make firm recommendations about the advisability of periodic withdrawal of medication difficult. If medication is to be stopped, it should be withdrawn gradually to prevent rebound psychiatric symptoms. Withdrawal dyskinesias are relatively common.

Management of Side Effects

Sedation, weight gain, and hypersalivation are the most common side effects. Weight gain may be especially problematic in the long-term use of the low-potency neuroleptics and risperidone. Neutropenia and seizures at rates significantly higher than seen in adults may limit the usefulness of clozapine (Kumra et al. 1996).

Acute extrapyramidal side effects (EPS), including dystonic reactions, parkinsonian tremor and rigidity, drooling, and akathisia, occur as in adults. Laryngeal dystonia is potentially fatal. Acute dystonia may be treated with oral or intramuscular diphenhydramine, 25 or 50 mg, or benztropine, 0.5–2.0 mg. When medication is initiated for an outpatient, the clinician should instruct a responsible adult to watch for a dystonic reaction and should provide a supply of medication for dystonia to be given to the patient if needed. Adolescent boys seem to be more vulnerable to acute dystonic reactions than are adult patients, so the physician may be more inclined to use prophylactic antiparkinsonian medication. Clinical experience suggests that children do not respond well to anticholinergics, and reduction of neuroleptic dose is therefore preferable (Campbell et al. 1985). For treatment or prevention of parkinsonian symptoms, adolescents may be given benztropine, 1–2 mg/day, in divided doses. Chronic parkinsonian symptoms are often drastically underrecognized by clinicians (Richardson et al. 1991). The neuromuscular consequences may impair performance of age-appropriate activities, and the subjective effects may lead to noncompliance with medication. Akathisia may be especially difficult to identify in very young patients or those with limited verbal ability. It may be misinterpreted as anxiety or agitation and mistakenly exacerbated with an increase in neuroleptic dose. Clonazepam (0.5 mg/day) may reduce neuroleptic-induced akathisia (Kutcher et al. 1987) in adolescents.

Potentially fatal neuroleptic malignant syndrome (NMS) has been reported in children and adolescents (Silva et al. 1999). Adolescents may present with serious medical complications (S. E. Peterson et al. 1995) or may have NMS without fever (Hynes and Vickar 1996). NMS is treated by discontinuation of the neuroleptic and aggressive supportive measures. The use of specific medications to treat NMS has not been studied in adolescents.

Abnormal laboratory findings are less often reported in studies of children than in studies of adults, but the clinician should be alert to their possibility, especially agranulocytosis or hepatic dysfunction. If an acute febrile illness or easy bruising occurs, medication should be withheld, and a CBC with differential and liver enzymes should be obtained (Campbell et al. 1985). Children may be at greater risk for neuroleptic-induced seizures than are adults because of their immature nervous systems and the very high prevalence of abnormal EEG findings in seriously disturbed children.

Of particular concern is behavioral toxicity, which is manifested as worsening of preexisting symptoms or development of new symptoms such as hyper- or hypoactivity, irritability, apathy, withdrawal, stereotypies, tics, or hallucinations (Campbell et al. 1985). Children and adolescents are more sensitive than adults are to cognitive dulling and sedation resulting from low-potency antipsychotic drugs (e.g., chlorpromazine and thioridazine) that interfere with ability to benefit from school (Campbell et al. 1985; Realmuto et al. 1984).

Anticholinergic side effects are unusual.

Miscellaneous side effects include abdominal pain, enuresis (Realmuto et al. 1984), photosensitivity, and various neuroendocrine effects that may be especially distressing to adolescents. For a more detailed discussion of neuroleptic side effects and their management, see Findling et al. (1998).

Discontinuation

Withdrawal dyskinesias, which are usually transient but potentially irreversible, are seen in 8%–51% of neuroleptic-treated children and adolescents (Campbell et al. 1985). Other withdrawal-emergent symptoms include nausea, vomiting, loss of appetite, diaphoresis, and hyperactivity (Gualtieri and Hawk 1980). A variety of behavioral symptoms may appear up to several weeks after neuroleptic withdrawal and persist for as long as 8 weeks (Gualtieri et al. 1984). These must be distinguished from a return of manifestations of the original disorder. A prolonged drug-free trial may be indicated, if possible, to determine whether neuroleptics are truly needed.

Treatment Resistance

Neuroleptic resistance is common in young schizophrenic patients, although a child whose symptoms have not responded to one neuroleptic may respond to another. If the response is insufficient after a 6-week trial at adequate doses (and assured compliance), another neuroleptic (usually in a different class) should be tried (McClellan and Werry 1994). In open trials and case studies, clozapine has been reported to be effective in a substantial proportion of neuroleptic-resistant adolescents and several children with schizophrenia (Blanz and Schmidt 1993; Frazier et al. 1994; Kowatch et al. 1995; Mozes et al. 1994; Remschmidt et al. 1994). (See Towbin et al. 1994 for suggestions regarding informed consent.)

Common therapeutic errors leading to the perception of neuroleptic resistance include incorrect diagnosis, subtherapeutic or excessive medication doses, premature changes in medication before efficacy can appear, failure to monitor target symptoms or ensure patient compliance, hasty or irrational polypharmacy, and failure to provide psychosocial therapies (McClellan and Werry 1992).

AGGRESSION

Assessment for Treatment

Many aggressive patients have a primary or secondary diagnosis of conduct disorder. When aggression is secondary to another psychiatric diagnosis, such as ADHD (impulsivity, low frustration tolerance), depression (increased irritability), mania (psychosis, irritability), schizophrenia (paranoid delusions or hallucinations), pervasive developmental disorder (decreased ability to communicate verbally), or substance abuse (intoxication or withdrawal), the primary disorder is the appropriate focus of treatment. Adults such as parents, teachers, juvenile justice authorities, and child care and nursing staff are quick to report verbal or physical aggression and demand its elimination. The physician's first duty is to perform a careful evaluation to identify any primary medical or psychiatric disorders. The frequency of brain damage is high in patients with violent conduct disorders, and a focused history may disclose symptoms suggestive of temporal lobe, psychomotor, or complex partial seizures (Lewis et al. 1982).

The youth's environment must be considered in detail, because aggression is often a response to the dynamics or reinforcement structure of a family, school, neighborhood, group home, or inpatient unit. Psychodynamic, systems, cognitive, and behavioral theories may all be useful in understanding the conditions that precipitate and maintain aggressive behavior and in reducing its frequency and severity. Parents and school personnel are likely to be unsophisticated regarding behavior modification, and they may require strong encouragement to institute appropriate contingency management programs. The physician should guard against being persuaded to use medication alone when other interventions instead of or in addition to medication would be more appropriate (e.g., aggression secondary to frustration at overly high academic demands or in response to peer bullying). No evidence indicates that premeditated, predatory aggression (Vitiello et al. 1990) will respond to any drug, unless the patient is so sedated that virtually all activities are limited. On the other hand, medication is preferable to a physical restraint and may facilitate other forms of treatment or permit the child to be placed in a less restrictive environment. A wide variety of medications are used on an as-needed basis in hospital settings to control aggressive behavior. Empirical data on the efficacy of this practice are essentially lacking.

Selection of Treatment

Various classes of medication may be prescribed in an attempt to reduce aggression. If the aggression is impulsive and the youth also has a diagnosis of ADHD, the first choice is a stimulant. In children with ADHD that responds positively to stimulants, oppositional and defiant behavior and aggression are reduced, and activity level and attention improve (Amery et al. 1984; Hinshaw 1991; Hinshaw et al. 1989; Klorman et al. 1989; Murphy et al. 1992; Whalen et al. 1987). Although stimulants have been suggested for the treatment of conduct disorder without ADHD, no data are yet available to support this strategy.

Lithium may be considered in the treatment of children with severe aggression, especially when such aggression is impulsive and accompanied by explosive affect and poor self-control. Although studies have not had consistent results (see Campbell et al. 1995b for a discussion), efficacy has been reported for some hospitalized prepubertal explosively aggressive children with conduct disorder in a double-blind, placebo-controlled trial (Campbell et al. 1995a). Lithium may be the first pharmacological choice for an aggressive child with a family history of bipolar mood disorder (especially if a family member has responded to lithium). (The use of lithium in children is described in the section, "Mood Disorders," earlier in this chapter.)

In patients with severe impulsive aggression with emotional lability and irritability who have abnormal EEG findings or a strong clinical suggestion of episodic phenomena, a trial of carbamazepine may be warranted, although deliberate aggression is rarely part of a frank seizure (R. W. Evans et al. 1987). Preliminary data suggest efficacy in children younger than 12 years with severe explosive aggression, even in the absence of neurological findings (Kafantaris et al. 1992). Efficacy was not shown, however, in a placebo-controlled trial of 22 hospitalized children with a DSM-III-R (American Psychiatric Association 1987) diagnosis of conduct disorder, solitary aggressive type (Cueva et al. 1996). Valproic acid appears to be effective in impulsive forms of aggression (Donovan et al. 2000; Steiner et al. 1998).

β-Adrenergic blockers may be useful in patients with otherwise uncontrollable rage reactions and impulsive aggression, especially those with evidence of organicity (Kuperman and Stewart 1987; Williams et al. 1982). Evidence of organicity does not appear to be a prerequisite for efficacy, however (Grizenko and Vida 1988).

Historically, neuroleptics have been used to control aggression. In view of the risk of cognitive dulling and TD, neuroleptics should be low on the list of medication options. Studies of hospitalized severely aggressive children ages 6–12 years have reported the short-term efficacy of haloperidol (1–6 mg/day or 0.04–0.21 mg/kg/day), thioridazine (mean 170 mg/day), and molindone (mean 26.8 mg/day) compared with placebo in reducing, although not eliminating, aggression, hostility, negativism, and explosiveness (Campbell et al. 1985; Greenhill et al. 1985). There are anecdotal reports of the use of atypical neuroleptics. (The use of neuroleptics in children is discussed in the section, "Schizophrenia," earlier in this chapter.)

Use of many other drugs is speculative at present. One pilot study found that bupropion reduced symptoms of conduct disorder regardless of whether ADHD was also present (Simeon et al. 1986). (The use of bupropion is discussed in the section, "Attention-Deficit/Hyperactivity Disorder," earlier in this chapter.) Trazodone may be useful in decreasing aggression in children with disruptive behavior disorders (Ghaziuddin and Alessi 1992). Clonidine may reduce aggression even in the absence of ADHD (Kemph et al. 1993). (See the earlier section on ADHD regarding the use of clonidine.) A small open-case series suggested that venlafaxine might be useful in conduct disorder, with or without ADHD (Derivan et al. 1995). Reports of several clinical cases noted reduction in aggression in nonpsychotic youngsters after initiation of risperidone (Fras and Major 1995). Based on data from adults and from animal studies, buspirone has been suggested as an option when aggression is presumed to result from anxiety.

Assessment of Response

Careful documentation of precipitants, severity, frequency, type (predatory vs. affective; verbal vs. physical), and targets (property, self, animals, children, adults) of aggression is necessary for evaluating efficacy of treatment. An instrument such as the Overt Aggression Scale (Kafantaris et al. 1996) or the Modified Overt Aggression Scale (Kay et al. 1988) can facilitate this process. Baseline measures are important. Even in samples of children with severe aggression resistant to outpatient treatment, 20%–45% respond (at least temporarily) to hospitalization alone or hospitalization plus a placebo with an immediate and significant decrease in aggressive behavior (Campbell et al. 1995b; Cueva et al. 1996; Malone et al. 1995a).

Use of Carbamazepine

Initiation of Treatment

Baseline hemoglobin, hematocrit, CBC with differential, and liver functions should be measured before starting carbamazepine in a child. The initial dose is 100 mg/day, with food. Use of the brand Tegretol is advised because of reports of both reduced serum levels and toxicity when generic formulations are substituted (Gilman et al. 1993). Children eliminate carbamazepine more rapidly than do adults (Jatlow 1987). Plasma levels (drawn approximately 12 hours after the last dose) are crucial because dosage calculated by weight correlates poorly with plasma concentration. The half-life is approximately 9 hours. Titration is gradual (increased weekly by 100 mg/day), guided by plasma levels, to a usual plateau of 8–12 mEq/mL. Therapeutic levels have not been empirically determined for psychiatric symptoms, but those established for epilepsy help define guides to compliance and toxicity. The usual daily dose range is 10–50 mg/kg, divided into three doses for children and two for older adolescents. Slow-release carbamazepine may be given twice a day for more consistent blood levels. Autoinduction of hepatic enzymes may lead to declining plasma concentration (especially in the first 6 weeks) requiring periodic increases in dose. Carbamazepine lowers the plasma levels of neuroleptics, imipramine, and valproic acid and may reduce the effectiveness of oral contraceptives. Erythromycin causes a clinically significant increase in carbamazepine levels and may result in toxicity.

Continuation, Maintenance, and Monitoring

The degree of ongoing laboratory monitoring necessary is controversial. A conservative recommendation includes CBC and liver function studies weekly for the first 4 weeks, monthly for 4 months, and every 3 months thereafter (Silverstein et al. 1983). A more modest regimen is CBC (with differential and platelet count), serum iron, BUN, and creatinine measurements after the first month and every 3–6 months thereafter (Trimble 1990). Routine monitoring is likely to be ineffective in detecting life-threatening idiosyncratic toxicity. Parents should be instructed to notify the physician, and tests should be ordered if a rash, sore throat, skin infection, facial or periorbital edema, fever, malaise, lethargy, weakness, vomiting, increased urinary frequency, anorexia, jaundice, easy bruising, bleeding, or mouth ulcers develop. If the neutrophil count drops below 1,000 or hepatitis occurs, the drug should be stopped (Silverstein et al. 1983).

Management of Side Effects

The most common adverse effects are drowsiness, headache, incoordination, vertigo, rash, and reversible dose-related leukopenia (especially when carbamazepine is started). Less common side effects include abdominal pain, nausea, vomiting, diplopia, nystagmus, ataxia, tics, muscle cramps, and exacerbation of seizures. Very rare but serious effects are blood dyscrasias (such as thrombocytopenia, agranulocytosis, or aplastic anemia), hepatotoxicity, severe skin reactions (e.g., Stevens-Johnson or systemic lupuslike syndromes), hypersensitivity syndrome (Bellman et al. 1995), and inappropriate secretion of antidiuretic hormone (in rare cases leading to acute renal failure) (Pellock 1987; Trimble 1990). Teratogenic effects have been reported. Adverse behavioral reactions (e.g., extreme irritability, agitation, insomnia, obsessive thinking, hyperactivity, aggression, mania, and psychosis or delirium with hallucinations and/or paranoia) may be seen during the first 1–4 weeks of treatment (R. W. Evans et al. 1987; Herskowitz 1987; Pleak et al. 1988).

Use of β-Adrenergic Blockers

In the drug class of β-adrenergic blockers (see Connor 1993 for a review), the most clinical experience has been accumulated with propranolol. Pindolol and nadolol have been suggested as alternatives with fewer side effects and longer half-lives. Pindolol was modestly effective in a double-blind, placebo-controlled study of children with comorbid ADHD and conduct problems but resulted in frequent paresthesias and distressing nightmares and hallucinations (Buitelaar et al. 1996).

Initiation of Treatment

The premedication workup should include a recent history and physical examination, with particular attention to medical contraindications: asthma, diabetes, bradycardia, heart block, cardiac failure, and hypothyroidism. Fasting blood sugar and a glucose tolerance test may be indicated if the patient is at risk for diabetes. An ECG may be considered.

In children and adolescents, the initial dose of propranolol is 10 mg three times a day, increasing by 10–20 mg every 3–4 days, monitoring pulse and blood pressure (minimum pulse 50 beats/minute, blood pressure 80/50 mm Hg). The standard daily dose range is 10–120 mg for children and 20–300 mg for adolescents, divided into three doses (2–8 mg/kg/day) (Coffey 1990). The short elimination half-life in children (2–4 hours) may necessitate four daily doses. Dose is titrated to clinical effect or side effects. Maximum improvement at a given dose may not be seen for up to 12 weeks. When propranolol or pindolol is used together with chlorpromazine or thioridazine (but not haloperidol), blood levels of both drugs are elevated.

Side Effects

Side effects are generally the same as those in adults. Tiredness, mild hypotension, and bradycardia are the most common side effects.

Discontinuation

β-Blockers should be tapered gradually to avoid rebound hypertension and tachycardia.

Use of Trazodone

The dose of trazodone used in the few reported cases has been 75 mg/day (mean 0.35 mg/kg/day) (Ghaziuddin and Alessi 1992). Reported side effects in youths include mild sedation and increased penile erections. Priapism is possible, with the potential for severe irreversible consequences.

Treatment Resistance

If aggression is not reduced at the highest appropriate drug dose, a different class of drug should be considered. A closer look at the family and school environment is indicated, with initiation of more intensive psychosocial treatment, perhaps including hospitalization.

ANXIETY DISORDERS

Anxiety disorders are one of the most prevalent categories of psychiatric disorders in children and adolescents. Prevalence in community samples is as high as 10% by self-report. Although symptoms of anxiety are widespread in children and often resolve spontaneously or with supportive treatment, when severity and chronicity are sufficient to lead to impairment of functioning and a brief trial of psychosocial intervention is ineffective, pharmacotherapy may be considered. Unfortunately, few controlled trials exist (except in patients with obsessive-compulsive disorder), and establishment of efficacy is confounded by extensive comorbidity and high placebo response rates.

Symptoms of the anxiety disorders overlap, and several trials have included subjects with heterogeneous disorders. A case series review of open clinical trials of fluoxetine (mean dose 25.7 mg/day) for children and adolescents with overanxious disorder, social phobia, or separation disorder ($N = 21$) found moderate to marked improvement in a substantial majority of patients (Birmaher et al. 1994). Interestingly, improvement typically did not begin until after 6–8 weeks of treatment. All patients had been unresponsive to psychotherapy before the drug trial.

A small open trial of buspirone in children and adolescents with various anxiety disorders, some of which were comorbid with other anxiety disorders or with ADHD, was promising in the reduction of anxiety, mood, and behavioral symptoms (Simeon et al. 1994).

Separation Anxiety Disorder

Assessment for Treatment

In separation anxiety disorder, cognitive, affective, somatic, or behavioral symptoms appear in response to genuine or fantasied separation from attachment figures. Common presenting problems are school refusal and insomnia. The differential diagnosis of school avoidance (formerly called *school phobia*) includes medical illness, realistic fear of something at school (e.g., bullies or a punitive teacher), simple phobia, social phobia, agoraphobia, mood disorder, schizophrenia, truancy (secondary to conduct or oppositional defiant disorder), or substance abuse. Certain medications, such as propranolol (prescribed for headache) or haloperidol (prescribed for Tourette's disorder), may produce symptoms of separation anxiety and school refusal.

Selection of Treatment

Psychological interventions such as family therapy, collaboration with school personnel, and behavior modification using contingencies and systematic desensitization are primary (American Academy of Child and Adolescent Psychiatry 1997b). If the child's separation anxiety is being exacerbated by a parent's anxiety or mood disorder, then the parent should also receive direct psychiatric treatment (possibly including medication) as well as guidance in child management. Medication for the child or adolescent may be useful as an adjunct if psychosocial treatment is ineffective after 3–4 weeks.

The efficacy of imipramine in separation anxiety disorder is controversial (Bernstein et al. 1990; Klein et al. 1992), although a recent study found that imipramine adds to the efficacy of cognitive-behavioral therapy (Bernstein et al. 2000). Typical starting doses are low: for example, for children ages 6–8 years, 10 mg at bedtime; for older children, 25 mg at bedtime (McDaniel 1986). The dose may be increased by 10–50 mg/week, depending on the age of the child. Clinical experience suggests that some children respond at a low dose, whereas others

may require the antidepressant dose range. As long as 6–8 weeks may be required for response. Medication is continued for at least another 8 weeks and then gradually withdrawn. (See section "Mood Disorders" earlier in this chapter for more detail on the use of imipramine.)

Benzodiazepines may be used in the short-term treatment of children with severe anticipatory anxiety. Alprazolam (0.03 mg/kg or 0.5–6.0 mg/day) may be useful in the treatment of separation anxiety disorder or school avoidance (Bernstein et al. 1990; Kutcher et al. 1992). In a small ($N = 15$) double-blind, placebo-controlled study of clonazepam (up to 2 mg/day) in children with separation anxiety disorder (and a variety of comorbid anxiety and behavior disorders), some patients appeared to improve, but the results were not statistically significant (Graae et al. 1994). Two subjects experienced serious disinhibition with irritability, tantrums, aggression, and attempted self-injury.

Assessment of Response

Response is measured behaviorally (e.g., return to school, ability to sleep alone) and by questions about subjective distress.

Overanxious Disorder and Generalized Anxiety Disorder

Assessment for Treatment

Overanxious disorder has been eliminated from DSM-IV, and the adult category—generalized anxiety disorder—is now used. Existing studies have used a variety of DSM and non-DSM criteria to select anxious children who experience a variety of worries, almost always including unrealistic worry about future events. These children often appear shy, self-doubting, and self-deprecating and have multiple somatic complaints. They may show habit disturbances, such as nail-biting, hair-pulling, or thumb-sucking.

Selection of Treatment

Several treatment modalities are typically used, although systematic data exist only for behavioral interventions. Behavioral methods include relaxation, desensitization by progressive exposure or in imagination, and contingent reinforcement of approach to feared objects or situations. Psychotherapy is often oriented toward promoting psychological individuation and autonomy in the child and family. Cognitive therapy is directed at changing self-defeating and pessimistic attitudes. Assertiveness training can be helpful, especially in a group setting. Treatment of any parental anxiety disorder is important.

Controlled drug studies of children who have only anxiety disorders are lacking. Benzodiazepines may be used in the short-term treatment of severe anticipatory anxiety in children. Although an open trial of alprazolam (0.5–1.5 mg/day) for children with avoidant and overanxious disorders was promising (Simeon and Ferguson 1987), a double-blind study did not find that alprazolam was superior to placebo in the context of an intensive treatment program (Simeon et al. 1992). Efficacy may have been limited by low doses and the short duration of treatment. Antihistamines are commonly prescribed, but no empirical data exist regarding their use. Anecdotal reports suggest the efficacy of buspirone (15–30 mg/day divided into three doses) in the treatment of overanxious disorder in adolescents (Kranzler 1988; Kutcher et al. 1992).

Assessment of Response

Both behavioral reports from parents and patient ratings of anxiety in target domains are useful.

Use of Benzodiazepines

Initiation of Treatment

Children absorb diazepam faster and metabolize it more quickly than adults do (Simeon and Ferguson 1985). The usual daily dose ranges for children and adolescents are lorazepam, 0.25–6.0 mg; diazepam, 1–20 mg; and alprazolam, 0.25–4.0 mg. The dosage schedule de-

pends on age (i.e., more frequent dosing in young children) and the specific drug (Coffey 1990; Kutcher et al. 1992).

Continuation, Maintenance, and Monitoring

Generally, benzodiazepines should be used for relatively brief periods.

Management of Side Effects

In addition to the risks of substance abuse and physical or psychological dependence, side effects include sedation, cognitive dulling, ataxia, confusion, and emotional lability. Paradoxical or disinhibition reactions may occur, manifested by acute excitation, irritability, increased anxiety, hallucinations, increased aggression and hostility, rage reactions, insomnia, euphoria, and/or incoordination (Coffey 1990; Reiter and Kutcher 1991; Simeon and Ferguson 1985).

Discontinuation

When treatment with benzodiazepines is being discontinued, the dose should be tapered gradually to avoid withdrawal seizures or rebound anxiety.

Use of Antihistamines

Initiation of Treatment

The initial dose of diphenhydramine or hydroxyzine in children and adolescents is 10 or 25 mg/day. Either drug is titrated gradually up to a maximum of 200–300 mg/day (5 mg/kg/day) (Coffey 1990).

Side Effects

The most common side effects are dizziness and oversedation. Some children become paradoxically agitated. Occasionally, incoordination, blurred vision, dry mouth, nausea, or abdominal pain may occur. At high doses, the seizure threshold is lowered. Leukopenia and agranulocytosis are extremely rare. Antihistamines have been reported to cause acute dystonic reactions, tics, and possibly (with chronic administration)

TD. They should not be prescribed for children with asthma because anticholinergic effects dry the mucous membranes.

Use of Buspirone

Initiation of Treatment

Tentative guidelines for use of buspirone in children and adolescents suggest a starting dose of 2.5–5.0 mg/day, increasing to three times a day over 2–3 days (Kutcher et al. 1992). The therapeutic effects may be delayed for 1–2 weeks after reaching the proper dose, with maximal effects not seen for an additional 2 weeks (Coffey 1990). After a 10-day interval to assess efficacy, the dose may be increased gradually to a maximum of 10 mg twice a day in children and 10 mg three times a day in adolescents.

Management of Side Effects and Discontinuation

Reported adverse effects of buspirone in adults include insomnia, dizziness, anxiety, nausea, headache, restlessness, agitation, depression, and confusion (Coffey 1990). Clinical experience with children and adolescents is limited, but side effects appear to be minimal. It is important to distinguish preexisting somatic complaints related to the generalized anxiety disorder from medication side effects. Buspirone can be discontinued relatively rapidly (i.e., over 4 days; Kutcher et al. 1992).

Selective Mutism

Selective mutism, a rare disorder characterized by the child's refusal to speak to certain people and in certain situations, despite the ability to do so, is considered by some to be related to social phobia in adolescents and adults. Psychosocial interventions typically include behavior modification and family therapy. Following several anecdotal reports and open trials, a 12-week

double-blind, placebo-controlled study ($N = 15$) of fluoxetine (0.6 mg/kg/day) reported modest efficacy over placebo according to parent ratings but not clinician or teacher ratings (Black and Uhde 1994). Subjects in both the placebo and the fluoxetine groups showed improvement over baseline ratings, but most subjects remained very symptomatic.

Obsessive-Compulsive Disorder

Assessment for Treatment

Obsessive-compulsive disorder is a chronic and often disabling disorder in childhood and adolescence. In community samples, the point prevalence is 3%–4% (Valleni-Basile et al. 1994; Zohar et al. 1992). Subclinical obsessive-compulsive symptomatology has been reported to occur in approximately 8% of adolescents (Apter et al. 1996; Valleni-Basile et al. 1996). Between one-third and one-half of adult patients with obsessive-compulsive disorder report an onset of the disorder early in life. The clinical manifestations of obsessive-compulsive disorder are similar at all ages, although in children rituals are more common than obsessions (Rapoport et al. 1992).

Selection of Treatment[2]

Pharmacotherapy plays a central role in the treatment of obsessive-compulsive disorder, although patients with childhood onset have a lower response rate to medications (Ackerman et al. 1994). *Within* the child and adolescent population, however, age does not appear to predict treatment response (D. A. Geller et al. 1995). Clinical experience suggests that individual children respond to one medication but not to others. No factors predicting differential response have yet been identified.

Successful treatment often requires the implementation of combined modalities. Cognitive-behavioral techniques have been reported

---

[2] See the American Academy of Child and Adolescent Psychiatry (1998a) practice parameters for a review.

to be efficacious for children with obsessive-compulsive disorder (March et al. 1994), often in combination with medication. Family and individual psychotherapy may be useful for residual symptoms that do not respond to pharmacotherapy.

Double-blind, placebo-controlled studies of clomipramine in youths have reported a 35%–75% reduction in obsessive-compulsive disorder symptoms in 60% of subjects, independent of depression (DeVeaugh-Geiss et al. 1992; Flament et al. 1985; Leonard et al. 1989). Plasma levels of clomipramine and its metabolites correlated with the presence of side effects but not with clinical response. Efficacy appears to be specific for serotonin reuptake blockade because desipramine failed to reduce obsessive-compulsive symptomatology.

Both open and double-blind, placebo-controlled studies of fluoxetine (20–80 mg/day) alone or in combination with low doses of clomipramine have found moderate to marked improvement in obsessive-compulsive symptomatology, including reductions of more than 50% in the level of functional impairment (Riddle et al. 1990, 1992; Simeon et al. 1990). Approximately half of subjects are responders, regardless of the presence of comorbid Tourette's disorder. Preliminary findings from a retrospective study suggest that higher doses of fluoxetine (i.e., 1 mg/kg/day) may result in response rates as high as 74% among both children and adolescents with obsessive-compulsive disorder (D. A. Geller et al. 1995). Other serotonin reuptake inhibitors (SRIs) also may be effective in the treatment of obsessive-compulsive disorder in children and adolescents. Apter et al. (1994) reported that fluvoxamine in doses of 100–300 mg/day resulted in a significant reduction in obsessive-compulsive severity, based on scores on the Yale-Brown Obsessive-Compulsive Scale (Y-BOCS; Goodman et al. 1989) in 14 adolescents with obsessive-compulsive disorder who were treated for 8 weeks. Efficacy did not become apparent until week 6. Neither comorbid disorders (present in 11 subjects) nor

the use of other psychotropic medications influenced treatment response to fluvoxamine. Multicenter controlled trials supported both safety and efficacy of fluvoxamine and sertraline in the treatment of obsessive-compulsive disorder in children and adolescents (March et al. 1998; Riddle and Pediatric OCD Research Group 1996).

In a substantial minority of children with obsessive-compulsive disorder, response to medication is delayed for 8 or even 12 weeks after reaching the expected therapeutic dose. Therefore, the physician should wait at least 10–12 weeks before changing drugs, adding an augmenting drug, or using a high-dose strategy. Early in treatment, some patients experience an exacerbation of obsessive-compulsive symptoms or complain of feeling agitated or "jittery." This phenomenon usually subsides after a few weeks.

Strategies developed for the treatment of treatment-resistant obsessive-compulsive disorder in adults are largely untested in children and adolescents. In general, trials of sufficient dose and duration of two or three different drugs used alone should precede the use of drug combinations to augment response.

Clomipramine. A starting dose of clomipramine, 25 mg/day, has been recommended with increases of 25–50 mg/day every 4–7 days. The maximum recommended dose is 3 mg/kg/day, up to 200 mg/day, although 50 mg/day (1 mg/kg/day) may be sufficient. Response is delayed for 10 days to 2 weeks (as in the treatment of depression), unlike the immediate response seen in the treatment of ADHD or enuresis (Rapoport 1986).

Children's experience of side effects is similar to that of adults, including tremor, fatigue, anticholinergic effects, dizziness, and sweating. Dose-dependent paranoia and aggression have been reported in two case studies. Cardiovascular monitoring (see Table 22–5) is necessary, given the potential for tachycardia, hypertension (and rarely, hypotension), and arrhythmias related to the use of TCAs in children. (See section, "Mood Disorders," for more detail on the use of TCAs.)

Fluoxetine. Fluoxetine is begun at a dose of 5–20 mg/day, usually in the morning. Although early reports cited higher doses, clinical experience suggests that relatively few youths require a dose greater than 20 mg/day for the treatment of obsessive-compulsive disorder, and some may respond to as low as 5 mg/day. Dose adjustments may require alternate-day regimens, use of the liquid formulation, or dissolving medication in juice and dispensing aliquots.

Although children have relatively few somatic side effects (anorexia, weight loss, headaches, nausea, vomiting, tremor), behavioral toxicity is common, perhaps related in part to akathisia. Symptoms include restlessness, insomnia, social disinhibition, agitation (Riddle et al. 1990/1991), and mania (Venkataraman et al. 1992). Suicidal ideation, self-destructive behavior, aggression, and psychotic symptoms have also been reported, although many children with these symptoms had preexisting risk factors for the development of these clinical features (King et al. 1991). Fluoxetine may interfere with sleep architecture, resulting in daytime tiredness.

Treatment typically is required for years. Relapse is common when fluoxetine is discontinued (Leonard et al. 1991).

Fluvoxamine. A typical starting dose of fluvoxamine is 25 mg/day, with a usual treatment range of 100–175 mg/day. Side effects most commonly seen in children are insomnia, agitation, somnolence, and upset stomach.

Assessment of Response

The Leyton Obsessional Inventory—Child Version (Berg et al. 1988) or the Children's Version of the Y-BOCS (Goodman et al. 1989) may be used to quantify symptom severity.

Panic Disorder

Assessment for Treatment

Both panic disorder and agoraphobia occur in children and adolescents (Ballenger et al. 1989). The diagnostic criteria and physical symptom profile are the same as those in adults. Cognitive immaturity may preclude anticipatory anxiety or the characteristic cognitions during an attack (i.e., fear of dying, going crazy, or doing something uncontrolled) (Nelles and Barlow 1988).

Selection of Treatment

There are virtually no systematic data on the treatment of panic disorder in youths. Treatment strategies that have proven successful in adults may be cautiously tried in children and adolescents. Medication doses used are typically conservative to avoid sedation that would impede the patient's academic learning. Supportive and educational individual and family psychotherapy may be useful. Case reports suggest that alprazolam (0.25–2.5 mg/day divided into three or four doses) or imipramine may be effective (Ballenger et al. 1989; Biederman 1987; Kutcher et al. 1992). Clonazepam efficacy (at 1–4 mg/day divided into two or three doses) is supported by preliminary controlled data (Reiter et al. 1992). The benzodiazepines can cause disinhibition and angry outbursts, however (Reiter and Kutcher 1991). Initial titration should be slow. If the patient responds, a maintenance period of 4–6 months should be followed by a drug-free trial to assess continuing need for medication. When discontinuing benzodiazepines, the dose should be tapered gradually (e.g., decreasing by 25% of the initial amount every 3–5 days) to avoid withdrawal symptoms. Other medications that have been used in adults (e.g., SSRIs) may be considered.

Posttraumatic Stress Disorder

Assessment for Treatment

Although the diagnostic criteria for posttraumatic stress disorder (PTSD) are essentially the same at all ages, the symptoms in children differ in some ways from those seen in adults (Terr 1987). Immediate effects include fear of separation from parent(s), of death, and of further fear, leading to withdrawal from new experiences. Perceptual distortions occur, most commonly in time sense and in vision, but auditory, touch, and olfactory misperceptions have been described. Children are likely to reexperience the event in the form of nightmares, daydreams, and/or repetitive, potentially dangerous reenactment in symbolic play or in actual behavior, rather than in intrusive flashbacks. They may later develop a variety of fears, such as fear of repetition of the experience and fear of other situations that may involve separation or danger or may remind the child of the event. Children may experience somatic symptoms, such as headaches and stomachaches. Increased arousal in children is most often manifested as sleep disturbances, which may add to functional impairment in other areas (Pynoos et al. 1987). Regression and guilt are common. Key items in the assessment include preexisting stressors; previous loss, anxiety, or depression; the nature and degree of exposure to the threat; and life changes secondary to the stressor itself.

Selection of Treatment

Controlled trials of any treatments are lacking (see American Academy of Child and Adolescent Psychiatry 1998b for a review). Individual or group insight-oriented play or verbal psychotherapy have been used most often. Systematic desensitization of specific trauma-related fears may be useful in conjunction with other interventions. Supportive therapy for parents and siblings to help them deal with the trauma can reduce contagion. Parents may require therapeutic attention for their own posttraumatic symptoms and/or to help them deal appropriately with their child's symptoms and reenactment.

The use of psychotropic medication to treat PTSD in children has not been systematically evaluated. Anecdotal reports suggest that pro-

pranolol may be effective in the treatment of agitated, hyperaroused children and adolescents with PTSD (Famularo et al. 1988). Propranolol was started at 0.8 mg/kg/day, divided into three doses, with titration to 2.5 mg/kg/day, unless limited by hypotension, bradycardia, or sedation. Case reports suggest the use of carbamazepine (Looff et al. 1995) or guanfacine (Horrigan 1996).

TOURETTE'S DISORDER

Assessment for Treatment

Tourette's disorder (or Tourette's syndrome) is a chronic motor and vocal tic disorder with a duration of more than 1 year, an onset during childhood or adolescence, and a prevalence of 0.03%–1.6%. The tics wax and wane over time and vary in complexity from simple movements or vocalizations (e.g., eye blinks, coughs) to complex, seemingly purposeful behaviors or verbalizations (e.g., facial expressions, coprolalia) (D. Cohen et al. 1992). Genetic studies suggest that Tourette's disorder is an autosomal dominant condition with incomplete, gender-specific penetrance and variable expression (Pauls and Leckman 1986). Linkage studies point to a clinical spectrum that includes Tourette's disorder proper, chronic tic disorder (CTD), obsessive-compulsive disorder, and probably transient tic disorder (TTD). Tourette's disorder is complicated by obsessive-compulsive disorder in 40% of cases. Although about half of the children with Tourette's disorder referred for treatment have ADHD, a genetic association with Tourette's disorder appears unlikely (Pauls and Leckman 1986).

Selection of Treatment

The treatment of Tourette's disorder and associated conditions should be comprehensive and directed toward fostering adaptive development and improving overall functioning rather than simply reducing tic symptoms. Psychopharmacological treatment can be quite effective. Careful monitoring for several months before starting medication is possible because Tourette's disorder is chronic and not usually an emergency. Monitoring permits establishing a baseline of symptoms and assessing the need for psychological and educational interventions.

Neuroleptics

Studies have focused primarily on blockade of dopamine D_2 and α-adrenergic receptors, because hypersensitivity of these neurochemical systems has been hypothesized to underlie Tourette's disorder. Dopamine antagonists have been the mainstay of treatment and are effective in 60%–70% of cases, reducing tic symptoms by approximately 60%–70% (Regeur et al. 1986; A. K. Shapiro and Shapiro 1984; E. Shapiro et al. 1989). Double-blind, placebo-controlled crossover studies using standardized assessments have found that both haloperidol and pimozide (which also acts as a calcium channel blocker) are effective in reducing tics (A. K. Shapiro and Shapiro 1984; E. Shapiro et al. 1989). In a double-blind, placebo-controlled head-to-head comparison, at equivalent doses, pimozide was more effective and had fewer side effects than haloperidol in children and adolescents with Tourette's disorder (Sallee et al. 1997). Other dopamine antagonists, including fluphenazine and piquindone, have been reported to be effective in open clinical trials.

Risperidone, which has both serotonin-2 (5-HT_2) and D_2 receptor antagonism, has undergone preliminary study in the treatment of Tourette's disorder. In open trials of adults with Tourette's disorder, risperidone was effective in decreasing the frequency and severity of both motor and phonic tics in more than half of the patients, including some for whom neuroleptics and/or clonidine were ineffective or poorly tolerated (Bruun and Budman 1996; Van der Linden et al. 1994). Side effects leading patients to discontinue medication were relatively common, however. Clinically and statistically significant reductions in tic frequency and intensity

were reported in an open-label study of seven children and adolescents (age 11–16 years) with Tourette's disorder whose symptoms had not responded to treatment with haloperidol or clonidine (Lombroso et al. 1995). Five patients were receiving concurrent clonidine or an SSRI.

Unfortunately, the neuroleptics have a troublesome side-effect profile. In one clinical sample, 81% of consecutive patients treated with haloperidol for Tourette's disorder discontinued treatment because of side effects (Silva et al. 1996).

α-*Adrenergic Agonists*

Clonidine is effective in ameliorating Tourette's disorder symptoms in a subgroup of patients. Some studies report a 35%–50% reduction in both tic and behavioral symptoms in a substantial minority of patients (Leckman et al. 1991), although other studies report no benefit (Goetz et al. 1987). Vocal tics and associated behavioral manifestations such as impulsivity and restlessness are the most responsive symptoms. Obsessive-compulsive symptoms do not improve. Because of side effects often associated with clonidine (particularly sedation and hypotension), guanfacine, a selective $α_{2a}$-receptor agonist, has been considered as a possible alternative (Chappell et al. 1995). Guanfacine differs from clonidine in having a longer half-life (17 vs. 12.7 hours) and in producing less sedation and hypotension at clinically comparable doses. In one study, 10 subjects with Tourette's disorder and comorbid ADHD experienced a significant reduction in the severity of motor and phonic tics when treated with approximately 1.5 mg/day of guanfacine (in two to three divided doses) (Chappell et al. 1995). The authors noted that guanfacine produced less fatigue and sedation than did clonidine.

Alternative Drugs

Preliminary reports regarding the use of calcium channel blockers and opioid antagonists have been promising, although findings have been inconsistent (Micheli et al. 1990). In one study, clonazepam (when added to clonidine) further reduced tic frequency and severity among seven children with Tourette's disorder, without affecting comorbid ADHD symptomatology (Steingard et al. 1994). In addition, anticholinergic stimulation through the use of nicotine gum has been reported to augment the efficacy of neuroleptics (McConville et al. 1991). Novel treatments are being considered, particularly for refractory cases. Nonsteroidal androgen receptor blocking agents (e.g., flutamide) have yielded modest benefits for some patients with Tourette's disorder (B. S. Peterson et al. 1994).

Treatment of Tourette's Disorder With Comorbidity

Several studies have focused on the treatment of comorbid neuropsychiatric conditions that frequently complicate Tourette's disorder. More than one-half of patients with Tourette's disorder also have obsessive-compulsive disorder. In an open trial, fluoxetine significantly reduced obsessive-compulsive symptomatology (Riddle et al. 1990). Tic frequency and severity were unaffected. These findings were not replicated, however, in a very small controlled trial with less symptomatic patients (Kurlan et al. 1993). Clomipramine, with or without a neuroleptic, has also been advocated for the treatment of Tourette's disorder and obsessive-compulsive disorder (D. Cohen et al. 1992). Patients with Tourette's disorder and obsessive-compulsive symptoms that are refractory to SRIs (e.g., fluvoxamine) may derive substantial benefit from the addition of neuroleptics (e.g., haloperidol) (McDougle et al. 1996). Depression is common among children and adults with Tourette's disorder. If pharmacological treatment is elected, an antidepressant may be used in conjunction with clonidine or a neuroleptic.

For children and adolescents with Tourette's disorder, symptoms of hyperactivity, impulsivity, and distractibility may be more impairing than the tics themselves. Accordingly, treatment is often focused on reducing ADHD

symptomatology. The treatment of comorbid ADHD is complicated and controversial. Stimulant medications have been reported to exacerbate or precipitate tics in as many as half of children with Tourette's disorder (Riddle et al. 1995; see Robertson and Eapen 1992 for a review). Other studies report no change in tics or actual reduction in tic frequency and/or severity among children with Tourette's disorder. In a double-blind study, Gadow et al. (1995a, 1995b) found that 34 prepubertal children with Tourette's disorder and ADHD had a marked reduction in hyperactivity, disruptive behavior, and aggression during methylphenidate treatment phases, without an exacerbation of tics. Although all three dosages (0.1 mg/kg, 0.3 mg/kg, 0.5 mg/kg) were beneficial, 0.3 mg/kg was the optimum minimum effective dose. The severity of either motor or phonic tics across all three observational settings (classroom, lunchroom, and playground) did not increase. Although a small but statistically significant increase in motor tic frequency occurred during classroom observations, vocal tics decreased during lunchroom observations. Current practice suggests that clinicians can give stimulants to children with comorbid ADHD and Tourette's disorder with informed consent and careful observation when behavioral symptoms cause more impairment than the tics and when other drugs are insufficiently effective or have problematic side effects.

Clonidine and desipramine (alone or in combination with neuroleptics) have been suggested as useful treatments for children with Tourette's disorder and comorbid ADHD (D. Cohen et al. 1992). In a double-blind, placebo-controlled, crossover study of 37 children with Tourette's disorder and ADHD (age 7–13 years), 25 mg four times a day of desipramine was superior to 0.05 mg four times a day of clonidine as shown by reductions in parent and teacher ratings of ADHD symptomatology (Singer et al. 1995). Clinical response was not correlated with blood levels of desipramine. Neither medication affected tics. Clinical observation suggests efficacy of nortriptyline in reducing both tics and ADHD symptoms (T. Spencer et al. 1993). Guanfacine has been reported to significantly reduce errors of commission and omission on vigilance tasks and to decrease ADHD symptoms in some patients with Tourette's disorder (Chappell et al. 1995).

Pimozide appears to have less risk than other neuroleptics of cognitive dulling (except at high doses) and may even enhance attention and memory in Tourette's disorder with comorbid ADHD (Sallee et al. 1994). Some clinicians advocate the combination of a neuroleptic and a stimulant (with careful monitoring).

Assessment of Response

The natural waxing and waning course of Tourette's disorder makes evaluation of medication efficacy difficult. A variety of symptom rating scales may be used to quantify the number and severity of tics as well as the patient's school and social impairment (Walkup et al. 1992).

Use of Neuroleptics

Initiation of Treatment

The initial dose of haloperidol is 0.5 mg/day. It may be slowly increased up to 1–3 mg/day, divided into twice-daily doses (D. Cohen et al. 1992). Pimozide, which may be given in a single daily dose, is started at 1 mg/day and may be gradually increased to a maximum of 6–8 mg/day (0.2 mg/kg). Risperidone doses are typically 0.5–9.0 mg/day.

Management of Side Effects

Neuroleptic side effects in children include akathisia, sedation, lethargy, feelings of being like a "zombie," intellectual dulling, weight gain, anxiety, irritability, dysphoria, parkinsonian symptoms, and TD (D. Cohen et al. 1992). In patients with Tourette's disorder, it may be especially difficult to distinguish medication-induced movements from those characteristic of the disorder. Dysphoria and school avoidance have also been reported (Mikkelsen et al. 1981). The side-effect profiles of haloperidol

and pimozide are generally similar, although pimozide may cause less sedation and EPS. Pimozide can affect cardiac electrophysiological functioning, including lengthening of the Q-T$_c$ interval. ECGs should, therefore, be monitored before and during pimozide treatment. Risperidone side effects in children include increased appetite, fatigue, dystonia, muscle stiffness, and almost universal weight gain (8–14 pounds) (Lombroso et al. 1995).

Discontinuation

When haloperidol (and sometimes pimozide) is withdrawn, severe exacerbation of symptoms lasting for up to several months may occur.

Use of α-Adrenergic Agonists

Initiation of Treatment

For clonidine, a gradual increase in dosage to a maximum of approximately 5 μg/kg/day (or 0.25 mg/day) is recommended. A typical guanfacine regimen is 0.5 mg three times per day, titrated up from a starting dose of 0.5 mg/day. (See section, "Attention-Deficit/Hyperactivity Disorder," earlier in this chapter for more information on the use of clonidine and guanfacine.)

Management of Side Effects

Among youths with Tourette's disorder treated with clonidine, 90% experienced transient sedation, and one-third to one-half reported dry mouth, dizziness, and irritability (Goetz et al. 1987; Leckman et al. 1991). Guanfacine has a similar side-effect profile, although it is generally better tolerated than clonidine. In an open-label study, side effects included fatigue, headache, insomnia, sedation, and dizziness/light-headedness (Chappell et al. 1995).

Discontinuation

If the α-adrenergic agonists are to be discontinued, gradual tapering off is recommended to avoid rebound tic symptoms and elevations in blood pressure and pulse.

AUTISTIC DISORDERS

Assessment for Treatment

Autism is a relatively rare developmental disorder of early onset that involves significant deficits in social reciprocity, pragmatic (social) communication, and the range and nature of preferred interests and activities. Autism differs from mental retardation in that there are qualitative deviations of development, not simply delays. Behavioral exacerbations in patients with autism may be a result of changes in routine, environmental stressors, an occult medical problem, or a comorbid psychiatric disorder. Evaluation is made more difficult by the limited communication abilities of many children with autism. Before starting medication, target symptoms should be selected and their baseline level measured. The core symptoms of autism are not generally drug responsive.

Selection of Treatment

Clinicians have used virtually all of the psychotropic medications in attempts to ameliorate the developmental deficits and behavioral difficulties associated with autism. Unfortunately, no medication has yet been identified that fundamentally changes the core social and linguistic deficits. However, medications can often reduce the frequency and intensity of associated behavioral disturbances, which include hyperactivity, agitation, mood instability, aggression, self-injury, and stereotypy, as well as comorbid Axis I disorders. Treatment selection is complicated by the tendency of persons with autism to experience idiosyncratic reactions to psychotropic medications.

Neuroleptics

Drugs such as haloperidol, trifluoperazine, or pimozide result in behavioral improvement in most cases. For example, haloperidol has been evaluated in a series of elegant placebo-controlled studies involving more than 100 autistic children (Anderson et al. 1984, 1989; Campbell et al. 1978). In doses of 0.5–4.0 mg/day, haloperidol significantly reduced hyperactivity, stereotypy, and withdrawal, without adversely affecting cognitive performance. In addition, haloperidol improved discrimination learning and language acquisition when used in combination with positive reinforcement and behavioral interventions (Campbell et al. 1982). The more sedating neuroleptics such as chlorpromazine often cause excessive sedation without significant clinical improvement, however. Case reports show risperidone to be helpful in pervasive developmental disorders (Demb 1996; McDougle et al. 1997).

The use of neuroleptics is discussed in the section, "Schizophrenia," earlier in this chapter. The trial must be of sufficient length to determine whether the drug is efficacious, barring serious side effects requiring immediate discontinuation. If the drug appears to be helpful, it should be continued for at least several months. Although few short-term side effects occur, prospective studies have indicated that withdrawal dyskinesias develop in 25%–30% of children, leading to concern about the potential for development of TD. Birth complications (during delivery) are associated with increased risk of withdrawal dyskinesias and TD in children with autism (Armenteros et al. 1995). Dyskinesias may be difficult to distinguish from the stereotyped movements characteristic of autism. Baseline and periodic follow-up AIMS ratings (and perhaps even videotaping) are indicated (Shay et al. 1993). At 3- to 6-month intervals, the drug should be discontinued so that the child may be observed for withdrawal dyskinesias and to determine whether the drug is still necessary. Some children may have physical withdrawal symptoms or a rebound phenomenon consisting of worsening of behavior for up to 8 weeks after the medication is stopped (Campbell et al. 1985).

Stimulants

Methylphenidate may reduce target symptoms of inattention, impulsivity, and overactivity in some higher-functioning children and adolescents with autistic disorder (Birmaher et al. 1988; Strayhorn et al. 1988). Although preoccupation, withdrawal, and stereotypy may increase, this is not always the case. In a double-blind, crossover study of 10 children ages 7–11 years with autistic disorder and mild cognitive impairment, methylphenidate resulted in modest but statistically significant reductions in hyperactivity without worsening behavior or increasing stereotypy (Quintana et al. 1995). On the basis of behavioral checklist data, hyperactivity decreased in the classroom but not at home. Other behavioral problems (e.g., aggression and self-injury) did not respond. No differences were found between dosages of 10 and 20 mg twice daily. (See section "Attention-Deficit/Hyperactivity Disorder" earlier in this chapter for information on the use of stimulants.)

Opioid Antagonists

Opioid antagonists have been studied in autism because of their possible involvement in attachment behavior and suggestions that endogenous opioid levels may be abnormal in some autistic individuals. Several controlled, acute-dose trials of naltrexone found modest improvements in activity level, attention, and irritability but no significant changes in social behavior (Willemsen-Swinkels et al. 1995b). A longer-term controlled study reported improvements in activity level, social withdrawal, and communication on global assessments but not on more systematic measures (Campbell et al. 1990). In two double-blind, placebo-controlled crossover studies of naltrexone (mean daily dose 1 mg/kg) administration in children (ages 3–8 years) with autism, results were mixed. Hyperactivity and restlessness improved most consistently (Kolmen et al. 1995). Another study found positive effects of naltrexone on teacher reports of hyperactivity and irritability but no effect on parent ratings or playroom observations. Social behaviors and stereotypies did not change (Willemsen-Swinkels et al. 1995b). Plasma naltrexone levels do not correlate with clinical response (Gonzalez et al. 1994). Some children experience mild sedation, but no significant side effects have been reported. Reversible hepatic inflammation may occur at higher doses.

Other Drugs

Several other medications have received preliminary study. Two small controlled trials of clonidine reported modest reductions in hyperactivity, overstimulation, and irritability (Frankhauser et al. 1992). Clinical experience suggests that tolerance often develops to the positive effects of clonidine. Lithium has been reported to reduce symptomatology among autistic individuals with cyclic mood disturbances.

The SRIs have attracted attention because of the frequent occurrence of compulsive, ritualistic behavior among autistic individuals. Two small controlled studies of clomipramine (Gordon et al. 1992, 1993) and several case reports of clomipramine, fluoxetine, and fluvoxamine suggested improvement in compulsive behavior, withdrawal, and irritability. However, in an open-label study of eight autistic children (ages 3–8 years), clomipramine was not effective in ameliorating symptoms associated with autism (based on evaluation with several standard instruments) despite optimal doses (50–175 mg/day or 2.5–4.64 mg/kg/day). In fact, six children were rated as worse on the CGI Consensus Ratings (Sanchez et al. 1996). In a double-blind, placebo-controlled study of adults with autistic disorder, half of the subjects who received fluvoxamine were positive responders (compared with none who received placebo), with reductions in repetitive thoughts and behavior, maladaptive behavior, and aggression and improvement in language use. Several of the fluvoxamine responders had significant improvements in overall adaptive functioning (e.g., moving from a group home to a supervised apartment or obtaining and maintaining full-time employment). Side effects were limited to mild sedation and nausea (McDougle et al. 1996). Sedation may become problematic if it limits energy available for communication or learning.

Studies of the combination of vitamin B_6 and magnesium have serious methodological problems, including small sample sizes, imprecise outcome measures, no adjustments for regression effects, and no long-term follow-up (Pfeiffer et al. 1995). Finally, several case reports suggest that β-blockers, buspirone, and trazodone may reduce agitation and explosive outbursts in some autistic individuals (Ratey et al. 1987).

ENURESIS

Assessment for Treatment

Functional enuresis is diagnosed when the frequency of medically unexplained urinary incontinence exceeds developmental (age-specific) expected norms. Enuresis is strongly familial, especially in males. Neurodevelopmental delays are common in enuretic boys, whereas frequent physiological causes of diurnal enuresis in girls include vaginal reflux of urine, "giggle incontinence," and urgency incontinence. Enuresis is occasionally caused by psychiatric disorders. Anxious children may experience urinary frequency, resulting in daytime incontinence if toilet facilities are not readily available or if the child is fearful of certain bathrooms. In oppositional defiant disorder, refusal to use the toilet may be part of the child's battle for control. Many children with ADHD wait until the last minute to urinate and then lose continence on the way to the bathroom. Secondary enuresis may be related to stress, trauma, or a psychosocial or developmental crisis.

Before starting any treatment, the clinician should obtain baseline measures of frequency of wetting.

Selection of Treatment

For younger children with nocturnal enuresis, the most useful strategy is to minimize second-ary symptoms by discouraging the parents from punishing or ridiculing the child while awaiting the child's maturation. For older children who are motivated to stop bed-wetting, a monitoring and reward procedure may be effective. "Bladder training" exercises may be helpful. If these simple interventions are unsuccessful, a urine alarm combined with behavior modification may be useful. Children may need treatment of comorbid psychiatric disorders and management of psychosocial stressors before they are motivated to participate in or respond to behavioral techniques.

Low doses of a TCA or desmopressin (DDAVP) can be helpful if behavioral interventions are ineffective, an associated mood or anxiety disorder is present, or special occasions (such as overnight camp) arise. Behavioral treatments are the first choice, however, because they avoid medication side effects and last longer. The combination of DDAVP with the urine alarm has been shown to increase the rate of dryness in children with severe wetting and those with family and behavioral problems (Bradbury and Meadow 1995).

All of the TCAs are equally effective in the treatment of nocturnal enuresis. The mechanism is unclear, but they do not seem to work by altering sleep architecture, by treating depression, or via peripheral anticholinergic activity. In 80% of patients, TCAs reduce the frequency of bed-wetting within the first week. Total remission, however, occurs in relatively few. Wetting returns when the drug is discontinued.

DDAVP is an analogue of antidiuretic hormone administered as a nasal spray to treat nocturnal enuresis (see Thompson and Rey 1995 for a review). A major drawback is its expense. A minority of patients become completely dry but usually relapse when medication is stopped (Klauber 1989).

Assessment of Response

Daily charts are used to monitor progress.

Use of Tricyclic Antidepressants

Initiation of Treatment

The treatment of enuresis requires much lower doses of TCAs than does the treatment of depression. As a result, ECG monitoring is not necessary. Imipramine is started at 10–25 mg at bedtime and increased by 10- to 25-mg increments weekly to 50 mg (75 mg in preadolescents), if necessary. Maximum dose is 2.5 mg/kg/day (Ryan 1990). At these doses, side effects are rare.

Treatment Resistance

Tolerance to TCAs may develop, requiring a dose increase. For some children, TCAs lose their effect entirely.

Use of Desmopressin

Onset of action of DDAVP is rapid (several days), and side effects are negligible (rare headache or nasal mucosa dryness or irritation) in patients with normal electrolyte regulation. It acts by increasing water absorption in the kidneys, thereby reducing the volume of urine. Evening fluid restriction is advised, to avoid hyponatremia (possibly resulting in seizures; Beach et al. 1992). The usual dose is 5–40 μg intranasally at bedtime. The likelihood of relapse may be decreased by tapering the drug slowly.

Discontinuation

Because enuresis has a high spontaneous remission rate, children and adolescents taking chronic medication should have a drug-free trial at least every 6 months.

SLEEP DISORDERS

Insomnia

Assessment for Treatment

Chronic insomnia is much more frequent in children with psychiatric disorders than in children without psychiatric disorders. What parents report as the child's insomnia is often related to behavioral or habit problems in settling down for the night, especially in the child with ADHD, oppositional defiant disorder, or separation anxiety disorder. Difficulty falling asleep, sleep continuity disturbance, and/or early-morning awakening can be secondary to depression, psychosis, or separation anxiety. A decreased need for sleep can be a symptom of mania. Insomnia may also be secondary to prescribed or over-the-counter medication (e.g., phenobarbital, theophylline, decongestants, or stimulants) or to substance abuse. A detailed sleep diary is needed before initiating any treatment. Sleep laboratory studies may be useful in complex cases.

Selection of Treatment

The first step is treatment of any primary psychiatric disorder. To address true insomnia, parents or adolescents are taught to remove environmental factors interfering with sleep and to develop a bedtime routine, which may include the use of a transitional object or a night-light. Behavioral treatment removes the secondary gain of parental attention for night wakening and provides positive reinforcement for appropriate sleep behavior, or at least for staying quietly in the child's own room. Older children and adolescents may benefit from hypnosis or systematic instruction in relaxation techniques. Short-term medication may facilitate faster results of a behavioral program with less distress to parent and child or may provide parents with a respite to regain enough energy to pursue other solutions.

Many children respond with paradoxical agitation to sedatives. Hypnotic medications are not recommended for chronic use. Chloral hydrate (25–50 mg/kg 30 minutes before bedtime with a maximum dose of 1,000 mg) or diazepam (0.2 mg/kg in preschool-aged children or 1–2 mg in school-aged children) may be indicated for short-term (3–5 days) use in a crisis or for severe insomnia that has not responded to psychological interventions (Dahl 1995).

Sleep Terror Disorder (Pavor Nocturnus) and Sleepwalking Disorder (Somnambulism)

Assessment for Treatment

Episodes of sleep terror typically occur during the first third of the night, in non–rapid eye movement (REM) sleep Stages 3 and 4, lasting 1–10 minutes. The child appears terrified, screams, stares, has dilated pupils, sweats, and has rapid pulse and hyperventilation. He or she is agitated and confused and cannot be comforted. When alert, the child most commonly has no memory of the episode. Return to sleep is rapid when the episode is over, with complete amnesia in the morning. Stress, anxiety, change in sleep schedule, exhaustion, or a febrile illness may increase the frequency of episodes. In children, no associated psychopathology is usually found. Various sedative, neuroleptic, and antidepressant medications, alone or in combination, have been reported to cause night terrors and/or somnambulism (Nino-Murcia and Dement 1987).

Sleepwalking is characterized by repeated episodes of arising from bed and engaging in motor activities while still asleep. Episodes (which last a few minutes to a half-hour) typically occur 1–3 hours after falling asleep, during Stage 3 and 4 delta (non-REM) sleep. The child or adolescent engages in perseverative, stereotyped movements (e.g., picking at blankets) that may progress to walking and other complex behaviors. The child is difficult to awaken, and his or her coordination is poor. Speech, when present, is usually incomprehensible. The youngster may awaken and be confused, may return to bed, or may lie down somewhere else and continue sleeping. The risk of injury is high. Morning amnesia is typical. Sleepwalking is often seen in children who had night terrors when younger. Likelihood of sleepwalking is increased when the child is overtired or under stress.

Selection of Treatment

For both sleep terror disorder and sleepwalking, restricting fluids prior to bedtime may avoid episodes that are triggered by a full bladder (Nino-Murcia and Dement 1987). Most cases of both disorders respond to support and education while waiting for the child to outgrow the problem. An adequate sleep schedule should be arranged and any specific anxieties or fears addressed. Parents of sleepwalkers should be guided to remove hazards in the environment, and they may need to lock the child's door. Medication (i.e., low doses of imipramine, diazepam, or clonazepam at bedtime) is used only if the episodes are frequent, are dangerous, severely disrupt the family, or interfere with the child's daytime functioning (Nino-Murcia and Dement 1987; Pesikoff and Davis 1971). Imipramine may be given at a dose of 10–50 mg (depending on weight) at bedtime.

EMOTIONAL AND BEHAVIORAL SYMPTOMS IN MENTALLY RETARDED CHILDREN AND ADOLESCENTS

Assessment for Treatment

Mental retardation is a developmental condition that includes subaverage intellectual functioning, impairments in adaptive behavior, and an onset during the developmental period. As such, mental retardation is not amenable to pharmacological treatment. Most people with mental retardation do not have emotional and behavioral difficulties. If such difficulties do occur, the clinician should conduct a thorough assessment to identify a psychiatric disorder and/or psychosocial stressors responsible for the symptoms and then should develop a comprehensive treatment plan. Community-based epidemiological studies indicate that the prevalence of psychiatric disorders among people with mental retardation is higher than in the general population (Gillberg et al. 1986). The full range of psychopathology is present. To improve the validity and reliability of psychiatric diagnosis, standardized assessment instruments can be used, such as the BDI, the CDI, the Aberrant Behavior Checklist (Aman et al. 1985), the Psychopathology Instrument for Mentally Retarded Adults (Aman et al. 1986), and others (Sturmey et al. 1991).

Selection of Treatment

Psychotropic medications can play an important role in the treatment of psychiatric disorders affecting individuals with mental retardation (Aman and Singh 1988; Bregman 1991). Drug selection is made according to the specific disorder that is comorbid with mental retardation.

ADHD

About 10%–20% of children with mental retardation manifest symptoms of ADHD. Well-controlled studies involving more than 100 subjects indicated that methylphenidate significantly reduces hyperactivity, impulsivity, and inattention and improves performance on laboratory measures of attention and memory (Handen et al. 1990, 1992). Responders (60%–75% of those studied) tend to have milder cognitive deficits and to be free from comorbid disorders such as autism and schizophrenia. Other predictors of a positive response to methylphenidate include higher baseline parent and teacher ratings of impulsivity and activity level, higher baseline teacher ratings of inattention and conduct problems, male gender, higher socioeconomic status, and Caucasian heritage (Handen et al. 1994). Children with mental retardation may be particularly prone to side effects such as irritability, social withdrawal, stereotypy, and overinclusive attention.

Schizophrenia

Schizophrenia affects 1%–2% of the mentally retarded population. Neuroleptic medications appear to be as efficacious among patients with mental retardation as they are among those in the general population (Menolascino et al. 1986). Treatment-resistant schizophrenia with cognitive impairments may respond to atypical neuroleptics.

Mood Disorders

Major and minor depression are common among mentally retarded individuals, and case reports documented the efficacy of antidepressants. However, double-blind studies are greatly needed. Mood-stabilizing agents (e.g., lithium carbonate, anticonvulsants) have received preliminary study for the treatment of bipolar disorder and aggressive behavior among individuals with mental retardation. For example, clinical reports and two placebo-controlled trials found that lithium was useful in reducing the frequency and severity of affective cycles and of aggressive and self-injurious behavior in as many as two-thirds to three-quarters of patients (Craft et al. 1987).

Obsessive-Compulsive Disorder

Obsessive-compulsive disorder has been reported among persons with mental retardation. An open-label trial of sustained-release clomipramine was reported for the treatment of disabling cleaning and collecting compulsions affecting 11 young adults with mild mental retardation (Barak et al. 1995). An 8-week trial of sustained-release clomipramine, 75 mg/day, resulted in a statistically significant decrease in the severity of compulsive rituals as assessed by several standardized obsessive-compulsive disorder instruments.

Behavioral Symptoms

Most medication studies that have targeted the treatment of stereotypy and destructive behavior in patients with mental retardation have not considered psychiatric diagnosis. Researchers have tried psychotropic medications of various classes, with inconsistent results. The neuroleptics have been studied most extensively. Some reports have been very favorable; however, several well-controlled studies have been discouraging. Risperidone has been promising in open trials (Hardan et al. 1996). The use of neuroleptics for behavioral difficulties must be weighed against their potential side effects, which include impairment in cognitive performance and the development of akathisia or TD (affecting 15%–35% of mentally retarded patients receiving chronic typical neuroleptic treatment). Low-potency neuroleptics may actually increase aggression. When discontinuing neuroleptics, gradual tapering off is recommended because withdrawal-induced symptomatic deterioration (e.g., anxiety, insomnia) may occur. Clonidine has been reported to reduce these symptoms, suggesting that withdrawal symptoms are caused by adrenergic hyperactivity (Sovner 1995).

Medications that enhance serotonergic activity, including lithium, buspirone, trazodone, and fluoxetine, have been reported to decrease aggressive behavior toward self and others. However, only lithium has been evaluated in controlled studies. The endogenous opioid system has been implicated in at least some forms of self-injury and stereotypy. Preliminary studies (some well controlled) of the opioid antagonists naloxone and naltrexone have reported favorable results; however, others have not. In a double-blind, placebo-controlled study of mentally retarded adults with self-injurious behavior, dosages of 50 mg/day for 4 weeks (six subjects) and 150 mg/day for 4 weeks (three subjects) did not have any clinical benefit (Willemsen-Swinkels et al. 1995a). Self-injurious behavior tended to increase with the higher dose. In another double-blind study, 0.5 mg/kg/day of naltrexone administered for 1 month was marginally superior to placebo in decreasing self-injurious behavior (Bouvard et al. 1995).

Some investigators have suggested that heightened noradrenergic activity may result in hyperarousal and may lead to explosive, destructive behavior. Several open clinical trials have reported that β-blockers such as propranolol or nadolol are effective in some cases (Connor et al. 1997; Ratey et al. 1987). Propranolol increases levels of Thorazine and imipramine (Gillette and Tannery 1994). Although benzodiazepines and other sedative-hypnotics are often prescribed for the treatment of destructive behavior among people with mental retardation, exacerbation of aggression and self-injurious behavior and paradoxical excitement may occur. Buspirone has been suggested for reducing anxiety (Ratey et al. 1991) and self-injurious behavior (Ricketts et al. 1994) among patients with mental retardation.

CONCLUSION

Psychopharmacological agents that are used carefully can be powerful additions to the therapeutic armamentarium for children and adolescents. Far more empirical work is required, however, to identify and document optimal treatments.

REFERENCES

Abikoff H, Gittelman R: Does behavior therapy normalize the classroom behavior of hyperactive children? Arch Gen Psychiatry 41:449–454, 1984

Achenbach TM: Integrative Guide for the 1991 CBCL/4–18, YSR, and TRF profiles. Burlington, VT, University of Vermont Department of Psychiatry, 1991

Ackerman DL, Greenland S, Bystritsky A, et al: Predictors of treatment response in obsessive-compulsive disorder: multivariate analyses from a multicenter trial of clomipramine. J Clin Psychopharmacol 14:247–254, 1994

Alessi N, Naylor MW, Ghaziuddin M, et al: Update on lithium carbonate therapy in children and adolescents. J Am Acad Child Adolesc Psychiatry 33:291–304, 1994

Aman MG: Monitoring and measuring drug effects, II: behavioral, emotional, and cognitive effects, in Practitioner's Guide to Psychoactive Drugs for Children and Adolescents, 2nd Edition. Edited by Werry JS, Aman MG. New York, Plenum Medical Book, 1999, pp 99–164

Aman MG, Singh NN (eds): Psychopharmacology of the Developmental Disabilities. New York, Springer-Verlag, 1988

Aman MG, Singh NN, Stewart AW, et al: The Aberrant Behavior Checklist: a behavior rating scale for the assessment of treatment effects. American Journal of Mental Deficiency 89: 485–491, 1985

Aman MG, Watson JE, Singh NN, et al: Psychometric and demographic characteristics of the Psychopathology Instrument for Mentally Retarded Adults. Psychopharmacol Bull 22:1072–1076, 1986

Ambrosini PJ, Emslie GJ, Greenhill LL, et al: Selecting a sequence of antidepressants for treating depression in youth. J Child Adolesc Psychopharmacol 5:233–240, 1995

Ambrosini PJ, Wagner KD, Biederman J, et al: Multicenter open-label sertraline study in adolescent outpatients with major depression. J Am Acad Child Adolesc Psychiatry 38:566–572, 1999

American Academy of Child and Adolescent Psychiatry: Practice parameters for the assessment and treatment of children, adolescents, and adults with attention-deficit/hyperactivity disorder. J Am Acad Child Adolesc Psychiatry 36: 85S–121S, 1997a

American Academy of Child and Adolescent Psychiatry: Practice parameters for the assessment and treatment of children and adolescents with anxiety disorders. J Am Acad Child Adolesc Psychiatry 36:69S–84S, 1997b

American Academy of Child and Adolescent Psychiatry: Practice parameters for the assessment and treatment of children and adolescents with obsessive-compulsive disorder. J Am Acad Child Adolesc Psychiatry 37:27S–45S, 1998a

American Academy of Child and Adolescent Psychiatry: Practice parameters for the assessment and treatment of children and adolescents with posttraumatic stress disorder. J Am Acad Child Adolesc Psychiatry 37:4S–26S, 1998b

American Academy of Pediatrics: Unapproved uses of approved drugs: the physician, the package insert, and the Food and Drug Administration: subject review. Pediatrics 98:143–145, 1996

American Psychiatric Association: Diagnostic and Statistical Manual of Mental Disorders, 3rd Edition, Revised. Washington, DC, American Psychiatric Association, 1987

American Psychiatric Association: Diagnostic and Statistical Manual of Mental Disorders, 4th Edition. Washington, DC, American Psychiatric Association, 1994

Amery B, Minichiello MD, Brown GL: Aggression in hyperactive boys: response to *d*-amphetamine. J Am Acad Child Adolesc Psychiatry 23: 291–294, 1984

Anderson LT, Campbell M, Grega DM, et al: Haloperidol in the treatment of infantile autism: effects on learning and behavioral symptoms. Am J Psychiatry 141:1195–1202, 1984

Anderson LT, Campbell M, Adams P, et al: The effects of haloperidol on discrimination learning and behavioral symptoms in autistic children. J Autism Dev Disord 19:227–239, 1989

Appler WD, McMann GL: Off-label uses of approved drugs: limits on physicians' prescribing behavior. J Clin Psychopharmacol 9:368–370, 1989

Apter A, Ratzoni G, King RA, et al: Fluvoxamine open-label treatment of adolescent inpatients with obsessive-compulsive disorder or depression. J Am Acad Child Adolesc Psychiatry 33: 342–348, 1994

Apter A, Fallon TJ, King RA, et al: Obsessive-compulsive characteristics: from symptoms to syndrome. J Am Acad Child Adolesc Psychiatry 35: 907–912, 1996

Armenteros JL, Adams PB, Campbell M, et al: Haloperidol-related dyskinesias and pre- and perinatal complications in autistic children. Psychopharmacol Bull 31:363–369, 1995

Armenteros JL, Whitaker AH, Welikson M, et al: Risperidone in adolescents with schizophrenia: an open pilot study. J Am Acad Child Adolesc Psychiatry 36:694–700, 1997

Arredondo DE, Docherty JP, Streeter BA: Bupropion treatment of adolescent depression. Paper presented at the 146th annual meeting of the American Psychiatric Association, San Francisco, CA, May 22–27, 1993

Ballenger JC, Carek DJ, Steele JJ, et al: Three cases of panic disorder with agoraphobia in children. Am J Psychiatry 146:922–924, 1989

Barak Y, Ring A, Levy D, et al: Disabling compulsions in 11 mentally retarded adults: an open trial of clomipramine SR. J Clin Psychiatry 56: 526–528, 1995

Barkley RA: The effects of methylphenidate on the interactions of preschool ADHD children with their mothers. J Am Acad Child Adolesc Psychiatry 27:336–341, 1988

Barkley RA: Attention Deficit Hyperactivity Disorder: A Handbook for Diagnosis and Treatment. New York, Guilford, 1990

Barkley RA: Attention Deficit Hyperactivity Disorder: A Handbook for Diagnosis and Treatment, 2nd Edition. New York, Guilford, 1998

Barkley RA, Fischer M, Newby RF, et al: Development of a multimethod clinical protocol for assessing stimulant drug response in children with attention deficit disorder. J Clin Child Psychol 17:14–24, 1988

Barrickman LL, Perry PJ, Allen AJ, et al: Bupropion versus methylphenidate in the treatment of attention-deficit hyperactivity disorder. J Am Acad Child Adolesc Psychiatry 34:649–657, 1995

Bartels MG, Varley CK, Mitchell J, et al: Pediatric cardiovascular effects of imipramine and desipramine. J Am Acad Child Adolesc Psychiatry 30:100–103, 1991

Bastiaens L: The impact of an intensive educational program on knowledge, attitudes, and side effects of psychotropic medications among adolescent inpatients. J Child Adolesc Psychopharmacol 2:249–258, 1992

Bastiaens L, Bastiaens DK: A manual of psychiatric medications for teenagers. J Child Adolesc Psychopharmacol 3:M1–M59, 1993

Beach PS, Beach RE, Smith LR: Hyponatremic seizures in a child treated with desmopressin to control enuresis: a rational approach to fluid intake. Clin Pediatr (Phila) 31:566–569, 1992

Beck AT, Ward CH, Mendelson M, et al: An inventory for measuring depression. Arch Gen Psychiatry 4:561–571, 1961

Beigel A, Murphy DL, Bunney WE Jr: The Manic-State Rating Scale. Arch Gen Psychiatry 25:256–262, 1971

Bellman B, Schachner LA, Pravder L, et al: Carbamazepine hypersensitivity. J Am Acad Child Adolesc Psychiatry 34:1405–1406, 1995

Berg CZ, Whitaker A, Davies M, et al: The survey form of the Leyton Obsessional Inventory—Child Version: norms from an epidemiological study. J Am Acad Child Adolesc Psychiatry 27:759–763, 1988

Bernstein GA, Garfinkel BD, Borchardt CM: Comparative studies of pharmacotherapy for school refusal. J Am Acad Child Adolesc Psychiatry 29: 773–781, 1990

Bernstein GA, Borchardt CM, Perwien AR, et al: Imipramine plus cognitive-behavioral therapy in the treatment of school refusal. J Am Acad Child Adolesc Psychiatry 39:276–283, 2000

Biederman J: Clonazepam in the treatment of prepubertal children with panic-like symptoms. J Clin Psychiatry 48 (suppl):38–41, 1987

Biederman J: Sudden death in children treated with a tricyclic antidepressant. J Am Acad Child Adolesc Psychiatry 30:495–498, 1991

Biederman J, Baldessarini RJ, Wright V, et al: A double-blind placebo controlled study of desipramine in the treatment of ADD, I: efficacy. J Am Acad Child Adolesc Psychiatry 28: 777–784, 1989a

Biederman J, Baldessarini RJ, Wright V, et al: A double-blind placebo controlled study of desipramine in the treatment of ADD, II: serum drug levels and cardiovascular findings. J Am Acad Child Adolesc Psychiatry 28:903–911, 1989b

Biederman J, Baldessarini RJ, Goldblatt A: A naturalistic study of 24-hour electrocardiographic recordings and echocardiographic findings in children and adolescents treated with desipramine. J Am Acad Child Adolesc Psychiatry 32:805–813, 1993

Biederman J, Thisted RA, Greenhill LL, et al: Estimation of the association between desipramine and the risk for sudden death in 5- to 14-year-old children. J Clin Psychiatry 56:87–93, 1995

Biederman J, Klein RG, Pine DS, et al: Debate forum: resolved: mania is mistaken for ADHD in prepubertal children. J Am Acad Child Adolesc Psychiatry 37:1091–1099, 1998

Birmaher B, Quintana H, Greenhill LL: Methylphenidate treatment of hyperactive autistic children. J Am Acad Child Adolesc Psychiatry 27:248–251, 1988

Birmaher B, Greenhill L, Cooper T, et al: Sustained release methylphenidate: pharmacokinetic studies in ADHD males. J Am Acad Child Adolesc Psychiatry 28:768–772, 1989

Birmaher B, Waterman GS, Ryan N, et al: Fluoxetine for childhood anxiety disorders. J Am Acad Child Adolesc Psychiatry 33:993–999, 1994

Black B, Uhde TW: Treatment of elective mutism with fluoxetine: a double-blind, placebo-controlled study. J Am Acad Child Adolesc Psychiatry 33:1000–1006, 1994

Blanz B, Schmidt MH: Clozapine for schizophrenia (letter). J Am Acad Child Adolesc Psychiatry 32:223, 1993

Bouvard MP, Leboyer M, Launay JM, et al: Low dose naltrexone effects on plasma chemistries and clinical symptoms in autism: a double-blind, placebo-controlled study. Psychiatry Res 58:191–201, 1995

Bradbury MG, Meadow SR: Combined treatment with enuresis alarm and desmopressin for nocturnal enuresis. Acta Paediatr 84:1014–1018, 1995

Bregman JD: Current developments in the understanding of mental retardation, part II: psychopathology. J Am Acad Child Adolesc Psychiatry 30:861–872, 1991

Briant RH: An introduction to clinical pharmacology, in Pediatric Psychopharmacology: The Use of Behavior Modifying Drugs in Children. Edited by Werry JS. New York, Brunner/Mazel, 1978, pp 3–28

Brown RT, Sexson SB: Effects of methylphenidate on cardiovascular responses in attention deficit hyperactivity disordered adolescents. J Adolesc Health 10:179–183, 1989

Brown TE, Gammon GD: ADHD-associated difficulties falling asleep and awakening: clonidine and methylphenidate treatments. Paper presented at the annual meeting of the American Academy of Child and Adolescent Psychiatry, Washington, DC, October 1992

Bruun RD, Budman CL: Risperidone as a treatment for Tourette's syndrome. J Clin Psychiatry 57:29–31, 1996

Buitelaar JK, van der Gaag RJ, Swaab-Barneveld H, et al: Pindolol and methylphenidate in children with attention-deficit hyperactivity disorder: clinical efficacy and side-effects. J Child Psychol Psychiatry 37:587–595, 1996

Campbell M, Anderson LT, Meier M, et al: A comparison of haloperidol, behavior therapy, and their interaction in autistic children. Journal of the American Academy of Child Psychiatry 17:640–655, 1978

Campbell M, Anderson LT, Small AM, et al: The effects of haloperidol on learning and behavior in autistic children. J Autism Dev Disord 12:167–175, 1982

Campbell M, Green WH, Deutsch SI (eds): Child and Adolescent Psychopharmacology. Beverly Hills, CA, Sage, 1985

Campbell M, Anderson LT, Small AM, et al: Naltrexone in autistic children: a double-blind and placebo-controlled study. Psychopharmacol Bull 26:130–135, 1990

Campbell M, Adams PB, Small AM, et al: Lithium in hospitalized aggressive children with conduct disorder: a double-blind and placebo-controlled study. J Am Acad Child Adolesc Psychiatry 34:445–453, 1995a

Campbell M, Kafantaris V, Cueva JE: An update on the use of lithium carbonate in aggressive children and adolescents with conduct disorder. Psychopharmacol Bull 31:93–102, 1995b

Campbell M, Rapoport JL, Simpson GM: Antipsychotics in children and adolescents. J Am Acad Child Adolesc Psychiatry 38:537–545, 1999

Cantwell DP, Swanson J, Connor DF: Case study: adverse response to clonidine. J Am Acad Child Adolesc Psychiatry 36:539–544, 1997

Carlson CL, Pelham WE, Milich R, et al: Single and combined effects of methylphenidate and behavior therapy on the classroom performance of children with attention-deficit hyperactivity disorder. J Abnorm Child Psychol 20:213–232, 1992

Chappell PB, Riddle MA, Scahill L, et al: Guanfacine treatment of comorbid attention-deficit hyperactivity disorder and Tourette's syndrome: preliminary clinical experience. J Am Acad Child Adolesc Psychiatry 34:1140–1146, 1995

Coffey BJ: Anxiolytics for children and adolescents: traditional and new drugs. J Child Adolesc Psychopharmacol 1:57–83, 1990

Cohen D, Riddle M, Leckman J: Pharmacotherapy of Tourette's syndrome and associated disorders. Psychiatr Clin North Am 15:109–129, 1992

Cohen NJ, Sullivan J, Minde K, et al: Evaluation of the relative effectiveness of methylphenidate and cognitive behavior modification in the treatment of kindergarten-aged hyperactive children. J Abnorm Child Psychol 9:43–54, 1981

Conners CK: A teacher rating scale for use in drug studies with children. Am J Psychiatry 126:884–888, 1969

Conners CK: Controlled trial of methylphenidate in preschool children with minimal brain dysfunction. International Journal of Mental Health 4:61–74, 1975

Conners CK: Methodology of antidepressant drug trials for treating depression in adolescents. J Child Adolesc Psychopharmacol 2:11–22, 1992

Conners CK, Casat CD, Gualtieri CT, et al: Bupropion hydrochloride in attention deficit disorder with hyperactivity. J Am Acad Child Adolesc Psychiatry 35:1314–1321, 1996

Connor DF: Beta blockers for aggression: a review of the pediatric experience. J Child Adolesc Psychopharmacol 3:99–114, 1993

Connor DF, Ozbayrak KR, Benjamin S, et al: A pilot study of nadolol for overt aggression in developmentally delayed individuals. J Am Acad Child Adolesc Psychiatry 36:826–834, 1997

Connor DF, Fletcher KE, Swanson JM: A meta-analysis of clonidine for symptoms of attention-deficit hyperactivity disorder. J Am Acad Child Adolesc Psychiatry 38:1551–1559, 1999

Coté CJ, Kauffman RE, Troendle GJ, et al: Is the "therapeutic orphan" about to be adopted? Pediatrics 98:118–123, 1996

Craft M, Ismail IA, Krishnamurti D, et al: Lithium in the treatment of aggression in mentally handicapped patients: a double-blind trial. Br J Psychiatry 150:685–689, 1987

Cueva JE, Overall JE, Small AM, et al: Carbamazepine in aggressive children with conduct disorder: a double-blind and placebo-controlled study. J Am Acad Child Adolesc Psychiatry 35:480–490, 1996

Dahl RE: Child and adolescent sleep disorders. Child Adolesc Psychiatr Clin North Am 4:323–341, 1995

Demb HB: Risperidone in young children with pervasive developmental disorders and other developmental disabilities. J Child Adolesc Psychopharmacol 6:79–80, 1996

Derivan A, Agular L, Upton GV, et al: A study of venlafaxine in children and adolescents with conduct disorder. Paper presented at the 42nd annual meeting of the American Academy of Child and Adolescent Psychiatry, New Orleans, LA, October 1995

DeVeaugh-Geiss J, Moroz G, Biederman J, et al: Clomipramine hydrochloride in childhood and adolescent obsessive compulsive disorder: multicenter trial. J Am Acad Child Adolesc Psychiatry 31:45–49, 1992

Diamond JM, Deane FP: Conners Teacher's Questionnaire: is frequent administration clinically useful? Paper presented at annual meeting of the American Academy of Child and Adolescent Psychiatry, Seattle, WA, October 1988

Doherty M, Gordon A, Brown J, et al: Placebo substitution during medication reductions: controlling for expectancies. Paper presented at the annual meeting of the American Academy of Child and Adolescent Psychiatry, October 1987

Donnelly M, Zametkin AJ, Rapoport JL, et al: Treatment of childhood hyperactivity with desipramine: plasma drug concentration, cardiovascular effects, plasma and urinary catecholamine levels, and clinical response. Clin Pharmacol Ther 39:72–81, 1986

Donovan ST, Stewart JW, Nunes EV, et al: Divalproex treatment for youth with explosive temper and mood lability: a double-blind, placebo-controlled crossover design. Am J Psychiatry 157:818–820, 2000

Dulcan MK (ed): Information for Parents, Youth, and Teachers on Medications for Feelings and Behavior. Washington, DC, American Psychiatric Press, 1999

Dulcan MK, Martini DR: Concise Guide to Child and Adolescent Psychiatry. Washington, DC, American Psychiatric Press, 1999

DuPaul GJ, Rapport MD: Does methylphenidate normalize the classroom performance of children with attention deficit disorder? J Am Acad Child Adolesc Psychiatry 32:190–198, 1993

DuPaul GJ, Rapport MD, Perriello LM: Teacher ratings of academic skills: the development of the Academic Performance Rating Scale. School Psychology Review 20:284–300, 1991

Edelbrock C, Costello AJ, Kessler MK: Empirical corroboration of attention deficit disorder. Journal of the American Academy of Child Psychiatry 23:285–290, 1984

Elia J, Borcherding BG, Rapoport JL, et al: Methylphenidate and dextroamphetamine treatments of hyperactivity: are there true nonresponders? Psychiatry Res 36:141–155, 1991

Emslie GJ, Rush AJ, Weinberg WA: A double-blind, randomized placebo-controlled trial of fluoxetine in depressed children and adolescents. Arch Gen Psychiatry 54:1031–1037, 1997

Emslie GJ, Walkup JT, Pliszka SR, et al: Nontricyclic antidepressants: current trends in children and adolescents. J Am Acad Child Adolesc Psychiatry 38:517–528, 1999

Evans RW, Clay TH, Gualtieri CT: Carbamazepine in pediatric psychiatry. J Am Acad Child Psychiatry 26:2–8, 1987

Evans SW, Pelham WE: Psychostimulant effects on academic and behavioral measures for ADHD junior high school students in a lecture format classroom. J Abnorm Child Psychol 19:537–552, 1991

Famularo R, Fenton T: The effect of methylphenidate on school grades in children with attention deficit disorder without hyperactivity. J Clin Psychiatry 48:112–114, 1987

Famularo R, Kinscherff R, Fenton T: Propranolol treatment for childhood posttraumatic stress disorder, acute type. American Journal of Diseases of Children 142:1244–1247, 1988

Findling RL, Blumer JL (eds): Child and adolescent psychopharmacology. Pediatr Clin North Am 45(5), 1998

Findling RL, Schulz SC, Reed MD, et al: The antipsychotics: a pediatric perspective. Pediatr Clin North Am 45:1205–1232, 1998

Fine S, Jewesson B: Active drug placebo trial of methylphenidate: a clinical service for children with an attention deficit disorder. Can J Psychiatry 34:447–449, 1989

Firestone P: Factors associated with children's adherence to stimulant medication. Am J Orthopsychiatry 52:447–457, 1982

Fitzpatrick PA, Klorman F, Brumaghim JT, et al: Effects of sustained-release and standard preparations of methylphenidate on attention deficit disorder. J Am Acad Child Adolesc Psychiatry 31:226–234, 1992

Flament MF, Rapoport JL, Berg CZ, et al: Clomipramine treatment of childhood obsessive-compulsive disorder. Arch Gen Psychiatry 42:977–983, 1985

Fletcher SE, Case CL, Sallee FR, et al: Prospective study of the electrocardiographic effects of imipramine in children. J Pediatr 122:652–654, 1993

Frankhauser M, Karumanchi V, German M, et al: A double-blind, placebo-controlled study of the efficacy of transdermal clonidine in autism. J Clin Psychiatry 53:77–82, 1992

Fras I, Major LF: Clinical experience with risperidone (letter). J Am Acad Child Adolesc Psychiatry 34:833, 1995

Frazier JA, Gordon CT, McKenna K, et al: An open trial of clozapine in 11 adolescents with childhood-onset schizophrenia. J Am Acad Child Adolesc Psychiatry 33:658–663, 1994

Fristad MA, Weller EB, Weller RA, et al: Self-report vs. biological markers in assessment of childhood depression. J Affect Disord 15:339–345, 1988

Fristad MA, Weller RA, Weller EB: The Mania Rating Scale (MRS): further reliability and validity studies with children. Ann Clin Psychiatry 7:127–132, 1995

Gadow KD: Pediatric psychopharmacology: a review of recent research. J Child Psychol Psychiatry 33:153–195, 1992

Gadow KD, Swanson HL: Assessing drug effects on academic performance. Psychopharmacol Bull 21:877–886, 1985

Gadow KD, Nolan EE, Sprafkin J, et al: School observations of children with attention-deficit hyperactivity disorder and comorbid tic disorder: effects of methylphenidate treatment. J Dev Behav Pediatr 16:167–176, 1995a

Gadow KD, Sverd J, Sprafkin J, et al: Efficacy of methylphenidate for attention-deficit hyperactivity disorder in children with tic disorder. Arch Gen Psychiatry 52:444–455, 1995b

Gammon GD, Brown TE: Fluoxetine and methylphenidate in combination for treatment of attention deficit disorder and comorbid depressive disorder. J Child Adolesc Psychopharmacol 3:1–10, 1993

Geller B: Valproate and polycystic ovaries: reply. J Am Acad Child Adolesc Psychiatry 37:9–10, 1998

Geller B, Fetner HH: Children's 24-hour serum lithium level after a single dose predicts initial dose and steady state plasma levels (letter). J Clin Psychopharmacol 9:155, 1989

Geller B, Fox LW, Fletcher M: Effect of tricyclic antidepressants on switching to mania and on the onset of bipolarity in depressed 6- to 12-year-olds. J Am Acad Child Adolesc Psychiatry 32:43–50, 1993

Geller DA, Biederman J, Reed ED, et al: Similarities in response to fluoxetine in the treatment of children and adolescents with obsessive-compulsive disorder. J Am Acad Child Adolesc Psychiatry 34:36–44, 1995

Geller JL, Gaulin BD, Barreira PJ: A practitioner's guide to use of psychotropic medication in liquid form. Hospital and Community Psychiatry 43:969–971, 1992

Ghaziuddin N, Alessi NE: An open clinical trial of trazodone in aggressive children. J Child Adolesc Psychopharmacol 2:291–297, 1992

Gillberg C, Persson E, Grufman M, et al: Psychiatric disorders in mildly and severely mentally retarded urban children and adolescents: epidemiological aspects. Br J Psychiatry 149:68–74, 1986

Gillette DW, Tannery LP: Beta blocker inhibits tricyclic metabolism. J Am Acad Child Adolesc Psychiatry 33:223–224, 1994

Gilman JT, Alvarez LA, Duchowny M: Carbamazepine toxicity resulting from generic substitution. Neurology 43:2696–2697, 1993

Gittelman R, Abikoff H, Pollack E, et al: A controlled trial of behavior modification and methylphenidate in hyperactive children, in Hyperactive Children: The Social Ecology of Identification and Treatment. Edited by Whalen CK, Henker B. New York, Academic Press, 1980, pp 221–243

Goetz CG, Tanner CM, Wilson RS, et al: Clonidine and Gilles de la Tourette's syndrome: double-blind study using objective rating methods. Ann Neurol 21:307–310, 1987

Gonzalez NM, Campbell M, Small AM, et al: Naltrexone plasma levels, clinical response and effect on weight in autistic children. Psychopharmacol Bull 30:203–208, 1994

Goodman WK, Price LH, Rasmussen SA, et al: The Yale-Brown Obsessive Compulsive Scale, I: development, use, and reliability. Arch Gen Psychiatry 46:1006–1011, 1989

Gordon C, Rapoport J, Hamburger S, et al: Differential response of seven subjects with autistic disorder to clomipramine and desipramine. Am J Psychiatry 149:363–366, 1992

Gordon CT, State RC, Nelson JE, et al: A double-blind comparison of clomipramine, desipramine, and placebo in the treatment of autistic disorder. Arch Gen Psychiatry 50:441–447, 1993

Goyette CH, Conners CK, Ulrich RF: Normative data on revised Conners Parent and Teacher Rating Scales. J Abnorm Child Psychol 6:221–236, 1978

Graae F, Milner J, Rizzotto L, et al: Clonazepam in childhood anxiety disorders. J Am Acad Child Adolesc Psychiatry 33:372–376, 1994

Greenhill LL: Stimulant-related growth inhibition in children: a review, in Strategic Interventions for Hyperactive Children. Edited by Gittleman M. New York, ME Sharpe, 1981, pp 39–63

Greenhill LL, Osman BB (eds): Ritalin: Theory and Patient Management, 2nd Edition. New York, Mary Ann Liebert, 2000

Greenhill LL, Solomon M, Pleak R, et al: Molindone hydrochloride treatment of hospitalized children with conduct disorder. J Clin Psychiatry 46:20–25, 1985

Greenhill LL, Abikoff HB, Arnold LE, et al: Medication treatment strategies in the MTA study: relevance to clinicians and researchers. J Am Acad Child Adolesc Psychiatry 35:1304–1313, 1996

Grizenko N, Vida S: Propranolol treatment of episodic dyscontrol and aggressive behavior in children. Can J Psychiatry 33:776–778, 1988

Grob CS, Coyle JT: Suspected adverse methylphenidate-imipramine interactions in children. Dev Behav Pediatr 7:265–267, 1986

Gualtieri CT, Hawk B: Tardive dyskinesia and other drug-induced movement disorders among handicapped children and youth. Applied Research in Mental Retardation 1:55–69, 1980

Gualtieri CT, Quade D, Hicks RE, et al: Tardive dyskinesia and other clinical consequences of neuroleptic treatment in children and adolescents. Am J Psychiatry 141:20–23, 1984

Hagino OR, Weller EB, Weller RA, et al: Untoward effects of lithium treatment in children aged four through six years. J Am Acad Child Adolesc Psychiatry 34:1584–1590, 1995

Halperin JM, Gittelman R, Katz S, et al: Relationship between stimulant effect, electroencephalogram, and clinical neurological findings in hyperactive children. J Am Acad Child Adolesc Psychiatry 25:820–825, 1986

Hamilton M: Development of a rating scale for primary depressive illness. British Journal of Social and Clinical Psychology 6:278–296, 1967

Handen BL, Breaux AM, Gosling A, et al: Efficacy of Ritalin among mentally retarded children with ADHD. Pediatrics 86:922–930, 1990

Handen B, Breaux A, Janosky J, et al: Effects and noneffects of methylphenidate in children with mental retardation and ADHD. J Am Acad Child Adolesc Psychiatry 31:455–461, 1992

Handen BL, Janosky J, McAuliffe S, et al: Prediction of response to methylphenidate among children with ADHD and mental retardation. J Am Acad Child Adolesc Psychiatry 33:1185–1193, 1994

Hardan A, Johnson K, Johnson C, et al: Case study: risperidone treatment of children and adolescents with developmental disorders. J Am Acad Child Adolesc Psychiatry 35:1551–1556, 1996

Herskowitz J: Developmental toxicology, in Psychiatric Pharmacosciences of Children and Adolescents. Edited by Popper C. Washington, DC, American Psychiatric Press, 1987, pp 81–123

Hinshaw SP: Stimulant medication and the treatment of aggression in children with attentional deficits. J Clin Child Psychol 20:301–312, 1991

Hinshaw SP, Henker B, Whalen CK, et al: Aggressive, prosocial, and nonsocial behavior in hyperactive boys: dose effects of methylphenidate in naturalistic settings. J Consult Clin Psychol 57:636–643, 1989

Horrigan JP: Guanfacine for PTSD nightmares (letter). J Am Acad Child Adolesc Psychiatry 35:975, 1996

Horrigan JP, Barnhill LJ: Guanfacine for treatment of attention-deficit hyperactivity disorder in boys. J Child Adolesc Psychopharmacol 5:215–223, 1995

Hughes CW, Emslie GJ, Crismon ML, et al: The Texas Children's Medication Algorithm Project: report of the Texas Consensus Conference Panel on Medication Treatment of Childhood Major Depressive Disorder. J Am Acad Child Adolesc Psychiatry 38:1442–1454, 1999

Hunt RD, Capper S, O'Connell P: Clonidine in child and adolescent psychiatry. J Child Adolesc Psychopharmacol 1:87–102, 1990

Hunt RD, Lau S, Ryu J: Alternative therapies for ADHD, in Ritalin: Theory and Patient Management. Edited by Greenhill LL, Osman BB. New York, Mary Ann Liebert, 1991, pp 75–95

Hunt RD, Arnsten AFT, Asbell MD: An open trial of guanfacine in the treatment of attention-deficit hyperactivity disorder. J Am Acad Child Adolesc Psychiatry 34:50–54, 1995

Hynes AFM, Vickar EL: Case study: neuroleptic malignant syndrome without pyrexia. J Am Acad Child Adolesc Psychiatry 35:959–962, 1996

Jatlow PI: Psychotropic drug disposition during development, in Psychiatric Pharmacosciences of Children and Adolescents. Edited by Popper C. Washington, DC, American Psychiatric Press, 1987, pp 27–44

Johnston HF, Fruehling JJ: Using antidepressant medication in depressed children: an algorithm. Psychiatric Annals 24:348–356, 1994

Kafantaris V, Campbell M, Padron-Gayol MV, et al: Carbamazepine in hospitalized aggressive conduct disorder children: an open pilot study. Psychopharmacol Bull 28:193–199, 1992

Kafantaris V, Lee DO, Magee H, et al: Assessment of children with the Overt Aggression Scale. J Neuropsychiatry Clin Neurosci 8:186–193, 1996

Kay SR, Wolkenfeld F, Murrill LM: Profiles of aggression among psychiatric patients. J Nerv Ment Dis 176:539–546, 1988

Kemph JP, DeVane CL, Levin GM, et al: Treatment of aggressive children with clonidine: results of an open pilot study. J Am Acad Child Adolesc Psychiatry 32:577–581, 1993

Kent JD, Bladfer JC, Koplewicz HS, et al: Effects of late-afternoon methylphenidate administration on behavior and sleep in attention-deficit hyperactivity disorder. Pediatrics 96:320–325, 1995

King RA, Riddle MA, Chappell PB, et al: Emergence of self-destructive phenomena in children and adolescents during fluoxetine treatment. J Am Acad Child Adolesc Psychiatry 30:179–186, 1991

Klauber GT: Clinical efficacy and safety of desmopressin in the treatment of nocturnal enuresis. J Pediatr 114:719–722, 1989

Klein RG, Mannuzza S: Hyperactive boys almost grown up, III: methylphenidate effects on ultimate height. Arch Gen Psychiatry 45:1131–1134, 1988

Klein RG, Landa B, Mattes JA, et al: Methylphenidate and growth in hyperactive children. Arch Gen Psychiatry 45:1127–1130, 1988

Klein RG, Koplewicz HS, Kanner A: Imipramine treatment of children with separation anxiety disorder. J Am Acad Child Adolesc Psychiatry 31:21–28, 1992

Klein RG, Abikoff H, Barkley RA, et al: Clinical trials in children and adolescents, in Clinical Evaluation of Psychotropic Drugs: Principles and Guidelines. Edited by Prien RF, Robinson DS. New York, Raven, 1994, pp 501–546

Klorman R, Brumaghim JT, Salzman LF, et al: Comparative effects of methylphenidate on attention-deficit hyperactivity disorder with and without aggressive/noncompliant features. Psychopharmacol Bull 25:109–113, 1989

Klorman R, Brumaghim JT, Fitzpatrick P, et al: Clinical effects of a controlled trial of methylphenidate on adolescents with attention deficit disorder. J Am Acad Child Adolesc Psychiatry 29:702–709, 1990

Knight MM, Wigder KS, Fortsch MM, et al: Medication education for children: is it worthwhile? Journal of Child Psychiatric Nursing 3:25–28, 1990

Kolmen BK, Feldman HM, Handen BL, et al: Naltrexone in young autistic children: a double-blind, placebo-controlled cross-over study. J Am Acad Child Adolesc Psychiatry 34:223–231, 1995

Kovacs M: The Children's Depression Inventory (CDI). Psychopharmacol Bull 21:995–998, 1985

Kowatch RA, Suppes T, Gilfillan SK, et al: Clozapine treatment of children and adolescents with bipolar disorder and schizophrenia: a clinical case series. J Child Adolesc Psychopharmacol 5:241–253, 1995

Kranzler HR: Use of buspirone in an adolescent with overanxious disorder. J Am Acad Child Adolesc Psychiatry 27:789–790, 1988

Kumra S, Frazier JA, Jacobsen LK, et al: Childhood-onset schizophrenia: A double-blind clozapine-haloperidol comparison. Arch Gen Psychiatry 53:1090–1097, 1996

Kuperman S, Stewart MA: Use of propranolol to decrease aggressive outbursts in younger patients. Psychosomatics 28:315–319, 1987

Kurlan R, Como PG, Deeley C, et al: A pilot controlled study of fluoxetine for obsessive-compulsive symptoms in children with Tourette's syndrome. Clin Neuropharmacol 16:167–172, 1993

Kutcher SP: Child and Adolescent Psychopharmacology. Philadelphia, PA, WB Saunders, 1997

Kutcher SP, MacKenzie S, Galarraga W, et al: Clonazepam treatment of adolescents with neuroleptic-induced akathisia. Am J Psychiatry 144:823–824, 1987

Kutcher SP, Reiter S, Gardner DM, et al: The pharmacotherapy of anxiety disorders in children and adolescents. Psychiatr Clin North Am 15:41–67, 1992

Leckman JF, Ort S, Caruso KA, et al: Rebound phenomena in Tourette's syndrome after abrupt withdrawal of clonidine. Arch Gen Psychiatry 43:1168–1176, 1986

Leckman J, Hardin M, Riddle M, et al: Clonidine treatment of Gilles de la Tourette's syndrome. Arch Gen Psychiatry 48:324–328, 1991

Leonard HL, Swedo SE, Rapoport JL, et al: Treatment of obsessive compulsive disorder with clomipramine and desipramine in children and adolescents. Arch Gen Psychiatry 46:1088–1092, 1989

Leonard HL, Swedo SE, Lenane MC, et al: A double-blind desipramine substitution during long-term clomipramine treatment in children and adolescents with obsessive-compulsive disorder. Arch Gen Psychiatry 48:922–927, 1991

Leonard HL, Meyer MC, Swedo SE, et al: Electrocardiographic changes during desipramine and clomipramine treatment in children and adolescents. J Am Acad Child Adolesc Psychiatry 34:1460–1468, 1995

Lewis DW, Pincus JH, Shanok SS, et al: Psychomotor epilepsy and violence in a group of incarcerated adolescent boys. Am J Psychiatry 139:882–887, 1982

Liberthson RR: Sudden death from cardiac causes in children and young adults. N Engl J Med 334:1039–1044, 1996

Lombroso PJ, Scahill L, King RA, et al: Risperidone treatment of children and adolescents with chronic tic disorders: a preliminary report. J Am Acad Child Adolesc Psychiatry 34:1147–1152, 1995

Loney J, Milich R: Hyperactivity, inattention, and aggression in clinical practice. Advances in Developmental and Behavioral Pediatrics 3:113–147, 1982

Looff D, Grimley P, Kuller F, et al: Carbamazepine for PTSD. J Am Acad Child Adolesc Psychiatry 34:703–704, 1995

Malone RP, Biesecker KA, Luebbert JF, et al: Importance of placebo baseline in clinical drug trials involving aggressive children (abstract). Psychopharmacol Bull 31:593, 1995a

Malone RP, Delaney MA, Luebbert JF, et al: The lithium test dose prediction method in aggressive children. Psychopharmacol Bull 31:379–381, 1995b

Mandoki MW: Risperidone treatment of children and adolescents: increased risk of extrapyramidal side effects? J Child Adolesc Psychopharmacol 5:49–67, 1995

March JS, Mulle K, Herbel B: Behavioral psychotherapy for children and adolescents with obsessive-compulsive disorder: an open trial of a new protocol-driven treatment package. J Am Acad Child Adolesc Psychiatry 33:333–341, 1994

March JS, Biederman J, Wolkow R, et al: Sertraline in children and adolescents with obsessive-compulsive disorder: a multicenter randomized controlled trial. JAMA 280:1752–1756, 1998

McBride MC: An individual double-blind cross-over trial for assessing methylphenidate response in children with attention deficit disorder. J Pediatr 113:137–145, 1988

McClellan JM, Werry JS: Schizophrenia. Psychiatr Clin North Am 15:131–148, 1992

McClellan J, Werry J: Practice parameters for the assessment and treatment of children and adolescents with schizophrenia. J Am Acad Child Adolesc Psychiatry 33:616–635, 1994

McConville BJ, Fogelson MH, Norman AB, et al: Nicotine potentiation of haloperidol in reducing tic frequency in Tourette's disorder. Am J Psychiatry 148:793–794, 1991

McConville BJ, Minnery KL, Sorter MT, et al: An open study of the effects of sertraline on adolescent major depression. J Child Adolesc Psychopharmacol 6:41–51, 1996

McDaniel KD: Pharmacologic treatment of psychiatric and neurodevelopmental disorders in children and adolescents (part 1). Clin Pediatr (Phila) 25:65–71, 1986

McDougle CJ, Naylor ST, Cohen DJ, et al: A double-blind, placebo-controlled study of fluvoxamine in adults with autistic disorder. Arch Gen Psychiatry 53:1001–1008, 1996

McDougle CJ, Holmes JP, Bronson MR, et al: Risperidone treatment of children and adolescents with pervasive developmental disorders: a prospective, open-label study. J Am Acad Child Adolesc Psychiatry 36:685–693, 1997

Menolascino F, Wilson J, Golden C, et al: Medication and treatment of schizophrenia in persons with mental retardation. Ment Retard 24:277–283, 1986

Micheli F, Gatto M, Lekhuniec E, et al: Treatment of Tourette's syndrome with calcium antagonists. Clin Neuropharmacol 13:77–83, 1990

Mikkelsen EJ, Detlor J, Cohen DJ: School avoidance and social phobia triggered by haloperidol in patients with Tourette's disorder. Am J Psychiatry 138:1572–1576, 1981

Mozes T, Toren P, Chernauzan N, et al: Clozapine treatment in very early onset schizophrenia. J Am Acad Child Adolesc Psychiatry 33:65–70, 1994

MTA Cooperative Group: A 14-month randomized clinical trial of treatment strategies for attention-deficit/hyperactivity disorder. Arch Gen Psychiatry 56:1073–1086, 1999a

MTA Cooperative Group: Moderators and mediators of treatment response for children with attention-deficit/hyperactivity disorder. Arch Gen Psychiatry 56:1088–1096, 1999b

Munetz MR, Benjamin S: How to examine patients using the Abnormal Involuntary Movement Scale. Hospital and Community Psychiatry 39:1172–1177, 1988

Murphy DA, Pelham WE, Lang AR: Aggression in boys with attention deficit-hyperactivity disorder: methylphenidate effects on naturalistically observed aggression, response to provocation, and social information processing. J Abnorm Child Psychol 20:451–466, 1992

Nehra A, Mullick F, Ishak KG, et al: Pemoline-associated hepatic injury. Gastroenterology 99:1517–1519, 1990

Nelles WB, Barlow DH: Do children panic? Clin Psychol Rev 8:359–372, 1988

Nino-Murcia G, Dement WC: Psychophysiological and pharmacological aspects of somnambulism and night terrors in children, in Psychopharmacology: The Third Generation of Progress. Edited by Meltzer HY. New York, Raven, 1987, pp 873–879

Overholser JC, Brinkman DC, Lehnert KL, et al: Children's Depression Rating Scale—Revised: development of a short form. J Clin Child Psychol 24:443–452, 1995

Patterson JF: Hepatitis associated with pemoline (letter). South Med J 77:938, 1984

Pauls DL, Leckman JF: The inheritance of Gilles de la Tourette syndrome and associated behaviors: evidence for an autosomal dominant transmission. N Engl J Med 315:993–997, 1986

Pelco LE, Kissel RC, Parrish JM, et al: Behavioral management of oral medication administration difficulties among children: a review of literature with case illustrations. Dev Behav Pediatr 8:90–96, 1987

Pelham WE: The effects of stimulant drugs on learning and achievement in hyperactive and learning disabled children, in Psychological and Educational Perspectives on Learning Disabilities. Edited by Torgesen JK, Wong B. New York, Academic Press, 1985, pp 259–295

Pelham WE, Bender ME: Peer relationships in hyperactive children: description and treatment. Advances in Learning and Behavioral Disabilities 1:365–436, 1982

Pelham WE, Murphy HA: Attention deficit and conduct disorders, in Pharmacological and Behavioral Treatment: An Integrative Approach. Edited by Hersen M. New York, Wiley, 1986, pp 108–148

Pelham WE, Schnedler RW, Bologna NC, et al: Behavioral and stimulant treatment of hyperactive children: a therapy study with methylphenidate probes in a within-subject design. J Appl Behav Anal 13:221–236, 1980

Pelham WE, Milich R, Walker JL: Effects of continuous and partial reinforcement and methylphenidate on learning in children with attention deficit disorder. J Abnorm Psychol 95:319–325, 1986

Pelham WE, Milich R, Murphy DA, et al: Normative data on the IOWA Conners Teacher Rating Scale. J Clin Child Psychol 18:259–262, 1989

Pelham WE, Midlam JK, Gnagy EM, et al: A comparison of Ritalin and Adderall: efficacy and time-course in children with attention deficit hyperactivity disorder. Pediatrics 103:e43, 1999

Pellock JM: Carbamazepine side effects in children and adults. Epilepsia 28 (suppl 3):564–570, 1987

Pesikoff RB, Davis PC: Treatment of pavor nocturnus and somnambulism in children. Am J Psychiatry 128:778–781, 1971

Peterson BS, Leckman JF, Scahill L, et al: Steroid hormones and Tourette's syndrome: early experience with antiandrogen therapy. J Clin Psychopharmacol 14:131–135, 1994

Peterson SE, Myers KM, McClellan J, et al: Neuroleptic malignant syndrome: three adolescents with complicated courses. J Child Adolesc Psychopharmacol 5:139–149, 1995

Petti TA, Law W: Abrupt cessation of high-dose imipramine treatment in children. JAMA 246:768–769, 1981

Pfeiffer SI, Norton J, Nelson L, et al: Efficacy of vitamin B6 and magnesium in the treatment of autism: a methodological review and summary of outcomes. J Autism Dev Disord 25:481–493, 1995

Pleak RR, Birmaher B, Gavrilescu A, et al: Mania and neuropsychiatric excitation following carbamazepine. J Am Acad Child Adolesc Psychiatry 27:500–503, 1988

Pliszka SR: Tricyclic antidepressants in the treatment of children with attention deficit disorder. J Am Acad Child Adolesc Psychiatry 26:127–132, 1987

Popper C: Medical unknowns and ethical consent, in Psychiatric Pharmacosciences of Children and Adolescents. Edited by Popper C. Washington, DC, American Psychiatric Press, 1987, pp 127–161

Popper CW, Zimnitzky B: Sudden death putatively related to desipramine treatment in youth: a fifth case and a review of speculative mechanisms. J Child Adolesc Psychopharmacol 5:283–300, 1995

Poznanski EO, Freeman LN, Mokros HB: Children's Depression Rating Scale—Revised. Psychopharmacol Bull 21:979–989, 1985

Preskorn SH, Weller E, Hughes CW, et al: Depression in prepubertal children: dexamethasone nonsuppression predicts differential response to imipramine vs. placebo. Psychopharmacol Bull 23:128–133, 1987

Preskorn SH, Weller E, Jerkovich G, et al: Depression in children: concentration-dependent CNS toxicity of tricyclic antidepressants. Psychopharmacol Bull 24:140–142, 1988

Pynoos RS, Frederick C, Nader K, et al: Life threat and posttraumatic stress in school-age children. Arch Gen Psychiatry 44:1057–1063, 1987

Quintana H, Keshavan M: Case study: risperidone in children and adolescents with schizophrenia. J Am Acad Child Adolesc Psychiatry 34:1292–1296, 1995

Quintana H, Birmaher B, Stedge D, et al: Use of methylphenidate in the treatment of children with autistic disorder. J Autism Dev Disord 25:283–294, 1995

Rapoport JL: Antidepressants in childhood attention deficit disorder and obsessive-compulsive disorder. Psychosomatics 27:30–36, 1986

Rapoport JL, Swedo SE, Leonard HL: Childhood obsessive compulsive disorder. J Clin Psychiatry 53 (suppl):11–16, 1992

Rapport MD, Jones JT, DuPaul GJ, et al: Attention deficit disorder and methylphenidate: group and single-subject analyses of dose effects on attention in clinic and classroom settings. J Clin Child Psychol 16:329–338, 1987

Rapport MD, Carlson GA, Kelly KL, et al: Methylphenidate and desipramine in hospitalized children, I: separate and combined effects on cognitive function. J Am Acad Child Adolesc Psychiatry 32:333–342, 1993

Ratey J, Bemporad J, Sorgi P, et al: Brief report: open trial effects of beta-blockers on speech and social behaviors in 8 autistic adults. J Autism Dev Disord 17:439–446, 1987

Ratey J, Sovner R, Parks A, et al: Buspirone treatment of aggression and anxiety in mentally retarded patients: a multiple-baseline, placebo lead-in study. J Clin Psychiatry 52:159–162, 1991

Realmuto GM, Erickson WD, Yellin AM, et al: Clinical comparison of thiothixene and thioridazine in schizophrenic adolescents. Am J Psychiatry 141:440–442, 1984

Regeur L, Pakkenberg B, Fog R, et al: Clinical features and long-term treatment with pimozide in 65 patients with Gilles de la Tourette's syndrome. J Neurol Neurosurg Psychiatry 49:791–795, 1986

Reiter S, Kutcher SP: Disinhibition and anger outbursts in adolescents treated with clonazepam (letter). J Clin Psychopharmacol 11:268, 1991

Reiter S, Kutcher S, Gardner D: Anxiety disorders in children and adolescents: clinical and related issues in pharmacological treatment. Can J Psychiatry 37:432–438, 1992

Remschmidt H, Schulz E, Martin PDM: An open trial of clozapine in thirty-six adolescents with schizophrenia. J Child Adolesc Psychopharmacol 4:31–41, 1994

Richardson MA, Haugland G, Craig TJ: Neuroleptic use, parkinsonian symptoms, tardive dyskinesia, and associated factors in child and adolescent psychiatric patients. Am J Psychiatry 148:1322–1328, 1991

Ricketts RW, Goza AB, Ellis CR, et al: Clinical effects of buspirone on intractable self-injury in adults with mental retardation. J Am Acad Child Adolesc Psychiatry 33:270–276, 1994

Riddle MA (guest ed): Pediatric psychopharmacology I. Child Adolesc Psychiatr Clin North Am 4(1), 1995a

Riddle MA (guest ed): Pediatric psychopharmacology II. Child Adolesc Psychiatr Clin North Am 4(2), 1995b

Riddle MA, Pediatric OCD Research Group: Fluvoxamine in the treatment of OCD in children and adolescents: a multicenter, double-blind, placebo-controlled trial. American Psychiatric Association 1996 Annual Meeting New Research Program and Abstracts (NR 197). Washington, DC, American Psychiatric Association, 1996, p 121

Riddle MA, Hardin MT, Cho SC, et al: Desipramine treatment of boys with attention-deficit hyperactivity disorder and tics: preliminary clinical experience. J Am Acad Child Adolesc Psychiatry 27:811–814, 1988

Riddle MA, Hardin MT, King RA, et al: Fluoxetine treatment of children and adolescents with Tourette's and obsessive compulsive disorders: preliminary clinical experience. J Am Acad Child Adolesc Psychiatry 29:45–48, 1990

Riddle MA, King RA, Hardin MT, et al: Behavioral side effects of fluoxetine in children and adolescents. J Child Adolesc Psychopharmacol 1:193–198, 1990/1991

Riddle MA, Scahill L, King RA, et al: Double-blind, cross-over trial of fluoxetine and placebo in children and adolescents with obsessive compulsive disorder. J Am Acad Child Adolesc Psychiatry 31:1062–1069, 1992

Riddle MA, Geller B, Ryan N: Another sudden death in a child treated with desipramine. J Am Acad Child Adolesc Psychiatry 32:792–797, 1993

Riddle MA, Lynch KA, Scahill L, et al: Methylphenidate discontinuation and reinitiation during long-term treatment of children with Tourette's disorder and attention-deficit hyperactivity disorder: a pilot study. J Child Adolesc Psychopharmacol 5:205–214, 1995

Rivera-Calimlim L, Griesbach PH, Perlmutter R: Plasma chlorpromazine concentrations in children with behavioral disorders and mental illness. Clin Pharmacol Ther 26:114–121, 1979

Robertson MM, Eapen V: Pharmacologic controversy of CNS stimulants in Gilles de la Tourette's syndrome. Clin Neuropharmacol 15:408–425, 1992

Ryan ND: Heterocyclic antidepressants in children and adolescents. J Child Adolesc Psychopharmacol 1:21–31, 1990

Ryan ND: The pharmacologic treatment of child and adolescent depression. Psychiatr Clin North Am 15:29–40, 1992

Ryan ND, Puig-Antioch J, Cooper T, et al: Imipramine in adolescent major depression: plasma level and clinical response. Acta Psychiatr Scand 73:275–288, 1986

Safer DJ: Relative cardiovascular safety of psychostimulants used to treat attention-deficit hyperactivity disorder. J Child Adolesc Psychopharmacol 2:279–290, 1992

Sallee F, Stiller R, Perel J, et al: Targeting imipramine dose in children with depression. Clin Pharmacol Ther 40:8–13, 1986

Sallee FR, Sethuraman G, Rock CM: Effects of pimozide on cognition in children with Tourette syndrome: interaction with comorbid attention deficit disorder. Acta Psychiatr Scand 90:4–9, 1994

Sallee FR, Nesbitt L, Jackson C, et al: Relative efficacy of haloperidol and pimozide in children and adolescents with Tourette's disorder. Am J Psychiatry 154:1057–1062, 1997

Sanchez LE, Campbell M, Small AM, et al: A pilot study of clomipramine in young autistic children. J Am Acad Child Adolesc Psychiatry 35:537–544, 1996

Schleifer M, Weiss G, Cohen N, et al: Hyperactivity in preschoolers and the effect of methylphenidate. Am J Orthopsychiatry 45:38–50, 1975

Schouten R, Duckworth KS: Medicolegal and ethical issues in the pharmacologic treatment of children, in Practitioner's Guide to Psychoactive Drugs for Children and Adolescents. Edited by Werry JS, Aman MG. New York, Plenum Medical Book, 1993, pp 161–178

Schroeder JS, Mullin AV, Elliott GR, et al: Cardio-vascular effects of desipramine in children. J Am Acad Child Adolesc Psychiatry 28:376–379, 1989

Shapiro AK, Shapiro E: Controlled study of pimozide vs. placebo in Tourette's syndrome. J Am Acad Child Adolesc Psychiatry 23:161–173, 1984

Shapiro E, Shapiro A, Fulop G, et al: Controlled study of haloperidol, pimozide, and placebo for the treatment of Gilles de la Tourette's syndrome. Arch Gen Psychiatry 46:722–730, 1989

Shay J, Sanchez LE, Cueva JE, et al: Neuroleptic-related dyskinesias and stereotypies in autistic children: videotaped ratings. Psychopharmacol Bull 29:359–363, 1993

Sheth RD, Wesolowski CA, Jacob JC, et al: Effect of carbamazepine and valproate on bone mineral density. J Pediatr 127:256–262, 1995

Silva RR, Munoz DM, Daniel W, et al: Causes of haloperidol discontinuation in patients with Tourette's syndrome. J Clin Psychiatry 57:129–135, 1996

Silva RR, Munoz DM, Alpert M, et al: Neuroleptic malignant syndrome in children and adolescents. J Am Acad Child Adolesc Psychiatry 38:187–194, 1999

Silverstein FS, Boxer L, Johnston MV: Hematological monitoring during therapy with carbamazepine in children. Ann Neurol 13:685–686, 1983

Simeon JG, Ferguson HB: Recent developments in the use of antidepressant and anxiolytic medications. Psychiatr Clin North Am 8:893–907, 1985

Simeon JG, Ferguson HB: Alprazolam effects in children with anxiety disorders. Can J Psychiatry 32:570–574, 1987

Simeon JG, Ferguson HB, Fleet JVW: Bupropion exacerbates tics in children with attention-deficit hyperactivity disorder and Tourette's syndrome. J Am Acad Child Adolesc Psychiatry 32:211–214, 1986

Simeon JG, Thatte S, Wiggins D: Treatment of adolescent obsessive-compulsive disorder with a clomipramine-fluoxetine combination. Psychopharmacol Bull 26:285–290, 1990

Simeon JG, Ferguson HB, Knott V, et al: Clinical, cognitive, and neurophysiological effects of alprazolam in children and adolescents with overanxious and avoidant disorders. J Am Acad Child Adolesc Psychiatry 31:29–33, 1992

Simeon JG, Knott VJ, Dubois C, et al: Buspirone therapy of mixed anxiety disorders in childhood and adolescence: a pilot study. J Child Adolesc Psychopharmacol 4:159–170, 1994

Simeon JG, Carrey NJ, Wiggins DM, et al: Risperidone effects in treatment-resistant adolescents: preliminary case reports. J Child Adolesc Psychopharmacol 5:69–79, 1995

Singer HS, Brown J, Quaskey S, et al: The treatment of attention deficit hyperactivity disorder in Tourette's syndrome: a double-blind placebo-controlled study with clonidine and desipramine. Pediatrics 95:74–81, 1995

Sovner R: Thioridazine withdrawal-induced behavioral deterioration treated with clonidine: two case reports. Ment Retard 33:221–225, 1995

Speltz ML, Varley CK, Peterson K, et al: Effects of dextroamphetamine and contingency management on a preschooler with ADHD and oppositional defiant disorder. J Am Acad Child Adolesc Psychiatry 27:175–178, 1987

Spencer EK, Alpert M, Pouget ER: Scales for the assessment of neuroleptic response in schizophrenic children: specific measures derived from the CPRS. Psychopharmacol Bull 30:199–202, 1994

Spencer T, Biederman J, Steingard R, et al: Bupropion exacerbates tics in children with attention-deficit hyperactivity disorder and Tourette's syndrome. J Am Acad Child Adolesc Psychiatry 32:211–214, 1993

Steiner H, Petersen M, Ford S, et al: Valproate and related compounds in the treatment of conduct disorder, in Scientific Proceedings of the Annual Meeting of the American Academy of Child and Adolescent Psychiatry, Vol 14. 1998, p 4

Steingard RJ, Goldberg M, Lee D, et al: Adjunctive clonazepam treatment of tic symptoms in children with comorbid tic disorders and ADHD. J Am Acad Child Adolesc Psychiatry 33:394–399, 1994

Strayhorn JM, Rapp N, Donina W, et al: Randomized trial of methylphenidate for an autistic child. J Am Acad Child Adolesc Psychiatry 27:244–247, 1988

Strober M, Morrell W, Lampert C, et al: A family study of bipolar I illness in adolescence: early onset of symptoms linked to increased familial loading and lithium resistance. J Affect Disord 15:255–268, 1988

Strober M, Morrell W, Lampert C, et al: Relapse following discontinuation of lithium maintenance therapy in adolescents with bipolar I illness: a naturalistic study. Am J Psychiatry 147: 457–461, 1990

Strober M, Freeman R, Rigali J, et al: The pharmacotherapy of depressive illness in adolescence, II: effects of lithium augmentation in nonresponders to imipramine. J Am Acad Child Adolesc Psychiatry 31:16–20, 1992

Sturmey P, Reed J, Corbett J: Psychometric assessment of psychiatric disorders in people with learning difficulties (mental handicap): a review of measures. Psychol Med 21:143–155, 1991

Tannock R, Ickowicz A, Schachar R: Differential effects of methylphenidate on working memory in ADHD children with and without comorbid anxiety. J Am Acad Child Adolesc Psychiatry 7:886–896, 1995

Teicher MH, Glod CA: Neuroleptic drugs: indications and guidelines for their rational use in children and adolescents. J Child Adolesc Psychopharmacol 1:33–56, 1990

Terr LC: Childhood psychic trauma, in Basic Handbook of Child Psychiatry, Vol V. Edited by Call JD, Cohen RL, Harrison SI, et al. New York, Basic Books, 1987, pp 262–272

Thompson S, Rey JM: Functional enuresis: is desmopressin the answer? J Am Acad Child Adolesc Psychiatry 34:266–271, 1995

Towbin KE, Dykens EM, Pugliese RG: Clozapine for early developmental delays with childhood-onset schizophrenia: protocol and 15-month outcome. J Am Acad Child Adolesc Psychiatry 33:651–657, 1994

Trimble MR: Anticonvulsants in children and adolescents. J Child Adolesc Psychopharmacol 1:107–124, 1990

Ullmann RK, Sleator EK: Attention deficit disorder children with or without hyperactivity: which behaviors are helped by stimulants? Clin Pediatr (Phila) 24:547–551, 1985

Ullmann RK, Sleator EK: Responders, nonresponders, and placebo responders among children with attention deficit disorder. Clin Pediatr (Phila) 25:594–599, 1986

Ullmann RK, Sleator EK, Sprague RL: A change of mind: the Conners abbreviated rating scales reconsidered. J Abnorm Child Psychol 13: 553–565, 1985

Urman R, Ickowicz A, Fulford P, et al: An exaggerated cardiovascular response to methylphenidate in ADHD children with anxiety. J Child Adolesc Psychopharmacol 2:29–37, 1995

Valleni-Basile LA, Garrison CZ, Jackson KL, et al: Frequency of obsessive-compulsive disorder in a community sample of young adolescents. J Am Acad Child Adolesc Psychiatry 33:782–791, 1994

Valleni-Basile LA, Garrison CZ, Waller JL, et al: Incidence of obsessive-compulsive disorder in a community sample of young adolescents. J Am Acad Child Adolesc Psychiatry 35:898–906, 1996

Van der Linden C, Bruggeman R, Van Woerkom T: Serotonin-dopamine antagonist and Gilles de La Tourette's syndrome: an open pilot dose-titration study with risperidone. Mov Disord 9:687–688, 1994

Varley CK, Trupin EW: Double-blind assessment of stimulant medication for attention deficit disorder: a model for clinical application. Am J Orthopsychiatry 53:542–547, 1983

Venkataraman S, Naylor MW, King CA: Mania associated with fluoxetine treatment in adolescents. J Am Acad Child Adolesc Psychiatry 31: 276–281, 1992

Vitiello B, Behar D, Hunt J, et al: Subtyping aggression in children and adolescents. J Neuropsychiatry Clin Neurosci 2:189–192, 1990

Walkup JT, Rosenberg LA, Brown J, et al: The validity of instruments measuring tic severity in Tourette's syndrome. J Am Acad Child Adolesc Psychiatry 31:472–477, 1992

Weller E, Weller R, Fristad M: Lithium dosage guide for prepubertal children: a preliminary report. Journal of the American Academy of Child Psychiatry 25:92–95, 1986

Weller E, Weller R, Fristad M, et al: Saliva monitoring in prepubertal children. J Am Acad Child Adolesc Psychiatry 26:173–175, 1987

Wender PH: Attention-Deficit Hyperactivity Disorder in Adults. New York, Oxford University Press, 1995

Werry JS, Aman MG: Practitioner's Guide to Psychoactive Drugs for Children and Adolescents, 2nd Edition. New York, Plenum Medical Book, 1999

West SA, Keck PE, McElroy SL, et al: Open trial of valproate in the treatment of adolescent mania. J Child Adolesc Psychopharmacol 4:263–267, 1994

Whalen CK, Henker B, Castro J, et al: Peer perceptions of hyperactivity and medication effects. Child Dev 58:816–828, 1987

Whalen CK, Henker B, Buhrmester D, et al: Does stimulant medication improve the peer status of hyperactive children? J Consult Clin Psychol 57:545–549, 1989

Wilens TE, Biederman J, Geist DE, et al: Nortriptyline in the treatment of ADHD: a chart review of 58 cases. J Am Acad Child Adolesc Psychiatry 32:343–349, 1993

Wilens TE, Biederman J, Baldessarini RJ, et al: Cardiovascular effects of therapeutic doses of tricyclic antidepressants in children and adolescents. J Am Acad Child Adolesc Psychiatry 35:1491–1501, 1996

Wilens TE, Spencer TJ, Swanson JM, et al: Debate forum: combining methylphenidate and clonidine. J Am Acad Child Adolesc Psychiatry 38:614–622, 1999

Willemsen-Swinkels SH, Buitelaar JK, Nijhof GJ, et al: Failure of naltrexone hydrochloride to reduce self-injurious and autistic behavior in mentally retarded adults. Arch Gen Psychiatry 52:766–773, 1995a

Willemsen-Swinkels SH, Buitelaar JK, Weijnen FG, et al: Placebo-controlled acute dosage naltrexone study in young autistic children. Psychiatry Res 16:203–215, 1995b

Williams DT, Mehl R, Yudofsky S, et al: The effect of propranolol on uncontrolled rage outbursts in children and adolescents with organic brain dysfunction. Journal of the American Academy of Child Psychiatry 21:129–135, 1982

Winsberg BG, Perel JM, Hurwic MJ, et al: Imipramine protein binding and pharmacokinetics in children, in The Phenothiazines and Structurally Related Drugs. Edited by Forrest IS, Carr CJ, Usdin E. New York, Raven, 1974, pp 425–431

Winsberg BG, Goldstein S, Yepes LE, et al: Imipramine and electrocardiographic abnormalities in hyperactive children. Am J Psychiatry 132:542–545, 1975

Wolf DV, Wagner KD: Tardive dyskinesia, tardive dystonia, and tardive Tourette's syndrome in children and adolescents. J Child Adolesc Psychopharmacol 3:175–198, 1993

Youngerman J, Canino IA: Lithium carbonate use in children and adolescents. Arch Gen Psychiatry 35:216–224, 1978

Zahn TP, Rapoport JL, Thompson CL: Autonomic and behavioral effects of dextroamphetamine and placebo in normal and hyperactive prepubertal boys. J Abnorm Child Psychol 8:145–160, 1980

Zametkin A, Yamada EM: Monitoring and measuring drug effects, I: physical effects, in Practitioner's Guide to Psychoactive Drugs for Children and Adolescents, 2nd Edition. Edited by Werry JS, Aman MG. New York, Plenum Medical Book, 1999, pp 69–98

Zametkin AJ, Linnoila M, Karoum F, et al: Pemoline and urinary excretion of catecholamines and indoleamines in children with attention deficit disorder. Am J Psychiatry 143:359–362, 1986

Zohar AH, Ratzoni G, Paul DL, et al: An epidemiological study of obsessive compulsive disorder and related disorders in Israeli adolescents. J Am Acad Child Adolesc Psychiatry 31:1057–1061, 1992

TWENTY-THREE

Treatment of Substance-Related Disorders

James W. Cornish, M.D.,
Laura F. McNicholas, M.D., Ph.D., and
Charles P. O'Brien, M.D., Ph.D.

ALCOHOL

Alcoholism is the most prevalent substance use disorder in the United States, affecting approximately 14% of the population at some point in their lifetime (Robins et al. 1984). The magnitude of this problem is huge, involving the loss of 65,000 lives and costs of $136 billion per year (National Institute of Alcoholism and Alcohol Abuse 1990). The amount and pattern of alcohol consumption and the harmful effects of drinking are associated in a predictable manner (Kranzler et al. 1990).

The principal forms of treatment for alcoholism have been self-help/support groups, such as Alcoholics Anonymous (see section "Self-Help Groups" later in this chapter), or psychosocial treatments in inpatient or outpatient rehabilitation programs or sheltered living situations. Unfortunately, psychosocial treatments for alcohol-dependent persons have had only limited success in reducing alcohol use (Holder et al. 1991). Pharmacotherapy has been directed at specific indications that often occur during the course of treatment for alcoholism. Studies have been conducted involving alcohol detoxification treatments, alcohol sensitization agents, anticraving agents, and agents to diminish drinking by treating associated psychiatric disorders.

Alcohol Detoxification

Detoxification refers to the clearing of alcohol from the body and the readjustment of all systems to functioning in the absence of alcohol. The alcohol withdrawal syndrome at the mild end may include only headache and irritability, but about 5% of alcoholic patients have severe withdrawal symptoms (Schuckit 1991) manifested by tremulousness, tachycardia, perspiration, and even seizures (rum fits). The presence of malnutrition, electrolyte imbalance, or infection increases the possibility of cardiovascular collapse.

Pharmacotherapy with a benzodiazepine is the treatment of choice for the prevention and treatment of the signs and symptoms of alcohol withdrawal (Nutt et al. 1989). Many patients detoxify from alcohol without specific treatment or medications. However, it is difficult to determine accurately which patients require medication for alcohol withdrawal. Patients in good physical condition with uncomplicated, mild to moderate alcohol withdrawal symptoms can usually be treated as outpatients (Hayashida et al. 1989).

A typical regimen requires the patient to attend the clinic daily for 5–10 days to receive clinical evaluations, multiple vitamins, and benzodiazepine pharmacotherapy. A typical medication dosing regimen involves giving enough benzodiazepine on the first day of treatment to relieve withdrawal symptoms; the dose should be adjusted if withdrawal symptoms increase or if the patient complains of excessive sedation. Over the next 5–7 days, the dose of benzodiazepine is tapered to zero. Most clinicians use longer-acting benzodiazepines such as clonazepam, chlordiazepoxide, or diazepam. The usual starting dose of medication on the first day is 25–50 mg of chlordiazepoxide or 10 mg of diazepam given every 6 hours (Schuckit 1991). The diagnosis of delirium tremens is given to patients who have marked confusion and severe agitation in addition to the usual alcohol withdrawal symptoms (Goodwin 1992).

It is important to remember that the risk of mortality is 5% in patients with severe alcohol withdrawal symptoms (Schuckit 1987). Patients who have medically complicated or severe alcoholic withdrawal must be treated in a hospital. Benzodiazepines will usually be sufficient to calm agitated patients; however, some patients may require intravenous barbiturates to control extreme agitation (Goodwin 1992).

Alcohol Sensitizing Agents

Disulfiram inhibits a key enzyme, aldehyde dehydrogenase, involved in breakdown of ethyl alcohol. After drinking, the alcohol-disulfiram reaction produces excess blood levels of acetaldehyde, which is toxic in that it produces facial flushing, tachycardia, hypotension, nausea

and vomiting, and physical discomfort. The usual maintenance dose of disulfiram is 250 mg/day.

There have been only a few randomized controlled trials, and these trials have had mixed results for drug efficacy (Peachy and Naranjo 1984). The most comprehensive trial was the Veterans Administration (VA) Cooperative Study of disulfiram treatment of alcoholism. This study was conducted with male veterans and found no differences between disulfiram, 250 mg/day and 1 mg/day (an ineffective dose), and placebo groups in total abstinence, time to first drink, employment, or social stability. Among patients who drank, those in the 250-mg disulfiram group reported significantly fewer drinking days (Fuller et al. 1986).

The main problem with disulfiram is that frequently patients stop taking it and relapse to drinking (Goodwin 1992). Disulfiram is most effective when it is used in a clinical setting that emphasizes abstinence and offers a mechanism to ensure that the medication is taken. Drug compliance may be successfully ensured by giving the medication at 3- to 4-day intervals in the physician's office, or at the treatment center, or by having a spouse or family member administer it.

Alcohol Anticraving Agents

According to Volpicelli et al. (1992), an ideal pharmacotherapy has few, if any, side effects; decreases patients' craving for alcohol so that they have less motivation to drink; and blocks the reinforcing effects of alcohol so that if they resume drinking, they experience neither pleasant nor unpleasant effects.

Several animal models have implicated the involvement of neurotransmitter systems, including endogenous opioid peptides, catecholamine, serotonin, dopamine, and γ-aminobutyric acid (GABA), in alcohol craving and consumption. The only pharmacological intervention that has thus far shown substantial promise involves blocking opioid receptors. Opioid antagonists, such as naloxone and naltrexone, that block opioid receptors have been found to decrease alcohol consumption in animal models (Altshuler et al. 1980; Myers et al. 1986; Volpicelli et al. 1986). Conversely, rats pretreated with small doses of an opioid agonist, such as morphine, show increased alcohol drinking (Hubbell et al. 1986), whereas higher doses reduce alcohol drinking. Rats bred for alcohol preference have not only high alcohol consumption but also high endogenous opioid activity, and naltrexone blocks alcohol drinking in these rodents in a dose-related fashion (Froehlich et al. 1990). Collectively, these findings suggest that alcohol consumption is reinforced by an interaction with the endogenous opioid system and that blocking opioid receptors with specific antagonists lessens behavioral reinforcement, which decreases drinking. This hypothesis also explains why higher doses of opioids, which are an external supply of opioid activity, can reduce drinking.

The first human study of the efficacy and safety of naltrexone in the treatment of alcoholism was a 12-week double-blind trial conducted by Volpicelli et al. (1992), in which 72 subjects were randomly assigned to receive either naltrexone 50 mg/day or placebo in addition to standard psychosocial treatment. The naltrexone group had lower rates of relapse, fewer drinking days, and reduced alcohol craving compared with the placebo group. The results indicated that half as many naltrexone-treated patients (23%) relapsed as those receiving placebo (54.3%). The most striking effects were seen in those who sampled alcohol. Of the 20 placebo patients, 19 (95%) relapsed after they sampled alcohol, compared with only 8 of 16 (50%) of the naltrexone patients. In the other double-blind, placebo-controlled study, 97 alcohol-dependent subjects were randomized to receive either naltrexone or placebo and either coping skills/relapse prevention therapy or a supportive therapy (O'Malley et al. 1992). Compared with the placebo group, the naltrexone-treated patients drank on half as many days, drank one-third as much alcohol

during occasions of drinking, and had less severe alcohol-related problems. As in the prior study, those randomly assigned to naltrexone had significantly fewer relapses during the 3-month treatment period, and this difference was still present at follow-up 6 months later. In a series of laboratory studies involving social drinkers, Swift and associates (1994) found that naltrexone altered human alcohol intoxication. They reported that following a standard dose of alcohol, subjects who were treated with naltrexone had less euphoria than did placebo-treated subjects. In addition to studies on naltrexone, research has been done with the opiate antagonist nalmefene as a treatment for alcohol dependence. In a preliminary 12-week study, Mason and associates (1994) reported that nalmefene-treated subjects had a significantly better outcome than that of the placebo-treated subjects.

The evidence so far suggests that naltrexone is most likely to improve relapse rates when combined with a strong psychosocial rehabilitation program.

Another promising pharmacotherapy for alcohol dependence is acamprosate, whose chemical name is calcium acetyl homotaurinate. Structurally, acamprosate is similar to the amino acid taurine and is believed to act as a GABA receptor agonist. Acamprosate has been reported as a safe and effective treatment for alcoholism in several controlled studies. In 1985, Lhuintre et al. published the results of a double-blind study in which 85 subjects, described as severely alcoholic, were randomized to 3 months of treatment with either acamprosate or placebo. Seventy subjects completed the trial, and of these, 20 of 33 (60%) acamprosate-treated subjects and 12 of 37 (32%) placebo-treated subjects were abstinent during the study. Positive results were reported for two subsequent placebo-controlled trials (Lhuintre et al. 1990; Paille et al. 1995) in which the total number of abstinent days was lower for acamprosate-treated subjects compared with placebo-treated subjects. In 1996, the reports of two German double-blind, placebo-controlled studies were published. In the first trial, Sass et al. (1996) studied 272 subjects randomly assigned to a year of treatment with either acamprosate or placebo and evaluated for an additional 12 months following the discontinuation of study medication. Compared with placebo-treated subjects, the subjects who received acamprosate had a significantly lower dropout rate, a greater number of days before their first drink, and a greater number of days of total abstinence during the study.

The second study, which had a similar design, involved 455 subjects and was conducted by Whitworth and colleagues (1996). The results of this trial were that acamprosate was superior to placebo with respect to the number of dropouts, relapse rate, and total days of abstinence. Interestingly, 18% of the acamprosate-treated subjects compared with 7% of the placebo-treated subjects remained continuously abstinent a year after discontinuation of study medication. These impressive clinical results for acamprosate warrant further study of this potentially beneficial medication.

Less encouraging results have been reported for two drugs that target the serotonin system. Kranzler and colleagues (1995b) studied fluoxetine, a serotonin reuptake inhibitor, as a treatment for alcoholism. There were no differences in outcomes measures between the fluoxetine-treated and placebo-treated subjects. B. A. Johnson et al. (1996) studied ritanserin, a serotonin type 2 receptor antagonist, in a large multicenter trial. In this study, ritanserin showed no advantage over placebo as a pharmacotherapy for alcohol dependence.

Agents Used to Diminish Drinking by Treating Associated Psychiatric Disorders

Depressed alcoholic patients treated with lithium showed no difference compared with those treated with placebo in a multiple center VA study (Dorus et al. 1989). In a study in which desipramine was the pharmacotherapy for alco-

holism, the results indicate a trend toward decreased drinking in both depressed and nondepressed subjects (Mason and Kocsis 1991).

McGrath et al. (1993) studied alcoholic patients (93% met DSM-III-R [American Psychiatric Association 1987] criteria for dependence) who had an antecedent history of depression (>90%) or who continued to have depressive symptoms after 6 months of abstinence. Eighty patients were randomly assigned to 12 weeks of treatment with either imipramine or placebo. Of the imipramine-treated patients, 65% had a significant reduction in depressive symptoms and alcoholic consumption compared with 25% for the placebo-treated group.

Summary

Benzodiazepines are the pharmacotherapeutic agents of choice for prevention and treatment of the signs and symptoms of alcohol withdrawal. Although disulfiram was no better than placebo when tested in large controlled studies of alcoholism, it is effective when used in clinical settings that stress abstinence and ensure medication compliance. The opioid antagonist naltrexone, approved a few years ago by the Food and Drug Administration (FDA) for treatment of alcoholism, appears to markedly decrease relapse rates in abstinent patients who sample alcohol. Encouraging results from several clinical studies indicate that acamprosate is a potentially useful medication.

BENZODIAZEPINES AND OTHER SEDATIVES

The benzodiazepines have largely replaced older sedative-hypnotic agents, such as barbiturates and meprobamate, in clinical use. Clinical experience and scientific study have shown that although the benzodiazepines, as a class of drugs, are safer in isolated overdose situations than the older agents, physiological dependence is certainly possible and occurs with long-term use, even at therapeutic doses. These findings have touched off a controversy that has yet to be settled. Most patients who are, in fact, physiologically dependent on benzodiazepines do not increase the dose of medication above the physician's prescription or in any other way abuse the prescribed medication. However, if the benzodiazepine were to be abruptly discontinued, the patient would, in all probability, experience a withdrawal abstinence syndrome that could be extremely severe. Thus, any patient treated with a benzodiazepine for a significant length of time, that is, longer than 3–6 months, should be slowly tapered off his or her medication; this does not preclude the possibility of re-emergence of the patient's symptoms, which may necessitate continued use of the medication. The fact that patients become physiologically dependent on therapeutic doses of benzodiazepines has led some people in the field to equate any use of benzodiazepines in any patient for long-term treatment with abuse of the drug. This is undoubtedly an overstatement of the abuse of these agents. Significant abuse of benzodiazepines does, in fact, occur but is usually seen in patients abusing other drugs also, *not* in the patient who is carefully monitored and is stable on therapeutically indicated benzodiazepines.

In general, patients who abuse only benzodiazepines are rare; benzodiazepine abuse in combination with abuse of other drugs is much more common. Alcoholic patients will not infrequently abuse benzodiazepines if the opportunity presents, and patients who abuse cocaine and opioids are also likely to use benzodiazepines concomitantly. Studies in alcoholic patients admitted for detoxification have shown that the rate of benzodiazepine use among these patients is between 28% and 41%, as determined by urinalysis (Crane et al. 1988; Ogborne and Kapur 1987; Soyka et al. 1989); generally only about one-third of patients with a positive urine test for benzodiazepines admitted to using the drugs.

Methadone-maintained patients often use benzodiazepines but frequently on a sporadic basis. Magura et al. (1987) showed that 40% of patients in four methadone programs in New York had urine tests that were positive for benzodiazepines, whereas studies in England show rates of benzodiazepine-positive urine tests of 54% (Lipsedge and Cook 1987) and 59% (Beary et al. 1987) in methadone patients. In patients who use benzodiazepines in conjunction with other drugs, the issues of abuse and physiological dependence take on a much different meaning than in stable patients on long-term prescribed benzodiazepines. If these patients use or abuse more than one substance, the use or abuse of benzodiazepines can seriously interfere with drug abuse treatment for other substances.

COCAINE

Cocaine abuse in the United States has maintained an epidemic status since the early 1980s. Highly purified, low-priced cocaine is widely available. The consequences and by-products of this epidemic have touched most American communities. The National Household Survey on Drug Abuse (Substance Abuse and Mental Health Services Administration 1995), which is based on a sample of 22,181 people representative of the United States population, estimated that in 1994 there were 1.4 million current cocaine users. When compared with the 1985 survey, the more recent survey showed that weekly (chronic) users have remained constant at approximately 640,000 persons. Furthermore, the chronic cocaine users are developing a significant number of medical and psychosocial problems. According to data from the Drug Abuse Warning Network, DAWN (Substance Abuse and Mental Health Services Administration 1993), cocaine-related hospital emergencies, especially among patients aged 35 and older, continue to increase (see Figure 23–1).

The selection of potential pharmaco-

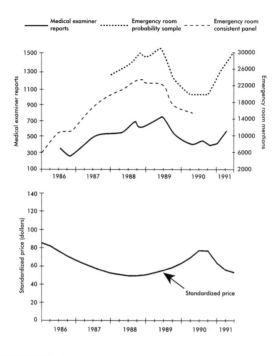

Figure 23–1.   Emergency room mentions and medical examiner reports involving cocaine and standardized price of cocaine by quarter, 1986–1991.
Source.   Price and Purity of Cocaine, A White Paper, October 1992. Office of National Drug Control Policy.

therapies has been based on the current understanding of the neurochemical changes that result from chronic stimulant use. Cocaine administration results in increased levels of dopamine in the region of the nucleus accumbens in rats, which is an important part of the brain reward pathways. Cocaine and other abused substances that increase nucleus accumbens dopamine also decrease the threshold for brain-stimulation reward (Kornetsky and Porrino 1992).

Pharmacotherapy of cocaine dependence must be considered separately from pharmacotherapy used to treat complications involved in cocaine abuse such as depression and psychotic reactions. Although a withdrawal syndrome for cocaine dependence has been proposed (Gawin and Kleber 1986), this withdrawal generally consists simply of somnolence, lack of energy, craving for cocaine, and periods of depression. It usually resolves spontaneously over several

days, but there is evidence from imaging studies that receptor changes and even brain metabolic effects from chronic cocaine use may persist for weeks or months after the last dose of cocaine. A variety of medications have been used to deal with these biochemical changes that are thought to play a role in relapse to compulsive cocaine use. Antidepressant medications have been used based on the theory that they too block reuptake of biogenic amines and thus may repair some of the deficit produced by the abrupt withdrawal of cocaine. The best data have been obtained with desipramine, which is also the medication most studied. The results from several double-blind studies with desipramine (Arndt et al. 1992; Gawin et al. 1989; Kosten et al. 1992) indicate that it has a modest effect, at best, in inducing abstinence from cocaine. The studies of Arndt et al. (1992) and Kosten et al. (1992) both involved methadone maintenance subjects who were abusing cocaine, mainly intravenously. Patients who abuse only cocaine, primarily not by intravenous administration, may have a better prognosis than cocaine-abusing, methadone-maintained patients. Further research is needed, particularly in nonintravenous abusers, in order to determine which population of cocaine abusers benefits most from desipramine pharmacotherapy.

The list of medications found to be ineffective as cocaine treatments continues to grow. Grabowski et al. (1995) reported negative results for the serotonin reuptake inhibitor fluoxetine in two controlled clinical trials. Bupropion was studied in a multicenter trial (Margolin et al. 1995) and found to have no advantage over placebo treatment. Kampman et al. (1996) completed a trial for amantadine but were unable to replicate the positive findings of a prior study (Alterman et al. 1992).

Another approach has been based on animal studies that indicate that cocaine can produce kindling of seizure activity. *Kindling* is an electrical phenomenon that refers to the increase in seizure activity when a standard subthreshold stimulus is applied repeatedly to certain brain structures, especially the amygdaloid nucleus. Small doses of cocaine applied to the amygdala have also been shown to produce kindling, and thus the drug carbamazepine, which blocks kindling (Post 1988), might have a role in the treatment of cocaine dependence. Unfortunately, double-blind studies thus far have not shown any benefit from carbamazepine in preventing relapse to cocaine use (Cornish et al. 1995; Halikas et al. 1992; Kranzler et al. 1995a; Montoya et al. 1995).

The lack of success in identifying an effective medication for treating cocaine dependence has not dampened scientific enthusiasm or impeded further research. On the contrary, there is renewed interest in studying various methods of altering the physiological effects of cocaine. Some of the most exciting work involves schemes for either blocking the effects of cocaine or hastening the destruction of cocaine.

The first area of research is based on the fact that cocaine must attach to its binding site on the dopamine transporter in order to produce pharmacological effects. Researchers (Bagasra et al. 1992; Fox et al. 1996) have focused on making anticocaine antibodies for this specific cocaine-binding site with the hope of developing a cocaine vaccine.

The second area involves the catabolism of cocaine. The strategy is to accelerate the inactivation of cocaine by augmenting the natural cholinesterase activity (Hoffman et al. 1996; Schwartz and Johnson 1996). If successful, the resultant medication regimen would be crucial to the treatment of cocaine overdose (Gorelick 1997; Mattes et al. 1996) and would be a possible pharmacological adjunct to the psychosocial treatment for cocaine dependence.

Summary

No medication is clearly identified as an effective pharmacotherapeutic agent for cocaine-dependent persons. Desipramine, which has been studied in several double-blind studies, appears to be moderately effective at inducing abstinence. Research to develop a cocaine vaccine as well as to find methods of accelerating the catabolism of cocaine offers innovative approaches in the search for a medication treatment for cocaine dependence.

OPIOIDS

Pharmacotherapy of opioid dependence has a long history, in part because "heroinism" was one of the first recognized drug problems in the United States and because therapeutically used congeners of the drug of abuse, heroin, were readily available. Later studies have shown only limited success with nonpharmacological treatment.

Detoxification From Opioid Dependence

The classical method of opioid detoxification was, and remains, short-term substitution therapy. The medication traditionally used has been methadone, at a sufficient dose to suppress signs and symptoms of heroin withdrawal abstinence; the methadone is then tapered over a period ranging from 1 week to 6 months. The idea behind a rapid (i.e., 1- to 2-week) detoxification regimen is to achieve total opioid abstinence quickly so that treatment can be continued in a drug-free setting. Most practitioners consider 21 days sufficient for short-term outpatient detoxification. However, many patients have very chaotic lives when presenting for treatment and require a period of stabilization before they can hope to maintain a drug-free lifestyle. The 6-month stabilization/detoxification regimen (see subsection "Methadone" later in this chapter, for regulations) allows these patients to work on the most acute personal and employment problems while they are stabilized on a relatively low dose (30–40 mg/day) of methadone and then are detoxified from methadone to continue treatment in a drug-free setting.

More recently, a partial agonist, buprenorphine, has been studied for efficacy in suppressing withdrawal abstinence signs and symptoms. In outpatient trials, Bickel et al. (1988) showed that buprenorphine is as effective as methadone in a 10-week double-blind trial. In an open trial, Kosten and Kleber (1988) compared three doses of buprenorphine and found that 4 mg, administered sublingually, was superior to 2 or 8 mg of buprenorphine in suppressing signs and symptoms of withdrawal abstinence.

There has always been concern about substitution detoxification on the basis that the physician is prolonging the problem by prescribing an addictive medication, even with a tapering regimen. Many of the symptoms of opioid withdrawal abstinence appear to be mediated by overactivity in the sympathetic nervous system. This led Gold and his associates (1978, 1980) to attempt to depress this overactivity and thereby ameliorate the withdrawal abstinence syndrome by using adrenergic agents that have no abuse potential. Clonidine, an α-adrenergic agonist with inhibitory action primarily at the locus coeruleus, was effective in inpatient populations in decreasing the signs and symptoms of opioid withdrawal abstinence. Outpatient detoxification with clonidine has not been as successful as inpatient treatment. Inpatient studies reported an 80%–90% success rate, whereas outpatient studies have reported success rates as low as 31% in detoxifying patients from methadone and 36% in detoxifying patients from heroin. The problems identified in outpatient clonidine detoxification include 1) access to heroin and other opioids, 2) lethargy, 3) insomnia, 4) dizziness, and 5) oversedation. The last four adverse effects were noted in inpatient populations during detoxification with clonidine but were easily managed in the hospital setting.

Because clonidine was much less successful in the outpatient setting, various approaches were studied in efforts to improve the efficacy of this agent. One of the major reasons clonidine was less successful in the outpatient setting was that heroin and other opioids were available to the patient. Naltrexone, a competitive opioid antagonist, was added to the clonidine regimen in efforts both to speed up the time course of withdrawal and to block the effect of any opioid used illicitly by the patient. As reported by Stine and Kosten (1992), Kosten showed that 82% of patients were successfully detoxified, as outpatients, in 4–5 days using a single daily dose regimen of clonidine and 12.5 mg of naltrexone.

Loimer and colleagues have studied very rapid opioid detoxification. These methods have involved anesthetizing patients with either methohexital (Loimer et al. 1990) or midazolam (Loimer et al. 1991) and then using naltrexone to precipitate abstinence. These protocols successfully detoxified patients in 48 hours but required major medical intervention (intubation, mechanical ventilation, and intravenous fluids) and exposed the patient to the risks of general anesthesia. No follow-up studies of patients undergoing rapid detoxification, to determine the patients' drug use or adherence to outpatient therapy, have been done.

Two major problems with detoxification

have been identified. The first is that all regimens must be individualized; this eliminates the possibility of standard protocols for opioid detoxification. The second problem is more serious in terms of patient management: opioid-abusing and -dependent patients in drug-free treatment have an extremely high relapse rate. Maddux and Desmond (1992) reported on six long-term (3 years or longer) follow-up studies of drug-free treatment of opiate abuse and dependence. Abstinence rates at follow-up in these studies ranged from 10% to 19%; the percentage of patients with unknown status at follow-up ranged from 10% to 32%. Because drug-free treatment of opioid users has such high relapse rates, other modalities of treatment have been developed.

Maintenance Treatment of Opioid Dependence

Methadone maintenance has been the mainstay of the pharmacotherapy of opioid dependence since its introduction by Dole and Nyswander (1965). Levomethadyl acetate (LAAM), a long-acting congener of methadone, was approved by the FDA for maintenance treatment in 1993 and is available in opioid-dependence treatment programs. More recently, buprenorphine has been studied in clinical trials as a maintenance therapy in opioid-dependent patients; it has not yet received FDA approval but does show a great deal of promise as an alternative to methadone maintenance.

Methadone.   As discussed earlier in this chapter, methadone has been used for both short- and long-term detoxification from opioids. Methadone maintenance, however, is designed to support patients with opioid dependence for months or years while the patient engages in counseling and other therapy to change his or her lifestyle. Extensive clinical experience has shown that methadone is safe and effective. Further, this experience has shown that although patients on methadone mainte-

nance show physiological signs of opioid tolerance, there are minimal side effects, and patients' general health and nutritional status improve.

This approach to the treatment of opioid dependence has been controversial since its beginning. Physicians and other treatment professionals who regard opioid dependence using a disease model have little or no problem treating patients with an active drug for long periods of time, especially in light of repeated treatment failures in the absence of active medication therapy. However, many people view methadone maintenance as simply substituting a legal drug for an illegal one and refuse to accept any outcome other than total abstinence from all drugs. These people point to long-term follow-up studies of methadone maintenance patients (see Maddux and Desmond 1992) that show that 5 years after discharge from the maintenance program, only 10%–20% of the patients are completely abstinent, which is defined as not being enrolled in methadone maintenance and not using illicit opioids. However, long-term follow-up studies of patients discharged from drug-free treatment programs show that only 10%–19% of opioid-dependent patients are abstinent at 3- or 5-year time points (see Maddux and Desmond 1992) using the same definition.

Despite these results of patients discharged from programs, studies of outcome measures other than total abstinence done on patients in maintenance treatment consistently show that these patients have marked improvement in various measures. Investigators have shown up to an 85% decrease in criminal behavior, measured by self-report or arrest records, in patients in treatment, whereas employment among maintenance patients ranges from 40% to 80%. Gerstein (1992) quoted a Swedish study published in 1984 showing the results over 5 years in 34 patients who applied for treatment to the only methadone clinic in Sweden at the time. The 34 patients were randomly assigned to either methadone maintenance or outpatient drug-free therapy; those patients in drug-free treatment could not apply for methadone for a minimum of 24 months after being accepted into the study. After 2 years, 71% of methadone patients were doing well, compared with 6% of patients admitted to drug-free treatment. After 5 years, 13 of 17 patients remained on methadone and were free of illicit drugs, whereas 4 of 17 patients had been discharged from treatment for continued drug use. Of the 17 drug-free treatment patients, 9 had subsequently been switched to methadone treatment, were free of illicit drug use, and were "socially productive." Of the remaining 8 patients, 5 were dead (allegedly from overdose), 2 were in prison, and 1 was drug-free.

Furthermore, although previous generations of drug abusers had hepatitis B, endocarditis, and other infections, in this age when intravenous drug use and concomitant sharing of needles and syringes place a patient at risk for human immunodeficiency virus (HIV) infection, the medical consequences of heroin dependence must be taken into account when determining appropriate therapy for a patient. These issues are currently being studied by a variety of methods, but the overall clinical impression of increased general health in methadone maintenance patients is very strong. Additionally, Metzger et al. (1993) studied HIV seroconversion rates in opioid-dependent subjects. In this study, 152 subjects were in methadone maintenance treatment, and 103 subjects were out of treatment. At baseline, 12% of the subjects were HIV positive (10% of in-treatment and 16% of out-of-treatment subjects); follow-up of HIV-negative subjects over 18 months showed conversion rates of 3.5% for in-treatment subjects and 22% for those remaining out of treatment. These data suggest that although transmission of HIV still occurs, opioid-abusing intravenous drug users in methadone maintenance programs have a significantly lower likelihood of becoming infected than do patients who are not in treatment.

Methadone maintenance programs are licensed and regulated by the FDA and the Drug Enforcement Agency (DEA). A program and its physician must be licensed for a methadone maintenance program in order to prescribe or dispense more than a 2-week supply of any opioid to a patient known or suspected to be dependent on opioids. Most clinics are ambulatory and open 6–7 days per week, requiring patients to come into the clinic daily to receive medication unless and until a patient has "earned" privileges (take-home medication) by compliance with the clinic rules and abstinence from illicit substances. For a person to be eligible for methadone maintenance, she or he must be at least 18 years old (or have consent of the legal guardian) and must be physiologically dependent on heroin or other opioids for at least 1 year. The treatment regulations define a 1-year history of addiction to mean that the patient was addicted to an opioid narcotic at some time at least 1 year before admission and was addicted, either continuously or episodically, for most of the year immediately before admission to the methadone maintenance program. A physician must document evidence of current physiological dependence on opioids before a patient can be admitted to the program; such evidence may be a precipitated abstinence syndrome in response to a naloxone challenge or, more commonly, signs and symptoms of opioid withdrawal, evidence of intravenous injections, or evidence of medical complications of intravenous injections. Exceptions to these requirements are patients who have recently been in penal or chronic care, previously treated patients, or pregnant patients; in these cases, patients need not show evidence of current physiological dependence, but the physician must justify their enrollment in methadone maintenance. A person younger than 18 years must have documented evidence of at least two attempts at short-term detoxification or drug-free treatment (the episodes must be separated by at least 1 week) and have the consent of his or her parent or legal guardian.

The variability in clinic practice is widespread and, as with the issue of limiting doses, sometimes mandated by state regulators. These practices continue despite studies showing that doses of at least 60 mg/day were associated with longer retention in treatment, decreased use of illicit drugs, and a lower incidence of HIV infection (Hartel et al. 1988, 1989). Among patients receiving at least 71 mg/day of methadone, no heroin use was detected, whereas patients receiving doses of 46 mg/day of methadone or lower were five times more likely to use heroin than those receiving higher doses (Ball and Ross 1991).

Yet another issue that has engendered a great deal of controversy is the treatment of opioid-dependent pregnant women. It is currently estimated that up to 2%–3% of babies born each year have had intrauterine exposure to opioids. The complications and treatment of maternal opioid addiction and the effects on the fetus and neonate have been discussed by Finnegan (1991) and Finnegan and Kandall (1992). For the purposes of this chapter, it should be noted that current evidence shows that pregnant women who wish to be detoxified from opioids (either heroin or methadone) should *not* be detoxified before the 14th week of gestation because of the potential risk of inducing abortion or after the 32nd week of gestation because of possible withdrawal-induced fetal stress (see Finnegan 1991).

LAAM. LAAM is a long-acting opioid agonist for treatment of opioid dependence. The major difference between methadone and LAAM is the duration of action, which is based on the metabolism of the two drugs. Methadone is slowly metabolized to inactive metabolites; LAAM, on the other hand, is metabolized to two congeners, nor-LAAM and dinor-LAAM, both of which are more potent opioid agonists than LAAM itself. Further, the plasma half-life of methadone is about 35 hours (Gilman et al. 1990), whereas the half-lives for LAAM, nor-LAAM, and dinor-LAAM are estimated to be 47, 62, and 162 hours, respectively (Finkle et al. 1982). These prolonged half-lives of LAAM

and its active metabolites allow for every-other-day dosing or three times a week dosing, without the problem of diverted take-home medication that is inherent in methadone maintenance programs that allow take-home medication. It is also crucial to remember that LAAM will not reach steady-state plasma levels for 2–3 weeks after the medication is started or the dose changed and that too rapid an escalation in LAAM dose may result in an unintentional overdose because of drug accumulation, whereas too slow an escalation may result in the patient having withdrawal symptoms and using illicit opioids.

Buprenorphine. Buprenorphine is a partial agonist of μ-opioid type and is a clinically effective analgesic agent with an estimated potency of 25–40 times that of morphine (Cowan et al. 1977). Buprenorphine is currently approved only for use as an analgesic agent and not yet for treatment of opioid dependence. Human pharmacology studies have shown buprenorphine to be 25–30 times as potent as morphine in producing pupillary constriction, but buprenorphine was less effective in producing morphinelike subjective effects (Jasinski et al. 1978). Further, these studies showed that the physiological and subjective effects of morphine (15–120 mg) were significantly attenuated when morphine was administered 3 hours after buprenorphine in patients maintained on 8 mg/day of buprenorphine; the physiological and subjective effects of 30 mg of morphine were also tested at 29.5 hours after the last dose of chronically administered buprenorphine and were again significantly attenuated. In early clinical trials with opioid-dependent patients, it was found that patients would tolerate the sublingual route and that the dose of buprenorphine could be rapidly escalated to effective doses without significant side effects or toxicity (R. E. Johnson et al. 1989) and that detoxification from heroin dependence using buprenorphine was as effective as methadone (Bickel et al. 1988) or clonidine (Kosten and

Kleber 1988). R. E. Johnson et al. (1992) compared buprenorphine, 8 mg/day sublingually, and methadone, 20 mg/day or 60 mg/day, in a 25-week maintenance study and found that buprenorphine was as effective as 60 mg/day of methadone in reducing illicit opioid use and keeping patients in treatment. Both buprenorphine and methadone, 60 mg/day, were superior to methadone, 20 mg/day, in this study. A multicenter study compared sublingual doses of 1 mg of buprenorphine with 8 mg of buprenorphine; more than 700 patients were studied. Preliminary results show that the 8-mg dose was significantly better than the 1-mg dose on outcome measures of opiate-free urine tests and retention in treatment (W. Ling, personal communication, June 1997). Both detoxification and maintenance studies have shown that the abrupt discontinuation of buprenorphine in a blind fashion causes only very minor elevations in withdrawal scores on any withdrawal scale (Bickel et al. 1988; Fudala et al. 1990; Jasinski et al. 1978; R. E. Johnson et al. 1989; Kosten and Kleber 1988).

Relapse Prevention

As noted earlier in this chapter, various methods of detoxifying patients from opioids have been developed. These methodologies were, by and large, unsuccessful in achieving permanent opioid abstinence in patients. It has long been thought that both conditioned reactivity to drug-associated cues (Wikler 1973) and protracted withdrawal symptoms (Martin and Jasinski 1969) contribute to the high rate of opioid relapse. The use of a blocking dose of a pure opioid antagonist would block the positive reinforcing effects of the illicit drugs. Naltrexone was shown to be orally effective in blocking the subjective effects of morphine for up to 24 hours (Martin et al. 1973). Patients using naltrexone maintenance for relapse prevention need to be carefully screened as they *must* be opioid-free at the start of naltrexone administration. Many practitioners administer a naloxone

challenge, which must be negative, before starting naltrexone. Naltrexone is usually administered either daily (50 mg) or three times weekly (100 mg, 100 mg, and 150 mg).

Many opioid-addicted patients have very little motivation to take naltrexone and to remain abstinent. However, patients with better identified motivation, among them groups of recovering professionals (e.g., physicians, attorneys) and federal probationers, who face loss of license to practice a profession or legal consequences, have significantly better success with naltrexone.

SELF-HELP GROUPS

Self-help groups, such as Alcoholics Anonymous, Narcotics Anonymous, and Cocaine Anonymous among others, which are based on a 12-step method of recovery, can be a valuable source of support for the recovering patient. These groups are a fellowship of recovering people interested in helping themselves and others lead drug-free lives. Self-help groups are also available to non-drug-abusing family members to help them understand the addictive process and how family member dynamics can affect the drug-abusing or recovering family member.

HALLUCINOGENS

The use and abuse of hallucinogens wax and wane much more than the use of some other drugs, such as alcohol and opioids. The major drugs of abuse that fall into this classification are cannabis and related compounds, lysergic acid diethylamide (LSD) and other indolealkylamines (psilocybin), and phencyclidine (PCP) and its congeners. Cannabis has a relatively constant rate of use, but its use alone almost never causes the user to seek medical attention. LSD use today occurs in isolated groups, polysubstance abusers, and adolescents and young adults who frequent "rave" clubs. Most users of LSD and related compounds are not seen in emergency rooms, but occasionally patients experiencing acute adverse reactions to these drugs are brought to medical attention. The most frequent adverse effects of LSD and related compounds are acute panic reactions. Most acute panic reactions require only a calm atmosphere and reassurance; occasionally a patient will be seen who benefits from a low dose of benzodiazepine.

PCP intoxication, however, can have serious psychiatric and medical complications. A schizophrenic-like psychotic state can be produced by very low doses of PCP, but behavioral disinhibition, frequently accompanied by anxiety, rage, aggression, and panic, rather than the core psychotic effects, necessitates treatment in most cases in which treatment is mandated. There is no convincing evidence of the superiority of either benzodiazepines or neuroleptics in treating the acute reaction to PCP. Benzodiazepines are frequently used because of their rapid onset of action and because they can be titrated intravenously. There is a paucity of information on chronic use of PCP and treatment, if indicated, in the chronic user.

NICOTINE

According to the Department of Health and Human Services, there are 51 million smokers in the United States, and tobacco accounts for approximately 400,000 deaths per year (U.S. Department of Health and Human Services 1990). Since the mid-1960s, the incidence of smoking in the United States has progressively decreased by about 1% per year (U.S. Department of Health and Human Services 1989). This remarkable change in tobacco use is a consequence of the realization by society that tobacco-related mortality and morbidity are entirely preventable. Most of these smokers have symptoms that meet the DSM-IV (American Psychiatric Association 1994) criteria for the

substance use disorder nicotine dependence. The behavioral aspects of nicotine dependence are similar to those for alcohol and opiate dependence, as well as the production of tolerance and physical dependence. In about 80% of smokers (Gross and Stitzer 1989), nicotine abstinence leads to well-described withdrawal signs and symptoms (Hughes and Hatsukami 1986).

Pharmacotherapy in the form of nicotine replacement has been a key element in reducing withdrawal symptoms and initiating smoking cessation.

Nicotine Replacement

Nicotine polacrilex gum is typically prescribed so that patients have free access to it for periods up to 4 months. Transdermal nicotine is initially administered in 15- to 21-mg patches for 4–12 weeks, followed by lower-dose patches for up to another 8 weeks. The results from several well-controlled studies (Gross and Stitzer 1989; Schneider et al. 1983) confirm that nicotine gum reduces irritability and withdrawal symptoms such as sleep disturbance, difficulty concentrating, and restlessness. Interestingly, nicotine gum does not appear to reduce craving for cigarettes. Transdermal nicotine also has excellent documentation for its ability to decrease the severity of withdrawal symptoms and also to decrease craving for tobacco (Daughton et al. 1991; Tonnesen et al. 1991).

Neither gum nor transdermal nicotine has any long-term effect on weight gain. Both nicotine preparations provide a significant advantage over placebo in smoking cessation. Stitzer (1991) reviewed seven double-blind, placebo-controlled smoking cessation trials using nicotine gum. Abstinence rates at 4–6 weeks were 73% for nicotine gum compared with 49% for placebo gum. Most of the transdermal nicotine double-blind studies were reviewed by Palmer et al. (1992), who found that quit rates at 4–6 weeks were 39%–71% for nicotine compared with 13%–41% for the placebo patches. The

FDA approved nicotine gum in 1981 and transdermal nicotine in 1991 as prescription medications, and in 1996, both were approved for over-the-counter (nonprescription) use.

Beyond the initiation of abstinence, both preparations are associated with a progressive relapse to smoking. After 1 year, abstinence rates are about 25% for the nicotine gum and patch compared with 12% for placebo (Benowitz 1993).

The nasal spray and the inhaler are two newer preparations that provide rapid release forms of nicotine. The potential advantage of these rapid release preparations is that they closely simulate smoking by providing a rapid plasma concentration and oral and sensory stimulation. The results from the initial trials for the nasal spray (Sutherland et al. 1992) and the inhaler (Tonnesen et al. 1993) are similar to those for the gum and patch.

Nonnicotine Pharmacotherapies

Propranolol was studied in a placebo-controlled, double-blind trial and found to be no better than placebo for smoking cessation (Farebrother et al. 1980).

The antihypertensive agent clonidine is an α_2-adrenergic agonist that has been used for its nonhypertensive effects to treat opiate and alcohol withdrawal symptoms. It has also been studied in the treatment of smokers and found to decrease both nicotine withdrawal symptoms and tobacco craving (Glassman et al. 1984). Glassman et al. (1990) reviewed six placebo-controlled trials of clonidine for smoking. Five of the trials reported that clonidine-treated patients had significantly improved quit rates at 4–6 weeks, compared with those treated with placebo. One trial (Franks et al. 1989) reported that clonidine and placebo treatments were equal.

Antidepressant treatment of nicotine dependence has also been investigated. Imipramine was studied in a controlled trial as a treatment for nicotine withdrawal symptoms and smoking cessation but was no better than pla-

cebo (Jacobs et al. 1971). Doxepin was compared with placebo in two studies (Edwards et al. 1988, 1989). In both trials, the doxepin-treated subjects performed better, but because these studies contained small numbers of subjects, the investigators consider the findings to be preliminary.

Bupropion, a monocyclic antidepressant that has serotonergic, noradrenergic, and dopaminergic effects, was approved by the FDA as a pharmacotherapeutic agent for smoking cessation. In a double-blind trial (Ferry et al. 1992) in which 42 men were randomly assigned to 12 weeks of treatment with either bupropion, 300 mg/day, or placebo, the results showed significantly longer continuous abstinence for bupropion-treated subjects at the end of treatment, as well as 6 and 12 months after treatment. Several trials have examined the efficacy and dose response of bupropion for smoking cessation (Hurt et al. 1997; Jorenby et al. 1999).

Psychological Interventions

It is well recognized that smoking is maintained by both behavioral and pharmacological aspects (Jaffe and Kranzler 1979; Leventhal and Cleary 1980). It is not surprising that the combination of nicotine gum replacement and behavioral modification therapy is superior to either treatment alone (Hall et al. 1985; Killen et al. 1984). Hall and Killen (1985) each conducted a controlled combined treatment trial for smoking cessation. They found that the abstinence rates from these studies, 44% at 12 months and 50% at 10.5 months, were "some of the highest abstinence rates ever reported" (Hall and Killen 1985, p. 139). In order to determine the minimum behavioral treatment necessary to optimize abstinence, we need more controlled trials involving combined therapy.

Smoking and Psychiatric Disorders

The incidence of smoking in persons who abuse alcohol, stimulants, and opiates is about 90%;

however, compared with the other two groups, alcoholic patients smoke the most cigarettes (Burling and Ziff 1988).

Research supports clinical observations that cigarette smoking is extremely common among patients with schizophrenia. Goff et al. (1992) studied schizophrenic outpatients and found that 74% smoked compared with a national average of approximately 30%. Between 80% and 90% of a group of institutionalized schizophrenic patients were found to smoke (Matherson and O'Shea 1984). There is no known reason for the high rate of nicotine use by schizophrenic patients. Some have speculated that the dopamine-augmenting effect of nicotine may counterbalance a relative dopamine deficiency that exists in schizophrenic patients (Glassman 1993). However, nicotine-induced changes in other neurotransmitters (e.g., serotonin) (Benwell and Balfour 1982) may help to explain why so many schizophrenic patients smoke.

Glassman and colleagues (1988) conducted pioneering research establishing the link between major depression and cigarette smoking. Using data from the Epidemiological Catchment Area survey (Regier et al. 1984), they found that 76% of persons with a lifetime history of major depression "had ever smoked" compared with 52% of persons without a depression history. Similarly, the incidence of depression was 6.6% in smokers compared with 2.9% in nonsmokers, and smokers with a history of depression had a low rate of cessation. These findings have been replicated by several investigators, and the association between depression and smoking is well supported. Another observation is that depressive symptoms appear during smoking cessation in persons with a history of depression (Covey et al. 1990). These researchers also found that alcoholism had the highest association with smoking. Last, depressed mood may lead to relapse in smoking among subjects without major depression (Killen et al. 1996), and bupropion appears to be effective in promoting cessation. Smoking rates among persons with anxiety disorders are also at least twice that of persons without a psychiatric diagnosis.

It is unclear what role smoking plays in psychopathology of these disorders. There is some information supporting smoking in these populations as a maladaptive coping strategy (Revell et al. 1985). Future research on smoking in these targeted populations may indicate the most efficient treatment approaches for patients who have both nicotine dependence and a psychiatric disorder.

Summary

Nicotine replacement combined with behavior modification therapy is very effective in relieving nicotine withdrawal symptoms and in initiating smoking cessation. The antidepressant bupropion has been approved by the FDA as a treatment for smoking cessation. We must await the results of future research in order to establish methods of improving long-term nicotine abstinence.

REFERENCES

Alterman AI, Droba M, Antelo RE, et al: Amantadine may facilitate detoxification of cocaine addicts. Drug Alcohol Depend 31:19–29, 1992

Altshuler HL, Phillips PE, Feinhandler DA: Alteration of ethanol self-administration by naltrexone. Life Sci 26:679–688, 1980

American Psychiatric Association: Diagnostic and Statistical Manual of Mental Disorders, 3rd Edition, Revised. Washington, DC, American Psychiatric Association, 1987

American Psychiatric Association: Diagnostic and Statistical Manual of Mental Disorders, 4th Edition. Washington, DC, American Psychiatric Association, 1994

Arndt IO, Dorozynsky L, Woody GE, et al: Desipramine treatment of cocaine dependence in methadone-maintained patients. Arch Gen Psychiatry 49:888–893, 1992

Bagasra O, Forman LJ, Howeedy A, et al: A potential vaccine for cocaine abuse prophylaxis [see comments]. Immunopharmacology 23(3): 173–179, 1992

Ball JC, Ross A: The Effectiveness of Methadone Maintenance Treatment. New York, Springer-Verlag, 1991

Beary MD, Christofides J, Fry D, et al: The benzodiazepines as substances of abuse. Practitioner 231:19–20, 1987

Benowitz NL: Nicotine replacement therapy: what has been accomplished—can we do better? Drugs 45:157–170, 1993

Benwell ME, Balfour DJ: The effects of nicotine administration on 5-HT uptake and biosynthesis in rat brain. Eur J Pharmacol 84:71–77, 1982

Bickel WE, Stitzer ML, Bigelow GE, et al: A clinical trial of buprenorphine: comparison with methadone in the detoxification of heroin addicts. Clin Pharmacol Ther 43:72–78, 1988

Burling TA, Ziff DC: Tobacco smoking: a comparison between alcohol and drug abuse in patients. Addict Behav 13:185–190, 1988

Cornish JW, Maany I, Fudala PJ, et al: Carbamazepine treatment for cocaine dependence. Drug Alcohol Depend 38:221–227, 1995

Covey LS, Glassman AH, Stetner F: Depression and depressive symptoms in smoking cessation. Compr Psychiatry 31:350–354, 1990

Cowan A, Lewis JW, Macfarlane IR: Agonist and antagonist properties of buprenorphine, a new antinociceptive agent. Br J Pharmacol 60: 537–545, 1977

Crane M, Sereny G, Gordis E: Drug use among alcoholism detoxification patients: prevalence and impact on alcoholism treatment. Drug Alcohol Depend 22:33–36, 1988

Daughton DM, Heatley SA, Pendergast JJ, et al: Effect of transdermal nicotine delivery as an adjunct to low-intervention smoking cessation therapy. Arch Intern Med 151:749–752, 1991

Dole VP, Nyswander M: A medical treatment for diacetylmorphine (heroin) addiction: a clinical trial with methadone hydrochloride. JAMA 193:646–650, 1965

Dorus W, Ostrow DG, Anton R, et al: Lithium treatment of depressed and nondepressed alcoholics. JAMA 262:1646–1652, 1989

Edwards NB, Simmons RC, Rosenthal TL, et al: Doxepin in the treatment of nicotine withdrawal. Psychosomatics 29:203–206, 1988

Edwards NB, Murphy JK, Downs AD, et al: Doxepin as an adjunct to smoking cessation. Am J Psychiatry 146:373–376, 1989

Farebrother MJB, Pearce SJ, Turner P, et al: Propranolol and giving up smoking. British Journal of Diseases of the Chest 74:95–96, 1980

Ferry LH, Robbins AS, Scariati PD, et al: Enhancement of smoking cessation using the antidepressant bupropion hydrochloride. Abstract from the 65th Scientific Sessions of the American Heart Association, New Orleans, LA. Circulation 86 (suppl 1):671, 1992

Finkle BS, Jennison TA, Chinn DM, et al: Plasma and urine disposition of 1-alpha-acetylmethadol and its principal metabolites in man. J Anal Toxicol 6:100–105, 1982

Finnegan LP: Treatment issues for opioid-dependent women during the perinatal period. J Psychoactive Drugs 23:191–201, 1991

Finnegan LP, Kandall SR: Maternal and neonatal effects of alcohol and drugs, in Substance Abuse: A Comprehensive Textbook. Edited by Lowinson JH, Ruiz P, Millman RB, et al. Baltimore, MD, Williams & Wilkins, 1992, pp 628–656

Fox BS, Kantak KM, Edwards MA, et al: Efficacy of a therapeutic cocaine vaccine in rodent models [see comments]. Nat Med 2(10):1129–1132, 1996

Franks P, Harp J, Bell B: Randomized controlled trial of clonidine for smoking cessation in a primary care setting. JAMA 262:3011–3013, 1989

Froehlich JC, Harts J, Lumeng L, et al: Naloxone attenuates voluntary ethanol intake in rats selectively bred for high ethanol preference. Pharmacol Biochem Behav 35:385–390, 1990

Fudala PJ, Jaffe JH, Dax EM, et al: Use of buprenorphine in the treatment of opiate addiction, II: physiologic and behavioral effects of daily and alternate-day administration and abrupt withdrawal. Clin Pharmacol Ther 47:525–534, 1990

Fuller RK, Branchey L, Brightwell DR, et al: Disulfiram treatment of alcoholism: a Veterans Administration cooperative study. JAMA 256:1449–1455, 1986

Gawin FH, Kleber HD: Abstinence symptomatology and psychiatric diagnosis in cocaine abusers. Arch Gen Psychiatry 43:107–113, 1986

Gawin FH, Kleber HD, Byck R, et al: Desipramine facilitation of initial cocaine abstinence. Arch Gen Psychiatry 46:117–121, 1989

Gerstein DR: The effectiveness of drug treatment, in Addictive States, Vol 70. Edited by O'Brien CP, Jaffe JH. New York, Raven, 1992, pp 253–282

Gilman AG, Rall TW, Nies AS, et al (eds): Goodman and Gilman's The Pharmacological Basis of Therapeutics, 8th Edition. New York, Pergamon, 1990

Glassman AH: Cigarette smoking: implications for psychiatric illness. Am J Psychiatry 150:546–553, 1993

Glassman AH, Jackson WK, Walsh BT, et al: Cigarette craving, smoking withdrawal, and clonidine. Science 226:864–866, 1984

Glassman AH, Stetner F, Walsh Raizman PS, et al: Heavy smokers, smoking cessation, and clonidine: results of a double-blind, randomized trial. JAMA 259:2863–2866, 1988

Glassman AH, Helzer JE, Covey LS, et al: Smoking, smoking cessation, and major depression. JAMA 264:1546–1549, 1990

Goff DC, Henderson DC, Amico E: Cigarette smoking in schizophrenia: relationship to psychopathology and medication side effects. Am J Psychiatry 149:1189–1194, 1992

Gold MS, Redmond DE, Kleber HD: Clonidine blocks acute opiate withdrawal symptoms. Lancet 2:599–602, 1978

Gold MS, Pottach AC, Sweeney DR, et al: Opiate withdrawal using clonidine. JAMA 243:343–346, 1980

Goodwin DW: Alcohol: clinical aspects, in Substance Abuse—A Comprehensive Textbook. Edited by Lowinson JH, Ruiz P, Millman RB. Baltimore, MD, Williams & Wilkins, 1992, pp 144–151

Gorelick DA: Enhancing cocaine metabolism with butyrylcholinesterase as a treatment strategy. Drug Alcohol Depend 48:159–165, 1997

Grabowski J, Rhoades H, Elk R, et al: Fluoxetine is ineffective for treatment of cocaine dependence or concurrent opiate and cocaine dependence: two placebo controlled double-blind trials. J Clin Psychopharmacol 15:163–173, 1995

Gross J, Stitzer ML: Nicotine replacement: ten-week effects on tobacco withdrawal symptoms. Psychopharmacology 93:334–341, 1989

Halikas J, Crosby RD, Graves N: Double-blind carbamazepine enhancement in the treatment of cocaine abuse, in Abstracts: Annual Meeting of the American College of Neuropsychopharmacology, San Juan, Puerto Rico, 1992, p 231

Hall SM, Killen JD: Psychological and pharmacological approaches to smoking relapse prevention. NIDA Res Monogr 53:131–143, 1985

Hall SM, Tunstall C, Rugg D, et al: Nicotine gum and behavioral treatment in smoking cessation. J Consult Clin Psychol 53:256–258, 1985

Hartel D, Selwyn PA, Schoenbaum EE: Methadone maintenance and reduced risk of AIDS and AIDS-specific mortality in intravenous drug users, in Fourth International Conference on AIDS. Stockholm, Sweden, Abstract 8526, 1988

Hartel D, Schoenbaum EE, Selwyn PA: Temporal patterns of cocaine use and AIDS in intravenous drug users in methadone maintenance, in Fifth International Conference on AIDS. Montreal, Canada, Abstract, 1989

Hayashida M, Alterman AI, McLellan AT, et al: Comparative effectiveness and costs of inpatient and outpatient detoxification of patients with mild-to-moderate alcohol withdrawal syndrome. N Engl J Med 320:358–365, 1989

Hoffman RS, Morasco R, Goldfrank LR: Administration of purified human plasma cholinesterase protects against cocaine toxicity in mice. J Toxicol Clin Toxicol 34:259–266, 1996

Holder H, Longabaugh R, Miller W, et al: The cost effectiveness of treatment for alcoholism: a first approximation. J Stud Alcohol 52:517–540, 1991

Hubbell CL, Czirr SA, Hunter GA, et al: Consumption of ethanol solution is potentiated by morphine and attenuated by naloxone persistently across repeated daily administrations. Alcohol 3:39–54, 1986

Hughes JR, Hatsukami D: Signs and symptoms of tobacco withdrawal. Arch Gen Psychiatry 43:289–294, 1986

Hurt RD, Sachs DPL, Glover ED, et al: A comparison of sustained-release bupropion and placebo for smoking cessation. N Engl J Med 337:1195–1202, 1997

Jacobs MA, Spilken AA, Norman MM, et al: Interaction of personality and treatment conditions associated with success in a smoking control program. Psychosom Med 33:545–546, 1971

Jaffe JH, Kranzler M: Smoking as an addictive disorder. NIDA Res Monogr 23:4–23, 1979

Jasinski DR, Pevnick JS, Griffith JD: Human pharmacology and abuse potential of the analgesic buprenorphine. Arch Gen Psychiatry 35:501–516, 1978

Johnson BA, Jasinski DR, Galloway GP, et al: Ritanserin in the treatment of alcohol dependence—a multi-center clinical trial. Ritanserin Study Group. Psychopharmacology (Berl) 128:206–215, 1996

Johnson RE, Cone EJ, Henningfield JE, et al: Use of buprenorphine in the treatment of opiate addiction, I: physiologic and behavioral effects during a rapid dose induction. Clin Pharmacol Ther 46:335–343, 1989

Johnson RE, Jaffe JH, Fudala PJ: A controlled trial of buprenorphine treatment for opioid dependence. JAMA 267:2750–2755, 1992

Jorenby DE, Leischow SJ, Nides MA, et al: A controlled trial of sustained-release bupropion, a nicotine patch, or both for smoking cessation. N Engl J Med 340:685–691, 1999

Kampman K, Volpicelli JR, Alterman A, et al: Amantadine in the early treatment of cocaine dependence: a double-blind, placebo-controlled trial. Drug Alcohol Depend 41:25–33, 1996

Killen JD, Maccoby N, Taylor CB: Nicotine gum and self-regulation training in smoking relapse prevention. Behav Res Ther 15:234–248, 1984

Killen JD, Fortmann SP, Kraemer HC, et al: Interactive effects of depression symptoms, nicotine dependence, and weight change on late smoking relapse. J Consult Clin Psychol 64:1060–1067, 1996

Kornetsky C, Porrino LJ: Brain mechanisms of drug-induced reinforcement, in Addictive States, Vol 70. Edited by O'Brien CP, Jaffe JH. New York, Raven, 1992, pp 59–78

Kosten TR, Kleber HD: Buprenorphine detoxification from opioid dependence: a pilot study. Life Sci 42:635–641, 1988

Kosten TR, Morgan CM, Falcione J, et al: Pharmacotherapy for cocaine-abusing methadone-maintained patients using amantadine or desipramine. Arch Gen Psychiatry 49:894–898, 1992

Kranzler HR, Babor TF, Laureman RJ: Problems associated with average alcohol consumption and frequency of intoxication in a medical population. Alcohol Clin Exp Res 14:119–126, 1990

Kranzler HR, Bauer LO, Hersh D, et al: Carbamazepine treatment of cocaine dependence: a placebo-controlled trial. Drug Alcohol Depend 38:203–211, 1995a

Kranzler HR, Burleson JA, Korner P, et al: Placebo-controlled trial of fluoxetine as an adjunct to relapse prevention in alcoholics. Am J Psychiatry 152:391–397, 1995b

Leventhal H, Cleary P: The smoking problem: a review of the research and theory in behavioral risk modification. Psychol Bull 88:370–405, 1980

Lhuintre JP, Daoust M, Moore ND, et al: Ability of calcium bis acetyl homotaurine, a GABA agonist, to prevent relapse in weaned alcoholics. Lancet 1(8436):1014–1016, 1985

Lhuintre JP, Moore N, Tran G, et al: Acamprosate appears to decrease alcohol intake in weaned alcoholics. Alcohol Alcohol 25:613–622, 1990

Lipsedge MS, Cook CCH: Prescribing for drug addicts. Lancet 2:451–452, 1987

Loimer N, Schmid R, Lenz K, et al: Acute blocking of naloxone-precipitated opiate withdrawal symptoms by methohexitone. Br J Psychiatry 157:748–752, 1990

Loimer N, Lenz K, Schmid R, et al: Technique for greatly shortening the transition from methadone to naltrexone maintenance of patients addicted to opiates. Am J Psychiatry 148:933–935, 1991

Maddux JF, Desmond DP: Methadone maintenance and recovery from opioid dependence. Am J Drug Alcohol Abuse 18:63–74, 1992

Magura S, Goldsmith D, Casriel C, et al: The validity of methadone clients' self-reported drug use. Int J Addict 22:727–750, 1987

Margolin A, Kosten TR, Avants SK, et al: A multicenter trial of bupropion for cocaine dependence in methadone-maintained patients. Drug Alcohol Depend 40:125–131, 1995

Martin WR, Jasinski DR: Physical parameters of morphine dependence in man: tolerance, early abstinence, protracted abstinence. J Psychiatr Res 7:9–17, 1969

Martin WR, Jasinski D, Mansky P: Naltrexone, an antagonist for the treatment of heroin dependence. Arch Gen Psychiatry 28:784–791, 1973

Mason BJ, Kocsis JH: Desipramine treatment of alcoholism. Psychopharmacol Bull 27:155–161, 1991

Mason BJ, Ritvo EC, Morgan RO, et al: A double-blind, placebo-controlled pilot study to evaluate the efficacy and safety of oral nalmefene HCl for alcohol dependence. Alcohol Clin Exp Res 18:1162–1167, 1994

Matherson E, O'Shea B: Smoking and malignancy in schizophrenia. Br J Psychiatry 145:429–432, 1984

Mattes C, Bradley R, Slaughter E, et al: Cocaine and butyrylcholinesterase (BChE): determination of enzymatic parameters. Life Sci 58:L257–L261, 1996

McGrath PJ, Nunes EV, Delivannides D, et al: Imipramine treatment of depressed alcoholics. Paper presented at the 33rd annual meeting of the New Clinical Drug Evaluation Unit Program (NCDEU), Boca Raton, FL, June 1993

Metzger DS, Woody GE, McLellan AT, et al: Human immunodeficiency virus seroconversion among in- and out-of-treatment intravenous drug users: an 18-month prospective follow-up. J Acquir Immune Defic Syndr Hum Retrovirol 6:1049–1056, 1993

Montoya ID, Levin FR, Fudala PJ, et al: Double-blind comparison of carbamazepine and placebo for treatment of cocaine dependence. Drug Alcohol Depend 38:213–219, 1995

Myers RD, Borg S, Mossberg R: Antagonism by naltrexone of voluntary alcohol selection in the chronically drinking macaque monkey. Alcohol 3:383–388, 1986

National Institute of Alcoholism and Alcohol Abuse: Seventh Special Report to the US Congress on Alcohol and Health. Rockville, MD, U.S. Department of Health and Human Services, 1990

Nutt D, Adinoff B, Linnoila M: Benzodiazepines in the treatment of alcoholism, in Recent Developments in Alcoholism, Treatment Research, Vol 7. Edited by Galanter M. New York, Plenum, 1989, pp 283–313

Ogborne AC, Kapur BM: Drug use among a sample of males admitted to an alcohol detoxification center. Alcohol Clin Exp Res 11:183–185, 1987

O'Malley SS, Jaffe AJ, Chang G, et al: Naltrexone and coping skills therapy for alcohol dependence. Arch Gen Psychiatry 49:881–887, 1992

Paille FM, Guelfi JD, Perkins AC, et al: Double-blind randomized multicentre trial of acamprosate in maintaining abstinence from alcohol. Alcohol Alcohol 30:239–247, 1995

Palmer KJ, Buckley MM, Faulds D: Transdermal nicotine: a review of its pharmacodynamic and pharmacokinetic properties and therapeutic efficacy as an aid to smoking cessation. Drugs 44:498–529, 1992

Peachy JE, Naranjo CA: The role of drugs in the treatment of alcoholism. Drugs 27:171–182, 1984

Post R: Time course of clinical effects of carbamazepine: implications for mechanisms of action. J Clin Psychiatry 49 (suppl 1):35–46, 1988

Regier DA, Myers JK, Kramer M, et al: The NIMH Epidemiologic Catchment Area Program: historical context, major objectives, and study population characteristics. Arch Gen Psychiatry 41:934–941, 1984

Revell AD, Warburton DM, Wesnes K: Smoking as a coping strategy. Addict Behav 10:209–224, 1985

Robins LN, Helzer JE, Weissman MM, et al: Lifetime prevalence of specific psychiatric disorders in three sites. Arch Gen Psychiatry 41:949–958, 1984

Sass H, Soyka M, Mann K, et al: Relapse prevention by acamprosate: results from a placebo-controlled study on alcohol dependence. Arch Gen Psychiatry 53:673–680, 1996

Schneider NG, Jarvik ME, Forsythe AB, et al: Nicotine gum in smoking cessation: a placebo controlled, double-blind trial. Addict Behav 8: 253–261, 1983

Schuckit MA: Alcohol and alcoholism, in Harrison's Principles of Internal Medicine. Edited by Braunwald E, Isselbacher KJ, Petersdorf RG, et al. New York, McGraw-Hill, 1987, pp 2106–2111

Schuckit MA: Alcohol and alcoholism, in Harrison's Principles of Internal Medicine, Vol 2. Edited by Wilson JD, Braunwald E, Isselbacher KJ, et al. New York, McGraw-Hill, 1991, pp 2149–2151

Schwartz HJ, Johnson D: In vitro competitive inhibition of plasma cholinesterase by cocaine: normal and variant genotypes. J Toxicol Clin Toxicol 34:77–81, 1996

Soyka M, Lutz W, Kauert G, et al: Epileptic seizures and alcohol withdrawal: significance of additional use (and misuse) of drugs and electro-encephalographic findings. Epilepsy 2:109–113, 1989

Stine SM, Kosten TR: Use of drug combinations in treatment of opioid withdrawal. J Clin Psychopharmacol 12:203–209, 1992

Stitzer ML: Nicotine-delivery products: demonstrated and desirable effects, in New Developments in Nicotine-Delivery Systems. Edited by Henningfield JE, Stitzer ML. Ossining, NY, Cortland Communications, 1991, pp 35–45

Substance Abuse and Mental Health Services Administration: Preliminary Estimates From the Drug Abuse Warning Network—Third Quarter 1992 Estimates of Drug-Related Emergency Room Episodes (Advance Report No 2). Washington, DC, U.S. Government Printing Office, 1993

Substance Abuse and Mental Health Services Administration: Preliminary Estimates From the 1994 National Household Survey on Drug Abuse (Advance Report No 3). Washington, DC, U.S. Government Printing Office, 1995

Sutherland G, Stapleton JA, Russell MAH, et al: Randomised controlled trial of nasal nicotine spray in smoking cessation. Lancet 340:324–329, 1992

Swift RM, Whelihan W, Kuznetsov O, et al: Naltrexone-induced alterations in human ethanol intoxication. Am J Psychiatry 151:1463–1467, 1994

Tonnesen P, Norregaard J, Simonsen K, et al: A double-blind trial of a 16-hour transdermal nicotine patch in smoking cessation. N Engl J Med 325:311–315, 1991

Tonnesen P, Norregaard J, Mikkelson K, et al: A double-blind trial of a nicotine inhaler for smoking cessation. JAMA 269:1268–1271, 1993

U.S. Department of Health and Human Services: Reducing the health consequences of smoking: 25 years of progress: a report of the Surgeon General. Washington, DC, U.S. Government Printing Office, 1989

U.S. Department of Health and Human Services: The health benefits of smoking cessation: a report of the Surgeon General. Washington, DC, U.S. Government Printing Office, 1990

Volpicelli JR, Davis MA, Olgin JE: Naltrexone blocks the post-shock increase of ethanol consumption. Life Sci 38:841–847, 1986

Volpicelli JR, Alterman AI, Hayashida MD, et al: Naltrexone in the treatment of alcohol dependence. Arch Gen Psychiatry 49:886–880, 1992

Whitworth AB, Fischer F, Lesch OM, et al: Comparison of acamprosate and placebo in long-term treatment of alcohol dependence [see comments]. Lancet 347(9013):1438–1442, 1996

Wikler A: Dynamics of drug dependence. Arch Gen Psychiatry 28:611–616, 1973

TWENTY-FOUR

Treatment of Eating Disorders

W. Stewart Agras, M.D.

In this chapter, the pharmacological treatment of two classic eating disorders—anorexia nervosa (AN) and bulimia nervosa (BN)—is considered, together with that of binge-eating disorder, which is included as a new entity in DSM-IV (American Psychiatric Association 1994).

BULIMIA NERVOSA

BN is a relatively common disorder affecting some 1%–2% of young women (Fairburn and Beglin 1990). The disorder usually has an onset in late adolescence or early adult life, with a prodromal period characterized by dissatisfaction with body shape and a fear of becoming overweight, followed by marked dietary restriction. Sooner or later periods of dietary restriction are followed by episodes of binge eating experienced as a loss of control over dietary intake, often accompanied by the consumption of large amounts of food. This, in turn, further aggravates both the dissatisfaction with body shape and the fear of weight gain. Ultimately, the bulimic person discovers purging, usually in the form of self-induced vomiting, with or without laxative use, or (in rare cases) by chewing food and spitting it out.

DSM-IV distinguishes two forms of BN—namely, purging and nonpurging types, the latter characterized by the use of exercise or fasting rather than other types of compensatory behavior (American Psychiatric Association 1994). The implications of this classification for treatment are unknown. Medical complications of BN are relatively rare; the most frequent are potassium depletion and dental caries. Comorbid psychopathology includes major depression; various anxiety disorders, including generalized anxiety disorder, social phobia, and panic disorder; alcoholism; and personality disorders, particularly those in the Cluster B spectrum. It is now recognized that the natural history of the disorder is frequently one of chronicity (Keller et al. 1992), which emphasizes the importance of adequate and early treatment.

Binge Eating

The form and content of binge-eating episodes have been studied in two ways: 1) in the natural environment by self-monitoring and 2) in the laboratory. Despite reports by bulimic patients that their binges are typically very large, often greater than 5,000 kcal (Johnson et al. 1982), self-monitoring studies of patients with BN reported a different picture. In the first of these studies, binge-eating episodes averaged 1,459 calories (range 45–5,138 kcal) compared with 321 calories (range 10–1,652 kcal) in non-binge-eating episodes (Rosen et al. 1986). Sixty-five percent of binge episodes were within the range of nonbinge episodes. Subsequent self-monitoring studies essentially confirmed the findings.

Laboratory studies have reported a somewhat different picture. The average binge is larger than that found in the self-monitoring studies; caloric consumption varies from a mean of 3,031 kcal to 7,774 kcal across studies, with a range of 83–25,755 kcal for binge episodes (Hadigan et al. 1989; Mitchell and Laine 1985). These differences between laboratory and field studies may be partly a result of differences in sample selection, because many of the participants in laboratory studies were inpatients with more severe BN. Self-monitoring is also likely to underestimate the caloric content of binges because of deficiencies in recording. Laboratory studies may overestimate caloric consumption during binge episodes, whereas field studies may underestimate such consumption.

Factors maintaining binge eating.   Differentiating between factors that cause and those that maintain binge eating is important, because the latter may be more critical in the treatment of BN. Two factors—dietary restraint and transient negative moods—appear to be important in maintaining binge eating and subsequent purging. Chronic dietary restraint is often accompanied by long periods between meals (e.g., skipping breakfast and lunch), after which the bulimic person loses control over eating and begins to binge eat. This pattern of restraint is fueled by cognitive distortions regarding food intake and an exaggerated sense of the importance of body shape and weight.

The effects of negative mood on binge eating have been suggested by the fact that bulimic patients report negative mood to be the most frequent trigger of binge eating (Bruce and

Agras 1992). Laboratory studies have confirmed this observation: negative mood leads to loss of control over eating, provokes binge eating, and leads bulimic patients to classify their eating episodes as binges (Telch and Agras 1996).

Etiology of Bulimia Nervosa

Relatively little is known about the etiology of BN. Studies suggest that the disorder is heritable and that familial aggregation is most likely explained in part by heritability and in part by familial psychological influences specific to the affected individual (Kendler et al. 1991). Various neurochemical hypotheses have been proposed; the most frequent is reduction in brain serotonin (5-hydroxytryptamine [5-HT]) synthesis. Dietary restriction has been shown to lead to decreased plasma tryptophan levels, which would likely reduce 5-HT synthesis. It is possible that bulimic patients may be particularly sensitive to such changes and become locked in a vicious circle of neurochemical changes once they begin dieting, resulting in an effect on satiety. On the other hand, it must be remembered that food intake is controlled by several neurochemical systems, including norepinephrine and peptide YY, both of which potentiate eating; hence, it may be too early to implicate one particular system. In addition, nutritional state markedly affects these neurochemical systems, making the task of detailing the abnormalities in BN even more complicated.

Social factors are also implicated in BN. During the 1980s, the number of cases of BN seen in clinics around the world increased dramatically (Garner et al. 1985). This increase occurred concurrently with the portrayal of a thin body shape as the ideal for women, despite the fact that few women can meet this social demand (Brownell 1991). Such social pressure may have led more young women to diet, increasing the risk of binge eating and purging in the biologically susceptible individual. Patton et al. (1990), in a 1-year follow-up study of schoolgirls in London, found that dieting was associated with a relative risk eight times higher than that of nondieters for the development of an eating disorder. However, even though the vast majority of female adolescents diet, only 2%–3% develop an eating disorder. This finding poses an interesting dilemma for public health policy. On the one hand, the prevalence of obesity is increasing, which suggests that dietary interventions are important, but on the other hand, a small proportion of women may respond to dieting by developing an eating disorder. Education about healthy eating habits would seem important, particularly in adolescents, in an effort to stop the development of highly restrictive dieting.

Psychopharmacological Treatment of Bulimia Nervosa

Antidepressant treatment. The use of antidepressants in the treatment of BN was sparked by the observation that depression is often a comorbid feature of the disorder (Pope and Hudson 1982). In 1982, two groups of researchers conducted small-scale uncontrolled studies indicating that both monoamine oxidase inhibitors and tricyclic antidepressants reduced binge eating and purging (Pope and Hudson 1982; Walsh et al. 1982). These observations were followed by a series of double-blind, placebo-controlled studies confirming the utility of antidepressants in treating BN, at least in the short term. A wide range of antidepressant drugs have been found effective, including imipramine (Agras et al. 1987; Mitchell et al. 1990; Pope et al. 1983), desipramine (Agras et al. 1991; Barlow et al. 1988; Blouin et al. 1989; Hughes et al. 1986), phenelzine (Walsh et al. 1984, 1988), bromofarin (Kennedy et al. 1993), trazodone (Pope et al. 1989), bupropion (Horne et al. 1988), and fluoxetine (Fluoxetine Bulimia Nervosa Collaborative Study Group 1992). In these studies, the rate of decrease in binge eating and purging ranged from 30% to 91% (median 69%). Complete recovery from binge eating and purging ranged from 10% to 60% (median 32%), and the dropout rate from the medication

groups ranged from 0% to 48% (median 23%). In other words, of 100 patients with BN, about 77 will continue taking medication, and 25 will be in remission at the end of treatment with a single antidepressant.

Antidepressants are prescribed for BN in the same dosage used for treating depression, with the exception of fluoxetine, because a dosage of 60 mg/day was found to be more effective than 20 mg/day in reducing binge eating and purging in a placebo-controlled trial involving 387 bulimic women (Fluoxetine Bulimia Nervosa Collaborative Study Group 1992). One problem with medication given at times other than bedtime is that a significant amount of medication may be purged through subsequent vomiting. Side effects and reasons for dropout from the various medications were similar to those observed in the treatment of depression, with the exception of bupropion, for which a higher than expected proportion of patients with BN had a grand mal seizure (Horne et al. 1988). The authors concluded that bupropion should not be used in patients with BN until the reason for the high proportion of seizures in these patients was established.

Overall, most antidepressants appear to be effective in the short-term treatment of BN, but the effects are limited, with about one-quarter to one-third of patients achieving remission on average. Less is known about the long-term effectiveness of antidepressants. In one uncontrolled study (Pope et al. 1985) in which a variety of antidepressants were used over the course of a 2-year follow-up, 50% of patients achieved and maintained remission from binge eating and purging. The only controlled longer-term follow-up studies have been plagued by sample size problems, with relatively few participants' symptoms meeting criteria for entry into the follow-up phase of treatment (Pyle et al. 1990; Walsh et al. 1991). Even with continued medication treatment, about one-third of patients in these studies relapsed. Little evidence indicated that continued treatment with a single antidepressant was more effective than the placebo condition. This outcome raises the question of whether treatment with a different antidepressant for patients who do not respond initially (or who relapse) would be more effective. One open-label study suggested that about half of such patients will respond to a different antidepressant, with complete remission of symptoms (Mitchell et al. 1989). This would raise the remission rate for the hypothetical cohort of 100 patients to 50. Hence, sequential trials of different antidepressants would seem useful in the treatment of BN.

Combined treatment.   Cognitive-behavior therapy for BN was developed in parallel with the use of antidepressants, and numerous controlled studies suggest that such treatment is effective (Fairburn et al. 1992). Cognitive-behavior therapy has four distinct phases. First, the extent of the problem is examined by careful history taking and the use of self-monitoring of food intake, binge eating, and purging. Second, dietary intake is slowly normalized by shaping at least three adequate meals each day. This diet shortens the long intervals between eating episodes that are typical of patients with bulimia and lessens dietary restraint; thus, the probability of binge eating is reduced. Third, distorted cognitions regarding caloric intake and body shape and weight are corrected. Finally, relapse prevention procedures (e.g., coping with high-risk situations) are practiced. Treatment usually extends over a 6-month period, averaging about 20 sessions.

Cognitive-behavior therapy in either individual or group format has been shown to be more effective in reducing binge eating and/or purging than placebo (Mitchell et al. 1990), supportive psychotherapy plus self-monitoring of eating behavior (Agras et al. 1989), stress management (Laessle et al. 1991), behavior therapy (Fairburn et al. 1993), and psychodynamic forms of psychotherapy (Garner et al. 1993; Walsh et al. 1997).

The existence of two different and effective treatments—antidepressant medications and cognitive-behavior therapy—naturally leads to the question of whether the combination of such treatments would be more effective than either treatment alone.

The first study of this question used a randomized 2 × 2 design with four experimental groups: 1) imipramine combined with group psychosocial treatment, 2) imipramine with no psychosocial treatment, 3) placebo combined with group psychosocial treatment, and 4) placebo with no psychosocial treatment (Mitchell et al. 1990). The treatment phase was preceded by a single-blind placebo washout phase. One hundred and seventy-one women with BN entered the treatment phase, which lasted for 10 weeks. The psychosocial treatment was an intensive group variant of cognitive-behavior therapy, with 5 daily sessions in the first week and 22 treatment sessions overall. The mean daily dose of imipramine was 217 mg for the psychosocial treatment group and 266 mg for the group receiving medication alone. As might be expected, the dropout rate was significantly higher for those in the medication groups (34%) compared with those taking placebo (15%). The results for reductions in binge eating and purging were quite straightforward. Imipramine was found to be superior to placebo, which confirmed previous study results. However, cognitive-behavioral treatment, with a remission rate of 51%, was superior to imipramine, with a remission rate of 16%, and combining the two treatments did not result in any additional advantage in reducing binge eating and purging. The combined treatment was, however, significantly superior to cognitive-behavioral treatment in reducing depression.

In the second study (Agras et al. 1991, 1994), 71 participants were randomly allocated to one of three groups: 1) desipramine (mean dose 168 mg), 2) cognitive-behavioral treatment, and 3) combined treatment. In half of the desipramine participants, medication was withdrawn at 16 weeks, and in the remaining half, desipramine was discontinued at 24 weeks. Cognitive-behavioral treatment lasted for 24 weeks. Eighteen percent of participants stopped taking desipramine before medication was withdrawn compared with 4.3% of subjects receiving cognitive-behavior therapy. Cognitive-behavioral treatment, with a 48% remission rate, was significantly superior to desipramine, with a 33% remission rate, in reducing the frequency of binge eating and purging, and the combined treatment was no more effective than cognitive-behavioral treatment alone. However, the group receiving desipramine alone for 24 weeks was the most cost-effective in terms of the cost of treatment per recovered patient at 1-year follow-up (Koran et al. 1995).

A more recent study involved 120 women with BN and used a more sophisticated medication regimen consisting of desipramine followed by fluoxetine if the first medication was either ineffective or poorly tolerated (Walsh et al. 1997). It is important to note that the two-medication combination was used by two-thirds of the patients assigned to active medication, which suggests that a two-medication combination is an experimental design closer to clinical reality than a single medication is. This study used a five-cell design: cognitive-behavior therapy combined with placebo or active medication, psychodynamically oriented therapy combined with placebo or active medication, and medication alone. Cognitive-behavior therapy (plus placebo) was more effective than psychodynamic therapy (plus placebo) in reducing both binge eating and purging. The average dose of desipramine was 188 mg/day and of fluoxetine was 55 mg/day. Of patients receiving medication, 43% dropped out of the study compared with 32% of those receiving psychotherapy, which is a nonsignificant difference. Patients receiving active medication (in combination with psychological treatments) reduced binge eating significantly more than those receiving placebo. Finally, antidepressant medication combined with cognitive-behavior therapy was superior to medication alone in reducing purging frequency. Of those receiving cognitive-behavior therapy plus medication,

50% were in remission compared with 25% of those receiving medication alone.

Comprehensive Treatment of Bulimia Nervosa

For the most part, patients with BN are best treated as outpatients, unless there are either medical or psychiatric reasons for hospitalization (e.g., an intercurrent physical illness or comorbid psychiatric disorder requiring hospitalization, such as major depression with suicidality). One reason that outpatient treatment is useful is that gains made in the hospital may not carry over to the patient's home, where more complex food stimuli and greater stress than in the hospital are present.

At present, no clear guidelines exist for the sequence of pharmacological and psychological therapies. It can be argued that because cognitive-behavior therapy is superior to medication, psychological treatment might be the best initial approach in uncomplicated cases of BN, and medication could be added if the response to cognitive-behavior therapy were unsatisfactory. On the other hand, antidepressant medication appears to be more cost-effective than cognitive-behavior therapy. Patients should be advised of these facts so that they can make an informed choice. When marked depression accompanies the bulimic symptoms, antidepressant therapy should be used either alone or in combination with cognitive-behavior therapy, because depressive symptoms have a superior response to antidepressants used in the treatment of BN. If the first antidepressant does not lead to therapeutic gains in a reasonable time, the use of alternative antidepressants should be considered, followed by the addition of cognitive-behavior therapy if the response is not satisfactory.

BINGE-EATING DISORDER

About 2% of women in the general population have symptoms that meet criteria for binge-eating disorder (Bruce and Agras 1992). In clinical populations, the ratio of women to men with binge-eating disorder is approximately 3:2, the highest rate for men for any eating disorder. Although obesity is not a requirement for the diagnosis of binge-eating disorder, a substantial overlap exists between binge-eating disorder and obesity. Studies have shown that more than one-quarter of obese subjects have symptoms that meet criteria for binge-eating disorder and that the prevalence of binge eating increases as body mass index increases (Marcus et al. 1985; Telch et al. 1988). Because binge eating often precedes the onset of becoming overweight, binge eating may be a risk factor for obesity and the multiple health problems associated with being overweight. Moreover, the syndrome is associated with comorbid psychopathology similar to that of BN and causes much distress; hence, it is an entity deserving of treatment in its own right. One study that compared individuals with binge-eating disorder with weight-matched non-binge-eating obese individuals found that subjects with binge-eating disorder were significantly more likely to receive diagnoses of major depression (51%), panic disorder (9%), and borderline personality disorder (9%) than those without binge-eating disorder (Yanovski et al. 1992).

Antidepressant Treatment

Because of the similarity between BN and binge-eating disorder, investigators have suggested that treatments effective for BN should also be effective for binge-eating disorder. To date, three double-blind, placebo-controlled studies of the use of antidepressants in binge-eating disorder have been done (Alger et al. 1991; Hudson et al. 1998; McCann and Agras 1990). One of these studies involved 23 women with binge-eating disorder; patients who received desipramine reduced their binge eating significantly more than those who received placebo, and 60% of the desipramine group was abstinent at the end of 12 weeks' treatment

(McCann and Agras 1990). In addition, hunger was significantly reduced and dietary restraint was increased in those assigned to the active drug condition. When medication was withdrawn, rapid relapse across all parameters occurred. The second study had a large placebo effect with no differences between imipramine and placebo in reducing binge eating (Alger et al. 1991). The third study, involving 85 patients with binge-eating disorder, found that fluvoxamine was superior to placebo in reducing binge eating (Hudson et al. 1998).

Although the McCann and Agras (1990) study suggested that antidepressants are useful in the treatment of binge-eating disorder, patients who stopped binge eating did not lose weight in this short-term study. This finding is in accord with the two controlled psychological treatment studies of this disorder (Telch et al. 1990; Wilfley et al. 1993), neither of which reported significant weight loss in the treated group. Hence, a comprehensive treatment approach would of necessity require combining antidepressants with weight loss therapy. In one controlled study, 108 overweight women with binge-eating disorder were treated for 3 months with cognitive-behavior therapy, followed by 6 months of weight loss treatment combined with desipramine. No additive effect of desipramine on binge eating was found, although the medication group lost significantly more weight (10.5 lb) than the comparison group (Agras et al. 1994).

ANOREXIA NERVOSA

AN is a relatively rare disorder characterized by marked weight loss (at least 15% below ideal body weight), an intense fear of gaining weight, a disturbance in the experience of body shape (i.e., feeling fat in the face of marked weight loss), and (in females) amenorrhea. Because the disorder is rare, it is difficult in any one center to acquire an adequate sample size in a reasonable time; thus, satisfactory randomized, double-blind medication trials are difficult to accomplish. Moreover, medication trials should be long enough and use sufficient medication dosages to adequately show effects in this chronic relapsing disorder. Unfortunately, few trials to date meet these criteria; many are of short duration or use very small doses of medication.

The first medication to be evaluated in the treatment of AN was chlorpromazine, given in high doses of up to 1,000 mg/day (Dally and Sargant 1960). Unfortunately, the control group involved a retrospective comparison with patients admitted to the same center several years earlier. It is thus impossible to determine whether the findings were due to cohort or medication effects, particularly because the duration of illness was markedly different between the two cohorts. In further studies of antipsychotic agents in the treatment of AN, neither pimozide nor sulpiride (both selective dopamine antagonists) showed clear-cut efficacy (Vandereycken 1984; Vandereycken and Pierloot 1982). Therefore, little evidence exists for the utility of antipsychotic agents in the treatment of AN.

One of the best studies to date investigated the use of cyproheptadine (up to 32 mg/day) and amitriptyline (up to 160 mg/day) with a placebo control involving 72 hospitalized anorexic patients (Halmi et al. 1986). Eighty percent of patients were able to tolerate the maximum dose of cyproheptadine, and 70% tolerated the maximum dose of amitriptyline; in both groups, weight gain was related to the ability to tolerate the maximum dose. Overall, neither cyproheptadine nor amitriptyline was found to be effective in increasing the rate of weight gain or decreasing the number of days required to reach target weight. However, an interesting interaction was observed between cyproheptadine and the subtype of AN (bulimic or nonbulimic). In nonbulimic anorexic patients, cyproheptadine significantly decreased the number of days required to reach target weight as compared with amitriptyline. However, in bulimic anorexic pa-

tients, cyproheptadine appeared to have a deleterious effect on weight gain. This study suggests that the subtyping of AN into bulimic and nonbulimic variants is valid and that cyproheptadine in doses of 32 mg/day may be of some use in treatment of patients with the nonbulimic subtype. Few side effects of this medication are observed in patients with AN. Other studies of tricyclic antidepressants, including amitriptyline and clomipramine, have reported a lack of efficacy in the acute treatment phase, although the dosage of clomipramine used was very low (Biederman et al. 1985; Crisp et al. 1987). Similarly, lithium carbonate did not appear effective in promoting weight gain, although the study duration was only 4 weeks (Gross et al. 1981).

Two uncontrolled studies suggested that fluoxetine may be useful in the treatment of AN (Gwirtsman et al. 1990; Kaye et al. 1991). In the larger of these studies, Gwirtsman et al. (1990) followed up 31 patients with AN treated with fluoxetine for about a year after discharge from the hospital and found that 29 patients had maintained their weight at or above 85% of ideal body weight. Dose varied from 20 to 80 mg, with an average dose for good responders of 26 mg/day. Given the high relapse rate usually associated with AN, these findings are encouraging and certainly worthy of follow-up in a double-blind, placebo-controlled trial.

Overall, apart from the treatment of comorbid psychiatric disorders, such as obsessive-compulsive disorder or major depression, psychopharmacological agents have a limited role in the treatment of AN. For the nonpurging anorexic patient, cyproheptadine may prove useful in accelerating weight gain during the initial refeeding phase of treatment. In addition, tentative evidence suggests that fluoxetine may be of use in the maintenance phase of treatment. This latter finding may assume greater importance if it is confirmed in a placebo-controlled study, based on the finding that outpatient therapy may be as effective as inpatient treatment for AN (Crisp et al. 1991).

CONCLUSION

The place of psychopharmacological agents in the treatment of BN has been well worked out. Adequate treatment with sequential trials of different antidepressants should result in abstinence rates of about 40%. The addition of cognitive-behavioral treatment appears to enhance the effectiveness of the antidepressants. In the case of AN, many clinicians believe that medication does not significantly affect outcome. However, there are encouraging results from the use of fluoxetine in the maintenance phase of treatment of this disabling disorder.

Finally, it is too early to detail the role of pharmacological agents in the treatment of binge-eating disorder. However, sequential trials of antidepressants may be expected to yield results in binge-eating disorder similar to those in BN, with the possible added advantage of small additional weight losses.

REFERENCES

Agras WS, Dorian B, Kirkley BG, et al: Imipramine in the treatment of bulimia: a double-blind controlled study. Int J Eat Disord 6:29–38, 1987

Agras WS, Rossiter EM, Arnow B, et al: Cognitive-behavioral and response prevention treatment for bulimia nervosa. J Consult Clin Psychol 57:215–221, 1989

Agras WS, Rossiter EM, Arnow B, et al: Pharmacologic and cognitive-behavioral treatment for bulimia nervosa: a controlled comparison. Am J Psychiatry 159:325–333, 1991

Agras WS, Telch CF, Arnow B, et al: Weight loss, cognitive-behavioral, and desipramine treatments in binge-eating disorder: an additive design. Behavior Therapy 25:225–238, 1994

Alger A, Schwalberg D, Bigaouette JM, et al: Effect of a tricyclic antidepressant and opiate antagonist on binge-eating behavior in normoweight bulimic and obese, binge-eating subjects. Am J Clin Nutr 53:865–871, 1991

American Psychiatric Association: Diagnostic and Statistical Manual of Mental Disorders, 4th Edition. Washington, DC, American Psychiatric Association, 1994

Barlow J, Blouin J, Blouin A, et al: Treatment of bulimia with desipramine: a double-blind crossover study. Can J Psychiatry 33:129–133, 1988

Biederman J, Herzog DB, Rivinus TM, et al: Amitriptyline in the treatment of anorexia nervosa: a double-blind, placebo-controlled study. J Clin Psychopharmacol 5:10–16, 1985

Blouin J, Blouin A, Perez E: Bulimia: independence of antibulimic and antidepressant properties of desipramine. Can J Psychiatry 34:24–29, 1989

Brownell KD: Dieting and the search for the perfect body: where physiology and culture collide. Behavior Therapy 22:1–12, 1991

Bruce B, Agras WS: Binge-eating in females: a population-based investigation. Int J Eat Disord 12:365–373, 1992

Crisp AH, Lacey JH, Crutchfield M: Clomipramine and drive in people with anorexia nervosa: an inpatient study. Br J Psychiatry 150:355–358, 1987

Crisp AH, Norton K, Gowers S, et al: A controlled study of the effects of therapies aimed at adolescent and family psychopathology in anorexia nervosa. Br J Psychiatry 149:82–87, 1991

Dally PJ, Sargant W: A new treatment of anorexia nervosa. BMJ 1:1770–1773, 1960

Fairburn CG, Beglin SJ: Studies of the epidemiology of bulimia nervosa. Am J Psychiatry 147:401–408, 1990

Fairburn CG, Agras WS, Wilson GT: The research on the treatment of bulimia nervosa: practical and theoretical implications, in The Biology of Feast and Famine: Relevance to Eating Disorders. Edited by Anderson GH, Kennedy SH. New York, Academic Press, 1992, pp 317–340

Fairburn CG, Jones R, Peveler RC, et al: Psychotherapy and bulimia nervosa: longer-term effects of interpersonal psychotherapy, behavior therapy, and cognitive behavior therapy. Arch Gen Psychiatry 50:419–428, 1993

Fluoxetine Bulimia Nervosa Collaborative Study Group: Fluoxetine in the treatment of bulimia nervosa. Arch Gen Psychiatry 49:139–147, 1992

Garner DM, Olmsted MP, Garfinkel PE: Similarities among bulimic groups selected by weight and weight history. J Psychiatr Res 19:129–134, 1985

Garner DM, Rockert W, Davis R, et al: Comparison between cognitive-behavioral and supportive-expressive therapy for bulimia nervosa. Am J Psychiatry 150:37–46, 1993

Gross HA, Ebert MH, Faden VB, et al: A double-blind controlled trial of lithium carbonate in primary anorexia nervosa. J Clin Psychopharmacol 1:376–381, 1981

Gwirtsman HE, Guze BH, Yager J, et al: Fluoxetine treatment of anorexia nervosa: an open clinical trial. J Clin Psychiatry 51:378–382, 1990

Hadigan C, Kissileff HR, Walsh BT: Patterns of food selection during meals in women with bulimia. Am J Clin Nutr 50:759–766, 1989

Halmi CA, Eckert E, LaDu TJ, et al: Treatment efficacy of cyproheptadine and amitriptyline. Arch Gen Psychiatry 43:177–181, 1986

Horne RL, Ferguson JM, Pope HG, et al: Treatment of bulimia with bupropion: a multicenter controlled trial. J Clin Psychiatry 49:262–266, 1988

Hudson JI, McElroy SL, Raymond NC, et al: Fluvoxamine in the treatment of binge-eating disorder: a multicenter placebo-controlled, double-blind trial. Am J Psychiatry 155:1956–1962, 1998

Hughes PL, Wells LA, Cunningham CJ, et al: Treating bulimia with desipramine. Arch Gen Psychiatry 43:182–187, 1986

Johnson WG, Stuckey MK, Lewis LD, et al: Bulimia: a descriptive survey of 316 cases. Int J Eat Disord 2:3–16, 1982

Kaye WH, Weltzin TE, Hsu G, et al: An open trial of fluoxetine in patients with anorexia nervosa. J Clin Psychiatry 52:464–471, 1991

Keller MB, Herzog DB, Lavori PW, et al: The naturalistic history of bulimia nervosa: extraordinarily high rates of chronicity, relapse, recurrence, and psychosocial morbidity. Int J Eat Disord 12:1–10, 1992

Kendler KS, MacLean C, Neale M, et al: The genetic epidemiology of bulimia nervosa. Am J Psychiatry 148:1627–1637, 1991

Kennedy SH, Goldbloom DS, Ralevski E, et al: Is there a role for selective monoamine oxidase inhibitor therapy in bulimia nervosa? A placebo-controlled trial. J Clin Psychopharmacol 13:415–422, 1993

Koran LM, Agras WS, Rossiter E, et al: Comparing the cost-effectiveness of psychiatric treatments: bulimia nervosa. Psychiatry Res 58:13–21, 1995

Laessle PJ, Beumont PJV, Butow P, et al: A comparison of nutritional management with stress management in the treatment of bulimia nervosa. Br J Psychiatry 159:250–261, 1991

Marcus MD, Wing RR, Lamparski DM: Binge-eating and dietary restraint in obese patients. Addict Behav 10:163–168, 1985

McCann UD, Agras WS: Successful treatment of compulsive binge-eating with desipramine: a double-blind placebo-controlled study. Am J Psychiatry 147:1509–1513, 1990

Mitchell JE, Laine DC: Monitored binge-eating behavior in patients with bulimia. Int J Eat Disord 4:177–183, 1985

Mitchell JE, Pyle RL, Eckert ED, et al: Response to alternative antidepressants in imipramine nonresponders with bulimia nervosa. J Clin Psychopharmacol 9:291–293, 1989

Mitchell JE, Pyle RL, Eckert ED, et al: A comparison study of antidepressants and structured intensive group psychotherapy in the treatment of bulimia nervosa. Arch Gen Psychiatry 47:149–160, 1990

Patton E, Johnson-Sabine E, Wood A, et al: Abnormal eating attitudes in London schoolgirls—a prospective epidemiological study: outcome at twelve-month follow-up. Psychol Med 20:383–394, 1990

Pope HG, Hudson JI: Treatment of bulimia with antidepressants. Psychopharmacology (Berl) 78:176–179, 1982

Pope HG, Hudson JI, Jonas JM, et al: Bulimia treated with imipramine: a placebo-controlled double-blind study. Am J Psychiatry 140:554–558, 1983

Pope HG, Hudson JI, Jonas JM, et al: Antidepressant treatment of bulimia: a two-year follow-up study. J Clin Psychopharmacol 5:320–327, 1985

Pope HG, Keck PE, McElroy SL, et al: A placebo-controlled study of trazodone in bulimia nervosa. J Clin Psychopharmacol 9:254–259, 1989

Pyle RL, Mitchell JE, Eckert ED, et al: Maintenance treatment and 6-month outcome for bulimic patients who respond to initial treatment. Am J Psychiatry 147:871–875, 1990

Rosen JC, Leitenberg H, Fisher C, et al: Binge-eating episodes in bulimia nervosa: the amount and type of food consumed. Int J Eat Disord 5:255–267, 1986

Telch CF, Agras WS: Do emotional states influence binge eating in the obese? Int J Eat Disord 20:271–280, 1996

Telch CF, Agras WS, Rossiter EM: Binge-eating increases with increasing adiposity. Int J Eat Disord 7:115–119, 1988

Telch CF, Agras WS, Rossiter EM, et al: Group cognitive-behavioral treatment for the non-purging bulimic: an initial evaluation. J Consult Clin Psychol 58:629–635, 1990

Vandereycken W: Neuroleptics in the short-term treatment of anorexia nervosa: a double-blind placebo-controlled study with sulpiride. Br J Psychiatry 144:288–292, 1984

Vandereycken W, Pierloot R: Pimozide combined with behavior therapy in the short-term treatment of anorexia nervosa: a double-blind placebo-controlled cross over study. Acta Psychiatr Scand 66:445–450, 1982

Walsh BT, Stewart JW, Wright L, et al: Treatment of bulimia with monoamine oxidase inhibitors. Am J Psychiatry 139:1629–1630, 1982

Walsh BT, Stewart JW, Roose SP, et al: Treatment of bulimia with phenelzine: a double-blind, placebo-controlled study. Arch Gen Psychiatry 41:1105–1109, 1984

Walsh BT, Gladis M, Roose SP, et al: Phenelzine vs placebo in 50 patients with bulimia. Arch Gen Psychiatry 45:471–475, 1988

Walsh BT, Hadigan CM, Devlin MJ, et al: Long-term outcome of antidepressant treatment for bulimia nervosa. Am J Psychiatry 148:1206–1212, 1991

Walsh BT, Wilson GT, Loeb KL, et al: Medication and psychotherapy in the treatment of bulimia nervosa. Am J Psychiatry 154:523–531, 1997

Wilfley DE, Agras WS, Telch CF, et al: Group cognitive-behavioral therapy and group interpersonal psychotherapy for the non-purging bulimic: a controlled comparison. J Consult Clin Psychol 61:296–305, 1993

Yanovski SZ, Nelson JE, Dubbert BK, et al: Association of binge-eating disorder and psychiatric comorbidity in the obese. Am J Psychiatry 150:1472–1479, 1992

TWENTY-FIVE

Treatment of Agitation and Aggression

Stuart C. Yudofsky, M.D.,
Jonathan M. Silver, M.D., and
Robert E. Hales, M.D., M.B.A.

PREVALENCE OF AGITATION AND AGGRESSION AMONG PSYCHIATRIC AND OTHER MEDICAL PATIENTS

Psychiatrists are frequently called on to assess and treat agitation and aggression in psychiatric patients. Violence occurs at higher rates among patients with psychiatric illnesses just prior to their admissions to and discharges from psychiatric facilities than in the general population (Monahan 1992). Overall, approximately 10% of patients with chronic psychiatric disorders admitted to psychiatric services in both the private and the not-for-profit sectors acted violently toward others just prior to their admissions (Tardiff 1983; Tardiff and Sweillam 1982). Among patients with neuropsychiatric disease, such as posttraumatic brain injury, delirium, Alzheimer's disease, and other dementias, the incidence of agitation and aggression is much higher than for hospitalized patients with chronic psychiatric disorders (Elliott 1992). For example, among a sample of outpatients with Alzheimer's disease, Reisberg and co-workers (1987) reported that 48% had agitation, 30% had violent behavior, and 24% had verbal outbursts, which, together, accounted for the most common of all behavioral symptomatologies in this population.

Rovner et al. (1986) found that 90% of a sample of nursing home residents had symptoms that met DSM-III (American Psychiatric Association 1980) criteria for organic mental disorders. Of this sample, 48% exhibited behavioral agitation, which constituted the most common behavioral problem. Similarly, Chandler and Chandler (1988) reported that the most common behavioral problems in a sample of 65 nursing home residents were agitation and aggression, which affected 48% of their sample. These behaviors are also highly prevalent in the acute and chronic recovery stages of traumatic brain injury (Silver and Yudofsky 1994a). Rao et al. (1985) reported that 96% of 26 patients had acute agitation following traumatic brain injury. However, Brooke et al. (1992a), in a prospective study of 100 patients who sustained acute brain injury, documented—with the Overt Aggression Scale (OAS; Yudofsky et al. 1986)—that

11% were agitated and aggressive and that 35% were restless. Agitation and aggression may occur in patients months to many years after head injury, as is the case in posttraumatic seizure disorders. Oddy et al. (1985) followed up 44 patients for 7 years after severe traumatic brain injury and determined that agitation occurred in 31% of this population, whereas an additional 43% had severe irritability, temper outbursts, and aggression.

In this chapter, we review nosological, diagnostic, and pathophysiological aspects of agitation and aggression and, thereafter, focus on the pharmacotherapy of agitation and aggression in the context of a comprehensive treatment plan.

DIFFERENTIATING AGGRESSION, AGITATION, AND ANXIETY

Agitation and aggression most often occur as consequences of experiential and biological predispositions in the context of current evocative situations or environments. Far more attention has been devoted to the neurobiology and neuropathology of aggression than to those of agitation. (A review of the brain pathways involved in aggression and the ways in which neuropathology and psychopathology combine to provoke aggression can be found in a chapter by Ovsiew and Yudofsky 1993.) Table 25–1 summarizes brain loci that are associated with aggressive behaviors, and Table 25–2 reviews the work of Valzelli (1981) on brain regions that trigger or suppress agitation and aggression. As we discuss later in this chapter, a broad range of conditions and disorders that affect the brain can result in symptoms of agitation and aggression. Unfortunately, these aggressive symptoms are often not afforded diagnostic primacy and are, therefore, either not treated at all or "mistreated" with agents that do not have anti-aggressive properties.

We developed a rating scale, the OAS (Yudofsky et al. 1986; see Figure 25–1 and the

next section of this chapter), which encompasses the definition, diagnosis, and operationalization of aggression. Figure 25–2 shows a newer rating scale, the Overt Agitation Severity Scale (OASS; Yudofsky et al. 1997). The reader, by briefly reviewing this scale and comparing it with the OAS, can be helped to differentiate between agitation and aggression. Anxiety and neuropsychiatric syndromes or side effects such as akathisia also must be differentiated from agitation and aggression. When the clinician confuses akathisia with agitation or aggression, he or she may increase the patient's antipsychotic dose. Apart from the increased sedation from

Table 25–1. Neuropathology of aggression

Locus	Activity
Hypothalamus	Orchestrates neuro-endocrine response via sympathetic arousal
	Monitors and regulates somatic status
Limbic system	
Amygdala	Activates and/or suppresses hypothalamus
	Receives input from neocortex
Temporal cortex	Associated with aggression in both ictal and interictal states; associated with experiential memory for pain and danger
Frontal neocortex	Modulates limbic and hypothalamic states
	Associated with social and judgment aspects of aggression

Source.   Reprinted from Silver JM, Hales RE, Yudofsky SC: "Neuropsychiatric Aspects of Traumatic Brain Injury," in *The American Psychiatric Press Textbook of Neuropsychiatry,* 2nd Edition. Edited by Yudofsky SC, Hales RE. Washington, DC, American Psychiatric Press, 1992, pp. 363–395. Copyright 1992, American Psychiatric Press. Used with permission.

Table 25–2. Areas of the brain that mediate aggressive behaviors

Triggers	Suppressors
Medial hypothalamus	Frontal lobes
Posteromedial hypothalamus	Septal nuclei
Thalamic center median	Cerebellar lobes
Thalamic lamella medialis	Cerebellar fastigium
Dorsomedial thalamus	
Anterior cingulum	
Anterior (ventral) hypothalamus	
Centromedial amygdala	

the antipsychotic, the misuse of a neuroleptic in this circumstance ultimately will aggravate the akathisia and result in a vicious cycle of ever-increasing doses of antipsychotic drug and consequent intensification of the akathisia. We advise clinicians to use standardized rating scales such as the OAS and the OASS to help diagnose, document, distinguish, and monitor aggression, agitation, and anxiety.

DOCUMENTATION AND RATING OF AGITATION AND AGGRESSION

Aggression

Accurate documentation of episodes of agitation and aggression is critical to recording characteristics of such episodes when they occur, to assessing the effectiveness of interventions in the treatment of agitated and aggressive patients, and to conducting research related to disorders of agitation and aggression. The OAS and the OASS are 1-page rating scales that were developed to assess the effects of pharmacological agents in the treatment of agitation and aggression (Silver and Yudofsky 1991). In the OAS, aggressive behaviors are divided into four categories: verbal aggression, physical aggres-

sion against objects, physical aggression against self, and physical aggression against other people. Within each category, descriptive statements and numerical scores are used to define and rate four levels of severity. All behaviors shown by a patient during an aggressive episode are checked off by an observer (such as routine hospital staff or a family member). Therapeutic interventions used in response to these aggressive episodes are also listed, rated on the OAS, and checked off by the rater. These interventions are documented because they may indicate the observer's interpretation of the relative severity of the aggressive behaviors.

Our research, which evaluated more than 5,000 episodes of aggression in chronically hospitalized psychiatric inpatients, indicated that hospital records and other official communications and documentation did not include descriptions of most aggressive behaviors that occurred. Simultaneous use of the OAS ensured that a significantly greater percentage of aggressive episodes and behaviors was documented (Silver and Yudofsky 1987b).

Agitation

The OASS includes 47 observable characteristics of agitation that are subcategorized into 12 behaviorally related units. The characteristics were identified as representative of the full content domain of agitation from the clinical and theoretical literature. Further subcategorization, for the purposes of enhancing its ease of use, are anatomically based: 1) vocalizations and oral/facial movements, 2) upper torso and upper extremity movements, and 3) lower extremity movements.

Each behavioral subgroup is rated with a Likert-type frequency score from 1 (mild signs) to 4 (very severe signs). For each subgroup, a corresponding 5-point Likert-type frequency score is selected by the rater from 0 (behavior is not present) to 4 (behavior is always present). The total OASS score is obtained by multiplying each item's frequency response by a weight

Overt Aggression Scale (OAS)

Stuart Yudofsky, M.D., Jonathan Silver, M.D., Wynn Jackson M.D., and Jean Endicott, Ph.D.

Identifying Data

Name of patient	Name of rater
Sex of patient: 1 male 2 female	Date / / (mo/da/yr) Shift: 1 night 2 day 3 evening

☐ No aggressive incident(s) (verbal or physical) against self, others, or objects during the shift (check here).

Aggressive Behavior (check all that apply)

Verbal aggression	Physical aggression against self
☐ Makes loud noises, shouts angrily	☐ Picks or scratches skin, hits self, pulls hair (with no or minor injury only)
☐ Yells mild personal insults (e.g., "You're stupid!")	☐ Bangs head, hits fist into objects, throws self onto floor or into objects (hurts self without serious injury)
☐ Curses viciously, uses foul language in anger, makes moderate threats to others or self	☐ Small cuts or bruises, minor burns
☐ Makes clear threats of violence toward others or self (I'm going to kill you.) or requests to help to control self	☐ Mutilates self, makes deep cuts, bites that bleed, internal injury, fracture, loss of consciousness, loss of teeth

Physical aggression against objects	Physical aggression against other people
☐ Slams door, scatters clothing, makes a mess	☐ Makes threatening gesture, swings at people, grabs at clothes
☐ Throws objects down, kicks furniture without breaking it, marks the wall	☐ Strikes, kicks, pushes, pulls hair (without injury to them)
☐ Breaks objects, smashes windows	☐ Attacks others, causing mild to moderate physical injury (bruises, sprain, welts)
☐ Sets fires, throws objects dangerously	☐ Attacks others, causing severe physical injury (broken bones, deep lacerations, internal injury)

Time incident began: ___ ___ : ___ ___ am/pm	Duration of incident: ___ ___ : ___ ___ (hours/minutes)

Intervention (check all that apply)

☐ None	☐ Immediate medication given by mouth	☐ Use of restraints
☐ Talking to patient	☐ Immediate medication given by injection	☐ Injury requires immediate medical treatment for patient
☐ Closer observation	☐ Isolation without seclusion (time out)	☐ Injury requires immediate treatment for other person
☐ Holding patient	☐ Seclusion	

Comments

Figure 25–1. Overt Aggression Scale. *Source.* Reprinted from Yudofsky SC, Silver JM, Jackson W, et al.: "The Overt Aggression Scale for the Objective Rating of Verbal and Physical Aggression." *American Journal of Psychiatry* 143:35–39, 1986. Copyright 1986, American Psychiatric Association. Used with permission.

Overt Agitation Severity Scale (OASS)

Intensity (I)	Behavior	Not present	Rarely	Some of the time	Most of the time	Always present	Severity score (SS) (I × F = SS)
				Frequency (F)			
A.	**Vocalizations and oral/facial movements**						
1	Whimpering, whining, moaning, grunting, crying	0	1	2	3	4	= _____
2	Smacking or licking of lips, chewing, clenching jaw, licking, grimacing, spitting	0	1	2	3	4	= _____
3	Rocking, twisting, banging of head	0	1	2	3	4	= _____
4	Vocal perseverating, screaming, cursing, threatening, wailing	0	1	2	3	4	= _____
B.	**Upper torso and upper extremity movements**						
1	Tapping fingers, fidgeting, wringing of hands, swinging or flailing arms	0	1	2	3	4	= _____
2	Task perseverating (e.g., opening and closing drawers, folding and unfolding clothes, picking at objects, clothes, or self)	0	1	2	3	4	= _____
3	Rocking (back and forth), bobbing (up and down), twisting or writhing of torso, rubbing or masturbating self	0	1	2	3	4	= _____
4	Slapping, swatting, hitting at objects or others	0	1	2	3	4	= _____
C.	**Lower extremity movements**						
1	Tapping toes, clenching toes, tapping heel, extending, flexing, or twisting foot	0	1	2	3	4	= _____
2	Shaking legs, tapping knees and/or thighs, thrusting pelvis, stomping	0	1	2	3	4	= _____
3	Pacing, wandering	0	1	2	3	4	= _____
4	Thrashing legs, kicking at objects or others	0	1	2	3	4	= _____

Total OASS = _____

Subtract baseline OASS = _____

Revised OASS = _____

(continued)

Figure 25–2. Overt Agitation Severity Scale.

Instructions for completing form

Step one: For each behavior, circle the corresponding frequency.

Step two: For every behavior *exhibited*, multiply the intensity score (I) by the frequency (F) and record as the severity score (SS).

Step three: For the Overt Agitation Severity Score (OASS), total all severity scores and record as total OASS.

Step four: Does this patient have a neuromuscular disorder (i.e., Parkinson's disease, tardive dyskinesia) affecting total OASS?   Yes   No

Step five: If yes, please establish a baseline OASS in nonagitated state and subtract from above total OASS for revised OASS.

Comments: _____

_____

_____

Diagnosis: _____   **Name of rater:** _____

Sex of patient: Male   (1); Female   (2)   **Time of observation:** _____

Age: _____   **Date:** _____

Current medication:

Name: Dose: Frequency:

Name: Dose: Frequency:

Name: Dose: Frequency:

Name: Dose: Frequency:

Name: Dose: Frequency:

Figure 25–2.   Overt Agitation Severity Scale *(continued)*. *Source.*   Reprinted from Yudofsky SC, Kopecky HJ, Kunik M, et al.: "The Overt Agitation Severity Scale for the Objective Rating of Agitation." *Journal of Neuropsychiatry and Clinical Neurosciences* 9:541–548, 1997. Copyright 1997, American Psychiatric Press. Used with permission.

that corresponds to the intensity of the symptom being measured. The total of the weighted responses indicates the severity of agitation. For patients with neuromuscular disorders (e.g., Parkinson's disease, akathisia, tardive dyskinesia), in which impaired motor activity can mimic agitation, a baseline nonagitated OASS score is obtained and subtracted from the score obtained during an agitated state to determine the revised OASS score.

Maintenance and Compliance

We encourage practitioners to utilize the OAS and OASS to establish baseline scores for ag-

gression before initiating psychopharmacological intervention and, thereafter, to document the efficacy (or lack thereof) of any therapeutic intervention. The documentation of aggression and agitation through the rating scales is often essential to *maintaining* a psychopharmacological treatment plan. We are often consulted by other physicians or by family members who contend that the psychopharmacological intervention "has stopped working." In these circumstances, professionals and family members are so alarmed by the patient's single episode of violence or agitation and its implications that they demand significant revisions in the treatment plan, which often entail the abrupt discontinuation of the current pharmacological agent and the initiation of another medication. In a significant percentage of these cases, the pharmacological agent has been highly, but not entirely, effective; however, for a variety of reasons (such as increased stress, poor compliance, concomitant use of alcohol or illicit substances), the agitation and aggression have "broken through" the pharmacological intervention. Documentation of agitation and aggression with rating scales is very useful in proving to patients, their families, and caregivers that a pharmacological intervention has been partially effective (e.g., the number of events may have been reduced by 80%, and the intensity of the events may have diminished by 94%). These data from rating scales may obviate a potentially deleterious "overreaction" by caregivers to a single extreme event and the discontinuation of an effective pharmacological regimen.

NEUROTRANSMITTER INVOLVEMENT IN AGITATION AND AGGRESSION

Multiple neurotransmitters and neurotransmitter systems are involved in the mediation of agitation and aggression; serotonin, norepinephrine, dopamine, acetylcholine, and γ-aminobutyric acid (GABA) play important roles. In neuropsychiatric disorders, it is the rule rather than the exception that multiple neurotransmitter systems are involved simultaneously in diffuse regions of the brain. In addition, different transmitters may affect one another in influencing agitation and aggression, which we have learned from the roles of neurotransmitters in depression. Most frequently, the critical factor relative to the role of neurotransmitters in agitation and aggression is the *relationship* among the neurotransmitters in both function and dysfunction.

Norepinephrine tracks originate in the locus coeruleus in the lateral tegmental system

and course to the forebrain—an area frequently involved in traumatic brain injury and associated with dyscontrol of rage and violent behavior. The β_1-adrenergic receptors have been implicated through their localization in this region (limbic forebrain and cerebral cortex) and have been judged to be involved in the mediation of aggressive behavior (Alexander et al. 1979). Animal studies suggest that norepinephrine is involved in many aspects of aggressive behavior, including sham rage, affective aggression, and shock-induced fighting (Eichelman 1987). Higley et al. (1992) documented an association between aggression in free-ranging rhesus monkeys and cerebrospinal fluid (CSF) norepinephrine levels. Brown et al. (1979) reported that humans who have aggressive or impulsive behavior have increased levels of the norepinephrine metabolite 3-methoxy-4-hydroxyphenylglycol (MHPG).

Currently, dysfunction in serotonergic systems is receiving the most scientific attention with regard to the roles these systems play in agitation and aggression (Coccaro 1992; Wetzler et al. 1991). Serotonergic neurons originate in the raphe, are located in the pons and upper brain stem, and project to the frontal cortex. Clinical studies have implicated the role of lowered levels of serotonin in the central nervous system in the expression of aggression and impulsivity, particularly violent self-destructive acts, in humans (Coccaro et al. 1992; Kruesi et al. 1992; Linnoila and Virkkunen 1992). Dopamine systems are prominent in both mesolimbic and mesocortical regions of the brain. A variety of indirect evidence indicates that increased dopamine in the brain—particularly the release of dopamine after brain lesions—leads to increased agitation and aggression in animal models and in humans (Bareggi et al. 1975; Blackburn et al. 1992; Hamill et al. 1987; Kruesi et al. 1990). The profound increases in aggressive behavior after severe traumatic brain injury are thought to be closely associated with subsequent changes in dopaminergic systems (Eichelman et al. 1972).

DIFFERENTIAL DIAGNOSIS OF AGITATION AND AGGRESSION

In establishing a treatment plan for patients with agitation or aggression, the overarching principle is that diagnosis precedes treatment. The history of the development of the symptoms in a biopsychosocial context is usually the most critical part of the evaluation.

As stated earlier in this chapter, brain disorders are strongly associated with agitation and the dyscontrol of rage and violence. Table 25–3 includes common etiologies of neurologically induced agitation and aggression, and Table 25–4 lists categories of medications and drugs that are associated with engendering agitation and aggression (Yudofsky et al. 1990). Characteristic features that alert the clinician to the po-

---

Table 25–3. Common etiologies of neurologically induced agitation and aggression

Traumatic brain injury

Stroke and other cerebrovascular disease

Medications, alcohol and other abused substances, over-the-counter drugs

Delirium (e.g., hypoxia, electrolyte imbalance, anesthesia and surgery, uremia)

Alzheimer's disease

Chronic neurological disorders: Huntington's disease, Wilson's disease, Parkinson's disease, multiple sclerosis, systemic lupus erythematosus

Brain tumors

Infectious diseases: encephalitis, meningitis, acquired immunodeficiency syndrome (AIDS)

Epilepsy (ictal, postictal, and interictal)

Metabolic disorders: hyperthyroidism or hypothyroidism, hypoglycemia, vitamin deficiencies, porphyria

---

Source. Reprinted from Yudofsky SC, Silver JM, Hales RE: "Pharmacologic Management of Aggression in the Elderly." *Journal of Clinical Psychiatry* 51 (10 suppl):22–28, 1990. Copyright 1990, Physicians Postgraduate Press. Used with permission.

Table 25–4. Categories of medications and drugs associated with agitation and aggression

Sedative, hypnotic, and antianxiety agents

Alcohol

Central nervous system depressants

Barbiturates

Benzodiazepines (intoxication and withdrawal states)

Analgesics

Opiates and other narcotics (intoxication and withdrawal states)

Steroids

Prednisone

Cortisone

Anabolic steroids (therapeutic doses and withdrawal states)

Antidepressants

All categories (especially in initial phases of treatment)

Stimulants

Amphetamines

Cocaine (associated with manic excitement in early stages of abuse and secondary to paranoid ideation in later stages of use)

Caffeine (in high doses)

Antipsychotics

Phenothiazines

Butyrophenones (high-potency dopamine antagonists that lead to akathisia)

Anticholinergics

Over-the-counter sedatives (associated with delirium and central anticholinergic syndrome)

Hallucinogens

Lysergic diethylamide (LSD)

Phencyclidine

Psilocybin (intoxication states)

Source. Reprinted from Yudofsky SC, Silver JM, Hales RE: "Pharmacologic Management of Aggression in the Elderly." *Journal of Clinical Psychiatry* 51 (10 suppl):22–28, 1990. Copyright 1990, Physicians Postgraduate Press. Used with permission.

Table 25–5. **Characteristic features of neuroaggressive disorder**

Reactive	Triggered by modest or trivial stimuli
Nonreflective	Usually does not involve premeditation or planning
Nonpurposeful	Aggression serves no obvious long-term goals
Explosive	Buildup is *not* gradual
Periodic	Brief outbursts of rage and aggression; punctuated by long periods of relative calm
Ego-dystonic	After outbursts, patients are upset, concerned, and embarrassed as opposed to blaming others or justifying behavior

Source. Reprinted from Yudofsky SC, Silver JM, Hales RE: "Pharmacologic Management of Aggression in the Elderly." *Journal of Clinical Psychiatry* 51 (10 suppl):22–28, 1990. Copyright 1990, Physicians Postgraduate Press. Used with permission.

tential presence of neurologically induced aggression are summarized in Table 25–5.

In soliciting the patient's history of agitation and aggression, the clinician must interview family members, teachers, friends, work associates, and others because patients with these symptoms—as opposed to their families—tend to minimize the presence and importance of these behaviors (Silver and Yudofsky 1994a). In addition, in crafting a multifaceted treatment plan, the clinician must secure from the patient and observers the context in which agitation or aggression occurs. Determination of the mental status of the patient *before* the agitated or aggressive event, the nature of the precipitant, the physical and social environment in which the behavior occurs, the ways in which the event is mitigated, and the primary and secondary gains related to agitation and aggression is essential. If the agitation or aggression occurs in the context of a psychiatric disorder, a review of both the individual's and the family's psychiatric history

should be emphasized. For *all* patients with agitation or aggression, the clinician must obtain a history of physical illness, review neurological signs and symptoms in detail, and conduct a thorough physical examination. Special focus should be placed on the neurological evaluation and on relevant laboratory testing as guided by information from the history and physical and neurological examinations. We find neuropsychological tests such as the Halstead-Reitan Battery and the Luria-Nebraska Neuropsychological Battery more useful than standard psychological tests such as the Minnesota Multiphasic Personality Inventory (MMPI) or projective psychological tests in evaluating patients with agitated and/or aggressive symptoms and disorders.

TREATMENT OF AGITATION AND AGGRESSION

Overview

Treatment of agitation and aggression is guided by the following four *D's*:

1. **D**etermining the etiologies of the psychological and/or organic disorder(s) that may contribute to the agitation or aggression
2. **D**elineating the biopsychosocial context in which the behaviors occur
3. **D**ocumenting and rating the agitation or aggression with the OAS and/or the OASS
4. **D**eveloping a multifaceted treatment plan

Almost without exception, treatment of agitation or aggression requires a multifaceted approach that often combines pharmacological treatments, behavioral treatments, psychodynamically informed psychotherapy, family treatment, and (as indicated) other specific approaches such as spiritual counseling, occupational therapy, and couples treatment.

The review of the psychopharmacological management of agitation and aggression is the focus of this chapter; therefore, we do not expand on the other therapeutic approaches that also have been shown to have efficacy in the treatment of agitation and aggression. For a comprehensive review of behavioral treatments of aggression in psychiatric patients, the reader is referred to a review article published in collaboration with us (Corrigan et al. 1993). A sum-

mary of the behavioral treatments of aggression that may be used in combination with pharmacological interventions is shown in Table 25–6 (Corrigan et al. 1993).

In conceptualizing an approach to the pharmacological treatment of agitation and aggression, we differentiate between the management of acute agitation and aggression (often consti-

Table 25–6. Behavioral treatment of aggression

Strategy	Indications	Special considerations
Token economy	Provides both proactive and reactive strategies for aggressive behaviors	A strict format for implementing contingency management
Aggression replacement		
Differential reinforcement schedules	Replace punishing contingency for previolent behavior	Differential reinforcement of other behaviors is resource-intensive; differential reinforcement of incompatible behaviors requires identification of suitable interfering behaviors
Assertiveness training	Effective for patients who become angry when their needs are not met	Patients must work well in skills training groups
Activity programming	Diminishes opportunities for unstructured, frustrating interactions	Activities that patients find reinforcing should be identified
Decelerative techniques		
Social extinction	Effective with previolent patients who respond to social reinforcements	May not work with schizoid patients
Contingent observation	Effective with previolent patients who respond to social reinforcements	Patients must be sufficiently organized to perceive models accurately
Self-controlled timeout	Effective with violent patients immediately after incidents	May diminish risky attempts to seclude or restrain
Overcorrection	Effective with relatively docile patients	Stop if patient struggles with guided practice
Contingent restraint	Effective with violent patients who do not comply with self-controlled timeout and are resistant to guided practice	Decreases inadvertent reinforcement of behaviors that covary with seclusion and restraint

Source. Reprinted from Corrigan PW, Yudofsky SC, Silver JM: "Pharmacological and Behavioral Treatments for Aggressive Psychiatric Inpatients." *Hospital and Community Psychiatry* 44(2):125–133, 1993. Copyright 1993, American Psychiatric Association. Used with permission.

tutes a medical emergency) and the pharmacological treatment of chronic agitation and aggression (often constitutes a prophylactic and maintenance approach). Currently, no medication has U.S. Food and Drug Administration (FDA) approval for the treatment of these behaviors. Most frequently, when medications are used (and often misused), it is their sedating side effects that are sought. Although this may be appropriate in emergency or specific situations, such as using antipsychotics to treat both psychosis and agitation in a patient with delusional depression, prolonged use of sedation to "cover over" agitation or aggression has disadvantages. For example, when neuroleptics are used to manage agitation or aggression, side effects, including oversedation, hypotension, confusion, neuroleptic malignant syndrome, parkinsonism, akathisia, dystonia, and tardive dyskinesia, may emerge. When benzodiazepines are administered for prolonged periods to manage agitation or aggression, side effects, such as oversedation, motor disturbances including poor coordination, mood disturbances, memory impairment, confusion, dependency, overdoses, withdrawal syndromes, and paradoxical violence, often complicate treatment.

Pharmacological Management of Acute Agitation and Aggression

Antipsychotic medications. Antipsychotics are the most commonly prescribed medications for the treatment of both acute and chronic agitation and aggression. These agents are appropriate and effective in the treatment of agitation or aggression that derives from psychosis. An example would be to use an antipsychotic drug in a manic patient who appeared at the gates of the White House in an angry and agitated state after she had sent hundreds of letters to the president detailing his scheme to redecorate the White House "in a more vivid color scheme." Another example would be to use an antipsychotic in a patient with paranoid schizophrenia who hears voices commanding him to use

physical force to protect himself from a neighbor "who is monitoring my thoughts through a dental device that was surgically implanted during my sleep."

Unfortunately, however, in our experience, the most common use of antipsychotic medications is in the treatment of chronic agitation or aggression associated with brain disorders (including schizophrenia). Over time (i.e., days to months), tolerance to the sedative side effects of the neuroleptics develops, and the clinician must increase the dose to maintain the sedation. A vicious cycle often emerges—neuroleptics are increased to "treat" akathisias that are mistaken for increased irritability and agitation of the associated illness. Herrera et al. (1988) noted a marked increase in violent behavior when patients with schizophrenia were treated with haloperidol in doses ranging to 60 mg/day, when compared with violent behaviors that occurred during treatment with chlorpromazine in doses up to 1,800 mg/day or with clozapine in doses ranging to 900 mg/day. We interpret these findings to be the result of haloperidol's increased risk of causing akathisia as compared with chlorpromazine or clozapine. These complications and side effects can be avoided by establishing, before initiating neuroleptics to treat acute agitation or aggression, a treatment plan that includes 1) operationalized ratings of agitation and aggression with the OAS and OASS, 2) the reduction of neuroleptics when symptoms remit, and 3) prospectively specified dates when the antipsychotic agent will be tapered and discontinued.

Unless agitation or aggression is clearly related to psychotic ideation that is responding to treatment with antipsychotic agents, we limit the use of both antipsychotics and benzodiazepines for "sedating" agitation or aggression to a maximum period of 4 weeks. Beyond this time, clinicians must consider whether the agitation or aggression is chronic and alter the treatment plan accordingly to utilize medications that are recommended for treatment of chronic behaviors (see next section).

The essence of managing acute episodes of agitation or aggression by using neuroleptics for sedation is to increase the dose of the neuroleptic, often every 1–2 hours, to achieve the lowest dose that will produce the sedation necessary to "control" the violent behaviors. Despite the aforementioned disadvantages of haloperidol in the management of chronic agitation or aggression, this medication—because it can be taken orally, intramuscularly, and intravenously, and because it has a low level of cardiovascular side effects compared with other classes of neuroleptics—is used most often. Summarized guidelines for the use of haloperidol in the management of acute agitation or aggression are provided in Table 25–7.

Clozapine has been used to treat agitation and aggression in patients with a broad variety of neuropsychiatric disorders, including traumatic

---

Table 25–7. **Use of haloperidol in the acute management of agitation or aggression**

---

1. Initiate haloperidol—1 mg orally or 0.5 mg intravenously or intramuscularly every hour.

2. Increase dose by 1 mg every hour until agitation or aggression is controlled.

3. Administer haloperidol as 2 mg orally or 1 mg intravenously or intramuscularly every 8 hours.

4. When patient is not agitated or violent for at least 48 hours, taper at rate of 25% of highest daily dose.

5. If agitation or violent behavior reemerges while tapering drug, reevaluate etiology and consider switching to a more specific medication to manage chronic behavioral dysfunction.

6. Do not continue haloperidol administration for more than 6 weeks—unless agitation or aggression is secondary to psychosis.

Source. Adapted from Yudofsky SC, Silver JM, Hales RE: "Pharmacologic Management of Aggression in the Elderly." *Journal of Clinical Psychiatry* 51 (10 suppl): 22–28, 1990. Copyright 1990, Physicians Postgraduate Press. Used with permission.

brain injury (Michals et al. 1993) and mental retardation (Cohen and Underwood 1994). These and other similar studies used open trial methodologies to report that clozapine reduced agitated, aggressive, and self-injurious behaviors. The clinician must be cautioned, however, that clozapine significantly lowers seizure thresholds, which is an especially dangerous side effect in patients with brain disorders. Seizures occurred in two of nine brain-injured patients who received clozapine to treat refractory aggression (Michals et al. 1993).

Benzodiazepines. Benzodiazepines may also be indicated for the management of acute agitation and aggression. Intramuscular lorazepam has advantages over other benzodiazepines as an effective medication for the emergency treatment of agitated or aggressive patients (Bick and Hannah 1986). In the management of acute agitation or aggression, lorazepam's advantages are similar to those of haloperidol, including flexible routes of administration (intravenous, intramuscular, or oral). In addition, lorazepam has a relatively brief half-life compared with other benzodiazepines such as diazepam or chlordiazepoxide, which can result in oversedation of the patient through the buildup of overly high plasma levels of the respective benzodiazepine. Table 25–8 contains guidelines for the use of lorazepam in the acute management of agitation or aggression.

In a randomized, double-blind study, Lenox et al. (1992) compared lorazepam with haloperidol in the treatment of manic agitation in 20 hospitalized patients with bipolar disorder who were also taking lithium. The investigators found no significant difference in the treatment groups in the degree of or time to response.

Other categories of medication. Other medications such as paraldehyde, chloral hydrate, and diphenhydramine may also be prescribed to sedate patients with acute agitation or aggression. However, in general, benzodiazepines and neuroleptics are the preferred medi-

Table 25–8. Use of lorazepam in the acute management of agitation or aggression

1. Initiate lorazepam—1–2 mg orally or intramuscularly.

2. Repeat dose every hour until agitation or aggression is controlled.

3. If intravenous dose must be given, push slowly! Do not exceed 2 mg (1 mL) per minute to avoid respiratory depression and laryngospasm; may be repeated in 30 minutes if required.

4. When patient is no longer agitated or violent, maintain dose at maximum of 2 mg orally or intramuscularly every 4 hours.

5. When patient is not agitated or violent for 48 hours, taper at rate of 10% of highest total daily dose.

6. If agitation or violent behavior reemerges while tapering drug, reevaluate etiology and consider switching to a more specific medication to manage chronic aggression.

7. After 6 weeks, if lorazepam cannot be tapered without reemergence of agitation or aggression, reevaluate and revise treatment plan to include a more specific medication to manage chronic behavioral dysfunction.

Source. Adapted from Yudofsky SC, Silver JM, Hales RE: "Pharmacologic Management of Aggression in the Elderly." *Journal of Clinical Psychiatry* 51 (10 suppl): 22–28, 1990. Copyright 1990, Physicians Postgraduate Press. Used with permission.

cations because they are safe and convenient and because their use, benefits, and risks are familiar to psychiatrists and hospital staff.

The scientific literature is replete with case reports of a broad range of medications that mitigate acute agitation or aggression in special clinical circumstances. For example, a study by Gualtieri et al. (1989) reported that amantadine, a dopamine agonist, reduced aggressive behavior in patients recovering from traumatic brain injury. Intensive care specialists who treat the medical sequelae of trauma may use succinylcholine with requisite ventilatory support to induce pharmacological paralysis in patients in intensive care units who have severe agitation following traumatic brain injury or surgical procedures. Clearly, the application of such interventions is best limited to those professionals who, by virtue of their subspecialty focus, have sufficient experience and resources necessary to use these novel approaches safely in the treatment of acute agitation and aggression.

Pharmacological Management of Chronic Agitation and Aggression

When patients' agitation and aggression persist beyond several weeks, *maintenance approaches* should be considered. We advocate that the decision about the choice of the specific psychopharmacological agent be guided by the determination of the underlying illness that causes the chronic behavior and by the co-occurrence of other psychiatric symptoms such as anxiety, mania, or depression. Table 25–9 outlines our approach to the pharmacological treatment of chronic agitation or aggression.

Antipsychotic medications. As we discussed earlier in this chapter, restricting the use of antipsychotic medications to the treatment of agitation or aggression that is directly related to psychotic ideation or perception, such as paranoid delusions or command hallucinations, is generally clinically indicated. The clinician should attempt to taper the antipsychotic agent at regular intervals to gauge its efficacy in treating both the psychosis and the attendant agitation and aggression in such patients. If the agitated or aggressive behavior persists in the absence of psychosis, or if the psychosis is unaffected by the discontinuation of the antipsychotic medication, other approaches to the pharmacotherapy of agitation and aggression must be considered.

Antianxiety medications. Various case reports and prospective studies have reported that buspirone, a serotonin-1A (5-HT$_{1A}$) agonist,

Table 25–9.   Psychopharmacological treatment of chronic agitation or aggression

Medication class	Indications	Side effects and special clinical considerations
Antipsychotic	Agitation or aggression secondary to psychotic symptoms	Oversedation, akathisias, multiple extrapyramidal side effects
Antianxiety	Comorbid anxiety symptoms	Oversedation, confusion, paradoxical rage, dependency
Benzodiazepines		
Buspirone	Comorbid anxiety and/or depression	Delayed onset of action (3–5 weeks)
Anticonvulsant	Seizure disorder, organic brain syndrome, manic states	Bone marrow suppression, hepatoxicity
Carbamazepine		
Valproate		
Antimanic	Manic excitement, bipolar disorder, cyclothymia	Neurotoxicity and confusion
Lithium		
Valproate		
Cardiovascular	Organic brain syndromes	Delayed onset of action (4–6 weeks)
Propranolol (and other β-blockers)		
Antidepressant		
SSRIs	Depression; mood lability; irritability	Require standard doses for treatment of depression
Trazodone	Depression with insomnia	Oversedation, brief half-life

Note.   SSRIs = selective serotonin reuptake inhibitors.
Source.   Adapted from Yudofsky SC, Silver JM, Hales RE: "Pharmacologic Management of Aggression in the Elderly." *Journal of Clinical Psychiatry* 51 (10 suppl):22–28, 1990. Copyright 1990, Physicians Postgraduate Press. Used with permission.

was effective in the management of aggression and agitation associated with brain disorders (Colenda 1988; Gualtieri 1991; Ratey et al. 1992a; Stanislav et al. 1994; Tiller et al. 1988) and developmental disabilities and autism (Ratey et al. 1989, 1991; Realmuto et al. 1989). Because we have observed that some patients become more agitated or aggressive in the initial phases of treatment with buspirone, we advocate beginning treatment at low doses (e.g., 5 mg twice a day) and increasing the dose by 5 mg every 3–5 days. Doses ranging from 45 to 60 mg/day and a latency of 3–5 weeks may be required before therapeutic effects are observed.

Although no double-blind, controlled studies of clonazepam in the management of chronic agitation or aggression have been done, several case reports indicate that it was beneficial in the treatment of agitation in elderly persons (Freinhar and Alvarez 1986) and in a patient with schizophrenia and seizures (Keats and Mukherjee 1988). We also prescribe clonazepam when agitation or aggression occurs in patients with pronounced anxiety or with neurologically induced tics and disinhibited motor behavior. Initial dosages are 0.5 mg twice a day and rarely exceed a total daily dose of 6 mg. Oversedation is the most common side effect, and daytime sedation may be mitigated by prescribing a single dose before bedtime.

Anticonvulsant medications.   Overall, we prioritize the use of anticonvulsant medications, particularly carbamazepine and valproate, for the treatment of chronic agitation or aggression that is associated with seizure disorders or manic affects. Anticonvulsants are our second choice to β-blockers for disruptive behaviors related to diffuse neuronal destruction (e.g., those that occur subsequent to traumatic brain injury, middle cerebral artery stroke, and Alzheimer's disease).

One nonrandomized, placebo-controlled crossover study of 25 patients with dementia showed that low doses of carbamazepine (modal dose of 300 mg/day) reduced agitated behavior in some patients (Tariot et al. 1994). Several open studies indicated that carbamazepine may be effective in reducing aggressive behavior associated with organic brain disorders (Mattes 1988), schizophrenia (Hakoloa and Laulumaa 1982; Luchins 1983), developmental disabilities (Folks et al. 1982; Yatham and McHale 1988), and dementia (Gleason and Schneider 1990; Leibovici and Tariot 1988; Lemke 1995). Carbamazepine has also been used in combination with other medications to treat agitation and aggression. Lemke (1995) conducted an open, prospective study of 15 elderly patients with Alzheimer's disease whose severe agitation had not responded to neuroleptics. When carbamazepine was combined with haloperidol, a "significant improvement" was reported after 4 weeks of treatment. We use carbamazepine to treat agitation and aggression in the same doses and with the same blood levels that we use in the treatment of bipolar disorder.

Several studies have reported that valproate is efficacious in the treatment of agitation and aggression in patients with a wide variety of medical disorders. Most of these studies were published as case reports of valproate's usefulness in reducing agitation and aggression in patients with dementias and other organic brain syndromes (Giakas et al. 1990; Kahn et al. 1988; Lemke 1995; Mattes 1992; Mellow et al. 1993). Lott et al. (1995) conducted an open-label trial of 10 elderly nursing home patients with dementia and agitation. These patients were prospectively treated with valproate at doses ranging from 375 to 750 mg/day. Eight of the patients had a 50% or greater reduction in the frequency of agitation, and the intensity of the behavioral outbursts also diminished in many of these patients. Valproate was well tolerated by all patients in this study. Because of valproate's favorable side-effect profile (e.g., lower incidence of ataxia, rashes, behavioral changes), we prefer to use valproate rather than carbamazepine in the treatment of agitation and aggression.

Antimanic medications.   Because aggressive behavior may be present in the manic state of bipolar disorder and because agitation is a frequent concomitant of both manic and depressed states, mood-stabilizing medications such as lithium and valproate (Wilcox 1994) treat these behaviors by treating the underlying illness. In addition, many reports suggest that lithium is of value in the treatment of agitation and aggression in patients without bipolar illness but with other specific underlying medical disorders. Included in this group are patients who have mental retardation with self-directed aggression (Luchins and Dojka 1989) or aggression toward others (Dale 1980) and patients who have traumatic brain injury (Haas and Cope 1985). Aggressive people from special segments of the population such as children and adolescents (Vetro et al. 1976) or prison inmates (Sheard et al. 1976) also have been reported to respond to lithium. Our clinical group limits the use of lithium to the treatment of agitation and aggression in patients with mania. The dosages and blood levels of lithium we use are the same as those recommended for nonagitated patients with bipolar disorder. One caveat, however, is that many patients with brain injury have increased sensitivity to the neurotoxic effects of lithium (Hornstein and Seliger 1989; Moskowitz and Altshuler 1991) and, therefore, must be followed up very closely with neuropsychiatric examinations and serum lithium level measurements.

Antidepressant medications. Although many antidepressants have been suggested for the treatment of agitation and aggression in patients with a wide range of neuropsychiatric disorders, most of these medications act either preferentially or specifically on the serotonergic system of the brain. Amitriptyline (Jackson et al. 1985; Szlabowicz and Stewart 1990) and trazodone (Lebert et al. 1994; Pinner and Rich 1988) have been reported to be useful in the treatment of agitation and aggression; however, most recent reports focus on the use of the selective serotonin reuptake inhibitors (SSRIs) (Albritton and Borison 1995; Bass and Beltis 1991; Coccaro et al. 1990; Fava et al. 1993). We have used SSRIs to treat agitation and aggression associated with brain lesions successfully and have found this category of antidepressant to be especially effective in patients with concomitant depression or dysthymia. We initiate treatment with relatively low doses (e.g., 10 mg of fluoxetine, 25 mg of sertraline, 50 mg of nefazodone). If effects are not achieved over a period of several weeks, we gradually increase the dose to relatively high ranges (e.g., 80–100 mg/day of fluoxetine, up to 200–300 mg/day of sertraline, 400 mg/day of nefazodone). For patients without comorbid depression, we prefer to prescribe β-blockers or anticonvulsants before initiating a trial of antidepressants.

Although we just reviewed the use of antidepressants to treat agitation that stems from disorders other than depression, clinicians should be aware that depression is underdiagnosed, occurs in all age groups, and presents in atypical ways that include symptoms of agitation and aggression. For these patients, the accurate diagnosis of and a multifaceted treatment approach to depression are more critical than the specific agent chosen. Friedman et al. (1992) identified 17 of 154 elderly patients in a Canadian chronic-care facility who had disruptive vocalizations. Eight had a previous diagnosis of depression but were not taking antidepressants. Five of these patients who were given the antidepressant doxepin had significant reductions in their noisiness and agitation. We interpret the results of this study to mean that the agitation and disruptive vocalizations of patients with untreated depression are best addressed by treating the underlying mood disorder with antidepressants.

β-Blockers. More than 15 years have passed since β-blockers were first reported to be effective in treating chronic aggression in adults and children with organic brain syndromes (Yudofsky et al. 1981, 1984). Subsequently, more than 25 papers have been published in the neurological and psychiatric literature that report on the use of β-blockers to treat aggression (Silver and Yudofsky 1994b). The β-blockers that have been shown to have therapeutic effects in prospective, placebo-controlled studies include propranolol (a lipid-soluble, nonselective receptor antagonist) (Brooke et al. 1992b; Greendyke et al. 1986; Mattes 1988), nadolol (a water-soluble, nonselective receptor antagonist) (Brooke et al. 1992b; Greendyke et al. 1986; Mattes 1988; Ratey et al. 1992b), and pindolol (a lipid-soluble, nonselective antagonist with partial sympathomimetic activity) (Greendyke and Kanter 1986). Because much of this evidence from the scientific literature suggests that β-adrenergic receptor antagonists are specific and effective agents for the treatment of agitation and aggression in patients with organic brain syndromes, and because of our own extensive clinical experience with β-blockers to treat aggressive patients with neuropsychiatric disorders, this approach has become our "first line" of treatment of neurologically induced agitation and aggression.

Our guidelines for the clinical use of propranolol for treatment of agitation and aggression are summarized in Table 25–10 (Silver and Yudofsky 1987a). Several key clinical points are related to the use of propranolol:

- Peripheral effects of β-blockade (e.g., lowered blood pressure, bradycardia) are frequently saturated when the patient

---

Table 25–10. **Clinical use of propranolol in the management of chronic agitation or aggression**

1. Conduct a thorough medical examination.
2. Exclude patients with bronchial asthma, chronic obstructive pulmonary disease, insulin-dependent diabetes mellitus, congestive heart failure, persistent angina, significant peripheral vascular disease, and hyperthyroidism.
3. Avoid sudden discontinuation of propranolol (particularly in patients with hypertension).
4. Begin with a single test dose of 20 mg/day in patients in whom hypotension or bradycardia are clinical concerns. Increase the dose by 20 mg/day every 3 days.
5. Administer 20 mg of propranolol three times a day in patients without cardiovascular or cardiopulmonary disorder.
6. Increase the dose of propranolol by 60 mg/day every 3 days.
7. Increase medication unless the pulse rate declines to less than 50 beats per minute or systolic blood pressure is lower than 90 mm Hg.
8. Do not administer medication if severe dizziness, ataxia, or wheezing occurs. Reduce or discontinue propranolol if such symptoms persist.
9. Increase the dose of propranolol to 12 mg/kg or until agitated or aggressive behavior is controlled.
10. Doses of greater than 800 mg are not usually required to control aggressive behavior.
11. Continue administration of the highest dose of propranolol for at least 8 weeks before concluding that the patient is not responding to the medication. Some patients, however, may respond rapidly to propranolol.
12. Use caution when prescribing concurrent medications. Monitor plasma levels of all antipsychotic and anticonvulsant medications.

Source.   Reprinted from Silver JM, Hales RE, Yudofsky SC: "Neuropsychiatric Aspects of Traumatic Brain Injury," in *The American Psychiatric Press Textbook of Neuropsychiatry,* 3rd Edition. Edited by Yudofsky SC, Hales RE. Washington, DC, American Psychiatric Press, 1997, p. 546. Copyright 1997, American Psychiatric Press. Used with permission.

achieves a dose of approximately 280 mg/day. If orthostatic hypotension occurs, one measure should be to ensure that the patient's salt intake is adequate because many contemporary diets encourage the avoidance of salt. Thereafter, increasing the β-blocker dose is not usually associated with cardiovascular side effects.

■ Encouragement and support of the family and other members of the treatment team by the clinician are an essential component of care because of the long latency of 6–8 weeks before a therapeutic response occurs.

■ Controlled trials and our own extensive clinical experience indicate that depression is a rare side effect of use of β-blockers, despite reports that depression is commonly associated with their use (Yudofsky 1992).

■ The combination of propranolol and thioridazine should be avoided whenever possible because the use of propranolol is associated with a significant increase in plasma levels of thioridazine, which has an absolute dosage ceiling of 800 mg/day (Silver et al. 1986). The pharmacological characteristics of β-blockers are summarized in Table 25–11.

CONCLUSION

Agitation and aggression occur commonly and have serious and far-reaching consequences for

Table 25–11.　Pharmacological characteristics of β-adrenergic receptor antagonists

Drug name (by receptor selectivity)	Trade name	Potency[a]	Local anesthetic activity	Intrinsic sympathomimetic activity	Lipid solubility	Plasma half-life (hours)
Nonselective (β_1 and β_2) antagonists						
Alprenolol	Aptine	0.3–1.0	+	++	++	2–3
Nadolol	Corgard	0.5	0	0	0	14–18
Pindolol	Visken	5.0–10.0	±	++	+	3–4
Propranolol	Inderal	1.0	++	0	++	3–5
Sotalol	Sotalex	0.3	0	0	0	5–12
Timolol	Blocadren	5.0–10.0	0	±	0	4
Selective (β_1) antagonists						
Acebutolol	Sectral	0.3	+	+	0	3
Atenolol	Tenormin	1.0	0	0	0	6–8
Metoprolol	Lopressor	0.5–2.0	±	0	+	3–4

Note.　0 = none; ± = questionable; + = intermediate; ++ = significant.
[a]Propranolol = 1.
Source.　Data from Hoffman and Lefkowitz 1990 and American Medical Association Division of Drugs 1986.

patients with respect to their functioning at home, at work, and in other social settings. When assessing patients who have these behaviors, the clinician should focus on careful history taking, thorough physical examination, and relevant laboratory testing to diagnose any medical condition that could underlie and/or aggravate the symptoms.

Although pharmacological treatment of agitation and aggression may be highly effective, medications for this purpose should be used in the context of a carefully crafted treatment plan involving the full range of biopsychosocial approaches. When medications are used to treat acute agitation or aggression, the sedative side effects of antipsychotics or benzodiazepines are commonly required. However, prolonged use of neuroleptics or benzodiazepines frequently leads to disabling side effects and, therefore, should be avoided for the treatment of chronic disruptive behaviors. A wide range of medications are helpful in the prophylaxis of chronic agitation and aggression. The underlying etiology of the symptomatologies guides the choice of the specific pharmacological agent for the treatment of chronic behavioral disturbances.

REFERENCES

Albritton J, Borison R: Paroxetine treatment of anger associated with depression. J Nerv Ment Dis 183:666–667, 1995

Alexander RW, Davis JN, Lefkowitz RJ: Direct identification and characterization of β-adrenergic receptors in rat brain. Nature 258:437–440, 1979

American Psychiatric Association: Diagnostic and Statistical Manual of Mental Disorders, 3rd Edition. Washington, DC, American Psychiatric Association, 1980

Bareggi SR, Porta M, Selentati A, et al: Homovanillic acid and 5-hydroxyindole-acetic acid in the CSF of patients after a severe head injury, I: lumbar CSF concentration in chronic brain post-traumatic syndromes. Eur Neurol 13:528–544, 1975

Bass JN, Beltis J: Therapeutic effect of fluoxetine on naltrexone-resistant self-injurious behavior in an adolescent with mental retardation. J Child Adolesc Psychopharmacol 1:331–340, 1991

Bick PA, Hannah AL: Intramuscular lorazepam to restrain violent patients (letter). Lancet 1:206, 1986

Blackburn JR, Pfaus JG, Phillips AG: Dopamine functions in appetitive and defensive behaviors. Prog Neurobiol 39:247–279, 1992

Brooke MM, Questad KA, Patterson R, et al: Agitation and restlessness after closed head injury: a prospective study of 100 consecutive admissions. Arch Phys Med Rehabil 73:320–323, 1992a

Brooke MM, Patterson DR, Questad KA, et al: The treatment of agitation during initial hospitalization after traumatic brain injury. Arch Phys Med Rehabil 73:917–921, 1992b

Brown GL, Goodwin FK, Ballenger JC, et al: Aggression in human correlates with cerebrospinal fluid amine metabolites. Psychiatry Res 1:131–139, 1979

Chandler JD, Chandler JE: The prevalence of neuropsychiatric disorders in a nursing home population. J Geriatr Psychiatry Neurol 1:71–76, 1988

Coccaro EF: Impulsive aggression and central serotonergic system function in humans: an example of a dimensional brain-behavioral relationship. International Journal of Clinical Psychopharmacology 7:3–12, 1992

Coccaro EF, Astill JL, Herbert JL, et al: Fluoxetine treatment of impulsive aggression in DSM-III-R personality disorder patients. J Clin Psychopharmacol 10:373–375, 1990

Coccaro EF, Kavoussi RJ, Lesser J: Self- and other-directed human aggression: the role of the central serotonergic system. Int J Clin Psychopharmacol 6 (suppl 6):70–83, 1992

Cohen SA, Underwood MT: The use of clozapine in a mentally retarded and aggressive population. J Clin Psychiatry 55:440–444, 1994

Colenda CC: Buspirone in treatment of agitated demented patients (letter). Lancet 1:1169, 1988

Corrigan PW, Yudofsky SC, Silver JM: Pharmacological and behavioral treatments for aggressive psychiatric inpatients. Hospital and Community Psychiatry 44:125–133, 1993

Dale PG: Lithium therapy in aggressive mentally subnormal patients. Br J Psychiatry 137:469–474, 1980

Eichelman B: Neurochemical and psychopharmacologic aspects of aggressive behavior, in Psychopharmacology: The Third Generation of Progress. Edited by Meltzer HY. New York, Raven, 1987, pp 697–704

Eichelman B, Thoa NB, Ng KY: Facilitated aggression in the rat following 6-hydroxydopamine administration. Physiol Behav 8:1–3, 1972

Elliott FA: Violence: the neurologic contribution: an overview. Arch Neurol 49:595–603, 1992

Fava M, Rosenbaum JF, Pava JA, et al: Anger attacks in unipolar depression, part 1: clinical correlates and response to fluoxetine treatment. Am J Psychiatry 150:1158–1163, 1993

Folks DG, King LD, Dowdy SB, et al: Carbamazepine treatment of selective affectively disordered inpatients. Am J Psychiatry 139:115–117, 1982

Freinhar JP, Alvarez WA: Clonazepam treatment of organic brain syndromes in three elderly patients. J Clin Psychiatry 47:525–526, 1986

Friedman R, Gryfe CI, Tal DT, et al: The noisy elderly patient: prevalence, assessment, and response to the antidepressant doxepin. J Geriatr Psychiatry Neurol 5:187–191, 1992

Giakas WJ, Seibyl JP, Mazure CM: Valproate in the treatment of temper outbursts (letter). J Clin Psychiatry 51:525, 1990

Gleason RP, Schneider LS: Carbamazepine treatment of agitation in Alzheimer's outpatients refractory to neuroleptics. J Clin Psychiatry 51:115–118, 1990

Greendyke RM, Kanter DR: Therapeutic effects of pindolol on behavioral disturbances associated with organic brain disease: a double-blind study. J Clin Psychiatry 47:423–426, 1986

Greendyke RM, Kanter DR, Schuster DB, et al: Propranolol treatment of assaultive patients with organic brain disease: a double-blind crossover, placebo-controlled study. J Nerv Ment Dis 174:290–294, 1986

Gualtieri CT: Buspirone for the behavior problems of patients with organic brain disorders. J Clin Psychopharmacol 11:280–281, 1991

Gualtieri CT, Chandler M, Coons TB, et al: Amantadine: a new clinical profile for traumatic brain injury. Clin Neuropharmacol 12:258–270, 1989

Haas JF, Cope N: Neuropharmacologic management of behavior sequelae in head injury: a case report. Arch Phys Med Rehabil 66:472–474, 1985

Hakoloa HP, Laulumaa VA: Carbamazepine in treatment of violent schizophrenics (letter). Lancet 1:1358, 1982

Hamill RW, Woolf PD, McDonald JV, et al: Catecholamines predict outcome in traumatic brain injury. Ann Neurol 21:438–443, 1987

Herrera JN, Sramek JJ, Costa JF, et al: High potency neuroleptics and violence in schizophrenics. J Nerv Ment Dis 176:558–561, 1988

Higley JD, Mehlman PT, Taum DM, et al: Cerebrospinal fluid monoamine and adrenal correlates of aggression in free-ranging rhesus monkeys. Arch Gen Psychiatry 49:436–441, 1992

Hoffman BB, Lefkowitz RJ: Adrenergic receptor antagonists, in Goodman and Gilman's The Pharmacological Basis of Therapeutics, 8th Edition. Edited by Gilman AG, Rall TW, Neiw AS, et al. New York, Pergamon, 1990, pp 221–243

Hornstein A, Seliger G: Cognitive side effects of lithium in closed head injury (letter). J Neuropsychiatry Clin Neurosci 1:446–447, 1989

Jackson RD, Corrigan JD, Arnett JA: Amitriptyline for agitation in head injury. Arch Phys Med Rehabil 66:180–181, 1985

Kahn D, Stevenson E, Douglas CJ: Effect of sodium valproate in three patients with organic brain syndromes. Am J Psychiatry 145:1010–1011, 1988

Keats MM, Mukherjee S: Antiaggressive effect of adjunctive clonazepam in schizophrenia associated with seizure disorder. J Clin Psychiatry 49:117–118, 1988

Kruesi MJ, Rapoport JL, Hamburger S, et al: Cerebrospinal fluid monoamine metabolites, aggression, and impulsivity in disruptive behavior disorders of children and adolescents. Arch Gen Psychiatry 47:419–426, 1990

Kruesi MJP, Hibbs ED, Zahn TP, et al: A 2-year prospective follow-up study of children and adolescents with disruptive behavior disorders: prediction by cerebrospinal fluid 5-hydroxyindoleacetic acid, homovanillic acid, and autonomic measures. Arch Gen Psychiatry 49: 429–435, 1992

Lebert F, Pasquier F, Petit H: Behavioral effects of trazodone in Alzheimer's disease. J Clin Psychiatry 55:536–538, 1994

Leibovici A, Tariot PN: Carbamazepine treatment of agitation associated with dementia. J Geriatr Psychiatry Neurol 1:110–112, 1988

Lemke MR: Effect of carbamazepine on agitation in Alzheimer's inpatients refractory to neuroleptics. J Clin Psychiatry 56:354–357, 1995

Lenox RH, Newhouse PA, Creelman WL, et al: Adjunctive treatment of manic agitation with lorazepam versus haloperidol: a double-blind study. J Clin Psychiatry 53:47–52, 1992

Linnoila VMI, Virkkunen M: Aggression, suicidality, and serotonin. J Clin Psychiatry 53 (10 suppl):46–51, 1992

Lott AD, McElroy SL, Keys MA: Valproate in the treatment of behavioral agitation in elderly patients with dementia. J Neuropsychiatry Clin Neurosci 7:314–319, 1995

Luchins DJ: Carbamazepine for the violent psychiatric patient (letter). Lancet 2:755, 1983

Luchins DJ, Dojka D: Lithium and propranolol in aggression and self-injurious behavior in the mentally retarded. Psychopharmacol Bull 25:372–375, 1989

Mattes JA: Carbamazepine vs propranolol for rage outbursts. Psychopharmacol Bull 24:179–182, 1988

Mattes JA: Valproic acid for nonaffective aggression in the mentally retarded. J Nerv Ment Dis 180:601–602, 1992

Mellow AM, Solano-Lopez C, Davis S: Sodium valproate in the treatment of behavioral disturbance in dementia. J Geriatr Psychiatry Neurol 6:205–209, 1993

Michals ML, Crismon ML, Roberts S, et al: Clozapine response and adverse affects in nine brain-injured patients. J Clin Psychopharmacol 13:198–203, 1993

Monahan J: Mental disorder and violent behavior: perceptions and evidence. Am Psychol 47: 511–521, 1992

Moskowitz AS, Altshuler L: Increased sensitivity to lithium-induced neurotoxicity after stroke: a case report. J Clin Psychopharmacol 11: 272–273, 1991

Oddy M, Caughlan T, Tyerman A, et al: Social adjustment after closed head injury: a further follow-up seven years after injury. J Neurol Neurosurg Psychiatry 44:564–568, 1985

Ovsiew F, Yudofsky SC: Aggression: a neuropsychiatric perspective, in Rage, Power and Aggression. Edited by Glick RA, Roose SP. New Haven, CT, Yale University Press, 1993, pp 213–230

Pinner E, Rich CL: Effects of trazodone on aggressive behavior in seven patients with organic mental disorders. Am J Psychiatry 145:1295–1296, 1988

Rao N, Jellinek HM, Woolson DC: Agitation in closed head injury: haloperidol effects on rehabilitation outcome. Arch Phys Med Rehabil 66:30–34, 1985

Ratey J, Sovner R, Mikkelsen E, et al: Buspirone therapy for maladaptive behavior and anxiety in developmentally disabled persons. J Clin Psychiatry 50:382–384, 1989

Ratey J, Sovner R, Parks A, et al: Buspirone treatment of aggression and anxiety in mentally retarded patients: a multiple-baseline, placebo lead-in study. J Clin Psychiatry 52:159–162, 1991

Ratey JJ, Leveroni CL, Miller AC, et al: Low-dose buspirone to treat agitation and maladaptive behavior in brain-injured patients: two case reports. J Clin Psychopharmacol 12:362–364, 1992a

Ratey JJ, Sorgi P, O'Driscoll GA, et al: Nadolol to treat aggression and psychiatric symptomatology in chronic psychiatric inpatients: a double-blind, placebo-controlled study. J Clin Psychiatry 53:41–46, 1992b

Realmuto FM, August GJ, Garfinkel BD: Clinical effect of buspirone in autistic children. J Clin Psychopharmacol 9:122–124, 1989

Reisberg B, Borenstein J, Salob SP, et al: Behavioral symptoms in Alzheimer's disease: phenomenology and treatment. J Clin Psychiatry 48 (5 suppl):9–15, 1987

Rovner BW, Kavonek S, Filipp L, et al: Prevalence of mental illness in a community nursing home. Am J Psychiatry 143:1446–1449, 1986

Sheard MH, Marini JL, Bridges C, et al: The effects of lithium in impulsive aggressive behavior in man. Am J Psychiatry 133:1409–1413, 1976

Silver JM, Yudofsky SC: Aggressive behavior in patients with neuropsychiatric disorders: the scope of the problem. Psychiatric Annals 17:367–370, 1987a

Silver JM, Yudofsky SC: Documentation of aggression in the assessment of the violent patient. Psychiatric Annals 17:375–384, 1987b

Silver JM, Yudofsky SC: The Overt Aggression Scale: overview and guiding principles. J Neuropsychiatry Clin Neurosci 3 (suppl 1): S22–S29, 1991

Silver JM, Yudofsky SC: Aggressive disorders, in Neuropsychiatry of Traumatic Brain Injury. Edited by Silver JM, Yudofsky SC, Hales RE. Washington, DC, American Psychiatric Press, 1994a, pp 313–353

Silver JM, Yudofsky SC: Pharmacology, in Neuropsychiatry of Traumatic Brain Injury. Edited by Silver JM, Yudofsky SC, Hales RE. Washington, DC, American Psychiatric Press, 1994b, pp 631–670

Silver JM, Yudofsky S, Kogan M, et al: Elevation of thioridazine plasma levels by propranolol. Am J Psychiatry 143:1290–1292, 1986

Stanislav SW, Fabre T, Crismon ML, et al: Buspirone's efficacy in organic-induced aggression. J Clin Psychopharmacol 14:126–130, 1994

Szlabowicz JW, Stewart JT: Amitriptyline treatment of agitation associated with anoxic encephalopathy. Arch Phys Med Rehabil 71:612–613, 1990

Tardiff K: A survey of assault by chronic patients, in Assaults Within Psychiatric Facilities. Edited by Lion JR, Reid WH. New York, Grune & Stratton, 1983, pp 3–19

Tardiff K, Sweillam A: The occurrence of assaultive behavior among chronic psychiatric inpatients. Am J Psychiatry 139:212–215, 1982

Tariot PN, Erb R, Leibovici A, et al: Carbamazepine treatment of agitation in nursing home patients with dementia: a preliminary study. J Am Geriatr Soc 42:1160–1166, 1994

Tiller JWG, Dakis JA, Shaw JM: Short-term buspirone treatment in disinhibition with dementia (letter). Lancet 2:510, 1988

Valzelli L: Psychobiology of Aggression and Violence. New York, Raven, 1981

Vetro A, Szentistvanyi L, Pallag M, et al: Therapeutic experience with lithium in childhood aggressivity. Pharmacopsychiatry 133:1409–1413, 1976

Wetzler S, Kahn RS, Asnis GM, et al: Serotonin receptor sensitivity and aggression. Psychiatry Res 37:271–279, 1991

Wilcox J: Divalproex sodium in the treatment of aggressive behavior. Ann Clin Psychiatry 6(1): 17–20, 1994

Yatham LN, McHale PA: Carbamazepine in the treatment of aggression: a case report and a review of the literature. Acta Psychiatr Scand 78:188–190, 1988

Yudofsky SC: β-Blockers and depression: the clinician's dilemma. JAMA 267:1826–1827, 1992

Yudofsky SC, Williams D, Gorman J: Propranolol in the treatment of rage and violent behavior in patients with organic brain syndromes. Am J Psychiatry 138:218–220, 1981

Yudofsky SC, Stevens L, Silver J, et al: Propranolol in the treatment of rage and violent behavior associated with 5 patients with Korsakoff's psychosis. Am J Psychiatry 141:114–115, 1984

Yudofsky SC, Silver JM, Jackson M, et al: The Overt Aggression Scale: an operationalized rating scale for verbal and physical aggression. Am J Psychiatry 143:35–39, 1986

Yudofsky SC, Silver JM, Hales RE: Pharmacologic management of aggression in the elderly. J Clin Psychiatry 51 (10 suppl):1–58, 1990

Yudofsky SC, Kopecky HJ, Kunik M, et al: The Overt Agitation Severity Scale for the objective rating of agitation. J Neuropsychiatry Clin Neurosci 9:541–548, 1997

TWENTY-SIX

Treatment of Personality Disorders

Robert L. Trestman, Ph.D., M.D.,
Ann Marie Woo-Ming, M.D.,
Marie deVegvar, M.D., and
Larry J. Siever, M.D.

Although pharmacotherapy has long been a therapeutic mainstay of the major Axis I syndromes, more recently, psychopharmacology has gained acceptance as a treatment option for severe personality disorders. By definition, a *personality disorder* is constituted by enduring maladaptive symptoms or behaviors that have an early onset and persist without periods of remission. More recently, it has been viewed that this very pattern may actually represent chronic disorders in mood, impulsivity, aggression, cognition, or anxiety. This so-called dimensional approach to character disorders has been supported by research suggesting biological correlates of these various dimensions. Psychopharmacology has more fully emerged as a treatment of personality disorders, for example, by targeting affective instability as one would in a chronic affective disorder.

Pioneering studies of patients with personality disorders showed that pharmacological interventions used in affective and schizophrenic disorders might be of benefit (Klein 1968; Klein and Greenberg 1967; Liebowitz and Klein 1981; Rifkin et al. 1972b). However, years passed before the field made use of these early findings; for example, disorders such as cyclothymia were still considered personality disorders. More recent studies that categorized syndromes with DSM-III-R or DSM-IV (American Psychiatric Association 1987, 1994) criteria, in conjunction with work focused on clinical dimensions, suggested that pharmacological intervention may be beneficial in personality disorders for affective symptoms, including affective instability or transient depression, impulsivity/aggression, psychotic-like symptoms or cognitive/perceptual distortions, and anxiety. These results are complemented by evi-

The authors' research was supported in part by grants from the National Institutes of Health, National Center for Research Resources (RR00071) to the Mt. Sinai Medical Center, National Institutes of Mental Health (R01-MH41131), and Department of Veterans Affairs Merit Award (7609004).

dence implicating both genetic and biological factors in the pathogenesis of these disorders. A growing body of studies suggests that genetic factors play an important role in the development of normal personality (Goldsmith 1982; Tellegen et al. 1988). Although the heritability of the personality disorders has been less extensively studied, twin studies (Torgersen 1984), adoptive studies (Cloninger et al. 1978), and family studies (Siever et al. 1990; Silverman et al., in press) suggest that underlying dimensions of personality may be heritable. Developmental studies demonstrate a long-term continuity of behavioral traits such as fearfulness or shyness, which may have specific psychophysiological correlates (Kagan et al. 1988). Comparable studies in primates also suggest behavioral and biological continuity for behavioral dimensions such as aggression or affective sensitivity to separation (Suomi 1991).

In this chapter, we discuss issues of pharmacotherapy for patients with personality disorders. Appropriate selection and assessment of patients for pharmacotherapy are initially addressed, as are issues of initiating and maintaining psychopharmacological treatment in this population. Subsequent sections focus on specific syndromes and behavioral dimensions that have received adequate research interest to tentatively suggest appropriate psychopharmacological intervention. However, many Axis II syndromes do not lend themselves to pharmacological treatment and have not been the focus of controlled treatment studies (e.g., schizoid, narcissistic, histrionic, dependent, and obsessive-compulsive personality disorders); therefore, they are not discussed in this chapter.

ASSESSMENT FOR TREATMENT

Before considering psychopharmacological treatment of signs and symptoms of a presumed personality disorder, the clinician should conduct a formal assessment to evaluate the differential diagnosis and possible complicating medical factors. A proposed sequence for this assessment is a detailed psychiatric history, substance abuse history, family history, medical history, and physical and laboratory examination. Specific issues of differential diagnosis are addressed in subsequent sections of this chapter.

Psychiatric History

Axis I and Axis II diagnoses must be differentiated initially. In general, Axis I disorders such as schizophrenia, major depression, and bipolar disorder take precedence in the differential diagnosis and treatment priority. For example, if bipolar disorder, type I, is diagnosed, it will usually be the initial target of treatment. When the bipolar disorder is optimally treated and residual mood disturbances ruled out, personality disorder disturbances may then appropriately be addressed.

In the process of obtaining a detailed past and present psychiatric history, the clinician must pay careful attention not only to the signs and symptoms of psychiatric illness per se but also to the pattern and timing of their presentation. One explicit example is the presence of impulsive-aggressive behavior, sexual promiscuity, and labile affect. If this symptom cluster is stable over time and has been present since adolescence, dramatic cluster personality disorders might head the differential diagnosis list. However, if the symptoms are episodic and associated with increased energy and decreased sleep, Axis I disorders such as bipolar disorder (mania) or organic mental disorder associated with substance intoxication or withdrawal become more probable as primary diagnoses.

Medication history is critical in this assessment. Optimally, for each psychotropic medication taken, the target symptoms, dose, duration, and efficacy should be determined. Given the frequent ambiguity of the behavioral, affective, and cognitive complaints, it is particularly important to operationally define each of the target symptoms assessed.

Substance Abuse and Dependence History

Drug and alcohol use must be carefully assessed and monitored. Before attempting to diagnose and treat personality disorders, the clinician should determine whether the patient has substance abuse and/or dependence and, when it is found, should treat it. Symptoms such as affective lability, impulsivity, and aggression that might otherwise be ascribed to personality disorders may remit with the resolution of substance abuse or dependence.

Interviewing of Family Members

Because of the nature of personality disorder diagnoses, it is frequently difficult for these patients to describe adequately the extent and severity of interpersonal difficulties. It is therefore important in this population to interview family members, with the knowledge and permission of the patient, to improve the database from which therapeutic interventions will be made. This is especially relevant regarding a history of substance abuse, which can have a profound effect on symptomatology and is frequently an area of patient denial. Patient refusal of family interviews should raise the question of the reliability of the patient's stated information.

Family History

A thorough family history is of the utmost importance because it may suggest the existence of biological vulnerabilities to mood disorders, drug or alcohol abuse, and perhaps personality disorders. It may prove valuable to speak with family members directly (again, with the permission of the patient) to evaluate more fully the potential presence of psychiatric illness in relatives of the proband.

Medical History

Many medical illnesses may present as psychiatric illness. Examples include endocrine, neuro-

logical, rheumatological, and metabolic disorders that have been reviewed elsewhere (Horvath et al. 1989). Further, medications prescribed for the treatment of other disorders may have cognitive, behavioral, or affective consequences. One common example is the use of steroids in the treatment of severe asthma, chronic obstructive pulmonary disease, or systemic lupus erythematosus. Some of the potential complications arising from the use of high-dose steroids may include agitation, aggressive behavior, and affective lability.

Physical and Laboratory Examinations

A complete physical examination and routine laboratory studies, including blood counts and chemistries, thyroid function tests, serology (for syphilis and human immunodeficiency virus [HIV]), and computed tomography (CT)/magnetic resonance imaging (MRI) of the head, if indicated, should be obtained. Clinical indications should be used to guide the clinician in selecting further tests. Treatment of underlying conditions may not completely correct the disorder but may at least ameliorate the symptoms.

TREATMENT INITIATION AND MANAGEMENT OF TOXIC EFFECTS

When beginning any psychotropic medication in a patient with a personality disorder diagnosis, the clinician should discuss the treatment in detail with the patient and, when possible, the patient's family. Given the frequent sensitivity to medication side, or toxic, effects in patients with personality disorders and the chronic nature of the disturbances to be treated, a recommended treatment algorithm is to begin with a minimal dose of medication and incrementally and gradually increase to a therapeutic level.

ASSESSMENT OF RESPONSE

With any patient, it is important to define desired target symptoms and to operationalize the outcome measures. Although this may sound more like a research paradigm than a clinical treatment plan, this approach to the treatment of behavioral, cognitive, anxiety, and/or affective symptoms in patients with personality disorders will reduce the risk of inappropriate expectations, ambiguous results, and power struggles between the patient and the clinician. For example, if the target symptom is reduction of affective instability, a simple 10-cm visual analogue scale might be used: one end might be behaviorally anchored with "most erratic, unstable emotions I have ever experienced," whereas the other might be anchored with "most stable I have ever experienced my emotions to be." The patient would place a mark on this scale to describe his or her experience for the preceding week at baseline and at each subsequent office visit.

MAINTENANCE AND MONITORING

Many of the symptoms in patients with personality disorders that are a target for pharmacotherapy (such as affective lability or impulsivity) are themselves inconstant. It may then be necessary for the clinician to be willing to work with the patient to modify the dosing of medications appropriately.

Blood levels of medications, if available, may be monitored to ensure appropriate adherence to the medication regimen and to confirm that therapeutic levels are being maintained.

TREATMENT RESISTANCE

Given that, by definition, interpersonal relationships are disturbed in patients with personality disorders, these disturbances will likely intrude on the therapeutic relationship. Issues involving patients' adherence to a prescribed medication regimen, consistently and accurately reporting missed doses or side effects, and a willingness to discuss potential problems with medication all may evolve in the psychopharmacological management of any individual patient. Such discussions should be held at the outset of treatment and at appropriate intervals to ensure each other of concern on the clinician's part and cooperation and collaboration on the patient's part.

SPECIFIC SYNDROMAL TREATMENT

Not all personality disorder syndromes have received psychopharmacological research attention; indeed, even the most carefully studied of the syndromes is lacking in adequate numbers of well-defined, full-scale, placebo-controlled, double-blind studies. What follows are discussions of the psychobiology and psychopharmacological treatment of syndromes that, in our opinion, have received enough attention to support even tentative psychopharmacological treatment recommendations.

ECCENTRIC PERSONALITY DISORDERS: SCHIZOTYPAL PERSONALITY DISORDER

Regarded as part of the schizophrenia spectrum, the Cluster A ("odd cluster") personality disorders include schizotypal, schizoid, and paranoid types. Of the three, schizotypal personality disorder (SPD) has been the most clearly defined from clinical, psychobiological, and genetic perspectives. For example, in common with schizophrenic patients, SPD subjects have neuropsychological abnormalities, impairment in attention and information processing (Siever et al. 1990, 1993b). In comparison with relatives of healthy volunteers, the relatives of schizophrenic patients have significantly higher rates of SPD (Silverman et al. 1986, 1993). Similarly, assessments of the siblings of schizophrenic patients have found them to be at higher risk for both schizophrenia and SPD if either or both parents had SPD (Baron et al. 1985).

From a phenomenological viewpoint, psychotic-like and deficit-like symptoms are two central dimensions of SPD, paralleling the positive and negative symptomatology of the schizophrenia. Magical thinking, ideas of reference, and perceptual disorders are included in the psychotic-like aspect of SPD, whereas poor interpersonal relatedness and social isolation are descriptive of the deficit-like syndrome. Plasma levels of the dopamine metabolite homovanillic acid (HVA) have been found to correlate with psychotic-like symptoms in patients with SPD (Amin et al. 1997; Siever et al. 1993a), as in schizophrenia (M. Davidson and Davis 1988; Davis et al. 1985). Furthermore, the dopaminergic agent amphetamine exacerbated these positive-like symptoms among patients with SPD and borderline personality disorder (BPD) (Schulz et al. 1988). On the other hand, decreased plasma HVA levels may be associated with deficit-like symptoms in relatives of schizophrenic patients (Amin et al. 1997), as well as diminished cognitive performance on neuropsychological testing of patients with SPD (Siever et al. 1993b), and both cognitive and negative symptoms may improve following amphetamine in SPD patients (Kirrane 2000).

These psychobiological, genetic, and clinical perspectives support the concept of SPD as a schizophrenia-related disorder and suggest a role for psychopharmacological treatments for SPD as for schizophrenia. The agents most studied to date have been the antipsychotic drugs.

Differential Diagnoses

Other diagnoses to be considered include schizophrenia, residual schizophrenia, delusional disorder, and the interictal personality sometimes associated with temporal-lobe epilepsy. It is also important to consider the social context of the patient. The patient may come from a culture in which superstitiousness and forms of magical thinking are accepted; if so, it must be determined that the signs and symptoms go beyond that person's cultural norms. Interviews with family members may often be helpful in making this distinction.

Treatment Selection

Antipsychotics. Low-dose antipsychotic medications have received the most attention in studies conducted over the past 25 years in patients with personality disorders. Seventeen patients with SPD were given haloperidol (maximum 12 mg/day) in a 6-week open-label study (Hymowitz et al. 1986). Mild to moderate improvement in target symptoms of social isolation, odd communication, and ideas of reference was observed in the 50% of patients who remained in the study. This high attrition rate speaks to the intolerance of, and sensitivity to, side effects in this patient population.

Low doses of thiothixene (mean dose 9 mg/day) or haloperidol (mean dose 3 mg/day) were used in a blinded comparison study of 52 patients with histories of recent transient psychotic episodes whose symptoms met DSM-III-R BPD or SPD criteria (Serban and Siegel 1984); 84% of the patients were moderately to markedly improved at 3-month follow up, with decreased derealization, paranoid ideation, anxiety, and depression.

In a 12-week double-blind, placebo-controlled study, 50 patients with BPD or SPD received thiothixene (mean dose 8.7 mg/day) (Goldberg et al. 1986). In the group receiving the drug, significant decreases were observed in measures of illusions, psychoticism, phobic anxiety, and ideas of reference; depressive symptoms were unaffected; and no improvement was noted in measures of global functioning.

Although these results appear promising, note that all but one of these studies were uncontrolled, and the single double-blind, placebo-controlled study (Goldberg et al. 1986) used a heterogeneous sample. Furthermore, there is no evidence that any given agent or class of antipsychotic agent is more effective than another.

In summary, preliminary evidence indicates that low doses of antipsychotic medication (1–2 mg/day of haloperidol equivalent) are effective in at least temporarily reducing or relieving the symptoms of cognitive/perceptual dysfunction in patients with personality disorders. There are no studies of which we are aware that have examined long-term, chronic use of antipsychotic medications in SPD or related personality disorders. Concerns for the development of tardive dyskinesia or dystonia argue that if antipsychotic medications are to be used in this population, they should be administered for short-term use (months) with subsequent medication withdrawal and reassessment. Recent studies suggest that atypical antipsychotic medications may be of value in these patients.

Given the high rates of comorbidity—30%–50% in clinic settings—between SPD and major depression, antidepressants may be useful in the treatment of SPD. Clinical trials using antidepressants in subjects with personality disorders have also suggested a role for these drugs among patients with SPD. So far, however, mixed samples of subjects with only a limited number of actual patients with SPD have been described (Markovitz et al. 1991; Soloff et al. 1989).

Thus, controlled clinical trials in groups of patients with primarily SPD are needed to evaluate 1) antipsychotic and antidepressant efficacy, 2) optimal dosing regimens, 3) treatment duration, and 4) risk-benefit ratios.

Treatment Initiation

It is recommended that antipsychotic medication in this population be started at the level of 1 mg/day or less of haloperidol equivalent. After 1–2 weeks, if no untoward effects emerge, this treatment dose may be increased to 2 mg/day of haloperidol equivalent. Before initiating treat-

ment, it is advisable to document any evidence of dyskinesias or dystonias at baseline to determine whether any subsequent changes occur.

Management of Side Effects

At low antipsychotic doses, minimal side effects are expected. However, side effects such as akinesia, akathisia, and dystonia or dyskinesia are possible. These would be treated as usual. Periodic assessment should be made for occurrence of or change in medication-induced movement disorders.

Assessment of Response

Beyond global assessment of functioning, the clinician may operationalize target symptoms and follow them up at each visit to determine treatment efficacy. Although commonly conducted during an unstructured clinical interview, this may also be done with relevant sections of brief standardized instruments (e.g., the Brief Psychiatric Rating Scale [BPRS]) or with patient-specific visual analogue scales as described earlier in this chapter.

Treatment Resistance

Some patients with SPD are uncomfortable even taking low doses of antipsychotic medication, primarily because of behavioral toxicity: dysphoria or a worsening of some of the deficit-like symptoms. If such symptoms arise in the context of otherwise successful pharmacotherapy, the clinician should consider reducing the dose of antipsychotic to the lowest effective level.

IMPULSIVE AND AFFECTIVELY UNSTABLE PERSONALITY DISORDERS: BORDERLINE PERSONALITY DISORDER

Cluster B ("dramatic cluster") personality disorders, particularly BPD, can be conceptualized as including two dimensions: impulsive aggression and affective lability. The diagnosis of BPD, for example, is defined in DSM-IV (p. 650) as "a pervasive pattern of instability of interpersonal relationships, self-image, and affects" and characterized by criteria that include potentially self-damaging impulsivity, inappropriate or uncontrolled anger, recurrent suicidal threats or gestures, and physically self-damaging acts. Impulsive aggression is also characteristic of other personality disorders, although it is expressed somewhat differently in each. For example, in antisocial personality disorder, a disregard for social norms coupled with impulsive aggression may lead to behaviors such as lying, stealing, and destruction of property. This suggests that impulsivity/aggression may be a dimension of behavior that is not restricted to a single psychiatric diagnosis but may occur in both the Cluster B personality disorders and certain Axis I disorders (i.e., intermittent explosive disorder; bipolar disorder, manic type; and conduct disorder). A number of biological determinants can be associated with impulsive aggression, further supporting the notion of this dimension as a final common pathway to a variety of distinct categorical causes.

Family studies, for example, show significantly greater occurrences of impulsive-aggressive behaviors in first-degree relatives of patients with BPD than in relatives of other patients with personality disorders (Silverman et al. 1991); whereas preliminary results from a twin study point to genetic heritability for BPD criteria such as impulsivity and anger (Torgersen 1992).

Serotonin is thought to be a modulatory neurotransmitter with inhibitory effects on a variety of functions, including mood, arousal, cognition, and feeding behavior. There is evidence of an association between increased aggression toward self and/or others and reduced serotonergic function. Both reduced metabolites and reduced responses to serotonergic agents have been reported (Coccaro et al. 1989; Linnoila et al. 1983).

Another key aspect of BPD is affective instability, which may be characterized as rapid, exaggerated shifts in affect in response to emotionally charged environmental stimuli such as criticism, separation from a significant person, or frustration (American Psychiatric Association 1987; Siever and Davis 1991). Affective instability may impair the ability to maintain a stable sense of self and thus disrupt interpersonal relationships. The inability to consistently modulate these mood shifts may also impair learning and the development of cognitive processes, as affective states may influence state-dependent learning (Bartlett and Santruck 1979), and selective memory may be the result of inadequate memory storage and recall (Kalus and Siever 1993).

There is evidence of an increased prevalence of affectively labile subjects in the first-degree relatives of patients with BPD, suggesting a heritable component to the dimensional characteristic (Silverman et al. 1991). Some of our preliminary studies demonstrate that patients with personality disorders who have affective instability have a heightened depressive response to the acetylcholinesterase inhibitor physostigmine, when compared with patients with personality disorders without this descriptive characteristic, suggesting that the cholinergic system may play a role in the modulation of affective instability in patients with personality disorders (Steinberg et al. 1994).

The noradrenergic system may also play a part in the regulation of affective instability. One study of compulsive gamblers, for example, observed an increase in noradrenergic function associated with extroversion (Roy et al. 1989). In a preliminary study, we examined 31 patients with DSM-III (American Psychiatric Association 1980) personality disorder and found positive correlations between increased measures of noradrenergic function and measures of irritability and verbal hostility (Trestman et al. 1993). Psychopharmacological interventions might therefore logically target serotonergic or catecholaminergic systems in an attempt to treat patients with BPD who are impulsive, aggressive, or affectively labile.

Differential Diagnoses of Impulsivity

Other diagnoses to consider in the differential include the Axis I impulse dyscontrol disorders; bipolar disorder, rapid-cycling or mixed subtypes; and organic syndromes secondary to epilepsy, trauma, or substance abuse.

Differential Diagnoses of Affective Lability

Clinically, it is important to distinguish affective lability from a major mood disorder such as major depression or rapid-cycling bipolar disorder (Coccaro and Siever 1995). The diagnosis of major mood disorder is further complicated by the potential presence of comorbid atypical depression or of hysteroid dysphoria (Liebowitz and Klein 1981) in patients with personality disorders and affective lability.

Atypical depression is not uncommon in patients with personality disorder who have affective lability and is characterized by dysphoria with prominent mood reactivity, anxiety, rejection hypersensitivity and markedly decreased energy sometimes described as *leaden paralysis*. Other features of this disorder include hypersomnia and hyperphagia (especially carbohydrate craving or binge eating; Coccaro and Siever 1995). It is potentially valuable to probe for these symptoms during the initial evaluation given the benefits of monoamine oxidase inhibitors (MAOIs) for atypical depressive features (Coccaro 1993; Parsons et al. 1989).

Substance abuse, intoxication, and withdrawal syndromes may also present initially with affective lability, as may connective tissue disorders such as systemic lupus erythematosus, infectious diseases such as HIV-associated encephalopathy, or neurological disorders such as multiple sclerosis or the dementias.

Treatment Selection

Serotonin reuptake inhibitors. The serotonin reuptake inhibitor fluoxetine has been used in several studies with dramatic cluster patients. In a double-blind, placebo-controlled study, 20–60 mg of fluoxetine given for 12 weeks reduced scores of overt aggression and irritability among a group of patients with personality disorders with histories of impulsive-aggressive behavior (Coccaro and Kavoussi 1995). In 22 volunteers with BPD symptoms without a history of suicidal behavior, significant reductions in impulsive-aggressive behavior, irritability, and anger occurred in a 12-week fluoxetine double-blind, placebo-controlled study (Salzman et al. 1992). An analysis of covariance demonstrated significant decreases in anger that did not correlate with depression scores, a finding consistent with other studies (Coccaro et al. 1990; Markovitz et al. 1991). Furthermore, a preliminary study of patients with BPD suggested that fluoxetine may decrease affective lability per se (Teicher et al. 1989).

Although many other studies are preliminary, have a small sample size, or are not double blind, the general results seem to also support the efficacy of fluoxetine in patients with BPD in a nonspecific manner or for symptoms of impulsive aggression or affective instability (Coccaro et al. 1990; Cornelius et al. 1991; Norden 1989).

Twenty-two patients whose symptoms met DSM-III criteria for BPD and/or SPD were treated in an open-label trial of fluoxetine (12 weeks duration, 80 mg/day) (Markovitz et al. 1991). Both affective and impulsive symptoms and the frequency of self-mutilation decreased significantly; self-injurious behavior did not decrease significantly until 9 weeks into the trial. Given the high dosing schedule of 80 mg/day, the delayed response is unlikely attributable to an "underdosing" effect and raises the possibility that the full effects of the drug, regardless of dose, may not be apparent until 9 weeks or longer. In addition, the presence or absence of depression did not appear to influence the outcome with regard to impulsive-aggressive behavior, suggesting the possibility of a differential effect of fluoxetine on depression and on impulsive-aggressive behavior.

The effect of open-label sertraline on impulsive aggression was examined among 11 patients meeting criteria for at least one personality disorder (Kavoussi et al. 1994). After 4 weeks, significant decreases in irritability and overt aggression were noted, suggesting a role for the serotonin uptake inhibitors as a group in this dimension of behavior.

Two double-blind, placebo-controlled studies indicated that fluoxetine is effective in the treatment of BPD symptoms. Fluoxetine treatment reduced anger in symptomatic volunteers (Salzman et al. 1995) and impulsive aggression in patients with personality disorder. In the second study, 40 patients with irritable aggression, meeting criteria for a personality disorder, who were not currently depressed were started on 20 mg of fluoxetine. Fluoxetine was superior to placebo in reducing irritability and aggression; treatment response was first apparent during the second month of treatment for irritability and third month for aggression. These results were not due to secondary measures such as anxiety or alcohol use (Coccaro and Kavoussi 1997).

Overall, fluoxetine is a reasonable first choice for the treatment of impulsive-aggressive behavior, because it is relatively safe in overdose and may also treat depression and affective lability. Controlled treatment trials have not as yet been conducted with the newer alternative selective serotonin reuptake inhibitors sertraline and paroxetine. Such trials may prove these agents to be useful alternatives to fluoxetine, given the differing pharmacokinetics and pharmacodynamics of these agents.

Tricyclic antidepressants. Studies conducted in patients with BPD using tricyclic antidepressants have generally shown a poor response to treatment (Cole et al. 1984; Soloff et al. 1986a, 1986b, 1989). Coupled with the lethal potential of overdose and the anticholinergic

toxicity of these medications, tricyclic antidepressants are not generally recommended for the treatment of BPD.

Monoamine oxidase inhibitors. MAOIs are a class of antidepressants that alter the noradrenergic system (Cowdry and Gardner 1982; Liebowitz and Klein 1981). One relevant study targeted the treatment of hysteroid dysphoria, a disorder with characteristics of affective lability and rejection sensitivity similar to those seen in patients with BPD (Liebowitz and Klein 1981). The results of this preliminary study marginally supported the use of MAOIs in this condition; 40% taking active medication relapsed compared with 66% taking placebo who relapsed (Liebowitz and Klein 1981). Consistent with these early findings, a more recent treatment trial of BPD (Cowdry and Gardner 1988) demonstrated that patients taking tranylcypromine, even without current major depression, significantly improved with regard to the target symptoms of impulsivity and affective lability. Furthermore, one study has found that phenelzine may be more effective in the treatment of atypical depression even when patients have a comorbid diagnosis of BPD (Parsons et al. 1989). However, more recently, phenelzine was found to be less effective than haloperidol in decreasing impulsivity/hostile belligerence among a group of patients with BPD, although hostility scores were overall decreased with phenelzine (Soloff et al. 1993).

Given the available, if limited, evidence of MAOI efficacy, one of the practical concerns limiting their more widespread use is the risk of a hypertensive crisis. Patients who may also have difficulties with impulse regulation may still be liable to overdose on the MAOI. Reversible inhibitors of MAO-A, which are less likely to induce a hypertensive crisis, may therefore provide an excellent alternative if proven to be as effective as the present nonselective MAOIs for the treatment of affective instability (Liebowitz et al. 1990).

Lithium carbonate.   Beyond its role in the treatment of bipolar disorder, lithium may treat affective lability (Van der Kolk 1986), regardless of the syndrome per se. Further, lithium may be effective in decreasing impulsivity in general (Shader et al. 1974), impulsivity associated with affective lability (Rifkin et al. 1972a), and episodic violence, especially in patients with antisocial personality disorder (Schiff et al. 1982). Impulsive-aggressive prison inmates were treated with lithium carbonate for 3 months in a double-blind, placebo-controlled study; a significant reduction in the number of aggressive acts was observed (Sheard et al. 1976). A more recent controlled trial also found lithium to decrease therapist perceptions of irritability, anger, and suicidality among borderline patients (Links et al. 1990). The antiaggressive effects of lithium carbonate may be due to its enhancement of serotonergic postsynaptic receptors and/or its possible inhibition of catecholaminergic function (Coccaro et al. 1990) and a decrease in mood lability often associated with impulsivity.

Lithium carbonate has also been shown to have mood-stabilizing effects in patients with "emotionally unstable personality disorder," a diagnosis that is characterized by significant affective lability (Rifkin et al. 1972b). An additional indication for the use of lithium may be the presence of bipolar disorder in a first-degree relative of a proband with affective lability.

Anticonvulsants.   The presence of mood lability, rage episodes, brief psychotic disturbances, and soft neurological signs in some patients with BPD suggested similarities with temporal-lobe epilepsy (despite a normal electroencephalogram result) and led to trials of anticonvulsants (Klein and Greenberg 1967; Gardner and Cowdry 1986b). One comprehensive 6-week double-blind, placebo-controlled study with a crossover design was conducted to examine the effects of four medications, including carbamazepine, in 16 female patients with DSM-III-R BPD (Cowdry and Gardner 1988). Target symptoms included impulsive self-inju-

rious behavior and severe dysphoria. The average dose of carbamazepine was 820 mg/day, and those receiving the medication had a significant decrease in behavioral dyscontrol. Reduction of impulsive-aggressive behavior was associated with the capacity to delay action and "reflect." Although the mechanism of action is not yet understood, this study, along with other preliminary trials (Gardner and Cowdry 1986b; Luchins 1984), suggests that carbamazepine may be useful, either alone or as an adjunct to a serotonin reuptake inhibitor, for the control of impulsive aggression. Overall, carbamazepine's most significant effect has been demonstrated with behavioral dyscontrol (Cowdry and Gardner 1988).

Valproic acid has gained popularity in clinical practice as a mood stabilizer and has also been recently investigated in BPD. Modest reductions in irritability, anger, and impulsivity were noted for some among 8 outpatients with BPD who were given open-label valproate, up to 500 mg/day for 8 weeks (Stein et al. 1995). Similarly, 10 adolescents with mood lability/temper outbursts were all found to have clear improvement in frequency and severity of their symptoms with the use of divalproex sodium up to 1 g/day orally for 5 weeks, administered in an open-label fashion (Donovan et al. 1997). A more recent controlled study supports these conclusions (Hollander 1999).

Adrenergic antagonists.   Propranolol has been shown to diminish explosive behaviors among a diverse group of patients including adolescents with rage outbursts or destructive behavior, among mentally retarded patients, or in Huntington's disease patients (Campbell et al. 1992; Stewart 1993). Formal investigations with patients who have personality disorders remain to be carried out.

Antipsychotics.   A number of studies have suggested the general benefits of low-dose antipsychotics in individuals with impulsivity, depression, paranoid and schizotypal features, and rejection sensitivity. For example, haloperidol was found to be more effective than phenelzine in decreasing impulsivity/hostile belligerence among a group of 92 subjects with BPD (Soloff et al. 1993). The use of 4–16 mg/day of haloperidol for 5 weeks among a large sample of inpatients with BPD led to global improvements in hostile depression and impulsive ward behaviors (Soloff et al. 1989).

Support for the efficacy of these medications comes from other trials as well. Patients with BPD (*N* = 80) were treated with loxapine (mean dose 14 mg/day) compared with chlorpromazine (mean dose 110 mg/day) in a 6-week double-blind protocol. A decrease in suspiciousness, hostility, and anxiety, as well as improvement in depressed mood, was reported with both agents (Leone 1982). One double-blind, placebo-controlled crossover study of the effects of carbamazepine, tranylcypromine, trifluoperazine, and alprazolam on 16 patients with DSM-III-defined BPD noted improvement in suicidality and anxiety (Cowdry and Gardner 1988).

A significant improvement in hostility, depression, and cognitive/perceptual disturbances was observed in a 12-week thioridazine (mean dose 92 mg/day) open-label study of 11 patients with DSM-III-R BPD (Teicher et al. 1989). Six of the 11 patients who completed the study showed decreased symptomatology on the impulse action patterns and psychosis subscales of the Diagnostic Interview for Borderline Personality Disorder. In addition, anxiety, interpersonal sensitivity, and paranoid ideation diminished.

Low-dose antipsychotics, in summary, appear potentially useful in the treatment of patients with BPD who are more severely impaired, regardless of specific symptoms (Goldberg et al. 1986; Soloff et al. 1986b). It must be kept in mind, however, that these agents have been tested in patients with BPD only for relatively short periods (less than 4 months). Because of the potential for tardive dyskinesia, it may be most prudent to minimize both dose and duration of antipsychotic treatment in patients with BPD. Also, because of common antipsychotic side effects, compliance is often a problem. As with most medications, a careful risk-benefit assessment must be made for the specific indication and individual being treated.

Stimulants. One case report using methylphenidate has described improvement of mood lability and impulsivity in an adult with a diagnosis of BPD and comorbid attention-deficit disorder (Hooberman and Stern 1984). One finding associated with BPD improvement on tranylcypromine (an MAOI with psychostimulant actions) is a history of childhood attention-deficit/hyperactivity disorder (ADHD) (Cowdry and Gardner 1988). Adult residual ADHD may be characterized by impulsivity, irritability, mood lability, difficulty in focusing, and subtle learning disabilities.

Psychostimulants such as methylphenidate may be considered for the treatment of carefully selected adult patients with BPD who had well-documented cases of childhood ADHD and no significant history of drug or alcohol dependence. Carefully controlled studies are needed to evaluate this possibility.

Benzodiazepines. Benzodiazepines have received little controlled attention in the treatment of BPD. In a double-blind, placebo-controlled study, 7 of 12 patients (58%) developed serious behavioral dyscontrol (self-mutilation, drug overdoses, aggression) while taking alprazolam compared with 1 of 12 (8%) taking placebo (Gardner and Cowdry 1986a). Given the potential dyscontrol problem and the risk of drug dependency, therapy with alprazolam or other benzodiazepines is not currently indicated in this population.

Treatment Initiation

It may help the patient cooperate fully with treatment if it is specified 1) that only limited success from psychopharmacological intervention is expected and 2) that a logical progression of medication interventions will be made, based on the responses of the individual to treatment.

Assessment of Response

Given that several symptoms may be targeted, it will benefit both patient and clinician to define objectively each of the target symptoms with either visual analogue scales or structured instruments (self-report or interview) at baseline and at each session and to record a clinical global impression at these same visits to balance general progress with symptom-specific progress.

Treatment Resistance

Patients with BPD may often, intentionally or unintentionally, resist treatment. As many, if not all, of the targeted symptoms fluctuate, patients may benefit from specific psychoeducation as to the nature of the disturbances and the expected response to treatment to help them tolerate the occasional problems without discontinuing treatment.

ANXIOUS PERSONALITY DISORDERS: AVOIDANT PERSONALITY DISORDER

Anxiety is an alerting signal that warns of threats to safety, but it can also become maladaptive as reflected in personality characteristics such as shyness, rejection sensitivity, and a diminished ability to take advantage of opportunities. Shyness is a trait that appears to be rather stable during childhood development. As youngsters, shy toddlers avoid strangers; as adults, they continue to be uncomfortable and anxious in new situations and social gatherings (Kagan et al. 1988).

People who have a low threshold for physiological arousal in anticipation of threatening consequences might develop avoidant behavior (Kalus and Siever 1993). Although anxiety is a prominent feature of several Axis I disorders, hyperarousal as a concomitant of a low stimulation threshold may also contribute to the pa-

thology of the anxious cluster diagnoses.

Anxious individuals have increased tonic levels of sympathetic activity and cortical arousal, slower habituation to new stimuli, and lower sedation thresholds than do nonanxious individuals (Claridge 1967, 1985; Gray 1982). Studies of the noradrenergic system in social phobia yield equivocal results in the growth hormone response to clonidine (Tancer 1993; Uhde 1994). Preliminary evidence of serotonergic involvement may be reflected in the increased cortisol response to fenfluramine among subjects with social phobia (Uhde 1994). Stimulation of the locus coeruleus in primates is associated with responses that closely mimic anxiety in people (Redmond 1987). One hypothesis suggests a role for serotonergic function in harm avoidance, with a positive correlation between serotonin activity and increased avoidance behavior (Cloninger 1986). Consistent with this hypothesis, the postsynaptic serotonin agonist m-chlorophenylpiperazine (m-CPP) increases hormonal release as well as measures of anxiety in patients with panic disorder as compared with control subjects or patients with major depressive disorder (Kahn et al. 1988).

Differential Diagnoses

Axis I anxiety disorders constitute most of the potentially confounding diagnoses. When identified, these Axis I disorders may take priority in treatment. Furthermore, avoidant and dependent personality disorders may be secondary to a major depressive disorder or obsessive-compulsive disorder; following their treatment, these apparent personality disorders may also resolve (Ricciardi et al. 1992). Thus, what is viewed as a personality disorder with associated affective symptoms may in actuality be an affective disorder with associated personality problems.

Treatment Selection

By extension to their use in related Axis I disorders, medications such as β-adrenergic receptor antagonists (Gorman et al. 1985), the benzo-diazepine alprazolam, and the MAOI phenelzine (Liebowitz et al. 1986) may each be effective in the treatment of some patients with personality disorders with anxiety.

In a study by Cowdry and Gardner (1988), the MAOI tranylcypromine was helpful in alleviating anxiety in most patients who had avoidant personality disorder. Phenelzine led to a significant decrease in avoidant personality features among subjects with social phobia in two controlled situations (Liebowitz et al. 1992; Versiani et al. 1992). Alprazolam, used for the treatment of social phobia, also diminished specific symptoms of avoidant personality disorder (being fearful of saying something foolish or avoiding social and occupational situations requiring interpersonal contact) (Cowdry and Gardner 1988). Similar results were produced with the use of clonazepam (J. T. Davidson et al. 1993).

Patients with avoidant personality disorder who were treated with tranylcypromine (30 mg/day), phenelzine (60 mg/day), or fluoxetine (20 mg/day) for a period of 2–3 months (Deltito and Stam 1989) showed marked improvement in case reports with regard to increased assertiveness, improved occupational and social functioning, and decreased social sensitivity. Increased self-confidence, assertiveness, and socialization within several weeks were also described with the use of fluoxetine in case reports of patients with avoidant personality and social phobia (Goldman and Grinspoon 1990; Sternbach 1990). Double-blind, placebo-controlled studies are needed to confirm these observations.

CONCLUSION

Substantial evidence now suggests that biological components contribute to some of the more severe personality disorder syndromes such as SPD and BPD and to some of the troubling characteristics of personality disorders. These areas include, but may not be limited to, cognitive and perceptual dysfunction, impulsivity and aggression, affective instability, and anxiety/excessive inhibition. Furthermore, there is growing evidence from controlled treatment trials demonstrating the efficacy of psychopharmacological interventions in the treatment of these signs and symptoms.

REFERENCES

American Psychiatric Association: Diagnostic and Statistical Manual of Mental Disorders, 3rd Edition. Washington, DC, American Psychiatric Association, 1980

American Psychiatric Association: Diagnostic and Statistical Manual of Mental Disorders, 3rd Edition, Revised. Washington, DC, American Psychiatric Association, 1987

American Psychiatric Association: Diagnostic and Statistical Manual of Mental Disorders, 4th Edition. Washington, DC, American Psychiatric Association, 1994

Amin F, Siever LJ, Silverman J, et al: Plasma HVA in schizotypal personality disorder, in Plasma Homovanillic Acid in Schizophrenia: Implications for Presynaptic Dopamine Dysfunction. Edited by Friedhoff AJ, Amin F. Washington, DC, American Psychiatric Press, 1997, pp 133–180

Baron M, Gruen R, Asnis L: Familial transmission of schizotypal and borderline personality disorders. Am J Psychiatry 142:927–933, 1985

Bartlett JC, Santruck JW: Affect-dependent episodic memory in young children. Child Dev 50:513–518, 1979

Campbell M, Gonzalez NM, Silva RR: The pharmacologic treatment of conduct disorders and rage outbursts. Psychiatr Clin North Am 15:69–85, 1992

Claridge G: Personality and Arousal. Oxford, England, Pergamon, 1967

Claridge G: Origins of Mental Illness. New York, Blackwell, 1985

Cloninger CR: A unified theory of personality and its role in the development of anxiety states. Psychiatric Developments 3:167–226, 1986

Cloninger CR, Christiansen KO, Reich T, et al: Implications of sex differences in the prevalence of antisocial personality, alcoholism, and criminality for familial transmission. Arch Gen Psychiatry 35:941–951, 1978

Coccaro EF: Psychopharmacologic studies in patients with personality disorders: review and perspective. Journal of Personality Disorders 7 (suppl):181–192, 1993

Coccaro EF, Kavoussi RJ: Fluoxetine in aggression in personality disorders. American Psychiatric Association 1995 Annual Meeting New Research Program and Abstracts. Washington, DC, American Psychiatric Association, 1995

Coccaro EF, Kavoussi RJ: Fluoxetine and impulsive aggressive behavior in personality disordered subjects. Arch Gen Psychiatry 54:1081–1088, 1997

Coccaro EF, Siever LJ: The neuropsychopharmacology of personality disorders, in Psychopharmacology: The Fourth Generation of Progress. Edited by Bloom F, Kupfer D. New York, Raven, 1995, pp 1567–1579

Coccaro EF, Siever LJ, Klar H: Serotonergic studies in patients with affective and personality disorders: correlates with suicidal and impulsive aggressive behavior. Arch Gen Psychiatry 45: 177–185, 1989

Coccaro EF, Astill JL, Herbert JA, et al: Fluoxetine treatment of impulsive aggression in DSM-III-R personality disorder patients. J Clin Psychopharmacol 10:373–375, 1990

Cole JO, Salomon M, Gunderson J: Drug therapy in borderline patients. Compr Psychiatry 25: 249–254, 1984

Cornelius JR, Soloff PH, Perel JM, et al: A preliminary trial of fluoxetine in refractory borderline patients. J Clin Psychopharmacol 11:116–120, 1991

Cowdry RW, Gardner DL: Pharmacology of borderline personality disorder. Arch Gen Psychiatry 139:741–746, 1982

Cowdry RW, Gardner DL: Pharmacotherapy of borderline personality disorder: alprazolam, carbamazepine, trifluoperazine, and tranylcypromine. Arch Gen Psychiatry 45:111–119, 1988

Davidson JT, Potts NS, Richichi EA, et al: Treatment of social phobia with clonazepam and placebo. J Clin Psychopharmacol 13:423–428, 1993

Davidson M, Davis KL: A comparison of plasma homovanillic acid concentrations in schizophrenic patients and normal controls. Arch Gen Psychiatry 45:561–563, 1988

Davis KL, Davidson M, Mohs RC, et al: Plasma homovanillic acid concentration and the severity of schizophrenic illness. Science 227:1601–1602, 1985

Deltito JA, Stam M: Psychopharmacological treatment of avoidant personality disorder. Compr Psychiatry 30:498–504, 1989

Donovan SJ, Susser ES, Nunes EV, et al: Divalproex treatment of disruptive adolescents: a report of ten cases. J Clin Psychiatry 58:1, 12–15, 1997

Gardner DL, Cowdry RW: Alprazolam induced discontrol in borderline personality disorder. Am J Psychiatry 142:98–100, 1986a

Gardner DL, Cowdry RW: Positive effects of carbamazepine on behavioral dyscontrol in borderline personality disorder. Am J Psychiatry 143:519–522, 1986b

Goldberg SC, Schulz SC, Schulz PM, et al: Borderline and schizotypal personality disorders treated with low-dose thiothixene versus placebo. Arch Gen Psychiatry 43:680–686, 1986

Goldman MJ, Grinspoon L: Ritualistic use of fluoxetine by a former substance abuser (letter). Am J Psychiatry 147:1377, 1990

Goldsmith HH: Genetic influences on personality from infancy to adulthood. Child Dev 54:331–355, 1982

Gorman JM, Liebowitz MR, Fyer AJ, et al: Treatment of social phobia with atenolol. J Clin Psychopharmacol 5:298–301, 1985

Gray JA: The Neuropsychology of Anxiety. Oxford, England, Oxford University Press, 1982

Hollander E: Managing aggressive behavior in patients with obsessive-compulsive disorder and borderline personality disorder. J Clin Psychiatry 60 (suppl 15):38–44, 1999

Hooberman D, Stern TA: Treatment of attention deficit and borderline personality disorders with psychostimulants: case report. J Clin Psychiatry 45:441–442, 1984

Horvath TB, Siever LJ, Mohs RC, et al: Organic mental syndromes and disorders, in Comprehensive Textbook of Psychiatry/V. Edited by Kaplan HI, Sadock BJ. Baltimore, MD, Williams & Wilkins, 1989, pp 599–641

Hymowitz P, Frances A, Jacobsberg LB, et al: Neuroleptic treatment of schizotypal personality disorders. Compr Psychiatry 27:267–271, 1986

Kagan J, Reznick S, Snidman N, et al: Childhood derivatives of inhibition and lack of inhibition to the unfamiliar. Child Dev 59:1580–1589, 1988

Kahn RS, Wetzler S, Van Praag H, et al: Behavioral indications for serotonin receptor hypersensitivity in panic disorder. Psychiatry Res 25:101–104, 1988

Kalus O, Siever LJ: The biology of personality disorders, in An Examination of Illness Subtypes: State vs Trait and Comorbid Psychiatric Disorders. Edited by Mann JJ, Kupfer DJ. New York, Plenum, 1993, pp 89–107

Kavoussi RJ, Liu J, Coccaro EF: An open trial of sertraline in personality disordered patients with impulsive aggression. J Clin Psychiatry 55:137–141, 1994

Kirrane RM, Mitropoulou V, Nunn M, et al: Effects of amphetamine on visuospatial working memory performance in schizophrenia spectrum personality disorder. Neuropsychopharmacology 22:14–18, 2000

Klein DF: Psychiatric diagnosis and a typology of clinical drug effects. Psychopharmacology 13:359–386, 1968

Klein DF, Greenberg IM: Behavioral effects of diphenylhydantoin in severe psychiatric disorders. Am J Psychiatry 124:847–849, 1967

Leone NF: Response of borderline patients to loxapine and chlorpromazine. J Clin Psychiatry 43:148–150, 1982

Liebowitz MR, Klein DF: Interrelationship of hysteroid dysphoria and borderline personality disorder. Psychiatr Clin North Am 4:67–87, 1981

Liebowitz MR, Fyer AJ, Gorman JM, et al: Phenelzine in social phobia. J Clin Psychopharmacol 6:93–98, 1986

Liebowitz MR, Hollander E, Schneier F, et al: Reversible and irreversible monoamine oxidase inhibitors in other psychiatric disorders. Acta Psychiatr Scand Suppl 360:29–34, 1990

Liebowitz MR, Schneier FR, Campeas R, et al: Phenelzine vs. atenolol in social phobia: a placebo-controlled comparison. Arch Gen Psychiatry 49:290–300, 1992

Links PS, Steiner M, Boiago I, et al: Lithium therapy for borderline patients: preliminary findings. Journal of Personality Disorders 4:173–181, 1990

Linnoila M, Virkunnen M, Scheinin M, et al: Low cerebrospinal fluid 5-hydroxyindoleacetic acid concentration differentiates impulsive from nonimpulsive violent behavior. Life Sci 33:2609–2614, 1983

Luchins DJ: Carbamazepine in violent non-epileptic schizophrenics. Psychopharmacol Bull 20:569–571, 1984

Markovitz PJ, Calabrese JR, Schulz SC, et al: Fluoxetine in the treatment of borderline and schizotypal personality disorders. Am J Psychiatry 148:1064–1067, 1991

Norden MJ: Fluoxetine in borderline personality disorder. Prog Neuropsychopharmacol Biol Psychiatry 13:885–893, 1989

Parsons B, Quitkin FM, McGrath PJ: Phenylzine, imipramine, and placebo in borderline patients meeting criteria for atypical depression. Psychopharmacol Bull 25:524–534, 1989

Redmond DE: Studies of the nucleus locus coeruleus in monkeys and hypotheses for neuropsychopharmacology, in Neuropsychopharmacology: The Third Generation of Progress. Edited by Meltzer H. New York, Raven, 1987, pp 967–975

Ricciardi JN, Baer L, Jenike MA, et al: Changes in DSM-III-R Axis II diagnoses following treatment of obsessive-compulsive disorder. Am J Psychiatry 149:829–831, 1992

Rifkin A, Levitan SJ, Galewski J, et al: Emotionally unstable personality disorder—a follow-up study. Biol Psychiatry 4:65–79, 1972a

Rifkin A, Quitkin F, Curillo C, et al: Lithium carbonate in emotionally unstable character disorders. Arch Gen Psychiatry 27:519–523, 1972b

Roy A, DeJong J, Linnoila M: Extraversion in pathological gamblers correlates with indices of noradrenergic function. Arch Gen Psychiatry 46:679–681, 1989

Salzman C, Wolfson AN, Miyawaki E, et al: Fluoxetine treatment of anger in borderline personality disorder (abstract). Proceedings of the American College of Neuropsychopharmacology, 1992, p 24

Salzman C, Wolfson AN, Schatzberg A, et al: Effect of fluoxetine on anger in symptomatic volunteers with borderline personality disorder. J Clin Psychopharmacol 15:23–29, 1995

Schiff HB, Sabin TD, Geller A, et al: Lithium in aggressive behavior. Am J Psychiatry 139:1346–1348, 1982

Schulz SC, Cornelius J, Schulz PM, et al: The amphetamine challenge test in patients with borderline personality disorder. Am J Psychiatry 145:809–814, 1988

Serban G, Siegel S: Response of borderline and schizotypal patients to small doses of thiothixene and haloperidol. Am J Psychiatry 141:1455–1458, 1984

Shader RI, Jackson AH, Dodes LM: The antiaggressive effects of lithium in man. Psychopharmacologia 40:17–24, 1974

Sheard MH, Marini JL, Bridges DL, et al: The effect of lithium on impulsive aggressive behavior in man. Am J Psychiatry 133:1409–1413, 1976

Siever LJ, Davis KL: A psychobiological perspective on the personality disorders. Am J Psychiatry 148:1647–1658, 1991

Siever LJ, Silverman JM, Horvath T, et al: Increased morbid risk for schizophrenia-related disorders in relatives of schizotypal personality disordered patients. Arch Gen Psychiatry 47:634–640, 1990

Siever LJ, Amin F, Coccaro EF, et al: Cerebrospinal fluid homovanillic acid in schizotypal personality disorder. Am J Psychiatry 150:149–151, 1993a

Siever LJ, Kalus OF, Keefe RSE: The boundaries of schizophrenia. Psychiatr Clin North Am 16:217–244, 1993b

Silverman JM, Mohs RC, Siever LJ, et al: Heritability for schizophrenia-spectrum disorder in schizophrenic and schizophrenia related personality disorder patients. Clinical Neuropsychopharmacology 9:271–273, 1986

Silverman JM, Pinkham L, Horvath TB, et al: Affective and impulsive personality disorder traits in the relatives of borderline personality disorder patients. Am J Psychiatry 148:1378–1385, 1991

Silverman JM, Siever LJ, Horvath TB, et al: Schizophrenia-related and affective personality disorder traits in relatives of probands with schizophrenia and personality disorders. Am J Psychiatry 150:435–442, 1993

Silverman JM, Greenberg DA, Altsteil LD, et al: Evidence of a locus for schizophrenia and related disorders on the short arm of chromosome 5 in a large pedigree. Am J Med Genet (in press)

Soloff PH, George A, Nathan RS, et al: Paradoxical effects of amitriptyline in borderline patients. Am J Psychiatry 143:1603–1605, 1986a

Soloff PH, George A, Nathan RS, et al: Progress in pharmacotherapy of borderline disorders. Arch Gen Psychiatry 43:691–697, 1986b

Soloff PH, George A, Nathan RS, et al: Amitriptyline vs haloperidol in borderlines: final outcomes and predictors of response. J Clin Psychopharmacol 9:238–246, 1989

Soloff PH, Cornelius JR, George A, et al: Efficacy of phenelzine and haloperidol in borderline personality disorder. Arch Gen Psychiatry 50:377–385, 1993

Stein DJ, Simeon D, Frenkel M, et al: An open trial of valproate in borderline personality disorder. J Clin Psychiatry 56:506–510, 1995

Steinberg BJ, Trestman RL, Siever LJ: The cholinergic and noradrenergic neurotransmitter systems and affective instability in borderline personality disorder, in Biological and Neurobehavioral Studies in Borderline Personality Disorder. Edited by Silk KR. Washington, DC, American Psychiatric Press, 1994, pp 41–62

Sternbach HA: Fluoxetine treatment in social phobia (letter). J Clin Psychopharmacol 10:230, 1990

Stewart JT: Huntington's disease and propranolol. Am J Psychiatry 150:166–167, 1993

Suomi SJ: Primate separation models of affective disorders, in Neurobiology of Learning, Emotion and Affect. Edited by Madden J. New York, Raven, 1991, pp 321–334

Tancer ME: Neurobiology of social phobia. J Clin Psychiatry 54 (suppl 12):26–30, 1993

Teicher MH, Glod CA, Aaronson ST, et al: Open assessment of the safety and efficacy of thioridazine in the treatment of patients with borderline personality disorder. Psychopharmacol Bull 25:535–549, 1989

Tellegen A, Lykken DT, Bouchard TJ, et al: Personality similarity in twins reared apart and together. J Pers Soc Psychol 54:1031–1039, 1988

Torgersen S: Genetic and nosological aspects of schizotypal and borderline personality disorders. Arch Gen Psychiatry 41:546–554, 1984

Torgersen S: The genetic transmission of borderline personality features displays multidimensionality. Abstract presented at the annual meeting of the American College of Neuropsychopharmacology, San Juan, Puerto Rico, December 14–18, 1992

Trestman RL, deVegvar M-L, Coccaro EF, et al: The differential biology of impulsivity, suicide, and aggression in depression and in personality disorders. Biol Psychiatry 33:46A–47A, 1993

Uhde TW: A review of biological studies in social phobia. J Clin Psychiatry 55 (suppl 6):17–27, 1994

Van der Kolk BA: Uses of lithium in patients without major affective illness (letter). Hospital and Community Psychiatry 37:675, 1986

Versiani M, Nardi AE, Mundim FD, et al: Pharmacotherapy of social phobia: a controlled study with moclobemide and phenelzine. Br J Psychiatry 161:353–360, 1992

TWENTY-SEVEN

Treatment of Psychiatric Emergencies

Michael J. Tueth, M.D.,
C. Lindsay DeVane, Pharm.D., and
Dwight L. Evans, M.D.

In this chapter, we discuss the treatment of psychiatric emergencies from the standpoint of requirements for nonpharmacological, limited pharmacological, and primarily pharmacological intervention. Although most psychiatric emergencies require both pharmacological and psychotherapeutic intervention, many also require that legal action or procedures be followed. In addition, the psychiatrist must decide which level of restrictive environment is appropriate for the patient (see Table 27–1).

PSYCHIATRIC EMERGENCIES REQUIRING NONPHARMACOLOGICAL INTERVENTION

Areas of nonpharmacological interventions include decisions regarding admission to the hospital versus discharge to the community, involuntary versus voluntary admission to a psychiatric facility, and legal action requiring involvement or notification of third parties.

Involuntary or Voluntary Admissions

Involuntary confinement in a psychiatric facility necessitates that the patient be judged suicidal or homicidal based on the presence of a mental disorder. Patients who are determined to be dangerous but who do not have a mental disorder should be referred to the appropriate law enforcement agency. Any patient who is judged by the clinician to be actively suicidal, homicidal, or dangerously psychotic should be admitted to a psychiatric inpatient unit. In addition, patients who are experiencing self-neglect or deterioration in well-being secondary to a psychiatric disorder should be strongly considered for hospitalization even if they are not actually suicidal, homicidal, or psychotic. Although most of these patients can be voluntarily admitted, a subset of patients who exercise poor judgment and refuse

Table 27–1. Levels of restrictive environments for psychiatric patients

Out-of-hospital environment

Out of hospital, alone

Out of hospital, with family or friends

Community residence (i.e., halfway house, boarding home, or nursing home)

In-hospital environment

Medical or surgical floor

Intensive care unit

Unlocked psychiatric unit

Locked psychiatric unit

Constant one-to-one observation

Unlocked seclusion room with observation

Locked seclusion room with observation

Leather and chemical restraints in seclusion room with observation

admission secondary to their psychosis or a self-destructive state of mind should be admitted involuntarily.

Suicidal State

Most suicides occur secondary to a mental disorder. The most common mental disorders leading to suicide include major depression, substance abuse, schizophrenia, and severe personality disorders. Various factors have been identified as increasing suicidal risk. These factors include increasing age, history of violence, previous suicidal behavior, male gender, loss of physical health, long duration of depression, and unwillingness to accept help. However, hopelessness is recognized as the emotional state that best identifies suicidal risk.

Published data have further shown that statistically derived risk factors alone cannot predict suicide mainly because the sensitivity of these valid risk factors is high, but specificity is low (i.e., many false positives). Although it is not possible to accurately predict suicide among psychiatric patients, the clinician's knowledge and judgment and the patient's communicated intentions remain the most important factors in identifying suicidal risks (Goldstein et al. 1991). Risk factors among alcoholic individuals who commit suicide include continued drinking, major depressive episodes, suicidal communication, poor social support, serious medical illness, unemployment, and living alone (Murphy et al. 1992). Patients with panic disorder and comorbid major depression, substance abuse, or borderline personality disorder are particularly at risk for committing suicide. For instance, although 2% of the patients with panic disorder have been reported to attempt suicide, this percentage increased to 25% in panic disorder patients with a comorbid diagnosis of borderline personality disorder (Friedman et al. 1992). Suicide prevalence in elderly people is at least four times higher than in other adult populations (Spar and LaRue 1990). The second highest prevalence for suicide is in the adolescent population. Comorbidity has been found in most adolescent suicides, including depression, antisocial behavior, and alcohol abuse (Marttunen et al. 1991).

Although the no harm or no suicide contract is helpful in the inpatient evaluation of the suicidal patient, it should be used with caution. The contract may help in defining risk and establishing trust, but it provides no medicolegal protection if the patient commits suicide. Furthermore, this contract should not replace a comprehensive assessment of the patient (Stanford et al. 1994).

Homicidal State

Although the vast majority of patients who attempt suicide have a mental disorder, many patients who commit murder or who have homicidal intentions do not have a specific mental disorder. A high correlation exists between sadness and attempted suicide, but there is no correlation between sadness and violence toward others (Apter et al. 1991). The best predictor of violence is a history of violence. However, it has been suggested that clinical decisions regarding dangerousness to others are best determined by the patient's mental state and the need for restraints in the emergency room (Beck et al. 1991).

Self-Neglect and Nonagitated Psychotic State

Patients who do not take care of their physical needs secondary to a mental disorder and patients who are psychotic but nonviolent may not represent a direct threat to themselves or others. Nevertheless, their condition will sometimes deteriorate without psychiatric intervention. These patients do not usually require involuntary hospitalization, but a decision to commit them involuntarily is occasionally necessary. Rational judgment and consultation with a patient's family is often the best approach in making this decision. Bagby and colleagues (1991) showed that involuntary commitments are generally based on legally mandated factors (e.g., psychosis or dangerousness), but there was some reliance on other factors (e.g., treatability and availability of alternative resources). However, discharge planning, including long-term disposition, should be pursued early in the hospital course.

Although psychiatric patients who are considered dangerous can be legally detained against their will, they cannot be medicated without their consent unless a court order is obtained. The exception is when the patient is considered an immediate risk to self or others as demonstrated by verbal or behavioral signs. In this situation, a patient can be given medication to control the immediate life-threatening situation, but not after the crisis has passed. Most patients who initially refuse psychiatric medication later voluntarily take medication. Also, patients who are taken to court to determine competency are almost always declared incompetent to make their medication decisions. It has therefore been suggested that the judicial process might be changed—for example, to an in-house clinical review preceding judicial review to make the process more efficient and fair (Hoge et al. 1990; Zito et al. 1991).

PSYCHIATRIC EMERGENCIES USUALLY REQUIRING MINIMAL PHARMACOLOGICAL INTERVENTION

Some psychiatric emergency situations should emphasize diagnosis because identifying a physical cause for the behavioral change is crucial. These situations include first occurrence of panic attack, dissociative episode, catatonia, conversion symptoms, and mania. Other emergencies require primarily psychotherapeutic intervention: such situations may involve patients with adjustment disorders or acute grief reactions, victims of rape and assault, and unstable patients with personality disorders. Use of a benzodiazepine on a short-term basis should be considered together with psychotherapy in these patients. Low to moderate doses of lorazepam or diazepam are recommended (Table 27–2). For more long-term management of personality disorders in unstable patients, the use of mood stabilizers can lead to fewer emotional fluctuations.

Adjustment Disorders

The essential feature of adjustment disorder is a maladaptive reaction to an identifiable psychosocial stressor or stressors that occurred within 3 months of the onset of the stressor and that has persisted for no longer than 6 months. Symptoms associated with adjustment disorder include anxiety, depression, disturbance of conduct, and mixed symptoms (American Psychiatric Association 1994). However, the usual presentation is an adjustment disorder with mixed emotional features. Crisis intervention psychotherapy has proven to be the best treatment for an adjustment disorder. Most crises are self-limited and resolve naturally, but they can definitely be helped by skilled psychotherapeutic intervention. The essential elements of this intervention include establishing rapport with the patient, demonstrating empathy, listening, obtaining a thorough history, and constructing

Table 27–2. Recommended psychopharmacological drug use in psychiatric emergencies

For healthy adult psychiatric patients

For agitation or substance withdrawal

Lorazepam 1–2 mg po, im, or iv every 1–2 hours as needed or

Diazepam 5–10 mg po, im, or iv every 1–2 hours as needed

For psychotic symptoms

Haloperidol 10–20 mg/day po or im as needed (higher dosages usually are not needed)

For medically ill, delirious, or elderly psychiatric patients

For agitation or substance withdrawal

Lorazepam 0.25–1.0 mg po, im, or iv every 1–2 hours as needed

For psychotic symptoms

Haloperidol 1–5 mg/day as needed (higher dosages usually are not needed)

Note. po = orally; im = intramuscularly; iv = intravenously.

a plan to deal with the reality of the situation. The therapist helps the patient reestablish his or her defenses, draws on the patient's own resources as well as social support resources, and attempts to increase the patient's confidence and self-esteem (Hyman 1988).

Borderline Personality Disorder

Patients undergoing acute adjustment disorders who also have a borderline personality disorder usually have much difficulty with recovery. Sometimes they experience intermittent psychotic symptoms, suicidal urges, and loss of emotional control. These patients often need a brief psychiatric admission to prevent further deterioration. Borderline personalities often deteriorate along three lines: affective instability, transient psychotic phenomenon, and impulsive-aggressive behavior. Affective instability

has responded to mood stabilizers such as carbamazepine and valproate or antidepressants. The role of monoamine oxidase inhibitors (MAOIs) or tricyclic antidepressants (TCAs) is not completely understood. Liebowitz and Klein (1981) suggested that core borderline features might respond to MAOIs. Within the context of atypical depression, such patients respond better to phenelzine than to imipramine (McGrath et al. 1993; Parsons et al. 1989). Transient psychotic symptoms often respond to low-dose neuroleptic medication, and impulsive-aggressive behavior has responded to serotonergic agents (Coccaro and Kavoussi 1991).

Conditions Requiring Organic Workup

Panic Attack

When for the first time a patient develops signs and symptoms consistent with the diagnosis of panic disorder, he or she should be evaluated medically (by an internist if necessary) to rule out physical causes. The symptoms of a panic attack (including shortness of breath, tachycardia, sweating, and chest pain) are consistent with many medical illnesses, including hypoglycemia, hyperthyroidism, and myocardial infarction or angina. Not until medical conditions have been excluded should a psychiatrist make a diagnosis of panic disorder. Following an initial panic attack, a patient may need a short course of a benzodiazepine to treat the accompanying anxiety and fear before obtaining a medical evaluation.

Dissociative Episodes

Dissociative amnesia is a relatively rare condition compared with physical causes for the amnestic syndrome. Amnesia is a frequent accompaniment of medical-surgical abnormalities such as head injury, brain tumor, cardiovascular incidents, and substance use. Not until organic amnestic disorder has been ruled out should the psychiatrist assume a psychogenic basis for memory loss. Any other dissociative episodes occurring for the first time, such as dissociative fugue or depersonalization experiences, need an organic evaluation to rule out physical causes.

Catatonia

Although major depression and schizophrenia (catatonic type) are the most common psychiatric disorders that are associated with catatonia, some medical and neurological conditions also cause this syndrome. Medical causes include hypercalcemia and hepatic encephalopathy. Catatonia may also appear as an adverse drug side effect from neuroleptic medication and phencyclidine (PCP). Neurological causes for catatonia include parkinsonism and encephalitis. Unless the patient has had a previous episode of catatonia with an established causative psychiatric diagnosis, he or she should be fully evaluated by medical and/or neurological consultants. After eliminating physical causes, the clinician may find that catatonia improves temporarily through intravenous administration of amobarbital or lorazepam as in conversion states (Perry and Jacobs 1982; Rosebush et al. 1990).

Mania

In patients older than 50, the initial onset of mania is relatively uncommon. Any patient with an initial onset of mania (but especially a patient who is older than 50) should be evaluated for organic causes. Various drugs, medical illness, and neurological disease can cause this syndrome.

Conversion Disorder

A patient with a rather sudden onset of unexplained neurological symptoms should have a full neurological workup before the diagnosis of "conversion hysteria" can be made. Traditionally, the amobarbital interview has been useful for assessment, initial management, and recovery of function in conversion disorders (Perry and Jacobs 1982). It has been reported that intravenous administration of lorazepam accompanied by repeated hypnotic suggestions resulted in full recovery in conversion disorder (Stevens 1990).

PSYCHIATRIC EMERGENCIES USUALLY REQUIRING PHARMACOLOGICAL INTERVENTION

Many psychiatric patients require pharmacological intervention as the primary treatment of their condition. These patients include most assaultive or aggressive patients, agitated psychotic patients, patients undergoing substance withdrawal, and substance-intoxicated patients with aggressivity.

Assaultive Behavior From Any Cause

On initial presentation, it is often impossible to accurately diagnose psychiatrically an assaultive or aggressive individual. Treatment usually precedes a definitive diagnosis. When a patient is assessed to be actively or potentially violent, then quick, decisive, and well-planned action is mandatory. The level of restriction that the psychiatrist chooses for each patient is based on good medical judgment, making use of the least restrictive environment (Table 27–1). However, when a patient is judged to be eminently violent, often a more restrictive environment is needed to minimize potential injury to the patient and others. Every emergency room and psychiatric unit in which potentially violent patients are treated should have a seclusion room with leather restraints available. In implementing the decision to restrain a violent patient, staff must act decisively with sufficient strength to fully control the situation. This usually requires at least five strong assistants. Often, when patients see a sufficient show of force, they will voluntarily allow themselves to be restrained.

Most patients who are physically restrained will also require psychopharmacological treatment. Intramuscular or intravenous medication can be used without a patient's consent to treat a life-threatening emergency. The three drugs most often used in this situation are lorazepam, diazepam, and haloperidol (Table 27–2). Any of these drugs can be given intravenously but are usually given intramuscularly. They are well absorbed if given in a deltoid muscle, but absorption of benzodiazepines may occasionally be erratic (Arana and Hyman 1991). For a healthy adult, the recommended dosage of lorazepam is 1–2 mg every hour as needed; of diazepam, 5–10 mg every hour as needed; and of haloperidol, 5–10 mg twice a day. Haloperidol is usually only required for patients who are clearly psychotic. However, haloperidol can worsen certain substance intoxications (e.g., PCP), and it frequently causes acute dystonia early in the course of treatment especially in younger adult patients. In these cases, chlorpromazine, 900 mg two or three times a day, might be substituted for haloperidol. An alternative is intramuscular chlorpromazine (30–150 mg/day), which is associated with fewer extrapyramidal side effects (EPS) than haloperidol but greater anticholinergic effects and orthostatic hypotension. Unless the patient is clearly delusional or hallucinating, lorazepam or diazepam is the recommended medication for emergency use.

Bipolar Disorder

Agitated psychosis can occur in bipolar disorder in two forms: major depression and mania. Electroconvulsive therapy (ECT) is quite effective in the treatment of major depression, especially with catatonia, as well as in severe mania. Moreover, these disorders are more commonly managed psychopharmacologically. Although these disorders have traditionally been treated with neuroleptic medication, more recently, alternative therapies have been suggested. Studies have shown that lithium and valproate are both effective in reducing manic symptoms. However, valproate has a broader spectrum of response and has approximately equal benefit for patients with pure mania as for those with mixed mania, rapid cycling, comorbid substance abuse, and secondary bipolar disorder (Bowden 1995;

Bowden et al. 1994; Freeman et al. 1992). Pope and colleagues (1991) concluded that valproate was an effective alternative for manic patients who did not tolerate or respond to lithium. Divalproex oral loading in the treatment of acute mania is often effective. It can be given at 20 mg/kg/day orally in divided doses for 5 days, resulting in therapeutic blood levels and rapid onset of antimanic response in some patients (Keck et al. 1993). Furthermore, it has been reported that oral loading with divalproex is as effective as haloperidol in treating acute psychotic mania (McElroy et al. 1996).

Schizophrenia

Treatment of schizophrenic exacerbation has changed markedly in the past 5 years. Rapid neuroleptization (tranquilization) with antipsychotics such as haloperidol in 5-mg doses administered every hour as needed has been replaced by 10–20 mg/day of haloperidol in combination with a benzodiazepine (usually lorazepam) as needed. Several studies have clearly shown that 10–20 mg/day of haloperidol, or the equivalent dose of another antipsychotic, is sufficient as an antipsychotic dose (McEvoy et al. 1991; Rifkin et al. 1991; Van Putten et al. 1990; Volavka et al. 1992). Likewise, benzodiazepine augmentation of neuroleptic medication has been shown to control agitation during exacerbations of schizophrenia (Barbee et al. 1992; Bodkin 1990; Salzman et al. 1991).

Delirium

Delirium is defined as a mental disorder with a physical cause that develops over a short period of time and fluctuates over the course of a day. Patients have disturbances of consciousness, poor attention, and a change in cognition or development of perceptual disturbances (American Psychiatric Association 1994). Delirium must always be considered as a cause of agitated psychotic behavior, especially in medically ill and elderly patients.

In addition to treating underlying organic causes of delirium and protecting the patient and others from harm while he or she is in a delirious state, medications can help to calm the patient's agitation. Low doses of haloperidol or lorazepam are usually employed. If the delirium is thought to be due to a substance withdrawal state, lorazepam is the drug of choice. It is important to remember that delirium can be accurately diagnosed by electroencephalogram (EEG). An abnormal EEG finding is virtually always present in delirium (Boutros 1992; Engel and Romano 1959).

Dementia

A patient with dementia can become agitatedly psychotic for various reasons, including delirium, catastrophic reaction, or a reaction to delusions and/or hallucinations. The best treatment for a patient with dementia is nonpharmacological—that is, behavior modification and supportive approaches. However, pharmacotherapy may be indicated, but very low doses of neuroleptics and/or benzodiazepines are recommended because of the high incidence of side effects including delirium, pseudoparkinsonism, and increased falls. Aggressive behavior in elderly patients with brain damage and dementia can respond to other medications, including serotonin reuptake inhibitors, propranolol, and carbamazepine (Deutsch et al. 1991; Maletta 1990). In addition, buspirone in daily doses of 15–45 mg has been reported to be effective in reducing aggressive behavior in brain-damaged patients (Ratey et al. 1991).

Substance Withdrawal

Withdrawal signs and symptoms from alcohol, sedatives and hypnotics, and benzodiazepines are similar. The major signs include tremulousness and autonomic instability (American Psychiatric Association 1994). Also, insomnia and weakness that are not commonly caused by anxiety often present as symptoms of alcohol or sedative withdrawal. The treatment of withdrawal and prevention of Wernicke-Korsakoff syndrome are important considerations. Alcohol

withdrawal is probably best treated with benzodiazepines, although barbiturates might have advantages such as preferential renal excretion. Diazepam, because of its relatively long duration of action, has the advantage of providing a smoother tapering-off period. However, lorazepam is recommended for patients with significant liver disease because its metabolism is less impaired in these patients.

Alcohol withdrawal delirium is a life-threatening illness that usually should be treated in an intensive care unit. It is characterized by delirium developing within a week of the cessation of or reduction of alcohol consumption, usually accompanied by excessive autonomic activity, fever, perceptual disturbances, and agitation. The presence of a concomitant physical illness predisposes to the syndrome (American Psychiatric Association 1994). Administration of intramuscular thiamine before administration of an intravenous or oral carbohydrate load is necessary in an alcohol-dependent patient to prevent the development of Wernicke-Korsakoff syndrome (Hyman 1988). Although use of benzodiazepines to treat agitation is recommended, neuroleptic medication should not be used because of the frequency of adverse events.

Substance Intoxication With Violent Behavior

The major substances that lead to violent behavior are cocaine and PCP and, to a lesser extent, amphetamines, hallucinogens, and cannabis. The treatment of psychosis in substance intoxication is similar to the treatment of agitated psychosis (Tables 27–1 and 27–2).

Psychoactive Drug Side Effects

Adverse drug effects necessitating prompt remedial action can occur at any time during pharmacotherapy with psychoactive drugs. One basis for selection of initial therapy is to avoid those drugs producing a high incidence of certain side effects. Informing patients and family of expected side effects can be comforting. Nevertheless, the clinician can expect patients who experience unanticipated and untoward drug reactions to be frightened and to often require immediate intervention.

Antipsychotic Agents

Extrapyramidal side effects. Because all currently available antipsychotic drugs (with the relative exception of clozapine) block the dopamine, subtype 2 (D_2), receptor in the nigrostriatal tract, EPS may emerge during therapy (Goetz and Klawans 1981). Symptoms include acute dystonic reactions, akathisias, and parkinsonism (i.e., akinesia, tremor, rigidity). Antipsychotic drug-induced laryngeal and/or pharyngeal dystonia can precipitate cardiac arrhythmias, presumably through vagal reflexes. In addition, akathisia can be distressing and may result in maladaptive reactions, even contributing to suicidal behavior. These reactions require that antipsychotic dosage be kept as low as possible, but EPS are not consistently dose-related. When EPS appear, anticholinergic agents (e.g., benztropine, 0.5–4.0 mg/day; trihexyphenidyl, 2–10 mg/day; or diphenhydramine, 25–100 mg/day) may be used in treatment. Acute dystonias respond most rapidly to intravenous administration. Caution should be exercised to follow up adequately, because the duration of therapeutic effects following parenteral administration may be brief, and acute EPS can reoccur. There is no consistent evidence that one antiparkinsonian drug is consistently superior to another for treatment of EPS.

Neuroleptic malignant syndrome. An increasingly recognized adverse effect of antipsychotic drugs is the neuroleptic malignant syndrome (NMS). This is an acute and potentially lethal reaction manifested by fever, muscular rigidity, central nervous system abnormalities, and autonomic dysfunction (Caroff 1980).

It may occur at any time during antipsychotic drug treatment, even after the drug has been recently discontinued. The treatment consists of discontinuing the suspected drug and providing supportive treatment and pharmacotherapy with such dopaminergic agents as bromocriptine.

Cardiovascular side effects. Antipsychotics produce a variety of cardiovascular effects. In addition to orthostasis, hypotension, and tachycardia, electrocardiogram (ECG) changes are common. The risk of hypotension is increased in elderly patients, with parenteral administration, or with large changes in dosage. General recommendations to prevent hypotensive episodes would include making gradual dose increments, instructing patients to stand slowly when they rise from a reclining position, or recommending that elderly patients wear elastic stockings. Many of these patients are voluntarily salt deprived, and salt supplementation of their diet is often very useful. If systolic pressure falls below 90 mm Hg, the dosage should be held or reduced. It may be necessary to position the patient with legs elevated. In cases in which shock develops, drug treatment may be necessary. The unopposed β-agonist activity of epinephrine can lead to further decreases in blood pressure, and this drug is therefore not recommended. Preferred pressor treatment would be norepinephrine, phenylephrine, or metaraminol.

ECG changes can include prolongation of Q-T interval; S-T segment depression; blunted, notched, or inverted T waves; or appearance of U waves. The occurrence of serious arrhythmias is rare but can be life threatening. Factors that predispose to ECG changes include hypokalemia, recent food intake, heavy exercise, and alcohol abuse (Nasrallah 1978). Taking a baseline and follow-up ECGs on patients with increased risk factors is recommended. Avoiding the use of strongly anticholinergic phenothiazines, especially in elderly patients, may minimize the risk of causing cardiac effects of antipsychotics (Risch et al. 1982).

Anticholinergic side effects. Anticholinergic side effects may be prominent with the antipsychotics and can include dry mouth, blurred vision, urinary retention, and constipation. Many of these side effects can be distressing to patients. The avoidance of drugs with high degrees of muscarinic receptor-binding properties is a useful guide in drug selection. A patient with urinary retention may present with overdistension of the bladder, discomfort, or pain. Reducing drug dosage is usually helpful, or a trial of bethanechol (10–50 mg three or four times per day) can be considered. Constipation can be accompanied by pain, abdominal rigidity, and vomiting. Mild cases can be treated with diet, increased fluid intake, and exercise. Laxatives should be used in the lowest effective dose. Constipation may be a symptom of paralytic ileus, which (if left untreated) may be fatal. Treatment consists of lowering the drug dose when possible, correcting fluid and electrolyte balance, and (if necessary) restoring bowel continuity and function by intubation of the gut and relief of abdominal distension and pressure.

The anticholinergic effects of the antipsychotics and antidepressants may aggravate glaucoma, especially the narrow-angle type. Blurred vision from these drugs results from relaxation of the ciliary muscle and loss of accommodation for near vision. Complaints of eye pain, especially in patients older than 40, should prompt an ophthalmic examination. It may be necessary to decrease the dose of the offending drug or to change to another agent with lower anticholinergic properties. The short-term use of 1% pilocarpine eyedrops may be beneficial for treatment of mydriasis and cycloplegia (Malone et al. 1992).

Clozapine-specific effects. Patients taking clozapine may experience profound hypotension with or without syncope shortly following initiation of therapy, as early as the first or second dose. Although the documented incidence is less than 0.03%, respiratory and/or cardiac arrest has occurred. The most serious reaction to clozapine is agranulocytosis, which can be fatal. Most cases of bone marrow suppression occur between 6 weeks and 6 months after therapy begins, but weekly monitoring of the blood count is justified for the duration of treatment. Prodromal signs of bone marrow suppression include sore throat, low-grade fever, or flulike symptoms. If the white blood cell (WBC) count is below 3,500, then it should be rechecked biweekly. If the WBC count falls below 3,000 or the granulocyte count below 1,500, then the drug should be discontinued. Preventive measures against infection may be necessary, including isolation and antibiotic therapy. Most patients will need hospitalization for close monitoring while bone marrow function returns to normal.

Cyclic Antidepressants

Anticholinergic toxicity (i.e., a delirium or psychosis) can occur from use of any anticholinergic drug, including many of the cyclic antidepressants, antipsychotics, and the antiparkinsonian drugs used to treat EPS. The syndrome results from competitive inhibition of acetylcholine at central and peripheral cholinergic muscarinic receptors. Elderly patients are believed to be especially vulnerable, as well as patients in whom combinations or high doses of anticholinergic agents are used.

Hypertensive crisis. The most serious adverse effect of MAOIs is the precipitation of a hypertensive crisis, usually following ingestion of dietary products containing large amounts of tyramine or other substances coadministered with sympathomimetic properties. Management includes discontinuing the MAOI and treating the hypertension. The recommended treatment is intravenous administration of an α-adrenergic blocker. Phentolamine (up to 5 mg intravenously) has been used. An alternative would be chlorpromazine (25–50 mg intramuscularly or orally), which has the advantage of being routinely available in emergency rooms and psychiatric units. Oral nifedipine has been recommended for patients to carry with them to treat a hypertensive crisis, but it is important to be aware of the potential risk of hypotension following ingestion of nifedipine if the patient is not actually hypertensive (Hesselink 1991). An early indication of the need for oral nifedipine is the sudden onset of a severe bilateral pounding occipital headache.

Priapism.   Priapism may appear in male patients receiving trazodone (often after 1 or 2 weeks of therapy) and, to a much lesser extent, with antipsychotic drugs (Scher et al. 1983). This situation constitutes an emergency, because if left untreated, permanent erectile dysfunction may result. Immediate urological consultation should be sought, as surgical intervention may be necessary. Complaints of unusual erectile activity should be viewed with suspicion as a prodromal symptom of priapism and the drug immediately discontinued.

REFERENCES

American Psychiatric Association: Diagnostic and Statistical Manual of Mental Disorders, 4th Edition. Washington, DC, American Psychiatric Association, 1994

Apter A, Kotler M, Sevy S, et al: Correlates of risk of suicide in violent and nonviolent psychiatric patients. Am J Psychiatry 148:833–877, 1991

Arana GW, Hyman SE: Handbook of Psychiatric Drug Therapy, 2nd Edition. Boston, MA, Little, Brown, 1991

Bagby RM, Thompson JS, Dickens SE, et al: Decision making in psychiatric civil commitment: an experimental analysis. Am J Psychiatry 148: 28–33, 1991

Barbee JG, Mancuso DM, Freed CR, et al: Alprazolam as a neuroleptic adjunct in the emergency treatment of schizophrenia. Am J Psychiatry 149:506–510, 1992

Beck JC, White KA, Gage B: Emergency psychiatric assessment of violence. Am J Psychiatry 148: 1562–1565, 1991

Bodkin JA: Emerging uses for high-potency benzodiazepines in psychotic disorders. J Clin Psychiatry 51 (suppl):41–46, 1990

Boutros NN: A review of indications for routine EEG in clinical psychiatry. Hospital and Community Psychiatry 43:716–719, 1992

Bowden CL: Predictors of response to divalproex and lithium. J Clin Psychiatry 56 (suppl 3): 25–30, 1995

Bowden CL, Brugger AM, Swann AC, et al: Efficacy of divalproex vs. Lithium and placebo in the treatment of mania. JAMA 271:918–924, 1994

Caroff SN: The neuroleptic malignant syndrome. J Clin Psychiatry 41:79–82, 1980

Coccaro EF, Kavoussi RJ: Biological and pharmacological aspects of borderline personality disorder. Hospital and Community Psychiatry 42: 1029–1033, 1991

Coté TR, Biggar RJ, Dannenberg AL: Risk of suicide among persons with AIDS: a national assessment. JAMA 268:2066–2068, 1992

Deutsch LH, Bylsma FW, Rovner BW, et al: Psychosis and physical aggression in probable Alzheimer's disease. Am J Psychiatry 148:1159–1163, 1991

Engel GL, Romano J: Delirium: a syndrome of cerebral insufficiency. Journal of Chronic Disease 9:260–277, 1959

Freeman TW, Clothier JL, Pazzaglia P, et al: A double-blind comparison of valproate and lithium in the treatment of acute mania. Am J Psychiatry 149:108–111, 1992

Friedman S, Jones JC, Chernen L, et al: Suicidal ideation and suicide attempts among patients with panic disorder: a survey of two outpatient clinics. Am J Psychiatry 149:680–685, 1992

Goetz CG, Klawans HL: Drug-induced extrapyramidal disorders—a neuropsychiatric interface. J Clin Psychopharmacol 1:297–303, 1981

Goldstein RB, Black DW, Nasrallah A, et al: The prediction of suicide. Arch Gen Psychiatry 48: 418–422, 1991

Hesselink JMK: Safer use of MAOIs with nifedipine to counteract potential hypertensive crisis (letter). Am J Psychiatry 148:1616, 1991

Hoge SK, Appelbaum PS, Lawlor T, et al: A prospective, multicenter study of patients' refusal of antipsychotic medication. Arch Gen Psychiatry 47:949–956, 1990

Hyman SE: Manual of Psychiatric Emergencies, 2nd Edition. Boston, MA, Little, Brown, 1988

Keck PE, McElroy SL, Tugrul KC, et al: Valproate oral loading in the treatment of acute mania. J Clin Psychiatry 54:305– 308, 1993

Liebowitz MR, Klein DF: Interrelationship of hysteroid dysphoria and borderline personality disorder. Psychiatr Clin North Am 4:67–87, 1981.

Maletta GJ: Pharmacologic treatment and management of the aggressive demented patient. Psychiatric Annals 20:446–455, 1990

Malone DA Jr, Camara EG, Krug JH Jr: Ophthalmologic effects of psychotropic medications. Psychosomatics 33:271–277, 1992

Marttunen MJ, Aro HM, Henriksson MM, et al: Mental disorders in adolescent suicide. Arch Gen Psychiatry 48:834–839, 1991

McElroy SL, Keck PE, Stanton SP, et al: A randomized comparison of divalproex oral loading versus haloperidol in the initial treatment of acute psychotic mania. J Clin Psychiatry 57:142–146, 1996

McEvoy JP, Hogarty GE, Steingard S: Optimal dose of neuroleptic in acute schizophrenia: a controlled study of the neuroleptic threshold and higher haloperidol dose. Arch Gen Psychiatry 48:739–745, 1991

McGrath PJ, Stewart JW, Nunes EV, et al: A double-blind crossover trial of imipramine and phenelzine for outpatients with treatment-refractory depression. Am J Psychiatry 150:118–123, 1993

Murphy GE, Wetzel RD, Robins E, et al: Multiple risk factors predict suicide in alcoholism. Arch Gen Psychiatry 49:459–463, 1992

Nasrallah HA: Factors influencing phenothiazine-induced ECG changes. Am J Psychiatry 135:118–199, 1978

Parsons B, Quitkin FM, McGrath PJ, et al: Phenelzine, imipramine, and placebo in borderline patients meeting criteria for atypical depression. Psychopharmacol Bull 25:524–534, 1989

Perry JC, Jacobs D: Overview: clinical applications of the amytal interview in psychiatric emergency settings. Am J Psychiatry 139:552–559, 1982

Pope HG, McElroy SL, Keck PE, et al: Valproate in the treatment of acute mania: a placebo-controlled study. Arch Gen Psychiatry 48:62–68, 1991

Ratey J, Sovner R, Parks A, et al: Buspirone treatment of aggression and anxiety in mentally retarded patients: a multiple-baseline, placebo lead-in study. J Clin Psychiatry 52:159–162, 1991

Rifkin A, Doddi S, Karajgi B, et al: Dosage of haloperidol for schizophrenia. Arch Gen Psychiatry 48:166–170, 1991

Risch SC, Groom GP, Janowsky DS: The effects of psychotropic drugs on the cardiovascular system. J Clin Psychiatry 43 (5, sect 2):16–26, 1982

Rosebush PI, Hildebrand AM, Fulong BG, et al: Catatonic syndrome in a general psychiatric inpatient population: frequency, clinical presentation, and response to lorazepam. J Clin Psychiatry 51:357–362, 1990

Salzman C, Solomon D, Miyawaki E, et al: Parenteral lorazepam versus parenteral haloperidol for the control of psychotic disruptive behavior. J Clin Psychiatry 52:177–180, 1991

Scher M, Drieger JN, Juergens S: Trazodone and priapism. Am J Psychiatry 140:1362–1363, 1983

Spar JE, LaRue A: Geriatric Psychiatry. Washington, DC, American Psychiatric Press, 1990

Stanford EJ, Goetz RR, Bloom JD: The no harm contract in the emergency room assessment of suicidal risk. J Clin Psychiatry 55:344–348, 1994

Stevens CB: Lorazepam in the treatment of acute conversion disorder. Hospital and Community Psychiatry 41:1255–1257, 1990

Van Putten T, Marder SR, Mintz J: A controlled dose comparison of haloperidol in newly admitted schizophrenic patients. Arch Gen Psychiatry 47:754–758, 1990

Volavka J, Cooper T, Czobor P, et al: Haloperidol blood levels and clinical effects. Arch Gen Psychiatry 49:354–361, 1992

Zito JM, Craig TJ, Wanderling J: New York under the Rivers decision: an epidemiologic study of drug treatment refusal. Am J Psychiatry 48:904–909, 1991

TWENTY-EIGHT

Psychopharmacology in the Medically Ill Patient

Alan Stoudemire, M.D., and
Michael G. Moran, M.D.

Prescribing psychotropic medications in medically ill patients requires careful risk-benefit assessment. In this chapter, the special psychopharmacological considerations that are required in making such risk-benefit assessments for the medical-psychiatric population are reviewed, including 1) potential interactions between psychotropic medications and drugs used for primary medical disorders; 2) effects of impaired renal, hepatic, or gastrointestinal functioning on psychotropic drug metabolism; and 3) side effects of psychotropic drugs that may complicate preexisting medical conditions.

A WORD ON NOMENCLATURE

The most consistent definition of *heterocyclic* compounds is that they are "cyclic compounds in which the rings include at least one atom of an element different from the rest"—in contrast to *homocyclic* compounds, in which all the ring atoms are the same (Parker 1993, p. 472). Richelson (1993, p. 232) stated that heterocyclic "describes any ring compound that contains within one or more rings an atom different from carbon," which is consistent with other definitions of the term (Grant and Grant 1987). The breakdown of heterocyclic and homocyclic antidepressants according to these definitions is shown in Table 28–1 (Jefferson 1995). Following the recommendation of Jefferson, we use the general term *cyclic antidepressants* (CyADs) to refer to non–monoamine oxidase inhibitor (MAOI) antidepressants; specific antidepressant classes, such as tricyclic antidepressants (TCAs) or selective serotonin reuptake inhibitors (SSRIs), are designated more specifically.

CYCLIC ANTIDEPRESSANTS IN PATIENTS WITH CARDIAC DISEASE

At therapeutic doses, the cardiovascular risks involved in prescribing CyADs are relatively small in the vast majority of patients. TCAs (e.g., imipramine, amitriptyline) have quinidine-like properties that can increase the P-R interval, QRS duration, and Q-T interval and "flatten" the T wave on the electrocardiogram (ECG). These effects are almost never of major clinical

Table 28–1. **Breakdown of heterocyclic and homocyclic antidepressants**

Heterocyclic	Homocyclic
Amoxapine	Amitriptyline
Desipramine	Bupropion
Doxepin	Fluoxetine
Imipramine	Maprotiline
Paroxetine	Nortriptyline
Trazodone	Sertraline
	Venlafaxine

Source. Adapted from Jefferson 1995.

significance unless patients have preexisting or latent cardiac conduction defects, congestive heart failure, or experienced a recent myocardial infarction (Jefferson 1975).

TCAs may cause ECG changes at therapeutic serum levels in patients with preexisting conduction delays such as atrioventricular (AV) block. Patients with preexisting intraventricular conduction delays (defined as a QRS interval greater than 0.11 seconds), sick sinus syndrome, second-degree heart block, bifascicular heart block, and prolonged Q-T$_c$ intervals are at higher risk for arrhythmias (Roose et al. 1987). Patients with relatively benign types of heart block, such as uncomplicated left bundle branch block, isolated left anterior or left posterior fascicular block, or right bundle branch block, are at a relatively lower risk for aggravation of heart block by TCAs (Stoudemire and Atkinson 1988).

A prolonged Q-T interval presents a relative contraindication to TCA treatment because of the hazard of malignant ventricular arrhythmias (torsades de pointes; an approximate guideline for the relatively safe use of TCAs is a Q-T interval of no more than 0.440 seconds). Prolonged Q-T intervals may also occur on a congenital basis and present problems in using TCAs. Such patients may not be symptomatic and may only be detected with a routine ECG. In patients without cardiac disease, dangerous prolongations of the Q-T interval (i.e., beyond

0.440 seconds) occur most often in situations involving TCA overdose (Fricchione and Vlay 1986; Schwartz and Wolf 1978). The Q-T interval may also be prolonged iatrogenically from use of antiarrhythmic agents, often in combination, that prolong the Q-T interval over the 0.440-second limit. Note that trazodone, fluoxetine, sertraline, paroxetine, nefazodone, venlafaxine, and bupropion have few, if any, quinidine-like side effects compared with TCAs (Fisch 1985; Preskorn and Othmer 1984; Sommi et al. 1987). These drugs are much safer than tricyclic agents in patients with cardiac conduction disease.

Although haloperidol is not an antidepressant, a series of reports have identified intravenous haloperidol as a rare potential cause of torsades de pointes (Hunt and Stern 1995). Oral haloperidol has not been reported to have clinically significant effects on the ECG, but the use of relatively high intravenous doses for severe agitation in intensive care settings can precipitate this arrhythmia. Most patients in intensive care settings can, from the cardiovascular standpoint, be treated with intravenous haloperidol, although more attention should likely be given to monitoring the duration of the Q-T interval during aggressive haloperidol therapy.

Fluoxetine, sertraline, paroxetine, fluvoxamine, venlafaxine, and bupropion have a low affinity for α-adrenergic receptors. Thus, they have minimal effects on pulse and blood pressure and therefore may offer significant advantages in elderly medically ill patients.

Venlafaxine has been reported to raise diastolic blood pressure in about 5%–13% of patients when used in doses greater than 200–225 mg/day, but in patients with preexisting propensity for hypertension, pressor effects may occur at lower doses (Feighner 1995). Bupropion may also elevate blood pressure. Both of these drugs may be used safely in patients with preexisting hypertension, but monitoring of blood pressure should be more frequent (weekly) until stable maintenance doses are reached.

MAOIs, which do not have quinidine-like

effects, may also be considered for patients with heart block, as can electroconvulsive therapy (ECT). The use of antidepressants in patients with cardiac conduction disease is reviewed in more detail elsewhere (Roose et al. 1987; Stoudemire and Atkinson 1988; Stoudemire and Fogel 1987; Stoudemire et al. 1993).

Myocardial Infarction

Whether a recent myocardial infarction (MI) in itself is a risk factor for cardiotoxicity from CyADs is not known definitively. Secondary complications of MI, such as heart failure, arrhythmias, orthostatic hypotension, and cardiac conduction abnormalities—and the potential influence of CyADs on cardiac rhythm, conduction, and blood pressure and the potential interactions with other drugs—are all important in assessing the relative safety of CyADs in the post-MI period (Stoudemire and Fogel 1987). No information is available from prospective studies to show increased morbidity or mortality associated with the use of TCAs by post-MI patients. Reports from studies of post-MI antiarrhythmic prophylaxis protocols, however, suggest a possible increased risk of morbidity and mortality after MI when drugs with properties similar to those of the tricyclics on cardiac conduction are used. In the Cardiac Arrhythmia Suppression Trials (CAST), which were designed to assess the prophylactic benefit of antiarrhythmics post-MI, two of the type IC antiarrhythmics being studied—flecainide and encainide—were discontinued less than 2 years into the study (A. H. Glassman et al. 1993). These two drugs appeared to increase rather than decrease mortality rates compared with placebo-treated patients (A. H. Glassman et al. 1993).

Flecainide and encainide were the first two antiarrhythmics examined. Moricizine eventually also was associated with increased mortality and was discontinued (Epstein et al. 1993). A meta-analysis of patients with ventricular arrhythmias treated with the type IA antiarrhythmic quinidine (Morganroth and Goin

1991; Teo et al. 1993) found an increased risk of mortality. Until more definitive data are available, a conservative approach would be to avoid tricyclics in the post-MI period, if possible, and to treat depression in such patients with SSRIs, venlafaxine, or bupropion.

Cardiac arrhythmias have been observed to emerge after TCAs are discontinued, particularly if the withdrawal is rapid (Regan et al. 1989; Van Sweden 1988). The decision to continue or discontinue TCAs after a cardiac event must be made on an individual basis and depends on multiple medical factors, such as the presence of heart block, orthostatic hypotension, and concurrent arrhythmias. Moreover, the complications caused by abrupt tricyclic withdrawal, or exacerbation or relapse of depression in the post-MI period, also should be considered. Hence, the use of antidepressants in the peri- and post-MI period must always be based on risk-benefit ratio assessment done in consultation with the patient's cardiologist.

The risk of depressive relapse in withdrawing a tricyclic after a cardiac event would have to be weighed against the extrapolated risk of their continued use based on their type IA quinidine-like (sodium channel blocking) effects. Most clinicians would likely opt to convert patients to an SSRI or bupropion post-MI or if significant cardiac conduction effects emerge.

Orthostatic Hypotension and Congestive Heart Failure

Orthostatic hypotension creates the most problems in medically ill patients treated with traditional tricyclics such as imipramine. Patients with preexisting hypotensive symptoms, impaired left ventricular functioning, or bundle branch block are at increased risk for orthostatic hypotension with tricyclic treatment (Rizos et al. 1988). Although in middle-aged and relatively healthy patients, the use of salt supplements and support hose can partially relieve orthostatic hypotension, these measures are of less benefit in elderly medical patients and, in the case of salt loading, may be contraindicated in patients with congestive heart failure or hypertension.

Imipramine has little or no effect on cardiac output in most patients, although it may produce orthostatic hypotension, a serious side effect that often prevents its use (A. H. Glassman et al. 1983). In patients with normal cardiac output and even in patients with stable or well-compensated congestive heart failure, nortriptyline usually has little or no effect on cardiac output and appears to have significantly fewer orthostatic hypotensive effects than does imipramine (Roose et al. 1981, 1986). At very low levels of cardiac output (20%–25% or less) or in decompensated heart failure, however, tricyclics may exacerbate congestive heart failure.

Bupropion appears to have minimal effects on the cardiovascular system, does not cause orthostatic hypotension, and, as noted earlier in this chapter, may actually cause an elevation in blood pressure, particularly in patients with preexisting hypertension. SSRIs appear to have little or no effect on blood pressure (Cooper 1988). Nefazodone has minimal effects on α-adrenergic receptors but can cause some degree of mild orthostatic hypotension (Taylor et al. 1995). Of the tricyclic agents, nortriptyline has been studied the most extensively in relation to blood pressure changes and has relatively less tendency to cause orthostatic hypotension than do tertiary tricyclic compounds such as imipramine and amitriptyline. In patients who have preexisting symptomatic orthostatic hypotension or who develop this condition, drugs such as fluoxetine, sertraline, paroxetine, venlafaxine, or bupropion should be used.

CYCLIC ANTIDEPRESSANTS IN PATIENTS WITH OTHER MEDICAL CONDITIONS

Glaucoma

Narrow-angle glaucoma can be exacerbated by antidepressants with high anticholinergic side effects, but patients with open-angle glaucoma generally can take TCAs with minimal risk. Patients with narrow-angle glaucoma may safely take TCAs if their glaucoma is being treated and monitored (E. Lieberman and Stoudemire 1987). In general, agents with low or no anticholinergic side effects would be preferred in treating this patient population.

Urogenital Tract Problems

Patients with known and untreated prostatic hypertrophy are at particular risk for urinary retention from traditional anticholinergic tricyclics. More typically, urinary retention that develops after use of a tricyclic often leads to the identification of latent prostatic disease. As with glaucoma, use of drugs with low or no anticholinergic effects would be the preferred choice in patients prone to urinary retention. Trazodone, which has low anticholinergic properties, can cause priapism, although the risk of this complication is low (about 1 in 7,000 men treated) (Falk 1987). Nefazodone, which has some similarities to trazodone, has not yet been reported to cause priapism.

Seizure Disorders

Human and animal reports vary in their conclusions as to the effects of CyADs on the seizure threshold (Edwards et al. 1986). Although antidepressants, particularly tricyclics, can cause seizures in overdose, their propensity to cause seizures in the general population and in patients with overt or latent epilepsy indicates some likelihood of lowering the seizure threshold. On the other hand, some antidepressants, such as doxepin, actually have been reported to have anticonvulsant effects on the electroencephalogram (EEG) when these drugs were given by injection to nonclinical volunteers (Simeon et al. 1969).

Some evidence suggests a higher rate of seizures for clomipramine than for the standard tricyclic imipramine (Burley 1977; Trimble

1978). It is relatively clear that maprotiline and bupropion should be avoided in patients prone to seizures. The data for bupropion indicate that—aside from certain groups at high risk for seizures—its effects on seizure threshold may not be significantly greater than those for other antidepressants. Nevertheless, bupropion should be avoided in patients with epilepsy and in other high-risk patients, such as those with a history of head trauma or patients with abnormal foci on the EEG, indicating potential enhanced central nervous system (CNS) irritability (Davidson 1989). The slow-release form of bupropion has been reported to have no increased risk for seizures. Among the traditional tricyclic agents, amitriptyline appears most likely to aggravate seizures (Edwards et al. 1986).

When CyADs are given to treated epileptic patients, anticonvulsant levels should be periodically checked and dosages adjusted to maintain the level in the therapeutic range because of possible drug interactions between CyADs and anticonvulsants (Table 28–2). For example, carbamazepine will *lower* tricyclic levels, and sodium valproate may *elevate* tricyclic levels.

Pharmacokinetic Considerations

When treating frail, medically ill elderly patients, starting dosages of TCAs should be low (e.g., 10 mg/day of nortriptyline). Dosage should be raised gradually, depending on a patient's toleration of side effects and response to treatment. Cases have been reported of toxic serum tricyclic levels in elderly patients taking as little as 25 mg/day (J. N. Glassman et al. 1985).

Plasma levels of the tertiary tricyclics amitriptyline and imipramine tend to be positively correlated with age (i.e., increased age equals increased serum level for a given dose; Nies et al. 1977). Metabolism of demethylated tricyclics such as nortriptyline and desipramine appears to be less affected by age than is metabolism of imipramine and amitriptyline (Abernethy et al. 1985; Antal et al. 1982; Cutler and

Narang 1984; Cutler et al. 1981; Neshkes et al. 1985; Nies et al. 1977).

Elderly and medically ill patients do not necessarily always need lower doses of TCAs, and elderly patients may show either great sensitivity or great tolerance to these drugs (J. N. Glassman et al. 1985; Rockwell et al. 1988; Stoudemire and Fogel 1987). Primary liver disease and hepatic dysfunction from diseases as well as congestive heart failure may result in slower metabolism of TCAs (and thus a longer half-life) compared with that in healthy patients.

A number of drugs may inhibit hepatic enzymes (e.g., SSRIs, antipsychotics, valproate, disulfiram, cimetidine, and methylphenidate) and may thereby increase plasma levels of TCAs (Table 28–2).

Cytochrome P450 (CYP) 3A3/4 is an isoenzyme that metabolizes the triazolobenzodiazepines triazolam, alprazolam, and midazolam; the antidepressant nefazodone; as well as erythromycin, cisapride, cyclosporine, lidocaine, nifedipine, quinidine, terfenadine, astemizole, and the protease inhibitors used to treat HIV infection (Table 28–3). CYP3A3/4 also participates in the *demethylation* of tricyclics such as imipramine and amitriptyline (Lemoine et al. 1993; Ohmori et al. 1993; von Moltke et al. 1994). Nefazodone increases the serum levels of alprazolam and triazolam, which are also metabolized by the CYP3A3/4 isoenzymes.

Nefazodone appears to be metabolized primarily via the CYP3A3/4 system. The package insert recommends that nefazodone not be used with the antihistamines terfenadine and astemizole because ventricular arrhythmias may occur by blocking their metabolism of CYP3A3/4.

Among the nonsedating antihistamines, astemizole (as well as the gastrointestinal medication cisapride, which promotes motility), even in recommended doses, can cause small increases in the Q-T$_c$ interval. This effect is of almost no clinical significance in normal dose ranges, but in overdose situations in patients with hepatic disease or when the medications

Table 28–2.   **Reported drug interactions with psychotropic agents: cyclic antidepressants (CyADs)**

Medication	Interactive effect
Type IA antiarrhythmics (quinidine, procainamide)	May prolong cardiac conduction time
Phenothiazines	May prolong Q-T interval and raise CyAD levels
Guanethidine	May decrease antihypertensive effect
Clonidine	
Prazosin and other α-adrenergic blocking agents	Potentiate hypotensive effect
Parenteral sympathomimetic pressor amines (e.g., epinephrine, norepinephrine, phenylephrine)	May cause slight increases in blood pressure
Disulfiram	Raise CyAD levels
Methylphenidate	
Cimetidine	
Warfarin	May increase prothrombin time (fluoxetine probably more likely to cause this effect)
Oral contraceptives	May lower CyAD levels
Ethanol	
Barbiturates	
Phenytoin	
Anticholinergic agents	TCA may potentiate side effects
Carbamazepine	Additive cardiotoxicity possible and lower tricyclic levels
Propafenone (type IC antiarrhythmic)	May elevate tricyclic levels
Digitoxin	Fluoxetine may displace digitoxin from protein-binding sites and increase bioactive levels of digitoxin; converse is also true
	May lower TCA serum levels

Note.   TCA = tricyclic antidepressant.

are used with drugs that impair their metabolism via CYP3A3/4 (e.g., erythromycin, ketoconazole, clarithromycin, troleandomycin), ventricular arrhythmias such as torsades de pointes may develop.

It should also be noted that the parent compound nefazodone is metabolized predominantly by CYP3A3/4, whereas a major metabolite of nefazodone, m-CPP (meta-chlorophenylpiperazine, a serotonin agonist), is metabolized predominantly by CYP2D6. If a patient is switched from an antidepressant (e.g., fluoxetine or paroxetine) that inhibits CYP2D6 to nefazodone, the metabolism of the m-CPP metabolite would be temporarily inhibited. This inhibition of m-CPP metabolism would increase the anxiogenic properties of this metabolite, possibly causing increased anxiety and agitation despite nefazodone's serotonin-2 (5-HT$_2$) receptor blockade effects. Hence, switching from a long-acting CYP2D6 inhibitor (such as fluoxetine) to nefazodone should al-

Table 28–3. **Substrates for and inhibitors of the cytochrome P450 (CYP) 3A3/4 isoenzyme**

Drugs metabolized by CYP3A4 isoenzyme

Alprazolam

Astemizole

Cyclosporine

Imipramine, amitriptyline (demethylation)

Lidocaine

Midazolam

Nefazodone

Nifedipine

Quinidine

Sertraline

Triazolam

Inhibitors of CYP3A4 activity

Cimetidine

Erythromycin (and other macrolide antibiotics)

Itraconazole

Ketoconazole

Selective serotonin reuptake inhibitors (weak effect)

Source. Reprinted from Stoudemire A, Fogel BS: "Psychopharmacology in Medical Patients: An Update," in *Medical-Psychiatric Practice*, Vol. 3. Washington, DC, American Psychiatric Press, 1995, pp. 79–149. Copyright 1995, American Psychiatric Press. Used with permission.

low sufficient time for fluoxetine to wash out (3–4 weeks), and starting doses of nefazodone should be conservative to prevent m-CPP toxicity.

Carbamazepine is metabolized by CYP3A3/4 and induces the enzyme's activity. Erythromycin and ketoconazole competitively inhibit CYP3A3/4 and therefore will inhibit the metabolism of carbamazepine.

The major metabolic pathway for sertraline is CYP3A3/4. Venlafaxine is metabolized (demethylated) by CYP2D6 and CYP3A3/4. Venlafaxine is weaker than the SSRIs in in-hibiting the 2D6 isoenzyme.

Table 28–4 summarizes drug interactions that have been reported over the past several years that appear to have the most clinical relevance. The mechanisms for these interactions vary: some may be related to direct metabolic effects on the cytochrome enzymatic systems, whereas others may be more related to pharmacodynamic interactions.

Because fluoxetine is tightly bound to plasma protein, the administration of fluoxetine to a patient taking another drug that is tightly bound to protein (e.g., warfarin, digitoxin) could theoretically cause a shift in plasma concentrations that results in an adverse effect. Conversely, adverse effects may result from displacement of protein-bound fluoxetine by other tightly bound drugs. (These qualities also apply to sertraline and paroxetine, which are also highly protein bound.) Interactions between SSRIs and warfarin may increase coagulation time (prothrombin time [PT], or INR). The potential interaction is theoretically based on SSRIs possibly displacing warfarin from protein-binding sites, leaving more unbound (free) warfarin to be biologically active. The most extensive studies have been done with fluoxetine, but fluoxetine does not appear to alter the pharmacological effects of warfarin (Rowe et al. 1978). In contrast, both fluvoxamine and sertraline (Wilner et al. 1991) *have* been reported to increase *total* warfarin levels and increase PTs presumably by enzyme inhibition. For example, fluvoxamine has been noted to increase warfarin levels by 60% and subsequently increase PTs (Benfield and Ward 1986). Although paroxetine has been reported to have no effect on total warfarin levels, bleeding time nevertheless increased when the two drugs were coadministered (Bannister et al. 1989). Little clinical evidence suggests these properties regarding protein binding are of major clinical significance; nevertheless, clinicians are advised to monitor clotting studies carefully when SSRIs are used with warfarin until steady-state levels are reached.

Table 28–4. Reported drug interactions with selective serotonin reuptake inhibitors

Drug	Effect	Reference(s)
	Fluvoxamine	
Propranolol	Fivefold increase in propranolol levels	Benfield and Ward 1986; van Harten et al. 1992b
Warfarin	Increase in warfarin concentrations by 60%; increased prothrombin time	Benfield and Ward 1986
Theophylline	Increase in theophylline levels by factor of three	Sperber 1991
Carbamazepine	Conflicting reports: increase in carbamazepine levels as well as stable carbamazepine levels reported when fluvoxamine added	Fritze et al. 1991; Spina et al. 1993a
Amitriptyline	Increase in tricyclic antidepressant serum levels	Bertschy et al. 1991
Clomipramine	No increase in demethylated metabolites of clomipramine	
Atenolol	Some decrease in clinical effect of atenolol	Benfield and Ward 1986
Bromazepam	Increase in bromazepam levels	van Harten et al. 1992a
Imipramine	Increase in imipramine levels	Spina et al. 1993b, 1993c
Desipramine	Slight increase in desipramine levels when fluvoxamine added to patients with stable serum levels of desipramine	Spina et al. 1993c
Lorazepam	No effect	van Harten et al. 1992a
	Fluoxetine	
Imipramine	Increase in imipramine levels	Bergstrom et al. 1992
Desipramine	Increase in desipramine levels	Bergstrom et al. 1992
Nortriptyline	Increase in nortriptyline levels	Ciraulo and Shader 1990
Haloperidol	Increase in haloperidol levels	Goff et al. 1991; Tate 1989
Perphenazine	Increase in perphenazine levels	Lock et al. 1990
Diazepam	Increase in diazepam levels	Lemberger et al. 1988
Alprazolam	Increase in alprazolam levels	Ciraulo and Shader 1990; Lasher et al. 1991
Terfenadine	Increase in terfenadine levels	von Moltke et al. 1996
Carbamazepine	Increase in both carbamazepine and carbamazepine 10,11-epoxide levels	Gidal et al. 1993; Grimsley et al. 1991
Warfarin	No effect on half-life of warfarin or the prothrombin time	Rowe et al. 1978

(continued)

Table 28–4.   **Reported drug interactions with selective serotonin reuptake inhibitors** *(continued)*

Drug	Effect	Reference
Fluoxetine *(continued)*		
Pimozide	Bradycardia when fluoxetine was added; delirium also reported, probably caused by increased pimozide levels	Ahmed et al. 1993; Hansen-Grant et al. 1993
Cyclosporine	No effect of fluoxetine on cyclosporine levels	Strouse et al. 1993
Valproic acid	Increase in valproate serum levels	Sovner and Davis 1991
Clozapine	Increase in clozapine levels	Centorrino et al. 1994
Clonazepam	No effect of fluoxetine on clonazepam levels	Greenblatt et al. 1992
Phenytoin	Possible increase in phenytoin levels	D. J. Woods et al. 1994
Metoprolol	Bradycardia when fluoxetine was added	Walley et al. 1993
Paroxetine		
Cimetidine	Increase in paroxetine levels by 50%	Bannister et al. 1989
Phenobarbital	Decrease in paroxetine levels by 25%	Greb et al. 1989
Carbamazepine, valproate, and phenytoin	No effect on carbamazepine serum levels when paroxetine coadministered with these anticonvulsants	Andersen et al. 1991
Phenytoin and carbamazepine	Possible decrease in paroxetine levels	Andersen et al. 1991
Molindone	Increase in extrapyramidal side effects	Malek-Ahmadi and Allen 1995
Drugs metabolized via CYP2D6 (includes tricyclics)	Increase in serum levels	See Table 28–3
Sertraline		
Tolbutamide	Decrease in tolbutamide levels	Warrington 1991
Warfarin	Increased prothrombin time	Wilner et al. 1991
Atenolol	No effect on atenolol level	Warrington 1991
Drugs metabolized by CYP2D6	Increase in serum levels	See Table 28–3
Tricyclics (including desipramine)	Elevation of tricyclic antidepressant levels	Barros and Asnis 1993

Source.   Reprinted from Stoudemire A, Fogel BS: "Psychopharmacology in Medical Patients: An Update," in *Medical-Psychiatric Practice*, Vol. 3. Washington, DC, American Psychiatric Press, 1995, pp. 79–149. Copyright 1995, American Psychiatric Press. Used with permission.

SSRIs and Hematological Effects

Fluoxetine may have hematological side effects. Fluoxetine diminishes granular storage of serotonin in platelets and has been reported to increase bleeding times. Petechiae, ecchymoses, and even melena have been reported rarely with fluoxetine treatment; evidence suggests that these hematological effects are dose related (Alderman et al. 1992). Impaired platelet aggregation has been described with fluoxetine in doses greater than 20 mg/day; platelet activity normalized several days after the drug was discontinued. This implies that the parent drug (fluoxetine) is responsible for hematological effects because the principal metabolite (norfluoxetine) would not be eliminated for at least several weeks. Whether other SSRIs clinically affect platelet functioning is not fully known. Based on the current state of knowledge, obtaining bleeding times in patients taking fluoxetine should be considered if these patients have planned elective surgery; however, screening of patients being treated with other SSRIs is not necessary.

A series of studies have investigated the use of sertraline with several drugs commonly used in general medicine. These studies have found the following results in healthy male volunteer subjects:

■ Sertraline does not alter the β-blocking activity of atenolol (Ziegler and Wilner 1996).

■ Sertraline does not appear to have a clinically significant effect on digoxin pharmacokinetics or ECG findings (Rapeport et al. 1996a).

■ Sertraline does not change levels of carbamazepine or levels of its intermediate (more toxic) metabolite 10,11-epoxide when these drugs are used together (Rapeport et al. 1996c). Sertraline does not have any significant effect on phenytoin levels (Rapeport et al. 1996b).

SSRIs and Extrapyramidal Side Effects

SSRIs can cause extrapyramidal side effects (EPS), including akathisia, dyskinesias, dystonias, and drug-induced parkinsonism (Arya and Szabadi 1993; Baldwin et al. 1991; Nicholson 1992; Wils 1992), via antidopaminergic effects. EPS are most likely to occur in older patients, particularly those whose histories or prior drug responses suggest preclinical Parkinson's disease (Dave 1994). Parkinsonian-like side effects may be caused by inhibition of neuronal production and release of dopamine caused by increases in synaptic serotonin. Inhibition of dopamine systems by serotonin and SSRIs has been demonstrated in animals (Baldessarini and Marsh 1990; Kapur and Remington 1996).

SSRIs have been reported to exacerbate symptoms of preexisting Parkinson's disease (Steur 1993), although some clinicians observe that such effects are rarely of clinical significance. Several of the reported cases of SSRIs causing EPS have occurred in patients treated with neuroleptics. Inhibition of neuroleptic metabolism by SSRIs may have played a role in the observed effect (Arya and Szabadi 1993; Nicholson 1992; Wils 1992).

Akathisia, however, is the most common neurological symptom caused by SSRIs. It may be seen in patients at any age. Akathisia can be managed by dose reduction of the SSRI or by treatment with low doses of propranolol (20–40 mg/day).

Renal Failure and Dialysis

The hydroxylated metabolites of TCAs have been found to be markedly elevated in patients with renal disease and on dialysis (Dawling et al. 1982; J. A. Lieberman et al. 1985) as compared with control subjects. Serum levels of the parent tricyclic compounds (amitriptyline and nortriptyline) after oral doses also tend to be somewhat higher in dialysis patients than in control subjects (J. A. Lieberman et al. 1985). However, no data indicate the need for routine measurement of the hydroxylated metabolites of TCAs in patients with chronic renal failure or in those on dialysis. Some toxicity may be accrued from these (unmeasured) hydroxylated tricyclic metabolites, but their effects are likely minimal unless patients have advanced end-stage organ failure. The fact that these hydroxylated metabolites contribute to side-effect hypersensitivity urges more conservative titration of doses in severely medically ill populations. In contrast, the serum levels of fluoxetine do not appear to be affected in the face of renal disease when patients are undergoing hemodialysis (Levy et al. 1996). Table 28–5 (Stoudemire et al. 1991) summarizes the side-effect profiles of the currently available non-MAOI CyADs.

MIRTAZAPINE

Mirtazapine, an antidepressant with a tetracyclic structure and a complex mechanism of action, was introduced into the United States in 1996. Mirtazapine blocks *presynaptic* noradrenergic α_2 autoreceptors that regulate biogenic amine release (deBoer 1996). This antagonism of central presynaptic α_2-adrenergic autoreceptors results in disinhibition of norepinephrine release and enhanced noradrenergic neurotransmission. Norepinephrine stimulation of α_1-adrenergic receptors increases serotonergic neurotransmission. Mirtazapine also blocks serotonin inhibiting α_2 adrenoreceptors located on serotonergic nerve terminals, which also causes an increase in serotonergic neurotransmission. Because $5\text{-}HT_2$ and $5\text{-}HT_3$ receptor subtypes are blocked by mirtazapine, the increased release of serotonin is exerted predominantly on $5\text{-}HT_1$ receptors. Mirtazapine does not block $5\text{-}HT_{1A}$ or $5\text{-}HT_{1B}$ receptors. Mirtazapine is a potent antagonist of H_1 receptors, which accounts for its sedating properties.

Mirtazapine follows linear pharmacokinetics in the therapeutic dose range of 15–45 mg/day; its average half-life of 20–40 hours makes it suitable for once-a-day (nocturnal) dosing (Hoyberg et al. 1996). Major metabolic pathways for mirtazapine are demethylation and hydroxylation followed by glucuronide conjugation. In vitro data from human liver microsomes indicate that CYP2D6 and CYP1A2 are involved in the hydroxylated 8-OH metabolites, and CYP3A forms the *N*-desmethyl and *N*-oxide metabolites (Package Insert, Organow, Inc., West Orange, NJ).

The manufacturer reports that the half-life of the drug is more extended in women than in men (mean 37 hours for women and 26 hours for men). The oral clearance of mirtazapine was decreased by 30% in patients with liver disease as compared with healthy control subjects. Compared with patients who have normal renal functioning, in patients with both moderate (glomerular filtration rate [GFR] 11–39 mL/min/1.73 m^2) and severe (GFR < 10 mL/min/1.73 m^2) renal impairment, the average oral clearance of mirtazapine was reduced by 30% and 50%, respectively (Package Insert data). Clearance of the drug is reduced in the elderly, with the most striking reductions in men (40% lower clearance in elderly men compared with younger men vs. only a 10% difference between older and younger women).

The overall clinical picture of mirtazapine could be summarized as follows:

- It is a relatively sedating drug that can be given once daily at night, although its sedative properties may diminish over time.
- Its side-effect profile has been associated with dry mouth, constipation, dizziness, and blurred vision (more than placebo) in some studies, particularly in elderly patients, as well as body weight gain.
- Its safety in patients with heart disease has not been studied, but ECG effects in persons without heart disease do not appear to be clinically significant.
- Its clearance is reduced in patients with liver and renal disease, and the drug rarely may cause agranulocytosis.

Table 28–5.   Side-effect profiles of antidepressants

	Effect on serotonin reuptake	Effect on norepinephrine reuptake	Sedating effect	Anticholinergic effect	Orthostatic effect	Dose range[d] (mg)
Amitriptyline[a]	++++	++	++++	++++	++++	75–300
Imipramine[a]	++++	++	+++	+++	++++	75–300
Nortriptyline	+++	+++	++	++	+	40–150
Protriptyline	+++	++++	+	+++	+	10–60
Trazodone	+++	+	+++	±[b]	++	200–600
Nefazodone	+	+	++	−	−	300–600
Desipramine	+	++++	+	+	++	75–300
Amoxapine[c]	++	+++	++	++	++	75–600
Maprotiline	−	++	++	+	++	150–200
Doxepin	+++	++	+++	++	++	75–300
Trimipramine[c]	+	+	++	++	++	50–300
Fluoxetine	++++	−	−	−	−	20–60
Paroxetine	++++	++	−	+	−	20–60
Sertraline	++++	−	−	−	−	50–200
Bupropion	−	−	−	±	−	150–450
Venlafaxine	++	++	−	−	−	75–450

Note.   Relative potencies (some ratings are approximated) based partly on affinities of these agents for brain receptors in competitive binding studies. − = none, + = slight, ++ = moderate, +++ = marked, ++++ = pronounced, ± = indeterminate.
[a]Available in injectable form.
[b]Most in vivo and clinical studies report the absence of anticholinergic effects (or no difference from placebo). There have been case reports, however, of apparent anticholinergic effects.
[c]Amoxapine and trimipramine have dopamine receptor blocking activity.
[d]Dose ranges are for treatment of major depression. Lower doses may be appropriate for other therapeutic uses.
Source.   Reprinted from Stoudemire A, Fogel BS, Gulley LR: "Psychopharmacology in the Medically Ill: An Update," in *Medical Psychiatric Practice*, Vol. 1. Edited by Stoudemire A, Fogel BS. Washington, DC, American Psychiatric Press, 1991, pp. 29–97. Copyright 1991, American Psychiatric Press. Used with permission.

■   Its mechanism of action is as a potent and highly selective presynaptic α_2-adrenoreceptor antagonist that increases noradrenergic neurotransmission by causing increased noradrenergic cell firing and norepinephrine release. Effects on serotonin are the result of norepinephrine-regulated stimulation of α_1 receptors that activate serotonin cells in the raphe nucleus (deBoer 1996). By blocking inhibitory α_2 adrenoreceptors that suppress serotonin activity, the overall effect is to enhance serotonin neurotransmission via this mechanism as well.

MAOIs IN MEDICALLY ILL PATIENTS

MAOIs may raise special problems in medically ill patients because of their effects on blood pressure and body weight as well as interactions with medications used in internal medicine. With respect to elderly medically ill patients, the most common effect of MAOIs is orthostatic hypotension. As compared with traditional tricyclics, there is relatively little difference between the orthostatic blood pressure effects of phenelzine compared with those of nortriptyline in patients age 55 and older (Georgotas et al. 1987). Effects on blood pressure may be ameliorated by slow, conservative dosing strategies. Divided-dose strategies also will help in minimizing blood pressure effects.

Hypertensive crises may be precipitated by drug interactions with MAOIs. The most consistent offenders are the *indirect* pressor amines (e.g., ephedrine, pseudoephedrine, and phenylpropanolamine; Table 28–6). *Direct* pressors (e.g., norepinephrine, epinephrine, and isoproterenol) are relatively safer, and in one well-designed animal study, they showed almost no pressor effects (Braverman et al. 1987). Nevertheless, close monitoring of blood pressure would be strongly advised if these drugs were administered to a patient taking MAOIs. Caution should be used in these situations because of possible hypertensive reactions (Feighner et al. 1985). Patients receiving bronchodilators are at a higher risk for side effects when taking MAOIs; however, at least theoretically, these patients should not have unusual problems as long as indirect sympathomimetics such as ephedrine are clearly avoided. Xanthines and cromolyn usually would be preferable to sympathomimetic drugs in asthmatic patients taking MAOIs.

Drug-induced hypertensive episodes would be particularly hazardous in patients with cardiovascular or cerebrovascular disease and in patients taking oral anticoagulants because of their greater risk for a cerebral hemorrhage. The first symptoms may include sudden fatigue or a pounding bilateral occipital headache. All patients treated with MAOIs (even those at relatively low risk) should carry 10-mg nifedipine tablets to be chewed or dissolved under the tongue at the first signs of a hypertensive reaction (Clary and Schweizer 1987). Nifedipine's hypotensive effect is relatively proportional to the degree of hypertension and has a direct antianginal effect that would be of benefit for patients with coronary insufficiency. Despite the U.S. Food and Drug Administration's (FDA) warning about nifedipine's capacity to produce hypotension, we believe that the risk is irrelevant to the danger of a sudden hypertensive episode during MAOI treatment.

All MAOIs—especially the hydrazines, such as phenelzine and isocarboxazid—are associated with carbohydrate craving and weight gain. Weight gain would be of particular importance in patients with diabetes mellitus and hyperlipidemia. For patients with these and other medical disorders that would be complicated by substantial weight gain, tranylcypromine typically would be the MAOI of choice. The "reversible" MAOI moclobemide is not manufactured in the United States but is often imported for use here. Moclobemide is not associated with weight gain and would theoretically be the preferred MAOI in a diabetic patient based on potential for weight gain. The use of the MAOI diet is not required for this drug, up to a dose of 900 mg/day.

Clinical tradition has usually mandated that MAOIs should always be discontinued prior to anesthesia and surgery. However, more recent evidence suggests that surgery or ECT can be safely performed during concurrent use of MAOIs (El Ganzouri et al. 1985; Stack et al. 1988; Wells and Bjorksten 1989), providing that there is no chance the patient would receive meperidine in the postoperative period. Sedation may occur when MAOIs are used in conjunction with benzodiazepines and may be misinterpreted as a worsening of depression.

OTHER SPECIAL CONSIDERATIONS IN THE USE OF MAOIs

MAOIs appear less likely than TCAs to aggravate seizures (Edwards 1985; Trinidad and Silver 1994), but their pharmacodynamic interactions with some anticonvulsants may create other problems, such as excessive sedation if barbiturate anticonvulsants are used. MAOIs, however, may be preferable in many situations to tricyclics in epileptic patients needing antidepressant therapy.

Table 28–6.   **Reported drug interactions with psychotropic agents: monoamine oxidase inhibitors (MAOIs)**

Medication	Interactive effect
Meperidine	Fatal reaction
L-Dopa, methyldopa, dopamine, buspirone, guanethidine, cyclic antidepressants, carbamazepine, cyclobenzaprine	Elevation of blood pressure
Direct-acting sympathomimetics	Elevation of blood pressure
Epinephrine, norepinephrine, isoproterenol, methoxamine	
Indirect-acting sympathomimetics	Severe hypertension
Cocaine, amphetamines, tyramine, methylphenidate, phenethylamine, metaraminol, ephedrine, phenylpropanolamine	
Direct- and indirect-acting sympathomimetics	Severe hypertension
Pseudoephedrine, metaraminol, phenylephrine	
Serotonergic agents	"Serotonin syndrome" (ataxia,
Fluoxetine, tryptophan	nystagmus, confusion, fever, tremor)
Caffeine	Mild elevation of blood pressure
Theophylline	
Aminophylline	
Hypoglycemic agents	Lower blood glucose
Anticoagulants	Prolonged prothrombin time
Succinylcholine	Phenelzine prolongs action
Diuretics	Increased hypotensive effect
Propranolol	
Prazosin	
Calcium channel blockers	
Midrin	Midrin contains isometheptene, a sympathomimetic (Kraft and Dore 1996), and can cause hypertension in combination with an MAOI.

MAOIs may cause a pyridoxine (vitamin B_6) deficiency manifested as peripheral polyneuropathy or as susceptibility to nerve entrapment neuropathy conditions such as carpal tunnel syndrome (Robinson and Kurtz 1987). Pyridoxine deficiency can be treated with 50–100 mg/day of vitamin B_6. The MAOIs also influence thiamine metabolism (decreasing erythrocyte transketolase; Ali 1985). In malnourished or alcoholic patients, this effect could theoretically increase the likelihood of clinical symptoms of thiamine deficiency.

Guidelines for more liberal dietary (tyramine) parameters for patients taking MAOIs have been published based on a critical literature review and a scientific assessment of the actual tyramine content of previously proscribed foods. These revised dietary recommendations are summarized in Table 28–7 (Gardner et al. 1996).

Table 28–7. Relative restrictions of foods and beverages with monoamine oxidase inhibitor (MAOI) use

Restriction	Foods
Absolute	Aged cheeses; aged and cured meats; banana peel; broad bean pods; improperly stored or spoiled meats, poultry, and fish; Marmite; sauerkraut; soy sauce and other soybean condiments; tap beer
Moderate	Red or white wine, bottled or canned beer (including nonalcoholic varieties)
Unnecessary	Avocados; bananas; beef/chicken bouillon; chocolate; fresh and mild cheeses (e.g., ricotta, cottage, cream cheese; processed slices); fresh meat, poultry, or fish; gravy (fresh); monosodium glutamate; peanuts; properly stored pickled or smoked fish (e.g., herring); raspberries; soy milk; yeast extracts (except Marmite)

Source. Reprinted from Gardner DM, Shulman KI, Walker SE, et al.: "The Making of a User Friendly MAOI Diet." *Journal of Clinical Psychiatry* 57:99–104, 1996. Copyright 1996, Physicians Postgraduate Press. Used with permission.

BENZODIAZEPINES

Complaints of anxiety and disturbed sleep are the most common indications for use of benzodiazepines among medically ill patients. However, when these complaints arise in medically ill patients who are taking several medications or who are in the hospital, care should be exercised in formulating the differential diagnosis.

Benzodiazepines in Medically Ill Elderly Patients

As with most psychotropics, benzodiazepines present greater risks for elderly patients than for younger ones (Meyer 1982; Thompson et al. 1983). The high prevalence of anxiety disorders among elderly patients means that they are likely to be prescribed these drugs frequently (Markovitz 1993). Although no benzodiazepines are especially safe for medically ill elderly patients, ultrashort-acting agents such as triazolam are more likely than longer-acting agents to cause confusion, dissociation, and anterograde amnesia (Morris and Estes 1987; Rickels et al. 1988).

Long half-life drugs accumulate and reach steady state slowly, tend to be highly lipophilic, and are cleared slowly after the drug is stopped. These drugs are generally metabolized by oxidation, a hepatic mechanism that decays in efficacy with age and hepatic dysfunction and, for those additional reasons, should be used cautiously in medically ill elderly patients. For example, adjustments downward in dose, greater time intervals between doses, and close follow-up assessment of cognitive functioning and mood would be indicated. Prototypical benzodiazepines in this group include diazepam, flurazepam, and quazepam.

Shorter-acting drugs are less lipophilic, accumulate less, and clear more rapidly after cessation than long-acting drugs. Rather than being oxidized, they are primarily conjugated and renally excreted in a metabolic process that is minimally affected by aging or hepatic disease. Although the adjustments necessary for medically ill elderly patients may be proportionately *less* among this group of conjugated benzodiazepines than for the longer-acting agents, adjustments are usually needed, and close follow-up is indicated (Grad 1995; Greenblatt et al. 1983). Drugs with a medium to short half-life include temazepam, oxazepam, and lorazepam. In patients with hepatic dysfunction due to cirrhosis, active hepatitis, or metabolic damage, one of these three drugs should be selected.

Benzodiazepines can induce ventilatory suppression in the setting of certain pulmonary conditions. Those patients who chronically retain CO_2 are at greatest risk, because benzodiazepines reduce the hypoxic response to ventilation—their only remaining ventilatory stimulus (Lakshminarayan et al. 1976; Modeo and Berry 1974). Another high-risk category is that of patients with sleep apnea (the periodic cessation of ventilation during sleep) caused by either obstruction or failure of central drive.

When using benzodiazepines as hypnotics or anxiolytics, a thorough differential diagnosis and evaluation of etiology should precede reflexive prescription of a drug (Mendelson 1992). Patients with hepatic or pulmonary disease and elderly patients should probably avoid drugs metabolized by oxidation, and, in general, shorter-acting drugs that are conjugated are preferable. Special attention should be given to the patient's need to get up at night, because some drugs, such as triazolam, can cause ataxia and confusion. A key strategy for the psychiatrist treating these patients is frequent follow-up in a manner that allows assessment of cognitive functioning, mood, gait, and (when indicated) ventilatory status with blood gases.

Newer Benzodiazepines

Estazolam's elimination half-life increases moderately in elderly patients from the usual range of 8–24 hours to a range of 13–34 hours. It is effective in elderly patients at half the usual 2-mg dose for younger patients. Little rebound insomnia occurs after abrupt cessation (Pierce and Shu 1990). Risk to elderly patients (of cognitive impairment) and chronic pulmonary patients (of ventilatory suppression) should be considered moderate to high.

Quazepam is a long-acting benzodiazepine that appears to have preferential BZ1 receptor affinity (Wamsley and Hunt 1991). Because the drug is highly lipophilic and rapidly absorbed, its onset of action is rapid. The duration of action of single doses is brief because of movement to fat stores, but repeated doses will result in accumulation there. The fact that quazepam and flurazepam share a major active metabolite argues for caution in the use of quazepam in medically ill elderly patients, patients with pulmonary disease, and patients with hepatic dysfunction.

Zolpidem has largely supplanted the use of triazolam as a short-acting sedative-hypnotic. Zolpidem does not seem to be associated with many of the problems with triazolam (rebound insomnia, anterograde amnesia); nevertheless, zolpidem may affect memory, and adverse reactions have been reported with this agent (Rush and Griffiths 1996), including possible interactions with SSRIs causing drug-induced delirium (Katz 1995). Acute psychotic reactions have also been reported, particularly when zolpidem has been taken with SSRIs (Markowitz and Brewerton 1996). One of the authors (A. S.) observed rebound daytime anxiety following acute discontinuation of zolpidem after prolonged use.

BUSPIRONE

The use of buspirone, a nonbenzodiazepine anxiolytic, has not been studied extensively in medically ill patients. Buspirone may have advantages in patients with chronic lung disease, because in animal studies it appears to stimulate respiratory drive, as opposed to the general depressant effect on respiration observed with benzodiazepines (Garner et al. 1989; Mendelson et al. 1989). Diazepam may markedly depress ventilatory response to exogenous CO_2 administration, whereas buspirone has no such overall effect (Rapoport 1989; Rapoport et al. 1988). In addition, buspirone does not depress ventilatory response to increasing CO_2 levels. Therefore, buspirone appears to be a potentially safe long-term anxiolytic for treatment of patients with respiratory disease.

Pharmacokinetic studies with buspirone indicate no clinically significant differences between young and elderly patients in standard pharmacokinetic measures with either acute or chronic dosing (Gammans et al. 1989). There appears to be no need to alter the initial doses of buspirone based solely on the patient's age.

NEUROLEPTICS

Apart from schizophrenia, delirium is perhaps the most common disorder treated with neuroleptics among elderly and medically ill patients. The therapeutic efficacy among the various available antipsychotics is essentially the same, and the choice of a particular agent is thus guided by the side-effect profile most likely to be tolerated or to cause the fewest problems in an individual patient. The antipsychotics can be arbitrarily divided into "high-potency" drugs (e.g., haloperidol and fluphenazine), which are relatively low in sedating and anticholinergic effects and high in EPS, and "low-potency" agents (e.g., chlorpromazine and thioridazine), which have opposite characteristics.

The same influences that merge to produce cerebral dysfunction in medically ill patients (i.e., electrolyte disturbances, hypoxemia, volume shifts, systemic infections, medications) make them vulnerable to side effects of any added medication, including neuroleptics. The neuroleptic alone may reduce symptoms in a delirium and thereby induce complacency about the underlying pathogenic cause. Thus, a careful differential diagnosis is necessary for the target syndrome (such as delirium) or symptom (such as agitation). Elderly and medically ill patients are generally more sensitive than younger patients to a given oral dose of low-potency agents, especially for chlorpromazine. As a result, most psychiatrists use high-potency agents, such as haloperidol, in the settings described.

Human data regarding the use of antipsychotic agents in the presence of epilepsy reveal few reliable guidelines for the clinician to follow. Among newer agents, clozapine has a well-documented seizure-inducing potential

(Trinidad and Silver 1994). Molindone may lower the seizure threshold less than other antipsychotics.

Neuroleptics in Patients With Cardiac Disease

Patients with cardiac conduction disease may be susceptible to quinidine-like effects of neuroleptics. The effects on the ECG and on the clinical examination are usually negligible. However, if the patient concurrently takes a type I antiarrhythmic—including a tricyclic—or has a significant preexisting conduction delay, the effect may be less benign and may require close monitoring or even cardiological consultation. If the $Q-T_c$ interval before starting the neuroleptic is 0.440 seconds or longer, added quinidine-like effects may result in fatal ventricular arrhythmias. Among antipsychotics, thioridazine appears to be the most dangerous drug in this regard (Stoudemire et al. 1993). Drug interactions with neuroleptics are listed in Table 28–8.

The psychiatrist should avoid prescribing low-potency agents such as chlorpromazine to patients with symptomatic orthostatic hypotension. These drugs cause a notable degree of α-adrenergic blockade and can worsen blood pressure regulation.

For the patient with an acute MI, the greatest risk again occurs among low-potency drugs, chiefly because of orthostatic hypotension but also because of tachycardia induced by vagolytic anticholinergic effects.

Neuroleptics in Patients With Other Medical Disorders

The anticholinergic effects of the lower-potency agents (e.g., thioridazine) may cause or exacerbate cognitive dysfunction in elderly patients and may also lead to increased intraocular pressure in patients with narrow-angle glaucoma. The antimuscarinic effects of these drugs may exacerbate prostatism and contribute to male

Table 28–8. Reported drug interactions with neuroleptics

Medication	Interactive effect
Type IA antiarrhythmics	Chlorpromazine or thioridazine may prolong cardiac conduction
Alprazolam Tricyclics β-Blockers Chloramphenicol Disulfiram MAOIs Acetaminophen Buspirone Fluoxetine	May increase neuroleptic levels
Barbiturates Hypnotics Rifampin Griseofulvin Phenylbutazone Carbamazepine Phenytoin	Lower neuroleptic levels through induction of hepatic enzymes
Gel-type antacids with Al^{3+} and Mg^{2+}	May interfere with neuroleptic absorption
Narcotics Epinephrine Enflurane Isoflurane	Potentiate hypotensive effects of neuroleptics
α-Methyldopa Prazosin ACE-inhibitors (captopril, enalapril)	Increase hypotensive effect
Narcotics Tricyclics Barbiturates	May increase sedative effects of neuroleptics
Iproniazid	May cause encephalopathy and hepatotoxicity when used with neuroleptics
Guanethidine Clonidine	Neuroleptics may decrease blood pressure control
Sodium valproate	Chlorpromazine increases valproate levels
Carbamazepine	Carbamazepine treatment lowers clozapine levels

Note. MAOI = monoamine oxidase inhibitor; ACE = angiotensin-converting enzyme.

sexual dysfunction. Thioridazine may induce impotence and retrograde ejaculation (Mitchell and Popkin 1983). The higher-potency drugs are less likely to cause these types of anticholinergic problems; however, these drugs are more likely to cause EPS.

Other Side Effects of Neuroleptics

EPS occur with all neuroleptics except clozapine and occur at a much lower rate with risperidone, olanzapine, and quetiapine. The high-potency agents produce EPS more commonly than do low-potency agents. Elderly patients are most susceptible to parkinsonian effects, and young male patients are most susceptible to dystonias. The hematological effects of clozapine will likely limit its general use, but the patient with Parkinson's disease and psychotic symptoms may be an ideal candidate for the drug.

Although all antipsychotics lower the seizure threshold, molindone, fluphenazine (Luchins et al. 1984), thioridazine, and mesoridazine (Edwards et al. 1986) appear to be the least proconvulsant. Reports suggest that chlorpromazine and clozapine are the most problematic in this regard.

Medically debilitated, dehydrated, and neurologically impaired patients appear to be at risk for two potentially catastrophic conditions: neuroleptic malignant syndrome and neuroleptic-induced catatonia. Patients with delirium who are taking antipsychotics thus require close monitoring of fluid status and vital signs (Harpe and Stoudemire 1987; Stoudemire and Luther 1984).

Increasing evidence indicates that antipsychotics have a therapeutic window of efficacy. Thus, in some patients, a dose increase may cause only more side effects and little therapeutic effect. However, in patients who have not yet responded, continued careful upward titration of the dose is indicated. Medically ill and elderly patients may respond to doses of haloperidol as low as 0.5–1.0 mg. Low doses of a benzodiazepine may act synergistically with neuroleptics, producing therapeutic effects without depressing the patient's level of consciousness (Levine 1994).

Clozapine

Clozapine is a novel antipsychotic with minimal EPS. Problems associated with its use include orthostatic hypotension, lowering of the seizure threshold, anticholinergic toxicity, and significant incidence of agranulocytosis (1%–2%). As a consequence, its FDA-approved indications

are restricted to psychosis in Parkinson's disease and refractory schizophrenia. Clozapine may reduce the symptoms of Parkinson's disease (Roberts et al. 1989) and may be useful in the treatment of refractory bipolar disorder. The danger of seizure increases with increasing dose. The hematological risk is so grave as to require complete blood counts weekly.

In patients with medical and neurological illness, the major side effects of concern for clozapine are its high anticholinergic profile, its propensity to cause orthostatic hypertension, its potential to lower the seizure threshold, and the development of clozapine-induced fever and leukopenia. The reported problems with agranulocytosis require weekly blood monitoring. Of these patients, 1%–2% taking low doses (below 300 mg/day) are at risk for seizure; this risk increases to 3%–4% for those patients taking intermediate doses and to about 5% at higher doses (600–900 mg/day). Nevertheless, clozapine may have advantages in treatment of patients who are prone to EPS and tardive dyskinesia because it has minimal EPS and has not been reported to cause tardive dyskinesia. The drug may in fact have some beneficial effect in the treatment of tardive dyskinesia caused by traditional neuroleptics.

Clozapine has been used to treat patients with psychosis in Parkinson's disease and has actually been found to reduce parkinsonian symptoms (Musser and Akil 1996; Roberts et al. 1989). Treatment of psychosis in Parkinson's disease should begin with low doses of clozapine (6.25–12.5 mg twice a day) and be titrated upward slowly if needed.

Risperidone

Risperidone is a relatively new high-potency antipsychotic that researchers initially hoped would offer some advantages for patients with Parkinson's-related psychotic symptoms and elderly patients prone to EPS. This drug has been reported to cause EPS in elderly patients even at relatively low doses of 1–2 mg, and reliable reports indicate that it causes neuroleptic malignant syndrome (Tarsy 1996). No evidence suggests that this agent necessarily offers major advantages in the treatment of psychosis in patients with Parkinson's disease.

Olanzapine

Olanzapine is an atypical antipsychotic agent. Its mechanism of antipsychotic activity is via combination of dopamine (D_{1-4}) and 5-HT_2 antagonism. The pharmacokinetics of the drug do not appear to be altered in the presence of advanced renal failure; its elimination half-life is increased by approximately 1.5 times in patients older than 65.

Mild elevations in the alanine aminotransferase (ALT; serum glutamic-pyruvic transaminase [SGPT]) levels were observed in about 2% of patients treated with olanzapine in placebo-controlled studies; none experienced jaundice or symptoms of hepatic impairment. These enzyme elevations tended to normalize as treatment continued.

Because olanzapine is metabolized by multiple enzyme systems, inhibition of a single cytochrome P450 isoenzyme is unlikely to appreciably decrease olanzapine clearance. Multiple doses of olanzapine do not appear to affect the pharmacokinetics of theophylline or its metabolites (predominantly metabolized by CYP1A2). Carbamazepine causes about a 50% *increase* in the clearance of olanzapine.

The most frequent treatment-emergent adverse side effects of olanzapine include postural hypotension, constipation, weight gain, new-onset diabetes, dizziness, and akathisia. Hence, the drug is not free of EPS; whether it offers advantages for the treatment of psychosis in Parkinson's disease is not known.

The effects on the ECG appear to be benign, and no clinically significant effects on the ECG have been observed. The primary cardiovascular effects of the drug appear to be the propensity for mild degrees of orthostatic hypotension. There have been no reports of

neutropenia with olanzapine. (Information supplied by Bruce Kinon, Eli Lilly Laboratories, 1996.)

LITHIUM IN PATIENTS WITH RENAL DISEASE

Because the kidney is the route for lithium excretion, renal competence and alterations in intravascular volume status are impediments to the prescription of the drug. Lithium occupies the "sodium space"; thus, any condition altering sodium movement will likely affect the body's handling of lithium. Volume depletion and traditional diuretic use are the most common clinical examples of conditions that raise serum lithium levels. Volume depletion occurs in conditions associated with vomiting, diarrhea, polyuria, and excessive sweating. Physical disability and diminished responsiveness to thirst could also hinder attempts at normal salt and water replacement. The result would be volume contraction and increased renal reabsorption of sodium and of lithium, with higher lithium levels on an unchanged oral dose. Among the diuretics, the thiazides have the most and furosemide the least effect on lithium concentration (Rizos et al. 1988). Indeed, the thiazides are used for the symptomatic treatment of lithium-induced diabetes insipidus. Potassium-sparing diuretics such as spironolactone may also reduce lithium clearance, but they have been less studied than other diuretics. Drug interactions with lithium are summarized in Table 28–9.

Renal failure patients on dialysis do not eliminate lithium between dialyses, and they therefore require only one dose in this interim. Levels are checked 2–3 hours after the dose, which is given after the dialysis. The dosage range is 300–600 mg/day (Levy 1993).

Advancing age itself generally brings a 30%–40% reduction in glomerular filtration rate and necessitates a proportional reduction in oral dose (Hardy et al. 1987). Older patients and others with CNS disease may show confusion

Table 28–9. Reported drug interactions with lithium (Li$^+$)

Medication	Interactive effect
Thiazide diuretics	Raise Li$^+$ levels
Spironolactone	
Triamterene	
Nonsteroidal antiinflammatants (e.g., indomethacin, ibuprofen, phenylbutazone, piroxicam)	
Acetazolamide	Lower Li$^+$ levels
Theophylline	
Aminophylline	
Calcium channel blockers	May either raise or lower Li$^+$ levels, effects not clear; verapamil may cause bradycardia when used with Li$^+$
Metronidazole	May raise Li$^+$ levels; may increase chances of nephrotoxicity
Tetracycline	Minor elevation of Li$^+$ levels
Enalapril and other angiotensin-converting enzyme (ACE) inhibitors	Anecdotally reported to raise Li$^+$ levels; systematic studies show little overall effect

and sedation at levels therapeutic for younger patients (DePaulo 1984). The psychiatrist should closely monitor lithium levels in these patients and aim for the lower end of the therapeutic range.

Almost all patients taking lithium experience some polyuria because of its effect in reducing the kidney's ability to concentrate urine. This symptom may be ameliorated by giving the lithium once daily, preferably early in the day. In some cases, the concomitant use of thiazide diuretics may be needed to control polyuria. In elderly or debilitated patients, dehydration may become significant (Minden et al. 1993).

Other Side Effects of Lithium

Lithium induces hypothyroidism in 2%–15% of patients and goiter in 3%–4%. People with pretreatment elevated levels of thyroid-stimulating hormone (TSH) are probably at greatest risk for these effects. Diminished effectiveness of antidepressant medication may be the clinical result. Monitoring of TSH and free thyroxine (T_4) levels may detect hypothyroidism and

prompt appropriate replacement treatment. Lithium cessation is rarely required.

Cardiac effects are generally quite benign and are restricted to nonspecific T-wave changes in the ECG and some increased susceptibility to digitalis toxicity (Mittal et al. 1985; Tilkian et al. 1976a, 1976b). Extreme sensitivity to side effects of lithium argues for consideration of alternative treatments, such as sodium valproate, for bipolar patients.

A significant risk in the use of lithium is its potential to exacerbate arrhythmias in patients with sinus node dysfunction (Steckler 1994). Although this condition is relatively rare, the propensity of lithium to unmask or aggravate sinus node dysfunction should prompt clinicians to be more judicious in the use of lithium in patients with this condition or who develop sinus arrhythmias in the context of lithium therapy. Pacemaker insertion would usually make the use of lithium safe in such patients, but if lithium actually precipitated sinus node dysfunction, use of valproic acid would be an alternative for an elderly bipolar patient requiring long-term prophylaxis.

PSYCHOSTIMULANTS

Psychostimulants such as methylphenidate, dextroamphetamine, and pemoline may be used for the treatment of depressed, medically debilitated patients (Kaufmann et al. 1982; Kayton and Raskind 1980; S. W. Woods 1986) and cancer patients (Olin and Masand 1996; Weitzner et al. 1995). In addition, methylphenidate has been reported to be effective in the treatment of depression in patients with acquired immunodeficiency syndrome (AIDS) (Fernandez et al. 1988). The dose ranges suggested for methylphenidate vary from 10 to 40 mg/day and for dextroamphetamine from 10 to 20 mg/day given in divided doses early in the day. The half-life for methylphenidate is much shorter than that for dextroamphetamine (2 vs. 12 hours).

Psychostimulants, particularly dextroamphetamine, may cause rebound depression, agitation, psychotic reactions, and dependency (Chiarello and Cole 1987). A less controversial indication for their use is in the treatment of pain in cancer patients to counteract the sedation of narcotics (Goldberg and Tull 1984). In this setting, problems with dependency are moot because most of these patients will have limited life expectancies. Drug interactions are summarized in Table 28–10.

Pemoline is a mild CNS psychostimulant with minimal sympathomimetic activity and a very low abuse potential. Pemoline is used primarily in the treatment of attention-deficit/hyperactivity disorder (ADHD) but also has been shown to have antidepressant (Conners and Taylor 1980) and cognitive-enhancing properties (Elizur et al. 1979; Small et al. 1968; Talland et al. 1967). Pemoline has been reported to be effective in depressed, debilitated cancer patients, with effects similar to those of methylphenidate and dextroamphetamine. The usual dose in adults with medical illness is initially 18.75 mg once or twice a day, which can be increased over several days to 37.5 mg twice a day. Reported side effects include agitation, an-

orexia, and manic behavior. Pemoline may also cause a reversible elevation in liver enzymes as well as more severe hepatic injury. Deaths have been reported (Nehra et al. 1990).

A major advantage of pemoline is that it can be given as a chewable tablet and is reliably absorbed through the buccal mucosa—a route for patients with gastrointestinal motility or absorptive dysfunction (Breitbart and Mermelstein 1992).

CARBAMAZEPINE

Carbamazepine's dose-related toxicities include ataxia, diplopia, and sedation. Several additional toxicities that are particularly relevant when carbamazepine is used in patients with concurrent medical illness include hematological toxicity, hepatic toxicity, hyponatremia, quinidine-like cardiac effects, and effects on the pituitary-thyroid axis.

Carbamazepine may produce a transient reduction in white blood cell (WBC) count in approximately 10% of patients during the first 4 months of treatment (Rall and Schleifer 1985) and in extremely rare cases produces potentially fatal agranulocytosis and aplastic anemia. The incidence of aplastic anemia has been estimated at 0.5 cases per 100,000 treatment-years (Hart and Easton 1982), but neither the age of the patient nor the duration of treatment predicts the development of aplastic anemia (Pisciotta 1975).

Because of the risk of early neutropenia, weekly or biweekly monitoring of WBC count is usually advised during the first few months of therapy. Carbamazepine should usually be discontinued if the WBC count declines to below 3,500. However, exceptions may be necessary if the indications for carbamazepine are very strong or if a concurrent medical problem or drug treatment might be contributing to the decreased blood count. In such situations, hematological consultation will help to determine the appropriate frequency of monitoring and cutoff

Table 28–10. Reported drug interactions with benzodiazepines and psychostimulants

Medication	Interactive effect
Benzodiazepines	
Cimetidine	May elevate serum levels of benzodiazepines metabolized predominantly by oxidation
Disulfiram	
Ethanol	
Isoniazid	
Estrogens	Tend to lower benzodiazepine levels
Cigarettes	
Methylxanthine derivatives	
Rifampin	
Sodium valproate	Enhanced sedative effect of benzodiazepines (not applicable to lorazepam)
Psychostimulants	
Guanethidine	Decreased antihypertensive effect
Vasopressors	Increased pressor effect
Oral anticoagulants	Increased prothrombin time
Anticonvulsants	Increased phenobarbital, primidone, phenytoin levels
Tricyclics	Increased blood levels of cyclic antidepressants
MAOIs	Hypertension

Note. MAOI = monoamine oxidase inhibitor.

point for drug discontinuation. Administration of lithium and carbamazepine lowers the risk for neutropenia because lithium stimulates WBC production. Therefore, the lithium-carbamazepine combination might be an option for patients who have concurrent medical or hematological problems that suppress the WBC count and who have bipolar disorder unresponsive to lithium alone (Brewerton 1986; Vieweg et al. 1986).

Hepatic toxicity from carbamazepine, like hematological toxicity, comes in benign and relatively benign forms as well as in a rare and malignant form. Mild asymptomatic elevations in serum glutamic-oxaloacetic transaminase (SGOT), SGPT, and γ-glutamyl transpeptidase (GGTP) occur in 5%–10% of patients treated with carbamazepine (Jeavons 1983; Pellock 1987). Life-threatening acute hepatitis with liver failure occurs on an allergic basis in fewer than 1 in 10,000 treated patients (Jeavons 1983). This toxicity most often occurs during the first month of therapy. In patients with preexisting liver disease, carbamazepine would be relatively (but not absolutely) contraindicated. However, frequent monitoring of liver enzymes and PT would be a reasonable precaution. In patients without liver disease, elevations of SGOT and SGPT to twice normal levels would generally be acceptable. The upper bounds of transaminase elevation might need to be higher in patients with preexisting hepatic disease who required carbamazepine therapy. Consultation with a gastroenterologist would be indicated to determine both an appropriate schedule for monitoring and criteria for drug discontinuation.

Hyponatremia is a relatively frequent side effect of carbamazepine for which advanced age and higher serum levels are risk factors (Kalff et al. 1984; Lahr 1985; Perucca et al. 1978) and may be aggravated by other conditions predisposing to hyponatremia such as diuretic use, congestive heart failure, and occult malignancy. Patients with risk factors for hyponatremia should have weekly electrolyte measurements during the first month of carbamazepine therapy. If hyponatremia develops, the clinician's response should depend on the severity of the condition, and sodium levels of less than 125 mEq/L would usually be a reason to discontinue carbamazepine. Lesser degrees of hyponatremia should be considered in relation to the necessity of the drug for the patient. In some cases, drugs aggravating hyponatremia, such as diuretics, can be discontinued instead. Persistent hyponatremia after discontinuation of carbamazepine would warrant a full evaluation for inappropriate antidiuretic hormone (ADH) secretion.

Carbamazepine has quinidine-like cardiac effects. Clinically significant aggravation of heart block has been reported (Beerman and Edhag 1978; Benassi et al. 1987). Patients older than 40 years or with known cardiac risk factors should have a pretreatment ECG before receiving carbamazepine.

A major effect of carbamazepine is related to its potent effect on inducing drug metabolism by the hepatic microsomal system (Perucca and Richens 1989), which causes lower serum levels of other drugs metabolized by the liver, including (among many others) TCAs, neuroleptics, propranolol, quinidine, phenytoin, valproic acid, and warfarin. Levels of drugs metabolized by the hepatic microsomal system should probably be obtained more often in patients taking carbamazepine, and repeated levels of the other medications may be needed if carbamazepine doses are significantly changed.

Because carbamazepine is metabolized by the liver, drugs that inhibit the hepatic metabolic enzymes may raise carbamazepine levels and lead to acute carbamazepine toxicity after a new drug is added. These types of clinically significant interactions have been reported for fluoxetine, cimetidine, verapamil (Beattie et al.

1988; MacPhee et al. 1986), diltiazem (Brodie and MacPhee 1986), danazol (Kramer et al. 1986), propoxyphene (Dam et al. 1977), and the antibiotic erythromycin (Wong et al. 1983) and are listed in Table 28–11.

Phenytoin- and carbamazepine-treated patients may have decreased free T_4 and triiodothyronine (T_3) concentrations but appear clinically euthyroid and have normal TSH levels. This effect is explained primarily by the fact that therapeutic levels of phenytoin and carbamazepine displace T_4 and T_3 from serum binding proteins. When added to serum, these drugs effect an *increase* in free hormone fractions and free T_4 and T_3 concentrations. The most likely sequence is that in patients beginning anticonvulsant therapy:

1. A transient *increase* in serum free T_4 concentration
2. A transient decrease in TSH
3. A decrease in total T_4 concentration
4. Normal serum free T_4 concentration
5. Normal steady-state TSH levels

The concentrations of serum free T_4 and free T_3 are essentially unchanged and remain in the normal ranges with long-term therapy with phenytoin and carbamazepine. These findings are based on special techniques using an ultrafiltration assay of free T_4 fractions in undiluted serum, a technique that is not used in most laboratories. Hence, routine measurement of free T_4 will likely show decreased free T_4 concentrations in patients taking phenytoin or carbamazepine. Clinicians should rely on the TSH level to confirm the euthyroid state of these patients (Surks and DeFesi 1996).

VALPROATE

Valproic acid is increasingly being given to patients with bipolar spectrum disorders. The drug's gastrointestinal effects are well known. These problems are markedly reduced by the

Table 28–11. **Reported drug interactions with carbamazepine**

Medication	Interactive effect
Erythromycin	May raise carbamazepine to toxic levels and precipitate heart block
Antiarrhythmics	May have additive effects on cardiac conduction time
Fluoxetine	May raise carbamazepine levels to toxic levels
Cimetidine	
Diltiazem	
Verapamil	
Danazol	
Propoxyphene	
Nefazodone	
Quinidine	Serum levels lowered by carbamazepine
Phenytoin	
Warfarin	
Tricyclic antidepressants	
Neuroleptics	
Propranolol	
Valproate	
Clonazepam	
Phenobarbital	Decreases serum levels of carbamazepine and increases concentrations of carbamazepine's epoxide metabolite
Phenytoin	Decreases levels of carbamazepine; phenytoin levels decrease when used with carbamazepine
Warfarin	Carbamazepine causes increased metabolism of anticoagulants due to hepatic enzyme induction
Oral contraceptives	Carbamazepine reduces efficacy; loss of contraceptive effect possible

availability of enteric-coated preparations and by patients taking the medications after meals. Although hepatic failure was a major concern with valproate in the past, this problem is encountered almost exclusively in children younger than 2 years. The incidence of valproate-related hepatic necrosis in adults is less than 1 in 10,000 (Eadie et al. 1988). In adults, serum ammonia may be elevated as a result of inhibition of urea synthesis, but this effect is almost always benign and is of concern only in patients with preexisting liver disease. Significant liver disease is a relative contraindication to valproate treatment. One review found that between 1987 and 1993, fatal hepatotoxicity from anticonvulsant *monotherapy* with valproate occurred in only one

patient older than 20; the chances of hepatotoxicity increase by a factor of 6 with anticonvulsant polytherapy. Risk factors for valproate hepatotoxicity include children younger than 10 years, polytherapy, developmental delays, and coincident metabolic disorders (such as cytochrome and oxidase deficiency) (Bryant and Dreifuss 1996). The drug appears to be safe and effective in the elderly (Puryear et al. 1995).

Valproate can increase the PT and decrease fibrinogen levels and platelet counts, but such effects very rarely lead to clinically significant bleeding (Stoudemire et al. 1991). Patients should have a coagulation panel (PT/partial thromboplastin time [PTT]) and a platelet count before undergoing surgery.

With respect to drug interactions, valproate tends to inhibit hepatic enzymes involved in drug metabolism. This effect is in contrast to that of carbamazepine, which is a hepatic enzyme inducer. Hence, the capacity for carbamazepine toxicity is increased when the two drugs are used together. In addition, valproate may displace carbamazepine from serum protein-binding sites, which increases the bioavailable fraction of carbamazepine but does not change the absolute blood level; thus, side effects may increase at a given carbamazepine level.

With valproate, protein-binding sites are readily saturated. Dose increases beyond the point of saturation may lead to enhanced side effects, even though dose increases are relatively small and absolute serum levels increase only slightly. Drug interactions with valproate are listed in Tables 28–12 and 28–13 (Abbott Laboratories data). More detailed discussions of the use of valproate in the medical patient may be found elsewhere (Fogel and Stoudemire 1993; Stoudemire et al. 1991, 1993).

ECT IN MEDICALLY ILL PATIENTS

ECT should be considered as a primary treatment for many severely depressed medically ill patients. In medically debilitated depressed patients and those with advanced cardiovascular disease, appropriate pharmacological management before and during anesthesia can usually attenuate the autonomic responses (i.e., hypertension and tachycardia) that pose the primary risks for elderly patients with cerebrovascular or cardiovascular disease. Advanced technical reviews of the use of ECT and special anesthetic considerations in medically ill patients may be found elsewhere (Knos and Sung 1991, 1993; Silver et al. 1986).

Table 28–12.   **Reported drug interactions with valproate**

Medication	Interactive effect
Benzodiazepines (except lorazepam)	Sedative effects and serum levels of benzodiazepine increased by valproate
Carbamazepine Phenytoin Phenobarbital	Lower levels of valproate
Phenobarbital	Phenobarbital levels increased by valproate
Phenytoin Carbamazepine	Bioavailable phenytoin and carbamazepine increased by valproate by displacing these drugs from serum protein-binding sites
10-11-Epoxide metabolite of carbamazepine	This metabolite's levels increased by valproate
Tricyclic antidepressants (TCAs)	TCA levels increased by valproate
Chlorpromazine Cimetidine Salicylates	Increase levels of valproate
Anticoagulants (warfarin)	Increase prothrombin times; valproate also inhibits secondary phase of platelet aggregation

Table 28–13. **Effects of valproate on other drugs: potentially important interactions**

Drug administered with divalproex sodium	Interaction
Carbamazepine	Serum levels of carbamazepine decreased by 17%
10,11-Epoxide	Levels of carbamazepine-10,11-epoxide increased by 45% in patients with epilepsy taking valproate and carbamazepine.
Clonazepam	Concomitant use with valproic acid may induce absence status in patients with a history of absence-type seizures.
Diazepam	Valproate displaced diazepam from plasma albumin-binding sites and inhibited its metabolism. Coadministration of valproate 1,500 mg/day to healthy volunteers increased the free fraction of diazepam (10 mg) by 90%; diazepam plasma clearance decreased by 25% and volume of distribution by 20%. Elimination half-life of diazepam did not change.
Ethosuximide	Valproate inhibited ethosuximide metabolism. Administration of a single 500-mg dose of ethosuximide with valproate (800–1,600 mg/day) to healthy volunteers increased ethosuximide elimination half-life by 25% and decreased its total clearance by 15%. Serum levels of both drugs should be monitored in patients receiving valproate and ethosuximide, especially with other anticonvulsants.
Lamotrigine	Coadministration of valproate to healthy volunteers increased lamotrigine elimination half-life from 26 to 70 hours. The dose of lamotrigine should be reduced when coadministered with valproate.
Phenobarbital	Valproate inhibited phenobarbital metabolism, resulting in a 50% increase in phenobarbital half-life and a 30% decrease in plasma clearance. The fraction of phenobarbital dose excreted unchanged increased by 50%. There is evidence for severe central nervous system depression, with or without significant elevations of barbiturate or valproate serum concentrations. All patients receiving concomitant barbiturate therapy should be monitored closely for neurological toxicity.
Primidone	Primidone is metabolized to a barbiturate and may be involved in a similar interaction with valproate.
Phenytoin	Valproate displaced phenytoin from its plasma albumin-binding sites and inhibited its hepatic metabolism. Coadministration of valproate 400 mg twice a day with phenytoin 250 mg to healthy volunteers increased the free fraction of phenytoin by 60%; total plasma clearance and apparent volume of distribution increased by 30%. Both the clearance and the apparent volume of distribution of free phenytoin were reduced by 25%. In patients with epilepsy, breakthrough seizures have occurred with the combination of valproate and phenytoin.
Tolbutamide	In vitro, the unbound fraction of tolbutamide was increased from 20% to 50% when added to plasma samples from patients treated with valproate. The clinical relevance of this displacement is unknown.

(continued)

Table 28–13.   **Effects of valproate on other drugs: potentially important interactions** *(continued)*

Drug administered with divalproex sodium	Interaction
Warfarin	The potential exists for valproate to displace warfarin from its plasma albumin-binding sites. The therapeutic relevance of this displacement is unknown; coagulation tests should be monitored if divalproex sodium is initiated in patients taking anticoagulants.
Zidovudine	In HIV-positive patients, the clearance of zidovudine 100 mg every 8 hours decreased by 38% after administration of valproate 250 or 500 mg every 8 hours; zidovudine half-life was unaffected.

Source.   Reprinted from "Advancing the Treatment of Mania Associated With Bipolar Disorder." North Chicago, IL, Abbott Laboratories, 1995.

REFERENCES

Abernethy DR, Greenblatt DJ, Shader RI: Imipramine and desipramine disposition in the elderly. J Pharmacol Exp Ther 232:183–188, 1985

Ahmed I, Dagincourt PG, Miller LG, et al: Possible interaction between fluoxetine and pimozide causing sinus bradycardia. Can J Psychiatry 38:62–63, 1993

Alderman CP, Moritz CK, Ben-Tovim DI: Abnormal platelet aggregation associated with fluoxetine therapy. Ann Pharmacother 26:1517–1519, 1992

Ali BH: Effect of some monoamine oxidase inhibitors on the thiamine status of rabbits. Br J Pharmacol 86:869–875, 1985

Andersen BB, Mikkelsen M, Vesterager A, et al: No influence of the antidepressant paroxetine on carbamazepine, valproate and phenytoin. Epilepsy Res 10:201–204, 1991

Antal EJ, Lawson IR, Alderson LM, et al: Estimating steady-state desipramine levels in noninstitutionalized elderly patients using single dose disposition parameters. J Clin Psychopharmacol 2:193–198, 1982

Arya DK, Szabadi E: Dyskinesia associated with fluvoxamine (letter). J Clin Psychopharmacol 13:365–366, 1993

Baldessarini R, Marsh E: Fluoxetine and side effects (letter). Arch Gen Psychiatry 47:191–192, 1990

Baldwin D, Fineberg N, Montgomery S: Fluoxetine, fluvoxamine and extrapyramidal tract disorders. Int Clin Psychopharmacol 6:51–58, 1991

Bannister SJ, Houser VP, Hulse JD, et al: Evaluation of the potential for interactions of paroxetine with diazepam, cimetidine, warfarin, and digoxin. Acta Psychiatr Scand 80 (suppl 350):102–106, 1989

Barros J, Asnis G: An interaction of sertraline and desipramine (letter). Am J Psychiatry 150:1751, 1993

Beattie B, Biller J, Mehlhaus B, et al: Verapamil-induced carbamazepine neurotoxicity: a report of two cases. Eur Neurol 28:104–105, 1988

Beerman B, Edhag O: Depressive effects of carbamazepine on idioventricular rhythm in man. BMJ 2:171–172, 1978

Benassi E, Bo GP, Cociot L, et al: Carbamazepine and cardiac conduction disturbances. Ann Neurol 22:280–281, 1987

Benfield P, Ward A: Fluvoxamine: a review of its pharmacodynamic and pharmacokinetic properties, and therapeutic efficacy in depressive illness. Drugs 32:313–334, 1986

Bergstrom RF, Peyton AL, Lemberger L: Quantification and mechanism of fluoxetine and tricyclic antidepressant interaction. Clin Pharmacol Ther 51:239–248, 1992

Bertschy G, Vandel S, Bandel B, et al: Fluvoxamine-tricyclic antidepressant interaction. Eur J Clin Pharmacol 40:119–120, 1991

Braverman B, McCarthy RJ, Ivankovich AD: Vasopressor challenges during chronic MAOI or TCA treatment in anesthetized dogs. Life Sci 40:2587–2595, 1987

Breitbart W, Mermelstein H: Pemoline: an alternative psychostimulant for the management of depressive disorders in cancer patients. Psychosomatics 33:352–356, 1992

Brewerton TD: Lithium counteracts carbamazepine-induced leukopenia while increasing its therapeutic effect. Biol Psychiatry 21:677–685, 1986

Brodie MM, MacPhee GJA: Carbamazepine neurotoxicity precipitated by diltiazem. BMJ 292:1170–1171, 1986

Bryant AE, Dreifuss FE: Valproic acid hepatic fatalities, III: U.S. experience since 1986. Neurology 46:465–469, 1996

Burley DM: A brief note on the problem of epilepsy in antidepressant treatment, in Depression—The Biochemical and Physiologic Role of Ludiomil. Edited by Jukes A. Newark, NJ, Ciba, 1977, pp 201–203

Centorrino F, Baldessarini RJ, Kando J, et al: Serum concentrations of clozapine and its major metabolites: effects of cotreatment with fluoxetine or valproate. Am J Psychiatry 151:123–125, 1994

Chiarello RJ, Cole JO: The use of psychostimulants in general psychiatry: a reconsideration. Arch Gen Psychiatry 44:286–295, 1987

Ciraulo DA, Shader RI: Fluoxetine drug-drug interactions, I: antidepressants and antipsychotics. J Clin Psychopharmacol 10:48–50, 1990

Clary C, Schweizer E: Treatment of MAOI hypertensive crisis with sublingual nifedipine. J Clin Psychiatry 48:249–250, 1987

Conners K, Taylor E: Pemoline, methylphenidate and placebo in children with minimal brain dysfunction. Arch Gen Psychiatry 37:923–930, 1980

Cooper GL: The safety of fluoxetine—an update. Br J Psychiatry 153 (suppl 3):77–86, 1988

Cutler NR, Narang PK: Implications of dosing tricyclic antidepressants and benzodiazepines in geriatrics. Psychiatr Clin North Am 7:845–861, 1984

Cutler NR, Zavadil AP III, Eisdorfer C: Concentrations of desipramine in elderly women are not elevated. Am J Psychiatry 138:1235–1237, 1981

Dam M, Kristensen CB, Hensen BS, et al: Interaction between carbamazepine and propoxyphene in man. Acta Neurol Scand 56:603–607, 1977

Dave M: Fluoxetine-associated dystonia (letter). Am J Psychiatry 151:149, 1994

Davidson J: Seizures and bupropion: a review. J Clin Psychiatry 50:256–261, 1989

Dawling S, Lynn K, Rosser R, et al: Nortriptyline metabolism in chronic renal failure: metabolite elimination. Clin Pharmacol Ther 32:322–329, 1982

deBoer T: The pharmacologic profile of mirtazapine. J Clin Psychiatry 57 (suppl 4): 19–25, 1996

DePaulo JR: Lithium. Psychiatr Clin North Am 7: 587–599, 1984

Eadie MJ, Hooper WD, Dickinson RG: Valproate-associated hepatotoxicity and its biochemical mechanisms. Medical Toxicology Adverse Drug Experience 3:85–106, 1988

Edwards JG: Antidepressants and seizures: epidemiological and clinical aspects, in The Psychopharmacology of Epilepsy. Edited by Trimble MR. Chichester, England, Wiley, 1985, pp 119–139

Edwards JG, Long SK, Sedgwick EM, et al: Antidepressants and convulsive seizures: clinical, electroencephalographic, and pharmacological aspects. Clin Neuropharmacol 9:329–360, 1986

El Ganzouri AR, Ivankovich AD, Braverman B, et al: Monoamine inhibitors: should they be discontinued pre-operatively? Anesth Analg 64: 592–596, 1985

Elizur A, Wintner I, Davidson S: The clinical and psychological effects of pemoline in depressed patients: a controlled study. International Pharmacopsychiatry 14:127–134, 1979

Epstein AE, Hallstrom AP, Rogers WJ, et al: Mortality following ventricular arrhythmia suppression by encainide, flecainide, and moricizine after myocardial infarction. JAMA 270: 2451–2455, 1993

Falk WE: Trazodone and priapism. Biological Therapies in Psychiatry 10:9–10, 1987

Feighner JP: Cardiovascular safety in depressed patients: focus on venlafaxine. J Clin Psychiatry 56:574–579, 1995

Feighner JP, Herbstein J, Damlouji N: Combined MAOI, TCA, and direct stimulant therapy of treatment-resistant depression. J Clin Psychiatry 46:206–209, 1985

Fernandez F, Adams F, Levy JK, et al: Cognitive impairment due to AIDS-related complex and its response to psychostimulants. Psychosomatics 29:38–46, 1988

Fisch C: Effect of fluoxetine on the electrocardiogram. J Clin Psychiatry 46:42–44, 1985

Fogel BS, Stoudemire A: New psychotropics in medically ill patients, in Medical-Psychiatric Practice, Vol 2. Edited by Stoudemire A, Fogel BS. Washington, DC, American Psychiatric Press, 1993, pp 69–111

Fricchione GL, Vlay SC: Psychiatric aspects of patients with malignant ventricular arrhythmias. Am J Psychiatry 143:1518–1526, 1986

Fritze J, Unsorg B, Lanczik M: Interaction between carbamazepine and fluvoxamine. Acta Psychiatr Scand 84:538–584, 1991

Gammans RE, Westrick ML, Shea JP, et al: Pharmacokinetics of buspirone in elderly subjects. J Clin Pharmacol 29:72–78, 1989

Gardner DM, Shulman KI, Walker SE, et al: The making of a user friendly MAOI diet. J Clin Psychiatry 57:99–104, 1996

Garner SJ, Eldridge FL, Wagner PG, et al: Buspirone, an anxiolytic drug that stimulates respiration. American Review of Respiratory Disease 139:946–950, 1989

Georgotas A, McCue RE, Friedman E, et al: A placebo-controlled comparison of the effect of nortriptyline and phenelzine on orthostatic hypotension in elderly depressed patients. J Clin Psychopharmacol 7:413–416, 1987

Gidal BE, Aderson GD, Seaton TL, et al: Evaluation of the effect of fluoxetine on the formation of carbamazepine epoxide. Ther Drug Monit 15:405–409, 1993

Glassman AH, Johnson LL, Giardina EV, et al: The use of imipramine in depressed patients with congestive heart failure. JAMA 250:1977–2001, 1983

Glassman AH, Roose SP, Bigger JT: The safety of tricyclic antidepressants in cardiac patients: risk-benefit reconsidered. JAMA 269:2673–2675, 1993

Glassman JN, Dugas JE, Tsuang MT: Idiosyncratic pharmacokinetics complicating treatment of major depression in an elderly woman. J Nerv Ment Dis 173:573–576, 1985

Goff DC, Midha KK, Brotman AW, et al: Elevation of plasma concentrations of haloperidol after the addition of fluoxetine. Am J Psychiatry 148:790–792, 1991

Goldberg RG, Tull RM: Psychosocial Dimensions of Cancer: A Practical Guide for Health Care Providers. New York, Free Press, 1984, pp 111–169

Grad RM: Benzodiazepines for insomnia in community-dwelling elderly: a review of benefit and risk. J Fam Pract 41:473–481, 1995

Grant R, Grant C (eds): Grant and Hackh's Chemical Dictionary, 5th Edition. New York, McGraw-Hill, 1987, p 282

Greb WH, Buscher G, Dierdorf H-D, et al: Effect of liver enzyme inhibition by cimetidine and enzyme induction by phenobarbitone on the pharmacokinetics of paroxetine. Acta Psychiatr Scand 80 (suppl 350):95–98, 1989

Greenblatt DJ, Divoll M, Abernethy DR, et al: Benzodiazepine kinetics: implications for therapeutics and pharmacogeriatrics. Drug Metab Rev 14:251–292, 1983

Greenblatt DJ, Preskorn SH, Cotreau MM, et al: Fluoxetine impairs clearance of alprazolam but not of clonazepam. Clin Pharmacol Ther 52:479–486, 1992

Grimsley SR, Jann MW, Carter JG, et al: Increased carbamazepine plasma concentrations after fluoxetine coadministration. Clin Pharmacol Ther 50:10–15, 1991

Hansen-Grant S, Silk KR, Guthrie S: Fluoxetine-pimozide interaction (letter). Am J Psychiatry 150:1751–1752, 1993

Hardy BG, Shulman KI, MacKenzie SE, et al: Pharmacokinetics of lithium in the elderly. J Clin Psychopharmacol 7:153–158, 1987

Harpe C, Stoudemire A: Aetiology and treatment of the neuroleptic malignant syndrome. Medical Toxicology Adverse Drug Experience 2:166–176, 1987

Hart RG, Easton JD: Carbamazepine and hematological monitoring. Ann Neurol 11:309–312, 1982

Hoyberg OJ, Maragakis B, Mullin J, et al: A double-blind multicentre comparison of mirtazapine and amitriptyline in elderly depressed patients. Acta Psychiatr Scand 93:184–190, 1996

Hunt N, Stern TA: The association between intravenous haloperidol and torsades de pointes. Psychosomatics 36:541–549, 1995

Jeavons PM: Hepatoxicity in antiepileptic drugs, in Chronic Toxicity of Antiepileptic Drugs. Edited by Oxley J, Janz D, Meinardi H. New York, Raven, 1983, pp 1–46

Jefferson JW: A review of the cardiovascular effects and toxicity of tricyclic antidepressants. Psychosom Med 37:160–179, 1975

Jefferson JW: Just what is a heterocyclic antidepressant? (letter) J Clin Psychiatry 56:433, 1995

Kalff R, Houtkooper HA, Meyer JWA, et al: Carbamazepine and sodium levels. Epilepsia 25:390–397, 1984

Kapur S, Remington G: Serotonin-dopamine interaction and its relevance to schizophrenia. Am J Psychiatry 153:466–476, 1996

Katz SE: Possible paroxetine-zolpidem interaction (letter). Am J Psychiatry 152:1689, 1995

Kaufmann MW, Murray GB, Cassem NH: Use of psychostimulants in medically ill depressed patients. Psychosomatics 23:817–819, 1982

Kayton W, Raskind M: Treatment of depression in the medically ill elderly with methylphenidate. Am J Psychiatry 137:963–965, 1980

Knos GB, Sung Y-F: Anesthetic management of the high-risk medical patient receiving electroconvulsive therapy, in Medical Psychiatric Practice, Vol 1. Edited by Stoudemire A, Fogel BS. Washington, DC, American Psychiatric Press, 1991, pp 99–144

Knos GB, Sung Y-F: ECT anesthesia strategies in the high risk medical patient, in Psychiatric Care of the Medical Patient. Edited by Stoudemire A, Fogel BS. New York, Oxford University Press, 1993, pp 225–240

Kraft K, Dore F: Computerized drug interaction programs: how reliable? (letter) JAMA 275:1087, 1996

Kramer G, Theisohn M, von Unruh GE, et al: Carbamazepine-danazol interaction: its mechanism examined by a stable isotope technique. Ther Drug Monit 8:387–392, 1986

Lahr MB: Hyponatremia during carbamazepine therapy. Clin Pharmacol Ther 37:693–696, 1985

Lakshminarayan S, Sahn SA, Hudson LD, et al: Effect of diazepam on ventilatory responses. Clin Pharmacol Ther 20:178–183, 1976

Lasher TA, Fleishaker JC, Steenwyk RC, et al: Pharmacokinetic pharmacodynamic evaluation of the combined administration of alprazolam and fluoxetine. Psychopharmacology 104:323–327, 1991

Lemberger L, Rowe H, Bosomworth JC, et al: The effect of fluoxetine on the pharmacokinetics and psychomotor responses of diazepam. Clin Pharmacol Ther 43:412–419, 1988

Lemoine A, Gautier JC, Azoulay D, et al: Major pathway of imipramine metabolism is catalyzed by cytochromes P-450 1A2 and P-450 3A4 in human liver. Mol Pharmacol 43:827–832, 1993

Levine RL: Pharmacology of intravenous sedatives and opioids in critically ill patients. Crit Care Clin 10:709–731, 1994

Levy NG: Chronic renal failure, in Psychiatric Care of the Medical Patient. Edited by Stoudemire A, Fogel BS. New York, Oxford University Press, 1993, pp 627–635

Levy NG, Blumenfield M, Beasley CM, et al: Fluoxetine in depressed patients with renal failure and in depressed patients with normal kidney function. Gen Hosp Psychiatry 18:8–13, 1996

Lieberman E, Stoudemire A: Use of tricyclic antidepressants in patients with glaucoma. Psychosomatics 28:145–148, 1987

Lieberman JA, Cooper TB, Suckow RF, et al: Tricyclic antidepressant and metabolite levels in chronic renal failure. Clin Pharmacol Ther 37:301–307, 1985

Lock JD, Gwirtsman HE, Targ EF: Possible adverse drug interactions between fluoxetine and other psychotropics. J Clin Psychopharmacol 10:383–384, 1990

Luchins DJ, Oliver AP, Wyatt RJ: Seizures with antidepressants: an in vitro technique to assess relative risk. Epilepsia 25:25–32, 1984

MacPhee GJ, McInnes GT, Thompson GG, et al: Verapamil potentiates carbamazepine neurotoxicity: a clinically important inhibitory interaction. Lancet 1(8483):700–703, 1986

Malek-Ahmadi P, Allen SA: Paroxetine-molindone interaction. J Clin Psychiatry 56:82–83, 1995

Markovitz PJ: Treatment of anxiety in the elderly. J Clin Psychiatry 54 (suppl):64–80, 1993

Markowitz J, Brewerton T: Zolpidem-induced psychosis. Ann Clin Psychiatry 8:89–91, 1996

Mendelson WB: Neuropharmacology of sleep induction by benzodiazepines. Crit Rev Neurobiol 6:221–232, 1992

Mendelson WB, Martin JV, Rapoport D, et al: Buspirone: stimulation of respiratory rate in freely moving rats (abstract). Sleep Research 18:62, 1989

Meyer BR: Benzodiazepines in the elderly. Med Clin North Am 66:1017–1035, 1982

Minden SL, Bassuk EL, Nadler SP: Lithium intoxication: a coordinated treatment approach. J Gen Intern Med 8:33–40, 1993

Mitchell J, Popkin M: The pathophysiology of sexual dysfunction associated with antipsychotic drug therapy in males: a review. Arch Sex Behav 12:173–183, 1983

Mittal SR, Mathur AK, Advani GB: Genesis of lithium-induced T wave flattening. Int J Cardiol 7:164–166, 1985

Modeo DG, Berry DJ: Effects of chlordiazepoxide in respiratory failure due to chronic bronchitis. Lancet 2:869–870, 1974

Morganroth J, Goin JE: Quinidine-related mortality in the short-to-medium-term treatment of ventricular arrhythmias: a meta-analysis. Circulation 84:1977–1983, 1991

Morris HH, Estes ML: Traveler's amnesia: transient global amnesia secondary to triazolam. JAMA 258:945–946, 1987

Musser WS, Akil M: Clozapine as a treatment for psychosis in Parkinson's disease: a review. J Neuropsychiatry Clin Neurosci 8:1–9, 1996

Nehra A, Mullick F, Ishak KG, et al: Pemoline-associated hepatic injury. Gastroenterology 99: 1517–1519, 1990

Neshkes RE, Gerner R, Jarvik LF, et al: Orthostatic effect of imipramine and doxepin in depressed geriatric outpatients. J Clin Psychopharmacol 5:102–106, 1985

Nicholson SD: Extra pyramidal side effects associated with paroxetine. West of England Medical Journal 7(3):90–91, 1992

Nies A, Robinson DS, Friedman MJ, et al: Relationship between age and tricyclic antidepressant plasma levels. Am J Psychiatry 134:790–793, 1977

Ohmori S, Takeda S, Rikihisa T, et al: Studies on cytochrome P450 responsible for oxidative metabolism of imipramine in human liver microsomes. Biol Pharm Bull 16:571–575, 1993

Olin J, Masand P: Psychostimulants for depression in hospitalized cancer patients. Psychosomatics 37:57–62, 1996

Parker SP (ed): McGraw-Hill Encyclopedia of Chemistry, 2nd Edition. New York, McGraw-Hill, 1993, p 472

Pellock JM: Carbamazepine side effects in children and adults. Epilepsia 28 (suppl 3):S64–S70, 1987

Perucca E, Richens A: General principles: biotransformation, in Antiepileptic Drugs, 3rd Edition. Edited by Levy R, Mattson R, Meldrum B, et al. New York, Raven, 1989, pp 23–48

Perucca E, Garratt A, Hebdige S, et al: Water intoxication in epileptic patients receiving carbamazepine. J Neurol Neurosurg Psychiatry 41: 713–718, 1978

Pierce MW, Shu VS: Efficacy of estazolam: the United States clinical experience. Am J Med 88 (suppl 3A):6S–11S, 1990

Pisciotta AV: Hematological toxicity of carbamazepine. Adv Neurol 11:355–368, 1975

Preskorn SH, Othmer SC: Evaluation of bupropion hydrochloride: the first of a new class of atypical antidepressants. Pharmacotherapy 4:20–34, 1984

Puryear LJ, Kunik ME, Workman R Jr: Tolerability of divalproex sodium in elderly psychiatric patients with mixed diagnoses. J Geriatr Psychiatry Neurol 8:234–237, 1995

Rall TW, Schleifer LS: Drugs effective in the therapy of the epilepsies, in The Pharmacological Basis of Therapeutics, 7th Edition. Edited by Gilman AG, Goodman LS, Rall TW, et al. New York, Macmillan, 1985, pp 446–472

Rapeport WG, Coates PE, Dewland PM, et al: Absence of a sertraline-mediated effect on digoxin pharmacokinetics and electrocardiographic findings. J Clin Psychiatry 57 (suppl 1):16–19, 1996a

Rapeport WG, Muirhead DC, Williams SA, et al: Absence of effect of sertraline on the pharmacokinetics and pharmacodynamics of phenytoin. J Clin Psychiatry 57 (suppl 1):24–28, 1996b

Rapeport WG, Williams SA, Muirhead DC, et al: Absence of a sertraline-mediated effect on the pharmacokinetics and pharmacodynamics of carbamazepine. J Clin Psychiatry 57 (suppl 1): 20–23, 1996c

Rapoport DM: Buspirone: anxiolytic therapy with respiratory implications. Family Practice Recertification 11 (suppl):33–41, 1989

Rapoport DM, Greenberg HE, Goldring RM: Comparison of the effects of buspirone and diazepam on control of breathing (abstract). Federation of American Societies for Experimental Biology 2:A1507, 1988

Regan WM, Margolin RA, Mathew RJ: Cardiac arrhythmia following rapid imipramine withdrawal. Biol Psychiatry 25:482–484, 1989

Richelson E: Review of antidepressants in the treatment of mood disorders, in Current Psychiatric Therapy. Edited by Dunner DL. Philadelphia, PA, WB Saunders, 1993, pp 232–238

Rickels K, Fox IL, Greenblatt DJ, et al: Clorazepate and lorazepam: clinical improvement and rebound anxiety. Am J Psychiatry 145:312–317, 1988

Rizos AL, Sargenti CJ, Jeste DV: Psychotropic drug interactions in the patient with late-onset depression or psychosis, part 2. Psychiatr Clin North Am 11:253–277, 1988

Roberts HE, Dean RC, Stoudemire A: Clozapine treatment of psychosis in Parkinson's disease. J Neuropsychiatry Clin Neurosci 1:190–192, 1989

Robinson DS, Kurtz NM: Question the experts: what is the degree of risk of hepatotoxicity for depressed patients receiving phenelzine therapy? J Clin Psychopharmacol 7:61–62, 1987

Rockwell E, Lam RW, Zisook S: Antidepressant drug studies in the elderly. Psychiatr Clin North Am 11:215–233, 1988

Roose SP, Glassman AH, Siris S, et al: Comparison of imipramine- and nortriptyline-induced orthostatic hypotension: a meaningful difference. J Clin Psychopharmacol 1:316–319, 1981

Roose SP, Glassman AH, Giardina EGV, et al: Nortriptyline in depressed patients with left ventricular impairment. JAMA 256:3253–3257, 1986

Roose SP, Glassman AH, Giardina EGV, et al: Tricyclic antidepressants in depressed patients with cardiac conduction disease. Arch Gen Psychiatry 44:273–275, 1987

Rowe H, Carmichael R, Lemberger L: The effect of fluoxetine on warfarin metabolism in the rat and man. Life Sci 23:807–812, 1978

Rush CR, Griffiths RR: Zolpidem, triazolam, and temazepam: behavioral and subject-rated effects in normal volunteers. J Clin Psychopharmacol 16:146–157, 1996

Schwartz P, Wolf S: QT interval prolongation as predictor of sudden death in patients with myocardial infarction. Circulation 57:1074–1077, 1978

Silver JM, Yudofsky SC, Kogan M, et al: Elevation of thioridazine plasma levels by propranolol. Am J Psychiatry 143:1290–1292, 1986

Simeon J, Spero M, Fink M: Clinical and EEG studies of doxepin. Psychosomatics 10:14–17, 1969

Small IF, Sharpley P, Small JG: Influence of Cylert upon memory changes with ECT. Am J Psychiatry 125:837–840, 1968

Sommi RW, Crismon ML, Bowden CL, et al: Fluoxetine: a serotonin-specific second-generation antidepressant. Pharmacotherapy 7:1–15, 1987

Sovner R, Davis JM: A potential drug interaction between fluoxetine and valproic acid (letter). J Clin Psychopharmacol 11:389, 1991

Sperber AD: Toxic interaction between fluvoxamine and sustained release theophylline in an 11-year-old boy. Drug Saf 6:460–462, 1991

Spina E, Avenoso A, Pollicino AM, et al: Carbamazepine coadministration with fluoxetine or fluvoxamine. Ther Drug Monit 15:247–250, 1993a

Spina E, Pollicino AM, Avenoso A, et al: Effect of fluvoxamine on the pharmacokinetics of imipramine and desipramine in healthy subjects. Ther Drug Monit 15:243–246, 1993b

Spina E, Pollicino AM, Avenoso A, et al: Fluvoxamine-induced alterations in plasma concentrations of imipramine and desipramine in depressed patients. Int J Clin Pharmacol Res 13:167–171, 1993c

Stack CG, Rogers P, Linter SPK: Monoamine oxidase inhibitors and anaesthesia. Br J Anaesth 60:222–227, 1988

Steckler TL: Lithium- and carbamazepine-associated sinus node dysfunction: nine-year experience in a psychiatric hospital. J Clin Psychopharmacol 14:336–339, 1994

Steur ENHJ: Increase of Parkinson disability after fluoxetine medication. Neurology 43:211–213, 1993

Stoudemire A, Atkinson P: Use of cyclic antidepressants in patients with cardiac conduction disturbances. Gen Hosp Psychiatry 10:389–397, 1988

Stoudemire A, Fogel BS: Psychopharmacology in the medically ill, in Principles of Medical Psychiatry. Edited by Stoudemire A, Fogel BS. Orlando, FL, Grune & Stratton, 1987, pp 79–112

Stoudemire A, Luther J: Neuroleptic malignant syndrome and neuroleptic-induced catatonia: differential diagnosis and treatment. Int J Psychiatry Med 14:57–63, 1984

Stoudemire A, Fogel BS, Gulley LR: Psychopharmacology in the medically ill: an update, in Medical Psychiatric Practice, Vol 1. Edited by Stoudemire A, Fogel BS. Washington, DC, American Psychiatric Press, 1991, pp 29–97

Stoudemire A, Fogel BS, Gulley LR, et al: Psychopharmacology in the medically ill, in Psychiatric Care of the Medical Patient. Edited by Stoudemire A, Fogel BS. New York, Oxford University Press, 1993, pp 155–206

Strouse TB, Skotzko CE, Fawzy FI: Absence of adverse drug interactions between fluoxetine and cyclosporine in organ transplant recipients (Abstract 46). Presented at the annual meeting of the Academy of Psychosomatic Medicine, New Orleans, LA, November 1993, p 19

Surks MI, DeFesi CR: Normal serum free thyroid hormone concentrations in patients treated with phenytoin or carbamazepine: a paradox resolved. JAMA 275:1495–1498, 1996

Talland GA, Hagen DQ, James M: Performance tests of amnestic patients with Cylert. J Nerv Ment Dis 144:421–429, 1967

Tarsy D: Risperidone and neuroleptic malignant syndrome (letter). JAMA 275:446, 1996

Tate JL: Extrapyramidal symptoms in a patient taking haloperidol and fluoxetine. Am J Psychiatry 146:399–400, 1989

Taylor DP, Carter RB, Eison AS, et al: Pharmacology and neurochemistry of nefazodone, a novel antidepressant drug. J Clin Psychiatry 56 (suppl 6):3–11, 1995

Teo KK, Yusuf S, Furberg CD: Effects of prophylactic antiarrhythmic drug therapy in acute myocardial infarction. JAMA 270:1589–1595, 1993

Thompson TL II, Moran MG, Nies AS: Psychotropic drug use in the elderly. N Engl J Med 308:134–138, 194–199, 1983

Tilkian JG, Schroeder JS, Kao JJ, et al: The cardiovascular effects of lithium in man. Am J Med 61:665–670, 1976a

Tilkian JG, Schroeder JS, Kao J, et al: Effect of lithium on cardiovascular performance: a report on extended ambulatory monitoring and exercise testing before and during lithium. Am J Cardiol 38:701–798, 1976b

Trimble M: Non-monoamine oxidase inhibitor antidepressants and epilepsy: a review. Epilepsia 19:241–250, 1978

Trinidad A, Silver PA: Use of psychotropic medication in the neurologically ill, in Psychotropic Drug Use in the Medically Ill. Edited by Silver PA. Adv Psychosom Med 21:61–89, 1994

van Harten J, Holland RL, Wesnes K: Influence of multiple-dose administration of fluvoxamine on the pharmacokinetics of the benzodiazepines bromazepam and lorazepam: a randomised, cross-over study (abstract). Eur Neuropsychopharmacol 2:381, 1992a

van Harten J, Holland RL, Wesnes K, et al: Kinetic and dynamic interaction study between fluvoxamine and benzodiazepines. Poster presented at the Second Jerusalem Conference on Pharmaceutical Sciences and Clinical Pharmacology, Jerusalem, Israel, May 24–29, 1992b

Van Sweden B: Rebound antidepressant cardiac arrhythmia. Biol Psychiatry 24:360–369, 1988

Vieweg WVR, Yank GR, Row WT, et al: Increase in white blood cell count and serum sodium level following the addition of lithium to carbamazepine treatment among three chronically psychotic male patients with disturbed affective states. Psychiatr Q 58:213–217, 1986

von Moltke LL, Greenblatt DJ, Harmatz JS, et al: Cytochromes in psychopharmacology (editorial). J Clin Psychopharmacol 14:1–4, 1994

Walley T, Pirmohamed M, Proudlove C, et al: Interaction of metoprolol and fluoxetine (letter). Lancet 341:967–968, 1993

Wamsley JK, Hunt ME: Relative affinity of quazepam for type-1 benzodiazepine receptors. J Clin Psychiatry 52 (suppl):15–20, 1991

Warrington SJ: Clinical implications of the pharmacology of sertraline. Int Clin Psychopharmacol 6 (suppl 2):11–21, 1991

Weitzner MA, Meyers CA, Valentine AD: Methylphenidate in the treatment of neurobehavioral slowing associated with cancer and cancer treatment. J Neuropsychiatry Clin Neurosci 7: 347–350, 1995

Wells DG, Bjorksten AR: Monoamine oxidase inhibitors revisited. Can J Anaesth 36:64–74, 1989

Wilner KD, Lazar JD, Apseloff G, et al: The effects of sertraline on the pharmacodynamics of warfarin in healthy volunteers (abstract). Biol Psychiatry 29:354S–355S, 1991

Wils V: Extrapyramidal symptoms in a patient treated with fluvoxamine (letter). J Neurol Neurosurg Psychiatry 55:330–331, 1992

Wong YY, Ludden TM, Bell RD: Effect of erythromycin on carbamazepine kinetics. Clin Pharmacol Ther 33:460–464, 1983

Woods DJ, Coulter DM, Pillans P: Interaction of phenytoin and fluoxetine (letter). N Z Med J 107(970):19, 1994

Woods SW: Psychostimulant treatment of depressive disorders secondary to medical illness. J Clin Psychiatry 47:12–15, 1986

Ziegler MG, Wilner KD: Sertraline does not alter the beta-adrenergic blocking activity of atenolol in healthy male volunteers. J Clin Psychiatry 57 (suppl 1):12–15, 1996

TWENTY-NINE

Geriatric Psychopharmacology

Carl Salzman, M.D.,
Andrew Satlin, M.D., and
Adam B. Burrows, M.D.

Psychotropic drugs play an important (but not exclusive) role in the treatment of late-life psychopathology. In this chapter, we review specific uses of psychotropic drugs to treat disorders characterized by disruptive behavior, depression, mania, anxiety, sleep dysfunction, and impaired cognition.

There are important differences in the use of psychoactive medications for elderly and younger adult patients. An appreciation of these differences is essential for optimal prescribing of these drugs. Before prescribing, the clinician must consider several processes: 1) physiological changes associated with aging, 2) physiological changes caused by disease, 3) the potential influence of concurrent medications, and 4) the social context of illness and treatment.

PHYSIOLOGICAL CHANGES ASSOCIATED WITH AGING

The aging process varies considerably, and the effects of aging and disease may be difficult to distinguish. Despite the clinical heterogeneity of the aging population, certain physiological changes are observed consistently. These include changes in nervous system structure and function, such as enhancement of some brain enzymes with aging and increased receptor site sensitivity in several neurotransmitter systems (Morgan et al. 1987; Oreland and Gottfries 1986; Robinson et al. 1977). Age-related changes are also evident in the sensory, respiratory, cardiovascular, gastrointestinal, genitourinary, endocrine, and neuromuscular systems.

A useful generalization often applied to age-related physiological changes is the concept of diminished physiological reserve. In this model, age-related changes in central nervous system (CNS) function may not become clinically apparent until an individual confronts a physiological challenge, such as an acute illness or medical intervention. Under the stress of these circumstances, clinical problems such as disruptive behavior, affective symptoms, and diminished sleep and cognition are revealed through symptoms in a vulnerable system. Thus, illness is typically expressed nonspecifically in elderly patients, and neuropsychiatric symptoms may represent the expression of diverse clinical problems.

DISEASE AND DISABILITY

Chronic disease and functional disability characterize the aging population. More than 80% of Americans older than 65 report at least one chronic medical condition, and most have multiple chronic problems (National Center for Health Statistics 1987). Chronic diseases impose functional limitations such that by age 85, half of all Americans have difficulty with at least one daily self-care activity (Dawson et al. 1987). Dementias impose growing challenges on individuals and the health care system. Community-based surveys suggest that 25%–50% of people age 85 and older have dementia, with 40%–70% of dementia cases attributed to Alzheimer's disease and the remainder primarily to vascular causes (Aronson et al. 1991; Evans et al. 1989; Skoog et al. 1993).

MEDICATIONS AND ELDERLY PATIENTS

It is not surprising that older individuals consume a disproportionate share of prescription drugs. Although elderly people constitute 12% of the American population, those older than 65 receive one-third of all prescriptions. Polypharmacy is common; community-dwelling Americans older than 65 fill, on average, 13 prescriptions each year and take twice as many medications as younger Americans (Institute of Medicine 1991; National Center for Health Statistics 1987; Office of Epidemiology and Biostatistics 1987; Stewart et al. 1989). After cardiovascular drugs and analgesics, psychotropic drugs are most frequently prescribed in the treatment of elderly patients.

The risks of medication use in elderly patients are well documented. Adverse drug reactions are more common among elderly people than among younger people and account for 10%–30% of their hospitalizations (Ancill et al. 1988; Antonijoan et al. 1990; Col et al. 1990; Grymonpre et al. 1988; Institute of Medicine

1991; Ives et al. 1987; Ray et al. 1992). It appears that the risk of adverse drug reactions is not simply a result of age-related vulnerability but rather is a function of complex interactions between medical frailty and the prescription of multiple medications (Avorn et al. 1989; Carbonin et al. 1991; Gurwitz and Avorn 1991). Medications that require monitoring of therapeutic levels, such as antidepressants, may be more likely than other drugs to cause adverse reactions in elderly outpatients (J. K. Schneider et al. 1992). Consultation-liaison by clinical pharmacists may reduce adverse drug effects (Kroenke and Pinholt 1990; J. K. Schneider et al. 1992).

THE SOCIAL CONTEXT OF AGING

Clinicians must consider the following questions: How and where will a drug be taken by an elderly patient? Will the cost of the drug be an issue? Will the drug be administered by a caregiver? Is the patient in a nursing home or other long-term care facility?

Approximately 5% of individuals older than 65 and more than 20% of those older than 85 live in nursing homes (National Center for Health Statistics 1987). Many other elderly persons receive formal and informal care and assistance with daily activities in community settings. As would be expected, nursing home residents have more disability, disease, and dependence than do community-dwelling elderly persons. Also, not surprisingly, polypharmacy is common in nursing homes; reports indicate an average of eight medications prescribed per resident (Beers et al. 1988). Psychotropic drugs are among the most frequently prescribed medications in nursing homes. Antipsychotic neuroleptics are prescribed for 20%–30% of residents (Avorn et al. 1992; Beardsley et al. 1989; Beers et al. 1988; Garrard et al. 1991).

Unfortunately, medications are commonly prescribed without clear documentation of an appropriate indication (Beardsley et al. 1989;

Garrard et al. 1991; Ray et al. 1980; Saban et al. 1982; Zimmer et al. 1986). This problem has been a particular concern with regard to psychotropic medications and was the subject of federal regulation through the Nursing Home Reform Amendments of the Omnibus Budget Reconciliation Act (OBRA) of 1987.

THERAPEUTIC CONSIDERATIONS: PSYCHOTROPIC MEDICATIONS

Effect of Aging and Disease

Aging and disease contribute to physiological changes that alter the effect and availability of medications. Pharmacodynamic changes affect the physiological effect produced by a given concentration of drug. Pharmacokinetic changes affect the amount of drug that is made available for clinical effect after a given dose. Aging is associated with both pharmacodynamic and pharmacokinetic changes, and the coexistence of chronic diseases can further alter the body's response to drugs.

Pharmacodynamics. Elderly patients are more sensitive than younger patients to the therapeutic and toxic effects of psychotropic agents. For a given concentration of drug, elderly patients usually experience more sedation, anticholinergic toxicity, extrapyramidal side effects (EPS), and orthostatic hypotension. In the setting of degenerative brain diseases, such as Alzheimer's disease and Parkinson's disease, drug sensitivities may increase as the amount of neuronal tissue in key brain areas declines. Patients with Alzheimer's disease and acetylcholine deficiency are more sensitive to anticholinergic side effects, whereas patients with Parkinson's disease are more sensitive to dopamine receptor blockade.

Pharmacokinetics. Four pharmacokinetic parameters determine the bioavailability of a drug after administration: absorption, distribution, metabolism, and clearance. Two significant changes occur with aging. First, distribution changes significantly. An almost universal decrease in lean body mass and a corresponding increase in body fat composition occur. Fat-soluble drugs such as benzodiazepine sedative-hypnotics, neuroleptics, and cyclic antidepressants distribute more widely in the body and will thus take longer to clear. Water-soluble drugs such as lithium distribute through a smaller volume and thus can reach higher tissue concentrations. Second, age-related changes in hepatic metabolism of psychotropic drugs occur. An age-related decrement in phase I oxidative biotransformation results. This process is generally controlled by the hepatic cytochrome P450 (CYP) drug-metabolizing system. The activity of several specific cytochromes, including CYP3A4, decreases in older as compared with younger patients. The extent of the impairment may be greater in elderly men than in women (von Moltke et al. 1998). The decrease in phase I oxidative biotransformation further delays hepatic metabolism and contributes to the prolonged half-lives of many psychotropic drugs and the delayed and prolonged appearance of active intermediate metabolites. The cumulative effect of large volumes of distribution for fat-soluble drugs and delayed hepatic metabolism results in a dramatic prolongation of clinical effect for many drugs, especially long-acting benzodiazepines.

Chronic diseases and the aging process alter the pharmacokinetic patterns of psychotropic drugs. Malnutrition or chronic inflammatory conditions can reduce the synthesis of plasma-binding proteins, resulting in higher free (or bioavailable) drug concentrations. Chronic liver disease or congestion will further delay clearance, leading to higher drug levels for even longer periods. Many older people have reduced glomerular filtration rates. For these individuals, renal clearance of drugs such as lithium will be impaired, and higher drug concentrations will result. Altogether, pharmacological changes associated with aging and disease mean that for a given dose of most psychoactive drugs, the bioavailable concentration at the target tissue will be higher, and for a given concentration at a CNS site of action, the physiological effect will be greater. These generalizations support the maxim to "start low and go slow" when prescribing drugs to geriatric patients.

Side effects.   In elderly patients, side effects typically occur in vulnerable physiological systems. In the cardiovascular system, for example, decreased baroreceptor sensitivity predisposes to orthostatic hypotension, and diminished reserve in the cardiac conduction system predisposes to heart block. Changes in bowel motility predispose to constipation and impaction, whereas bladder weakness and prostatic enlargement predispose to urinary retention. In the CNS, changes in the extrapyramidal and vestibular systems predispose to problems with gait, balance, and posture. Dementia (even early in the course) predisposes to delirium.

POLYPHARMACY: ISSUES IN PRESCRIBING PSYCHOACTIVE DRUGS

The high prevalence of polypharmacy in elderly patients leads to three common prescribing problems:

1. A correlation exists between an increasing number of medications prescribed and an increasing risk of medication noncompliance.
2. One drug can impair the absorption, metabolism, or clearance of another drug or displace it from a protein-binding site.
3. A confluence of adverse effects may result. For example, additive effects of vasodilators and antidepressants on blood pressure are common, as are the additive toxic effects from multiple drugs with anticholinergic properties. Monoamine oxidase inhibitors (MAOIs) present special problems with regard to potentially cata-

strophic interactions with sympathomimetic agents and catecholamine precursors.

TREATMENT OF PSYCHOSIS, AGITATION, AND BEHAVIORAL DISRUPTION

Elderly patients who have psychosis, severe illness, or dementia often manifest behavioral symptoms that require treatment. Prevalence rates of agitation are particularly high in nursing homes (Billig et al. 1991; Cohen-Mansfield et al. 1989; Peabody et al. 1987; Rovner et al. 1986; Wragg and Jeste 1988; Zimmer et al. 1984). Severe agitation, screaming, and assaultiveness are seen frequently in the moderate to severe stages of dementia (particularly Alzheimer's disease) as well as in late-life schizophrenia.

Treatment Guidelines

Although medications are commonly used to treat severe agitation and psychosis in elderly patients, they are not the only form of treatment. Agitation and psychosis may be caused by drug toxicity, medical illness, pain, frustration, loneliness, reduced sensory input, new environment, diminished nutritional status, and environmental factors. Treatment approaches include using orienting stimuli, avoiding patient isolation, and using nonpharmacological treatments such as music, exercise, pets, and social contact.

Medications that are commonly used to treat disruptive behavior include neuroleptics, β-blockers, drugs with serotonergic effects, mood stabilizers, and hormones.

Neuroleptics

Neuroleptics are the most commonly used drugs to treat severe disruptive behavior in elderly patients (Devanand et al. 1988; Helms 1985; Maletta 1984; Phillipson et al. 1990; Risse and Barnes 1986; Salzman 1987; L. S. Schneider et al. 1990b; Small 1988; Wragg and Jeste

1988). Neuroleptics undergo a complicated stepwise hepatic metabolism. The effects of the aging process on this metabolism have not been extensively studied. However, limited data suggest that blood levels of parent compounds and active metabolites are 1.5–2 times higher in older patients compared with younger adult control subjects (Aoba et al. 1985; Cohen and Sommer 1988; Forsman and Ohman 1977), but not in all patients.

No current data suggest that any one neuroleptic is better at controlling agitated behavior or psychotic thinking than any other, given comparable therapeutic doses. Selection of a particular neuroleptic (or subclass of neuroleptics) is guided by the side-effect profile of each drug or drug class in relation to the patient's history of drug response (or lack of response) and the nature of concomitant chronic illness and medication.

Three categories of neuroleptic side effects occur regularly and may be particularly troublesome for older patients. These side effects are sedation, orthostatic hypotension, and EPS. Low-potency neuroleptics, such as chlorpromazine and thioridazine, commonly cause sedation or orthostatic hypotension. Although sedation may be helpful at bedtime for disruptive elderly patients, the sedative effect often continues through the next day because of the medications' prolonged elimination half-lives. During the day, a sedated elderly person may actually become more agitated and disruptive. For this reason and because of the risk of orthostatic hypotension, low-potency neuroleptics may present a risk in this population. In clinical practice, however, low doses of thioridazine are still used with considerable success for the treatment of agitation. High-potency neuroleptics, such as haloperidol and fluphenazine, are a commonly used alternative to low-potency neuroleptics because high-potency medications lack sedating and orthostatic hypotensive properties. Unfortunately, these high-potency compounds are more likely to produce EPS than are the low-potency medications. Among the latter,

drug-induced parkinsonian-like EPS may be associated with a lack of behavioral improvement (Ganzini et al. 1991).

Therefore, the clinician must evaluate the risks and benefits of different neuroleptics when selecting one to treat behavioral disruption. Current clinical practice tends to favor the use of high-potency medications, with an attempt to prevent or minimize EPS by using exceedingly low doses (Devanand et al. 1988, 1989, 1992; Petrie et al. 1982). Clinical experience suggests, for example, that doses of haloperidol in the range of 0.25–1.0 mg one to four times a day may help diminish disruptive behavior without producing undue EPS.

In elderly patients who have not previously taken neuroleptics, tardive dyskinesia develops rapidly and at lower doses than in younger patients (Karson et al. 1990; Lieberman et al. 1984; Saltz et al. 1989; Yassa et al. 1988). Tardive dyskinesia is more common in patients with evidence of cortical atrophy (Sweet et al. 1992). When neuroleptics are discontinued, tardive dyskinesia symptoms are less likely to disappear in older patients than in younger adults (De Veaugh-Geiss 1988; Smith and Baldessarini 1980; Yassa et al. 1984). However, for some elderly patients with tardive dyskinesia who are given maintenance neuroleptics, the symptoms do not increase (Huang 1986; Yassa 1991).

Neuroleptic malignant syndrome may also occur in older patients taking neuroleptics. This syndrome was more common in elderly patients who had either dementia or Parkinson's disease while taking neuroleptics (Addonizio 1992). There is a burgeoning database on the utility of atypical antipsychotic drugs, including risperidone, olanzapine, quetiapine, and clozapine, in the elderly.

Nonneuroleptics

Clinical experience and anecdotal reports (summarized in Salzman 1990c) suggest that drugs such as β-blockers, trazodone, buspirone, serotonergic antidepressants, anticonvulsants, and lithium may help manage a variety of agitated behaviors refractory to more conventional treatment.

β-Blockers. β-Blockers, sometimes modestly helpful in reducing agitated and assaultive behavior in elderly patients, are given in low doses. Not all studies, however, are positive (Risse and Barnes 1986; Weiler et al. 1988). These drugs can be given only to those elderly patients without cardiovascular disorder and chronic obstructive pulmonary disease (particularly asthma). Side effects include sedation, orthostatic hypotension, and decreased cardiac output.

Trazodone. The antidepressant drug trazodone has been reported to be an effective treatment for agitation and severely disruptive behavior (Greenwald et al. 1986; Pinner and Rich 1988; Simpson and Foster 1986; Tingle 1986). Although no double-blind studies to date compare this drug with placebo or with neuroleptics, clinical experience suggests that it is effective in doses of 50–200 mg/day, with few side effects other than sedation.

Buspirone. Buspirone, a nonbenzodiazepine antianxiety agent, has been reported to be effective in controlling disruptive behavior in older patients in one study (Colenda 1988) but not in another (Strauss 1988). However, oral dyskinesia was reported in an elderly patient with dementia who was given buspirone, and this symptom persisted for at least 4 months after symptom onset (Strauss 1988). Research studies have not yet compared its effect with that of placebo or other drugs for treating agitation. The average daily dose range is 20–80 mg in divided doses; side effects are reported to be relatively mild.

Selective serotonin reuptake inhibitors.
Current clinical experience suggests that the antidepressant fluoxetine has some antiagitation properties in elderly patients. However, a study (Olafsson et al. 1992) failed to demonstrate effectiveness of fluvoxamine in the treatment of behavioral disruption in elderly patients with dementia. Careful research into the anti-agitation properties of the selective serotonin reuptake inhibitors (SSRIs) is essential, because these drugs also tend to be activating and may actually increase agitation in some older patients. Although the SSRIs may also be helpful in states of dementia-associated agitation, they often cause severe worsening of agitation in the late stages of a dementing illness.

Anticonvulsants and lithium carbonate.
In doses of 50–200 mg/day, carbamazepine has controlled chronic disruptive behavior and agitation in older patients, particularly those with dementia (Leibovici and Tariot 1988). Like carbamazepine, lithium carbonate is sometimes useful in managing disruptive behavior (Holton and George 1985). The therapeutic range is 150–900 mg in divided doses. Because both of these drugs may produce neurotoxicity characterized by increased agitation, confusion, and disorientation, the lowest possible therapeutic dosage should be given, and the drugs should be discontinued if behavior worsens.

Experience with valproate in managing disruptive behavior suggests that this drug, like carbamazepine, may be effective in controlling severe agitation.

Estrogen. A single case report (Kyomen et al. 1991) suggests that estrogen (e.g., diethylstilbestrol 1 mg/day or conjugated estrogen 0.625 mg/day) reduces the number of incidents of physical aggression but not of verbal aggression or physical or verbal repetitive behaviors in elderly male patients with dementia.

TREATMENT OF DEPRESSION

Depression is the most common psychiatric illness in the older population (Blazer and Williams 1980). Prevalence rates of depressive disorders in older people reach 20% for major depression and are even higher for milder forms. Suicide rates among depressed elderly people are particularly high (Alexopoulos et al. 1988). Research points to the high prevalence of diagnosed major depression in nursing home residents and the unusually high mortality (from causes other than suicide) of patients with depression (Parmelee et al. 1993; Rovner et al. 1991).

Although older people with depressive disorders can present with signs and symptoms similar to those in younger adults, late-life depression is characterized by diagnostic and symptomatic heterogeneity (Alexopoulos 1990). Ascribing diagnostic significance to individual depressive symptoms may be misleading. For example, early-morning awakening, appetite disturbance, and low energy level (which are characteristic vegetative signs of depression) may each result from the normal aging process, from drugs commonly taken by elderly patients, from medical conditions more common in elderly people, or from a combination of these factors (Salzman et al. 1992).

In addition to the heterogeneity of depressive symptom patterns, people older than 65 have remarkably diverse psychological functioning. Although precise age boundaries are lacking, elderly people are occasionally subdivided into the "young-old" (65 to 75 or 79) and the "old-old" (75 to 80+). Symptomatic presentation of depression may differ between these two groups, although considerable similarities and overlap of symptoms are also found. For example, the appearance of depression in very old (80+), frail nursing home residents may differ from that in younger, healthier nursing home residents and may confuse the diagnostician (Burrows et al. 1995). Factors of pharmacokinetic disposition and pharmacodynamic drug sensitivity may be quite different in old-old patients. Response to antidepressant treatment may also be different between these two general categories (Salzman et al. 1993), although, once again, similarities of response also exist, and

overlap between the two groups is common. Virtually all studies of the pharmacological treatment of late-life depression have focused on the young-old group. One review (Salzman et al. 1993) noted that only one controlled study of depressed patients who were older than 75 has been done, and just 171 identifiable patients older than 75 have been studied in all antidepressant studies of elderly subjects. Consequently, treatment guidelines for very old patients are based on treatment of young-old or even of young and middle-aged adults and may be misleading.

As a general principle, elderly patients (especially those who are old-old) are more sensitive to the effects of antidepressants than are younger adults, although wide interindividual variability is seen. Elderly patients are more likely than younger adults to experience the side effects of sedation, orthostatic hypotension, and anticholinergic symptoms. Orthostatic hypotension (due to reduced central and peripheral controls of blood pressure) may lead to falls and serious fractures. For unclear reasons, pretreatment systolic orthostatic blood pressure may predict clinical response: patients who have large pretreatment systolic orthostatic blood pressure changes in the morning before treatment with antidepressants have a significantly greater response to antidepressant or electroconvulsive therapy (ECT) (Jarvik et al. 1983; L. S. Schneider et al. 1986; Stack et al. 1988). In some older patients, sensitivity to anticholinergic side effects of tricyclic antidepressants (TCAs) may limit dosing levels and may cause CNS symptoms of delirium even at therapeutic doses. A review of anticholinergic side effects in elderly patients found that cognitive impairment, which occurs in normal aging, is enhanced and also may be associated with behavioral disturbances (Meyers 1992). Activation and insomnia resulting from SSRIs may be greater in older patients than in younger patients, although these differences have not been carefully defined by controlled research studies.

Antidepressants, like neuroleptics, undergo

complicated hepatic metabolism requiring both phase I (dealkylation, aromatic hydroxylation) and phase II (conjugation) reactions. The aging process may affect the first set of processes. As a general rule, dealkylation becomes less efficient, which leads to higher levels of tertiary tricyclic amines compared with the secondary amine metabolite and reduced clearance of these compounds, with accumulation and higher blood levels. For these reasons, older patients, on average, need lower doses of antidepressants to achieve therapeutic effect; old-old patients may need even lower doses than young-old patients. Pharmacokinetic data also suggest that for drugs with established therapeutic blood level ranges (e.g., nortriptyline and desipramine), older patients respond to the same levels as younger adult counterparts (Cutler et al. 1981; Dawling et al. 1980a, 1980b, 1981; Kanba et al. 1992; Katz et al. 1989; Kitanka et al. 1982; Nelson et al. 1985, 1988). However, the wide range of interindividual variability and limited research data design suggest that the pharmacokinetics of antidepressants in elderly patients have not yet been consistently characterized in comparison with younger patients (von Moltke et al. 1993).

Phase I metabolism of TCAs also produces a water-soluble hydroxymetabolite whose clearance depends on renal function. This metabolite was previously thought to be inactive; however, in some patients, it may be associated with quinidine-like cardiotoxicity (McCue et al. 1989; Nelson et al. 1988; L. S. Schneider et al. 1990a; Young et al. 1984, 1985). Impaired renal function in older patients or in very elderly individuals may lead to higher levels of hydroxymetabolites and the potential for cardiotoxicity (Kutcher et al. 1986).

Treatment Guidelines

Traditionally, treatment of the depressed elderly patient with antidepressants has followed recommendations for younger and middle-aged adults. ECT or TCAs plus neuroleptics are usually prescribed for patients with delusional de-

pression (Kroessler and Fogel 1993). TCAs have been the primary treatment for melancholic major depressive disorder, especially on an inpatient service, and MAOIs have been used for less severely depressed patients who do not require hospitalization. The new class of SSRIs has been studied primarily in depressed elderly outpatients and found to be useful for mild to moderately severe depression. These recommendations, however, are based on a small number of studies, with an age sample skewed toward young-old subjects.

Increased clinical experience and more recent studies have suggested that precise boundaries between these prescribing guidelines may not exist, and treatment recommendations for depressed elderly patients may be changing. For example, the combination of fluoxetine and perphenazine has been found effective in the treatment of psychotic depression in a study that included a few patients older than 60 (Rothschild et al. 1993). There are many reviews of antidepressant treatment in elderly patients (Alexopoulos 1992; Caine et al. 1993; Dewan et al. 1992; Kim 1988; Koenig and Breitner 1990; Magni et al. 1988; Peabody et al. 1986; Rockwell et al. 1988; Salzman 1990a, 1990c, 1993; Smith and Buckwalter 1992; Weissman et al. 1992).

Tricyclic Antidepressants

More than 400 studies of the treatment of serious major depression, nondelusional type, in elderly subjects have been done (Salzman 1994). In general, all TCAs are helpful for depressed elderly patients, although secondary amines are preferred. Regardless of the type of antidepressant used, however, one study suggested that elderly patients who have had major depression should continue taking their antidepressant to prevent relapse (Old Age Depression Interest Group 1993).

Although secondary amine TCAs are preferred to tertiary amines because side effects of secondary amines are usually less intense, the severity of tricyclic-related side effects in elderly patients may be correlated with dose. Because therapeutic blood levels of TCAs in elderly patients may be achieved with lower-than-usual doses, use of tertiary amines in elderly patients may be possible if doses remain low. A study of low-dose doxepin, for example, reported efficacy without serious side effects (Lakshmanan et al. 1986).

Before initiating treatment with TCAs in elderly patients, clinicians should do a physical examination and obtain an electrocardiogram (ECG). Starting doses should be extremely low (e.g., 10–25 mg/day), and dosage increments should be of a similar magnitude. The adage "start low and go slow" is applicable to the use of antidepressants in elderly patients. In addition, clinicians should try to prescribe the dose of antidepressant that produces the best therapeutic response with the fewest side effects, regardless of the final dose. Using the ECG to monitor potential cardiotoxicity will help determine the upper limit of doses.

Trazodone

The antidepressant effects of trazodone are unpredictable; thus, it is a less reliable first choice among the various available antidepressants. It is recommended, however, for older patients who have not responded to other compounds, and sometimes it has surprising therapeutic effects in the previously treatment-refractory older patient. Although trazodone causes sedation and orthostatic hypotension (Gerner et al. 1980), it has minimal anticholinergic properties and does not interfere with memory (Branconnier and Cole 1981).

Bupropion

Bupropion has been found to be effective for elderly subjects in research studies (Branconnier et al. 1983; Halaris 1986). A few elderly patients have reported an unusual side effect of falling backward that may be dose related (Szuba and Leuchter 1992).

Selective Serotonin Reuptake Inhibitors

SSRIs have been prescribed to elderly patients with major depression, less serious dysthymic disorders, and atypical depressions. The advantages of these drugs is the lack of anticholinergic side effects, cardiotoxicity, and orthostatic hypotension. In research studies, the efficacy of the SSRIs fluoxetine, paroxetine, sertraline, and fluvoxamine is equivalent to that of the TCAs (Dunner et al. 1992; Feighner and Cohn 1985; Feighner et al. 1988; Salzman 1994). For these reasons, the SSRIs have become the first choice among the various categories of antidepressants for elderly patients. However, in some elderly patients, these drugs cause unacceptable agitation and insomnia. Another report (Brymer and Winograd 1992) also noted that fluoxetine use may be associated with unacceptable weight loss in patients older than 75. Low starting doses and small dosage increments are recommended.

Monoamine Oxidase Inhibitors

MAOIs may be both safe and effective for some older patients with atypical depression characterized by withdrawal, lack of motivation, apathy, and lack of energy (Georgotas et al. 1981, 1983, 1986; Lazarus et al. 1986). Clinical overviews of the use of MAOIs include those of Jenike (1985), Zisook (1985), and Salzman (1992). These drugs are rarely the first-choice antidepressant for major depression. As with TCAs and SSRIs, older patients are likely to experience side effects. Lower doses (e.g., phenelzine 15–20 mg/day, tranylcypromine 10–40 mg/day) than those prescribed for younger adult patients are advised.

MAOIs can be given only to responsible, compliant elderly patients or to those whose medication is carefully supervised. The high risk of toxic drug interactions resulting from the large average number of drugs prescribed for the geriatric population may prevent these drugs from being recommended for many older outpatients.

TREATMENT OF MANIA

Elderly bipolar patients who have had many episodes tend to have rapid cycling and severe symptomatology, but bipolar disorder rarely appears for the first time in late life. Several studies suggest that first-onset mania in elderly patients is more likely to be associated with neurological impairment than is depression in this age group (Berrios and Bakshi 1991; Shulman et al. 1992; Snowdon 1991) and carries a greater risk for mortality than does depression (Dhingra and Rabins 1991; Shulman et al. 1992). Thus, late-onset mania may represent a different disorder from early-onset mania, or it may be secondary to other conditions.

Treatment Guidelines

Lithium is the primary treatment and prophylaxis for mania in elderly patients, as it is for younger adults. However, a review (Foster 1992) identified only five studies of antimanic efficacy of lithium in elderly subjects and concluded that the efficacy in elderly bipolar patients is not yet clearly established in the literature. Reviews of lithium effects in older patients include those of Foster (1992), Liptzin (1992), Stone (1989), Jefferson et al. (1987), and Glasser and Rabins (1984).

Age-associated reduction in renal clearance of lithium leads to accumulation and increased plasma levels in elderly patients more readily than in younger adults taking the same dosage. This effect is magnified by the reduction in the volume of distribution of lithium in elderly patients as a result of the relative loss of total body water. Therapeutic plasma levels for older patients with mania may need to be only 0.2–0.6 mEq/L. The daily dose necessary to achieve lower blood levels varies among older patients. As a general rule, starting lithium doses are low (e.g., 150–450 mg/day), with dosage increments of 150–300 mg at weekly intervals. However, it is important to recognize that some older patients with mania, particularly those with other psychiatric illnesses, may require doses and blood levels equivalent to those needed by younger patients. One prospective, double-blind, randomized lithium dose-reduction study found that dose reductions of 25%–50% to achieve serum levels of 0.45 mEq/L resulted in significantly increased affective symptoms in the elderly subjects (Abou-Saleh and Coppen 1989).

Older patients are more sensitive than younger patients to the therapeutic and toxic effects of lithium. The toxic profile of lithium in older patients differs in several important aspects from that of younger patients. Side effects of tremor and gastrointestinal upset occur in all age groups. In older patients, however, the first and often the most prominent side effects consist of a spectrum of neurotoxic symptoms, even at low therapeutic levels. In some patients, neurotoxicity may be associated with the presence of underlying neurological disease (Himmelhoch et al. 1980; Kemperman et al. 1989). Subtle but progressive impairment of recent recall (anterograde amnesia), disorientation, aphasia, restlessness, and irritability may appear as the first signs of excessive lithium dosage. This presents a double hazard: overdose and inaccurate interpretation of symptoms of cognitive impairment. Movement disorders also are early signs of toxicity—particularly EPS, dyskinesias, and cerebellar dysfunction, including irregular gait, decreased coordination, and dysarthria. Impaired consciousness also may develop at blood levels therapeutic for younger adults.

Other medical side effects may be common in elderly patients taking lithium. Cardiac effects include altered conduction due to sinus node dysfunction, sinoatrial block, bundle branch block, ventricular irritability, and possible myocardial injury. Lithium may impair urine concentration by the kidneys; this may be more severe in elderly patients with preexisting deficits in renal concentrating ability. Acute lithium toxicity may result in decreased glomerular filtration rate, and long-term use may be associated with tubular atrophy, glomerular sclerosis, and interstitial fibrosis. Hypothyroidism may be more common in elderly patients taking lithium and can present with more profound consequences such as myxedema coma.

Alternative medications for the treatment of mania in elderly patients have been less well studied than lithium. Neuroleptics are sometimes recommended for elderly patients as adjunctive treatment of severe agitation, insomnia, and potentially harmful behavior in patients with mania, particularly in the early stages of treatment before lithium exerts its effect. Among the alternatives to lithium, anticonvulsants have been used with increased frequency. Valproic acid is generally well tolerated in older patients (McFarland et al. 1990; Satlin and Liptzin 1998). Valproic acid pharmacokinetics are affected by the aging process; higher unbound fractions may be present in the cerebrospinal fluid. Thus, total concentrations as measured in blood may be misleading, and doses may need to be lower in elderly patients than in younger patients. The most common reported side effects are neurological symptoms (tremor, sedation, and ataxia), asymptomatic serum hepatic transaminase elevations, alopecia, increased appetite, and weight gain. The initial sedative effect, which generally lasts only about a week, may be helpful for elderly patients with mania who are agitated and have insomnia. Carbamazepine, like valproic acid, may be useful in the treatment and prevention of mania. In the elderly, however, fewer reports of use of carbamazepine are available than for valproic acid. Side effects of carbamazepine include bradycardia, confusion, ataxia, and impairment of water excretion. The most serious toxic effect of carbamazepine is depression of bone marrow function, which may result in leukopenia and potentially fatal infections, but this effect appears to be less common in the elderly. Other drugs that have been used to treat mania in younger adults include benzodiazepines and calcium channel blockers; these compounds have not been well studied in elderly patients. ECT is as useful for severe mania in elderly patients as in younger adults.

TREATMENT OF ANXIETY

In older patients, symptoms of anxiety are common, and the diagnosis of generalized anxiety disorder is not as clearly defined as in younger adults. Clinically significant anxiety symptoms commonly occur in states of depression and dementia as well as secondary to physical illness or as a result of drug treatment. Panic and phobic anxiety disorders may also occur in older people but are less prevalent than in younger adults and are often associated with physical illness and concomitant psychiatric disorder (Sheikh 1990). Various reviews of the pharmacological treatment of generalized anxiety in elderly patients have been conducted (Allen 1986; Hershey and Kim 1988; Salzman 1990b).

Treatment Guidelines

Benzodiazepines, the primary treatment of anxiety, are widely used in the treatment of anxious elderly patients (Beardsley et al. 1989; Beers et al. 1988; Buck 1988; Koepke et al. 1982; Pinsker and Suljaga-Petchel 1984). Elderly patients generally are more sensitive than younger patients to both the therapeutic and the toxic effects of benzodiazepines, or interindividual variability may be great. Low doses are generally recommended; side effects of sedation, impaired coordination, and cognitive impairment may result from higher doses that are commonly therapeutic for younger adults.

Like other psychotropic drugs, benzodiazepines undergo stepwise hepatic metabolism. The long-half-life benzodiazepines that are currently available in the United States undergo both phase I and phase II reactions. Phase I reactions tend to be prolonged in elderly patients and lead to drug accumulation and increased half-life. Phase II reactions are unaffected by age. Because short-half-life benzodiazepines undergo only phase II metabolism, they are preferred for older patients (Greenblatt and Shader 1990).

Benzodiazepines often cause four types of toxicity in older patients: 1) sedation, 2) ataxia and falls (Hale et al. 1988; Rashi and Logan 1986; Ray et al. 1987), 3) psychomotor slowing, and 4) cognitive impairment (Salzman 1990b). The last type—an increasing public health concern—is characterized by anterograde amnesia, diminished short-term recall, increased forgetfulness, and decreased attention. Discontinuing the drug is associated with improved memory and heightened concentration (Salzman et al. 1992).

Buspirone

Buspirone, a nonbenzodiazepine anxiolytic, has antianxiety properties in elderly patients. Although research data suggest that it is as effective as benzodiazepines (Napoliello 1986), clinical experience favors benzodiazepines as more rapid and reliable anxiolytics. Because research and clinical experience differ, recommendations for its use remain tentative: buspirone is recommended when benzodiazepines are ineffective or cannot be prescribed.

TREATMENT OF SLEEP DISORDERS

Disordered sleep is a common complaint among elderly people (Ancoli-Israel 1989; Pollack and Perlick 1991). Of people older than 65, 12% report persistent insomnia, and 1.6% report persistent daytime hypersomnia (Ford and Kamerow 1989). Although only about 12% of Americans are elderly, they receive 35%–40% of all prescriptions for sedative-hypnotics (Gottlieb 1990).

Treatment Guidelines

Sedative-hypnotic medications are indicated for the short-term treatment of insomnia associated

with situational, psychological, psychiatric, or medical conditions that are expected to be time limited or to respond to appropriate therapy. For some elderly patients, long-term use can be justified by the morbidity of chronic sleep deprivation. Regular nightly use, however, may cause significant worsening of cognition, disorientation, confusion, and socially inappropriate behavior in some older people (Regestein 1992). Selection of a particular drug to alleviate sleep problems (like the selection of an antianxiety drug) is guided by the drug's pharmacokinetic properties, the drug's side-effect profile, the patient's medical and emotional health, and the patient's history of sedative-hypnotic use. Reviews of psychotropic drugs to treat sleep disorders in older patients include those of Regestein (1992), Reynolds (1991), and Prinz and colleagues (1990).

Benzodiazepines are the most commonly prescribed sedative-hypnotics. Five are currently marketed for this indication: flurazepam, quazepam, triazolam, temazepam, and estazolam. In general, the benzodiazepines with a long half-life (e.g., flurazepam and, to a lesser extent, quazepam) accumulate and are likely to produce daytime sedation in elderly patients. Long-term use can gradually produce a dementia syndrome of cognitive loss, psychomotor retardation, and apathy. Drugs with a shorter half-life cause less daytime sedation and hangover. For example, triazolam, when used in the recommended dose of 0.125 mg, is effective in older patients with sleep fragmentation, daytime sleepiness, and periodic limb movements of sleep (PLMS) (Bonnet and Arand 1991). Withdrawal symptoms and interdose rebound are common. Use of benzodiazepines with an intermediate half-life may be especially useful in elderly patients. Temazepam, which has a half-life of 10–20 hours, has been found to be effective in elderly patients and to cause little hangover, but it has a slow onset of action. The anxiolytic drugs lorazepam and oxazepam are pharmacokinetically similar and are as effective as temazepam for inducing sleep. Estazolam, another benzodiazepine with an intermediate half-life of 12–15 hours, is an effective hypnotic in elderly patients (Vogel and Morris 1992). With intermediate-half-life benzodiazepines, daytime performance and memory are not adversely affected, and rebound insomnia rarely extends beyond one night after discontinuation.

Other classes of psychotropic drugs are also given to older patients to induce sleep. Sedating neuroleptics such as thioridazine in low doses or antidepressants with sedating side effects such as trazodone and doxepin may be beneficial. Antihistaminic drugs such as diphenhydramine and hydroxyzine also may be helpful in some patients, although these drugs have the potential for anticholinergic, hypotensive, and cardiac side effects. Chloral hydrate is also effective and safe for short-term use. Barbiturates should not be given to elderly patients.

Two hypnotics that increase delta sleep are available. Because delta sleep typically decreases with aging, these medications may be of particular benefit to older people. Zolpidem, a clinically effective imidazopyridine hypnotic, does not appear to impair memory (Frattola et al. 1990). Zaleplon, a recently marketed hypnotic with a short half-life (4 hours), also may not impair memory in old people.

TREATMENT OF DEMENTIA

Some degree of memory loss and a slowing of other cognitive processes are common with advancing age. Dementia is diagnosed when other cognitive impairments and impaired social or occupational functioning accompany the memory loss. Dementia due to neurodegenerative disorders typically follows a slowly progressive course, with worsening attention, orientation, ability to concentrate, visual recognition, and language function in addition to declining short-term and long-term memory. Clinical overviews of the diagnosis and treatment of memory loss include those of Foster and Martin (1990), Crook (1989), and Rosebush and Salzman (1988).

Alzheimer's disease is the most common cause of degenerative dementia in elderly people. This idiopathic condition, characterized pathologically by senile plaques and neurofibrillary tangles in the brain, may affect as many as 10% of all people older than 65 and nearly 50% of those older than 85 (Evans et al. 1989). Alzheimer's disease also may cause various psychiatric syndromes, including depression, anxiety, psychosis, and behavioral disturbances such as agitation, sleep-wake cycle disorders, and aggression. At present, no known effective treatment is available to ameliorate or reverse the cognitive impairment caused by Alzheimer's disease. Numerous drugs have been studied, based on their presumed effects on those aspects of brain neurochemistry that appear abnormal in Alzheimer's disease. Comprehensive reviews of this research include those of Tariot (1992), Miller and colleagues (1992), and Crook and colleagues (1990).

Evidence has suggested that the degree of cognitive impairment in patients with Alzheimer's disease is correlated with CNS cholinergic deficits (Perry et al. 1978). Restitutive therapies using choline or lecithin as cholinergic precursors have not yielded clinically significant results. Other approaches have used acetylcholinesterase inhibitors to block the enzyme that metabolizes acetylcholine. Three examples are physostigmine, tetrahydroaminoacridine (tacrine, THA), and velnacrine maleate. Most studies of physostigmine showed small improvements in cognition, but the effect was brief (Jenike et al. 1990; Stern et al. 1988). The effects of THA have been both negative and positive. Two trials showed no benefit, but the effect may have been compromised by low doses of the drug (Chatellier and Lacomblez 1990; Gauthier et al. 1990). Three other trials found improvements that ranged from modest to clinically noticeable by physicians and caregivers (Davis et al. 1992; Eagger et al. 1991; Farlow et al. 1992).

In all of these studies, high rates of liver enzyme elevations—often more than three times normal—were found. Overall, however, the modest therapeutic effects of THA seemed to outweigh the possible toxic consequences so that this compound will be available for clinical use in the United States. Other restitutive cholinergic approaches involve the use of muscarinic or nicotinic agonists, or agents that purportedly enhance the potassium-evoked release of acetylcholine (Lavretsky and Jarvik 1992; Spagnoli et al. 1991). Acetylcarnitine may have some direct cholinergic activity, although its mechanism of action is uncertain.

Donepezil (Aricept) is an acetylcholinesterase inhibitor that is now widely used to treat the cognitive impairment of mild to moderate states of dementia. Side effects are minimal, although occasional agitation has been noted and the drug is well tolerated. Its efficacy is variable; some patients experience a slowing of the progression of dementia. Other cholinesterase inhibitors will be released for clinical use shortly. Those that inhibit butylcholinesterase as well as acetylcholinesterase may have a therapeutic advantage.

Restitutive therapies based on known deficits of other neurotransmitters in Alzheimer's disease also have been tested. These include attempts to improve

- Noradrenergic transmission using clonidine or guanfacine
- Serotonergic function using alaproclate or minaprine
- γ-Aminobutyric acid (GABA)ergic function using tetrahydroisoxazolopyridinol (THIP)
- Peptide neurotransmission using somatostatin analogues, arginine vasopressin, adrenocorticotropic hormone (ACTH) agonists, thyrotropin-releasing hormone (TRH) analogues, and opiate receptor antagonists

No therapy improved cognition, although effects on mood were occasionally reported (Tariot 1992). Studies of selegiline, an MAOI that at low doses appears to be selective for MAO-B, have been encouraging.

Evidence indicates that neuronal death in neurodegenerative disorders such as Alzheimer's disease may be mediated by a sustained increase in cytosolic free calcium (Branconnier et al. 1992). Increased calcium influx into the cell may be a result of changes in the receptor for glutamate, which is part of the N-methyl-D-aspartate (NMDA) receptor complex. Newer therapeutic approaches to Alzheimer's disease involve attempts to block calcium channels with antagonists such as nimodipine. One study of nimodipine found significantly less deterioration on some cognitive measures than with placebo, but the short duration of the treatment period limited its clinical relevance (Tollefson 1990).

Another approach to the treatment of Alzheimer's disease involves attempts to enhance CNS cellular metabolism. Ergoloid mesylates is classified as a metabolic enhancer based on its ability to change levels of cyclic adenosine monophosphate. Although ergoloid mesylates has been studied for more than 20 years, evidence indicates that its efficacy is questionable (Thompson et al. 1990).

"Nootropics" are putative metabolic enhancers that were originally synthesized as GABA derivatives. The first of these was piracetam, and the class now includes oxiracetam, pramiracetam, aniracetam, and vinpocetine. Studies of these drugs indicate variable effects on mood and overall functional status but no clear cognitive effect (Tariot 1992).

Future research on treating the cognitive disorders of Alzheimer's disease may be directed at preventing the accumulation of β-amyloid protein fragments, which result from the abnormal processing of the amyloid precursor protein and constitute the core of the senile plaque. Additional research will be directed at targeted drug delivery systems to overcome the problems with drug delivery to the brain caused by peripheral metabolism, poor blood-brain barrier penetration, erratic drug absorption, serum protein binding, systemic adverse effects, and poor patient compliance (Miller et al. 1992).

SUMMARY AND CONCLUSION

Psychotropic drugs can benefit the older patient in acute emotional crisis or with chronic recurrent symptoms of severe mental distress that cannot be alleviated solely by other interventions. Regardless of the symptoms being treated or the class of drug being used, sound psychotropic treatment may be guided by the following principles:

- The clinician must carefully review the elderly patient's current physical illness and medication regimen before beginning treatment.
- The likelihood that concomitant medication for physical illness taken by an older patient may interact adversely with psychotropic drugs is increased.
- An older patient is more likely to develop toxic effects from psychotropic drugs, even at doses and blood levels usually considered nontoxic in younger adults.
- The average older patient's greater sensitivity to psychotropic drug effects (pharmacodynamics) and the tendency of psychotropic drugs to accumulate and exert greater effects for longer periods (pharmacokinetics) signify the need for low starting doses, low dosage increments, and low therapeutic and maintenance doses to avoid toxicity.
- Drug response varies greatly among elderly people. An old-old patient may be even more sensitive to drugs than would a young-old patient.
- As a corollary, fixed dosing guidelines are not useful when treating an elderly patient. Some older people require doses equal to those prescribed for younger adults.
- The clinician should maintain close contact and have frequent meetings with the older patient being treated to ensure optimal compliance and to monitor effects and reactions.

REFERENCES

Abou-Saleh MT, Coppen A: The efficacy of low-dose lithium: clinical, psychological and biological correlates. J Psychiatr Res 23:157–162, 1989

Addonizio G: Neuroleptic malignant syndrome in the elderly, in Psychopharmacological Treatment Complications in the Elderly. Edited by Shamoian CA. Washington, DC, American Psychiatric Press, 1992, pp 63–70

Alexopoulos GS: Clinical and biological findings in late-onset depression, in American Psychiatric Press Review of Psychiatry, Vol 9. Edited by Tasman A, Goldfinger SM, Kaufmann CA. Washington, DC, American Psychiatric Press, 1990, pp 249–262

Alexopoulos GS: Treatment of depression, in Clinical Geriatric Psychopharmacology, 2nd Edition. Edited by Salzman C. Baltimore, MD, Williams & Wilkins, 1992, pp 137–174

Alexopoulos GS, Young RC, Meyers BS, et al: Late-onset depression. Psychiatr Clin North Am 11:101–115, 1988

Allen RM: Tranquilizers and sedative/hypnotics: appropriate use in the elderly. Geriatrics 41:75–88, 1986

Ancill RJ, Embury GD, MacEwan GW, et al: The use and misuse of psychotropic prescribing for elderly psychiatric patients. Can J Psychiatry 33: 585–589, 1988

Ancoli-Israel S: Epidemiology of sleep disorders. Clin Geriatr Med 5:347–362, 1989

Antonijoan RM, Barbanoj MJ, Torrent J, et al: Evaluation of psychotropic drug consumption related to psychological distress in the elderly: hospitalized vs. nonhospitalized. Neuropsychobiology 23:25–30, 1990

Aoba A, Kakita Y, Yamaguchi N, et al: Absence of age effect on plasma haloperidol neuroleptic levels in psychiatric patients. Journal of Gerontology 40:303–308, 1985

Aronson MK, Ooi WL, Geva DL, et al: Dementia: age-dependent incidence, prevalence, and mortality in the old-old. Arch Intern Med 151: 989–992, 1991

Avorn J, Dreyer P, Connelly K, et al: Use of psychoactive medication and the quality of care in rest homes. N Engl J Med 320:227–232, 1989

Avorn J, Soumerai SB, Everett DE, et al: A randomized controlled trial of a program to reduce the use of psychoactive drugs in nursing homes. N Engl J Med 327:168–173, 1992

Beardsley RS, Larson DB, Burns BJ, et al: Prescribing of psychotropics in elderly nursing home residents. J Am Geriatr Soc 37:327–330, 1989

Beers M, Avorn J, Soumerai SB, et al: Psychoactive medication use in intermediate care facility residents. JAMA 260:3016–3020, 1988

Berrios GE, Bakshi N: Manic and depressive symptoms in the elderly: their relationships to treatment outcome, cognition and motor symptoms. Psychopathology 24:31–38, 1991

Billig N, Cohen-Mansfield J, Lipson S: Pharmacological treatment of agitation in a nursing home. J Am Geriatr Soc 39:1002–1005, 1991

Blazer D, Williams CD: Epidemiology of dysphoria and depression in an elderly population. Am J Psychiatry 137:439–444, 1980

Bonnet MH, Arand DL: Chronic use of triazolam in patients with periodic leg movements, fragmented sleep and daytime sleepiness. Aging 3: 313–324, 1991

Branconnier RJ, Cole JO: Effects of acute administration of trazodone and amitriptyline on cognition, cardiovascular function, and salivation in the normal geriatric subject. J Clin Psychopharmacol 1:82S–88S, 1981

Branconnier RJ, Cole JO, Ghazvinian S, et al: Clinical pharmacology of bupropion and imipramine in elderly depressives. J Clin Psychiatry 44: 130–133, 1983

Branconnier RJ, Branconnier ME, Walshe TM, et al: Blocking the Ca 2+-activated cytotoxic mechanisms of cholinergic neuronal death: a novel treatment strategy for Alzheimer's disease. Psychopharmacol Bull 28:175–181, 1992

Brymer C, Winograd CH: Fluoxetine in elderly patients: is there cause for concern? J Am Geriatr Soc 40:902–905, 1992

Buck JA: Psychotropic drug practice in nursing homes. J Am Geriatr Soc 36:409–418, 1988

Burrows AB, Satlin A, Salzman C, et al: Depression in a long-term care facility: clinical features and discordance between nursing assessment and patient interviews. J Am Geriatr Soc 43: 1118–1122, 1995

Caine ED, Lyness JM, King DA: Reconsidering depression in the elderly. Am J Geriatr Psychiatry 1:4–20, 1993

Carbonin R, Pahor M, Bernabei R: Is age an independent risk factor for adverse drug reactions in hospitalized medical patients? J Am Geriatr Soc 39:1093–1099, 1991

Chatellier G, Lacomblez L: Tacrine (tetrahydroaminoacridine; THA) and lecithin in senile dementia of the Alzheimer type: a multicentre trial. BMJ 300:495–499, 1990

Cohen BM, Sommer BR: Metabolism of thioridazine in the elderly. J Clin Psychopharmacol 8:336–339, 1988

Cohen-Mansfield J, Marx MS, Rosenthal AS: A description of agitation in a nursing home. Journal of Gerontology 44:77–84, 1989

Col N, Fanale JE, Kronholm P: The role of medication non-compliance and adverse drug reactions in hospitalizations of the elderly. Arch Intern Med 150:841–845, 1990

Colenda CC: Buspirone in treatment of agitated demented patient. Lancet 2:1169, 1988

Crook TH: Diagnosis and treatment of normal and pathologic memory impairment in later life. Semin Neurol 9:20–30, 1989

Crook TH, Johnson BA, Larrabee GJ: Evaluation of drugs in Alzheimer's disease and age-associated memory impairment. Psychopharmacology (Berl) 26:37–55, 1990

Cutler NR, Zavadil AP, Eisdorfer C, et al: Concentrations of desipramine in elderly women. Am J Psychiatry 138:1235–1237, 1981

Davis KL, Thal LJ, Gamzu ER, et al: A double-blind, placebo-controlled multicenter study of tacrine for Alzheimer's disease. N Engl J Med 327:1253–1259, 1992

Dawling S, Crome P, Braithwaite RA, et al: Nortriptyline therapy in elderly patients: dosage prediction after single dose pharmacokinetic study. Eur J Clin Pharmacol 18:147–150, 1980a

Dawling S, Crome P, Braithwaite RA: Pharmacokinetics of single oral doses of nortriptyline in depressed elderly hospital patients and young healthy volunteers. Clin Pharmacokinet 5: 394–401, 1980b

Dawling S, Crome P, Heyer EJ, et al: Nortriptyline therapy in elderly patients: dosage prediction from plasma concentration at 24 hours after a single 50mg dose. Br J Psychiatry 139:413–416, 1981

Dawson D, Hundershot G, Fulton J: Aging in the eighties: functional limitations of individuals age 65 and over (Advance Data No. 133, June 1987), in Aging America: Trends and Projections, 1986–1987. Washington, DC, U.S. Department of Health and Human Services, 1987

Devanand DP, Sackeim HA, Mayeux R: Psychosis, behavioral disturbance, and the use of neuroleptics in dementia. Compr Psychiatry 29:387–401, 1988

Devanand DP, Sackeim HA, Brown RP, et al: A pilot study of haloperidol treatment of psychosis and behavioral disturbance in Alzheimer's disease. Arch Neurol 46:854–857, 1989

Devanand DP, Cooper T, Sackeim HA, et al: Low dose oral haloperidol and blood levels in Alzheimer's disease: a preliminary study. Psychopharmacol Bull 28:169–173, 1992

De Veaugh-Geiss J: Clinical changes in tardive dyskinesia during long-term follow-up, in Tardive Dyskinesia: Biological Mechanisms and Clinical Aspects. Edited by Wolf ME, Mosnaim AD. Washington, DC, American Psychiatric Press, 1988, pp 89–105

Dewan MJ, Huszonek J, Koss M, et al: The use of antidepressants in the elderly: 1986 and 1989. J Geriatr Psychiatry Neurol 5:40–44, 1992

Dhingra U, Rabins PV: Mania in the elderly: a 5–7 year follow-up. J Am Geriatr Soc 39:581–583, 1991

Dunner DL, Cohn JB, Walshe T III, et al: Two combined, multicenter double-blind studies of paroxetine and doxepin in geriatric patients with major depression. J Clin Psychiatry 53:57–60, 1992

Eagger SA, Levy R, Sahakian BJ: Tacrine in Alzheimer's disease. Lancet 337:989–992, 1991

Evans DA, Funkenstein H, Albert MS, et al: Prevalence of Alzheimer's disease in a community population of older persons. JAMA 262: 2551–2556, 1989

Farlow M, Gracon SI, Hershey LA, et al: A controlled trial of tacrine in Alzheimer's disease. JAMA 268:2523–2529, 1992

Feighner JP, Cohn JB: Double-blind comparative trials of fluoxetine and doxepin in geriatric patients with major depressive disorder. J Clin Psychiatry 46:20–25, 1985

Feighner JP, Boyer WF, Meredith CH, et al: An overview of fluoxetine in geriatric depression. Br J Psychiatry 153 (suppl 3):105–108, 1988

Ford DE, Kamerow DB: Epidemiological studies of sleep disturbances and psychiatric disorders: an opportunity for prevention? JAMA 262: 1479–1484, 1989

Forsman A, Ohman R: Applied pharmacokinetics of haloperidol in man. Current Therapeutic Research 21:396–411, 1977

Foster JR: Use of lithium in elderly psychiatric patients: a review of the literature. Lithium 3: 77–93, 1992

Foster JR, Martin CE: Dementia, in Verwoerdt's Clinical Geropsychiatry, 3rd Edition. Edited by Bienenfeld D. Baltimore, MD, Williams & Wilkins, 1990, pp 66–84

Frattola L, Maggioni M, Cesana B, et al: Double blind comparison of zolpidem 20 mg versus flunitrazepam 2 mg in insomniac in-patients. Drugs Exp Clin Res 16:371–376, 1990

Ganzini L, Heintz R, Hoffman WF, et al: Acute extrapyramidal syndromes in neuroleptic-treated elders: a pilot study. J Geriatr Psychiatry Neurol 4:222–225, 1991

Garrard J, Makris L, Dunham T, et al: Evaluation of neuroleptic drug use under proposed Medicare and Medicaid regulations. JAMA 265:463–467, 1991

Gauthier S, Bouchard R, Lamontagne A, et al: Tetrahydroaminoacridine-lecithin combination treatment in patients with intermediate stage Alzheimer's disease. N Engl J Med 322:1272–1276, 1990

Georgotas A, Mann J, Friedman E: Platelet monoamine oxidase inhibitors as a potential indicator of favorable response to MAOIs in geriatric depression. Biol Psychiatry 16:997–1001, 1981

Georgotas A, Friedman E, McCarthy M, et al: Resistant geriatric depressions and therapeutic response to monoamine oxidase inhibitors. Biol Psychiatry 18:195–205, 1983

Georgotas A, McCue RE, Hapworth W, et al: Comparative efficacy and safety of MAOIs versus TCAs in treating depression in the elderly. Biol Psychiatry 21:1155–1166, 1986

Gerner R, Estabrook W, Steuer J, et al: Treatment of depression with trazodone, imipramine, and placebo: a double-blind study. J Clin Psychiatry 41:216–220, 1980

Glasser M, Rabins P: Mania in the elderly. Age Ageing 13:210–213, 1984

Gottlieb GL: Sleep disorders and their management: special considerations in the elderly. Am J Med 88 (3A):29S–33S, 1990

Greenblatt DJ, Shader RI: Benzodiazepines in the elderly: pharmacokinetics and drug sensitivity, in Anxiety in the Elderly. Edited by Salzman C, Lebowitz B. New York, Springer, 1990, pp 131–145

Greenwald BS, Marin DB, Silverman SM: Serotonergic treatment of screaming and banging in dementia (letter). Lancet 2:1464–1465, 1986

Grymonpre RE, Mitenko PA, Sitar DS, et al: Drug-associated hospital admissions in older medical patients. J Am Geriatr Soc 36:1092–1098, 1988

Gurwitz JH, Avorn J: The ambiguous relationship between aging and adverse drug reactions. Ann Intern Med 114:956–966, 1991

Halaris A: Antidepressant drug therapy in the elderly: enhancing safety and compliance. Int J Psychiatry Med 16:1986–1987, 1986

Hale WE, May FE, Moore MT, et al: Meprobamate use in the elderly. J Am Geriatr Soc 36:1003–1005, 1988

Helms PM: Efficacy of antipsychotics in the treatment of the behavioral complications of dementia: a review of the literature. J Am Geriatr Soc 33:206–209, 1985

Hershey LA, Kim KY: Diagnosis and treatment of anxiety in the elderly. Rational Drug Therapy 22:3–6, 1988

Himmelhoch JM, Neil JF, May F, et al: Age, dementia, dyskinesias, and lithium response. Am J Psychiatry 137:941–945, 1980

Holton A, George K: The use of lithium in severely demented patients with behavioral disturbance. Br J Psychiatry 146:99–104, 1985

Huang CC: Comparison of two groups of tardive dyskinesia patients. Psychiatry Res 19:335–336, 1986

Institute of Medicine: Extending Life, Enhancing Life: A National Research Agenda on Aging. Washington, DC, National Academy Press, 1991

Ives TJ, Bentz EJ, Gwyther RE: Drug-related admissions to a family medicine inpatient service. Arch Intern Med 147:1117–1120, 1987

Jarvik LF, Read SL, Mintz J, et al: Pretreatment orthostatic hypotension in geriatric depression: predictor of response to imipramine and doxepin. J Clin Psychopharmacol 3:368–372, 1983

Jefferson JW, Griest JH, Ackerman DL, et al: Lithium Encyclopedia for Clinical Practice. Washington, DC, American Psychiatric Press, 1987

Jenike MA: The use of monoamine oxidase inhibitors in the treatment of elderly depressed patients. J Am Geriatric Soc 32:571–575, 1985

Jenike MA, Albert M, Heller H, et al: Oral physostigmine treatment for patients with presenile and senile dementia of the Alzheimer's-type: a double-blind, placebo-controlled trial. J Clin Psychiatry 51:3–7, 1990

Kanba S, Matsumoto K, Nibuya M, et al: Nortriptyline response in elderly depressed patients. Prog Neuropsychopharmacol Biol Psychiatry 16:301–309, 1992

Karson CG, Bracha HS, Powell A, et al: Dyskinetic movements, cognitive impairment, and negative symptoms in elderly neuropsychiatric patients. Am J Psychiatry 147:1646–1649, 1990

Katz IR, Simpson GM, Jethanandani V, et al: Steady state pharmacokinetics of nortriptyline in the frail elderly. Neuropsychopharmacology 2:229–236, 1989

Kemperman CJF, Gerdes JH, De Rooij J, et al: Reversible lithium neurotoxicity at normal serum level may refer to intracranial pathology. J Neurol Neurosurg Psychiatry 52:679–680, 1989

Kim KY: Diagnosis and treatment of depression in the elderly. Int J Psychiatry Med 18:211–221, 1988

Kitanka I, Ross RJ, Cutler NR, et al: Altered hydroxydesipramine concentrations in elderly depressed patients. Clin Pharmacol Ther 31:51–55, 1982

Koenig HG, Breitner JCS: Use of antidepressants in medically ill older patients. Psychosomatics 31:22–32, 1990

Koepke HH, Gold RL, Linden ME, et al: Multicenter controlled study of oxazepam in anxious elderly outpatients. Psychosomatics 23:641–645, 1982

Kroenke K, Pinholt EM: Reducing polypharmacy in the elderly: a controlled trial of physician feedback. J Am Geriatr Soc 38:31–36, 1990

Kroessler D, Fogel BS: Electroconvulsive therapy for major depression in the oldest old: effects of medical comorbidity on post-treatment survival. Am J Geriatr Psychiatry 1:30–37, 1993

Kutcher SP, Reid K, Dubbin JD, et al: Electrocardiogram changes and therapeutic desipramine and 2-hydroxydesipramine concentrations in elderly depressives. Br J Psychiatry 148:676–679, 1986

Kyomen HH, Nobel KW, Wei JY: The use of estrogen to decrease aggressive physical behavior in elderly men with dementia. J Am Geriatr Soc 39:1110–1112, 1991

Lakshmanan EB, Mion CC, Frengley JD: Effective low dose tricyclic antidepressant treatment for depressed geriatric rehabilitation patients. J Am Geriatr Soc 34:421–426, 1986

Lavretsky EP, Jarvik LF: A group of potassium-channel blockers-acetylcholine releasers: new potentials for Alzheimer disease? A review. J Clin Psychopharmacol 12:110–118, 1992

Lazarus LW, Groves L, Gierl B, et al: Efficacy of phenelzine in geriatric depression. Biol Psychiatry 21:699–701, 1986

Leibovici A, Tariot N: Carbamazepine treatment of agitation associated with dementia. J Geriatr Psychiatry Neurol 1:110–112, 1988

Lieberman J, Kane JM, Woerner M, et al: Prevalence of tardive dyskinesia in elderly samples. Psychopharmacol Bull 20:22–26, 1984

Liptzin B: Treatment of mania, in Clinical Geriatric Psychopharmacology, 2nd Edition. Edited by Salzman C. Baltimore, MD, Williams & Wilkins, 1992, pp 175–188

Magni G, Palazzolo O, Bianchin G: The course of depression in elderly outpatients. Can J Psychiatry 33:21–24, 1988

Maletta GS: Use of antipsychotic medications, in Annual Review of Gerontology and Geriatrics, Vol 4. Edited by Eisdorfer C. New York, Springer, 1984, pp 175–220

McCue RE, Georgotas A, Nagachandran N, et al: Plasma levels of nortriptyline and 10-hydroxynortriptyline and treatment-related electrocardiographic changes in the elderly depressed. J Psychiatr Res 23:73–79, 1989

McFarland BH, Miller MR, Straumfjord AA: Valproate use in the older manic patient. J Clin Psychiatry 51:479–481, 1990

Meyers BS: Adverse cognitive effects of tricyclic antidepressants in the treatment of geriatric depression: fact or fiction?, in Psychopharmacological Treatment Complications in the Elderly. Edited by Shamoian CA. Washington, DC, American Psychiatric Press, 1992, pp 1–16

Miller SW, Mahoney JM, Jann MW: Therapeutic frontiers in Alzheimer's disease. Pharmacotherapy 12:217–231, 1992

Morgan DG, May PC, Finch LE: Dopamine and serotonin systems in human and rodent brain: effects of age and neurodegenerative disease. J Am Geriatr Soc 35:334–345, 1987

Napoliello MJ: An interim multicentre report on 677 anxious geriatric out-patients treated with buspirone. British Journal of Clinical Practice 40:71–73, 1986

National Center for Health Statistics: Current estimates from the National Health Interview Survey: Vital and Health Statistics 1987, No. 10, in Aging America: Trends and Projections, 1986–1987. Washington, DC, U.S. Government Printing Office, 1987, p 164

Nelson JC, Atillasoy E, Mazure C: Desipramine plasma levels and response in elderly melancholic patients. J Clin Psychopharmacol 5:217–220, 1985

Nelson JC, Atillasoy E, Mazure C, et al: Hydroxydesipramine in the elderly. J Clin Psychopharmacol 8:428–433, 1988

Office of Epidemiology and Biostatistics, Center for Drug Evaluation and Research: Drug Utilization in the United States, 1986. Washington, DC, National Technical Information Service, 1987

Olafsson K, Jorgensen S, Jensen HV, et al: Fluvoxamine in the treatment of demented elderly patients: a double-blind, placebo-controlled study. Acta Psychiatr Scand 85:453–456, 1992

Old Age Depression Interest Group: How long should the elderly take antidepressants? A double-blind placebo-controlled study of continuation/prophylaxis therapy with dothiepin. Br J Psychiatry 162:175–182, 1993

Oreland L, Gottfries CG: Brain monoamine oxidase in aging and in dementia of the Alzheimer type. Prog Neuropsychopharmacol Biol Psychiatry 10:533–540, 1986

Parmelee PA, Katz IR, Lawton MP: Anxiety and association with depression among institutionalized elderly. Am J Geriatr Psychiatry 1:46–58, 1993

Peabody CA, Whiteford HA, Hollister LE: Antidepressants and the elderly. J Am Geriatr Soc 34:869–874, 1986

Peabody CA, Warner MD, Whiteford HA, et al: Neuroleptics and the elderly. J Am Geriatr Soc 35:233–238, 1987

Perry E, Tomlinson B, Blessed G, et al: Correlation of cholinergic abnormalities with senile plaques and mental test scores in senile dementia. BMJ 2:1457–1459, 1978

Petrie WM, Ban TA, Berney S, et al: Loxapine in psychogeriatrics: a placebo and standard controlled clinical investigation. J Clin Psychopharmacol 2:122–126, 1982

Phillipson M, Moranville JT, Jeste DV, et al: Antipsychotics. Clin Geriatr Med 6:411–422, 1990

Pinner E, Rich CL: Effects of trazodone on aggressive behavior in seven patients with organic mental disorders. Am J Psychiatry 145:1295–1296, 1988

Pinsker H, Suljaga-Petchel K: Use of benzodiazepines in primary-care geriatric patients. J Am Geriatr Soc 32:595–598, 1984

Pollack CP, Perlick D: Sleep problems and institutionalization of the elderly. J Geriatr Psychiatry Neurol 4:204–210, 1991

Prinz PN, Vitiello MV, Raskind MA, et al: Geriatrics: sleep disorders and aging. N Engl J Med 323:520–526, 1990

Rashi S, Logan RFA: Role of drugs in fractures of the femoral neck. BMJ 292:86, 1986

Ray WA, Federspiel CF, Schaffner W: A study of anti-psychotic drug use in nursing homes: epidemiologic evidence suggesting misuse. Am J Public Health 70:485–491, 1980

Ray WA, Griffin MR, Shaffner W, et al: Psychotropic drug use and the risk of hip fracture. N Engl J Med 316:363–369, 1987

Ray WA, Fought RL, Decker MD: Psychoactive drugs and the risk of injurious motor vehicle crashes in elderly drivers. Am J Epidemiol 136:873–883, 1992

Regestein QR: Treatment of insomnia in the elderly, in Clinical Geriatric Psychopharmacology, 2nd Edition. Edited by Salzman C. Baltimore, MD, Williams & Wilkins, 1992, pp 235–253

Reynolds CF: Sleep disorders, in Comprehensive Review of Geriatric Psychiatry. Edited by Sadavoy J, Lazarus LW, Jarvik LF. Washington, DC, American Psychiatric Press, 1991, pp 403–418

Risse SC, Barnes R: Pharmacologic treatment of agitation associated with dementia. J Am Geriatr Soc 34:368–376, 1986

Robinson DS, Sourkes TL, Nies A, et al: Monoamine metabolism in human brain. Arch Gen Psychiatry 34:89–92, 1977

Rockwell E, Lam RW, Zisook S: Antidepressant drug studies in the elderly. Psychiatr Clin North Am 11:215–233, 1988

Rosebush PI, Salzman C: Memory disturbance and cognitive impairment in the elderly, in Handbook of Clinical Psychopharmacology. Edited by Tupin JP, Shader RI, Harnett DS. New York, Jason Aronson, 1988, pp 159–210

Rothschild AJ, Samson AJ, Bessette MP, et al: Efficacy of the combination of fluoxetine and perphenazine in the treatment of psychotic depression. J Clin Psychiatry 54:338–342, 1993

Rovner B, Kafonek S, Filipp L, et al: Prevalence of mental illness in a nursing home. Am J Psychiatry 143:1146–1149, 1986

Rovner BW, German PS, Brant LJ, et al: Depression and mortality in nursing homes. JAMA 265:993–996, 1991

Saban RJ, Vitug AJ, Mark VH: Are nursing home diagnosis and treatment inadequate? JAMA 243:321–322, 1982

Saltz BL, Kane JM, Woerner MG, et al: Prospective study of tardive dyskinesia in the elderly. Psychopharmacol Bull 25:52–56, 1989

Salzman C: Treatment of agitation in the elderly, in Psychopharmacology: The Third Generation of Progress. Edited by Meltzer HY. New York, Raven, 1987, pp 1167–1176

Salzman C: The American Psychiatric Association Task Force Report on Benzodiazepine Dependency, Toxicity, and Abuse. J Psychiatr Res 24: 35–37, 1990a

Salzman C: Practical considerations of the pharmacologic treatment of depression and anxiety in the elderly. J Clin Psychiatry 51 (1 suppl):40–43, 1990b

Salzman C: Recent advances in geriatric psychopharmacology, in American Psychiatric Press Review of Psychiatry, Vol 9. Edited by Tasman A, Goldfinger SM, Kaufmann C. Washington, DC, American Psychiatric Press, 1990c, pp 279–292

Salzman C: Monoamine oxidase inhibitors and atypical antidepressants. Clin Geriatr Med 8:335–348, 1992

Salzman C: Pharmacologic treatment of depression in the elderly. J Clin Psychiatry 54 (suppl): 23–28, 1993

Salzman C: Pharmacological treatment of depression in elderly patients, in Diagnosis and Treatment of Depression in Late Life: Results of the NIH Consensus Development Conference. Edited by Schneider LS, Reynolds CF, Lebowitz BD, et al. Washington, DC, American Psychiatric Press, 1994, pp 181–244

Salzman C, Fisher J, Nobel K, et al: Cognitive improvement following benzodiazepine discontinuation in elderly nursing home residents. Int J Geriatr Psychiatry 7:89–93, 1992

Salzman C, Schneider LS, Lebowitz BD: Antidepressant treatment of very old patients. Am J Geriatr Psychiatry 1:21–29, 1993

Satlin A, Liptzin B: Treatment of mania, in Clinical Geriatric Psychopharmacology, 3rd Edition. Edited by Salzman C. Baltimore, MD, Williams & Wilkins, 1998, pp 310–332

Schneider JK, Mion LC, Frengley JD: Adverse drug reactions in an elderly outpatient population. American Journal of Hospital Pharmacy 49:90–96, 1992

Schneider LS, Sloane RB, Staples FR, et al: Pretreatment orthostatic hypotension as a predictor of response to nortriptyline in geriatric depression. J Clin Psychopharmacol 6:172–176, 1986

Schneider LS, Cooper TB, Suckow RF, et al: Relationship of hydroxynortriptyline to nortriptyline concentration and creatinine clearance in depressed elderly outpatients. J Clin Psychopharmacol 10:333–337, 1990a

Schneider LS, Pollock VE, Lyness SA: A meta-analysis of controlled trials of neuroleptic treatment in dementia. J Am Geriatr Soc 38:553–563, 1990b

Sheikh JI: Panic disorder, in Anxiety in the Elderly. Edited by Salzman C, Lebowitz B. New York, Springer, 1990, pp 251–266

Shulman KI, Tohen M, Satlin A, et al: Mania compared with unipolar depression in old age. Am J Psychiatry 149:341–345, 1992

Simpson DM, Foster D: Improvement in organically disturbed behavior with trazodone treatment. J Clin Psychiatry 47:191–193, 1986

Skoog I, Nilsson L, Palmertz B, et al: A population-based study of dementia in 85-year-olds. N Engl J Med 328:153–158, 1993

Small GW: Psychopharmacological treatment of elderly demented patients. J Clin Psychiatry 49 (suppl):8–13, 1988

Smith JM, Baldessarini RJ: Changes in prevalence, severity and recovery in tardive dyskinesia with age. Arch Gen Psychiatry 37:1368–1373, 1980

Smith M, Buckwalter KC: Medication management, antidepressant drugs, and the elderly: an overview. Journal of Psychosocial Nursing 30: 30–36, 1992

Snowdon J: A retrospective case-note study of bipolar disorder in old age. Br J Psychiatry 158: 485–490, 1991

Spagnoli A, Lucca U, Menasce G, et al: Long-term acetyl-L-carnitine treatment in Alzheimer's disease. Neurology 41:1726–1732, 1991

Stack JA, Reynolds CF III, Perel JM, et al: Pretreatment systolic orthostatic blood pressure (PSOP) and treatment response in elderly depressed inpatients. J Clin Psychopharmacol 8:116–120, 1988

Stern Y, Sano M, Mayeux R: Long-term administration of oral physostigmine in Alzheimer's disease. Neurology 38:1837–1841, 1988

Stewart RB, May FE, Moore MY, et al: Changing patterns of psychotropic drug use in the elderly: a five-year update. Ann Pharmacother 23: 610–613, 1989

Stone K: Mania in the elderly. Br J Psychiatry 155: 220–229, 1989

Strauss A: Oral dyskinesia associated with buspirone use in an elderly woman. J Clin Psychiatry 49:322–323, 1988

Sweet RA, Benoit H, Mulsant MD, et al: Dyskinesia and neuroleptic exposure in elderly psychiatric inpatients. J Geriatr Psychiatry Neurol 5: 156–161, 1992

Szuba MP, Leuchter AF: Falling backward in two elderly patients taking bupropion. J Clin Psychiatry 53:157–159, 1992

Tariot PN: Neurobiology and treatment of dementia, in Clinical Geriatric Psychopharmacology, 2nd Edition. Edited by Salzman C. Baltimore, MD, Williams & Wilkins, 1992, pp 277–299

Thompson TL, Filley CM, Mitchell WD, et al: Lack of efficacy of hydergine in patients with Alzheimer's disease. N Engl J Med 323: 445–448, 1990

Tingle D: Trazodone in dementia (letter). J Clin Psychiatry 47:482, 1986

Tollefson GD: Short-term effects of the calcium channel blocker nimodipine (Bay-e-9736) in the management of primary degenerative dementia. Biol Psychiatry 27:1133–1142, 1990

Vogel GW, Morris D: The effects of estazolam on sleep, performance, and memory: a long-term sleep laboratory study of elderly insomniacs. J Clin Pharmacol 32:647–651, 1992

von Moltke LL, Greenblatt DJ, Shader RI: Clinical pharmacokinetics of antidepressants in the elderly. Clin Pharmacokinet 24:141–160, 1993

von Moltke LL, Abernethy DR, Greenblatt DJ: Kinetics and dynamics of psychotropic drugs in the elderly, in Clinical Geriatric Psychopharmacology, 3rd Edition. Edited by Salzman C. Baltimore, MD, Williams & Wilkins, 1998, pp 70–96

Weiler PG, Mungo D, Bernick C: Propranolol for the control of disruptive behavior in senile dementia. J Geriatr Psychiatry Neurol 1:226–230, 1988

Weissman MM, Prusoff B, Sholomskas AJ, et al: A double-blind clinical trial of alprazolam, imipramine, or placebo in the depressed elderly. J Clin Psychopharmacol 12:175–182, 1992

Wragg RE, Jeste DV: Neuroleptics and alternative treatments: management of behavioral symptoms and psychosis in Alzheimer's disease and related conditions. Psychiatr Clin North Am 11: 195–213, 1988

Yassa R: The course of tardive dyskinesia in newly treated psychogeriatric patients. Acta Psychiatr Scand 83:347–349, 1991

Yassa R, Nair V, Schwartz G: Tardive dyskinesia: a two-year follow-up study. Psychosomatics 25: 852–855, 1984

Yassa R, Nastase C, Camille Y, et al: Tardive dyskinesia in a psychogeriatric population, in Tardive Dyskinesia: Biological Mechanisms and Clinical Aspects. Edited by Wolf ME, Mosnaim AD. Washington, DC, American Psychiatric Press, 1988, pp 125–133

Young RC, Alexopoulos GS, Shamoian CA, et al: Plasma 10-hydroxynortriptyline in elderly depressed patients. Clin Pharmacol Ther 35: 540–544, 1984

Young RC, Alexopoulos GS, Shamoian CA, et al: Plasma 10-hydroxynortriptyline and ECG changes in elderly depressed patients. Am J Psychiatry 142:866–868, 1985

Zimmer JG, Watson N, Trent A: Behavior problems among patients in skilled nursing facilities. Am J Public Health 74:1118–1121, 1984

Zimmer JG, Bentley DW, Valente WM: Systemic antibiotic use in nursing homes: a quality assessment. J Am Geriatr Soc 34:703–710, 1986

Zisook S: A clinical overview of monoamine oxidase inhibitors. Psychosomatics 26:240–246, 1985

THIRTY

Psychopharmacology During Pregnancy and Lactation

Zachary N. Stowe, M.D.,
James R. Strader Jr., B.S., and
Charles B. Nemeroff, M.D., Ph.D.

The management of mental illness during pregnancy and lactation represents a unique and complex clinical situation. The use of psychotropic medications during pregnancy and lactation has been comprehensively reviewed by several groups (Altshuler et al. 1996; Cohen 1989; Cohen et al. 1989; Kerns 1986; Miller 1991, 1994; Robinson et al. 1986; Stowe and Nemeroff 1995; Wisner and Perel 1988). The most common situations that the clinician will encounter in patients who are pregnant or lactating include the following:

- New-onset mental illness
- Exacerbation of psychiatric symptoms in the presence of preexisting mental illness
- Inadvertent conception during treatment with psychotropic medications
- Prepregnancy consultation for women who have a history of mental illness and/or are currently taking psychotropic medications

- Prophylactic treatment planning for women at high risk for a postpartum mental illness who plan to nurse

The literature, although expanding rapidly, provides little definitive data to develop scientifically derived guidelines in such situations. The most prominent confounding factors in these studies include 1) the failure of adequate sample size to establish a significant causal relationship for teratogenic or toxic effects of psychotropic medications, 2) the reliance on case reports, and 3) limited methodological consistency.

The Collaborative Perinatal Project followed up a cohort of 50,282 mother-infant pairs from 12 medical centers and found an overall infant malformation rate of 6.5% (Heinonen et al. 1977). Studies on embryonic development have shown that most major malformations occur during the embryonic period (i.e., the third through the eighth week of gestation). After week 11 of gestation, most of the organ systems (except for the central nervous system, teeth, ears, eyes, and external genitalia) are developed

(Sadler 1985). A second major issue, noted in previous reviews (Cohen et al. 1989), is that up to 80% of pregnant women are prescribed medications, and more than one-third of pregnant women may take psychotropic medications at some point in their pregnancy (Doering and Stewart 1978). Most previous case reports fail to control for maternal age, tobacco use, alcohol and drug abuse, potential exposure to environmental toxins, duration and timing of exposure, and the extent of prenatal care received.

PHYSIOLOGY—PREGNANCY

Physiological changes during pregnancy that may alter maternal serum concentrations of psychotropic medications include the following:

- Delayed gastric emptying, which results in increased exposure to an acidic environment and degradative enzymes
- Decreased gastrointestinal motility, presumably related to increased progesterone, which potentially enhances complete absorption of medication
- Increased volume of distribution (increased body fat, plasma volume, total body water), which produces decreased serum concentrations for a given dose
- Decreased protein binding capacity, which increases serum free drug concentrations (Wood and Hytten 1981)
- Increased hepatic metabolism, which results in more rapid degradation of certain medications

All of these factors may alter the drug concentration to which the fetus is exposed.

Although no evidence of placental filtering of psychotropic medications exists, formal studies are lacking. All psychotropic medications are assumed to cross the blood-placental barrier. Our group (Stowe et al. 1997a) studied the placental passage of antidepressants in women treated during pregnancy and found significant differences among the selective serotonin reuptake inhibitors (SSRIs), a finding that warrants more formal study to minimize fetal exposure within a given class of medication. The mechanism of placental transport is thought to be simple diffusion that is dependent on several properties of the individual medication (molecular size, percentage of protein binding, polarity, lipid solubility) and, of course, duration of exposure (Rayburn and Andresen 1982). Although the fetus and mother are at equilibrium with respect to circulation, the fetus has several distinct physiological attributes that may result in its increased exposure to medications and potentially greater drug concentrations in the central nervous system. These attributes include increased cardiac output, increased blood-brain barrier permeability, decreased plasma protein and plasma protein binding affinity, and decreased hepatic enzyme activity.

PHYSIOLOGY—LACTATION

After childbirth, the neonate continues to exhibit unique physiological characteristics, including decreased activity of certain hepatic metabolic enzyme systems. Hepatic maturation in the infant appears to occur at a highly variable rate (Warner 1986) and is more delayed in premature infants. Both glucuronidation and oxidation systems are initially immature at birth (as low as 20% of adult levels). The latter system typically matures by age 3 months (Atkinson et al. 1988). In addition, rates of glomerular filtration and tubular secretion are relatively low in neonates—30%–40% and 20%–30% lower than adult levels, respectively (Welch and Findlay 1981). Hence, the potential for the infant to be exposed to higher serum concentrations of parent compounds and metabolites of any drug needs to be considered.

Neonates and infants are exposed to psychotropic medications when the mother breast-feeds during pharmacological treatment. The excretion of psychotropic medications in breast milk has been reviewed elsewhere (Buist et al. 1990; Wisner et al. 1996). The literature is again difficult to interpret because of differences in the methodology of drug concentration assays as well as an identified gradient in breast milk with respect to lipophilic characteristics and protein content (Kauffman et al. 1994; Vorherr 1974). Most data have not controlled for which aliquot of the breast milk was used for assay nor the time after maternal dose when the aliquot was obtained.

The physiochemical properties of an individual medication appear to be the best predictor of the amount of medication present in breast milk (see Kacew 1993 for review). These properties include the degree of ionization, molecular weight, protein binding, and lipid solubility. Maternal protein binding affects the quantity of free drug available for diffusion across the mammillary epithelium, and most medications have a higher affinity for maternal plasma proteins than for milk proteins (Kacew 1993).

The American Academy of Pediatrics (1994) published a committee report on the excretion of drugs and other chemicals into human breast milk. Although admittedly not complete, the report's list of psychotropic medications underscores the need to encourage further collaborative work with pediatricians. The academy's classification of individual psychotropic medications includes 1) drugs that are contraindicated during breast-feeding, 2) drugs whose effect on nursing infants is unknown but may be of concern (i.e., no adverse events have been reported, but the medications are present in human milk and thus conceivably alter development of the central nervous system), and 3) maternal medications usually compatible with breast-feeding. The information contained in the academy's report is included later in this chapter in our discussion of the individual classes of psychotropic medications.

ASSESSMENT OF RISK-BENEFIT RATIO

The morbidity and mortality of untreated mental illness during pregnancy and lactation have received limited attention. The sparse data that are available suggest some salient illness-specific features about the course of illness during pregnancy that should be considered in the risk-benefit assessment. Some psychiatric disorders, such as panic disorder, may improve or abate during pregnancy (Klein et al. 1994/1995). In contrast, obsessive-compulsive disorder appears to be more prevalent during pregnancy: in one study, more than 25% of women reported symptom onset during pregnancy (Neziroglu et al. 1992). Psychiatric disorders with a psychotic component (e.g., schizophrenia, schizoaffective disorder) were observed to generally worsen during pregnancy (McNeil et al. 1984a, 1984b). Finally, the rates and severity of depression during pregnancy span a wide range based on the diagnostic criteria employed (Buesching et al. 1986; Cutrona 1983; Kumar and Robson 1984; Manley et al. 1982; O'Hara et al. 1982, 1984; Raskin et al. 1990; Watson et al. 1984).

Furthermore, at least one group has assessed the rates of "normal depressive symptomatology" that accompany the somatic changes of pregnancy in women whose symptoms did not meet criteria for depression (Affonso et al. 1993). Their findings suggest that, to some extent, the epidemiology of depression during pregnancy may be confounded by the natural occurrence of symptoms inventoried on many depression screening tools and rating scales. Together, these data depict a much more complex relationship between psychiatric illness and pregnancy, making general guidelines difficult to establish.

The risk to the fetus of untreated psychiatric illness during pregnancy is unclear. Although untreated schizophrenia is known to be associated with an increased incidence of perinatal death (Rieder et al. 1975), little is known of the effects, if any, of other psychiatric disorders on the fetus. One group that administered the General Health Questionnaire (Perkin et al. 1993) concluded that depressive and anxiety symptoms did not adversely affect obstetrical outcome. In contrast, Steer et al. (1992) found a risk of 3.97 for lower birth weight (<2,500 g), a risk of 3.39 for preterm delivery (<37 weeks' gestation), and a risk of 3.02 for small for gestational age (<10th percentile) in a group of adult women derived from an inner-city population with Beck Depression Inventory (Beck 1978) scores of 21 or higher. Similarly, preclinical studies have found an adverse effect of both maternal stress and increased maternal glucocorticoid concentrations on brain development (Meaney et al. 1996).

The vast majority of studies focus on untreated maternal depression. These studies show deleterious effects on maternal-infant attachment and child development (Avant 1981; Brazelton 1975; Campbell et al. 1995; Cradon 1979; Cutrona 1983; Murray 1992; Teti et al. 1995; Zahn-Waxler et al. 1984).

Because the majority of women are not aware of their pregnancy until at least 6 weeks of gestation, psychotropic medications may be discontinued after the period of greatest potential risk to the fetus has passed. Abrupt discontinuation of medications may also carry an increased risk of relapse or development of withdrawal symptoms. Both situations may result in increased risk to the mother and/or greater fetal exposure to medication. Clinicians assessing the risks and benefits of treating pregnant women with concurrent psychiatric illness should take into account personal and family psychiatric histories; the possible course of illness; the effects of untreated illness on the fetus; and the teratogenic, perinatal, and neurobehavioral effects of individual psychotropic medications.

To date, the U.S. Food and Drug Administration (FDA) has not approved any psychotropic medication for use during pregnancy or lactation. The current classification system is presented in Table 30–1. One potential con-

founder of this system is that adverse case reports are more likely to have been filed for medications that have been available longer. The significance of these adverse case reports is difficult to evaluate.

Altshuler et al. (1996) determined the risk of psychotropic medication during pregnancy to fall into one of three categories: 1) somatic teratogenicity and organ malformation; 2) neonatal toxicity, including perinatal syndromes and withdrawal symptomatology; and 3) long-term neurobehavioral and developmental teratogenic effects. We address each of these issues in the discussions to follow as we describe the individual classes of psychotropic medications. It is important to note that little is known about how most psychotropic medications affect these three axes.

ANTIDEPRESSANTS

Tricyclic antidepressants (TCAs) have been available in the United States since 1963, and their use has extended well beyond treating depression. The development of non-TCAs has further broadened the spectrum of the clinical utility of antidepressants as a class to include obsessive-compulsive disorder (clomipramine, fluvoxamine, paroxetine, sertraline, fluoxetine), panic disorder (imipramine, fluoxetine, paroxetine, sertraline), pain syndromes (amitriptyline, nortriptyline, doxepin, paroxetine, venlafaxine), bulimia (fluoxetine), and premenstrual syndromes (fluoxetine, nortriptyline, clomipramine). Investigations indicate that 9%–18% of women have symptoms that meet criteria for a mood disorder (both minor and major) during pregnancy (Kumar and Robson 1984; O'Hara et al. 1984, 1990; Watson et al. 1984).

Despite the widespread use of TCAs during pregnancy, no clear association with congenital malformations has been demonstrated (see Table 30–2 for information on individual medications). Altshuler et al. (1996) reviewed 14 studies, both prospective and retrospective in

Table 30–1. U.S. Food and Drug Administration (FDA) use-in-pregnancy ratings

Category	Interpretation
A	**Controlled studies show no risk:** Adequate, well-controlled studies in pregnant women have failed to demonstrate a risk to the fetus in any trimester of pregnancy.
B	**No evidence of risk in humans:** Adequate, well-controlled studies in pregnant women have not shown increased risk of fetal abnormalities despite adverse findings in animals, or, in the absence of adequate human studies, animal studies show no fetal risk. The chance of fetal harm is remote, but remains a possibility.
C	**Risk cannot be ruled out:** Adequate, well-controlled human studies are lacking, and animal studies have shown a risk to the fetus or are lacking as well. There is a chance of fetal harm if the drug is administered during pregnancy; but the potential benefits may outweigh the potential risk.
D	**Positive evidence of risk:** Studies in humans, or investigational or postmarketing data, have demonstrated fetal risk. Nevertheless, potential benefits from the use of the drug may outweigh the potential risk. For example, the drug may be acceptable if needed in a life-threatening situation or serious disease for which safer drugs cannot be used or are ineffective.
X	**Contraindicated in pregnancy:** Studies in animals or humans, or investigational or postmarketing reports, have demonstrated positive evidence of fetal abnormalities or risk that clearly outweighs any possible benefit to the patient.

Source.   *Physicians' Desk Reference*, 55th Edition. Montvale, NJ, Medical Economics, 2001.

design, of in utero exposure to TCAs representing more than 300,000 total live births. Only 13 malformations were noted in 414 first-trimester exposures—an incidence of 3.14%. Similar rates were noted by McElhatton et al. (1996) in a review of data from the European Network of Teratology Information Services. This rate is within the normal baseline incidence of 2%–4%.

The issue of neonatal withdrawal is complicated by the lack of data about maternal dosing during labor. Symptoms reported include tachypnea, tachycardia, cyanosis, irritability, hypertonia, clonus, and spasm (Eggermont 1973; Miller 1991; Webster 1973). Wisner et al. (1993) reported that the TCA dosage for women with depression during pregnancy may need to be increased over the course of pregnancy to maintain adequate therapeutic serum concentrations and response.

Human data on the use of monoamine oxidase inhibitors (MAOIs) during pregnancy and lactation are limited. Although the MAOIs are all FDA category C medications, one prospective study in a small group of patients indicated that in utero tranylcypromine exposure is associated with fetal malformations. Studies in animals (Poulson and Robson 1964) have reported teratogenic effects associated with the MAOIs. The dietary constraints and potential for hypertensive crisis are relative contraindications to the use of MAOIs during pregnancy (Wisner and Perel 1988).

Data on the use of SSRIs during pregnancy are steadily accumulating. In one of the first investigations of first-trimester exposure to

Table 30–2. Antidepressant medications

Generic name	Trade name	Daily dose (mg/day)[a]	Half-life (hours)[b]	Risk category[c]	American Academy of Pediatrics rating[d]
Tricyclic/heterocyclic antidepressants					
Amitriptyline	Elavil, Endep	150–300	10–22	D	Unknown, but of concern
Amoxapine	Asendin	150–400	8–20	C_m	Unknown, but of concern
Clomipramine	Anafranil	150–250	19–37	C_m	Unknown, but of concern[e]
Desipramine	Norpramin	150–300	12–76	C	Unknown, but of concern
Doxepin	Sinequan, Adapin	150–300	11–23	C	Unknown, but of concern
Imipramine	Tofranil	150–300	11–25	D	Unknown, but of concern
Nortriptyline	Pamelor, Aventyl	75–150	15–93	D	N/A
Maprotiline	Ludiomil	140–225	21–66	B_m	N/A
Protriptyline	Vivactil	15–60	54–198	C	N/A
Monoamine oxidase inhibitors					
Isocarboxazid	Marplan	30–60	N/A	C	N/A
Phenelzine	Nardil	45–90	N/A	C	N/A
Tranylcypromine	Parnate	30–60	N/A	C	N/A
Selective serotonin reuptake inhibitors					
Fluoxetine	Prozac	20–60	24–96	C	Unknown, but of concern
Fluvoxamine[f]	Luvox	50–300	17–22	C	Unknown, but of concern
Paroxetine[f]	Paxil	20–50	24	C	N/A
Sertraline	Zoloft	50–200	26	C	N/A
Other antidepressants					
Bupropion	Wellbutrin	150–450	8–24	B_m	N/A
Mirtazapine	Remeron	15–45	20–40	C	N/A
Nefazodone	Serzone	300–600	2–4	C	N/A

| Trazodone | Desyrel | 200–300 | 4–13 | C_m | Unknown, but of concern |
| Venlafaxine[f] | Effexor | 150–375 | 5–11 | C_m | N/A |

Note. N/A = not applicable.

[a] Dosing strategies adapted from Schatzberg and Cole 1991; Kaplan and Sadock 1993; and, for newer medications, the manufacturers' package inserts.

[b] Half-life of elimination is listed for parent compound.

[c] Risk category adapted from Briggs et al. 1994; "m" subscript is for data taken from the manufacturer's package insert.

[d] American Academy of Pediatrics 1994.

[e] Original 1994 committee report listed as "compatible," and a correction was later published.

[f] Not listed in Briggs et al. 1994. Risk category taken from *Physicians' Desk Reference* 1992, 1993, 1994, 1996.

fluoxetine (mean dose 25.8 mg/day), no demonstrable increase in fetal anomalies was noted among 128 women (Pastuszak et al. 1993). The manufacturer's index currently lists more than 1,700 cases of first-trimester exposure to fluoxetine with no evidence of an increased incidence of congenital malformations or of a clustering of any particular anomaly (Eli Lilly, Inc., personal communication, January 1997). McElhatton et al. (1996) reported that of 92 women who received SSRI monotherapy during pregnancy, only two cases of infant major malformations were noted. The only study to date of known first-trimester exposure to paroxetine found no congenital malformations among 63 pregnancies (Inman et al. 1993). Most recent data report no evidence of a teratogenic effect resulting from SSRI exposure (Ericson et al. 1999; Kulin et al. 1998).

Obstetrical outcome is not confined to physical malformations. Pastuszak et al. (1993) noted that the rate of spontaneous abortion was higher among SSRI- and TCA-treated women than among control subjects (14.8%, 12.2%, and 7.8%, respectively). Two groups have found a slight increase in birth weight among neonates exposed to fluoxetine during pregnancy, but these differences did not achieve statistical significance (Chambers et al. 1993; Nulman et al. 1997). In one report, third-trimester fluoxetine exposure was associated with decreased birth weight and increased minor anomalies (Chambers et al. 1996). The numerous confounding factors present in this study, however, render definitive conclusions speculative at best.

In a landmark study, Nulman et al. (1997) conducted extensive neurodevelopmental assessment of children exposed in utero to antidepressant medications (TCA-treated subjects, *n* = 80; fluoxetine-treated subjects, *n* = 55; no exposure, *n* = 84). Children between ages 16 and 86 months were assessed with numerous study measures and diagnostic tools for factors such as global intelligence quotient (IQ), language development, temperament, mood, activity level, and behavior. The children whose mothers received antidepressants during pregnancy—either fluoxetine or a TCA—did not differ from the no-exposure control children on any measure of neurodevelopment. Furthermore, global IQ and language development scores were nearly identical among all groups. In conclusion, in utero exposure to fluoxetine or TCAs did not affect either neurodevelopment or behavior in preschool-aged children.

Studies on drug excretion in breast milk have demonstrated that antidepressants are present in breast milk with a milk-to-serum ratio that is typically ≥1.0 (Buist et al. 1990). Wisner et al. (1996) reviewed the extant literature on the serum concentrations of antidepressants and their metabolites in nursing infants. They found that, although TCAs readily enter breast milk, most parent compounds and metabolites are undetectable in infant serum by 10 weeks, and there is no evidence of drug or metabolite accumulation in the neonate. The only exception to this was doxepin, which was present in concentrations of 3 ng/mL. Doxepin was also the only TCA to be associated with an adverse outcome (respiratory depression) during lactation in one study (Matheson et al. 1985). Those authors concluded that most TCAs (amitriptyline, nortriptyline, desipramine, clomipramine, and dothiepin) are safe for use during breastfeeding. The data on SSRIs were somewhat less benign.

Two groups (Birnbaum et al. 1999; Kim et al. 1997) did not find evidence of accumulation of fluoxetine in breast-feeding infants. Only a single case report is available for fluvoxamine (Wright et al. 1991). Expanding experience with sertraline (Altshuler et al. 1995; DeVane 1992; Stowe et al. 1997b) has indicated predominantly undetectable concentrations in infant serum (Stowe et al. 2000). The follow-up data on infants exposed during breast-feeding are sparse. Llewellyn et al. (1997) found no adverse effects on growth and milestone achievement in 12 infants exposed to sertraline. What is most remarkable about this literature is the small number of patients and infants that constitute the total number of studies.

The elapsed time between maternal dosing and infant feeding has been shown to affect the amount of antidepressant medication to which the nursling is exposed. Amitriptyline (Pittard and O'Neal 1986), desipramine (Stancer and Reed 1986), and trazodone (Verbeeck et al. 1986) appear to reach a peak in breast milk at 4–6 hours after an oral dose. A detailed study (Stowe et al. 1997b) of sertraline excretion into breast milk identified both a concentration gradient from "fore" milk to "hind" milk and a time course of excretion that paralleled the gastrointestinal absorptive phase. Peak concentrations occurred 7–10 hours after maternal dose, and by simply discarding one feeding (at 7–8 hours after the maternal dose), we determined that the total daily dose to which an infant would be exposed could be decreased by nearly 25%. The clinical utility of such calculations is obvious and substantial. The ability to estimate accurate levels of medication in breast milk would allow the development of individually tailored therapeutic regimens that maximize maternal care while minimizing infant exposure.

In summary, most earlier reviews recommend using the secondary amine TCAs (nortriptyline and desipramine) (Miller 1991; Wisner et al. 1996). In light of the increasing data on SSRIs and the lack of adverse reports, however, these recommendations are likely to be revised.

ANTIPSYCHOTICS

In contrast with other classes of psychotropic medications, antipsychotic agents have a considerably larger database that addresses concerns of neurobehavioral teratogenicity. Chlorpromazine, haloperidol, and perphenazine have received the greatest scrutiny, and investigators have failed to find a significant association between the use of these drugs and major congenital malformations (Goldberg and DiMascio 1978; Hill and Stern 1979; Nurnberg and

Table 30–3. Antipsychotic medications

Generic name	Trade name	Daily dose (mg/day)[a]	Half-life (hours)[b]	Risk category[c]	American Academy of Pediatrics rating[d]
Chlorpromazine	Thorazine	200–800	8–35	C	Unknown, but of concern
Clozapine	Clozaril	100–800	4–66	B_m	N/A
Fluphenazine	Prolixin	5–10	14–24	C	N/A
Haloperidol	Haldol	5–10	12–36	C_m	Unknown, but of concern
Loxapine	Loxitane	20–80	4–12	C	N/A
Mesoridazine	Serentil	100–400	24–48	C	Unknown, but of concern
Molindone	Moban	20–80	24–36	C	N/A
Olanzapine	Zyprexa	5–20	21–54	C_m	N/A
Perphenazine	Trilafon	8–32	8–21	C	Unknown, but of concern
Pimozide[e]	Orap	1–10	50–70	C	N/A
Risperidone[e]	Risperdal	1–16	3–20	C	N/A
Thioridazine	Mellaril	200–600	9–30	C	N/A
Thiothixene	Navane	10–40	34	C	N/A
Trifluoperazine	Stelazine	10–40	18–30	C	N/A
Medications for antipsychotic side effects					
Amantadine	Symmetrel	100–400	15	C_m	N/A
Benztropine	Cogentin	0.5–6.0	10–12	C	N/A
Diphenhydramine	Benadryl	25–150	5–11	C	N/A
Propranolol	Inderal	20–120	3.5–4.5	C_m	Compatible
Trihexyphenidyl	Artane	2–15	10–12	C	N/A

Note. N/A = not applicable.
[a]Dosing strategies adapted from Schatzberg and Cole 1991; Kaplan and Sadock 1993; and, for newer medications, the manufacturers' package inserts.
[b]Half-life of elimination is listed for parent compounds.
[c]Risk category adapted from Briggs et al. 1994; "m" subscript is for data taken from the manufacturer's package insert.
[d]American Academy of Pediatrics 1994.
[e]Not listed in Briggs et al. 1994. Risk category taken from *Physicians' Desk Reference* 1992, 1993, 1994, 1996.

Prudic 1984). Commonly prescribed antipsychotic medications, as well as agents used to treat their side effects, are listed in Table 30–3.

In a study (Van Waes and Van de Velde 1969) of 100 women treated with haloperidol (mean dose 1.2 mg/day) for hyperemesis gravidarum, no differences in gestational duration, fetal viability, or birth weight were noted. In a large prospective study, Milkovich and Van den Berg (1976) followed up almost 20,000 women treated for emesis, mostly with phenothiazines. When maternal age, medication, and gestational age at exposure were controlled, the authors found no significant increase in severe anomalies or neonatal survival rates.

Similar results have been obtained in several retrospective studies of women treated with trifluoperazine for repeated abortions and emesis (Moriarty and Nance 1963; Rawlings et al. 1963). In contrast, Rumeau-Rouquette et al. (1977) reported a significant association of major anomalies with prenatal exposure to phenothiazines with an aliphatic side chain but not with piperazine or piperidine class agents. Reanalysis of the data obtained by Milkovich and Van den Berg (1976) did find a significant risk of malformations associated with phenothiazine exposure in week 4 through 10 of gestation (Edlund and Craig 1976).

Beyond the potential teratogenic risks of these agents is the potential for other side effects of antipsychotic drugs, such as neuroleptic malignant syndrome (James 1988) and extrapyramidal side effects. The symptoms of extrapyramidal side effects in the neonate may include increased muscle tone and increased rooting and tendon reflexes that may persist for several months (Cleary 1977; Hill et al. 1966; O'Connor et al. 1981). In addition, in utero exposure to antipsychotics may produce neonatal jaundice (Scokel and Jones 1962) and intestinal obstruction (Falterman and Richardson 1980) postnatally.

Several studies in animals (Hoffeld et al. 1968; Ordy et al. 1966; Robertson et al. 1980) have shown that prenatal exposure to antipsychotic medications can cause persistent abnormalities in learning and memory; others (e.g., Dallemagne and Weiss 1982) have not observed such drug-induced alterations. Studies in humans have not detected significant differences in IQ scores at age 4 years among children exposed to antipsychotic drugs and control subjects ($n = 52$ [Kris 1965] and $n = 151$ [Slone et al. 1977]). However, these studies included women exposed to relatively low doses of phenothiazines (Kris 1965).

Antipsychotic drugs, like other psychotropics, are excreted into breast milk (see Buist et al. 1990 for a review). The most widely studied of these drugs is chlorpromazine: seven infants exposed to chlorpromazine did not have any developmental deficits at 16-month and 5-year follow-up evaluations (Kris and Carmichael 1957). The concentrations of several other antipsychotics in breast milk have been measured, including haloperidol (Stewart et al. 1980; Whalley et al. 1981), trifluoperazine and perphenazine (J. T. Wilson et al. 1980), and thioxanthenes (Matheson and Skjaeraasen 1988); the milk-to-serum ratio was consistently ≤1.

Various agents are available for the treatment of extrapyramidal side effects. In utero exposure to diphenhydramine has been the most widely reported. The Collaborative Perinatal Project found an association between first-trimester exposure to diphenhydramine and major and minor anomalies (see Miller 1991 and Wisner and Perel 1988 for reviews). One study in which 599 children with oral clefts were compared with 590 control subjects found a significantly higher rate of exposure to diphenhydramine in the children with oral clefts (Saxen 1974). The cautious use of anticholinergic agents is warranted by case reports of intestinal obstruction after perinatal exposure to antipsychotic drugs and benztropine (Falterman and Richardson 1980), as well as the potential adverse effects on maternal gastrointestinal motility. Studies in animals have shown that amantadine is a known teratogen (Hirsch and Swartz 1980), but reports in humans are lacking.

In summary, antipsychotic medications have been widely used for more than three decades, and the paucity of data linking these agents to either congenital or neurobehavioral deficits suggests that the risk of these medications is minimal. There are virtually no available data on the newly introduced atypical antipsychotic quetiapine.

ANXIOLYTICS

Benzodiazepines and antidepressants are the most commonly used drugs for the treatment of anxiety disorders, and benzodiazepines are the most widely prescribed psychotropic medications. A retrospective survey of Medicaid records (1980–1983) of 104,339 pregnant women found that at least 2% received one or more prescriptions for a benzodiazepine (Bergman et al. 1992). As a class, benzodiazepines readily traverse the placenta, and the presence of benzodiazepines in umbilical cord plasma demonstrates that these drugs accumulate in the fetus after prolonged administration (Mandelli et al. 1975; Shannon et al. 1972). We know that these medications are found in fetal brain, lungs, and heart (Mandelli et al. 1975). Mandelli et al. (1975) also found that the metabolism of diazepam in the fetus is slower than in the adult; the half-life of the parent compound is 31 hours in the fetus.

In contrast to concentrations of other benzodiazepines that have been studied, lorazepam concentrations were found to be lower in cord blood than in maternal serum but were excreted at a slower rate; detectable levels were excreted 8 days after delivery (Whitelaw et al. 1981). Earlier studies reported an increased risk of oral clefts after in utero exposure to diazepam (Aarkog 1975; Saxen 1975; Saxen and Saxen 1974), but later studies failed to confirm this association (Entman and Vaughn 1984; Rosenberg et al. 1984; Shiono and Mills 1984). Altshuler et al. (1996) pooled data from several studies investigating the association of oral cleft with in utero exposure to benzodiazepines. They found that, although exposure does confer an increased risk of oral cleft, the absolute risk increased by only 0.01%, from 6 in 10,000 to 7 in 10,000.

Table 30–4 lists benzodiazepine and non-benzodiazepine anxiolytics and sedative-hypnotics used in the treatment of anxiety disorders and insomnia, respectively.

Long-term, longitudinal follow-up studies are urgently needed. One group described a "benzodiazepine exposure syndrome" that included growth retardation, dysmorphism, and both mental and psychomotor retardation in infants exposed in utero to benzodiazepines (Laegreid et al. 1987). The same group later reported predominantly neonatal sedation and withdrawal (Laegreid et al. 1989). A second group failed to find an increased incidence of behavioral abnormalities at age 8 months, and no difference in IQ scores at age 4 years, for children exposed to chlordiazepoxide in utero (Hartz et al. 1975).

Buist et al. (1990) concluded that benzodiazepines at relatively low doses present no contraindications to nursing. In contrast to other classes of psychotropic medications, benzodiazepines appear to have lower milk-to-maternal serum ratios. Wreitland (1987) found a ratio of 0.1:0.3 for oxazepam and estimated that the infant would be exposed to 1/1,000th of the maternal dose. The percentage of the maternal dose of lorazepam to which a nursing infant is exposed has been estimated to be 2.2% (Summerfield and Nielsen 1985).

In summary, benzodiazepines should not be abruptly withdrawn during pregnancy, and, if possible, these drugs should be tapered sufficiently before delivery to limit neonatal withdrawal. Evidence from umbilical cord sampling indicates that lorazepam may not cross the placenta to the same degree as other benzodiazepines. Lorazepam and oxazepam bypass hepatic metabolism and may therefore have less potential for accumulation in the neonate. Finally, as noted in the comprehensive review by Miller (1991), diazepam with sodium benzoate as a preservative may also present some potential difficulties. Clonazepam (FDA category C) appears to have minimal teratogenic risks (Sullivan and McElhatton 1977).

MOOD-STABILIZING MEDICATIONS

The management of bipolar disorder during pregnancy has received considerable attention. Unlike affective anxiety and formal thought disorders, the number of clinically efficacious medications for bipolar disorder is quite limited (Table 30–5).

Table 30–4. Anxiolytic medications

Generic name	Trade name	Daily dose (mg/day)[a]	Half-life (hours)[b]	Risk category[c]	American Academy of Pediatrics rating[d]
Benzodiazepines					
Alprazolam	Xanax	0.5–6.0	12	D_m	N/A
Chlordiazepoxide	Librium	15–100	>100	D	N/A
Clonazepam	Klonopin	0.5–10	34	C	N/A
Clorazepate	Tranxene	7.5–60	>100	D	N/A
Diazepam	Valium	2–60	>100	D	Unknown, but of concern
Halazepam[e]	Paxipam	60–160	>100	N/A	N/A
Lorazepam	Ativan	2–6	15	D_m	Unknown, but of concern
Oxazepam	Serax	30–120	8	D	N/A
Prazepam[e]	Centrax	20–60	>100	D	Unknown, but of concern
Benzodiazepines for insomnia					
Estazolam[e]	ProSom	1–2	1–2	X	N/A
Flurazepam	Dalmane	15–30	>100	X_m	N/A
Quazepam[e]	Doral	7.5–30	>100	X	Unknown, but of concern
Temazepam	Restoril	15–30	11	X_m	Unknown, but of concern
Triazolam	Halcion	0.125–0.25	2	X_m	N/A
Nonbenzodiazepine anxiolytics and hypnotics					
Buspirone[e]	BuSpar	20–30	2–3	B	N/A
Chloral hydrate	Noctec	500–1,500	4–8	C_m	Compatible
Zolpidem tartrate[e]	Ambien	5–10	2–3	C	N/A

Note. N/A = not applicable.
[a]Dosing strategies adapted from Kaplan and Sadock 1993; and, for newer medications, the manufacturers' package inserts.
[b]Average half-life of elimination is listed for major metabolites.
[c]Risk category adapted from Briggs et al. 1994; "m" subscript is for data taken from the manufacturer's package insert.
[d]American Academy of Pediatrics 1994.
[e]Not listed in Briggs et al. 1994. Risk category taken from *Physicians' Desk Reference* 1992, 1993, 1994, 1996.

Lithium carbonate remains the cornerstone of the available treatments for bipolar disorder. The Registry of Lithium Babies was established in 1969 for Danish women after case reports were made of congenital malformations after in utero exposure to lithium (Schou 1976; Schou and Amdisen 1973). Further registers were established in Canada and the United States, culminating in the International Register of Lithium Babies.

Initial studies suggested a marked increase in cardiovascular malformations, particularly

Table 30–5.   Mood-stabilizing medications

Generic name	Trade name	Daily dose (mg/day)[a]	Half-life (hours)[b]	Risk category[c]	American Academy of Pediatrics rating[d]
Carbamazepine	Tegretol	400–1,600	12–17	C_m	Compatible
Clonazepam	Klonopin	0.5–10	34	C	N/A
Gabapentin	Neurontin	900–1,800	5–7	C	N/A
Lamotrigine	Lamictal	300–500	25	C	N/A
Valproic acid	Depakote (divalproex sodium)	750–1,500	8–10	D	Compatible
Lithium carbonate	Eskalith, Lithobid, Lithonate	900–2,100	20	D	Contra-indicated

Note.   N/A = not applicable.
[a]Dosing strategies adapted from Kaplan and Sadock 1993; and, for newer medications, the manufacturers' package inserts.
[b]Average half-life of elimination is listed for parent compound.
[c]Risk category adapted from Briggs 1994; "m" subscript is for data taken from the manufacturer's package insert.
[d]American Academy of Pediatrics 1994.

Ebstein's anomaly (Nora et al. 1974; Weinstein and Goldfield 1975). However, Cohen et al. (1994) completed an extensive survey of the available information and found an increase in the relative risk ratio for cardiac malformations of 1.2–7.7 and an overall increase in the relative risk for congenital malformations of 1.5–3.0 for in utero lithium exposure. Altshuler et al. (1996) determined that the risk for Ebstein's anomaly after in utero lithium exposure rose from 1 in 20,000 to 1 in 1,000. In contrast to the results of studies in animals, a 5-year follow-up study failed to find any significant behavioral teratogenetic sequelae associated with lithium exposure antenatally (Schou 1976).

The outcome studies for lithium discontinuation and relapse rates for patients with bipolar disorder (Suppes et al. 1991; Tohen et al. 1990) underscore the need to carefully assess the severity of illness, as outlined by Cohen et al. (1994). Briefly, it is recommended that women receive prepregnancy counseling and that those with a single episode should have medication tapered gradually and an attempt at lithium-free

pregnancy or, if indicated, reinstitution of lithium after the first trimester. It is recommended that the clinician offer a fetal echocardiogram between week 16 and 18 of gestation for women who were treated with lithium during their first trimester of pregnancy.

The previously noted physiological alterations are of importance in the management of lithium therapy during pregnancy and parturition. The changes in glomerular filtration rate during parturition and the potential for dehydration at that time, along with the associated rapid changes in fluid status, warrant close monitoring of lithium levels at delivery. The neonate may be at risk for lithium toxicity at serum concentrations lower than maternal concentrations, and the clinician should avoid the use of nonsteroidal antiinflammatory drugs in both the mother and the infant during the early postpartum period. Symptoms of toxicity include flaccidity, lethargy, and poor suck reflexes that may persist for more than 7 days (Woody et al. 1971). Lithium can also produce reversible changes in thyroid function (Karlsson et al.

1975), cardiac arrhythmias (N. Wilson et al. 1983), hypoglycemia, and diabetes insipidus (Mizrahi et al. 1979).

Several anticonvulsants have also been shown to be effective in the treatment of bipolar disorder. These include carbamazepine, valproic acid, and perhaps clonazepam. The bulk of the literature on the teratogenic risk of these compounds is derived from studies on the treatment of epilepsy during pregnancy. As noted by Cohen et al. (1994), these agents have not yet been proven to provide comparable levels of prophylaxis for manic episodes.

In utero exposure to both carbamazepine and valproic acid increases the congenital malformation rate in infants of epileptic mothers (Jones et al. 1989; Lindhout and Schmidt 1986). Fetal serum concentrations of carbamazepine are approximately 50%–80% of the maternal concentrations (Nau et al. 1982). The risk for spina bifida associated with fetal exposure to carbamazepine is 1% (relative risk is about 13.7%) (Rosa 1991). Similarly, valproic acid is a known human teratogen and confers a 1%–2% risk of neural tube defects.

All of the commonly used mood-stabilizing medications except clonazepam appear to carry an increased risk of fetal malformations and a potentially deleterious effect on later cognitive development. Like other psychotropic medications, mood-stabilizing medications are present in breast milk. Nursing infants can achieve serum lithium concentrations that are 40%–50% of maternal levels (Kirksey and Groziak 1984; Schou and Amdisen 1973). Although no reports of toxic effects are associated with lithium and nursing, the potential for such toxicity warrants close observation of the infant's hydration status (Chaudron and Jefferson 2000). In contrast, both carbamazepine and valproic acid appear in low concentrations in human milk, and both are considered compatible with breast-feeding (American Academy of Pediatrics 1994). The clinician may consider avoiding medications that increase the potential for liver toxicity, such as acetaminophen, in these infants.

In summary, the management of bipolar disorder during pregnancy requires careful assessment of the disorder and its severity. The guidelines suggested by Cohen et al. (1994) underscore the potentially favorable risk-benefit ratio of lithium use during pregnancy.

SUMMARY

There is a paucity of clinical data supporting the view that psychotropic medications are teratogenic; in contrast, preclinical studies in laboratory animals, in which high doses of these agents are typically used, reveal definite physical and neurobehavioral teratogenetic effects (Elia et al. 1987). Pregnant and nursing women are generally excluded in clinical studies of novel pharmacological agents, and routine postmarketing registries are not maintained by most pharmaceutical companies, thereby limiting the available data. It is doubtful that well-controlled studies will ever be conducted. Although some investigators have suggested that conducting such studies in pregnant and nursing women is unethical (Kerns 1986), it could be argued that failure to conduct such studies increases the overall risk to women and infants over time and may deprive some women of adequate treatment. Several characteristics (route of metabolism, protein binding affinity, lipid partitioning) warrant further study to determine whether these physicochemical features affect placental transfer and excretion into breast milk.

In the light of the higher prevalence of depressive and anxiety disorders in women than in men and the particularly high rates of these disorders during the childbearing years, it is likely that the clinician will be presented with complex issues of prescribing psychotropic medications during pregnancy and lactation. A thorough risk-benefit analysis should be completed for each woman presenting with concerns of psychiatric illness during pregnancy and lactation. This risk-benefit analysis should take into account factors such as maternal psychiatric his-

Table 30–6. Risk-benefit assessment for pregnancy: summary of facts

Known

85% of all pregnancies result in live births.

7%–14% of deliveries are preterm.

2%–4% of live births result in infants with significant malformations, and up to 12% have minor anomalies.

>60% of all women take at least one prescription medication during pregnancy.

In the ideal pregnancy, as defined by the Centers for Disease Control and Prevention, maternal weight is ±15% of ideal body weight, and the mother was taking prenatal vitamins with folic acid for 6 weeks before conception.

Most women learn of pregnancy at 5–8 weeks' gestation and therefore may be past the window of risk for fetal anomalies associated with psychotropic medication.

Increasing data

Pregnancy is not protective against psychiatric illness.

Major depressive episodes occur with similar incidence during pregnancy as during nongravid periods.

Obsessive-compulsive disorder may have its onset or may worsen during pregnancy.

The incidence of psychotic disorders varies throughout pregnancy; there are limited data suggesting a need to decrease dosage of antipsychotic medications.

Panic disorder may improve during pregnancy for some women.

The teratogenic risk of psychotropic medications, if any, has been historically overestimated.

Increasing data on obstetrical outcome and follow-up of infants of mothers taking psychotropic medications are comparable in study sample sizes to data on most other prescription drugs.

Untreated maternal mental illness may adversely affect obstetrical outcome.

Unknown

The potential long-term effect of untreated maternal psychiatric illness during pregnancy on infant development is unknown.

The long-term neurobehavioral effects of in utero exposure to psychotropic medications are unknown, although initial studies have not reported adverse effects for several medications.

tory; potential deleterious effects of untreated illness on both the mother and the fetus; and what is known in regard to somatic, perinatal, and long-term neurobehavioral teratogenicity of the different classes of psychotropic medications. Tables 30–6 and 30–7 summarize the basic risk-benefit assessment that should be individualized based on the patient's history and treatment goals.

Included in the risk-benefit assessment is the need for infant monitoring. Although no guidelines have been established in this regard, the type and frequency of infant serum monitoring should be consistent with adult monitoring as a minimum and should be repeated with any adjustment in maternal daily dose.

In light of the lack of data demonstrating the superior clinical efficacy of a single medication within a given class, we offer the following general treatment recommendations. We assume that the clinician has already exhausted reasonable nonpharmacological interventions:

- *Informed consent*—It is not possible to provide a complete list of all the risks for any given psychotropic medication. It is important to discuss with the patient the risks of using or not using psychotropic medications and to document that other treatment options have been attempted or considered. It is equally important to document the risk of the untreated illness to both the mother and the infant.

- *Choice of medication*—The most important factor is treatment history. A novel agent should not be used during these periods if a history of positive response exists. Such a decision only increases the risk of exposure to a second medication and continued risk of the illness. In the absence of a treatment history, medications with the following characteristics should be sought:

Table 30–7.	Risk-benefit assessment for lactation: summary of facts

Known: Postpartum

>60% of women plan to breast-feed during the puerperium.

5%–17% of all nursing women take a prescription medication during breast-feeding.

12%–20% of nursing women smoke cigarettes.

Breast-feeding is beneficial for the infant.

Breast-feeding is supported by all professional organizations as the ideal form of nutrition for the infant.

The postnatal period is a high-risk time for onset or relapse of psychiatric illness.

All psychotropic medications studied to date are excreted in breast milk.

Increasing data

Untreated maternal mental illness has an adverse effect on mother-infant attachment and later infant development.

The adverse effects of psychotropic agents on infants are limited to case reports.

The nursing infant's daily dose of psychotropic agents is less than the maternal daily dose.

Psychotropic medications are excreted into breast milk with a specific individual time course, allowing the minimization of infant exposure with continuation of breast-feeding.

Unknown

The long-term neurobehavioral effects of infant exposure to psychotropic medications through breast-feeding are unknown.

- *Greatest documentation of prior use*—Medications with some published data on relative safety. Being the first to use a particular medication in pregnancy or lactation is not recommended. Medications that have been available for a longer time have a larger database, although this usually consists predominantly of case reports, in pregnancy and lactation.

- *Lower FDA risk category (B > C > D)*—The FDA is empirically conservative and has access to the most pre- and postmarketing data. Whereas this rating may be controversial for some medications, as evidenced by the reclassification of the SSRIs to category C in the absence of any new data, it is reasonable that medical-legal considerations would support this approach.

- *Few or no metabolites*—Data from both pregnancy and lactation suggest that drug metabolites, which typically have longer elimination half-lives, may achieve higher steady states in both fetal circulation and infant serum. The issue of active versus inactive metabolites is unresolved with respect to teratogenic effects.

- *Fewer side effects*—Medications with fewer hypotensive and anticholinergic side effects are preferable. Additionally, the effect on seizure threshold and potential interaction with commonly used obstetrical anesthetic and analgesic agents should be minimized.

- *Concordant data*—Medications with conflicting data should be avoided; a clinically comparable alternative should be used, if available. This recommendation should also reduce any potential legal liability.

- *Dosage*—In contrast to previous recommendations (Cohen 1989; Stowe and Nemeroff 1995), the goal of treatment during pregnancy and lactation should be adequate treatment for syndrome resolution. Partial treatment only enhances the risk by exposing mother and infant to both illness and medications. The minimum effective dose should be maintained throughout treatment, and the clinician should remain mindful that often dosage requirements may be increased during pregnancy. Such increases do not increase fetal exposure beyond the initial treatment decision because the fetal circulation is exposed to maternal serum, not maternal dose. Adjustments may be indicated later in pregnancy as the volume of distribution changes. To minimize the potential for neonatal withdrawal and maternal toxicity after delivery, careful monitoring of side effects and serum concentrations may be indicated. Exposure of nursing infants can be minimized by adjusting the feeding and dose schedule and discarding the peak breast milk concentrations for several agents.

■ *Communication with the pediatrician*—It is highly recommended that the psychiatric clinician discuss the medication and potential interactions with the infant's pediatrician. The delay in hepatic maturity may affect the metabolism of psychotropic agents and potentially alter the serum levels of other medications prescribed for the infant.

REFERENCES

Aarkog D: Association between maternal intake of diazepam and oral clefts (letter). Lancet 2:921, 1975

Affonso DD, Mayberry LJ, Lovett S, et al: Pregnancy and postpartum depressive symptoms. J Womens Health 2(2):157–164, 1993

Altshuler LL, Burt VK, McMullen M, et al: Breastfeeding and sertraline: a 24-hour analysis. J Clin Psychiatry 56:243–245, 1995

Altshuler LL, Cohen L, Szuba MP, et al: Pharmacologic management of psychiatric illness during pregnancy: dilemmas and guidelines. Am J Psychiatry 153:592–606, 1996

American Academy of Pediatrics, Committee on Drugs: The transfer of drugs and other chemicals into human breast milk. Pediatrics 93:137–150, 1994

Atkinson HC, Begg EJ, Darlow BA: Drugs in human milk: clinical pharmacokinetic considerations. Clin Pharmacokinet 14:217–240, 1988

Avant K: Anxiety as a potential factor affecting maternal attachment. J Obstet Gynecol Neonatal Nurs 10:416–419, 1981

Beck AT: Depression Inventory. Philadelphia, PA, Philadelphia Center for Cognitive Therapy, 1978

Bergman U, Rosa FW, Baum C, et al: Effects of exposure to benzodiazepine during fetal life. Lancet 340:694–696, 1992

Birnbaum CS, Cohen LS, Grush LR, et al: Serum concentrations of antidepressants and benzodiazepines in nursing infants: implications for treatment. Pediatrics (electronic) 140:e1–e6, 1999

Brazelton TB: Mother infant reciprocity, in Maternal Attachment and Mothering Disorders: A Roundtable. Edited by Klaus MH, Leger T, Trause MA. North Brunswick, NJ, Johnson and Johnson, 1975, pp 49–54

Briggs GG, Freeman RK, Yaffe SJ: Drugs in Pregnancy and Lactation, 4th Edition. Baltimore, MD, Williams & Wilkins, 1994

Buesching DP, Glasser ML, Frate DA: Progression of depression in the prenatal and postpartum periods. Women Health 11:61–77, 1986

Buist A, Norman TR, Dennerstein L: Breastfeeding and the use of psychotropic medication: a review. J Affect Disord 19:197–206, 1990

Campbell SB, Cohn JF, Meyers T: Depression in first-time mothers: mother-infant interaction and depression chronicity. Dev Psychol 31:349–357, 1995

Chambers CD, Johnson KA, Jones KL: Pregnancy outcome in women exposed to fluoxetine. Reprod Toxicol 7:155–156, 1993

Chambers CD, Johnson KA, Dick LM, et al: Birth outcomes in pregnant women taking fluoxetine. N Engl J Med 335:1010–1015, 1996

Chaudron L, Jefferson J: Mood stabilizers during breastfeeding: a review. J Clin Psychiatry 61:79–90, 2000

Cleary MF: Fluphenazine decanoate during pregnancy. Am J Psychiatry 134:815–816, 1977

Cohen LS: Psychotropic drug use in pregnancy. Hospital and Community Psychiatry 40:566–567, 1989

Cohen LS, Heller VL, Rosenbaum JF: Treatment guidelines for psychotropic drug use in pregnancy. Psychosomatics 30:25–33, 1989

Cohen LS, Friedman JM, Jefferson JW, et al: A re-evaluation of risk of in utero exposures to lithium. JAMA 271:146–150, 1994

Cradon AJ: Maternal anxiety and neonatal well-being. J Psychosom Res 23:113–115, 1979

Cutrona CE: Causal attributions and perinatal depression. J Abnorm Psychol 92:161–172, 1983

Dallemagne G, Weiss B: Altered behavior of mice following postnatal treatment with haloperidol. Pharmacol Biochem Behav 16:761–767, 1982

DeVane CL: Pharmacokinetics of the selective serotonin reuptake inhibitors. J Clin Psychiatry 53 (suppl):13–20, 1992

Doering JC, Stewart RB: The extent and character of drug consumption during pregnancy. JAMA 239:843–846, 1978

Edlund MJ, Craig TJ: Antipsychotic drug use and birth defects: an epidemiologic reassessment. Compr Psychiatry 25:244–248, 1976

Eggermont E: Withdrawal symptoms in neonates associated with maternal imipramine therapy. Lancet 2:680, 1973

Elia J, Katz IR, Simpson GM: Teratogenicity of psychotherapeutic medications. Psychopharmacol Bull 23:531–586, 1987

Entman SS, Vaughn WK: Lack of relation of oral clefts to diazepam use in pregnancy. N Engl J Med 310:1121–1122, 1984

Ericson A, Kallen B, Wilholm BE: Delivery outcome after the use of antidepressants in early pregnancy. Eur J Clin Pharmacol 55:503–508, 1999

Falterman CG, Richardson CJ: Small left colon syndrome associated with maternal ingestion of psychotropic drugs. J Pediatr 97:308–310, 1980

Goldberg HL, DiMascio A: Psychotropic drugs in pregnancy, in Psychopharmacology: A Generation of Progress. Edited by Lipton HL, DiMascio A, Killam KF. New York, Raven, 1978, pp 1047–1055

Hartz SC, Heinonen OP, Shapiro S, et al: Antenatal exposure to meprobamate and chlordiazepoxide in relation to malformations, mental development, and childhood mortality. N Engl J Med 292:726–728, 1975

Heinonen OP, Stone D, Shapiro S: Birth Defects and Drugs in Pregnancy. Littleton, MA, Publishing Sciences Group, 1977

Hill RM, Stern L: Drugs in pregnancy: effects on the fetus and newborn. Current Therapeutics 20:131–150, 1979

Hill RM, Desmond MM, Kay JL: Extrapyramidal dysfunction in an infant of a schizophrenic mother. J Pediatr 69:589–595, 1966

Hirsch MS, Swartz MN: Antiviral agents. N Engl J Med 302:903–907, 1980

Hoffeld DR, McNew J, Webster RL: Effect of tranquilizing drugs during pregnancy on activity of offspring. Nature 218:357–358, 1968

Inman W, Kubotu K, Pearce G: Prescription event monitoring of paroxetine. Prescription Event Monitoring Reports, 1–44, 1993

James ME: Neuroleptic malignant syndrome in pregnancy. Psychosomatics 29:112–119, 1988

Jones KL, Larco RV, Johnson KA, et al: Pattern of malformations in the children of women treated with carbamazepine during pregnancy. N Engl J Med 320:1661–1669, 1989

Kacew S: Adverse effects of drugs and chemicals in breast milk on the nursing infant. J Clin Pharmacol Ther 33:213–219, 1993

Kaplan HI, Sadock BJ: Pocket Handbook of Psychiatric Drug Treatment. Baltimore, MD, Williams & Wilkins, 1993

Karlsson K, Lindstedt G, Lundberg PA: Transplacental lithium poisoning: reversible inhibition of fetal thyroid (letter). Lancet 1:1295, 1975

Kauffman RE, Banner W Jr, Berline CM Jr: The transfer of drugs and other chemicals into human milk. Pediatrics 93:137–150, 1994

Kerns LL: Treatment of mental disorders in pregnancy: a review of psychotropic drug risks and benefits. J Nerv Ment Dis 174:652–659, 1986

Kim J, Misri S, Riggs KW, et al: Steroselective excretion of fluoxetine and norfluoxetine in breast milk and neonatal exposures. Paper presented at the 150th annual meeting of the American Psychiatric Association, San Diego, CA, May 17–22, 1997

Kirksey A, Groziak SM: Maternal drug use: evaluation of risks to breast-fed infants. World Rev Nutr Diet 43:60–79, 1984

Klein DF, Skrobala AM, Garfinkel RS: Preliminary look at the effects of pregnancy on panic disorder. Anxiety 1:227–232, 1994/1995

Kris EB: Children of mothers maintained on pharmacotherapy during pregnancy and post-partum. Current Therapeutic Research 7: 785–789, 1965

Kris E, Carmichael D: Chlorpromazine maintenance therapy during pregnancy and confinement. Psychiatr Q 31:690–695, 1957

Kulin N, Pastuszak A, Sage S, et al: Pregnancy outcome following maternal use of the new selective serotonin reuptake inhibitors: a prospective controlled multicenter study. JAMA 279: 609–610, 1998

Kumar R, Robson KM: A prospective study of emotional disorders in childbearing women. Br J Psychiatry 144:35–47, 1984

Laegreid L, Olegard R, Wahlstrom J, et al: Abnormalities in children exposed to benzodiazepines in utero. Lancet 1:108–109, 1987

Laegreid L, Olegard R, Walstrom J, et al: Teratogenic effects of benzodiazepine use during pregnancy. J Pediatr 114:126–131, 1989

Lindhout D, Schmidt D: In utero exposure to valproate and neural tube defects. Lancet 1: 329–333, 1986

Llewellyn AM, Stowe ZN, Nemeroff CB: Infant outcome after sertraline exposure. Paper presented at the 150th annual meeting of the American Psychiatric Association, San Diego, CA, May 17–22, 1997

Mandelli M, Morselli PL, Nordio S, et al: Placental transfer of diazepam and its disposition in the newborn. Clin Pharmacol Ther 17:564–572, 1975

Manley PC, McMahon RJ, Bradley CF, et al: Depressive attributional style and depression following childbirth. J Abnorm Psychol 91: 245–254, 1982

Matheson I, Skjaeraasen J: Milk concentrations of flupenthixol, nortriptyline and zuclopenthixol and between breast differences in two patients. Eur J Clin Pharmacol 35:217–220, 1988

Matheson I, Pande H, Alertson AR: Respiratory depression caused by N-desmethyldoxepin in breast milk. Lancet 2(8464):1124, 1985

McElhatton PR, Garbis HM, Elefant E, et al: The outcome of pregnancy in 689 women exposed to therapeutic doses of antidepressants: a collaborative study of the European Network of Teratology Information Services (ENTIS). Reprod Toxicol 10(4):285–294, 1996

McNeil TF, Kaij L, Malmquist-Larson A: Women with nonorganic psychosis: mental disturbance during pregnancy. Acta Psychiatr Scand 70: 127–139, 1984a

McNeil TF, Kaij L, Malmquist-Larson A: Women with nonorganic psychosis: pregnancy's effect on mental health during pregnancy. Acta Psychiatr Scand 70:140–148, 1984b

Meaney MJ, Diorio L, Francis D, et al: Early environmental regulation of forebrain glucocorticoid receptor gene expression: implications for adrenocortical responses to stress. Dev Neurosci 18:49–72, 1996

Milkovich L, Van den Berg BJ: An evaluation of the teratogenicity of certain antinauseant drugs. Am J Obstet Gynecol 125:244–248, 1976

Miller LJ: Clinical strategies for the use of psychotropic drugs during pregnancy. Psychiatry in Medicine 9:275–299, 1991

Miller LJ: Psychiatric medication during pregnancy: understanding and minimizing the risks. Psychiatric Annals 24(2):69–75, 1994

Mizrahi EM, Hobbs JF, Goldsmith DI: Nephrogenic diabetes insipidus in transplacental lithium intoxication. J Pediatr 94:493–495, 1979

Moriarty AJ, Nance NR: Trifluoperazine and pregnancy. Canadian Medical Association Journal 88:375–376, 1963

Murray L: The impact of postnatal depression on infant development. J Child Psychol Psychiatry 33:543–561, 1992

Nau H, Kuhnz W, Egger HJ, et al: Anticonvulsants during pregnancy and lactation: transplacental maternal and neonatal pharmacokinetics. Clin Pharmacokinet 7:508–543, 1982

Neziroglu FN, Anemone MA, Yaryura-Tobias JA: Onset of obsessive-compulsive disorder in pregnancy. Am J Psychiatry 149:947–950, 1992

Nora JJ, Nora AH, Toews WH: Lithium, Ebstein's anomaly, and other congenital heart defects. Lancet 2:594–595, 1974

Nulman I, Rovet J, Stewart DE, et al: Neurodevelopment of children exposed in utero to antidepressant drugs. N Engl J Med 336:258–262, 1997

Nurnberg HG, Prudic J: Guidelines for treatment of psychosis during pregnancy. Hospital and Community Psychiatry 35:67–71, 1984

O'Connor MO, Johnson GH, James DI: Intrauterine effect of phenothiazines. Med J Aust 1:416–417, 1981

O'Hara MW, Rehm LP, Campbell SB: Predicting depressive symptomatology: cognitive-behavioral models and postpartum depression. J Abnorm Psychol 91:457–461, 1982

O'Hara MW, Neunaber DJ, Zekoski EM: Prospective study of postpartum depression: prevalence, course, and predictive factors. J Abnorm Psychol 93:158–171, 1984

O'Hara MW, Zekoski EM, Phillips LH, et al: Controlled prospective study of postpartum mood disorders: comparison of childbearing and non-childbearing women. J Abnorm Psychol 99:3–15, 1990

Ordy JM, Samorajski T, Collins RL: Prenatal chlorpromazine effects on liver survival and behavior of mice offspring. J Pharmacol Exp Ther 151:110–125, 1966

Pastuszak A, Schick-Boschetto B, Zuber C, et al: Pregnancy outcome following first trimester exposure to fluoxetine (Prozac). JAMA 269:2246–2248, 1993

Perkin R, Bland JM, Peacock JL, et al: The effect of anxiety and depression during pregnancy on obstetrical complications. J Obstet Gynecol 100:629–634, 1993

Pittard WB, O'Neal W: Amitriptyline excretion in human milk. J Clin Psychopharmacol 6:383–384, 1986

Poulson E, Robson JM: Effect of phenelzine and some related compounds in pregnancy. J Endocrinol 30:205–215, 1964

Raskin VD, Richman JA, Gaines C: Patterns of depressive symptoms in expectant and new parents. Am J Psychiatry 147:658–660, 1990

Rawlings WJ, Ferguson R, Maddison TG: Phenmetrazine and trifluoperazine. Med J Aust 1:370, 1963

Rayburn WF, Andresen BD: Principles of perinatal pharmacology, in Drug Therapy in Obstetrics and Gynecology. Edited by Rayburn WF, Zuspan F. Norwalk, CT, Appleton-Century-Crofts, 1982, pp 1–8

Rieder RO, Rosenthal D, Wender P, et al: The offspring of schizophrenics: fetal and neonatal deaths. Arch Gen Psychiatry 32:200–211, 1975

Robertson RT, Majka JA, Peter CP, et al: Effects of prenatal exposure to chlorpromazine on postnatal development and behavior of rats. Toxicol Appl Pharmacol 53:541–549, 1980

Robinson HE, Stewart DE, Flak E: The rational use of psychotropic drugs in pregnancy and postpartum. Can J Psychiatry 31:183–190, 1986

Rosa FW: Spina bifida in infants of women treated with carbamazepine during pregnancy. N Engl J Med 324:674–677, 1991

Rosenberg L, Mitchell AA, Parsells JL, et al: Lack of relation of oral clefts to diazepam use during pregnancy. N Engl J Med 309:1281–1285, 1984

Rumeau-Rouquette C, Goujard J, Huel G: Possible teratogenic effect of phenothiazines in human beings. Teratology 15:57–64, 1977

Sadler TW (ed): Langman's Medical Embryology, 5th Edition. Baltimore, MD, Williams & Wilkins, 1985, pp 58–88

Saxen I: Cleft palate and maternal diphenhydramine intake. Lancet 1:407–408, 1974

Saxen I: Association between oral clefts and drugs taken during pregnancy. Int J Epidemiol 4:37–44, 1975

Saxen I, Saxen L: Association between maternal intake of diazepam and oral clefts (letter). Lancet 2:498, 1974

Schatzberg AF, Cole JO: Manual of Clinical Psychopharmacology. Washington, DC, American Psychiatric Press, 1991

Schou M: What happened later to the lithium babies? Follow-up study of children born without malformations. Acta Psychiatr Scand 54:193–197, 1976

Schou M, Amdisen A: Lithium and pregnancy, III: lithium ingestion by children breast-fed by women on lithium treatment. BMJ 2:138, 1973

Scokel PW, Jones WD: Infant jaundice after phenothiazine drugs for labor: an enigma. Obstet Gynecol 20:124–127, 1962

Shannon RW, Fraser GP, Aitken RG, et al: Diazepam in preeclamptic toxaemia with special reference to its effect on the newborn infant. British Journal of Clinical Practice 26:271–275, 1972

Shiono PH, Mills JL: Oral clefts and diazepam use during pregnancy (letter). N Engl J Med 311:919–920, 1984

Slone D, Siskind V, Heinonen OP, et al: Antenatal exposure to the phenothiazines in relation to congenital malformations, perinatal mortality rate, birth weight, and intelligence quotient score. Am J Obstet Gynecol 128:468–486, 1977

Stancer HC, Reed KL: Desipramine and 2-hydroxydesipramine in human breast milk and the nursing infant's serum. Am J Psychiatry 143:12, 1597–1600, 1986

Steer RA, Scholl TO, Hediger ML, et al: Self-reported depression and negative pregnancy outcomes. Epidemiology 45:1093–1099, 1992

Stewart R, Karas B, Springer P: Haloperidol excretion in human milk. Am J Psychiatry 137: 849–850, 1980

Stowe ZN, Nemeroff CB: Psychopharmacology during pregnancy and lactation, in The American Psychiatric Press Textbook of Psychopharmacology. Edited by Schatzberg AF, Nemeroff CB. Washington, DC, American Psychiatric Press, 1995, pp 823–837

Stowe ZN, Lllewellyn AM, Strader JR, et al: Placental passage of antidepressants. Paper presented at the 150th annual meeting of the American Psychiatric Association, San Diego, CA, May 17–22, 1997a

Stowe ZN, Owens M, Landry JC, et al: Sertraline and desmethylsertraline in human breast milk and nursing infants. Am J Psychiatry 154: 1255–1260, 1997b

Stowe ZN, Cohen L, Hostetter A, et al: Paroxetine in human breast milk and nursing infants. Am J Psychiatry 157:185–189, 2000

Sullivan FM, McElhatton PR: A comparison of the teratogenic activity of the antiepileptic drugs carbamazepine, clonazepam, ethosuximide, phenobarbital, phenytoin, and pyrimidone in mice. Toxicol Appl Pharmacol 40:365–378, 1977

Summerfield RJ, Nielsen MS: Excretion of lorazepam into breast milk. Br J Anaesth 57:1042–1043, 1985

Suppes T, Baldessarini RJ, Faedda GL, et al: Risk of recurrence following discontinuation of lithium treatment in bipolar disorder. Arch Gen Psychiatry 47:1082–1088, 1991

Teti DM, Messinger DS, Gelfand DM, et al: Maternal depression and the quality of early attachment: an examination of infants, preschoolers, and their mothers. Dev Psychol 31:364–376, 1995

Tohen M, Waternaux CM, Tsuang MT: Outcome in mania: a 4-year prospective follow-up of 75 patients utilizing survival analysis. Arch Gen Psychiatry 47:1106–1111, 1990

Van Waes A, Van de Velde EJ: Safety evaluation of haloperidol in the treatment of hyperemesis gravidarum. J Clin Pharmacol 9:224–227, 1969

Verbeeck RK, Ross SG, McKenna EA: Excretion of trazodone in breast milk. Br J Clin Pharmacol 22:367–370, 1986

Vorherr H: Drug excretion in breast milk. Postgrad Med 56:97–104, 1974

Warner A: Drug use in the neonate: inter-relationships of pharmacokinetics, toxicity and biochemical maturity. Clin Chem 32:721–727, 1986

Watson JP, Elliot SA, Rugg AJ, et al: Psychiatric disorder in pregnancy and the first postnatal year. Br J Psychiatry 147:453–462, 1984

Webster PAC: Withdrawal symptoms in neonates associated with maternal antidepressant therapy. Lancet 2:318–319, 1973

Weinstein MR, Goldfield MD: Cardiovascular malformations with lithium use during pregnancy. Am J Psychiatry 132:529–531, 1975

Welch R, Findlay J: Excretion of drugs in human breast milk. Drug Metab Rev 12:261–277, 1981

Whalley LJ, Blain PG, Prime JK: Haloperidol secreted in breast milk. BMJ 282:1746–1747, 1981

Whitelaw AGL, Cummings AJ, McFadyen IR: Effect of maternal lorazepam on the neonate. BMJ 282:1106–1108, 1981

Wilson JT, Brown RD, Cherek DR, et al: Drug excretion in human breast milk: principles, pharmacokinetics and projected consequences. Clin Pharmacokinet 5:1–66, 1980

Wilson N, Forfar JC, Godman MJ: Atrial flutter in the newborn resulting from maternal lithium ingestion. Arch Dis Child 58:538–549, 1983

Wisner KL, Perel JM: Psychopharmacologic agents and electroconvulsive therapy during pregnancy and the puerperium, in Psychiatric Consultation in Childbirth Settings: Parent- and Child-Oriented Approaches. Edited by Cohen RL. New York, Plenum, 1988, pp 165–206

Wisner KL, Perel JM, Wheeler SB: Tricyclic dosage requirements across pregnancy. Am J Psychiatry 150:1541–1542, 1993

Wisner KL, Perel JM, Findling RL: Antidepressant treatment during breast-feeding. Am J Psychiatry 153:1132–1137, 1996

Wood SM, Hytten FE: The fate of drugs in pregnancy. Clin Obstet Gynecol 8:255–259, 1981

Woody JN, London WL, Wilbanks GD: Lithium toxicity in a newborn. Pediatrics 47:94–96, 1971

Wreitland MA: Excretion of oxazepam in breastmilk. Eur J Clin Pharmacol 33:209–210, 1987

Wright S, Dawling S, Ashford JJ: Excretion of fluvoxamine in breast milk. Br J Clin Pharmacol 31:209, 1991

Zahn-Waxler C, Cummings EM, Ianoff RJ, et al: Young offspring of depressed patients: a population of risk for affective problems and childhood depression, in Childhood Depression. Edited by Cichetti D, Schneider-Rosen K. San Francisco, CA, Jossey-Bass, 1984, pp 81–105

THIRTY-ONE

Treatment of Insomnia

Martin Reite, M.D.

Three things should be remembered when considering treatment of an insomnia complaint. First, insomnia is a symptom, not a disease. Second, it is important to perform a systematic differential diagnosis, keeping in mind the possibility that there will very likely be more than one cause of an insomnia complaint. And finally, most patients complaining of insomnia can be helped significantly.

The complaint of insomnia is essentially that sleep is difficult to initiate or maintain or is nonrestorative or not refreshing. There will usually be some associated daytime consequences as well, such as fatigue, sleepiness, or performance difficulties. Insomnia is among the most frequent of complaints. A Gallup poll found that nearly 40% of the general population complained of intermittent or chronic insomnia (Gallup Organization 1995).

CONSEQUENCES OF SLEEP LOSS

Although insomnia usually is associated with a varying degree of sleep loss, the complaint is not identical to reduced sleep, and it is useful to consider as well the known effects of sleep loss or sleep restriction in normal sleepers as well as in those with insomnia.

Normal sleepers who undergo sleep loss, as well as potentially normal sleepers who have medical or other conditions that lead to sleep loss and result in insomnia complaints, can experience impairments in mood and in motor and cognitive performance (Pilcher and Huffcutt 1996; Singh et al. 1997). Sleep loss increases the likelihood of motor vehicle and other accidents (Leger 1994) and may contribute to impaired health.

Many individuals experience significant restriction of sleep as a consequence of job pressures and similar demands, and this restriction can have adverse consequences as well. Physician house staff members have been reported to fall asleep frequently while driving, seemingly as a direct result of sleep loss (Marcus and Loughlin 1996). A study by Dawson and Reid (1997) demonstrated that healthy persons with no sleep complaints who remained awake for as long as 17 hours had performance impairment equivalent to that seen after ingestion of sufficient alcohol to raise blood alcohol concentration to 0.05%, which is the level for legal intoxication in many Western industrialized nations. This may help explain the increase in accidents and performance decrements associated with prolonged wakefulness.

Persistent sleep difficulties have been found to be predictive of future health problems as well. In a long-term follow-up study of 1,053 men questioned about insomnia while in medical school and evaluated for incidence of depression about 34 years later, self-reported insomnia and difficulty with sleeping were associated with a higher incidence of depression in later life (Chang et al. 1997). Epidemiological studies have suggested that a complaint of sleep problems might help predict as many as 47% of new cases of depression in the following year (Eaton et al. 1995).

Although it is clear that normal sleepers (and potentially normal sleepers with insomnia complaints due to definable causes) deprived of sleep have performance decrements that are potentially dangerous, there appears to be a group of persons with chronic insomnia in whom the relationship between sleep loss and performance decrements is not as clear. Many individuals with chronic insomnia underestimate the amount of sleep they actually obtain (Edinger and Fins 1995), and in spite of obtaining less sleep on the whole than normal sleepers, those with chronic insomnia may not show similar objective evidence of excessive daytime sleepiness on the Multiple Sleep Latency Test (MSLT, a test that quantifies the degree of sleepiness; Lichstein et al. 1994). It has been suggested that they may exhibit a state of general hyperarousal, which in some sense may serve to protect them from other consequences of reduced sleep (Bonnet and Arand 1995). Thus, researchers do not yet understand well the relationship between the effects of sleep restriction or sleep loss in otherwise normal or potentially normal sleepers and the effects of sleep restriction in individuals with certain chronic insomnia complaints.

THE INSOMNIA COMPLAINT

Insomnia can include difficulty in getting to sleep (sleep onset insomnia), difficulty staying asleep (sleep maintenance insomnia), or early-morning awakening (terminal insomnia). It does not appear that such subtypes are stable over time, however, and therefore, this method of subtyping may have little clinical utility (Hohagen et al. 1994). As a rule, insomnia complaints are more frequent in women (Karacan and Williams 1983), elderly persons (Morin and Gramling 1989), and patients of lower socioeconomic status (Ford and Kamerow 1989).

Insomnia complaints are normally grouped into three types by duration of complaint. Transient insomnia lasts only a few days, short-term insomnia perhaps 2–3 weeks, and chronic insomnia from 3 weeks to many years.

Transient Insomnia

Transient insomnia is essentially ubiquitous and is caused by stressful events or experiences that are usually well defined and known to the subject. Anxiety about a forthcoming examination, job interview, or vacation departure, or even concern about having to get up early enough, are all common conditions that can result in a transient insomnia complaint. Physicians rarely see transient insomnias (although they experience them themselves), because these insomnias usually resolve with the event. Transient insomnia can be effectively managed with a short-half-life hypnotic agent, such as triazolam (0.125 mg), zolpidem (5 mg), or zaleplon (10 mg) at bedtime for one or perhaps several nights. It is not unreasonable for individuals whose sleep is easily and predictably disrupted by stress to keep a hypnotic agent on hand for situations likely to disrupt sleep. The risk of using an occasional hypnotic agent appears to be outweighed by the performance decrements induced by one or more nights of poor sleep.

Several physiological causes of transient insomnia are sleep disruptions associated with high altitude, jet lag, and shift work. Travel from sea level to higher altitude, even that of several North American ski areas, can be associated with disruptions in sleep. Altitude-induced changes include frequent awakenings, periodic breathing with associated arousals (Reite et al. 1975), and, in more severe cases, related symptoms of acute mountain sickness. The periodic breathing per se can fragment sleep and produce an insomnia complaint; acute mountain sickness also includes insomnia as a component. The pathophysiology of acute mountain sickness is not well understood, but it may include disturbances of fluid balance associated with tissue hypoxia. Short-half-life hypnotics (e.g., zolpidem, 5 mg) can temporarily relieve high-altitude insomnia. Perhaps a better choice is acetazolamide (125–250 mg twice a day), which prevents or reduces symptoms of acute mountain sickness and improves sleep (Roberts 1994).

Two other transient insomnias, those associated with jet lag and work shift change, can be considered disturbances in circadian biology. Jet lag is a syndrome endured by travelers who traverse several time zones quickly, then try to sleep at a time when their circadian system would normally be in the wakeful state and try to remain awake when their circadian system is timed for sleep. The body temperature and serum cortisol rhythms are normally synchronized with sleep rhythm so that the low point (or *nadir*) of the body temperature rhythm occurs in the early morning hours, typically between 3:00 and 5:00 A.M., and the high point in the late afternoon or evening. We typically arise in the morning as body temperature is rising and fall asleep in the evening after body temperature has begun to fall.

Cortisol also reaches the low point in the midpoint of the night and begins to rise and reach its high point in the early morning about the time of arising. Body temperature and cortisol rhythms appear to have a common pacemaker, and when desynchronized from the sleep rhythm, as for example after an 8-hour time zone change, slowly return to synchronization, moving about 1 hour per day. The time when they are out of normal synchronization with the sleep rhythm is termed *internal desynchrony;* it can be associated with the typical symptoms of jet lag, including increased daytime sleepiness and insomnia during the new sleep time. How much of the jet lag syndrome is due to a state of circadian desynchrony and how much is due to sleep loss is still unclear. Preservation of sleep clearly diminishes the symptoms, however.

Shift work can also be associated with sleep complaints, for reasons similar to those encountered with jet lag. A "shift workers' maladaptation syndrome" has been described; it includes impaired sleep, increases in gastrointestinal and cardiovascular complaints, excessive substance use, and social and family difficulties (Gordon et al. 1986). DSM-IV (American Psychiatric Association 1994) recognizes a circadian rhythm sleep disorder, shift work type (307.45).

Symptoms of both jet lag and work shift change can be effectively managed by appropriate use of bright light, as well as sedative-hypnotic agents, possibly including melatonin. Bright light is a potent synchronizer of the circadian system. Light exposure can either phase-advance or phase-delay the circadian system, depending on the time of exposure. It is most active near the nadir of the circadian temperature rhythm. Bright-light exposure prior to the temperature nadir can further phase-delay the system, whereas exposure shortly following the nadir can phase-advance the circadian system. An example of the human phase response curve to bright-light exposure is illustrated in Figure 31–1.

Appropriately timed bright-light exposure can also be useful for shift-work changes and for jet lag. Appropriate timing for light exposure to minimize jet lag should be based on knowledge of the phase response curve to light, considering the traveler's place of origin (Reite et al. 1997). Exposure should be timed to maximize phase shift in either an advanced or a delayed direction on the basis of the likely temperature nadir. An example of the use of light to minimize jet lag is provided in Figure 31–2.

The top panel of Figure 31–2 illustrates the

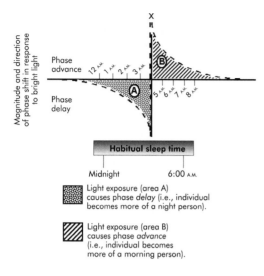

Figure 31–1. Type and magnitude of the response of the circadian rhythm to bright-light exposure. *Note.* Straight line represents time; period of habitual sleep is indicated at the bottom. Dashed line represents response of the circadian system to bright light, which is minimal during the midday hours. As the night progresses (and body temperature declines), light exposure progressively delays the circadian system. The effect is reversed at the time of the body temperature's lowest point (nadir); after this point, bright light causes an advancement of the circadian rhythm. The maximal response is found shortly before and shortly after the time of core body temperature minimum (✕).

use of light in travel from the eastern United States to Europe, for which a phase advance of the circadian system is desired. Typically, travelers depart the United States in the evening and arrive in Europe in the early morning (European time), which is the time when bright-light exposure will phase-delay the circadian system (not desired). Protection from light until about noon the first day will permit light exposure to phase-advance the circadian system in the desired direction. Subsequent days' light exposure can be advanced, further advancing the circadian system until it is entrained to the new time. The bottom panel of Figure 31–2 illustrates the use of natural light when it is desired to phase-delay the circadian system, as when trav-

eling from the United States to Asia. On arrival in Asia, light exposure at midday will have little effect, but light exposure in the late afternoon will most likely be in the phase-advance portion of the temperature rhythm, promoting the desired phase advance (postnadir) of the circadian system. On subsequent days, light exposure is encouraged later in the afternoon until entrainment is achieved.

Light exposure can also be manipulated to assist in adapting to shift work. Exposure to bright light (approximately 5,000 lux) during simulated night work for periods of 3–6 hours was experimentally shown to phase-shift the circadian temperature rhythm in the direction of circadian adaptation to the night work schedule (Eastman et al. 1995). Exposure to dim light (< 500 lux) had no such effect, and 6 hours of bright-light exposure were no better than 3 hours. Individuals with the greatest phase shifts also had more vigor, more sleep, and less mood disturbance, and overall they adapted better to night work. The timing of light exposure was thought to be important in inducing the reported phase shifts. Most subjects in the Eastman et al. study showed phase advance of temperature rhythms, possibly because the effective light exposure was maximum shortly after the time of the body temperature minimum, which is optimal sensitivity for phase advances. Manipulation of light exposure has been used successfully by the National Aeronautics and Space Administration (NASA) on space shuttle missions (Eastman et al. 1995), but this process has yet to be widely adopted in other industries.

The use of temazepam (20 mg) to facilitate daytime sleep in individuals required to stay awake at night in a simulated shift work condition demonstrated that temazepam increased daytime sleep and improved both performance and ability to stay awake at night (Porcu et al. 1997). The chronic use of a benzodiazepine agent to preserve sleep in shift workers, however, probably cannot be generally recommended.

Melatonin has been found useful in the alle-

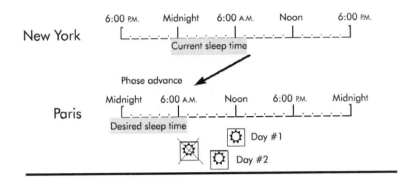

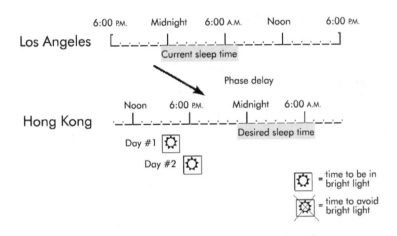

Figure 31–2. Examples of how to use bright light to reentrain the circadian system in west to east (phase advance) and east to west (phase delay) travel.

viation of jet lag (Arendt et al. 1986) and in improving accommodation to schedule changes in shift work (Dawson et al. 1995). Melatonin, or *N*-acetyl-5-methoxytryptamine, is synthesized from serotonin by two enzymes (arylalkylamine *N*-acetyltransferase and hydroxyindole-*O*-methyltransferase) that are largely confined to the pineal gland (Axelrod and Weissbach 1960; Coon et al. 1995). The hormone, secreted as light decreases, passively diffuses into the bloodstream, reaching maximum levels around 2:00–4:00 A.M. Normal young adults' average daytime and nighttime levels are about 10 and 60 pg/mL, respectively (Waldhauser and Dietzel 1985). Melatonin has not been approved for therapeutic use in humans by the U.S. Food and Drug Administration (FDA); thus, there is

little control over type of manufacture, relative purity, or accuracy of dosage, and there is relatively little information on optimal dosage, safety, and potential long-term side effects.

Short-Term Insomnia

Short-term insomnia is usually caused by stressful events of greater severity or duration than those associated with transient insomnia. Short-term insomnia can be effectively managed by hypnotic agents at bedtime for a week or two if necessary, or until the stress has subsided, although behavioral strategies such as attention to good sleep hygiene should also be invoked for these longer-lasting conditions. There is concern that if short-term insomnias do not resolve spontaneously, or are inadequately treated, they may lead, in susceptible individuals, to a more chronic insomnia complaint, such as a conditioned or psychophysiological insomnia.

Chronic Insomnias

Chronic insomnias last from many weeks to many years, and in these cases an accurate differential diagnosis is necessary for effective treatment. It is the rule rather than the exception that a given chronic insomnia condition has more than one cause; thus, it is important to examine systematically all possible causes, recognizing that several may be present and require treatment. It is sometimes helpful to conceptualize a chronic insomnia complaint as having two broad categories: 1) insomnia in potentially normal sleepers whose sleep is significantly disturbed by medical, psychiatric, circadian-rhythm, or other conditions that disrupt or limit sleep and therefore result in an insomnia complaint; and 2) psychophysiological or primary insomnia, representing a state of chronic physiological hyperarousal in susceptible individuals, thus leading to the insomnia complaints.

There is increasing evidence that there is a true primary insomnia disorder. Patients with this putative disorder present with impaired sleep, as well as associated symptoms such as increased body temperature (Adam et al. 1986), heart rate (Monroe 1967), and possibly metabolic rate (Bonnet and Arand 1995). These symptoms all reflect a state of central nervous system (CNS) hyperarousal, in which case the insomnia complaint is likely one symptom of a more complex underlying disorder.

Evaluation of Insomnia Complaint

The first issue when presented with a patient complaining of insomnia is to ensure that a sleep problem is indeed present and that the patient is not simply a short sleeper. Sleep need is likely genetically determined to a significant degree, and it approximates a normal distribution; most

individuals require about 7½–8 hours of sleep to feel rested the next day. There are, however, individuals on both ends of the distribution. Some short sleepers can seemingly get along fine on 4–5 hours of sleep, and some individuals habitually require 10 hours of sleep to feel rested the next day. Not infrequently, family members of a short sleeper think there must be something wrong with that individual because he or she is up and about while other family members are still sleeping, and they request that the person have a sleep evaluation.

In other situations, individuals who nap during the day may complain of not sleeping through the night. It is important to determine how many hours of sleep the person is getting. If, for example, he or she is napping 1½ hours in the afternoon, going to bed at 10:00 P.M., and awakening at 3:30 A.M., he or she is still getting a total of 7 hours of sleep, which might be all he or she requires. No physiological measure can predict a given individual's sleep need. We basically require sufficient sleep to feel rested and not excessively sleepy the next day.

Many patients do not inform their physicians of their sleep difficulty unless directly questioned. For this reason, it is worthwhile to include several brief questions about sleep during each new patient workup. In our experience, three routine questions will detect most significant sleep problems:

1. Are you content with your sleep? (This will identify most insomnia complaints.)
2. Are you excessively sleepy during the day? (This will identify most disorders of excessive sleepiness.)
3. Does your bed partner complain about your sleep? (This will identify most parasomnia disorders.)

A positive answer to any of these questions merits consideration of a more detailed sleep history to determine whether in fact a sleep disorder is likely present. Such a sleep history should include the following items:

- When did the symptoms begin?
- What has been their pattern since onset?
- Were there associated stress-related factors (e.g., job, school, family, health) at onset?
- What makes symptoms better or worse?
- What is a typical daily schedule (in detail—by the hour)
- What treatments and medications have been tried to date, and how did they work?

Sources of diagnostic information should include the bed partner whenever possible, because many sleep-related symptoms are apparent only to the bed partner. A sleep diary can also be useful at this stage of the evaluation, because it can provide a detailed daily description of sleep/wake/activity patterns.

SLEEP LABORATORY STUDIES

Laboratory studies useful in diagnosing sleep disturbances include all-night sleep recordings (polysomnography, or PSG), which monitor multiple physiological variables during sleep, either in the sleep laboratory or at home, and the MSLT.

The MSLT is usually performed the day after the PSG. The subject remains in the sleep laboratory and is asked to return to bed and try to go to sleep on four or five occasions (nap opportunities) at 2-hour intervals. Individuals with no sleep problems and who have obtained sufficient sleep the previous night will not go to sleep during these 20-minute nap opportunities or will have mean sleep latencies (for all nap opportunities) of greater than 15 minutes. Individuals who are excessively sleepy will have much shorter mean sleep latencies, often ranging down to less than 5 minutes for persons with narcolepsy or severe sleep apnea.

PSG studies are used most often in the evaluation of complaints of excessive daytime sleepiness, especially when sleep apnea or narcolepsy is being considered. PSG studies are rarely needed in the evaluation of insomnia complaints. Two exceptions, periodic limb movements of sleep (PLMS) and central apnea, are described below.

DIFFERENTIAL DIAGNOSIS

Assuming that a true chronic insomnia condition is present, the next step is to conduct a thorough differential diagnostic evaluation, which includes systematically considering the conditions that are most likely to result in insomnia complaints. Common causes (not necessarily listed in order of frequency) that should be systematically considered in the evaluation of a chronic insomnia complaint include the following:

- Medical conditions or treatments of medical conditions
- Psychiatric disorders
- Circadian rhythm disorders presenting as insomnia
- PLMS
- Substance abuse disorders
- Central sleep apnea
- Primary or conditioned (psychophysiological) insomnia

More than one cause may be present, and many if not most insomnia complaints will include a conditioned component that will likely require separate treatment. Most of these causes of insomnia (with the exception of PLMS and central apnea) do not require a PSG for diagnosis. A clinical assessment is usually adequate for establishing a diagnosis with a high degree of probability, at least to the extent that specific treatments can be tried.

Medical Conditions and Pharmacological Treatments of Medical Conditions

Medical conditions, or the pharmacological treatments of medical conditions, can result in insomnia complaints. The endocrinopathies are notorious for being associated with sleep-related complaints, as are conditions associated with chronic pain, breathing difficulties, cardiac arrhythmias, arthritis, fibromyalgia, and chronic fatigue syndrome. Similarly, a number of medications frequently used for treatment of medical conditions can, in susceptible patients, result in insomnia as a side effect. A list of the more commonly used medications that can result in insomnia complaints is provided in Table 31–1.

No specific sleep abnormalities are associated with medical disorders, other than usually a decrease in total sleep, an increase in awakenings, and perhaps decreases in rapid eye movement (REM) sleep. On occasion, fibromyalgia is associated with an alpha-delta type of sleep abnormality, in which alpha frequency activity is accentuated in the slow-wave-sleep background, with a complaint of nonrestorative sleep. Chronic fatigue syndrome is frequently accompanied by sleep complaints, but such complaints can include insomnia, hypersomnia, nonrestorative sleep, and sleeping at the wrong time of the 24-hour period. No PSG-based

sleep findings are specific to chronic fatigue syndrome as yet (Krupp et al. 1993).

The treatment of insomnia associated with medical conditions is first to isolate and appropriately treat the medical condition, and if the insomnia complaint persists, to evaluate the possibility of a separate additional sleep disorder. Conditioned insomnia can complicate insomnia complaints in this population, and it must be separately addressed (as outlined below).

Insomnia associated with acute medical conditions is appropriately treated with short-half-life hypnotic agents (e.g., zolpidem [5–10 mg], triazolam [0.125–0.25 mg], or zaleplon [10 mg] at bedtime) if no other contraindication to their use exists. Zolpidem might be safer for patients with compromised pulmonary function because it does not appear to significantly depress the respiratory system (Murciano et al. 1993). Insomnia complaints associated with fibromyalgia and chronic fatigue syndrome are frequently resistant to treatment, although small doses of amitriptyline (10–50 mg at bedtime) or cyclobenzaprine (10 mg three times a day) have been reported to be helpful, and occasionally zolpidem (5–10 mg) will help with the associated insomnia complaints.

Table 31–1.   Common drugs with insomnia as a side effect

β-Blockers

Stimulating tricyclics

Corticosteroids

Stimulants

Adrenocorticotropic hormone

Thyroid hormones

Monoamine oxidase inhibitors

Oral contraceptives

Diphenylhydantoin

Antimetabolites

Calcium channel blockers

Some decongestants

α-Methyldopa

Thiazides

Bronchodilators

Psychiatric Disorders

Psychiatric disorders, especially disorders associated with anxiety or depression, frequently include insomnia as an associated symptom. Chronic anxiety is not infrequently associated with sleep onset insomnia or sleep maintenance insomnia, whereas depression is not infrequently associated with early-morning awakening. These associations are not specific enough to be diagnostic, however, and a systematic psychiatric evaluation is necessary. Many depressive disorders appear to be accompanied by shortened REM latency, increased REM density during the first REM period of the night, and deficient slow-wave sleep. To date, however, such findings are not sufficiently specific to merit the cost of a PSG.

Antidepressant agents, although effective for the patient's depression, may have significantly different effects on sleep—a possibility that is useful to bear in mind. Table 31–2 shows sleep-related effects of the major antidepressant groups.

The choice of an antidepressant agent for a specific patient, all other things being equal, might well take into account the type of accompanying sleep complaint and the therapeutic effect on sleep desired. Typically, resolution of the depression will be accompanied by reduction in the sleep complaints. If, for a patient already complaining of insomnia, an antidepressant with a known high incidence of insomnia side effects is chosen, it may be useful to augment it with a hypnotic agent early in the course of treatment.

For patients with seasonal affective disorder (SAD), a disturbance in circadian rhythm control may underlie their symptoms. A study of 20 patients with SAD demonstrated evidence of a significant phase delay and relatively poor en-

Table 31–2. Overview of effects of antidepressant therapies on sleep

Drug	EEG sleep effects			Sedation
	Continuity	SWS	REM	
Tricyclics				
Amitriptyline	↑↑↑	↑	↓↓↓	++++
Doxepin	↑↑↑	↑↑	↓↓	++++
Imipramine	↔↑	↑	↓↓	++
Nortriptyline	↑	↑	↓↓	++
Desipramine	↔	↑	↓↓	+
Clomipramine	↑↔	↑	↓↓↓↓	±
MAOIs				
Phenelzine	↓	↔	↓↓↓↓	↔
Tranylcypromine	↓↓	↔	↓↓↓↓	↔
SSRIs				
Fluoxetine	↓	↔↓	↔↓	±
Paroxetine	↓↓	↔↓	↓↓	ND
Sertraline	↔	↔	↓↓	↔
Other antidepressants				
Bupropion	↓	↔	↑	↔
Venlafaxine	↓	↔	↓↓	++
SRMs				
Trazodone	↑↑↑	↔	↓	++++
Nefazodone	↑	↔	↑	↔

Note. ↑ = increased; ↓ = decreased; ↔ = no change; + = slight effect; ++ = small effect; +++ = moderate effect; ++++ = great effect; ± = no significant effect. EEG = electroencephalogram; SWS = slow-wave sleep; REM = rapid eye movement; MAOI = monoamine oxidase inhibitor; SSRI = selective serotonin reuptake inhibitor; ND = no data available; SRM = serotonin receptor modulator.

Source. Adapted from Winokur A, Reynolds C: "Overview of Effects of Antidepressant Therapies on Sleep," *Primary Psychiatry* 1:22–27, 1994. Used with permission of MBL Communications. Copyright 1994. All rights reserved.

trainment of the circadian system (Teicher et al. 1997). Such findings may explain the utility of bright-light treatment to reentrain the system and provide symptom relief.

Treatment of insomnia associated with anxiety can incorporate a benzodiazepine with sedative-hypnotic properties with a sufficient bedtime dose to augment sleep. Many antianxiety agents, such as sedative tricyclics, have sedative-hypnotic properties as well, which facilitates the management of the insomnia component. Panic attacks can occasionally arise exclusively from sleep (Rosenfeld and Furman 1994); treatment in such cases should probably follow conventional panic attack treatment strategies.

Bipolar disorder may be accompanied by prominent sleep disruption. Manic and hypomanic episodes may be accompanied by marked decreases in sleep, although not necessarily insomnia complaints. Sedative antidepressants have been shown to increase the risk of a shift to mania in treating insomnia complaints in bipolar depressed patients (Saiz-Ruiz et al. 1994), and the use of other hypnotic agents would therefore be more advisable in these patients. Milder cyclic mood disorders may also have associated insomnia complaints, which can be mistaken for a psychophysiological insomnia or conditioned arousal insofar as the patients find it difficult to turn off their thinking at sleep onset or after awakening during the night. If these patients are questioned carefully, evidence of a cyclic mood component will suggest that treatment with a mood stabilizer might be appropriate for the chronic insomnia complaint in these patients.

Posttraumatic stress disorder (PTSD) is a psychiatric disorder in which sleep disturbances are a hallmark. Patients with PTSD have increased sleep latency, decreased sleep efficiency, recurrent traumatic dreams, and evidence of increased REM density (Mellman et al. 1997), as well as evidence of impaired skeletal muscle inhibition during REM sleep (Ross et al. 1994). The treatment of disordered sleep accompany-ing PTSD is usually not separated from the treatment of the entire PTSD syndrome, but many medications used for PTSD have been described as helpful for the sleep complaints that accompany PTSD. These medications include tricyclic and monoamine oxidase inhibitor (MAOI) antidepressants, the presynaptic α-adrenergic agonist clonidine and the β-receptor agonist propranolol, the mood stabilizers lithium and carbamazepine, as well as benzodiazepines (Silver et al. 1990).

Circadian Rhythm Disorders

Circadian rhythm disorders usually present as sleep complaints. The most common is the *delayed sleep phase syndrome (DSPS)*, which presents as sleep onset insomnia. Typically, individuals with DSPS cannot get to sleep until 3:00–4:00 A.M. If they can then sleep until 10:00 A.M. or noon the next day, they can do fine, indicating that they have no trouble initiating or maintaining sleep, but if they are required to arise early to get to school or work, they complain of insomnia, and they are of course sleep deprived. They typically sleep in on weekends to recoup lost sleep. DSPS typically appears in adolescence or early adulthood, and it is frequently familial. In DSPS patients, evidence indicates that temperature rhythms and sleep rhythms are delayed and that possibly sleep persists for a longer time following the body temperature low point, suggesting that these patients may continue to sleep through the period when bright light would be most effective in phase-advancing their circadian system (Ozaki et al. 1988). About 50% of these cases presenting to sleep disorders clinics (presumably the more severe cases) respond favorably to treatment (Regestein and Monk 1995).

Other forms of circadian rhythm disorders presenting as sleep complaints include advanced sleep phase syndrome and non-24-hour sleep-wake syndrome, also known as hypernyctohemeral syndrome (Richardson and Malin 1996). Advanced sleep phase syndrome is accompanied by retiring very early in the evening and correspondingly arising very early in the morning, a schedule that sometimes mimics that of terminal insomnia. Patients with the hyper-nyctohemeral syndrome experience a failure of the circadian clock to entrain normally to the 24-hour day, and they sometimes experience a free-running 25-hour rhythm. This disorder is especially prevalent in blind persons, for whom light is unable to synchronize the circadian system. Some blind persons, however, are sensitive to light as an entrainer of the circadian system, so long as the retina and retinohypothalamic tract are normally functioning.

Treatment of circadian rhythm–based sleep disorders now most often includes both bright light and melatonin. Early-morning bright-light exposure, with restriction of light exposure in the evening, has been found to be effective for phase-advancing the circadian system in DSPS (Regestein and Pavlova 1995 [review]; Rosenthal et al. 1990). Evening bright-light treatment has been found to be effective in phase-delaying the circadian system and effectively treating advanced sleep phase syndrome. Bright light is usually ineffective in treating non-24-hour sleep-wake rhythms.

Melatonin has also been used successfully in the treatment of DSPS (Dahlitz et al. 1991; Lamberg 1996), and a case report indicated its successful use in entraining the circadian system in a blind retarded child who was unresponsive to bright light (Lapierre and Dumont 1995). Methylcobalamin (vitamin B_{12}) has also been reported to treat DSPS successfully, but well-controlled studies of its effectiveness have yet to be reported (Ohta et al. 1991; Yamadera et al. 1996).

Periodic Limb Movements of Sleep and Restless Legs Syndrome

PLMS and the related *restless legs syndrome* (RLS) are not infrequent causes of chronic insomnia complaints. PLMS can be transmitted as an autosomal dominant trait with onset in the second decade, and both PLMS and RLS can accompany a variety of medical illnesses, including peripheral neuropathies, anemia, uremia, and chronic pulmonary disease (Reite et al. 1997). The pathophysiology of the disorders remains unclear. RLS is not a true sleep disorder in that the uncomfortable sensations in the lower legs occur during wakefulness and that persons are aware of them. If RLS interferes with ability to sleep, however, it is perceived as an insomnia-like complaint. RLS is a common complaint, increasing in frequency with age and found in up to 23% of individuals older than 60 years (Montplaisir et al. 1997).

The involuntary limb movements, or leg (and occasionally arm) twitches or jerks, constituting PLMS are usually not recognized by the patient, because they occur during sleep. They may first be recognized as a problem by the bed partner, who complains of the patient's repeated bouts of kicking during the night. Patients who sleep alone may kick their bedcovers onto the floor during the night. PSG is required for accurate diagnosis of a PLMS disorder, quantifying both number of events and their association with awakenings or arousals. The isolated findings of PLMS (without associated arousals) during a sleep recording may have no clinical significance, but if occurrences of PLMS produce numerous short arousals during the night and so fragment sleep, they will likely be experienced as an insomnia complaint. Both RLS and PLMS have been associated with a variety of medical conditions, but they may occur in otherwise healthy individuals. They often but not always occur together, and, although most common in older individuals, they can have their onset in childhood.

Dopamine agonists such as carbidopa/levodopa and pergolide have been shown to be effective treatments in a large percentage of patients with RLS and PLMS. In general, patients with severe RLS have responded best to pergolide, whereas patients with PLMS but only mild to moderate RLS respond best to carbidopa/levodopa (Earley and Allen 1996).

Alternative treatments have included opioid agents and benzodiazepines (Silber 1997; Trenkwalder et al. 1996).

Substance Use Sleep Disorders

Substance use sleep disorders are disorders of sleep that include insomnia as a prominent component and that are associated with use or abuse of psychoactive substances, including nicotine (Phillips and Danner 1995). Now relatively infrequent, abuse of barbiturate hypnotic agents was formerly a frequent cause of chronic insomnia complaints. Alcohol remains a significant problem, as do stimulants and other drugs of abuse. Alcohol-dependent sleep disorder occurs in those who habitually "self-medicate" with alcohol to induce sleep. Alcohol does tend to decrease sleep latency and wakefulness during the first 3–4 hours of sleep. It also suppresses REM sleep and leads to REM rebound (with the possibility of vivid dreams or nightmares) with fragmented sleep the latter part of the night. Treatment includes withdrawal of alcohol, with long-term abstinence as the goal. When necessary, sedation can be provided by judicious use of antihistamines (e.g., diphenhydramine, 25–50 mg, or cyproheptadine, 4–24 mg).

Chronic use of stimulants leads to prolonged sleeplessness, and their withdrawal is followed by a period of hypersomnolence. A chronic insomnia complaint is often seen in long-term stimulant abusers even when they are not actively abusing the agents. Treatment is similar to that of alcohol-induced sleep disorder. Antikindling agents such as carbamazepine (100–600 mg/day) or divalproex (250–1,500 mg/day) may help when CNS hyperarousal/kindling is evident, as is sometimes seen in postcocaine panic disorder in polysubstance abusers.

Habituation to benzodiazepine agents does not usually result in insomnia unless they are too rapidly withdrawn, in which case the withdrawal syndrome may include insomnia. Doses should be tapered by one therapeutic dose per week.

In all cases of substance abuse sleep disorders, the insomnia complaint should emphasize behavioral treatment strategies to the fullest extent possible, because psychoactive agents have already proved to be a problem. A more detailed account of the treatment of substance abuse sleep disorders can be found in Chapter 3 of Reite et al. (1997).

Central Sleep Apnea

Central sleep apnea is a relatively rare cause of chronic insomnia and requires PSG for accurate diagnosis. This disorder can be missed because the typical presentation of sleep apnea (excessive daytime sleepiness, sonorous snoring, recent weight gain, hypertension) is not present. The patient may not be aware of the pauses in breathing and the arousals associated with resumption of breathing, although the bed partner will often be aware of the frequent breathing pauses. The frequent apneas cause sleep fragmentation, which results in insomnia complaints and often complaints of increased daytime sleepiness (Bonnet and Arand 1996). Central sleep apnea is frequently associated with medical and neurological disorders (Thalhofer and Dorow 1997), but it may also occur in otherwise healthy individuals. It is more frequently encountered in older individuals (Ancoli-Israel 1997). Both oxygen and continuous positive airway pressure (CPAP) can be used in the treatment of central apnea in patients with medical disorders (Franklin et al. 1997; Granton et al. 1996). The pharmacological treatment of central sleep apnea is less than optimal. Therapeutic options might include protriptyline (5–20 mg at bedtime), fluoxetine (10–20 mg/day), or theophylline (300–600 mg/day) (Ancoli-Israel 1997), although their efficacy has yet to be clearly established in well-controlled studies. Acetazolamide (250 mg twice a day) may be effective for high altitude–induced central apnea.

Primary Insomnia

Although there are several more rare causes of a chronic insomnia complaint, most often it is generally safe to assume that once the above specific causes have been systematically excluded, we are in all probability left with a possible primary insomnia diagnosis (DSM-IV 307.42). The nomenclature for this group is not clear, because specific pathophysiological mechanisms have yet to be identified. Whereas many individuals in these categories may experience a state of learned or conditioned arousal, there is likely another group of individuals with primary insomnia related to a state of chronic physiological hyperarousal of uncertain etiology, as outlined previously. The foregoing categories are often grouped under the term *psychophysiological insomnia*. These categories also include a group of individuals who complain of insomnia but who, when studied in the sleep laboratory, demonstrate normal sleep. This is termed the *sleep state misperception syndrome*.

Conditioned arousal (a term still sometimes used interchangeably with *psychophysiological insomnia*) characteristically begins when a susceptible individual experiences a stress-related transient insomnia and, after several nights of poor sleep, begins to fear going to bed because of concern that sleep will once again be difficult to initiate or maintain. This fear is associated with increased arousal, and soon a vicious circle is established in which merely going into the bedroom to prepare for sleep results in a conditioned arousal response sufficient to interfere with sleep. The conditioned arousal can persist long after the stress that caused the initial transient insomnia has resolved. Often, the conditioned arousal is limited to the individual's own bedroom and is not transferred to other sleeping locations. Such patients may be able to sleep on the living room couch, for example, and they may not necessarily have difficulty in napping during the day or sleeping well while on vacation in a new environment. They may also sleep normally if studied polysomnographically in the sleep laboratory, which is a new sleep environment in which they may not experience conditioned arousal. Thus, a normal PSG result does not mean that the patient does not experience

insomnia in his or her usual sleep environment. Conditioned insomnia appears to occur most often in individuals who have a history of *fragile sleep*, in which stressful events have been prone to interfere with their sleep.

Normal sleep on PSG also raises the question of a possible sleep state misperception syndrome. Patients with conditioned arousal insomnia who sleep normally in the laboratory, however, often comment that the laboratory sleep was an unusually good night of sleep, and they are able to differentiate it from their usual nighttime insomnia. Patients with sleep state misperception syndrome, on the other hand, still complain that the night spent in the sleep laboratory was illustrative of their usual poor sleep, even though the laboratory sleep may have been objectively normal.

COMBINED TREATMENT APPROACH FOR CHRONIC PSYCHOPHYSIOLOGICAL (PRIMARY) INSOMNIA

A treatment approach that combines both behavioral and pharmacological approaches is generally recommended for chronic psychophysiological or conditioned insomnia (Hajak et al. 1997; Mendelson and Jain 1995 [review]; Riemann 1996). Such approaches often work as well for sleep state misperception syndrome. Such a combined treatment approach offers the advantage of a pharmacological agent that can produce rapid relief of the sleep complaint, along with behavioral strategies, which take longer to become effective but provide long-term strategies that are under patients' control. It is important to avoid merely prescribing a hypnotic agent without also providing additional coping strategies for the patient. Morin and colleagues (1994), in a meta-analysis of treatment efficacy of nonpharmacological interventions, found that such treatments required on the average only 5 hours of therapy time and were effective in producing reliable changes in two of the four variables measured (sleep latency and time awake after sleep onset). Furthermore, these beneficial changes persisted at a 6-month follow-up.

BEHAVIORAL TREATMENTS

Behavioral treatment strategies are aimed at 1) breaking up bad sleep habits and replacing them with sleep-promoting habits, 2) directly decreasing physiological arousal levels, and 3) providing the patient with cognitive strategies to deal with sleep difficulties, thus promoting a sense of competence and diminishing anxiety about sleep.

First and foremost among the behavioral strategies is good *sleep hygiene:* the behaviors and habits that foster good sleep. Good sleep hygiene includes the following:

■ Establish a regular sleep schedule, ideally including early-morning arising that does not vary more than an hour on different days of the week.

■ Maintain a state of good aerobic fitness with regular exercise (but not within 3 hours of sleep onset).

■ Do not use caffeine or alcohol to excess. Caffeine can have a long-lasting effect on some individuals, and they should restrict it to mornings.

■ Ensure a quiet, dark, cool bedroom.

■ Provide a time to wind down in the evening before sleeping. Stop working 30 minutes before bedtime, and engage in a low-stress activity, such as reading or listening to music.

■ Consider a high-tryptophan snack (milk, cookies, banana) before bed.

■ Use the bedroom for sleep and sex but not for reviewing or thinking about the affairs of the day. If not asleep in 30 minutes, get up and read, or complete a task, returning to bed after sleepiness returns.

■ Minimize exposure to bright light to avoid phase-delaying the circadian system. Most reading lights and computer screens are not sufficiently bright to be troublesome in this regard.

Good sleep hygiene is appropriate for all, not just those with insomnia. Not infrequently, poor sleep hygiene contributes materially to an insomnia complaint. Careful questioning can identify such cases, and sometimes merely changing sleep habits in an appropriate manner is sufficient to significantly relieve the sleep complaint.

Several behavioral strategies discussed below are targeted directly at decreasing arousal level.

Biofeedback

Biofeedback involves monitoring physiological variables, such as electromyographic (EMG; muscle tension) responses, skin temperature, or electroencephalographic (EEG) activity patterns (alpha, theta, or sensorimotor rhythms); providing the patient with an auditory or visual cue that levels are not meeting a target threshold; and allowing the patient to develop strategies to modify the physiological indicators and so decrease arousal level. Biofeedback can be an important adjunct to the treatment of chronic insomnia, and it is especially useful for patients with high arousal levels.

Progressive Relaxation

Progressive relaxation is designed to make the patient aware of increased muscle tension and thus high arousal level. Patients contract muscle groups, become aware of the tense state, and then systematically relax them. Attention is paid to the feeling accompanying the relaxation response. As a result, patients can learn to avoid the high muscle tension that interferes with sleep onset, to lower their arousal level, and thus to permit (rather than induce) sleep (Jacobson 1974).

Sleep Restriction

Sleep restriction is useful for individuals who spend a considerable amount of time in bed but much of that time awake. Older patients are especially prone to spending more and more time in bed and achieving less and less sleep—for example, they may be spending 10 hours in bed yet claim to be sleeping only 6 hours. The essence of sleep restriction is to restrict the time in bed, which tends to consolidate sleep.

An increase in daytime sleepiness will accompany the early stages of sleep restriction, and patients may need considerable encouragement to complete the procedure, but it can be successful in consolidation of sleep in a sizable percentage of patients (Spielman et al. 1987 [review]).

Several other forms of cognitive therapy have been described as useful in the treatment of chronic insomnia, including stimulus control and paradoxical intention (Baillargeon 1997; Bootzin and Perlis 1992). Referral to a psychologist experienced in the various forms of cognitive therapy can be useful for these patients.

PHARMACOLOGICAL TREATMENT

Mendelson and Jain (1995) have suggested that the ideal hypnotic would have a therapeutic profile characterized by rapid sleep induction and no residual effects (including memory effects). Its pharmacokinetic profile would include rapid absorption and optimal half-life, as well as specific receptor binding and lack of active metabolites. Its pharmacodynamic profile would include lack of tolerance or physical dependence and no CNS or respiratory depression.

Although the ideal hypnotic agent has yet to be developed, these agents are being systematically improved with respect to most of the foregoing issues. Benzodiazepine compounds and nonbenzodiazepine agents active at the level of the benzodiazepine receptor are the most commonly used hypnotic agents today. These agents are relatively safe and have a good therapeutic profile; patients with insomnia do not appear to demonstrate short-term dose escalation (Roehrs et al. 1996). Older hypnotic agents (chloral hydrate, paraldehyde, barbiturates) may have a limited utility for very short-term use in specific patients, but they cannot be recommended for the treatment of chronic insomnia.

The benzodiazepine compounds differ substantially in terms of half-life, and the clinician can choose the agent with a half-life most appropriate for the clinical situation. A long-half-life hypnotic such as flurazepam (15–30 mg) or quazepam (7.5–15.0 mg) might be appropriate for an anxious patient in whom daytime anxiolytic effects are helpful, if the interference with psychomotor performance is acceptable and tolerable and if both patient and physician realize that considerable buildup in blood level can be expected. Patients with difficulty sleeping through the night might benefit from intermediate-half-life agents such as temazepam (15–30 mg) or estazolam (1–2 mg). Patients who must be alert in the morning without residual daytime sedation would best be managed by a short-half-life agent such as triazolam (0.125–0.25 mg) or zolpidem (5–10 mg). Zolpidem is an imidazopyridine agent active at the ω_1 benzodiazepine receptor but without the same degree of potential for tolerance or rebound as seen with conventional benzodiazepines. Zaleplon is a hypnotic from the pyrazolopyrimidine class. Like zolpidem, it is a nonbenzodiazepine ω_1 receptor agonist, but with a very short (1- to 1.5-hour) half-life. The usual dose is 10 mg.

Antidepressant agents, especially sedative tricyclics, are frequently used to manage chronic insomnia despite the relative lack of well-controlled double-blind studies demonstrating efficacy (Kupfer and Reynolds 1997). These agents are clearly indicated in insomnia that accompanies depressive disorders, where their effectiveness is clear. When used for other types of insomnia complaints, they are usually used at a dose lower than that of a typical antidepressant. Over-the-counter sleep agents, or various herbal remedies found in health food stores, have generally not been evaluated for hypnotic efficacy in well-controlled double-blind studies. Although some have modest sedative effects, consumers should be cautious, especially as concerns regular or excessive use of such agents.

INSOMNIA IN ELDERLY PERSONS

Sleep complaints are greater in elderly persons than in other age groups (Ganguli et al. 1996). More than 50% of persons older than 65 years complain of poor sleep (Ancoli-Israel 1997). Whereas it was once thought that elderly persons required less sleep, it now appears that they in fact get less sleep, but primarily because the conditions known to disrupt sleep and produce insomnia complaints increase with age. Sleep-related breathing disturbances (Ancoli-Israel et al. 1991b), depression, PLMS (Ancoli-Israel et al. 1991a), and medical conditions all increase with age, as do associated insomnia complaints. As a result of obtaining less sleep than needed, elderly persons tend to be sleepier during the day, as indicated by shorter mean sleep latencies on the MSLT (Dement et al. 1982).

The diagnosis and treatment of insomnia complaints in the elderly should proceed in a fashion no different from that outlined in this chapter. A systematic differential diagnosis, appropriate treatment of the specific medical, psychiatric, or other conditions that might adversely influence sleep, and a combined approach for the chronic insomnia component are indicated. Behavioral treatment should be emphasized, because many patients will be taking medications for other medical illnesses, thus increasing the possibility of drug interactions. Additionally, the metabolic breakdown of sedative-hypnotic agents might be diminished in elderly patients; thus, doses should begin lower, and caution should be exercised in the use of long-half-life agents (e.g., flurazepam) whose period of activity may be further prolonged.

Melatonin levels in elderly persons with insomnia have been found to be lower, with later onset of peak blood levels (Haimov et al. 1994). Some studies have suggested that melatonin replacement therapy might be a helpful treatment strategy for certain elderly individuals with sleep complaints (Garfinkel et al. 1995; Haimov et al. 1995). Elderly persons are at special risk for bereavement, and sleep disturbance associated with bereavement-related depression has been found to respond favorably to nortriptyline treatment in elderly individuals (Pasternak et al. 1994).

Especially important are good sleep hygiene, and reinforcing optimal circadian sleep/activity patterns. Often, elderly individuals are less active than their younger counterparts and are in less than optimal aerobic condition. Regular weight-lifting exercise in a cohort of 32 subjects ages 60–84 years was found to improve subjective sleep quality, depression, strength, and overall quality of life (Singh et al. 1997).

SUMMARY

Insomnia can be a complex symptom with a multifaceted causation. Careful attention to a systematic differential diagnostic procedure, keeping in mind the likelihood of comorbidity, contributes to accurate diagnosis and effective treatment.

Effective treatment is dependent on accurate diagnosis and tailoring the several behavioral and pharmacological treatment options to the specific patient. When this process is done with care, there is a high probability of a favorable outcome.

REFERENCES

Adam K, Tomeny M, Oswald I: Physiological and psychological differences between good and poor sleepers. J Psychiatr Res 20:301–316, 1986

American Psychiatric Association: Diagnostic and Statistical Manual of Mental Disorders, 4th Edition. Washington, DC, American Psychiatric Association, 1994

Ancoli-Israel S: Sleep problems in older adults: putting myths to bed. Geriatrics 52:20–30, 1997

Ancoli-Israel S, Kripke DF, Klauber MR, et al: Periodic limb movements in sleep in community-dwelling elderly. Sleep 14:496–500, 1991a

Ancoli-Israel S, Kripke DF, Klauber MR, et al: Sleep-disordered breathing in community-dwelling elderly. Sleep 14:486–495, 1991b

Arendt J, Aldhous M, Marks V: Alleviation of "jet lag" by melatonin: preliminary results of controlled double blind trial. BMJ 292:1170, 1986

Axelrod J, Weissbach H: Enzymatic O-methylation of N-acetylserotonin to melatonin. Science 131:1312–1313, 1960

Baillargeon L: Traitements cognitifs et comportementaux de l'insomnie: une alternative a la pharmacotherapie [Behavior and cognitive treatments for insomnia: an alternative to pharmacotherapy]. Can Fam Physician 43:290–296, 1997

Bonnet MH, Arand D: 24-hour metabolic rate in insomniacs and matched normal sleepers. Sleep 18:581–588, 1995

Bonnet MH, Arand DL: The consequences of a week of insomnia. Sleep 19:453–461, 1996

Bootzin RR, Perlis ML: Nonpharmacologic treatments of insomnia. J Clin Psychiatry 53 (suppl):37–41, 1992

Chang PP, Ford DE, Mead LA, et al: Insomnia in young men and subsequent depression. Am J Epidemiol 146:105–114, 1997

Coon SL, Roseboom PH, Baler R: Pineal serotonin N-acetyltransferase: expression cloning and molecular analysis. Science 270:1681–1683, 1995

Dahlitz M, Alvarez B, Vignau J, et al: Delayed sleep phase syndrome response to melatonin. Lancet 337:1121–1124, 1991

Dawson D, Reid K: Fatigue, alcohol and performance impairment (scientific correspondence). Nature 388:235, 1997

Dawson D, Encel N, Lushington K: Improving adaptation to simulated night shift: timed exposure to bright light versus daytime melatonin administration. Sleep 18:11–21, 1995

Dement WC, Seidel W, Carskadon MA: Daytime alertness, insomnia and benzodiazepines. Sleep 5:S28–S45, 1982

Earley CJ, Allen RP: Pergolide and carbidopa/levodopa treatment of the restless legs syndrome and periodic leg movements in sleep in a consecutive series of patients. Sleep 19:801–810, 1996

Eastman CI, Boulos Z, Terman M, et al: Light treatment for sleep disorders: consensus report, VI: shift work. J Biol Rhythms 10:157–164, 1995

Eaton WW, Badawi M, Melton B: Prodromes and precursors: epidemiologic data for primary prevention of disorders with slow onset. Am J Psychiatry 152:967–972, 1995

Edinger JD, Fins AI: The distribution and clinical significance of sleep time misperceptions among insomniacs. Sleep 18:232–239, 1995

Ford DE, Kamerow DB: Epidemiologic study of sleep disturbances and psychiatric disorders: an opportunity for prevention? JAMA 262:1479–1484, 1989

Franklin KA, Eriksson P, Sahlin C, et al: Reversal of central sleep apnea with oxygen. Chest 111:163–169, 1997

Gallup Organization: Sleep in America. Princeton, NJ, The Gallup Organization, 1995, pp 1–10

Ganguli M, Reynolds CF, Gilby JE: Prevalence and persistence of sleep complaints in a rural older community sample: the movies project. J Am Geriatr Soc 44:778–784, 1996

Garfinkel D, Laudon M, Nof D, et al: Improvement of sleep quality in elderly people by controlled-release melatonin. Lancet 346:541–544, 1995

Gordon NP, Cleary PD, Parker CE: The prevalence and health impact of shiftwork. Am J Public Health 76:1225–1228, 1986

Granton JT, Naughton MT, Benard DC, et al: CPAP improves inspiratory muscle strength in patients with heart failure and central sleep apnea. Am J Respir Crit Care Med 153:277–282, 1996

Haimov I, Laudon M, Zisapel N, et al: Sleep disorders and melatonin rhythms in elderly people. BMJ 309:167, 1994

Haimov I, Lavie P, Laudon M, et al: Melatonin replacement therapy of elderly insomniacs. Sleep 18:598–603, 1995

Hajak G, Muller-Popkes K, Riemann D, et al: Psychological, psychotherapeutic and other non-pharmacologic forms of therapy in treatment of insomnia. Fortschr Neurol Psychiatr 65: 133–144, 1997

Hohagen F, Kappler C, Schramm E, et al: Sleep onset insomnia, sleep maintaining insomnia and insomnia with early morning awakening—temporal stability of subtypes in a longitudinal study on general practice attenders. Sleep 17:551–554, 1994

Jacobson E: Progressive Relaxation. Chicago, IL, University of Chicago Press, Midway Reprint, 1974

Karacan I, Williams RL: Sleep disorders in the elderly. Am Fam Physician 27:143–152, 1983

Krupp LB, Jandorf L, Coyle PK, et al: Sleep disturbance in chronic fatigue syndrome. J Psychosom Res 37:325–331, 1993

Kupfer DJ, Reynolds CF: Management of insomnia. N Engl J Med 336:341–346, 1997

Lamberg L: Melatonin potentially useful but safety, efficacy remain uncertain. JAMA 276:1011–1014, 1996

Lapierre O, Dumont M: Melatonin treatment of a non-24-hour sleep-wake cycle in a blind retarded child. Biol Psychiatry 38:119–122, 1995

Leger D: The cost of sleep-related accidents: a report for the national commission on sleep disorders research. Sleep 17:84–93, 1994

Lichstein KL, Wilson NM, Noe SL, et al: Daytime sleepiness in insomnia: behavioral, biological and subjective indices. Sleep 17:693–702, 1994

Marcus CL, Loughlin GM: Effect of sleep deprivation on driving safety in housestaff. Sleep 19:763–766, 1996

Mellman TA, Nolan B, Hebding J, et al: A polysomnographic comparison of veterans with combat-related PTSD, depressed men, non-ill controls. Sleep 20:46–51, 1997

Mendelson WB, Jain B: An assessment of short-acting hypnotics. Drug Saf 13:257–270, 1995

Monroe LJ: Psychological and physiological differences between good and poor sleepers. J Abnorm Psychol 72:255–264, 1967

Montplaisir J, Boucher S, Poirer G, et al: Clinical, polysomnographic, and genetic characteristics of restless legs syndrome: a study of 133 patients diagnosed with new standards criteria. Mov Disord 12:61–65, 1997

Morin CM, Gramling SE: Sleep patterns and aging: comparison of older adults with and without insomnia complaints. Psychol Aging 4:290–294, 1989

Morin CM, Culbert JP, Schwartz SM: Non-pharmacological interventions for insomnia: a meta-analysis of treatment efficacy. Am J Psychiatry 151:1172–1180, 1994

Murciano D, Armengaud MH, Cramer PH, et al: Acute effects of zolpidem, triazolam, and flunitrazepam on arterial blood gases and control of breathing in severe COPD. Eur Respir J 6:625–629, 1993

Ohta T, Ando K, Iwata T, et al: Treatment of persistent sleep-wake schedule disorders in adolescents with methylcobalamin (vitamin B12). Sleep 14:414–418, 1991

Ozaki N, Iwata T, Itoh A, et al: Body temperature monitoring in subjects with delayed sleep phase syndrome. Neuropsychobiology 20:174–177, 1988

Pasternak RE, Reynolds CF, Houck PR, et al: Sleep in bereavement-related depression during and after pharmacotherapy with nortriptyline. J Geriatr Psychiatry Neurol 7:69–73, 1994

Phillips BA, Danner FJ: Cigarette smoking and sleep disturbance. Arch Intern Med 155:734–737, 1995

Pilcher JJ, Huffcutt AI: Effects of sleep deprivation on performance: a meta-analysis. Sleep 19:318–326, 1996

Porcu S, Bellatreccia A, Ferrara M, et al: Acutely shifting the sleep-wake cycle: nighttime sleepiness after diurnal administration of temazepam or placebo. Aviat Space Environ Med 68:688–694, 1997

Regestein QR, Monk TH: Delayed sleep phase syndrome: a review of its clinical aspects. Am J Psychiatry 152:602–608, 1995

Regestein QR, Pavlova M: Treatment of delayed sleep phase syndrome. Gen Hosp Psychiatry 17:335–345, 1995

Reite M, Jackson D, Cahoon R, et al: Sleep physiology at high altitude. Electroencephalogr Clin Neurophysiol 38:463–471, 1975

Reite M, Ruddy J, Nagel K: Concise Guide to the Evaluation and Management of Sleep Disorders, 2nd Edition. Washington, DC, American Psychiatric Press, 1997

Richardson GS, Malin HV: Circadian rhythm sleep disorders: pathophysiology and treatment. J Clin Neurophysiol 13:17–31, 1996

Riemann D: Insomnia: diagnostic and therapeutic procedure, 2: non-medicamentous and medicamentous therapy in general practice. Fortschr Med 114(30):399–401, 1996

Roberts MJ: Acute mountain sickness—experience on the roof of Africa expedition and military implications. J R Army Med Corps 140:49–51, 1994

Roehrs T, Shore E, Papineau K, et al: A two-week sleep extension in sleepy normals. Sleep 19:576–582, 1996

Rosenfeld DS, Furman Y: Pure sleep panic: two case reports and a review of the literature. Sleep 17:462–465, 1994

Rosenthal NE, Joseph-Vanderpool JR, Levendosky AA, et al: Phase-shifting effects of bright morning light as treatment for delayed sleep phase syndrome. Sleep 13:354–361, 1990

Ross RJ, Ball WA, Dinges DF: Rapid eye movement sleep disturbance in posttraumatic stress disorder. Biol Psychiatry 35:195–202, 1994

Saiz-Ruiz J, Cebollada A, Ibanez A: Sleep disorders in bipolar depression: hypnotics vs. sedative antidepressants. J Psychosom Res 38 (suppl): 55–60, 1994

Silber MH: Restless legs syndrome. Mayo Clin Proc 72:261–264, 1997

Silver JM, Sandberg DP, Hales RE: New approaches in the pharmacotherapy of posttraumatic stress disorder. J Clin Psychiatry 51 (10, suppl):33–38, 1990

Singh NA, Clements KM, Fiatarone MA: Sleep, sleep deprivation, and daytime activities: a randomized controlled trial of the effect of exercise on sleep. Sleep 20:95–101, 1997

Spielman AJ, Caruso LS, Glovinsky PB: A behavioral perspective on insomnia treatment. Psychiatr Clin North Am 10:541–553, 1987

Teicher MH, Glod CA, Magnus E, et al: Circadian rest-activity disturbances in seasonal affective disorder. Arch Gen Psychiatry 54:124–130, 1997

Thalhofer S, Dorow P: Central sleep apnea. Respiration 64:2–9, 1997

Trenkwalder C, Walters AS, Hening W: Periodic limb movements and restless legs syndrome. Neurol Clin 14:629–650, 1996

Waldhauser F, Dietzel M: Daily and annual rhythms in human melatonin secretion: role in puberty control. Ann N Y Acad Sci 453:205–214, 1985

Winokur A, Reynolds C: Overview of effects of antidepressant therapies on sleep. Primary Psychiatry 1:22–27, 1994

Yamadera H, Takahashi K, Okawa M: A multicenter study of sleep-wake rhythm disorders: therapeutic effects of vitamin B12, bright light therapy, chronotherapy and hypnotics. Psychiatry and Clinical Neurosciences 50:203–209, 1996

APPENDIX

New Psychotropic Drugs for Axis I Disorders

Recently Arrived, in Development, and Never Arrived

Joseph K. Belanoff, M.D., and
Ira D. Glick, M.D.

The vitality of the field of psychopharmacology depends on the continued introduction of new medications for treatment. In this chapter, we identify the current status of medications for schizophrenia, mood disorders, and anxiety. We discuss the mechanisms of these new drugs and compare them with drugs currently approved by the U.S. Food and Drug Administration (FDA). Table A–1 summarizes the clinical features of the new drugs.

Although this chapter is intended to be inclusive, a realistic caveat is that both medical and marketing decisions can dramatically influence the actual availability of any medication. We apologize in advance for any inadvertent omissions.

SCHIZOPHRENIA

Currently, a large number of new medications are being developed for the treatment of psychotic symptoms. One way to quickly grasp the overall picture is to characterize them on the basis of their (primary) receptor profile, as shown in Table A–2 (J. Lieberman, personal communication, August 1997).

Drugs That Recently Arrived

Risperidone and olanzapine are discussed by Marder in Chapter 8 of this volume.

Quetiapine. Quetiapine, a serotonin-dopamine antagonist, has shown efficacy in improving the positive and negative symptoms of schizophrenia (Casey 1996). It also appears to be comparable to haloperidol and chlorpromazine in acutely improving psychotic symptoms (Wetzel et al. 1995). Quetiapine has a favorable extrapyramidal side effects (EPS) profile and does not produce sustained increased levels of prolactin (Hirsch et al. 1996). In fact, the drug is generally well tolerated, complaints of mild somnolence and mild anticholinergic effects appearing most commonly.

Table A–1. Clinical features of new and most recent psychotropics

Drug (generic name)	Chemical classification	Presumed pharmacological effects	Comparison with standard drugs	Major side effects	Daily dose (mg)	Comment
Antipsychotics						
Risperidone	Benzisozole derivative	5-HT$_2$, D$_2$ blocker	Better than placebo and equal to standard	Anxiety, dizziness, rhinitis	3–6	? ↑ efficacy with negative symptoms; dose-related EPS
Olanzapine	Thieno-benzodiazepine	Complicated	Better than placebo and equal to standard	Sedation, orthostatic hypotension, anticholinergic	5–20	Low EPS, no agranulocytosis
Sertindole	Phenylindole	5-HT$_2$, D$_2$ blocker, α-blocker	Better than placebo and equal to standard	Nasal congestion, ↓ ejaculatory volume	20–24	Low EPS, ↑ Q-T interval?
Quetiapine	Dibenzothiazepine	Complicated	Better than placebo and equal to standard	Mild somnolence, mild constipation, dry mouth	200–400	? ↑ efficacy with negative symptoms, low EPS, no prolactinemia
Ziprasidone	Substituted benzisothiazolyl-piperazine	5-HT$_2$, D$_2$ blocker	Better than placebo and equal to standard	Mild orthostatic hypotension	?50–150	Low EPS, ? ↑ efficacy with negative symptoms and affective symptoms, ↑ Q-T interval?
MDL 100,907	Novel piperidine-methanol	5-HT$_{2A}$ blocker	Better than placebo and equal to standard	Mild sedation	?40–60	No EPS or prolactinemia

Drug	Class	Mechanism	Efficacy	Side effects	Dose	Comments
Aripiprazole	Quinolinone derivative	Postsynaptic D_2 blocker, presynaptic dopamine agonist	Better than placebo and equal to standard	Insomnia, headache	20–30	Low EPS
Zotepine	Dibenzothiophene	5-HT_2, D_2 blocker	Better than placebo and equal to standard	Moderate EPS, akathisia	250–350	Improvement in negative and positive symptoms, ? ↓ anxiety and depression
Nemonapride	Benzamide derivative	Selective D_2 antagonist	Better than placebo and equal to standard	Akathisia, drowsiness	15–25	Low EPS, ? improvement in negative symptoms
Antidepressants						
Nefazodone	Phenylpiperazine	5-HT reuptake inhibitor, 5-HT_2 blocker	Better than placebo and equal to standard	Sedation	300–600	? Useful in PMS, chronic pain, and social anxiety disorder
Mirtazapine	Tetracyclic	α_2 autoreceptor blocker, 5-HT_2 blocker, 5-HT_3 blocker, ↑ 5-HT release	Better than placebo and equal to standard	Sedation, dry mouth, weight gain	30–45	? Anxiolytic, sleep enhancer
Tianeptine	Tricyclic	5-HT reuptake enhancer	Better than placebo and equal to standard	Insomnia, ↑ anxiety	25–50	Few somatic complaints
Citalopram	Tertiary amine	SSRI	Better than placebo and equal to standard	Mild nausea, sedation	30–60	No cardiotoxicity
Flesinoxan	Piperazine derivative	5-HT_{1A} agonist	Better than placebo and equal to standard	Headache, dizziness, nausea	4–8	More study needed

Table A–1. Clinical features of new and most recent psychotropics *(continued)*

Drug (generic name)	Chemical classification	Presumed pharmacological effects	Comparison with standard drugs	Major side effects	Daily dose (mg)	Comment
Antidepressants *(continued)*						
Reboxetine	Methane-sulfonate salt	SNRI	Better than placebo and equal to standard	Somnolence, tremor, hypo-tension, dry mouth	8–10	Available in the U.K.
Moclobemide	Benzamide derivative	Reversible MAO$_A$-selective inhibitor	Better than placebo and equal to standard	Insomnia, headache, dry mouth, dizziness, fatigue, nausea, diarrhea	300–900	No dietary restrictions; not marketed in U.S.
Brofaromine	Piperidine derivative	Reversible MAO$_A$-selective inhibitor; 5-HT reuptake inhibitor	Better than placebo and equal to standard	Insomnia, dizziness, headache, dry mouth, anorexia	25–150	No dietary restrictions; not marketed in U.S.
Anxiolytics						
Abecarnil	β-Carboline	Benzodiazepine partial agonist	Better than placebo and equal to standard	Drowsiness, fatigue	3–9	Any interest?
Mood stabilizers						
Lamotrigine	Phenyltriazine	Inhibits release of glutamate	None so far	Dizziness, headache, rash	150–250	? Efficacy in bipolar depression
Gabapentin	GABA derivative	?	None so far	Somnolence, dizziness, ataxia	900–1,800	No interaction with CBZ or VPA
Tiagabine	Nipecotic acid derivative	GABA uptake inhibitor	None so far	Dizziness	800 divided	Short half-life

Topiramate	Sulfamate-substituted monosaccharide	Complicated	None so far	600 divided	Headache, somnolence, dizziness	Stops spread of seizures, as opposed to raising the seizure threshold, ? relevance to BAD
Vigabatrin	Gamma-vinyl GABA	Irreversible inhibitor of GABA-aminotransferase	None so far	1,500–3,000	Sedation, dizziness	? of increase in depression and psychosis in patients with epilepsy

Note. 5-HT = 5-hydroxytryptamine (serotonin); D_2 = dopamine type 2 [receptor]; EPS = extrapyramidal side effects; PMS = premenstrual syndrome; SSRI = selective serotonin reuptake inhibitor; SNRI = selective norepinephrine reuptake inhibitor; MAO = monoamine oxidase; GABA = γ-aminobutyric acid; CBZ = carbamazepine; VPA = valproic acid; BAD = bipolar affective disorder.

Drugs That Are in Development

Ziprasidone.　Ziprasidone, also a serotonin-dopamine antagonist, has proven efficacy in blocking dopaminergic behaviors in animal models without producing severe motor side effects (Reeves and Harrigan 1996). However, it is also a potent serotonin type 2 (5-HT$_{2A}$) receptor antagonist. Early studies report efficacy in positive and negative symptoms with few EPS in patients with schizophrenia. Clinical trials are now completed. Analysis of safety measures indicates that the agent is well tolerated and has a low incidence of EPS and orthostatic hypotension, only transient effects on prolactin levels, and no significant adverse effects on laboratory safety tests (Seeger et al. 1995). Questions have been raised about the effects of ziprasidone on the Q-T interval. This agent will likely be on the market when this volume is published.

MDL 100,907.　MDL 100,907 is a potent and selective 5-HT$_{2A}$ receptor antagonist with no dopamine effects (Sramek et al. 1996). In preclinical studies, it provided better ratings on central nervous system safety indices than did haloperidol, clozapine, risperidone, amperozide, and ritanserin. Early clinical trials have shown it to be well tolerated and to have no significant neurological side effects, no rise in serum prolactin levels, and very little orthostatic hypotension while significantly lowering scores on the Brief Psychiatric Rating Scale (Kehne et al. 1996; Overall and Gorham 1962). Phase 2 and 3 trials are in progress to determine efficacy.

Aripiprazole.　Aripiprazole (ORL-N597) is an antagonist at postsynaptic dopamine type 2 (D_2) receptors but an agonist at presynaptic dopamine autoreceptors. Animal models indicate that aripiprazole has less potential to cause EPS than do conventional antipsychotics. Early clinical studies show reduction in positive symptoms without significant neurological side effects (Otsuka Pharmaceuticals 1997).

Table A–2. Novel antipsychotic compounds

Compound	Pharmacological mechanism	Pharmaceutical company
Selective dopamine receptor agents		
SCH-39166	D_1 antagonist	Schering-Plough
NN22-0010	D_1 antagonist	Novo Nordisk
Remoxipride	D_2 antagonist	Astra
Raclopride	D_2 antagonist	Astra
NGD 94-1	D_4 antagonist	Neurogen
L-745,870	D_4 antagonist	Merck
SDZ-MAR-327	Partial D_2 agonist/antagonist	Sandoz
OPC-14597	D_2, D_3 antagonist, D_2 partial agonist 5-HT_{2A} antagonist	Otsuka
Mixed neuroreceptor antagonists		
Clozapine	D_2, D_1, 5-HT_{2A}, $NE\alpha_1$, α_2, H_1, ACH	Sandoz
Iloperidone (HP-873)	D_2, $NE\alpha_1$, α_2, 5-HT_{2A}	Roussel Uclaf SA
Mazapertine	D_2, D_3, $NE\alpha_1$, α_2, 5-HT_{1A}	Janssen
Olanzapine (LY 170053)	D_1, D_2, D_4, 5-HT_{2A}, $NE\alpha_1$, H_1	Lilly
Risperidone	D_2, 5-HT_{2A}, $NE\alpha_1$, α_2, H_1	Janssen
Quetiapine	D_2, D_1, 5-HT_{2A}, $NE\alpha_1$, α_2, ACH	Zeneca
Sertindole	D_2, D_1, 5-HT_{2A}, $NE\alpha_1$	Abbott/Lundbeck
Ziprasidone (CP-88059)	D_2, D_1, 5-HT_{2A}, $NE\alpha_1$	Pfizer
Serotonin antagonists		
Amperozide	$5\text{-HT}_{2A}/D_2$, D_1	Kabi-Pharmacia, Sandoz
MDL 100,907	5-HT_{2A} antagonist	Hoechst Merrell Dow

Note. Affinities for (the common) neuroreceptors for which all drugs have been tested. D_1, D_2, D_3, and D_4 refer to dopamine receptors; 5-HT_{1A} and 5-HT_{2A} refer to serotonin receptors; $NE\alpha_2$, α_1 are norepinephrine alpha receptors; ACH refers to muscarinic receptors; H_1 refers to histamine receptor. This list of neuroreceptor effects is not comprehensive and does not reflect the proportional affinity that the drugs have for respective neuroreceptors.
Source. Jeffrey Lieberman, M.D.

Zotepine. Zotepine is currently being marketed in Japan, the United Kingdom, and Germany (Ott 1992). It appears to show some efficacy in reducing anxiety, depression, and negative as well as positive symptoms of schizophrenia (Fleischhacker et al. 1989). It also appears to produce fewer EPS than standard antipsychotic agents do (Barnas et al. 1992; Fleischhacker et al. 1989). Its adverse effects include fatigue, dry mouth, and constipation (Kondo et al. 1994). Like risperidone, zotepine is a more potent D_2 receptor blocker at higher doses and has a similar propensity to cause neurological side effects.

Nemonapride. Nemonapride has been released in Japan. It is a benzamide derivative and a potent and highly selective D_2 receptor antagonist (Yamamoto et al. 1982). It has shown efficacy in treating both the positive and the negative symptoms of schizophrenia while maintaining a surprisingly favorable EPS profile. Its adverse effects include akathisia and drowsiness (Satoh et al. 1997).

Drugs That Never Arrived

Sertindole. Sertindole, a serotonin-dopamine antagonist, was shown to be effective in improving both the positive and the negative symptoms of schizophrenia. Like the other "atypicals," sertindole has a favorable EPS profile, although it is a more potent D_2 receptor blocker than clozapine and olanzapine. Sertindole appears to show greater selectivity for limbic as opposed to nigrostriatal D_2 receptors and has a relatively high affinity for 5-HT_2 receptors. Side effects include nasal congestion and decreased ejaculatory volume, which are probably related to α-adrenergic receptor blockade. Sertindole also appears to increase the Q-T interval on electrocardiogram. Data available as of this writing suggest that this side effect has little clinical significance (Borison 1995; Daniel et al. 1996), but the company has decided not to market the drug in the United States.

Remoxipride. Remoxipride was selected as a candidate atypical antipsychotic in 1978 (Lewander et al. 1990). It had a favorable EPS profile even though it was a potent D_2 receptor antagonist and had little effect on serotonin receptors. Remoxipride was not antihistaminergic and as a consequence was not sedating nor did it cause much weight gain. It had clear efficacy in treating the positive symptoms of schizophrenia, but in November 1993, it was dropped because of several cases of aplastic anemia (Lewander et al. 1992).

Raclopride. Raclopride had high affinity for D_2 and D_3 receptors compared with D_4 receptors. It had a favorable EPS profile compared with haloperidol. It was dropped because there was a suggestion that it increased tumor activity.

Amperozide. Amperozide had a significant effect on mesolimbic dopamine transmission as well as being a potent 5-HT_2 receptor antagonist (Svartengren and Celander 1994). It has been at least temporarily dropped from clinical trials.

Amisulpride. Amisulpride is available in Europe but was never marketed in the United States. It is a specific dopamine receptor antago-

nist with high affinity for D_2 and D_3 receptors. It seems to have selectivity for the limbic pathways. In clinical studies, patients showed improvement in negative symptoms of schizophrenia with amisulpride (Paillere-Martinot et al. 1995) while reporting fewer neurological side effects than with haloperidol (Perrault et al. 1997). It does produce galactorrhea. Clinicians report that it is particularly effective in helping patients with mild to moderate symptoms but not those with severe symptoms.

MAJOR DEPRESSION

Drugs That Recently Arrived

The three most recently released antidepressants in the United States are nefazodone, mirtazapine, and citalopram.

Nefazodone. Nefazodone is a phenylpiperazine analogue of trazodone. Like trazodone, nefazodone blocks serotonin reuptake but with less potency than either the tricyclic antidepressants or the selective serotonin reuptake inhibitors (SSRIs). Nefazodone (and trazodone) are, however, significant blockers of 5-HT_2 receptors. This combination may result in stimulation of 5-HT_{1A} receptors in the dorsal raphe nucleus (which in turn may help depression) while avoiding stimulation of 5-HT_2 receptors in the forebrain (avoiding agitation or anxiety) or in the spinal cord (avoiding sexual dysfunction).

Nefazodone (and trazodone) are readily absorbed from the gastrointestinal tract, reach peak plasma levels in 1–2 hours, and have half-lives of 6–12 hours. Both are metabolized in the liver, and 75% of their metabolites are excreted in the urine.

Nefazodone has three main metabolites. Hydroxynefazodone has a pharmacodynamic profile similar to that of nefazodone, with SSRI and 5-HT_2 receptor antagonism. A second metabolite, a triazoledione, is a weaker 5-HT_2 antagonist than nefazodone and does not inhibit serotonin reuptake. *m*-Chlorphenylpiperazide is a metabolite of nefazodone (and trazodone) and has some serotonin antagonist activity at the $5-HT_2$ receptor but agonist activity at serotonin receptor types 1A, 1B, 1C, and 1D (Cyr and Brown 1996).

Nefazodone has been shown to be effective in both first-episode and recurrent major depression. It may also be useful in premenstrual syndrome and pain management. Researchers are currently probing for a therapeutic window for nefazodone. It has a benign side-effect profile with much less sedation than trazodone.

Mirtazapine. Mirtazapine enhances both norepinephrine and serotonin release (de Boer 1995). It also blocks $5-HT_2$ and $5-HT_3$ receptors, an effect that directs the increase in serotonin function through the $5-HT_1$ class of receptors (Davis and Wilde 1996). Mirtazapine has a low to moderate affinity for histamine H_1 receptors, which may explain its sedating properties (Stimmel et al. 1997).

Analysis of all United States controlled studies involving mirtazapine reveals an efficacy equal to that of tricyclic antidepressants and a lower dropout rate (Kasper 1997). The most common side effects of mirtazapine ($\geq 5\%$, and twice placebo) were increased appetite, weight gain, somnolence, dry mouth, and dizziness. Nausea, vomiting, insomnia, and sexual dysfunction were equally or less frequently noted in mirtazapine-treated patients compared with tricyclic-treated patients (Montgomery 1995).

Citalopram. Citalopram is a potent SSRI (Lader 1996). Several studies have shown it to be better than placebo and equal in efficacy to standard antidepressant drugs (Montgomery and Djarv 1996). Citalopram is reported to have few side effects other than nausea, although one would presume that it also causes the type of sexual side effects that are seen with the other SSRIs (Muldoon 1996). It has few direct drug interactions but is an inhibitor of the cytochrome P450 (CYP) 2DC system (Brosen 1996).

Drugs That Are in Development

Tianeptine. Tianeptine is actually a serotonin uptake enhancer (Mitchell 1995). Although theoretically it might be presumed that tianeptine causes depression, it has actually been shown (in placebo-controlled studies) to be an effective antidepressant (Dalery et al. 1997; Invernizzi et al. 1994). It has few anticholinergic (Wilde and Benfield 1995) or cardiovascular side effects but does occasionally cause insomnia and nausea. Interestingly, it appears to have some efficacy in the treatment of chronic alcoholism.

Flesinoxan. Flesinoxan is a potent and selective $5-HT_{1A}$ agonist. No double-blind, placebo-controlled study of flesinoxan efficacy as an antidepressant has been published to date. In an open study of treatment-refractory depressed patients, flesinoxan was found to provide successful antidepressant effects (Grof et al. 1993). The most common side effects among patients in this study were headache, dizziness, and nausea.

Reboxetine. Reboxetine is a nontricyclic, selective norepinephrine reuptake inhibitor that is more potent than the older norepinephrine blocker desipramine. (However, it is not a cholinergic receptor blocker.) It does not significantly induce glucuronosyltransferase or the CYP3A4 system and has no interaction with the CYP2D6 system. As a consequence, reboxetine is unlikely to have any significant interaction with lorazepam, alprazolam, the tricyclic antidepressants, or the SSRIs. It has been released in the United Kingdom.

In early studies, reboxetine appeared to be significantly superior to placebo in treating major depression and dysthymia and may be as effective as imipramine in treating severe major depression (Berzewski et al. 1997). It tentatively appears that 8–10 mg/day is the optimum dosage. However, truly optimal doses have not yet been fully determined. Somnolence, tremor, hypotension, and dry mouth have been reported more frequently with reboxetine than with fluoxetine but not as frequently as with imipramine (Berzewski et al. 1997; Montgomery and Kasper 1995). Reboxetine does produce less gastrointestinal upset than does fluoxetine. Reboxetine is currently in early study in the United States.

Olanzapine. It has been suggested that olanzapine may be an effective monotherapy for psychotic major depression (DeBattista et al. 1997). The pharmacological properties of olanzapine include antagonism of dopamine (types 1–4) receptors, as well as 5-HT$_2$, muscarinic, α_1, and histamine receptors. It is conceivable that olanzapine, with its moderate 5-HT$_2$ antagonism and broad dopamine antagonism, has both primary antidepressant effects and antipsychotic effects. Interestingly, a number of case reports have suggested that clozapine, which has a similarly broad range of pharmacological activity, may also be useful in the monotherapy of psychotic depression (Ranjan and Meltzer 1996).

Drugs That Never Arrived

Reversible inhibitors of monoamine oxidase. The monoamine oxidase inhibitors currently available in the United States irreversibly bind their monoamine oxidase substrates. Reversible inhibitors of monoamine oxidase (RIMAs) are being developed. These drugs bind reversibly to monoamine oxidase, resulting in the full restoration of enzyme activity within 2–5 days after their discontinuation. Moreover, because RIMAs are competitive inhibitors, large amounts of ingested tyramine will displace the drug from the enzyme, limiting the potential for an extreme tyramine-induced reaction.

Moclobemide, an RIMA, has been shown to be better than placebo and equal to standard medication in treating major depression (Angst and Stabl 1992). Its adverse effects include nau-

sea and agitation, and, like irreversible monoamine oxidase inhibitors, it has a significant interaction with SSRIs, particularly in overdose (Rihmer et al. 1994). Unfortunately, moclobemide is not likely to be introduced in the United States any time soon. Similarly, **brofaromine,** another RIMA, has also been found to be an effective agent in depression (Chouinard et al. 1993) and even treatment-resistant depression (Volz et al. 1994). Its adverse effects include insomnia, dizziness, dry mouth, and anorexia.

Nomifensine. Nomifensine was available in the mid-1980s, but its manufacturer elected to stop its distribution. It had a reputation for being an effective stimulating antidepressant with good efficacy in treatment-resistant cases. Unfortunately, a few patients in England who were using nomifensine died from hemolytic anemia, and the company (perhaps fearful of the product liability litigation) withdrew the drug from the market (Cole 1988).

BIPOLAR DISORDER

Bipolar disorder is chronic, recurrent, often severely impairing, and usually present from adolescence or early adulthood (Bowden 1995). The established pharmacological treatments for bipolar disorder (lithium, carbamazepine, and valproic acid) have clear efficacy. Unfortunately, they also have multiple adverse effects ranging from the annoying to the potentially lethal, so the search for new agents is in full swing.

Drugs That Recently Arrived

Lamotrigine. Lamotrigine was approved by the FDA in December 1997 for use as adjunctive therapy in the treatment of partial seizures in adults with epilepsy (Gilman 1995). It is believed to inhibit the stimulated presynaptic release of glutamate and may have significant mood-stabilizing properties (Walden et al.

1996). Moreover, it may be effective in the treatment of bipolar depression (which is often difficult to treat with standard mood stabilizers). In order of decreasing frequency, the side effects associated with lamotrigine include dizziness, headaches, diplopia, ataxia, gastrointestinal upset, somnolence, and rash (Calabrese et al. 1996). (Slow titration may significantly reduce the chances of a rash.)

Gabapentin.   Gabapentin is a new antiseizure medication used as adjunctive therapy in patients with refractory partial seizures. The mechanism of action is unknown, and although it is structurally related to the neurotransmitter γ-aminobutyric acid (GABA), it does not interact with the GABA receptor (Singh et al. 1996). Gabapentin has a unique pharmacological profile for an anticonvulsant, including lack of binding to plasma proteins, primary elimination by the kidney, and no induction of hepatic enzymes (Andrews and Fischer 1994). Moreover, in clinical trials, no interactions have been observed between gabapentin and carbamazepine or valproic acid (Ramsay 1994). In a small inpatient study of patients with bipolar disorder that was refractory to standard treatment, gabapentin was used as adjunctive medicine with impressive results (Bennett et al. 1997). No serious side effects were seen, although somnolence, dizziness, and ataxia (usually resolving in 1–2 weeks) have been noted in earlier studies with epileptic patients (Andrews and Fischer 1994; Ramsay 1994). More recent studies suggest lack of efficacy of gabapentin in mania.

Tiagabine.   Tiagabine, a GABA uptake inhibitor (Gram 1994), has shown efficacy in a wide range of seizure models (Mengel 1994). Because it does not inhibit or induce drug metabolism, it does not alter the concentration of other antiseizure medications. Potential problems that have emerged in clinical studies include dizziness (which has been transient) and a short (5- to 8-hour) half-life (which could be offset by a controlled-release formulation) (Brodie 1995).

Topiramate.   Topiramate is an antiseizure medication that appears to have several possible mechanisms of action, including a modulation effect on voltage-dependent sodium conductance (Coulter et al. 1993) and enhancement of $GABA_A$ submediated C_1-flu (Brown et al. 1993). It appears to stop the spread of seizures as opposed to raising the seizure threshold. In both open trials (Rangel et al. 1988; Wilder et al. 1988) and controlled trials (Ben-Menachem et al. 1996; Tassinari et al. 1996) in patients with refractory partial seizures, it was quite effective. Side effects included dizziness, sedation, weight loss, and increased incidence of renal calculi.

Drug That Is in Development

Vigabatrin.   Vigabatrin is a specific, irreversible inhibitor of GABA-aminotransferase, the principal catabolic enzyme of GABA (Lippert et al. 1977). It has been shown to be effective in multiple double-blind, placebo-controlled studies of patients with refractory seizures (Gram et al. 1985; Loiseau et al. 1986; Tassinari et al. 1987). (Interestingly, by preventing the transmission of GABA to succinic semialdehyde, it is used to treat 4-hydroxybutyric aciduria, a rare inborn error of metabolism caused by the deficiency of succinic semialdehyde dehydrogenase [Rahbeeni et al. 1994].) It has few drug interactions but does cause sedation and dizziness in some patients (Tartara et al. 1986). There have been occasional reports of both psychosis and an increase in depressive symptoms in patients with epilepsy, so further clinical research is obviously needed.

ANXIETY DISORDERS

Anxiety disorders are almost always chronic and relapsing. It is probably necessary to find anxiolytics that may be used for long-term treatment. Effective anxiolytic medication that lacks the potential for abuse or dependence would be a major advance. The main choice today is between benzodiazepines, which are fast in onset but are associated with dependence, and antidepressants, which are effective and do not cause dependence but are slower in onset.

Drugs That Never Arrived

Abecarnil. Abecarnil is a β-carboline and a benzodiazepine partial agonist. Phase 1 studies in healthy volunteers have yielded findings typical of anxiolytic compounds while producing relatively few side effects. An extensive double-blind, placebo-controlled study in outpatients with generalized anxiety disorders found that abecarnil may be clinically efficacious at doses that produce few side effects (Ballenger et al. 1991). It is unclear whether the development of this drug will go forward.

Moclobemide and brofaromine. Both moclobemide and brofaromine have been shown to be effective in treating social phobia (Fahlen et al. 1995; Versiani et al. 1992). However, the data on moclobemide are somewhat less clear; one large study (Noyes et al. 1997) showed no difference from placebo. On the other hand, brofaromine produced a significant reduction in anxiety compared with placebo in patients with social phobia (Lott et al. 1997).

Brofaromine, in addition to inhibiting the A isoenzyme of monoamine oxidase, also inhibits the reuptake of serotonin. Because SSRIs, particularly fluvoxamine (van Vliet et al. 1994) and sertraline (Katzelnick et al. 1995), have been reported to be effective in treating social phobia, it is unclear which of brofaromine's qualities is most related to its efficacy in treating social phobia.

SUMMARY

In this chapter, we identify several medications that we believe show particular promise. However, there are a multitude of reasons, both medical and economic, that any or all of these medications may never be used as psycho-

pharmacological agents in the United States. Let us add these observations: Expert clinicians tend to be biased toward efficacy over safety. Because they are called on to treat the most difficult cases, and because of their own expert knowledge, they tend to be eager to have new agents available and are less troubled by potential hazards. Regulators are obligated to be biased in the direction of safety. Interestingly, pharmaceutical manufacturers are often in a middle ground, having strong economic incentives to provide new medications but keeping a serious eye toward the potential for hazard.

REFERENCES

Andrews CO, Fischer JH: Gabapentin: a new agent for the management of epilepsy. Ann Pharmacother 28:1188–1196, 1994

Angst J, Stabl M: Efficacy of moclobemide in different patient groups: a meta-analysis of studies. Psychopharmacology 106:S109–S113, 1992

Ballenger JC, McDonald S, Noyes R, et al: The first double-blind, placebo-controlled trial of a partial benzodiazepine agonist, abecarnil (ZK 112–119), in generalized anxiety disorder. Psychopharmacol Bull 27:171–179, 1991

Barnas C, Stuppack CH, Miller C, et al: Zotepine in the treatment of schizophrenic patients with prevailingly negative symptoms: a double-blind trial vs. haloperidol. Int Clin Psychopharmacol 7:23–27, 1992

Ben-Menachem E, Henriksen O, Dam M, et al: Double-blind, placebo-controlled trial of topiramate as add-on therapy in patients with refractory partial seizures. Epilepsia 37:539–543, 1996

Bennett J, Goldman WT, Suppes T: Gabapentin for treatment of bipolar and schizoaffective disorder. J Clin Psychopharmacol 17:141–142, 1997

Berzewski H, Van Joffaert M, Cagiano CA: Efficacy and tolerability of reboxetine compared with imipramine in a double-blind study in patients suffering from major depressive episodes. Eur Neuropsychopharmacol 7:S23, 1997

Borison RL: Clinical efficacy of serotonin-dopamine antagonists relative to classic neuroleptics. J Clin Psychopharmacol 15:24S–29S, 1995

Bowden CL: Treatment of bipolar disorder, in The American Psychiatric Press Textbook of Psychopharmacology. Edited by Schatzberg AF, Nemeroff CB. Washington, DC, American Psychiatric Press, 1995, pp 603–614

Brodie MJ: Tiagabine pharmacology in profile. Epilepsia 36:57–59, 1995

Brosen K: Are pharmacokinetic drug interactions with the SSRIs an issue? Int Clin Psychopharmacol 11:23–28, 1996

Brown SD, Wolf HH, Swinyard RE, et al: The novel anticonvulsant topiramate enhances GABA-mediated chloride flux (abstract). Epilepsia 34:122–123, 1993

Calabrese JR, Fatemi SH, Woyshville MJ: Antidepressant effects of lamotrigine in rapid cycling bipolar disorder. Am J Psychiatry 153:9, 1996

Casey DE: Seroquel (quetiapine): preclinical and clinical findings of a new atypical antipsychotic. Exp Opin Invest Drugs 5:939–957, 1996

Chouinard G, Saxena BM, Nair NPV, et al: Brofaromine in depression: a Canadian multicenter placebo trial and a review of standard drug comparative studies. Clin Neuropharmacol 16:S52–S54, 1993

Cole JO: Where are those new antidepressants we were promised? Arch Gen Psychiatry 45:193–197, 1988

Coulter DA, Sombati S, DeLorenzo RJ: Selective effects of topiramate on sustained repetitive firing and spontaneous bursting in hippocampal neurons (abstract). Epilepsia 34:123, 1993

Cyr M, Brown C: Nefazodone: its place among the antidepressants. Ann Pharmacother 30:1006–1012, 1996

Dalery J, Dagens-Lafant V, DeBodinat C: Value of tianeptine in treating major recurrent unipolar depression: study versus placebo for 16½ months of treatment. Encephale 23:56–64, 1997

Daniel D, Swann A, Silber C, et al: The long term cardiovascular safety of sertindole. Poster presented at the convention of the American College of Neuropsychopharmacology, San Juan, Puerto Rico, December 1996

Davis R, Wilde M: Mirtazapine: a review of its pharmacology and therapeutic potential in the management of major depression. CNS Drugs 5(5):384–402, 1996

DeBattista C, Solvason HB, Belanoff J, et al: Treatment in psychotic depression. Am J Psychiatry 154:1625–1626, 1997

de Boer T: The effects of mirtazapine on central noradrenergic and serotonergic neurotransmission. Int Clin Psychopharmacol 10:19–23, 1995

Fahlen T, Nilsson H, Borg K, et al: Social phobia: the clinical efficacy and tolerability of the monoamine oxidase A and serotonin uptake inhibitor brofaromine. Acta Psychiatr Scand 92:351–358, 1995

Fleischhacker WW, Barnas C, Stuppack CH: Zotepine vs. haloperidol in paranoid schizophrenia: a double-blind trial. Psychopharmacol Bull 25:97–100, 1989

Gilman JT: Lamotrigine: an antiepileptic agent for the treatment of partial seizures. Ann Pharmacother 29:144–151, 1995

Gram L: Tiagabine: a novel drug with a GABAergic mechanism of action. Epilepsia 35:585–587, 1994

Gram L, Koasterkov P, Dam M: Gamma-vinyl GABA: a double-blind, placebo-controlled trial in partial epilepsy. Ann Neurol 17:262–266, 1985

Grof P, Joffe R, Kennedy S, et al: An open study of oral flesinoxan, a 5-HT1A receptor agonist, in treatment-resistant depression. Int Clin Psychopharmacol 8:167–172, 1993

Hirsch SR, Link CGG, Goldstein JM, et al: ICI 204,636: a new atypical antipsychotic drug. Br J Psychiatry 168:45–56, 1996

Invernizzi G, Aguglia E, Bertolina A, et al: The efficacy and safety of tianeptine in the treatment of depressive disorder: results of a controlled double-blind multicentre study vs. amitriptyline. Neuropsychobiology 30:85–93, 1994

Kasper S: Efficacy of antidepressants in the treatment of severe depression: the place of mirtazapine. J Clin Psychopharmacol 17:19S–28S, 1997

Katzelnick DJ, Kobak KA, Greist MH, et al: Sertraline for social phobia: a double-blind, placebo-controlled crossover study. Am J Psychiatry 152:1368–1371, 1995

Kehne JH, Baron BM, Carr AA, et al: Preclinical characterization of the potential of the putative atypical antipsychotic MDL 100,907 as a potent 5-HT2A antagonist with a favorable CNS safety profile. J Pharmacol Exp Ther 277:968–981, 1996

Kondo T, Otani K, Ishida M, et al: Adverse effects of zotepine and their relationship to serum concentrations of the drug and prolactin. Ther Drug Monit 16:120–124, 1994

Lader M: Citalopram—a new antidepressant. Primary Care Psychiatry 2:49–58, 1996

Lewander T, Westerbergh S-E, Morrison D: Clinical profile of remoxipride—a combined analysis of a comparative, double blind multicentre trial programme. Acta Psychiatr Scand 358:92–98, 1990

Lewander T, Uppfeldt G, Kohler C, et al: Remoxipride and raclopride: pharmacological background and clinical outcome, in Novel Antipsychotics. Edited by Meltzer HY. New York, Raven, 1992, pp 67–78

Lippert B, Metcalf BW, Jung MJ, et al: 4-Aminohex-5-enoic acid, a selective catalytic inhibitor of 4-aminobutyric-acid aminotransferase in mammalian brain. Eur J Biochem 74:441–445, 1977

Loiseau P, Hardenberg JP, Pestre M, et al: Double-blind, placebo-controlled study of vigabatrin (gamma-vinyl GABA) in drug-resistant epilepsy. Epilepsia 27:115–120, 1986

Lott M, Greist JH, Jefferson JW, et al: Brofaromine for social phobia: a multicenter, placebo-controlled, double-blind study. J Clin Psychopharmacol 17:255–260, 1997

Mengel H: Tiagabine. Epilepsia 35:581–584, 1994

Mitchell PB: Novel antidepressants report: novel French antidepressants not available in the United States. Psychopharmacol Bull 31:509–519, 1995

Montgomery SA: Safety of mirtazapine: a review. Int Clin Psychopharmacol 10:37–45, 1995

Montgomery S, Djarv L: The antidepressant efficacy of citalopram. Int Clin Psychopharmacol 11:29–33, 1996

Montgomery S, Kasper S: Comparison of compliance between serotonin reuptake inhibitors and tricyclic antidepressants: a meta-analysis. Int Clin Psychopharmacol 9:33–40, 1995

Muldoon C: The safety and tolerability of citalopram. Int Clin Psychopharmacol 11:35–40, 1996

Noyes R, Moroz G, Davidson JRT, et al: Moclobemide in social phobia: a controlled dose-response trial. J Clin Psychopharmacol 17:247–254, 1997

Otsuka Pharmaceuticals: Investigator's Brochure. Rockville, MD, America Pharma, 1997

Ott C: Zotepin—ein Neuroleptikum mit neuartigem wirkungsmechanismus. Fundamenta Psychiatrica 6:216–224, 1992

Overall JE, Gorham DR: The Brief Psychiatric Rating Scale. Psychol Rep 10:799–812, 1962

Paillere-Martinot M-L, Lecrubier Y, Martinot J-L, et al: Improvement of some schizophrenic deficit symptoms with low doses of amisulpride. Am J Psychiatry 152:130–133, 1995

Perrault GH, Depoortere R, Morel E: Psychopharmacological profile of amisulpride: an antipsychotic drug with presynaptic D2/D3 dopamine receptor antagonist activity and limbic selectivity. J Pharmacol Exp Ther 280:73–82, 1997

Rahbeeni Z, Ozand PT, Rashed M: 4-Hydroxybutyric aciduria. Brain Dev 16 (suppl):64–71, 1994

Ramsay RE: Clinical efficacy and safety of gabapentin. Neurology 44:S23–S30, 1994

Rangel RJ, Penry JK, Wilder BJ, et al: Topiramate: a new antiepileptic drug for complex partial seizures—first use in epileptic patients (abstract). Neurology 38:234, 1988

Ranjan R, Meltzer H: Acute and long-term effectiveness of clozapine in treatment-resistant psychotic depression. Biol Psychiatry 40:253–258, 1996

Reeves K, Harrigan EP: Efficacy and safety of ziprasidone. Poster presented at the convention of the American College of Neuropsychopharmacology, San Juan, Puerto Rico, December 1996

Rihmer Z, Barsi J, Vad G, et al: Moclobemide (Aurorix) in primary major depression. Prog Neuropsychopharmacol Biol Psychiatry 18:367–372, 1994

Satoh K, Someya T, Shibasaki M: Nemonapride for the treatment of schizophrenia. Am J Psychiatry 154:292, 1997

Seeger TF, Seymour PA, Schmidt AW: Ziprasidone (CP-88,059): a new antipsychotic with combined dopamine and serotonin receptor antagonist activity. J Pharmacol Exp Ther 275: 101–103, 1995

Singh L, Field M, Oles R: Anxiolytic effects of gabapentin in preclinical tests. Poster presented at the convention of the American College of Neuropsychopharmacology, San Juan, Puerto Rico, December 1996

Sramek JJ, Elkins L, Church L: A bridging study of MDL 100,907 in schizophrenic patients. Poster presented at the convention of the American College of Neuropsychopharmacology, San Juan, Puerto Rico, December 1996

Stimmel GL, Dopheide JA, Stahl SM: Mirtazapine: an antidepressant with noradrenergic and specific serotonergic effects. Pharmacotherapy 17:10–12, 1997

Svartengren J, Celander M: The limbic functional selectivity of amperozide is not mediated by dopamine D2 receptors as assessed by in vitro and in vivo binding. Eur J Pharmacol 254:73–81, 1994

Tartara A, Manni R, Galimberti CA, et al: Vigabatrin in the treatment of epilepsy: a double-blind, placebo-controlled study. Epilepsia 27:717–223, 1986

Tassinari CA, Michelucci R, Ambrosetto G: Double-blind study of vigabatrin in the treatment of drug-resistant epilepsy. Arch Neurol 44: 907–910, 1987

Tassinari CA, Michelucci R, Chauvel P: Double-blind, placebo-controlled trial of topiramate (600 mg daily) for the treatment of refractory partial epilepsy. Epilepsia 37:763–768, 1996

van Vliet IM, den Boer JA, Westenberg HG: Psychopharmacological treatment of social phobia: a double-blind placebo-controlled study with fluvoxamine. Psychopharmacology 115: 128–134, 1994

Versiani M, Nardi AEW, Mundim FD, et al: Pharmacotherapy of social phobia, a controlled study with moclobemide and phenelzine. Br J Psychiatry 161:353–360, 1992

Volz HP, Faltus F, Magyar I, et al: Brofaromine in treatment-resistant depressed patients: a comparative trial versus tranylcypromine. J Affect Disord 30:209–217, 1994

Walden J, Hesslinger B, van Calker D, et al: Addition of lamotrigine to valproate may enhance efficacy in the treatment of bipolar affective disorder. Pharmacopsychiatry 29:193–195, 1996

Wetzel H, Szegedi A, Hain C, et al: Seroquel (ICI 204 636), a putative "atypical" antipsychotic, in schizophrenia with positive symptomatology: results of an open clinical trial and changes of neuroendocrinological and EEG parameters. Psychopharmacology 119:231–238, 1995

Wilde M, Benfield P: Tianeptine: a review of its pharmacodynamic and pharmacokinetic properties, and therapeutic efficacy in depression and coexisting anxiety and depression. Drugs 49: 411–439, 1995

Wilder BJ, Penry JK, Rangel RJ, et al: Topiramate: efficacy, toxicity and dose/plasma concentrations (abstract). Epilepsia 29:698, 1988

Yamamoto M, Usuda S, Tachikawa S, et al: Pharmacological studies on a new benzamide derivative, YM-09151–2, with potential neuroleptic properties. Neuropharmacology 21:945–951, 1982

Index

*Page numbers printed in **boldface** type refer to tables or figures.*